WOMEN'S HEALTH
A Primary Care Clinical Guide

WOMEN'S HEALTH
A Primary Care Clinical Guide

THIRD EDITION

Ellis Quinn Youngkin, PhD, RNC, ARNP
Professor and Associate Dean
Christine E. Lynn College of Nursing
Women's Health Care Nurse Practitioner
University Student Health Services
Florida Atlantic University
Boca Raton, Florida

Marcia Szmania Davis, MS, MS ED, RNC, WHCNP, ANP-BC
Women's Health Care Nurse Practitioner
Virginia Women's Center
Adjunct Clinical Assistant Professor
School of Nursing
Virginia Commonwealth University
Medical College of Virginia
Richmond, Virginia

PEARSON
Prentice
Hall

Upper Saddle River, New Jersey 07458

Library of Congress Cataloging-in-Publication Data
Women's health: a primary care clinical guide / [edited by] Ellis Quinn
Youngkin, Marcia Szmania Davis.—3rd ed.
    p. ; cm.
Includes bibliographical references and index.
    ISBN 0-13-110026-2 (alk. paper)
    1. Women—Health and hygiene—Sociological aspects. 2.
Women—Diseases. 3. Women's health services. 4. Gynecology. 5.
Obstetrics.
    [DNLM: 1. Women's health. 2. Primary Health Care. WA 309 W8712
2004] I. Youngkin, Ellis Quinn. II. Davis, Marcia Szmania.
    RA 564.85.W6668 2004
    613'.04244—dc21

                                                  2003008428

Publisher: Julie Levin Alexander
Assistant to Publisher: Regina Bruno
Executive Editor: Barbara Krawiec
Editorial Assistant: Sheba Jalaluddin
Director of Production and Manufacturing: Bruce Johnson
Managing Production Editor: Patrick Walsh
Production Liaison: Mary C. Treacy
Production Editor: Jessica Balch, Pine Tree Composition
Manufacturing Manager: Ilene Sanford

Manufacturing Buyer: Pat Brown
Design Director: Cheryl Asherman
Senior Marketing Manager: Nicole Benson
Marketing Assistant: Janet Ryerson
Channel Marketing Manager: Rachele Strober
Composition: Pine Tree Composition, Inc.
Printer/Binder: Courier Westford
Cover Printer: Phoenix Color Corp.

Notice: This volume is intended to educate students and health care providers, not to be a guide for any individual therapy. The authors and the publisher of this volume have taken care to make certain that the doses of drugs and schedules of treatments are correct and compatible with the standards generally accepted at the time of publication. Nevertheless, as new information becomes available, changes in treatment and in the use of drugs, devices, and other therapies become necessary. The reader is advised to carefully consult the instruction and information material included in the package insert of each drug, device, or therapy agent, as well as appropriate, current references before administration. This advice is especially important when using, administering, or recommending new or infrequently used drugs/devices/agents. The authors and publisher advise that an individual with a particular problem consult a primary care provider or a specialist in obstetrics, gynecology, or the field of medicine or advanced practice nursing appropriate for that problem. Under no circumstances should the reader use this volume in lieu of or to substitute for the judgment of the treating provider. The authors and the publisher disclaim all responsibility for any liability, loss, injury, or damage incurred as a consequence, directly or indirectly, of the use and application of any of the contents of this volume.

Pearson Education LTD.
Pearson Education Singapore, Pte. Ltd
Pearson Education, Canada, Ltd
Pearson Education–Japan
Pearson Education Australia PTY, Limited
Pearson Education North Asia Ltd
Pearson Educación de Mexico, S.A. de C.V.
Pearson Education Malaysia, Pte. Ltd
Pearson Education, Upper Saddle River, New Jersey

PEARSON
Prentice
Hall

10 9 8 7 6 5 4
ISBN 0-13-110026-2

DEDICATION

Cathy Anne James, RNC, MS, WHCNP, FAAN
January 16, 1953–October 17, 2001

Cathy was a beautiful, bright, caring, and inspiring woman, nurse, and friend, who loved life and was passionate about nursing. A true leader, she was a gifted women's health nurse practitioner with particular knowledge and skills in the field of infertility. One of the women she helped through the trials and tribulations of in vitro fertilization called Cathy an exceptional and wonderful human being. This description truly fits the fine person we knew as Cathy James. She was loved by all who had the honor to be her friend and colleague, and she is greatly missed.

Cathy received many awards, including election as a Fellow in the American Academy of Nursing, the most prestigious Society in the field of nursing, and Distinguished Practitioner in the Nursing Academy of the National Academies of Practice. She has published extensively and was the first U.S. nurse to be named to the international lectureship in reproductive endocrinology and infertility (REI) nursing. She was honored as the REI Nurse of the Year. She was a founder of the Nurses' Professional Group of the American Society for Reproductive Medicine.

We dedicate this third edition of *Women's Health: A Primary Care Clinical Guide* to Cathy. Cathy was the author for the chapter on infertility in the second edition of this book. She provided depth and breadth of then current information supported by state-of-the-art research. Her work added a very important strength to the book. It seems particularly fitting that a woman so visionary in nursing be remembered this way.

Ellis Quinn Youngkin
Marcia Szmania Davis

CONTENTS

CONTRIBUTORS

Kathleen M. Akridge, MS, RNC, WHNP
OB-GYN Associates of Hampton
A Division of Mid-Atlantic Women's Care, PLC
Hampton, Virginia
Adjunct Clinical Faculty
Virginia Commonwealth University
Medical College of Virginia
Richmond, Virginia

Lynette Galloway Branch, MS, RNC, FNP
Executive Director
Unity Intergenerational Center
Richmond, Virginia

Brenda T. Brickhouse, RNC, MS, WHCNP, CNM
Virginia Women's Center
Richmond, Virginia

Kathryn A. Caufield, MS, RN, CFNP
Old Hampton Family Practice
Sentara Medical Group
Hampton, Virginia

Joan Corder-Mabe, RNC, MS, WHCNP
Director, Division of Women's and Infant's Health
Virginia Department of Health
Richmond, Virginia

Valerie T. Cotter, MSN, CRNP
Associate Director
Adult Health and Gerontological Nurse Practitioner
  Program
School of Nursing
Education Director and Nurse Pracitioner
Alzheimer's Disease Center
University of Pennsylvania
Philadelphia, Pennsylvania

Leslie Fehan, MS, CNM, WHNP
Virginia Commonwealth University Health System
MCV Hospital
Richmond, Virginia

Elaine Ferrary, MS, RN, CFNP
Primary Care
Adjunct Clinical Faculty
Virginia Commonwealth University
Richmond, Virginia

Catherine Ingram Fogel, PhD, RNC, FAAN, WHCNP
Professor, School of Nursing
University of North Carolina
Chapel Hill, North Carolina

Donna E. Forrest, RNC, MS, FNP, WHCNP
Women's Health Care
Riverside Physician Associates
Newport News, Virginia

Marion Herndon Fuqua, MS, RNC, WHCNP
Formerly Women's Health Care Nurse Practitioner
Virginia and Kentucky

Jennifer R. Gardella, RNC, MSN
Egg Donation/Gestational Carrier Program Coordinator
Boston In Vitro Fertilization
Waltham, Massachusetts

Deborah Griswold, MSN, CFNP, ARNP
Coordinator for Clinical Programs
Florida Atlantic University
Student Health Services
Boca Raton, Florida

Janet C. Horton, MS, RN, APRN-BC
Family Nurse Practitioner
Henrico County Health System
and Bon Secours Care-A-Van
Richmond, Virginia

Rita A. Seeger Jablonski, PhD, RN, ANP-BC
Clinical Associate Professor
School of Nursing
Virginia Commonwealth University School of Nursing
Richmond, Virginia

Angela Carter Martin, MS, RN, CFNP, CS
Nurse Psychotherapist and Psychoanalyst
Chevy Chase, Maryland
Formerly Assistant Professor
Uniformed Services University of the Health Sciences
Associate Director, Postmaster's ANP Certificate Program
Washington, D.C.

Deborah A. Raines, PhD, RNC, CNS
Associate Professor
Christine E. Lynn College of Nursing
Florida Atlantic University
Boca Raton, Florida

Maryellen C. Remich, RNC, MS(N), OGNP
The Group for Women
Norfolk, Virginia

Jo Lynne W. Robins, RN, PhD, ANP-BC
Integrating Wellness, Inc.
Associate Professor School of Nursing
Virginia Commonwealth University
Richmond, Virginia

Kathleen J. Sawin, DNS, RN, CS, FAAN
Pediatric and Family Nurse Practitioner
Associate Professor, School of Nursing
Virginia Commonwealth University
Medical College of Virginia
Richmond, Virginia

Susan D. Schaffer, PhD, RN, CFNP
Associate Professor
University of Florida
College of Nursing
Gainesville, Florida

Barbara Peterson Sinclair, MN, OGNP, FAAN
Professor Emeritus
California State University - Los Angeles
Academic Specialist in Program Development
California State University - Northridge
Editor In Chief of *AWHONN Lifelines*
Washington, D.C.

Rachel Effolia Smith, MSN, FNP-CS
Formerly Clinical Assistant Professor
University of Florida
College of Nursing
Gainesville, Florida

Debera Jane Thomas, DNS, FNP/ANP, APRN
Associate Professor
University of Connecticut
School of Nursing
Hartford, Connecticut

Kelly L. Cokely Yeong, MS, WHNP
Virginia Women's Center
Adjunct Clinical Faculty
Virginia Commonwealth University
Richmond, Virginia

CONTRIBUTORS TO SECOND EDITION

A special thank you and recognition go to those who contributed to the second edition of this book:

Cynthia W. Bailey
Assessing Health During Pregnancy

Sharon Baker
Menstruation and Related Problems and Concerns

Judith B. Collins
Women and the Health Care System

Judy Parker-Falzoi
Common Medical Problems

Martha Edwards Hart
Immediate Assessment of the Newborn

Judith A. Lewis
Legal Issues in Primary Care of Women

Cathy James
Infertility

Mary Beth Bryant McGurin
Emergency Childbirth

Nancy Sharp
Women and the Health Care System

REVIEWERS

Elizabeth Abel, PhD, RNC, ANP, FNP
Associate Professor
University of Texas School of Nursing
Austin, TX

Nancy Alley, PhD, FNP
Associate Dean and Professor
East Tennessee State University
Johnson City, TN

Linda C. Andrist, PhD, RNC, WHNP
Associate Professor and Coordinator WHNP Specialty
MGH Institute of Health Professions
Boston, MA

Annette Bairan, PhD, APRN, BC, FNP
Professor of Nursing
School of Nursing
Kennesaw State University
Kennesaw, GA

Michele I. Bracken, MS, CRNP
Nursing Instructor
Salisbury University
Salisbury, MD

Ruth Brewer, PhD, RN, CS
Professor of Nursing
McNeese State University
Lake Charles, LA

Barbara L. Bridges, ARNP, EdD, FNP, WHNP
Associate Professor
University of Kansas Medical Center
Kansas City, KS

Carol L. Buck-Rolland, RN, MS, PNP, WHNP
Assistant Clinical Professor
University of Vermont School of Nursing
Burlington, VT

Barbara L. Cannella, MS, RNC, CNS
Clinical Instructor and Doctoral Candidate
Rutgers University College of Nursing
Newark, NJ

Anne P. Chien, MSN, RN, FNP
FNP Concentration Coordinator
University of Tennessee School of Nursing
Chattanooga, TN

Barbara Hansen Contrell, ARNP, MSN
Associate Professor
Florida State University
Tallahassee, FL

Michele Davidson, PhD, CNM, RN
Assistant Professor
George Mason University
Fairfax, VA

Angela Deneris, CNM, PhD
Associate Professor, Clinical
University of Utah College of Nursing
Salt Lake City, UT

Maureen Dever-Bumba, MSN, FNP-C, CPNP
Assistant Professor and Coordinator FNP Program
Medical College of Georgia
Augusta, GA

Linda Dumas, RN, PhD, RN, ANP
Associate Professor of Nursing
University of Massachusetts
Boston, MA

Sarah B. Freeman, PhD, RN, LS, FNP, FAANP
Associate Clinical Professor
Neil Hodgson Woodruff School of Nursing
Atlanta, GA

Jeanne Grace, RNC, WHC NP, PhD
Associate Professor of Clinical Nursing
University of Rochester School of Nursing
New York, NY

Dixie L. Harms, MSN, ARNP, RN, FNP-C
Coordinator, FNP Program
Drake University
Des Moines, IA

Loretta P. Higgins, RN, EdD
Associate Dean and Associate Professor
Boston College William F. Connell School of Nursing
Chestnut Hill, MA

Polly Hulme, APRN, PhD, FNP
Assistant Professor
University of Nebraska Medical Center
College of Nursing
Omaha, NE

Cecilia M. Jevitt, CNM, PhD
Assistant Professor Midwifery and Nursing
University of South Florida
Tampa, FL

Kathleen Utter King, CNM, MS, PhD
Senior Associate
University of Rochester School of Nursing
Rochester, NY

Judith A. Lewis, PhD, RNC, FAAN
Associate Professor and Director of Information Technology
School of Nursing
Virginia Commonwealth University
Richmond, VA

Gladys Mabunda, RN, PhD
Associate Professor and Coordinator
Public Health Nursing Specialization, School of Nursing

Southern Illinois University Edwardsville
Edwardsville, IL

Sally Mendelsohn, CNM, MS
Assistant Professor of Midwifery
New York University
New York, NY

Gretchen G. Mettler, CNM, MS
Instructor
Francis Payne Bolton School of Nursing
Cleveland, OH

Nancy E. Moss, CNM, FNP, PhD
Director of Nurse Midwifery
Interim Chair Adult Health Nursing
East Carolina University
Greenville, NC

Margaret Pierce, APRN, BC, MSN, MPH
Assistant Professor
University of Tennessee College of Nursing
Knoxville, TN

Janet Scoggin, CNM, PhD
Professor Emeritus
Arizona State University
Phoenix, AZ

Carol A. Smith, DSN, RN, CRNP
Associate Professor and Outreach Coordinator
School of Nursing
College of Health and Human Development
Pennsylvania State University
University Park, PA

Linda H. Snell, DNS, WHNP-C
Associate Professor
SUNY College of Brockport
Brockport, NY

Janice Twiss, PhD, APRN
Associate Professor
University of Nebraska Medical Center
Omaha, NE

Maria T. Wessel, EdD, CHES
Professor of Health Sciences
James Madison University
Harrisonburg, VA

PREFACE

Many women, by choice or by necessity, will seek out the women's health care provider as their source of primary care. This third edition of *Women's Health: A Primary Care Clinical Guide* is designed to help meet the needs of these providers who offer women more than basic reproductive health care. It covers the traditional reproductive and gynecologic content as well as selected common medical, psychosocial, developmental, and political problems, issues, and needs. We have updated every chapter, and, at the request of readers, included a new chapter: Chapter 5, Integrating Wellness: Complementary Therapies and Women's Health. To maintain a reasonable length of the book, we had to choose a chapter to omit, unfortunately. Since legal issues are covered well in most references on the role of the nurse practitioner, we now refer readers to such references for this topic. We hope to bring legal issues back in the future in an expanded manner with role and policy components specific to women's health.

Part I, Women, Health, and the Health Care System, begins with a chapter on the major historical and contemporary changes in health care relating to women, focusing on the important societal, economic, and political factors that will affect health needs for the end of this century and into the next. Chapter 2 discusses women's health and development through the life cycle, followed by Chapter 3, specific to the adolescent woman. Chapter 4 deals with incidences of diseases, general guidelines for health care screening, and interventions. Information on the revised 2001 Bethesda Guidelines for reporting and managing cervical cytology is included. Chapter 6 covers sexuality facts and issues. Chapter 7 concerns the health needs of lesbians.

Part II, Promotion of Gynecologic Health Care, delves into the more traditional health problems and needs of women related to the reproductive systems. Chapters 8 through 15 cover menstrual concerns, fertility management, infertility, sexually transmitted diseases and vaginitis, including the 2002 STD guidelines from the CDC, the special needs of women with HIV, pelvic and abdominal diseases, breast concerns, and the health concerns of perimenopausal and older women.

Part III, Promotion of Women's Health Care During Pregnancy, details uncomplicated and complicated pregnancy care, postpartum needs and problems, lactation issues, and fetal surveillance.

Primary Care Problems Affecting Women's Health, Part IV, was significantly expanded in the second edition to address even more of the medical problems frequently encountered in primary care of women such as headaches, anemia, hypertension, asthma, and dermatologic conditions. Chapters 21 and 22 are dedicated to current information on common medical problems. Selected psychosocial problems, such as violence, depression, and eating disorders and their impacts on women, with insights into related health care needs and therapies, are discussed in Chapter 23. Chapter 24 reviews unique care concerns of women with disabilities and chronic illness. The appendices address emergency childbirth (Appendix A), assessment of the newborn (Appendix B), and selected laboratory values commonly referenced in women's health (Appendix C).

We particularly intend this book to be a handbook, a resource that allows any primary health care provider to retrieve basic information easily. We see it as a reference with enough depth to be useful in a clinical setting, serving as a source of teaching advice for clients, including differential medical diagnoses, screening and early intervention measures, and guidelines for referral. Some of the chapters fit more easily into an outline format for diseases or other conditions, whereas many chapters conform to a more traditional text format or a combination format for presentation of issues.

We wish to remind the reader that the scope of advanced practice nursing varies from state to state, and the individual practitioner is responsible for knowing his or her legal limits of practice. Also, recognizing the rapidity with which new knowledge becomes available and standards change, the practitioner must stay ever alert.

Women's health care providers are continuously challenged to expand their knowledge and ability to help women fulfill a wide spectrum of needs, both physical and psychosocial. Women's health is no longer limited to reproductive organs. The broadening scope of women's health care is a critically important issue in this period of rapidly changing health care systems. Resources are burgeoning, empowering women to become more informed consumers in the health care arena, yet attaining holistic care to meet basic needs remains a struggle for many. We, with the contributing authors, hope that you as primary care providers in a rapidly changing world of health care will find this book a useful and an effective resource in your endeavors to provide women with the health care they need and deserve.

Our sincere thanks go to our excellent contributing authors. Their outstanding expertise and effort have made this book the useful clinical reference we envisioned. We also wish to thank the fine editors and staff at Prentice Hall Health and Pine Tree Composition, Inc., for their support and many hours of work on this project. Last, our deep appreciation goes to our families who encouraged us during the months of preparation and work. A special note goes to our inspiring "little women," Alicia, Valarie, Julianne, Emily, and Annie, who join the women of the twenty-first century in deserving the best health care of the new millennium.

Ellis Quinn Youngkin
Marcia Szmania Davis

I ❖ Women, Health, and the Health Care System

CHAPTER 1

WOMEN AND THE HEALTH CARE SYSTEM

Barbara Peterson Sinclair

T he field of women's health continues to evolve from a perspective that considered only the reproductive system to one that begins to incorporate the totality of a woman's experience across her life span. Doing this required support from the federal government and an interface with the health care system because the system itself faced great change and turmoil. It is an interesting journey.

Highlights

- Historical Perspective
- Societal Barriers to Quality Health Care
- Other Influences on Women's Health
- Political Action
- Federal Agencies Concerned with Women's Health
- Health Care Policy and Delivery
- System Issues for the Future
- The Future of Women's Health

❖ INTRODUCTION

Many women initially enter the health care system because of unique circumstances related to their reproductive organs. Historically, this focal point led to the emergence of a narrow definition of women's health care that centered primarily on pelvis and breasts. As a result, women's health was equated to reproductive health. This perspective is changing, even though a broader outlook has not yet been achieved in all situations. Today's philosophy of women's health care is beginning to evolve into a comprehensive approach that addresses physical, social, emotional, and spiritual needs—the totality of a woman's experience across the life span. This approach recognizes that health is more than the absence of disease or disability and is sensitive to the individual woman within the context of her particular circumstances.

However, the move toward a holistic approach must be tempered by viewing gender as a key variable in recognizing forces that impact women's health. Doing so allows for a wellness approach that:

◆ Emphasizes a women's assets and flexibility rather than just her problems.

◆ Includes a social perception that understands that women are routinely involved in overlapping and multiple roles.

◆ Recognizes that women have variable health and psychosocial needs as they transition through life and that health behaviors are based on cumulative experiences.

◆ Appreciates that both gender-specific experiences and individual diversity are normal in relation to health care needs and access to health resources (Grason, Hutchins, & Silver, 1999a).

One cannot generalize among all women but must view a woman as an individual within her total distinctive context—that is, age, family, culture, education, religion, society, emotional and physical status (Sinclair, 2000). Historically, women's reproductive systems were viewed from the perspective of women's health, whereas other systems in women were viewed from perspectives of men's health. As a result, norms of health, illness, and therapies for systems such as cardiac, respiratory, and metabolic were established for men but applied to women; however, women cannot be viewed as being the same as men because they respond differently physiologically, emotionally, and cognitively. The Institute of Medicine (2001a) reports that an individual's sex *does* matter in medical science and calls for more biomedical research to understand the many ways in which men and women differ within a broad range of diseases, conditions, and treatments. Attitudes are different, also. Women are concerned about quality health care not only for themselves but also for their families. They make approximately 70 percent of all health care decisions for the family—children, husbands, and parents—and over 80 percent of women have the sole or shared responsibility for financial decisions regarding their family's health (The National Women's Health Information Center [NWHIC], 2001a). Many women want the opportunity to be involved in decision making and self-care and be provided with appropriate information about achieving and maintaining the best possible health status for themselves and their loved ones (Sinclair, 1997).

HISTORICAL PERSPECTIVE

Throughout the ages, an evolution of the health care of women has occurred, often paralleling the changing roles of women in society. Women's consumer health activities began in the United States during the 1830s and 1840s. Suffrage during the mid-19th century was accomplished by the Popular Health Movement, which demanded a total redefinition of health and health care. In 1986, Abrums' historical perspective on women's health care discusses Naphey's 1870 work entitled *The Physical Life of Women: Advice to Maiden, Wife, and Mother*. Although the book was widely acclaimed as valuable scientific literature, it identified only three phases in a woman's life: maidenhood, matrimony, and maternity.

About the turn of the 20th century, it was believed that the ovaries and uterus were the controlling organs and the center of all disease in a woman's body, thus the etiology of most female complaints, including headaches, indigestion, and sore throats. Consequently, the stage was set for decades during which women's health care would be plagued with sexism and ageism. Women felt that they lacked control of their bodies, and many normal physiological processes were viewed by medicine and society as diseases. For example, menstruation was seen as a chronic problem, and pregnancy and menopause as disorders requiring intervention (Ehrenreich & English, 1973). Sexism in the health care system provided the basis for "oppression of women derived from her 'womanness': her biologic differences and her ability to bear children." These differences have been used to build social structures and a supportive ideology of female submissiveness and to "permit condescension toward women" (Marieskind, 1975). Further reinforcing this ideology, in 1905, the president of the Oregon State Medical Society stated, "Educated women could not bear children with ease because study arrested the development of the pelvis at the same time it increased the size of the child's brain, and therefore its head" (Bullough & Vought, 1973).

This ideology was also extended to mature women. In the popular 1970 book *Everything You Always Wanted to Know about Sex,* Dr. David Reuben described the menopausal woman:

> As the estrogen is shut off, a woman comes as close as she can to being a man. Increased facial hair, deepened voice, obesity, and the decline of breasts and female genitalia all contribute to a masculine appearance. Coarsened features, enlargement of the clitoris, and gradual baldness complete the picture. Not really a man but no longer a functional woman, these individuals live in a world of intersex . . . sex no longer interests them. To many women the menopause marks the end of their useful life. They see it as the onset of old age, the beginning of the end. They may be right. Having outlived their ovaries, they may have outlived their usefulness as human beings. The remaining years may be just marking time until they follow their glands into oblivion (Reuben, 1970).

THE 1960s AND 1970s

Many social changes erupted in the 1960s fueled by societal unrest about the lack of equality for all citizens. Most notable and visible was the civil rights movement. Major changes for women also evolved, catalyzed in 1963 by Betty Friedan's historic book *The Feminine Mystique,* which told of women's disenchantments with their relationships, both personal and institutional (Friedan, 1963). This disenchantment developed into the women's liberation movement, which addressed the cause of equal rights for women. Health care system change was strategic to women's liberation, because the system as an agent of so-

cial control was equally as restrictive as any political or economic system (Marieskind, 1975).

The women's health movement was an outgrowth of the women's liberation movement that preceded it. This grassroots effort challenged medical authority as a means of improving women's health and health care delivery and addressed a multitude of issues including childbirth reform, product safety, and self-help. It hoped to put an end to the sexism in the health care system.

"Activities that centered around abortion law reform provided the initial cohesion from which the women's health movement could emerge" (Marieskind, 1975). In January 1973, the landmark Supreme Court decision in *Roe v. Wade* provided women with a legal right to abortion.

The major thrust of the health movement was that women wanted to own and control their bodies, not just to be cured. In a landmark book published by the Boston Women's Health Collective, *Our Bodies, Ourselves,* women spoke out and asked for something different and better from health care providers (Boston Women's Health Collective, 1971). The publication encouraged open discussion about topics that were very difficult to talk about before this time (Olshansky, 2000).

The women's health movement also raised issues of childbirth education, natural methods of childbirth, and birthing options, including father participation in labor and delivery and home births. Spurred by consumer education in books, magazines, and networking meetings, women's requests from the health care system grew beyond childbearing issues. Hospitals, awakened to the fact that women were major customers, began to market women's services by establishing women's health resource centers (either within the hospital or as freestanding centers) to provide specialized care and education in homelike surroundings.

THE 1980s AND EARLY 1990s

Women have demanded participatory health care decision making, humanistic and holistic preventive care, and a wellness, rather than illness, orientation to care. In the sociopolitical arena women advocated for health services and policies that address reproductive freedom, contraceptive options, domestic violence, and research on women's special health problems (e.g., breast disease, menopause, osteoporosis, hormone replacement therapy, premenstrual syndrome, heart disease, human immunodeficiency virus/acquired immunodeficiency syndrome, depression, and stress-related illnesses). Even so, research on disease processes in women lagged far behind the knowledge that was identified for men. In many instances, findings from studies on men continued to be extrapolated and applied to women even though physiologic responses to pathological conditions were not the same.

Abortion rights remained a major emotional and legal issue for the nation. Since the *Roe v. Wade* decision in 1973, abortion has been legal in all 50 states. However, some states have implemented laws such as twenty-four-hour waiting periods, parental notification, and other restrictions. The court system used an undue burden measure to determine if such restrictions are legal. Access to abortion services was a critical issue. In many areas of the country, women had to travel hundreds of miles to find qualified abortion providers. These problems continue to exist.

Betty Friedan (1991), speaking out on the new feminine mystique, asserted that the women's movement had been halted by the general reversal of social progress in the United States during the 1980s and 1990s. She felt that the rights women had won during the past twenty years were in "grave danger."

Women were the preeminent consumers of health care in the United States, measured by standards such as doctors' visits, medication prescriptions, surgery, hospitalization, and nursing home care. Women were also responsible for spending two of every three health care dollars, and 60 to 70 percent of all hospital beds were filled by women (Day, 1997).

THE LATE 1990s AND EARLY 2000s

As the new century approached, health care for women continued to improve. Women began to make health a top priority for themselves as well as for their families. Of special consideration was the fact that women realized the importance of health in relation to productive and happy lives (Hankinson, Colditz, Manson, & Speizer, 2001). Women are living longer; their life span is approaching 80 years of age as compared to slightly over 48 years of age in 1900 (CDC, 2000). However, the quality of life as opposed to just longevity is recognized as a vital imperative; therefore, health behaviors take on a much larger role. Many of the chronic diseases seen in older women actually start much earlier, some during adolescence. This is especially true for frequently occurring life-threatening conditions such as heart disease, diabetes, and selected cancers. Healthy lifestyle choices have proven to be of great benefit and include well-balanced nutrition, maintenance of appropriate weight, reasonable exercise, not smoking, and a daily multiple vitamin (Hankinson et al., 2001) The need became evident to get out the message and encourage all women to undertake healthy behaviors and to initiate them at a young age.

Promoting health within the community was also undertaken. For example, bans on smoking in public locales, more nutritious choices of food in schools and workplaces, access to safe places to exercise, flexible work hours, and public health screening are all recognized as important, and attempts to implement them are quite common. Health education efforts are also more prevalent, but reliable information about health care has not been widely available. National studies demonstrate that women may not be as satisfied as men with the level of communication and health information given by the health care providers (NWHIC, 2001b).

Women's health has come along way from issues of reproduction and childbearing. Even so, healthier mothers and infants in the United States are considered one of the greatest public health achievements of the last century, and prenatal care has been attributed as the key factor in this accomplishment (Stubblefield, 1999). However, much remains to be done considering that the United States lags behind all other industrialized nations in ranking of infant mortality, especially with regard to disparity of access, care, and outcomes among minority populations. The overall fertility rate increased in 2000 after dropping each year in the preceding decade. It reached 2.1, which is considered to be the population's replacement level (National Center for Health Statistics [NCHS], 2001).

SOCIETAL BARRIERS TO QUALITY HEALTH CARE

Not all women are receiving comparable health care. Although positive strides have been made, many women still experience significant barriers. These include cost, availability of providers and services, lack of transportation, paternalism in the medical profession, poorly coordinated and disorganized methods for referral, and problems with access to insurance or inability to work within established health care delivery systems. Age is rapidly becoming another barrier as women are living longer and requiring greater health care resources.

RACIAL AND ETHNIC DISPARITY

A significant challenge for the 21st century is the elimination of disparity in health outcomes among racial and ethnic groups in the United States. The Institute of Medicine (2002) reports that minorities commonly receive poorer health care than whites, even when income, age, insurance, and medical conditions are similar. The greatest discrepancies in terms of mortality outcomes occur in the areas of cardiovascular disease, cancer, and diabetes. Although these outcomes reflect findings in both men and women, the situation for women of color is worse as they face barriers separate from and in addition to those of men. Another area of concern is the striking difference between the mortality rates of white and nonwhite infants. Infant mortality is a critical indicator of a nation's health and reflects the overall state of maternal health and the quality and accessibility of health care for women and infants (Henry, 2001).

Racial and ethnic disparity exists also in measures of morbidity. Fair or poor health status as reported by an individual or family is higher for nonwhite persons. Activity limitation due to chronic conditions is common among elderly persons and increases with age, at which time it is seen more often in women. Fewer services in total are available to older women (Institute of Medicine [IOM], 2002).

The IOM (2002) also reports that the bias among doctors and nurses, although not necessarily overt, may contribute to health disparities, as a result fostering distrust among minority patients that leads to aggravation of clinical problems. Physicians from the same ethnic or cultural group are relatively few, as evidenced by the percent of black physicians that has increased only from 3.5 percent to 3.9 percent since 1970. As a result, minorities are more likely to be treated by a white physician who may not fully understand the patients' language or customs. While the report found that some minority patients refused tests or treatments, it was more likely the provider's failure to present options clearly or the individual's lack of financial resources that interfered with the plan.

The Institute for the Future (2000) suggests that by 2011, fully one-third of the U.S. population will be ethnic and racial minorities due to higher birth rates among minorities and significant immigration.

MEDICAL RESEARCH

Until recently, medical research has largely ignored many health issues important to women, and women were underrepresented in clinical trials. In the past, research on women's health focused on fertility and reproduction, and too little research was aimed at women's unique response to disease and to common health issues. Even though women make up 51 percent of the U.S. population, research on major diseases and the drugs to treat them has been done mostly on mice and men. At present, most women still receive health assessments, outcomes, and recommendations based on what works for men.

Historically, many researchers excluded women, arguing that pregnancy and women's fluctuating hormone levels could alter study results, thereby negating findings, and that men were more convenient to the research plan. An interesting example of this is the study of aspirin as it relates to heart disease. Women were excluded from large clinical trials in this study, yet cardiovascular disease is the leading cause of death among U.S. women, and more women die of heart disease each year then do men (NWHIC, 2001b). Even when women were included in a few selected study sites, results were not routinely analyzed for gender differences. Results of the study, although primarily gathered from and intended for men, were then applied to women even though we now know that women develop heart disease later in life, are more likely to have co-existing conditions that mask symptoms, have symptoms that are actually different from those of men, and even respond to certain treatments in a different way.

During the 1990s, a time of major political activity and regulatory change, the national research agenda on women's health was invigorated. Through the efforts of women's health advocates and the unveiling of inequities in medical research, a broadened research agenda evolved and is beginning to yield insights into the health-related similarities and differences between men and women (NWHIC, 2001b). There is enormous support for more research in women's health issues in response to female demand for health information (Grason et al., 1999b). Although researchers have moved beyond the concept that women's health equates only reproductive health, reproductive health undoubtedly remains quite important, and it is expected that results of continued research on the total woman will have great consequences for all.

HEALTH CARE PRACTICES

It is very interesting that many health care providers treat women differently than they treat men. Compared to men, women often receive less thorough evaluations for similar complaints, are given less attention to their symptoms, and have fewer interventions for the same diagnoses.

Also, women tend not to get the same degree of explanation in response to questions and there may even be a difference in whether medications are prescribed (NWHIC, 2001b). Reasons for this vary from paternalistic perspectives on the part of some male physicians to the type of health care provider visited. Women using two physicians concurrently receive more clinical services than women using only one. In many cases, this occurs when women see both an obstetrician-gynecologist and a primary care physician. Advanced practice nurses also are starting to make positive impacts on the delivery of care to women, especially for those in managed care situations (Gonen, 1999).

While trying to meet needs for both reproductive and general health care, women often face fragmentation in the health care system. Even though they make more visits to the doctor and are more interested in and informed about health issues, women tend to have difficulties in getting or arranging to get all of the services needed for themselves and their children. The fragmentation and missed opportunities occur at three levels for reproductive aged women: between family planning and other reproductive health services, between reproductive and nonreproductive health services, and between reproductive health care and children's health care (Lu, Bragonier, Silver, & Bemis-Heys, 2000). Older women face the problem of having their reproductive systems somewhat ignored due to the greater incidence of chronic conditions—for example, cardiovascular disease or diabetes—and decreased musculoskeletal ability. In either situation, studies have shown that women are not as satisfied as men with the information they receive and the communication they have with their providers (McGlynn, 1998).

When the women's health movement of the 1960s and 1970s challenged the male-dominated medical profession's control over women's health practices and reproductive lives, reforms were undertaken and change was initiated. A side result of this action and of ensuing federal anti-discrimination laws was the increase of female physicians. In the late 1960s, 7.7 percent of all physicians were women. This number doubled by 1980, reached 34 percent by 1995, and estimates suggest that close to 50 percent of students entering medical school today are female (Grason et al., 1999b). It is anticipated that as more women enter the field of medicine less gender bias occurs, which bodes well for improvement in research and clinical practice for women.

Medical practice has resulted in the most common surgical procedures in the United States being hysterectomy and cesarean birth. Great attention was paid to the high rate of cesarean deliveries in the 1980s, suggesting that the procedure was not always based on absolute need. As a result, the numbers of cesareans steadily declined. However, the rate is again on the rise and now approximates 23 percent (NWHIC, 2001b).

ACCESS TO CARE AND INSURANCE

Access to care is greatly dependent upon:

- Economic status that dictates the type of insurance and discretionary dollars available for health.
- Educational levels that allow individuals to seek and understand information about health and health care systems.
- Availability of health care providers and facilities in a geographically desirable area.
- Health care providers that accept the individual's health plan and have time available for appropriate scheduling of appointments.

Women are more likely than men to have difficulty in financing health, twice as likely to be underinsured, and must face the additional burden of handling pregnancy-related and infant needs.

The Institute for the Future (2000) states that access to care will remain "tiered" and describes the tiers as follows. The top tier, or empowered consumers, have considerable discretionary income, subscribe to well-received insurance plans, and are educated to the point of being able to obtain information about their health from printed or electronic media or directly from a provider. These consumers engage in some shared decision making with their providers and include 38 percent of the population. The second tier, or worried consumers, consists of 34 percent of the population. They have access to some form of health insurance but have little or no choice of health plans. Members of this worried group may be temporary employees or early retirees or those in other circumstances that decrease their access to the discretionary income needed to assure health services. The third tier is composed of 28 percent of the population who are excluded consumers. In this group are the uninsured, Medicaid recipients, and others who do not have entry into market-based health insurance. Obviously, these three groups are affected in varying ways by different components and movements of the health care system. A report from The Center for Studying Health System Change (HSC) (2002) mentions that even in a strong economy, the number of Americans who did not seek or delayed receiving medical care failed to improve between 1997 and

2001, with the majority of those in the study citing cost as the primary reason. A 2002 Kaiser Family Foundation survey reported that about 25 percent of women missed care and 20 percent didn't fill prescriptions because of cost (California Healthline, 2002). This is perceived to be a bad omen because consumer concerns about cost are likely to increase in weaker economies. As head of the household, women outnumbered men in delaying or omitting health care.

Eighteen percent of all working age women in the United States are currently uninsured, and being employed does not solve the problem: Eight out of every ten uninsured women state that they are working or are married to a spouse who is working (Collins, 1999). Because women have longer life expectancy than men, they need a disproportionate share of long-term care resources. However, Medicare covers only short-term nursing home care and the elderly often need to pay for long-term needs out of savings or, in some situations, utilize Medicaid, if qualified to do so. The cost of prescription drugs is a major financial drain for the elderly. Drugs are not covered by Medicare, and even with other health plan coverage, seniors often must rely on out-of-pocket payments.

ACCESS TO PRENATAL CARE

Use of preventive health services contributes to the reduction of morbidity and mortality, and this is especially true for pregnant women and their offspring. Despite considerable advances in perinatal health, many women are still disadvantaged by not obtaining prenatal care early in their pregnancy. Based on the 17.2 percent of women who did not receive prenatal care in the first trimester in 1998, it appears that access to care must be improved, and additional programs are needed to alert and motivate women regarding the benefits of early care. Over one-fourth of the group who did not get care in the first trimester received very late care or no care whatsoever (NCHS, 2001).

Infant mortality in 1999 was 7.0 per 1,000. Although this number has significantly decreased in the last several decades, it is still higher than desired. The three major causes of infant deaths in the United States are congenital anomalies, preterm/low birth weight infants, and sudden infant death syndrome (NCHS, 2001). It is strongly believed that preconceptional care and early prenatal care will positively impact these conditions.

Multiple social and health problems contribute to the statistics mentioned above, but to a great extent, the results are due to problems in accessing prenatal care. The problem of access results from limitations in government

funding and by competition among managed care plans regarding who would care for women covered by Medicaid (Grason et al., 1999a). The poor health status of mothers and infants in central regions of large metropolitan areas and in rural locales may be indicative of nonfinancial barriers such as limited availability of obstetric providers, reduced access to specialized care, and lack of adequate education and health information. Women also must deal with limited enabling services, such as translators, babysitters, transportation, and culturally competent clinic environments (Lu et al., 2000).

OTHER INFLUENCES ON WOMEN'S HEALTH

POVERTY

Poverty and health are significantly interrelated. Low income women are in poorer health and have greater difficulty accessing health care services than do affluent women. Poor women face the inability to pay for care. About one-half of the nation's poor are either under 18 or over 65 years of age. Nearly three-fourths of the poor over 65 years of age are female; however, the group most likely to lack insurance coverage is 18- to 24-year-olds. Foreign-born populations are without health insurance almost twice as often as native-born people (Kelly & Joel, 1999). The medically indigent are in a special group who are either uninsured or have insufficient insurance once confronted with medical necessity. They are neither poor enough for Medicaid nor old enough for Medicare, but simply middle-class people with little savings who work at jobs that provide inadequate benefits. The group is often referred to as the working poor. The U.S. Census Bureau (2000) identified over 40 million Americans who fall within this group.

Inequities in income between men and women still persist. Although women's wages are still not commensurate with those of men, some improvement is being made, and the Bureau of Labor Statistics determined that women earn 75 cents to man's dollar when there is a comparison of like jobs. Even so, the majority of women still work in low-paying jobs because they are not sufficiently educated for other positions or such jobs tend to be more compatible with child rearing. Single women head of households are at particular economic disadvantage, yet such is the case in about one-fifth of our families (Kelly & Joel, 1999). Women and children are the fastest growing segment of the homeless population.

MARITAL STATUS

Marital status is also interrelated with standard of living and quality of health. Public policy is often developed on the outdated concept of the American family headed by a male wage earner with a spouse at home, even though this is no longer the case in a large majority of families. Unmarried and teen mothers are still of major concern. In 2000, the birth rate for unmarried women increased slightly, and the rate of teen pregnancy declined for the eighth consecutive year, reaching 48.5 births per 1,000 women aged 15 to 19 years (NCHS, 2001). Another major issue being examined is whether employment benefits such as health insurance will be extended to committed domestic or same sex partners.

LONGEVITY

Since the turn of the 20th century, women's life span continues to increase. While living longer, women are not necessarily living better. They represent 51 percent of the total U.S. population, 64 percent over age 65 and more than 75 percent above age 85. By living longer, women may have an increased incidence of chronic diseases that require long-term care. It is estimated that more than half of the women who have reached age 85 are living in nursing homes (IOM, 2001c).

MULTIPLE ROLES

In addition to being primary caregivers to children and aging parents, women work outside of the home and contribute significantly to the family income.

They provide the majority of paid and unpaid family care and have become the safety net for our health care system. Women make up three-fourths of the unpaid caregivers of the elderly (Raymond & Allshouse, n.d.). Without these family caregivers, many more individuals would be in health care institutions. A significant number of women find themselves in the "sandwich generation" by caring for both children and an elder. Women's multiple roles have raised issues concerning comparable worth, gender discrimination in the workforce, childcare, and the division of household chores. Stressful jobs, demands for care giving, household functions, and conflicting responsibilities can be linked to poor health—for example, increased stress that exacerbates chronic hypertension. Although success in multiple roles can produce increased self-esteem, the overall pressure may cancel the benefit.

POLITICAL ACTION

In response to issues raised by feminist leaders that health care services for women may not be adequately supported, a 1983 Public Health Services (PHS) task force was commissioned to investigate the status of women's health. The findings of the task force were published in 1985, and its fifteen recommendations focused on six major areas:

- Promoting physical and social environments that are safe and healthful.
- Providing services to prevent and treat disease.
- Conducting research and evaluation.
- Recruiting and training women health care personnel.
- Educating and informing the public and disseminating research information.
- Designing guidance for legislative and regulatory measures.

Based on the task force findings, academics and government policymakers agreed, for the first time, that women were disadvantaged in terms of health care (USPHS, 1985).

Despite the startling conclusions of the PHS report, little action was taken until 1989, when the Congressional Caucus on Women's Issues (CCWI) was formed. The CCWI included a bipartisan group of twenty-five members of Congress. In response to the PHS report, it officially requested an audit of National Institute of Health (NIH) clinical trials with regard to the number of women who were included. The audit was completed in 1990 and reported that NIH study results were not analyzed by gender, that NIH policy was not well communicated or understood, and that policy applied only to extramural, not intramural, research.

When the NIH, Congress, and the public reacted to this report, changes began to occur. Multimedia coverage showed women's omission from research, and reports focused on women's diseases. Meanwhile, the CCWI developed a women's health legislative agenda for research, prevention, and services. It was introduced in Congress in The Women's Health Equity Act (WHEA) in 1990 and has continued to the present.

The WHEA is a package of individual bills introduced as omnibus legislation that presents a forward-looking agenda for women's health. Title I addresses research on women's health, and Title II addresses the delivery of health services.

A significant number of WHEA provisions, including appropriate funding, have been enacted since the bill was introduced in 1990. This has resulted in meaningful progress toward rectifying the inequities in medical research and health care delivery for U.S. women.

The omnibus package also serves an important purpose in educational and health policy agenda setting. At the end of each congressional session, a review of the WHEA provides a means of measuring action on issues important to women (JAMWA, 2002; Women's Policy, 1996).

FEDERAL AGENCIES CONCERNED WITH WOMEN'S HEALTH

THE DEPARTMENT OF HEALTH AND HUMAN SERVICES (HHS)

HHS is the federal government's principal agency for protecting the health of all Americans and providing them with essential human services. As a result, both direct and indirect services are of benefit to women. Although the roots of health services can be traced to the earliest days of our country, the Department of Health, Education, and Welfare (HEW) came into a Cabinet-level existence in 1953. Education was made into a separate department in 1979, and HEW became the Department of Health and Human Services in 1980. The Department includes over 300 programs. Its operating divisions can be seen in Box 1–1. Several of the agencies listed are housed under various HHS divisions (HHS, 2002).

BOX 1–1. Department of Health and Human Services Operating Divisions

Public Health Service	Human Services
Agency for Healthcare Research and Quality (AHRQ)	Administration for Children and Families (ACF)
Centers for Disease Control and Prevention (CDC)	Administration on Aging (AoA)
Food and Drug Administration (FDA)	Centers for Medicare and Medicaid Services (CMS)
Health Resources and Services Administration (HRSA)	
Indian Health Service (IHS)	
National Institutes of Health (NIH)	
Substance Abuse and Mental Health Services Administration (SAMHSA)	

Office on Women's Health (OWH) of the U.S. Public Health Service

Established in 1991, the OWH is the government's focal point for women's health issues and works to rectify inequities in research, health care services, and education that have historically placed the health of women at risk. The Office on Women's Health coordinates women's health efforts in HHS to eliminate disparities in health status and supports culturally sensitive educational programs that encourage women to take personal responsibility for their own health and wellness. A large number of significant programs are incorporated in the office, such as the seventeen National Centers of Excellence in Women's Health and various outreach programs. Some of the specifics include Minority Women's Health, Girl and Adolescent Health, Older Women's Health, Reproductive Health, Violence Against Women, HIV/AIDS in Women, Breast Health, National Action Plan on Breast Cancer, Environmental Health, International Health, and OWH Publications (HHS, 2002).

National Women's Health Information Center

An additional service offered by the Office on Women's Health is the National Women's Health Information Center (NWHIC). NWHIC is a national information and referral service designed to provide women and their families with current, reliable, and cost-free health information and materials from federal agencies and respected private-sector organizations. This is accomplished through a comprehensive Web site and a toll-free call center. NWHIC has recently entered into a partnership agreement with the Academy of Nurse Practitioners to enhance dissemination of information by utilizing nurse practitioners to inform their patients about the Center and thus empower women to be better informed about health (NWHIC, 2001b).

Office of Research on Women's Health (ORWH) at the National Institutes of Health (NIH)

Established in 1990, the Office of Research on Women's Health serves as a focal point for women's health research at the NIH. The ORWH promotes, stimulates, and supports efforts to improve the health of women through biomedical and behavioral research. It works in partnership with NIH institutes and centers to ensure that women's health research is part of the scientific framework at NIH and throughout the scientific community. The ORWH (1996) has a threefold mandate:

1. To strengthen, develop, and increase research into diseases, disorders, and conditions that affect women and establish a research agenda for NIH based upon gaps in knowledge about women's health.
2. To ensure that women are appropriately represented as participants in NIH research.
3. To develop opportunities and support for recruitment, retention, reentry, and advancement of women in biomedical careers.

Since its inception, the new focus and resources dedicated to research on women have generated considerable new knowledge about women's health. For example, research has led to a better understanding of the interaction between life behaviors and health outcomes. A case in point is that women who take folic acid before pregnancy and especially during the first month following conception reduce the incidence of neural tube defects in their offspring.

Women's Health Initiative

The ORWH plays a collaborative role in the NIH's Women's Health Initiative (WHI), the largest clinical trial ever undertaken in the United States. The WHI, which is located within the National Heart, Lung and Blood Institute, is conducting a prospective observational study of over 161,000 women at forty clinical centers nationwide and focuses on strategies for preventing heart disease, breast cancer, colorectal cancer, and osteoporosis in postmenopausal women (NIH/NHLBI, 2002; Pinn, 1994). It is anticipated that a number of answers will be forthcoming from the WHI, including risk factors and biomarkers for disease, possible risks and benefits associated with hormone replacement therapy, dietary supplementation with calcium and vitamin D, and other interventions in preventing the conditions being studied (NIH/ORWH, 2002). The WHI spans approximately fifteen years and will cost more than $628 million.

Food and Drug Administration (FDA) Office of Women's Health (OWH)

The Food and Drug Administration has jurisdiction over drugs, medical devices, vaccines, blood and tissue products, foods, and cosmetics used by women and their families on a daily basis. The creation of the OWH in 1994 provided for the inclusion of patients of both genders in drug development and analyses of clinical data (women of childbearing potential were excluded from all drug re-

search prior to this time). The OWH has established itself as an effective voice for women's health concerns. According to OWH's published description, its mission is "to serve as a champion for women's health both within and outside the agency" (FDA, 2001). To meet its goals, OWH:

- Ensures that FDA functions remain gender sensitive and responsive.
- Works to correct gender disparities in drug, device, and biologics testing and regulation.
- Monitors progress of women's health initiatives with FDA.
- Promotes integrative and interactive approaches regarding women's health across all FDA components.
- Forms partnerships with governmental and nongovernmental entities to promote FDA's women's health objectives.

A number of programs have been conducted to meet stated goals. Premier among them is the Take Time To Care (TTTC) campaign that reaches millions of women of many cultures where they live and work to educate them about using medicines wisely. The program was developed in response to the finding that 30 to 50 percent of those who use medicines do not take them as directed, causing drain on health care delivery systems, absenteeism, and lost wages and costing Americans $76.6 billion each year (FDA, 2002).

The Agency for Healthcare Research and Quality (AHRQ)

The AHRQ is another HHS division that provides evidence-based information on health care outcomes; quality; and cost, use, and access. Information from AHRQ research helps people to make informed decisions and also improve the quality of health care services. In addition, it addresses medical errors. AHRQ research listings are extensive and currently include a variety of topics of concern to women, such as heart disease and stroke, breast and cervical cancer, hysterectomy, urinary incontinence, pelvic inflammatory disease, health care access, preventive services, domestic violence, HIV/AIDS, and alternative medicines (HHS, 2002).

Health Resources and Services Administration (HRSA) of the U.S. Public Health Service

HRSA directs programs that improve the nation's health by providing access to essential health services for people who are poor, uninsured, vulnerable; have special needs;

or who live in rural and urban areas where health care is scarce. Working in partnership with state and community organizations, HRSA ensures the availability of quality health services via its four key program areas: HIV/AIDS services, primary health care to the medically underserved, women and children, and availability of health professions in underserved areas.

Maternal Child Health Bureau (MCHB). HRSA's Maternal Child Health Bureau is an outgrowth of the 1912 Children's Bureau and the 1935 Social Security Act and is authorized to provide programs and foundations for maternal and child health services. The Bureau strengthens maternal child health infrastructures; assures availability of medical homes; and improves health, safety, and well-being of the mother and child population.

U.S. DEPARTMENT OF LABOR, WOMEN'S BUREAU

This Bureau is concerned with the women in the workforce and concentrates on the following programs: strengthening the family, women in high-technology jobs, women in apprenticeships and nontraditional occupations, and developing expertise for women in on-line distance learning.

ADDITIONAL HHS DIVISIONS

A number of other divisions under the Department of Health and Human Services offer programs that affect the health and safety of women. A brief list includes:

Substance Abuse and Mental Health Services Administration

SAMHSA works to improve the availability and quality of programs in substance abuse prevention, addiction treatment, and mental health services.

Centers for Disease Control and Prevention

CDC works with states and other partners to monitor disease outbreaks, implement prevention strategies, and maintain national health statistics.

Centers for Medicare and Medicaid Services

Formerly the Health Care Financing Administration (HICFA), the CMS administers programs that provide health care to about one-fourth of Americans. Medicare provides insurance for seniors and the disabled. Medicaid, a joint federal and state program, provides health coverage for low-income persons. CMS also administers the new Children's Health Insurance Program through approved state plans (S-CHIP).

Administration for Children and Families

ACF administers the state-federal welfare program as a means to promote the economic and social well-being of individuals and families. It also administers the Head Start Program and supports state activities in foster care and adoption services.

Administration on Aging

AoA is the federal focal point for older persons and their concerns. AoA administers key programs for seniors and works with state and regional agencies to provide services that meet the unique needs of older persons and their caregivers.

NON-FEDERAL ORGANIZATIONS

There are many state and local governmental agencies that provide significant services to women in conjunction with and independent of federal programs. Also, non-profit community and professional organizations make considerable contributions to the health and well-being of women and their families. Women's health has received significant attention since the early 1990s; however, there is a need to continue this directed focus to ensure that women's unique needs are understood and addressed. In addition to the continuation of research and therapeutic and educational efforts, it is vital that special consideration be given to distribution and application of newly derived evidence-based information.

HEALTH CARE POLICY AND DELIVERY

MANAGED CARE

The current health care system in the United States bears little resemblance to that of several decades ago. Change has been constant, particularly with third-party reimbursement (insurance coverage). The country found itself paying almost 14 percent of its gross national product for health, and, as cost increased, reform became a necessity. The marketplace looked to a system of managed care for help. The system was initially designed to organize (or manage) the care needed by individuals and groups. However, it became apparent that managed care was at least theoretically able to control the upward spiraling cost associated with health care. As a result, managed care programs came rushing into the marketplace to oppose the traditional fee-for-service plans that seemingly lacked built-in mechanisms to control cost problems. A dramatic paradigm shift occurred when large numbers of people—many in response to their employers' selections of health plan coverage—moved to managed care programs.

Managed care is an organizational structure that is predicated on the relationship between insurers and providers, in other words, cost (paid by the insurer) and utilization (use of services by the provider) are linked. Several linkage methods are possible, but the most common is the use of capitation or prepayment in which the financial risk is shifted away from the insurer to the provider or health plan. With capitation, a fixed amount of money is periodically paid to cover the services needed by individuals who are covered by the insurance. Prudent utilization of services can produce profit for the provider, whereas overutilization of services can create a financial liability.

The best managed care initiatives value a comprehensive approach with a focus on prevention, early intervention, and continuity of care. The worst managed care initiatives create incentives to provide inadequate care, less time with patients, frequent change of providers, very early discharge of hospitalized patients, and impingement on professional judgment. The goal of managed care is to consider the merit of services, procedures, and treatments in view of the resources available. In many instances, the primary provider is expected to be the "gatekeeper" who assures that care is timely and necessary. Some clinical control may be exercised over the physician and nurse providers with an ultimate goal of standardization.

Managed care includes three basic models: the health maintenance organization (HMO), preferred provider organization (PPO), and the point-of-service arrangement (POS), plus innumerable other small hybrid combinations. The HMO is both an insurer and provider that assesses a fixed prepaid fee for the services it provides. HMOs most often utilize either a staff model or an individual practice association (IPA). In the staff model, physician and nurse providers are employed directly and work in HMO-owned facilities. IPAs are community-based independent providers. In both situations, health plan members are assigned to primary physicians who function as gatekeepers and coordinators of care. Other provider models or combinations within HMOs are possible.

Large insurance companies, hospitals, and some physician groups formed preferred provider organizations. PPOs involve a plan or arrangement whereby volume is guaranteed to the provider in exchange for discounted fees to members of contracted plans. Members of plans are encouraged to see only providers selected from an approved list, and even with discounted fees, co-payments for services may result in the tendency not to seek care until health conditions become serious (Kelly & Joel, 1999). The POS model is a combination of HMO and PPO in which providers who are not members of the plan's network can be utilized but at increased cost to the insured at the time the service is delivered. The prepaid plan also permits the insured to access an assigned provider within the network at lower cost.

Enrollments and Costs

In 1999, 91 percent of employees covered by health insurance were in managed care plans, up from 27 percent in 1988 (Hurtado, Swift, & Corrigan, 2001). This shift brought about both opportunities and problems that affect how care is delivered and received. Some believe that managed care was too restrictive, and, as a consequence, more choice was sought, resulting in higher costs. Cost escalation per se somewhat flattened in the mid-1990s due to a strong economy, but by 2002, health care cost inflation returned with a vengeance. As a result of increased cost and decreased growth, managed care faces an uncertain future, although there seems to be no question that it will stay. The unknown is how will it change (Stoddard, Reschovsky, & Hargraves, 2001).

Implications for Women

According to the American College of Obstetricians and Gynecologists (1996), the shift to managed care has important implications for women, including the following:

◆ Cost-cutting strategies that influence the visible and measured cost of managed care may be based on hidden costs to women, i.e., decreased length of hospital stay for children and the elderly are often met by increased at-home care given by women as caregivers. In addition, with the gatekeeper referral system and the frequent need to go to multiple sites for diagnostic tests, an additional burden is placed on the patients and on women who are the principal care coordinators.

◆ Loss of continuity of care and an established trust relationship for a woman when her plan does not include the same provider.

◆ Potential prohibition of Ob/Gyn physicians from making referrals for services (i.e., surgical consult after abnormal mammography) if they are not classified as primary physicians.

◆ Constraining clinical judgment that may affect individualization of care and increase patient morbidity, i.e., dictating length of stay for mothers and newborns who may require more observation and nursing care.

◆ Attempts to cut costs by excluding the sickest or most troublesome populations from coverage, i.e., the uninsured with a high proportion of women and children.

HEALTH POLICY AND WOMEN'S HEALTH CARE

To understand health policy as it relates to women, the subject matter must be viewed within the context of all health policy, including major economic, social, and political forces that influence the field.

Health Care Costs

◆ At the present time, the problem surmounting all other considerations is one of cost. Annual spending on health care exceeds $4,800 per person nationally, up from $3,621 in 1994, primarily due to rising costs for prescription drug and hospitalization, and the introduction of new technologies that add to the complexity of medical services (Diede & Liliedahl, 2002).

◆ By 1999, national health care expenditures topped $1.1 trillion or 13.5 percent of the U.S. gross domestic product (Hurtado, Swift, & Corrigan, 2001). The United States spends more on health care than any other industrialized country in the world.

◆ Costs and the efforts to contain them are affecting the quality of the care delivered.

Corporate Influence on the Health Industry

◆ In today's market, a business approach is taken to health care delivery, with a focus on marketing services and the financial bottom line. Women's health care is viewed as a tremendous source of revenue for health care organizations. Exploitation of women's services as simply a hospital marketing strategy, without provision of quality services, must be guarded against.

◆ Economic good competes with social good; emphasis can be on paying for care or on providing care.

Competition

◆ Players in the health care marketplace—patients, providers, payers, purchasers, and policymakers—have competing objectives.

◆ Prices and costs of services should decrease with competition, but this principle is not reflected in the health care industry.

Safety

◆ Although cost containment is certainly important, a focus on cost alone will not suffice. The health care delivery system must also ensure that care is safe, effective, efficient, and tailored to an individual's specific needs. Safety, i.e., freedom from accidental injury during medical treatment, is a critical step in improving quality of care (IOM, 2001b).

◆ A report from the Institute of Medicine in 2000 cites alarming statistics: Each year there are an estimated 98,000 avoidable deaths among hospitalized patients. Adding nonfatal errors, the total comes to almost 1 million preventable injuries related to medical treatment every year. The deaths and injuries that are largely preventable are due more to system failures than to errors on the part of individuals.

◆ Changes to the system require a long-term commitment and motivation to succeed, but they can be accomplished. For example, researchers found that integrating computers, pharmacists, and physicians reduced medication errors by 66 percent (IOM, 2000).

Reproductive Freedom

◆ A public spotlight is on this women's issue.

◆ *Roe v. Wade,* which was the basis of the 1973 Supreme Court decision on abortion, is constantly challenged in test cases that seek to limit or reverse it.

◆ Title X, the nation's family planning program, faces challenges every year. Although the program has never funded abortion services, amendments that would require parental notification for contraception, gags on counseling concerning reproductive choices, and others are brought up at each appropriation cycle.

♦ Parental notification and/or consent for abortion is a national issue.

♦ Funding for and availability of abortion services are major health policy issues.

♦ Limited contraceptive options for women remain an issue, although several new alternatives and preparations have recently become available.

♦ Up to fifteen years and in excess of $50 million are required for a new contraceptive to move from the laboratory through the U.S. Food and Drug Administration (FDA) approval process.

♦ A study published in the *American Journal of Public Health* demonstrated that preventing unintended pregnancy saves a health care system at least $3,000 per woman per year (Trussell, 1995).

Technological Advances

Medical

♦ Advancing technology in areas such as bioengineering, transplantation, cloning, and use of fetal tissue raises issues of who shall live, who shall die, and who shall decide.

♦ The extraordinary success of the genome project sets the stage for additional ethical decision making in addition to significant need for increases in genetic counseling. In addition, stem cell research has become a major issue on the national scene.

♦ With increasing technological ability to save and prolong life, discussions of health care rationing arise, requiring explicit policy decisions of who receives advanced technology care.

Information Systems and Telemedicine

♦ Computers and electronic mail are now the current standard for transmitting messages and information. Computing is not just about computers, it is about living. In 1995, 35 percent of U.S. families had a personal computer at home; the number rose to 54 percent in 2000 (IDS Survey, 2002).

♦ By indicating a specific uniform resource locator (URL) or by utilizing a search engine such as Yahoo! or Google, health information can be accessed either on a specific disease such as breast cancer or diabetes or on health promotion activities such as exer-

cise or antismoking campaigns. An immense amount of information is now available on the World Wide Web to assist women so that they are appropriately prepared to be involved in their own health care.

♦ An effective way to gain overview of health resources on the Web is to use one of the Internet meta-directories that give categorized listings of relevant sites. For example, of particular interest for those desiring information regarding women's health is the Women's Health Information Resource at the Rosenthal Center, Columbia University (Rosenthal Center, 2002).

♦ Health care providers will have access to high-resolution x-ray transmission equipment that can send an image across town or across several states to consult with a clinical expert on a particular diagnosis. Pictures of skin conditions or EKG strips can be sent via high-speed telecommunications equipment for consultation with a specialist who has expertise not available in the patient's hometown.

♦ Computerized record keeping is seen as a method to increase necessary communication about patients, decrease superfluous paper charts, and maintain easily retrievable information. Many centers already use computerized records for portions of the chart and are moving towards totally electronic versions. Currently, it is possible for nursing notes to be entered at the bedside via handheld computers, and it is envisioned that elaboration on this methodology is within the foreseeable future. The need is great to protect electronic health information from falling into the wrong hands or being used injudiciously. Caution must be incorporated into this otherwise helpful methodology.

♦ Telemedicine is defined as removing distance and time barriers to the provision of health services or health information. In the United States, telemedicine systems continue to grow and have 206 functioning programs as of 2001. Telemedicine currently uses broader ranges of clinical specialties, and, although newer methods of technologies are utilized, the most common means of delivering care to isolated areas remains interactive television (Association of Telehealth Servce Providers [ATSP], 2001). Several pilot projects have been undertaken that involve nursing groups such as a Visiting Nurses' Association utilizing interactive video to frequently assess patients in their homes. New attitudes and evolving wireless technology will most likely alter existing healthcare patterns not only for those in remote areas but also for those needing specialized consultation and health information in any area.

- An implanted data chip is being used now by some people to store information about personal history. As hospitals gain technology to access the chip, it will become common practice.

Primary Care and Prevention

- The Institute of Medicine's Committee on the Future of Primary Care defines primary care as the provision of *integrated,* accessible health care services by *clinicians* who are *accountable* for addressing a large majority of personal health care needs, developing a *sustained partnership* with patients, and practicing in the context of *family and community.* A key term in this definition is *integration,* which encompasses the provision of *comprehensive, coordinated,* and *continuous* services (IOM, 1996).
- For women, having a primary care clinician means that they have a place to bring a wide range of health problems for appropriate attention—a place where they can expect, in most instances, that their problems will be resolved, or the primary care clinicians will guide women through the health system, referring them to specialists when appropriate. Primary care facilitates an ongoing relationship between women and their clinicians and fosters participation by women in decision making about their health care. Such continuing relationships provide opportunities for health promotion and disease prevention as well as for early detection of problems.
- The Bureau of Primary Health Care (BPHC) developed a program entitled "Pathways to Wellness: Women Centered Primary Health Care" as a means of demonstrating BPHC's vision to ensure access to health care and to eliminate health disparities for underserved women and women from racial, ethnic, and lifestyle minority groups. It reflects how communities across the country can translate the vision into practice and can share the lessons learned via the utilization of primary health care providers and community health care programs (BPHC, 2001).

Long-Term Care/Home Health Care

- Long-term care covers an array of services over ongoing periods of time to people of all ages with chronic conditions and functional limitations. Needs range from minimal personal assistance with activi-

ties of daily living to virtual total care. Care is delivered in a variety of settings: people's homes, residential care facilities, nursing homes, and skilled nursing facilities.

- Aging of the U.S. population in general and particularly the population of 85-year-olds and older (the oldest growing age group in the United States) has had a major effect on the demand for and supply of long-term care services and on the resources needed to provide them. The greatest increase is expected to occur when the baby boomers enter elderly ages, of which the first group reaches 65 in 2011 and the last around 2030 (IOM, 2001c). By this time, life expectancy will increase, with a considerable population living to 90 years and beyond.
- In 1999, there were approximately 1.5 million elderly nursing home residents who were 65 years of age or over, and more than half were 85 or older. The elderly represented over two-thirds of people in long-term care. Almost 75 percent of residents were female (IOM, 2001c).
- Women are the primary users of long-term care services in all settings.
- Women provide the significant majority of paid and unpaid family care in the home, especially for children and the elderly.

HIV/AIDS

- HIV/AIDS continues to be a major public health issue with an ongoing need for public policy and political forces to support funding for research, prevention, education, and treatment.
- In the United States an increasing proportion of AIDS cases occur in women. Females accounted for 26 percent of AIDS cases diagnosed in 2000 (there is no universal requirement for reporting HIV so data are not consistent or complete). Between 1998 and 1999, there were 10,841 new cases of AIDS reported in women. HIV/AIDS is the third leading cause of death in women ages 25 to 44 (CDC, 2001).
- The rate of HIV/AIDS is particularly high among African American women, who represent 64 percent of cases. Hispanic and white women each represent 18 percent of cases (National Institute of Allergy and Infectious Diseases [NIAID], 2002).
- Sixty-four percent of HIV in women occurs as a result of heterosexual contact, and approximately 33 percent are infected via injection drug use (CDC, 2001).

◆ Between the years of 1992 and 1998, perinatally acquired HIV decreased by 75 percent due to a targeted program for women who received services and programs to reduce or prevent perinatal HIV transmission, especially via increased screening and effective drug therapies. By 2001, the incidence of transmission by infected women dropped from 25 percent to about 8 percent (NIAID, 2002).

◆ Innovative strategies are needed to avert new infections, develop a more accurate surveillance system, create additional research endeavors, translate research and organizational findings to action at the community level, and continue to overcome social and policy barriers that impede HIV prevention.

Substance Abuse

◆ Substance abuse and its related problems are among society's most insidious health and social concerns. A report in *Healthy People 2010* reveals that seventy-two different conditions requiring hospitalization are wholly or partially attributable to substance abuse (USPHS, 2000).

◆ Large populations of substance abusers initiate use of alcohol and tobacco during or shortly after adolescence followed by progression to alcohol abuse or illicit drug use (USPHS, 2000). This speaks urgently to the need for intervention programs aimed at middle- and senior-high-school-aged students. A national awareness of the problem has led to raising the legal drinking age to 21 in all states and implementing tighter controls on advertising (Sinclair, 2000).

◆ Binge drinking has become a major concern involving almost seven million individuals between the ages of 12 and 20. Although males are more likely to engage in binge drinking than females, the numbers of females are increasing (SAMHSA, 2002).

◆ Alcohol use by women is prevalent but occurs less than in men. It is estimated that 3.8 million women are using alcohol inappropriately with 10 to 15 percent of that number being women over the age of 60 (SAMSHA, 2002).

◆ In 2000, 14 million Americans used illicit drugs (6.3% of population over the age of 12). Rates were higher among men than among women, 7.7 vs. 5.0. However, rates between the sexes were similar for nonmedical use of psychotherapeutics, e.g., pain relievers, tranquilizers, stimulants, and sedatives (SAMHSA, 2002).

◆ Smoking is the leading known cause of preventable death and disease among women (U.S. Surgeon General, 2001). According to SAMHSA, approximately 26 percent of women report tobacco use. There is no doubt that women have been extensively targeted in tobacco marketing. The health consequences of smoking are many, but in most instances they are reversible after some years of abstinence (Surgeon General, 2001).

◆ Substance abuse during pregnancy can cause severe outcomes for the offspring: fetal alcohol syndrome (alcohol), small-for-date babies (tobacco), and teratogenic effects (selected illicit and/or nonapproved prescription drugs). Children who have been exposed to second-hand smoke are at increased risk for Sudden Infant Death Syndrome (SIDS) and severe respiratory illnesses such as bronchitis or asthma. All women should be apprised of such deleterious effects before they actually become pregnant.

Violence and Abuse

◆ Violence is a major public health problem for U.S. women with two of every five women having experienced some form of violence in their lives. Further, it is estimated that 10 to 20 percent of young females are the victims of sexual abuse (NWHIC, 2001b).

◆ Violence against women cuts across socioeconomic lines and affects all races and classes. The incidence of domestic battery increases during pregnancy with estimates ranging from 40 to 60 percent of all pregnant women. Domestic violence is the single largest cause of injury to women in the United States (McFarlane, 1999).

◆ Professionals in the health field are in good positions to recognize abuse and intervene. However, physicians and nurses sometimes fail to notify legal authorities and to provide appropriate counseling to the woman. State laws vary regarding requirements that health care providers must report their suspicions.

Complementary and Alternative Medicine (CAM)

◆ In response to the perception that the modern health care system is disease-oriented with increasing reliance on newer technologies and specializations, consumers began using more and more alternatives to traditional western medicine. Although home remedies have been used for many years, a more directed holistic and integrated approach is espoused especially by and for women.

- Use of complementary and alternative medicine for prevention and healing is increasing, from 34 percent in 1990 to 42 percent in 1998 (NCCAM, 2002). CAMs are groups of diverse practices, products, and systems that are not presently part of conventional medicine, including acupuncture, reflexology, therapeutic touch, meditation, yoga, herbal therapies, nutritional supplements, homeopathy, naturopathic medicine, ayurveda, and many more.
- Regardless of the modality, the concept of individuals as bio-psycho-social-cultural-spiritual beings is shared, including the belief that the individual is capable of decision making and is an integral part of the health team (Olshansky, 2000).
- Integrative health care is a combination of the concepts and selected practices of CAM and Western medicine techniques and providers.
- In 1998, the National Center for Complementary and Alternative Medicine (NCCAM) evolved from the Office of Alternative Medicine at the National Institutes of Health. Its overriding mission is to give the U.S. public reliable information about the safety and effectiveness of complementary and alternative medicine practices (NCCAM, 2002). This is an extremely important function because there is no current law requiring CAMs to meet quality or review standards as with other foods, drugs, and systems of practice.

Liability Insurance

- Increased lawsuits have led to increased defensive medical practices by physicians to protect themselves. Hence, a major increase in the cost of liability insurance to providers has occurred.
- High liability insurance premiums have caused some obstetricians to eliminate maternity care or reduce services for high-risk women, leaving many women unserved.
- In the last several years a number of insurance companies have left the market, causing physicians to look for insurance coverage. Recent increases in insurance premiums, in response to increased malpractice awards, also have physicians looking at different options.
- Advanced practice nurses who function as direct care providers need to maintain individual liability insurance to be covered in the event of litigation. This is

true even when their employers insure them (Pearson, 2002).

- Many states have some type of tort reform, e.g., caps on malpractice awards. It is expected that national tort reform will be introduced into Congress in the near future; however, it is unlikely that stringent measures will be passed.

SYSTEM ISSUES FOR THE FUTURE

The health care system has been dominated by cost concerns for the better part of thirty years, and costs will continue to be of major importance. Currently, rising costs are putting pressure on health plans to develop and purchasers to buy health coverage with less comprehensive benefits and more cost sharing at the point of service. In addition, premiums for basic plans are increasing. Due to cost and administrative barriers, small businesses find it particularly challenging to provide health care coverage for employees. Even the very large group purchasers of health care have been hard hit by significant increases in cost. Both private and public sector initiatives are needed to improve affordability of health care coverage (California Healthline, 2002).

While cost is certainly important, focusing foremost on reducing cost will not meet the country's needs. The systems by which health care is delivered and financed must be designed to ensure that the care is safe, effective, efficient, and tailored to individuals' specific needs. As the Institute of Medicine (2001d) points out, the nation must be guided by a single organizing principle: imparting quality in health care. Overall, quality is deficient. Physician discontent and nurse shortage are widespread. Coverage for seniors is inconsistent, minimally responsive to need, and lacking in strategies for long-term care. Racial and ethnic minorities experience higher rates of mortality and morbidity than whites. The safety net for disadvantaged and underserved populations (Medicaid) must provide more efficient availability and access (45 million Americans are uninsured with 60 percent of families living below the 200% poverty line). Consumer attitudes must be changed regarding such concepts as care at end of life and mental health service. Health care must be available for young children via increases in the State Children's Health Insurance Program or other approaches. The list goes on. Each person's health and well-being are shaped by interaction of genetic endowments, environmental exposures, lifestyle and food choices, income, and medical care. This "total" person must be recognized in the health care each one receives.

The World Health Organization ranked quality of care among 191 nations. The United States ranked thirty-seventh, below Saudi Arabia, Morocco, and every industrialized nation in the world. Health reform must address quality and coverage with equal fervor (California Healthline, 2002).

THE FUTURE OF WOMEN'S HEALTH

The current field of women's health is one of the most rapidly evolving areas in health delivery. A major effort in the field during the next decade will take into account specific individual needs to the point of custom tailoring the care delivered. Research efforts during the next several decades will focus on basic differences between sexes at the clinical, cellular, and molecular levels (Future of Women's Health, 2000). In health care delivery, differences related to age and ethnicity of the individual woman will be considered as well as socio-behavioral issues such as caregiving roles, domestic violence, access to health information, lifestyle preferences, autonomy to make health decisions, and learning/motivation for health prevention and promotion.

It is likely that there will be more specific drug treatments for breast cancer, osteoporosis, inflammatory diseases, and menopause; better diagnostic procedures for heart disease; and less invasive surgery for fibroid removal, heart surgery, breast biopsy, and lumpectomy (Future of Women's Heath, 2000). Improved surveillance and quality assurance may allow for the development of better methods to gather and retrieve relevant data and a more consistent method to develop and measure standards of care. Women's and perinatal health must be better integrated to compensate for poor coordination of services; this may be achieved by increasing numbers of obstetricians'/gynecologists' being designated primary care providers (Grason et al., 1999a).

Programs to support entry of diverse and increased numbers of women into health fields will be undertaken in public and private sectors. These will involve new and expanded education programs at a variety of levels, improved capacity to provide care across the broad range of women-specific health needs, promoting women as leaders within the health professions, and developing new funding streams for women's health research and education.

REFERENCES

Abrums, M. (1986). Health care for women. *Journal of Obstetrics, Gynecologic and Neonatal Nursing, 3,* 250–255.

American College of Obstetricians and Gynecologists. (1996, April). *Committee opinion—Physician responsibility under managed care: Patient advocacy in a changing health environment.* Washington, DC: Author.

Association of Telehealth Service Providers (ATSP). (2001). *Report on U. S. telemedicine activity.* Retrieved May 23, 2002 from http://www/atsp.org/survey/telemed2001.asp.

Boston Women's Health Collective. (1971). *Our bodies, ourselves.* New York: Simon & Schuster.

Bullough, V., & Vought, M. (1973). Women, menstruation, and nineteenth-century medicine. *Bulletin of Historical Medicine, 47*(1).

Bureau of Primary Health Care (BPHC). (2001). *Pathways to wellness.* Retrieved May 23, 2002 from ftp://ftp.hrsa.gov/bphc/pdf/omwh/pathwaysBooktext.txt.

California Healthline. (2002). *The cost and quality of health care.* Retrieved March 22, 2002 from http://www.californiahealthline.org/members/printer_basecontent.asp?contentid.

The Center for Studying Health System Change (HSC). (2002). *Community tracking study.* Retrieved March 22, 2002 from http://www.nschange.org.

Centers for Disease Control (CDC). (2000). *Ten public health achievements: Healthier mothers and babies.* Retrieved March 13, 2002 from http://www.cdc.gov/phtn/tenachievements/mothers.

Centers for Disease Control (CDC). (2001). Division of HIV/AIDS Prevention. *HIV in women.* Retrieved May 14, 2002 from http://www.cdc.gov/hiv/graphics/images/1264/1264-9.htm.

Collins, K. S. (1999). *Health concerns across a woman's lifespan.* New York: The Commonwealth Fund.

Day, K. (1997, June 26). A fever for women's health care. Washingtonpost.com.

Diede, M. L., & Liliedahl, R. (2002). Getting on the right track. *American Journal of Managed Care, 8*(2), 172–181.

Ehrenreich, B., & English, D. (1973). *Complaints and disorders: The sexual politics of sickness.* New York: Feminist Press.

Food and Drug Administration (FDA). (2001). Office of Women's Health (OWH). Retrieved May 4, 2002 from http://www.fda.gov/womens/default.htm.

Food and Drug Administration (FDA). (2002). Office of Women's Health (OWH) overview. Retrieved May 4, 2002 from http://www.fda.gov/womens/programs.htm.

Freidan, B. J. (1963). *The feminine mystique.* New York: W. W. Norton.

Freidan, B. J. (1991, November). The dangers of the new feminine mystique. *McCall's,* 78–86.

Future of Women's Health. (2000). *Harvard Women's Health Watch, VII*(5), 4–6.

Gonen, J. S. (1999). Women's primary care in managed care: Clinical and provider issues. *Women's Health Issues, 9*(2 Suppl.), 55–145.

Grason, H., Hutchins, J., & Silver, G. (Eds.). (1999a). *Charting a course for the future of women's and perinatal health: Volume I—Concepts, findings, and recommendations.* Baltimore: Women's and Children's Health Policy Center, Johns Hopkins School of Public Health.

Grason, H., Hutchins, J., & Silver, G. (Eds.). (1999b). *Charting a course for the future of women's and perinatal health: Volume II—Reviews of key issues.* Baltimore: Women's and Children's Health Policy Center, Johns Hopkins School of Public Health.

Hankinson, S. E., Colditz, G. A., Manson, J. E. & Speizer, F. E. (Eds.). (2001). *Healthy women, healthy lives.* New York: Simon & Schuster Source.

Henry, J. K. (2001). Eliminating health inequities: National goals and developing programs. *Journal of Obstetric, Gynecologic, and Neonatal Nursing, Clinical Studies, 30*(5), 1–6.

Hurtado, M. P., Swift, E. K., & Corrigan, J. (Eds.). (2001). *Envisioning the national health care quality report.* Boardon Health Care Services. National Academy Press. Retrieved May 17, 2002 from http://books.edu/books/0308907343x/html.

IDS Consumer Computing Survey. (2002). Abstract. Retrieved May 4, 2002 from http://www.marketresearch.com/product/display.asp?ProductID.

The Institute for the Future. (2000). *Health and health care 2010: The forecast, the challenge.* San Francisco: Jossey-Bass Publishers.

Institute of Medicine (IOM). (1996). *Primary care: America's health in a new era.* Washington, DC: National Academy of Medicine.

Institute of Medicine (IOM). (2000). *To err is human: Building a safer health system.* Washington, DC: National Academy Press.

Institute of Medicine (IOM). (2001a). *Exploring the biological contribution to human health: Does sex matter?* Retrieved February 16, 2002 from http://www.iom.edu/iom/iomhome/nsf/wfiles/doessexmatter.

Institute of Medicine (IOM). (2001b). *Crossing the quality chasm: A new health system for the 21st century.* Washington, DC: National Academy Press.

Institute of Medicine (IOM). (2001c). *Improving quality of long-term care.* Retrieved March 15, 2002 from http://books.nap.edu/books/0309064988/htm/R1.html.

Institute of Medicine (IOM). (2001d). *Informing the future: Critical issues in health.* Retrieved March 15, 2002 from http://books.nap.edu/books/N1000335/html/17.html.

Institute of Medicine (IOM). (2002). *Unequal treatment: Confronting racial and ethnic disparities in health care.* Washington, DC: National Academy Press.

JAMWA Library of Links. (2002). *Women's Health Equity Act.* Retrieved May 4, 2002 from http://jamwa.amwa-doc.org/541-els.htm.

Kelly, L. Y., & Joel, L. A. (1999). *Dimensions of professional nursing* (8th ed.). New York: McGraw-Hill.

Lu, M. C., Bragonier, R., Silver, E. R., & Bemis-Heys, R. (2000). Where it all begins: The impact of preconceptional and prenatal care on early childhood development. In N. Halfon, E. Shulman, M. Hochstein, & M. Shannon (Eds.), *Building community systems for young children.* Los Angeles: UCLA Center for Healthier Children, Families and Communities.

Marieskind, H. (1975). The women's health movement. *International Journal of Health Services, 5*(2), 217–223.

McFarlane, J. (1999). Severity of abuse before and during pregnancy for African-American, Hispanic and Anglo women. *Journal of Nurse Midwifery, 44*(2), 139–144.

McGlynn, E. A. (1998). The effect of managed care on primary care services for women. *Women's Health Issues, 8*(1), 1–14.

National Center for Complementary and Alternative Medicine (NCCAM). (2002). NIH. Retrieved May 23, 2002 from http://nccam.nih.gov/health.

National Center for Health Statistics (NCHS). (2001). *Health: United States 2001.* Retrieved March 13, 2002 from http://www.cdc.gov/nchs.

National Institute of Allergy and Infectious Diseases (NIAID). (2002). *Fact sheet: Women with HIV/AIDS.* Retrieved May 18, 2002 from http://www/niaid.nih.gov/factsheets/womenhiv.htm.

National Institutes of Health (NIH)/National Heart, Lung, and Blood Institute (NHLBI). (2002a). *Women's health initiative.* Retrieved May 4, 2002 from http://www.nhlbi.nih.gov/whi/factsht.htm.

National Institutes of Health (NIH)/Office of Research on Women's Health (ORWH). (2002b). *Women's health initiative overview.* Retrieved May 4, 2002 from http://www4.od.nih.gov/orwh/overview.htm.

The National Women's Health Information Center (NWHIC). (2001a). *The history and future of women's health.* Retrieved February 16, 2002 from http://www.4women.gov/owh/pub/history.htm.

The National Women's Health Information Center (NWHIC). (2001b). *Women's health issues: An overview.* Retrieved March 12, 2002 from http://www.4women.gov/owh/pub/womhealth%20issues/index.htm.

Office of Research on Women's Health. (1996, March). *Overview statement on the women's health initiative.* National Institutes of Health, 1–2.

Olshansky, E. (2000). *Integrated women's health: Holistic approaches for comprehensive care.* Gaithersburg, MD: Aspen Publishers.

Pearson, L. (2002). NP legislative update. *The Nurse Practitioner, 27*(1), 10–22.

Pinn, V. (1994). The role of the NIH Office of Research on Women's Health. *Academic Medicine, 69*(9), 698–702.

Raymond, R., & Allshouse, K. (n.d.). *Resiliency amidst inequity: Older women workers in an aging U.S.* (pp. 1–4). Southport, CT: Southport Institute for Policy Analysis, Project for Women and Population Aging.

Reuben, D. (1971). *Everything you always wanted to know about sex.* New York: David McKay.

Rosenthal Center. (2002). *Women's health information resources.* Retrieved May 24, 2002 from http://www.rosenthal.hs.columbia.edu/women.html#Contents.

Sinclair, B. P. (1997). Advanced practice nurses in integrated heath care systems. *Journal of Obstetrics, Gynecologic and Neonatal Nursing, 26*(2), 217–223.

Sinclair, B. P. (2000). Health promotion and prevention. In D. Lowdermilk, S. Perry, & I. Bobak (Eds.), *Maternity and women's health care* (7th ed.; pp. 68–87). St. Louis: Mosby.

Stoddard, J., Reschovsky, J., & Hargraves, L. (2001). Trends in involvement of physicians with managed care. *American Journal of Managed Care, 7*(11), 1061–1067.

Stubblefield, P. G. (1999). Effect of prenatal care upon medical conditions in pregnancy. In M. C. McCormick & J. E. Siegel (Eds.), *Prenatal care: Effectiveness and implementation.* Cambridge, UK: Cambridge University Press.

Substance Abuse and Mental Health Services Administration (SAMHSA). (2002). *Topics in substance abuse.* Retrieved May 18, 2002 from http://www.samhsa.gov/oas/highlights.htm.

Trussell, J., Leveque, J. A., & Koenig, J. D. (1995). The economic value of contraception: A comparison of 15 methods. *The American Journal of Public Health, 85*(4), 494–503.

U.S. Census Bureau. (2000). *Health insurance coverage: 1999, current population survey.* Retrieved April 1, 2002 from http://www.census.gov/hhes/www/hlthin99.html.

U.S. Department of Health and Human Services (HHS). (2002). *HHS: What we do.* Retrieved April 1, 2002 from http://www.hhs.gov/news/press/2002pres/profile.html.

U.S. Public Health Service (USPHS). (1985). *Women's health: Report of the public health service task force on women's health issues: Volume II* (DHHS Publication No. PHS 85-50206). Washington, DC: U.S. Government Printing Office.

U.S. Public Health Service (USPHS). (2000). *Healthy people 2010.* Washington, DC: U.S. Department of Health and Human Services.

U.S. Surgeon General. (2001). *Women and smoking.* Retrieved May 18, 2002 from http://www/cdc.gov/tobacco/sgr_forwomen.htm.

Women's Policy, Inc. (1996). *The Women's Health Equity Act of 1996, Legislative summary and overview.* Washington, DC: Author.

CHAPTER 2

HEALTH AND DEVELOPMENT THROUGH THE LIFE CYCLE

Marcia Szmania Davis ◆ *Ellis Quinn Youngkin*

*P*erhaps as more emphasis is given to female perspectives, society can move toward more acceptance of power-with, rather than power-over, which would help facilitate a more peaceful environment on a larger scale (Lewis & Bernstein, 1996).

Highlights

- Growth and Development
- Adult Developmental Theories
    Erikson's Stages
    Levinson's Model
- Current Views on Women's Development
    A New Psychology of Women
- Major Periods and Tasks: The Women's Perspective

❖ INTRODUCTION

In order to define and understand women's development, one must address the societal norms that prevail over time (see Chapter 1). One important change during the late 1960s and early 1970s was women's realization that many important individual concerns they had previously been hesitant to discuss were actually widespread and political in nature. "The personal is political" slogan reflected an energy borne out in consciousness-raising groups where women talked about their lived experiences, learning that their innermost feelings were shared by women in general. A period of self-discovery began as women began to break out of socially constrictive stereotypes.

Earlier, in the 1950s, remarkable changes in women's lives were associated with fewer births, extended longevity, greater acceptance of lifestyle options in marriage and family formation, and attachment to the labor force (O'Rand & Henrette, 1982). Affirmative action movements eventually developed into academic programs in women's studies beginning in the 1960s, often with reluctant acceptance by universities (Grosskurth, 1991). These courses reflected limitations set on women by patriarchal societies, and

women contemplated the reasons. Recent history books celebrated women's influences that had largely been ignored or downplayed. In today's world, women, compared with their mothers, are better educated, spend more of their adult life living alone, and participate more consistently in the labor force (Woods, Lentz, & Mitchell, 1993).

Is the contemporary view of society toward women indeed different, however, from the past? The answer must be an equivocal yes, in part because traditional sex role stereotypes continue to pervade the thinking of many men and women. Women who do not marry and reproduce may be viewed as having failed to develop their fullest potential. Moreover, femininity has long been, and to a great extent continues to be, equated with passivity, looking attractive, making relationships work, and being unselfish and of service while being competent without complaint (Pipher, 1994; Woods et al., 1993). At the turn of the century, women are in state of flux where old expectations have broken down but have been replaced with new ideas that seem fragmentary, unrealistic, and often contradictory (Orenstein, 2001).

GROWTH AND DEVELOPMENT

Growth and development are often viewed according to a person's stage in the life cycle. Whereas *growth* refers to quantitative physical and physiological changes, *development* encompasses more qualitative changes, including functional, psychosocial, and cognitive behaviors. Both areas need to be assessed so that the health care provider can offer anticipatory guidance to women as they adapt to personal and environmental changes. Providers must also understand contemporary women's roles and expectations as well as their stressors within a social context in order to assist women in developing health promotion behaviors (Woods et al., 1993). The developmental theories most closely linked to sequential ages and life stages have frequently been used for clinical evaluation. Controversy exists, however, about the applicability of such theories to women, particularly because cultural biases may be a problem. For example, Erikson studied primarily white, middle-class males. Also, developmental norms may not apply to all cultural back-

grounds, and stage theories may promote ageism if one does not fulfill expectations, such as marriage, by a given point in life (Erikson, 1968; Norman, McCluskey-Fawcett, & Ashcroft, 2002).

Today, women's lives are very complex. Numbers of different life cycles and lines of development exist, overlap, conflict, and perhaps enhance each other. Seiden (1989) whimsically refers to a "life pretzel" where the biologic-reproductive circle, the family-marital circle, and the educational-vocational circle are all bound together. A simple circle tied to a reproductive life cycle will simply no longer suffice (if it ever did).

STAGE THEORIES OF DEVELOPMENT

Investigation of developmental change across the life span has gained prominence over the past fifty years, largely as a result of psychoanalytic influence. The resulting developmental theories emerged from the body of knowledge in child psychology. Although the life span developmental framework focused primarily on men, the resulting theories were generalized to apply to all adults. Women's development, which was seldom alluded to, was viewed narrowly and judged aberrant if gender development did not conform to the accepted male pattern (Kaschak, 1981).

Characteristics commonly attributed to women, such as being less aggressive, more emotional, and less independent, were seen to be less healthy. Although the majority of psychoanalytic clients were women, little was known about their experiences as women. Virtually no attention was directed towards the effects of the societal environment on women. Feminists thus came to view traditional psychotherapy as an agent of social control, reinforcing the traditional sex roles and traditional values that led to a devaluation of women.

HISTORICAL PSYCHOANALYTIC INFLUENCE

Freudian psychosexual theory and practice—the largest influence on psychotherapeutic knowledge—gave therapists a largely antifeminine orientation (Gilligan, 1982a; Hyde, 1985). Freud espoused that biological drives influence a person's psychological and personality development. In his view, superiority of men was largely derived from the possession of a penis. Penis envy purportedly led to feminine aggression. According to Freud, limitations of women inherent in their biology ("anatomy is destiny") included women's innate dependency, passivity, and masochism, which were required for their primary fulfilling role, successful motherhood. Compared with men, women were viewed as more narcissistic, more prone to jealousy, and having a weaker sense of justice (Strachey, 1961). Women were labeled "frigid" if they were incapable of mature (phallocentric) vaginal orgasm versus clitoral orgasm. The studies of Masters and Johnson proved this concept incorrect (Kaschak, 1981).

FEMINIST VIEWS ON PSYCHOANALYSIS

Critics condemned Freud for deriding women who displayed qualities that would be lauded in men, primarily boldness and independence (Grosskurth, 1991). Many women also voiced resentment toward the implied foreclosure on women's opportunities.

◆ Karen Horney (1920s and 1930s) proposed that if penis envy existed, it was because the penis symbol-

ized the social and political power of men (Hyde, 1985).
◆ Simone de Beauvoir (*The Second Sex,* 1949) caused a great deal of controversy by challenging the ideation of biological and psychological determination of roles for women.
◆ Betty Friedan (*The Feminine Mystique,* 1963) attempted to broaden society's narrow role of women's place being in the home.
◆ Kate Millet (*Sexual Politics,* 1969) continued to scorn Freud for upholding the male body as the norm and questioned the validity of Freud's concept of female fear of castration while ignoring issues such as rape.

ADULT DEVELOPMENTAL THEORIES

Although developmental changes during childhood and adolescence have been studied, relatively little attention has been paid to the adult years (Levinson, 1986), and the study of women's development is still in its infancy and is controversial. The climate exists for an interdisciplinary approach to the study of human development, and social scientists have shown us that societal issues must be closely addressed.

ERIKSON'S STAGES OF PSYCHOSOCIAL DEVELOPMENT (1950s TO 1960s)

One of the earliest contributors to the study of adult development, Erikson suggested the normalcy and necessity of growth and change during adult years and not just in childhood (Erikson, 1950, 1968). His theories, grounded in conceptions of the life cycle and the life course, addressed stages in ego development. According to Erikson,

◆ Each stage is primary at a particular age level, or segment of the life cycle, from infancy to old age.
◆ If a task that is appropriate to a given phase of life is not resolved, then development in subsequent phases of life may be impaired.
◆ A patterned sequence of stages occurs, each with appropriate physical, emotional, and cognitive tasks.
◆ A person who successfully passes through each stage eventually attains ego integrity, which is associated with high self-esteem and a positive outlook on life.

◆ A major difference for a woman is that her identity is enmeshed in a married state, wherein the task of her mate is to provide her with an adult identity, a necessary step in her mature integration of personality (see Chapter 1, Other Influences on Women's Health, Marital Status).

Erikson's eight stages of development, composed of bipolar tasks at various stages of life, include *Trust versus Mistrust,* infancy; *Autonomy versus Shame and Doubt,* early childhood; *Initiative versus Guilt,* preschool age; *Industry versus Inferiority,* school age; *Identity versus Identity Diffusion,* adolescence; *Intimacy versus Isolation or Self-Absorption,* young adulthood; *Generativity versus Stagnation,* middle adulthood; and *Integrity versus Despair and Disdain,* late adulthood.

LEVINSON'S MODEL OF ADULT DEVELOPMENT (1970s TO PRESENT)

This well-known model of adult development, which is grounded in psychoanalytic theory, is applied in research and psychotherapy (Levinson, 1978). Levinson believes that there is a single human life cycle through which both men and women evolve (the life structure). Tremendous variation exists related to gender, class, race, culture, historical epoch, specific circumstances, and genetics (Levinson, 1996). Levinson expanded on Erikson's notion of development and characterized each segment of adulthood in terms of intrinsic tasks (Erikson, 1950; Levinson, 1978, 1996). This theory proposes an underlying set of developmental periods and tasks along with transition crises that involve reassessment of one's life. Adult development is an evolving process of mutual interaction between self and the world, of which family and work are central components. Career choice and work are paramount in terms of goals, social roles, ethical standards and values, and development of self-concept. The assumption is that we desire self-actualization, which requires psychological and realistic change in controllable measures. To this extent, men and women are similar.

Levinson uses a central concept of gender splitting, which views a sharp division between feminine and masculine permeating every aspect of human life from cultural to individual. He also describes the current existence in the early stages of a vast historical transition where traditional patterns are eroding but satisfactory new ones have not been discovered and legitimized (Levinson, 1996). (Women's adult development is addressed later in this chapter in Major Periods and Tasks: The Women's Perspective.)

Theoretical models focusing particularly on women are developing. An extensive review of the literature by Caffarella and Olson (1993) shows women experiencing a nonlinear life course where discontinuities, periods of stability and transition, are the norm. Again, the importance of relationships, a need to maintain a fluid sense of self, and the ability to adapt to role changes are key throughout development.

Early Adult Transition (Ages 17 to 22)

The shaky start toward maturity involves taking new steps in individuation. Choices are made concerning career, lifestyle, and modification of existing family and social relationships. This is the adult era of greatest energy and abundance—and of greatest contradiction and stress.

Entering the Adult World (Ages 22 to 28)

Through the establishment of an independent living situation, exploration, and commitment to adult roles, the 20s reflect structure building.

Age 30 Transition (Ages 28 to 33)

During the transition period, the sense of being young, especially in terms of options, is given up. Current lifestyles, values, family situations, and career choices are evaluated. Biologically, the 20s and 30s are the peak years of life.

Settling Down (Ages 33 to 40)

Affirming personal integrity, realizing oneself as a full-fledged adult, and goal achievement are characteristic of this period.

Midlife Transition (Ages 40 to 45)

Lifestyle is critically examined, and the need arises to recognize time limitations for goal achievement. Polarities, including young—old and destruction—creation, are integrated. Levinson believes that the character of living always changes appreciably between early and middle adulthood.

Entering Middle Adulthood (Ages 45 to 50)

Undergoing restabilization after midlife transition, individuals in middle adulthood have biological capacities below earlier years but normally are still sufficiently fit for energetic, personally satisfying, and socially valuable lives.

Age 50 Transition (Ages 50 to 53)

Once more, lifestyle and major goals are reevaluated.

Middle Adulthood Culmination
(Ages 53 to 60)

Work continues toward achieving life goals and contributing to society.

Late Adulthood (Ages 60 to 80)
and the Late Adult Transition (60 to 65)

Although the character of one's life is fundamentally altered as a result of biological, psychological, and social changes, the individual recognizes that this period can be distinctive and fulfilling.

Late, Late Adulthood (Age 80
and Older)

At this time, the process of aging may be more obvious than the process of growth. The individual must make peace with dying; development occurs as one gives new meaning to life and death. These oldest adults may be an example for others by demonstrating wisdom and personal nobility.

CURRENT VIEWS
ON WOMEN'S DEVELOPMENT

WOMEN'S CONTRIBUTIONS

Women's influence has been largely absent in many areas, including art, literature, social sciences, and psychological research. Even though women have devoted their lives to supporting the lifelong development of others, their own development experiences are still essentially untold. Women's life experiences and viewpoints may indeed be different from men's as a result of complex factors such as social status, power and reproductive biology (Gilligan, 1982a; Miller, 1986). Indeed, the lives of women make up a complex web of economic, psychological, and social contradictions. Opportunities in one area are linked to constraints in others so that choices in one can have unexpected consequences (or benefits) many years later in another (Orenstein, 2000).

Gilligan's Theory of Moral Development

Gilligan, a clinical psychologist, traced women's voices as she studied the development of morality (Gilligan, 1982a). She found that existing psychological accounts failed to describe the progression of relationships toward a maturity of interdependence or trace the evolution of the capacity for responsible care. Gilligan challenged Freud, Piaget, and Kohlberg, who studied boys and men and then assumed that women's ability to make moral judgments was inferior (Gilligan, 1982b). Gilligan's work asserts that

◆ Women have learned, from their early socialization, to place priority on responsibility toward others in important relationships (the ethics of care) rather than on individual welfare and concerns. Identity and intimacy are not separate stages of development for women.

◆ When faced with a dilemma, women are interested in understanding individual circumstances and in obtaining the best possible solution for all concerned, rather than using more abstract universal justice principles employed by men.

◆ The standard of moral judgment that women use for self-assessment also has to do with relationships: the ability to nurture, to care for others, and to bear responsibility.

◆ Women's differing modes of moral reasoning lead to different forms of self-definition and different views of relationships (Gilligan, 1982a). Gilligan's work has been criticized as perpetuating gender stereotypes during the socially conservative 1980s (Mednick, 1989).

Bardwick's Model
of Human Development

Bardwick's model addresses women's adult development while incorporating much of Levinson's model of adult maturation. Bardwick maintains that psychological growth and change are intertwined and never cease (Bardwick, 1980). Moreover, the goals and values of one's life reflect changing societal and cultural values. The transition from one developmental stage to the next includes a process of self-evaluation. For women, transitions to new values and lifestyles are likely to be more extreme and more emotionally volatile than in previous generations, as options provided to women become more numerous.

Bardwick defines the self in terms of dependent, interdependent, and egocentric mental stances. A woman may maintain a *dependent* sense of self, which is basically relational, or move toward a more *interdependent* stance, in which a sense of self exists simultaneously with a keen awareness of being a contributing and receiving member of an affectional relationship. Bardwick, however, contends that for a woman to develop a permanent *egocentric* stance is rare, because socialization of women in our society and the definition of femininity tend much more toward an interdependent or dependent sense of self.

A NEW PSYCHOLOGY OF WOMEN

Equality

Caring for others is valued less in our society than are individuation and individual achievement; thus women's concern with relationships is often viewed as a weakness (Miller, 1986). The need for social equality is reflected in problems that arise when affiliation and relationships are molded by domination and subordination. A new language in psychology should describe the structuring of women's sense of self, that is, the need to make and then maintain relationships. Caring and connection must be separated from the resulting inequality and oppression. Women judge themselves in terms of their ability to care, so much so that professional and academic endeavors may be seen as jeopardizing their own sense of themselves (Gilligan 1982a). Personal conflict may arise when women have to choose between achievement and caring, if being successful is at the expense of another's failure.

Valuing Self

The psychology of women is distinct in relationships of temporary and permanent inequality (Gilligan, 1982b). A woman may be temporarily dominant in relationships of nurturance, yet subservient in relationships of permanently unequal social status and power. Women are subordinate in social position to men, yet at the same time entwined with them in the intimate and intense relationships of adult sexuality and family life. Feminist therapy involves the individual's recognition of the restrictive social binds that influence many women, including an overdependence on men for self-esteem and financial, psychological, and social needs. Women with less traditional sex role norms have reported better mental health and more health-promoting lifestyles (Woods et al., 1993).

In a small study, Hollis (1998) showed women, but not men, expressed regret and sometimes frustration toward perceived missed opportunities in life (e.g., career) due to confining social roles of wife and mother in decades ranging from the 1920s to the 1960s. Women traditionally have taken care of men, but men have tended to assume or devalue that care (Gilligan, 1982a). Women

need to learn to nurture and value themselves and other women, rather than nurturing only men and children. Women's psychology reflects both sides of relationships of interdependence.

Empowerment

Women need power to advance their own development and maintain an identity characterized by self-determination and a diminished need for continuous approval (Miller, 1986). Too often women find their lives being dominated by prevalent societal values. Often, women and men experience enormous differences in access to power and control of resources (Lott, 1987), and for women, a stance of less power may result in an emphasis on relatedness to others and compassion (Mednick, 1989). Powerlessness, or learned helplessness, in femininity may be exhibited in relationships of battering and more subtly as depression (Friedan, 1993; Kaschak, 1981). Perhaps as more emphasis is given to female perspectives, society can move toward more acceptance of power-with rather than power-over, which would help facilitate a more peaceful environment on a larger scale (Lewis & Bernstein, 1996). Mutuality in relationships would help foster efforts toward elimination of many social maladies such as violence against women and discrimination based on ethnicity and gender. Women could make significant steps toward healthier lives as stressors compromising many intimate affiliations diminish.

Many women have learned to demystify aspects of their lives, finding strength in the shared experiences of other women. Their strength is reflected in greater self-sufficiency, assertiveness, and self-knowledge. Consider the example of violence against women. Issues such as rape, battering of women, child sexual abuse, and incest were largely ignored, or their existence disbelieved, before the collected efforts of enraged women (Miller, 1986). Women have effected changes in medical/gynecologic care and will no longer accept care that is limited to their reproductive organs to the exclusion of concerns such as cardiac disease or to the discounting of entities such as premenstrual syndrome (PMS).

A Different Starting Point in Defining Women's Development/Tend and Befriend

Women essentially develop in a context of their attachment to others. The cornerstone of a new psychology of women is the appreciation of the power of relationship and connection in women's lives (Lewis & Bernstein, 1996). Women's sense of self, as well as their perceived strength, is based on the ability to form affiliations and relationships (Gilligan, 1982a; Lewis & Bernstein, 1996). Although this experience of attachment to others provides women with more opportunities for interpersonal pleasure, there is the concurrent fear of separation. Many women perceive the threat of a disrupted affiliation as a total loss of self. Perhaps there is a more ideal midpoint where affiliation is valued along with self-sufficiency. Possibilities exist for a more advanced approach to living and functioning in which affiliation is valued as highly, or more highly, than self-enhancement.

Along a similar vein, findings of a landmark study out of UCLA (Taylor et al., 2000) strengthen women's sense of value of friendship and affiliation. Women's response to stress may not be well characterized by the fight-or-flight response. Women's stress responses have developed to enhance survival of themselves and their offspring. Females create, maintain, and utilize social groups (befriend), particularly their female friends, in order to manage stressful situations, building on the attachment–care-giving process. Women also nurture their offspring (tend), while in turn reducing neuroendocrine responses that may compromise their health.

The tend-and-befriend behavior may be oxytocin-mediated, moderated by sex hormones and endogenous opioid peptide mechanisms. It is well known that animals as well as humans derive health benefits from social contact. Positive physical contact such as touching or hugging is known to release oxytocin, which further counters stress and produces a calming effect. The fact that men and women respond differently to stress has significant implication for health. Perhaps women need to find more time to partake of each other's nurturance and healing talk, rather than let other responsibilities close those ties (Apter & Josselson, 2000).

THE WAYS THAT WOMEN KNOW

The intellectual development of women has become another topic of study (Belenkey & Field, 1985; Belenkey et al., 1986). The inability of women to gain a voice reflects their image of being powerless, subjugated, and inadequate. Indeed, more women than men pose questions, listen to others, and refrain from speaking out, but women's pattern of discourse may be suitable for a maternal, caring, relationship-oriented role. For example, a mother may refrain from sharing ideas too quickly with her child in order to foster the child's own ability to form ideas. Thus, women may value drawing out the voices of others as a means of enhancing others' development. This mode

of discourse, similar to Socratic thinking, could serve as a model for promoting human development (Rosenblatt, 1995).

WOMEN'S ISSUES AND CONFLICTING VALUES

Value Changes

The value changes that occurred most dramatically during the 1970s redefined and expanded choices for women in their roles related to work and family (Bardwick, 1980). Many women must now address both modern and traditional patterns of lifestyle in their decision making. Facing conflicting life choices and societal norms, women grapple with cultural ambiguity and personal uncertainty. Traditional norms regarding femininity prevail, even for women in less traditional roles. For example, despite reduced gender separation of work and family roles in the 1990s, couples still tend to make decisions concerning geographical locations and timing of major family events according to the husband's career needs. On the other hand, women are choosing to have fewer children. This fact, combined with increasing longevity, means that a substantially shorter percentage of women's lives are spent childrearing. Also, with a lower marriage rate, later marriage, divorce, and widowhood, today's women will spend more of their lives alone than in any previous era (Orenstein, 2000).

Cultural Ambiguity and Personal Uncertainty

Although women's choices can create ambiguity and uncertainty, the freedom of choice is perhaps less frustrating than the restrictions of the recent past (Bardwick, 1980). Often, however, change may be an illusion for women; the reality of the social foundation of power still leans strongly toward enhanced status for traditional feminine values (Mednick, 1989; Orenstein, 2000). Modern women also face significant challenges to have it all because the social changes necessary to allow for ample choices have not been resolved. Barriers still exist to equitable pay, adequate childcare, and breaking through old boy networks. Women may have adequate drive to achieve; however, they may feel limited to a level of achievement that society deems appropriate for their gender difference or, some would argue, their social status. Conflict may arise between the need for affiliation or the desire for approval from other people and the pursuit of achievement for its own sake. Competition may be viewed as contrary to the traditional feminine ideal and may lead to social rejection. Although women and men tend to be compared favorably in neutral situations, women tend to have less internal hope for success in more competitive situations (Orenstein, 2000). A particular dilemma for women has been to achieve success in a traditionally male occupation or to achieve career success when contemplating motherhood. Economic and logistical demands (e.g., childcare) often find women slipping into more traditional roles (Orenstein, 2000).

Gender Issues

Levinson (1986, 1996) believes that the timing of developmental periods and tasks are similar for women and men, while giving weight to how men's and women's lives are affected by gender splitting issues, creating in human life a rigid division between male and female, masculine and feminine. To a much greater extent than we have previously been comfortable acknowledging, women and men have lived in different social worlds with very different social roles, identities, and psychological attributes.

The historical process within postindustrial conditions has included a gender revolution. Many social changes have reduced women's involvement in the family and have increased involvement in outside work. Some of these changes include (1) the sharp rise of human longevity; (2) the decreasing demand for women's work in the family, concomitant with smaller family size (contraception options); and (3) the growing incidence of divorce. More than 50 percent of all U.S. women are now in the labor force—part-time or full-time, paid or volunteer, continuously or sporadically (Levinson, 1996).

Other developmental themes hold that gender differences exist in movement through developmental periods (Bardwick, 1980; Caffarella & Olson, 1993; Hyde, 1985; Mercer, Nichols, & Doyle, 1989). Furthermore, women, more than men, tend to avoid evaluating their own lives. Perhaps this is because self-assessment may heighten women's awareness of their lack of self-determination and relative powerlessness, revealed in their tendency to respond to the directives and initiative of others (Bardwick, 1980). Women's self-esteem and identity also depend more heavily on validation by others.

Life Events, Options, and Stress

Along with more options, women may also experience discontent, as it is less clear what is expected of them. Stressors occur in traditional homemaker choices, in career options, and in attempts to combine the two. In addi-

tion, women may experience developmental periods at later ages and in more irregular sequences, while focusing on different aspects of their life structure (Mercer et al., 1989). Moreover, developmental tasks may be dealt with very differently at different times, as women themselves may change psychologically over time.

MAJOR PERIODS AND TASKS: THE WOMEN'S PERSPECTIVE

A well-formed body of knowledge on women's development does not exist; however, issues in women's development are discussed here, using Levinson's framework, where feasible, and other authors' contributions, especially those of Bardwick (1980). The novice phase of early adulthood—individuals as apprentice adults, ages 17 to 33—encompasses several large tasks, including forming a dream, a mentor relationship, an occupation, and an enduring relationship. Women and men may have significant differences in accomplishing these tasks (Roberts & Newton, 1987). Timing of major life events is not as important as understanding the importance in forming the life structure. A discussion of key transition periods follows.

EARLY ADULT TRANSITION (AGES 17 TO 22)

Major tasks for women in this period include value assessment; goal setting for education and work; formation of important peer relationships that focus on sex, love, commitment; formation of relationships to occupation; and separation from parents. Pipher (1994) describes young women's need to reject the person they most closely identify with as they grow up. They are socialized to have a tremendous fear of becoming like their mothers, and yet, if a young woman hates her mother, she hates herself. Strong girls may manage to stay close to their families and maintain some family loyalty, usually having someone in the family whom they love and trust. The task is not to end the relationship, but rather to reject certain aspects (e.g., submission, defiance), sustain more valued aspects, and build in new qualities such as mutual respect (Levinson, 1996). Individuation may be reflected in great differences in values between parents and young adults in areas such as politics and career choices. Values may more strongly reflect identification with peer groups, however, than true individuation or autonomy. Pipher (1994) notes girls may stay in adolescence longer now, taking about twelve years to make it through the crucible (age 22). Economics may be one reason; however, home may seem a safe haven in an increasingly dangerous world.

A major conflict exists between making commitments and avoiding them in order to keep options open (Erikson, 1968). Commitments are more easily made if one's peers are doing so. The early adult is often egocentric as she progresses through rapid emotional and physical changes. She may believe that she is invulnerable, unique, and immune, and hence be prone to misconceptions—for example, that sexual activity will not lead to pregnancy (Lichtman & Papera, 1990). In fact, approximately 95 percent of teenage pregnancies are unplanned (Johnson, 2000).

Gender Identity

A crucial task is to internalize a sense of gender, which encompasses a sense of one's body in relation to sexuality. To traditional young women, this focus may mean marriage, the prime example of moving into an adult sexual role. Women are essentially dependent at this time, and occasionally interdependent, as the need to form relationships dominates. A great deal of psychological fluidity exists with some sense of egocentrism. Men at this time exhibit comparatively less fluidity and interpersonal dependence and more egocentricity.

Traditional sex role expectations are still prominent in adolescence and early adulthood (Orenstein, 2000; Rosenblatt, 1995). For example, a woman may fear that her own ambitions will cost a relationship. A conflict exists between fulfillment of egocentric and interpersonal/dependent priorities as the early adult tries to define the sense of self.

Identity and Adult Commitments

Erikson describes the male adolescent as developing an autonomous, initiating, industrious self through the forging of an identity based on the ideal image—ability to support and justify adult commitments (Erikson, 1968). He describes the female adolescent as holding her identity in abeyance while preparing to attract the man she will marry and by whose status she will be defined. Such attitudes predominated well into the 1960s and, to a great degree, still exist. Pipher (1994) describes our culture as look-obsessed. Despite advances of feminism, escalating levels of sexism and violence against women and girls exist. Sexual harassment can begin in elementary school. Girls face undervaluement of their intelligence and low self-esteem. Girls remain prey to depression/suicide attempts and eating disorders as well as addictions now

more than ever. Many women, however, have begun to emerge as breadwinners in their own right, often choosing professions once thought of as strictly in the man's domain. These women may have more confusing choices as they struggle with career decisions that will affect their family's life (Orenstein, 2000).

Identity and Intimacy

For men, identity precedes intimacy and generativity in the traditional view of the optimum cycle of human separation and attachment. For women, these tasks are fused, developing together as the woman comes to know herself as she is known, primarily through her relationships with others (Gilligan, 1982a). Women struggle with priorities in career versus relationship, knowing that ambition and romance may be incompatible. Career/ambition requires assertion of self while romance encourages the suppression of it. A second-guessing of priorities is frequently present (Orenstein, 2000). Most men in their 20s are not ready to form loving, emotionally intimate relationships, or to make an enduring commitment to wives and families (Levinson, 1986). Whereas women resolve the intimacy issue by their 20s, men are still engaged in this task well into their 30s. Traditionally, men view attachment as a developmental impediment. Hence, married women may be intimacy mentors to their husbands.

Factors Influencing Identity

Identity development in women is influenced by communion, connection, relation (to friends and all significant others) embeddedness, spirituality, and affiliation (Josselson, 1987). In addition, in order to keep their true selves and grow into healthy adults, girls need the above as well as meaningful work, respect, challenges, and physical and psychological safety (Pipher, 1994). Men and women differ significantly in the separation–individuation process. Some women may never completely individuate from their mothers. Often they transfer their dependence onto a boyfriend because their vision of themselves is relational. A process of anchoring in the family of origin, with a partner and children, in a career, or with friends is critical to women's identity formation and provides the anchor for growth, change, or new directions in life. For women, identity and intimacy are developed at the same time (Gilligan, 1982a).

Identity and Parenthood

Motherhood has become increasingly central to women's sense of femininity, far more so than marriage (Orenstein, 2000). Safer (1996), a psychologist, finds most women see children as a source of fulfillment and not as an obstacle to it. Yet large studies show childless couples can be as happy as parents who have good relationships with their children and certainly happier that those whose relationships have distanced.

Women, especially working women or those with difficult infants, experience appreciably more change than do men in the transition to parenthood (McBride, 1990). Women tend to feel responsible for their children's success and happiness. They also experience the contagion of stress as they internalize the distress experienced by those to whom they are closest, particularly family members. During this period, however, if work serves as a visible marker of achievement, it may lessen stress. Indeed, women with multiple roles may be the most well adjusted. The supportive family buffers a woman from endless demands of childcare and other family responsibilities.

ENTRY LIFE STRUCTURE FOR EARLY ADULTHOOD (AGES 22 TO 28)

Life structures for women tend to be less stable than those for men, essentially because of more diverse concerns involving marriage, motherhood, and career. The primary tasks of this period are to build and maintain a first adult life structure and to enrich one's life within that structure.

AGE THIRTY TRANSITION AND THE SETTLING DOWN PERIOD OF EARLY ADULTHOOD (AGES 28 TO 39)

Both sexes in settling down must give up a youthful self-image and the idea that involvements are tentative and options still open. Priorities of the 20s may be reversed; choices and their consequences may be reassessed; and options regarding marriage and especially childbearing may not exist much longer (Hewlett, 2002; Levinson, 1986). A bewildering discovery occurring at about age 30 is that the life one has arduously constructed has major imperfections and that there is still some growing up to do (Levinson, 1996).

- *Men's Success.* Success in work is imperative to men's timetable. A shift in centrality by men—from work to family—may be a reaction to a combination of stress, age, or failure in work. Men sever ties with mentors in order to be seen as knowledgeable and successful in their own right of becoming one's own man (Levinson, 1986).

- *Women's Success.* In contrast, few women would define becoming one's own woman primarily through success in their work (Bardwick, 1980). Those who are successful in their careers may still be anxious about their femininity unless they are also involved in significant relationships and have experienced motherhood. Women may sacrifice success in careers and attain lower financial status as they compromise to maintain relationships while slipping into traditional roles (Orenstein, 2000). Sadness and depression may develop as women suppress their authentic selves and make repeated compromises (Jack, 1991). Factors leading to a sense of independence in men, such as career success, may instead highlight the dependent needs in women. Her success includes becoming more fully adult by dealing with the child in herself and with the cultural assumption that an adult female is still a girl (Levinson, 1996).

- *Prolonged Transition.* Women in their 30s are likely to experience a more prolonged and profound transition period than men are, perhaps most importantly linked to the age limits for childbearing (the biological clock). Current technology may permit some women to become pregnant well beyond their earlier expectations, however, these expectations may be unrealistic (Hewlett, 2002). The age 30 transition can be a time of increased individuation that is self-generated rather than relational. During the period of evaluation and reappraisal (ages 28 to 33), married women may demand that husbands recognize and accommodate their aspirations and interests outside of the home or postpone marriage for career (Orenstein, 2000; Roberts & Newton, 1987).

- *Career versus Family.* Women reappraise the relative importance of career and family, often adding the missing component rather than reversing priorities (e.g., a mother may begin a career). Women may attempt to lead a life in which they do it all. The mental health stressors of women's multiple roles may be influenced more by marital factors than by work factors. Work often buffers some marital stress, but parenthood exacerbates occupational stress, especially if responsibilities are not shared in the home (McBride, 1990).

Hewlett (2002) warns that when women embrace a male model of single-minded career focus they may encounter a "creeping nonchoice" in future motherhood. Women may be misinformed regarding their future of fertility options. A woman may see an epidemic of childlessness among professional women who find themselves past their peak fertility years. Unfortunately, women do not realize that after age 27 their chances of becoming pregnant begin to decline. Women may fear, often realistically, that by slowing down their careers to have children, they will run the risk of never catching up. Time to form meaningful relationships is limited by work factors.

Recent census data shows childlessness doubling in the last twenty years so that one in five women between the ages of 40 and 44 is childless. Forty-seven percent of those of the same age with professional degrees are childless. Certainly, many of these women choose not to have children. Hewlett's figures show that 14 percent made this choice, the others having the choice made for them.

- *Multiple Roles.* Having multiple roles may counterbalance some negative effects of a particular role. Thus, the healthiest women and men, may be those with multiple roles, including having a career, a spouse, and often children (Barnett & Hyde, 2001). Employment status accounted for most of the variance in psychological well-being for women aged 35 to 55. Married women with children and high prestige jobs reported the greatest well-being. However, "having it all" may mean "doing it all," and women may experience strain in attempting to fulfill multiple role obligations. U.S. society does not yet support working women with childcare options or pay that is comparable to men's. Often they must choose between family and career. Women's ability to cope with the stresses has been associated with having a high income and job satisfaction, marrying later, and arranging time for family activities (McBride, 1990).
- *American Values and Women's Sexuality.* The U.S. culture values youth and beauty, and often by age 35, a woman is no longer considered young. Women are labeled old ten to fifteen years earlier than men are, with resulting psychological, sexual, and economic disadvantages (Bell, 1979).
- *Confusing Choices.* Women in their 30s are facing the growing influence of feminist thinking and more egalitarian life patterns. At the same time, they are confronted by others who tell them that their behaviors should be more traditional. Women also struggle with their own psychological tendencies regarding more traditional values, which they internalized early in life. Orenstein (2000) describes our state of flux at the turn of the century. The demands and needs of motherhood in this half-changed world are extremely complicated whether a woman works full time, part

time, or stays at home. Over time, women talk less and less to those who have made choices different from their own, to their mutual loss.

- *Readjustment in the 30s.* Demographically, most women now in their 30s are married with school-age children. Those who are employed are not necessarily on a career path. Others who are unemployed have been out of school for about ten years (Bardwick, 1980). As women reach ages 35 to 40, their husbands' tremendous involvement in their own careers and children's decreasing dependence on them may provide the opportunity for personal change. Women may return to work or school or look for other relationships in the community. Family members may initially agree to change their lifestyles in order to accommodate the women's needs; however, when changes impact them directly, they may become resentful or confused.
- *Stress.* Stress is inherent in the reality or the illusion of choice. Some women may sacrifice personal relationships to achieve career success; others may be doing it all with very little support from their partners. Partners' expectations of each other in their relationship are not always clear. Many women who divorce in their 30s may become more confident and perhaps more angry. Anger may lead to egocentricism that enables women to formulate obtainable objectives. For married women, responsibilities outside the home—community and career involvement—may help them become less dependent economically, socially, and psychologically. Most women in this age group tend toward interdependence.

MIDLIFE TRANSITION AND MIDDLE ADULTHOOD (AGES 39 TO 60)

An appreciable change in the character of living occurs between early and middle adulthood. The main tasks of entering middle adulthood are making crucial choices, giving those choices meaning and commitment, and building a life structure around them (Levinson, 1986).

Midlife Transitions

- Assessment for both men and women may have a sense of urgency; they wish to accomplish their life goals as they confront mortality. Those who do not assess their lives at this point may feel frightened and unable to make changes in their lifestyles or careers. Men assess what they receive and what they give to work, family, friends, and community as they reach the symbolically powerful age of 40 (Levinson, 1978, 1986). Their established autonomy now allows greater compassion, more reflection, less tyranny by inner conflicts and external demands, and more genuine love of self and others. Middle-aged men may experience this as their fullest and most creative period.

By the end of middle adulthood, problems may include declining health, aging or death of parents, spousal death, and stagnation at work with no viable options. Although the relationship with one's spouse may only be comfortable, the option of ending it means losing crucial roots. Nonetheless, divorce has increased markedly for both men and women in their 40s. One may see a partner as a reason for discontent or as someone to blame for perceived losses. A new relationship may be viewed as a way to recoup the feelings and pleasure of youth.

◆ Women and men become more autonomous as they age, but women gain in larger increments (Goode, 1999). Becoming involved in a career after 40 can be an opportunity for real beginnings, but it also can be frightening. This may be a time for women to generate new values internally, reflecting who they are rather than what they do.

◆ Losses or adjustments in relationships may cause depression in women beginning the midlife phase; they may experience loneliness as children leave home or they become widowed or divorced. The empty nest concept is not totally supported by national data; a dependent woman who faces the loss of her children and her husband at this time may be more vulnerable. Women, but not men, tend to define their age status in terms of the timing of events within their family; even unmarried career women often discuss middle age in terms of the family they might have had (Orenstein, 2000). Women with more complex lives may experience sadness and joy in this time of readjustment as they face losses along with new beginnings. Many more men than women remarry at this age. The last three decades have seen a 40 percent decline in women's remarrying after divorce. They are now more economically independent and may no longer see marriage as their best option (Orenstein, 2000).

◆ *Change in Appearance.* Although women may feel dismay over excessive value placed on women's appearance, including its damaging impact on young girls, they may also feel invisible as their looks change and men may not notice them as they did in the past. Their cultural power is felt to be slipping away. Yet as women reach their 40s, they reach more towards something deeper: an authentic personal voice. At this time, women start viewing their life by how much is left to live (Lachman & James, 1997).

A majority of women have made a reality transition, as evidenced by a high employment rate. The expansion of activities, maturing, and increased self-confidence lead many of these women to be more interdependent rather than dependent, as compared with women in their 30s. This is perhaps the most complex of all developmental periods because women are given social permission to work at precisely the time their traditional responsibilities decline.

Middle Adulthood

Although Levinson's studies ended with men and women in their 40s, he believed that a major transition phase occurs from ages 50 to 55. A stable period follows from ages 55 to 60, during which rejuvenation in some can result in achieving significant fulfillment and enrichment (Levinson, 1978, 1986). For men especially whose connection with others depends largely on their jobs, retirement may be associated with a loss of prestige and decreased self-esteem. Women tend to face this loss much earlier if their primary role in life is that of mother, their secondary role that of homemaker, and their tertiary role that of sexual partner. As family becomes less central to women's lives, other sources of satisfaction can be significant. Often, the marital relationship has to be modified as women strive to create better lives for themselves. Career promotions are less common and may be disappointing compared with what was hoped for. Accomplishments in careers may not bring the same satisfaction or sense of accomplishment as in earlier years. The question "How successful am I in the eyes of the world?" may be less important than "What do I give and receive from my work? How satisfying is my relationship with work?" (Belensky, 1986; Orenstein, 2000).

◆ The aging process traditionally has been symbolized as retirement for men and menopause for women, although the formerly predominant all negative views regarding menopause have been challenged (Friedan, 1993). Anticipating menopause is often more dreadful than the difficulty experienced with its actual occurrence. Women often feel relief with the loss of menses as well as the loss of tasks associated with rearing young children. The real difficulty may be adjusting to the aging process—a continuum that does not just begin after menses ends. Other changes associated with aging are socially more apparent, such as graying hair and wrinkles. Bifocal glasses and hearing aids may be a threat to self-esteem and a visible admission of aging, which may cause problems in intimate relationships. Yet physical changes may be a liberating process, allowing women to reclaim lost parts of themselves, reviving connections to family, work, and community and finally, to a more authentic sense of self (Orenstein, 2000).

- "The sandwich generation" refers to the women who are caregivers for their children as well as for their aging parents. Depression, anxiety, and fatigue may result as women may neglect their own needs (Murray & Bachman, 2000).

    Aging is a gradual process, and changes of aging are adaptive across the life span. During middle age, women may to some extent lose their roles of mother and sex partner, especially through divorce or death. A partner's retirement may force another adaptation. Distancing from parents in the middle years is replaced by establishing a commitment for parents' care, which allows some women who see themselves primarily as homemakers to reestablish that lifestyle.

- Women in their 50s may feel the need to change or reassess values or direction at this stage in their lives; others will reject new values, believing themselves incapable of achieving different goals. Women most at risk for psychological dependence are traditional housewives who lack involvement or outside commitments. Interdependence is more likely to occur among older women who have found fulfillment in their traditional roles and who have assumed varied roles, whether through employment or other options. A few older women are egocentric as a result of being widows, divorced, displaced homemakers, or having never married.

- Societal views of aging women include negative stereotypes such as being inactive, unhealthy, asexual, unattractive, and ineffective—despite the diversity of older women who lead interesting, productive lives (Lott, 1987). Friedan (1993) addresses our denial of the personhood of age, with its definition ensuring the blackout of people over 50 as sexual beings, especially women. Widowed or divorced women may yearn for an intimate, sexual relationship. They may be hampered in moving beyond sexual measures of themselves in their youth. In fact, there may be an intimacy that may only be possible as we age. Revising expectations about advancing age requires that society move beyond these stereotypes and overcome ageist and sexual biases (Lichtman & Papera, 1990). Health care providers need to recognize the diversity among women as they age. Older women receive messages that growing older is a process to be prevented (with face lifts or antiaging facial creams) rather than to be enjoyed. Even professional women view aging as a serious impairment. Discrimination in employment is particularly harmful for women reentering the work force after their children leave home or when the loss of a spouse decreases their income and security. Throughout adulthood, women are increasingly threatened by poverty as a result of greater numbers of female-headed households and the continuing disparity in salaries between men and women. Older women are particularly affected by inadequate spousal retirement plans, especially if they themselves have a history of unemployment. As women live longer, they have more opportunity to develop illness, another stress on their finances.

LATE ADULT TRANSITION (AGES 60 TO 65)

Ages 60 to 65 mark the end of middle life and entry into the late adult transition (Levinson, 1996). Overall, women feel good about themselves and what they are accomplishing as they use time freed by retirement or other life changes to pursue creative activities, community work, and self-development (Mercer et al., 1989). Women's presence in the labor force has increased dramatically. In 1993, 8.2 percent of women over age 65 were working. More men than women leave the workforce early (Richardson, 1999). Yet higher poverty rates exist among older women. Women have substantial involvement in unpaid work, specifically caregiving and home labor, and suffer from discriminatory retirement policies. When women outlive their husbands, creativity may develop as a response to loss and loneliness, including social and emotional isolation. Women may also return to creative activities they enjoyed in earlier years. During their 60s women are most likely to experience transitions relating to their own illness and the illness and death of significant others.

LATE ADULTHOOD AND LATE, LATE ADULTHOOD

Women can expect to live well into their 70s and 80s. Ages 76 to 80 may represent a transition toward wisdom as women are challenged to adapt to a number of changes, including loss of health, friends, and family (Mercer et al., 1989). Women are more likely than men to experience chronic illness in later life. Bodily restrictions may impede social and personal activities leading to lowered self-esteem. Yet, importance of body image may decrease with age as women accept natural changes with aging (Hurd, 2000). A surge of creativity may continue as women find pleasurable ways to enrich their lives. Relationships and affiliation with others remain important for women, and their creativity may take the form of altruistic responses to the needs of others. Successful or creative aging may be associated with maintaining meaningful activities, keeping close relationships with persons of all ages, and remaining flexible and adaptable. Nonconformists who are willing to take risks and who sustain a positive outlook on life perhaps experience the greatest success in aging. Psychological development never ends as long as the individual engages in reality; thus the potential for growth and change is always present.

REFERENCES

Apter, T.E., & Josselson R. (2000). *Best friends: The pleasures and perils of girls' and women's friendships.* New York: Crown Publishing.

Bardwick, J.M. (1980). The seasons of a woman's life. In D.G. McGuigan (Ed.), *Women's lives: New theory, research, and policy.* Ann Arbor: University of Michigan, Center for Continuing Education of Women.

Barnett, R.C., & Hyde, J.S. (2001). Women, men, work, and family: An expansionist theory. *American Psychologist, 56* (10), 781–796.

Belenky, M.F., & Field, M. (1985). Epistemological development and the politics of talk in family life. *Journal of Education, 167*(3), 9–27.

Belenky, M.F., Clinchy, B., Goldberger, N., & Tarule, J. (1986). *Women's ways of knowing. The development of self, voice, and mind.* New York: Basic Books.

Bell, I.P. (1979). The double standard: Age. In Freeman (Ed.), *Women: A feminist perspective* (pp. 145–155). Palo Alto, CA: Mayfield.

Brehony, K.A. (1996). *Awakening at midlife: A guide to reviving your spirit, recreating your life, and returning to your truest self.* New York: Riverhead Books.

Caffarella, R.S., & Olson, S.K. (1993). Psychosocial development of women: A critical review of the literature. *Adult Education Quarterly, 43*(3), 125–151.

de Beauvoir, Simone (1949). *The Second Sex.* New York: Random House.

Erikson, E.H. (1950). *Childhood and society.* New York: Norton.

Erikson, E.H. (1968). *Identity, youth and crises.* New York: Norton.

Friedan, B. (1963) *The Feminine Mystique.* New York: Norton.

Friedan, B. (1993). *The fountain of age.* New York: Simon & Shuster.

Gilligan, C. (1982a). *In a different voice: Psychological theory and women's development.* Cambridge, MA: Harvard University Press.

Gilligan, C. (1982b). New maps of development: New visions of maturity. *American Journal of Orthopsychiatry, 52*(2), 199–212.

Goode, E. (1999, February 16). New study finds middle age is prime of life. *The New York Times,* D6.

Grosskurth, P. (1991). The new psychology of women. *New York Review of Books, 38*(17).

Hewlett, S.A. (2002). *Creating a life: Professional women and the quest for children.* New York: Talk Miramax Books.

Hollis, L.A. (1998). Sex comparisons in life satisfaction and psychosocial adjustment scores with an older adult sample: Examining the effect of sex role differences in older cohorts. *Journal of Women and Aging, 10*(3): 59–77.

Hurd, L.C. (2000). Older women's body image and embodied experience: An exploration. *Journal of Women and Aging, 12*(3/4), 77–97.

Hyde, J.S. (1985). *Half the human experience: The psychology of women* (3rd ed.). Lexington, MA: D.C. Heath.

Jack, D. (1991). *Silencing the self: Women and depression.* Cambridge, MA: Harvard University Press.

Johnson, B.E., Johnson, C.A., Murray, J.L., & Apgar, B.S. (2000). *Women's Health Care Handbook* (2nd ed.). Philadelphia: Hanley & Belfus, Inc.

Josselson, R. (1987). *Finding herself: Pathways to identity development in women.* San Francisco: Jossey-Bass.

Kaschak, E. (1981). Feminist psychotherapy: The first decade. In S. Cox (Ed.), *Female psychology* (pp. 387–401). New York: St. Martin's Press.

Lachman, M.E., & James, J.B. (Eds). (1997). *Multiple paths to midlife development.* Chicago: University of Chicago.

Levinson, D.J. (1978). *The seasons of a man's life.* New York: Alfred A. Knopf.

Levinson, D.J. (1986). A conception of adult development. *American Psychologist, 41*(1), 3–13.

Levinson, D.J. (1996). *The seasons of a woman's life.* New York: Alfred A. Knopf.

Lewis, J.A., & Bernstein, J. (1996). *Women's health: A relational perspective across the life cycle.* Sudbury, MA: Jones and Bartlett.

Lichtman, R., & Papera, S. (1990). *Gynecology: Well woman care.* Norwalk, CT: Appleton & Lange.

Lott, B. (1987). *Women's lives: Themes and variations in gender learning.* Pacific Grove, CA: Brooks/Cole.

McBride, A.B. (1990). Mental health effects of women's multiple roles. *American Psychologist, 45*(3), 381–384.

Mednick, M.T. (1989). On the politics of psychological constructs: Stop the bandwagon, I want to get off. *American Psychologist, 44*(8), 1118–1123.

Mercer, R.T., Nichols, E.G., & Doyle, G.C. (1989). *Transitions in a woman's life: Major life events in developmental context.* New York: Springer.

Miller, J.B. (1986). *Toward a new psychology of women* (2nd ed.). Boston: Beacon Press.

Millet, K. (1969). *Sexual Politics.* Chicago: University of Illinois Press.

Murray, J.L., & Bachman G. E. (2000). Sandwich generation. In B.E. Johnson, C.A. Johnson, J.L. Murray, & B.S. Apgar (Eds.), *Women's health care handbook* (2nd ed.). Philadelphia: Hanley & Belfus, Inc.

Norman, S.M., McCluskey-Fawcett, K., & Ashcroft, L. (2002). Older women's development: A comparison of women in their 60s and 80s on a measure of Erikson's developmental tasks. *International Journal of Aging and Human Development, 54*(1), 31–41.

O'Rand, A.M., & Henrette, J.C. (1982). Women at middle age: Development and transitions. *Annals of the American Academy of Political and Social Sciences.* Beverly Hills, CA: Sage.

Orenstein, P. (2000). *FLUX: Women on sex, work, love, kids and life in a self-changed world.* New York: Anchor Books.

Pipher, M. (1994). *Reviving Ophelia: Saving the selves of adolescent girls.* New York: Ballantine Books.

Richardson, V.E. (1999). Women and retirement. *Journal of Women and Aging, 11*(2–3), 49–66.

Roberts, P., & Newton, P.M. (1987). Levinsonian studies of women's adult development. *Psychology and Aging, 2*(2), 154–163.

Rosenblatt, E.A. (1995). Emerging concept of women's development. Implications for psychotherapy. *The Psychiatric Clinics of North America, 18*(1), 95–106.

Safer, J. (1996). *Beyond motherhood: Choosing a life without children.* New York: Pocket Books.

Strachey, J. (Ed. & Trans.). (1961). *The standard edition of the complete psychological works of Sigmund Freud.* London: Hogarth Press.

Woods, N.F., Lentz, M., & Mitchell, E. (1993). The new woman: Health promoting and health damaging behaviors. *Health Care for Women International, 14,* 389–405.

SELECTED BIBLIOGRAPHY

Bem, S.L. (1993). *The lenses of gender: Transforming the debate on sexual inequality.* New Haven: Yale University Press.

Brown, L., & Gilligan, C. (1992). *Meeting at the crossroads: Women's psychology and girls' development.* Cambridge, MA: Harvard University Press.

Eisler, R. (1988). *The chalice and the blade.* San Francisco: Harper.

Gilligan, C. (2002). *The birth of pleasure.* New York: Alfred A. Knopf.

Goodman, E., & O'Brien, P. (2001). *I know just what you mean: The power of friendship in women's lives.* New York: Simon & Schuster.

Sheehy, G. (1998). *Menopause: The silent passage.* New York: Pocket Books.

Sheehy, G. (1996). *New passages: Mapping your life across time.* New York: Random House.

Simmons, R. (2002). *Odd girl out: The hidden culture of aggression in girls.* New York: Harcourt.

Wiseman, R. (2002). *Queen Bees and Wannabes: Helping your daughter survive cliques, gossip, boyfriends and other realities of adolescence.* New York: Crown Publishers.

CHAPTER 3

ASSESSING ADOLESCENT WOMEN'S HEALTH

Deborah A. Raines

*A*dolescence offers unique opportunities for investment in the health and well-being of future generations.

Highlights

- Adolescence
- Hypothalamic-Pituitary-Gonadal Development
- Growth and Development of Puberty
- Developmental Tasks of Adolescence
- Health Issues and Risks
- Caring for Adolescents

❖ INTRODUCTION

Adolescence is considered a critical period in human development. The adolescent is an individual in transition between childhood and adulthood, and this transition is a complex process. Adolescent transitions include the completion of gender-specific physical growth and development resulting in reproductive maturity and the achievement of developmental tasks resulting in the establishment of a personal identity. Adolescence offers unique opportunities for investment in the health and well-being of future generations. Adolescence, however, is also a time of high-risk behaviors and involvement in conduct often disturbing to society. According to Hechinger (1992), the state of adolescent health in the United States has reached crisis proportions and adolescents' glaring need for health care is largely ignored. For example,

- In 2000, 10 percent of the U.S. population was made up of individuals ages 13 to 19.

- The birth rate was 34 percent for white teenagers, 83.7 percent for black teenagers, and 93.4 percent for Hispanic teenagers.
- Approximately 51 percent of twelfth-grade students reported having had sexual intercourse in the past three months.
- Condom use decreased by grade level with twelfth-graders being the least likely to use condoms.
- 312 new cases of adolescent AIDS were reported in 1999 (CDC, 2000).

As these data indicate, the adolescent's behavior has long-term implications for individual and societal health and well-being. In addition, lifelong health habits, such as diet, exercise, sexual practices, substance abuse, and use of health care resources, are formed during the adolescent years. Consequently, understanding the unique physical and developmental needs of the adolescent is important.

ADOLESCENCE

In the past, puberty and adolescence were considered synonymous. They are separate entities, however, encompassing the biological and psychological responses to this critical transition. Puberty is focused on physical changes culminating in the functional ability to engage in sexual reproduction. For the female, puberty begins with a physical growth spurt and ends with the onset of menstruation signifying the achievement of biological maturity. Adolescence is a broader concept based on the individual's progressive psychological maturation and readiness to assume adult responsibilities. Although chronologic age plays a role in definitions of adolescence and the anticipation of the events of puberty, the process of physical and psychological development is highly individualized and variable. Adolescence is typically defined as the period of life beginning with puberty and extending for an average of eight to ten years (Speroff, Glass, & Kase, 1999). Females experience the adolescent period an average of two years earlier than males, due in part to earlier onset of physical changes and development. The psychological responses of the adolescent are often delineated by chronologic age. Psychosocial development is frequently categorized as behaviors of early, middle, or late adolescence. Similar to the biological growth variation

during puberty, however, individual differences manifest themselves in the achievement of the developmental tasks of adolescence as well.

HYPOTHALAMIC-PITUITARY-GONADAL DEVELOPMENT

The growth and development changes evident in the adolescent are attributable to the hypothalamic-pituitary-gonadal (HPG) axis and the presence of sex hormones. The HPG axis is a cyclic phenomenon: the activity of gonadotrophic-releasing hormone, the pituitary secretion of gonadotropins, and the estradiol positive feedback triggering the preovulatory luteinizing hormone (LH) surge, follicular rupture, and corpus luteum formation (Speroff et al., 1999). The HPG axis is established during in utero development, becomes dormant or suspended during childhood, and is reactivated during the second decade of life by an as yet unidentified mechanism (Neinstein & Kaufman, 1996).

Gonadotropin-releasing hormone (GnRH), LH, follicle-stimulating hormone (FSH), and estrogen are detectable in the female fetus by 10 weeks' gestation. The episodic release of GnRH and gonadotropins (FSH and LH), with an intact negative feedback mechanism, demonstrates that the hypothalamic-pituitary-gonadal system is functional at a mature level prior to birth. The presence of the negative feedback response of the hypothalamus and pituitary in response to circulating estrogen prevents the development of mature, gender-specific sexual characteristics in the fetus.

During puberty, there is a resurgence of GnRH, LH and FSH, and sex steroid (estrogen) secretion. It has been suggested that the time frame of puberty is controlled by bloodborne substances that convey metabolic information related to carbohydrate or protein utilization as an indicator about the growth and nutrition of the body and that these signals influence the hormonal biochemistry of the body, thereby directing the activity of the GnRH secretory system (Baram, 1996). Although the exact mechanism of this reactivation of the HPG axis is not well explicated, sequential maturation of the central nervous system and decreased sensitivity of the hypothalamus and pituitary to circulating levels of estradiol are thought to play a significant role (Baram, 1996). Consequently, puberty is a brain-driven event controlled by maturation of the somatic component of the axis and not maturation of the gonad.

The increased secretion of hormones is initiated by release of GnRH in a pulsatile fashion coincident with sleep. Eventually, the pulsatile pattern increases in frequency and magnitude, extending beyond sleep time to encompass the entire 24-hour period (Baram, 1996). Gonadotrophic secretion causes progressive changes in the morphology of the ovarian follicles and an increase in estrogen secretion. In the female, the development of a positive feedback system, in which critical levels of estrogen trigger a large release of GnRH, stimulating LH to initiate ovulation, is the final stage of axis development during the adolescent years (Neinstein & Kaufman, 1996).

Reactivation of the HPG axis is responsible for the physical changes evident during puberty. After the completion of reproductive maturity, the HPG axis is replaced, however, as the mediator of hormone secretion. The mature ovary, with positive and negative feedback loops based on the secretion of estrogen and progesterone, takes over control of hormone levels. Thus, the gonadal component of the axis becomes the regulating force. The female gonad remains in control throughout the reproductive years.

GROWTH AND DEVELOPMENT OF PUBERTY

Physical changes during puberty are typified by growth spurts, development of secondary sexual characteristics, maturation of genital organs, and the onset of menstruation. These events occur in an orderly and sequential pattern. In the female, the onset of puberty is signaled by the initiation of rapid physical growth, and the end point of puberty is menarche. The age of pubertal growth and development spans from 8 to 14 years. Evidence of the physical changes prior to 8 years of age are considered precocious puberty and need further investigation. The age of puberty may be influenced by health status, genetics, and nutrition. Theories suggest that a minimum body weight and at least 17 percent body fat composition are necessary for the onset of menstruation (Speroff et al., 1999). The duration of puberty for the female ranges from 18 months to 5 years. The time of onset is not related to the duration of puberty.

Chronologic age and physical growth are closely linked with the concept of puberty. Age, height, and weight alone, however, are not the best indicators of physical maturity. To specifically classify the level of physical maturation and to determine normality of development, a sexual maturity rating (SMR) scale is essential. For females, sexual maturity rating scales are based on five stages of breast and genital hair development, correlating with prepubescent (stage 1) through adult characteristics (stage 5) (see Chapter 4).

GROWTH SPURT

After infancy, adolescence is the most rapid period of physical growth. In the female, onset of the growth spurt is between age 8 and 17 years. The mean age for peak height velocity growth is 12 years (Neinstein & Kaufman, 1996). The average duration of this growth spurt is three years in females (Murray & Zentner, 2001). Females grow approximately 2 1/2 to 5 inches (6–12.5 cm) in height per year and gain 8 to 20 pounds (3.5–4.5 kg) per year (Murray & Zentner, 2001). Consequently, the pubertal growth spurt contributes a significant proportion of adult body size. Initially, the increase in height is due to lengthening of the long bones in the legs and arms, often resulting in poor posture and decreased coordination. Later, growth is in trunk length resulting in adult body proportions. Following menarche, growth rate slows, due to epiphyseal fusion secondary to elevated estrogen levels. Females also experience growth and reshaping of the pelvis during puberty. The bony pelvis grows into the gynecoid shape characteristic of the mature female. Accelerated growth involves an interaction between the endocrine and skeletal systems. Human growth hormone (hGH), thyroxine, insulin, and corticosteroid are growth promoting, while parathyroid hormone,

1,25-dihydroxy-vitamin D, and calciton affect skeletal mineralization (Neinstein & Kaufman, 1996). HGH is the key hormone released by the pituitary gland and is the primary influence of adolescent growth. Activity of the pituitary gland is influenced by the multifocal effects of rising estrogen levels. The effect of hGH is modulated through somatomedins or a class of peptide hormones known as insulin-like growth factors (IGF I and IGF II) (Albertsson-Wikland, 1994) IGFs, as their names imply, have a biological effect similar to insulin, leading to stimulation of lipid and carbohydrate (CHO) metabolism, resulting in fat deposits and development of the female body form.

Weight gain is related to an increase in total body size but, more significantly, is attributable to an increase in the percent of body fat from 15.7 percent to 26.7 percent and a lower percentage of lean body mass (Speroff et al., 1999). In general, females add more adipose tissue as a result of estrogenic influence. Subcutaneous deposits of adipose tissue are evident in the female hips and breasts.

THELARCHE

Initiation of the female growth spurt precedes thelarche, or breast development, by approximately one year (Neinstein & Kaufman, 1996). The stimulus for breast development is estrogen. Breast growth is due to extensive fat depositions as well as growth and branching of the ductal system and development of small solid cell masses (potential alveoli) at the duct endings. During puberty, breast size varies and asymmetry is common.

The prepubertal breast has no glandular tissue, and the areola conforms to the general chest line. As puberty progresses, a breast bud with a small amount of glandular tissue and widening of the areola develops. The breast tissue grows larger and the elevation from the chest wall is more pronounced. In sexual maturity rating 4, the areola forms a projecting mound, also known as a double hump, from the contour of the breast. The final or adult stage of breast development is characterized by protrusion of the nipple, but the areola becomes congruent with the remainder of the breast tissue (see Chapter 4).

ADRENARCHE

Concurrent with breast development is pubic hair growth or adrenarche. Prepubescent females have no hair growth in the pubic area. Initial hair growth is a small amount of slightly pigmented, straight, vellus hair on the labia majora. As maturity progresses, the quantity of hair growth increases and the distribution spreads from the labia to the mons veris. The texture also becomes coarser, curlier, and more darkly pigmented. The final stage of pubic hair development is established in about two years and is characterized by an abundant quantity of coarse, curly hair in the typical female triangular distribution with a horizontal upper border. Approximately two years after the first appearance of pubic hair, axillary hair growth begins.

EXTERNAL AND INTERNAL GENITALIA

While thelarche and adrenarche are the most obvious of the physical changes associated with puberty, a number of maturational changes are occurring in other structures as well. In addition to pubic hair growth, the vulva is changing in shape and enlarging. The labia majora develop as fat is deposited in the subcutaneous tissue beneath them. Subcutaneous fat deposits also develop over the mons veris and the pubic symphysis. As the labia majora increase in size, they fall inward and tend to obscure the labia minora, which become more vascular and well rounded. The clitoris becomes larger and more erectile and the entire introitus appears larger.

Before puberty, the vaginal epithelium is only a few cells thick, is incapable of glycogen production, has scant secretions, and has an alkaline pH. With the influence of increasing estrogen levels, the vaginal lining is transformed to a layer of thick, stratified squamous epithelial cells containing glycogen. The thickness of the vaginal lining varies with the cyclic circulating levels of female sex hormones. With decreased hormone stimulation, the vaginal epithelium exfoliates, resulting in increased vaginal secretions. During early adolescence, the presence of leukorrhea, or a white mucoid discharge, often precedes menarche by approximately one year (Speroff et al., 1999). Cellular exfoliation results in the conversion of the intracellular glycogen to lactic acid. Lactic acid formation results in the establishment of Doderlein's bacilli as a component of the normal vaginal flora making the environment more hostile to foreign bacteria and viruses (Speroff et al., 1999).

The uterus changes from the tubular formation of childhood to a hollow, muscular adult organ. The uterus prior to puberty is characterized by an elongated cervix with a small fundus. Under estrogenic stimulation, both the cervix and the fundus enlarge, but the major change is seen in the fundus. The size of the fundus increases in all dimensions, so that eventually the fundus accounts for three-fourths of the total uterine size (Speroff et al., 1999). Concurrent with uterine growth, the endometrial lining proliferates, under the influence of cyclic circulating hormone levels, in preparation for menarche.

The ovaries and fallopian tubes also grow, but their growth is slower. The ovaries increase in size and the tubes enlarge and lose some of their tortuousness. The final stage of ovarian development, however, is attained only after the ovary is capable of reacting to both FSH and LH. While uterine and ovarian development begin in parallel, the ovary must develop an adequate vascular system to transport the stimulus for FSH to the follicle cell. The development of a vascular system begins with the onset of puberty but proceeds at a slower rate than does uterine development. Consequently, with increased FSH secretion, estrogen is produced, which leads to gradual proliferation of vascular channels. With fully developed vascular channels, ovarian estrogen secretion is elevated to levels adequate to trigger the release of luteinizing hormone and to initiate ovulation (Speroff et al., 1999). The slower development of ovarian function, as compared with endometrial function, is the rationale for early menstrual cycles being anovulatory.

MENARCHE

Menarche is the final major landmark of puberty. Menarche occurs after a series of the physical changes of puberty have occurred. In general, menarche occurs approximately one to three years after initiation of thelarche and during sexual maturity rating 3 or 4. The initial menstrual cycles may be irregular not only in frequency but in duration and quantity. Early menstrual cycles are frequently anovulatory, secondary to the immaturity of ovarian function. Immature ovarian function results in lack of progesterone secretions. Therefore, the endometrial lining is in the proliferative phase. For the first year after menarche, the intervals between periods vary widely. The variability decreases with time and establishment of pulsatile secretion of FSH and LH and mature ovarian response, including the secretion of estrogen and progesterone (Speroff et al., 1999). A woman's interval pattern is usually set about three or four years after menarche. Establishment of a rhythmic menstrual pattern is thought to be associated with the initiation of ovulation and ovarian control of hormone secretion (Speroff et al., 1999).

DEVELOPMENTAL TASKS OF ADOLESCENCE

Psychosocial development is a sequential process including the stages of early, middle, and late adolescence. Psychosocial developmental tasks are delineated by chronologic age, in part related to the influence of cultural and social norms that influence their resolution. The developmental tasks of adolescence include the following: accepting one's mature body and sexual identity, developing a personal value system, preparing for productive function, achieving independence from parents, and developing an adult identity. The achievement of psychological maturity is progressive as the individual attains greater physical, cognitive, and social skills. Erikson labeled adolescence the stage of identity versus role confusion, or a time when individuals face identity crisis from which they will emerge with either a clear sense of identity or a state of confusion about their future roles and purpose (Erikson, 1965).

EARLY ADOLESCENCE

Early adolescence is the period between ages 11 and 13 years. Interests focus on same gender peer group identification. Peer acceptance and conformity are important and are often the source of parental conflicts. At this stage, the adolescent wishes to be more grown-up and is concerned with developing into a physically mature adult and with being normal. The adolescent's definition of normal is in relation to the peer group. Therefore, individual variation in physical development can be a source of distress. Questions related to physical development are highly mechanistic in nature, focusing on concern and curiosity about their own and peers' bodies. During the early adolescent stage, the individual's thinking is concrete and lacks the ability for abstract thinking or introspection (Wadsworth, 1996). Because of the concrete thinking pattern and the limited reasoning capacities, the early adolescent is easily overwhelmed and overruled.

The early adolescent has an increased interest in sexual processes but has no direct sexual ambitions. She frequently finds sexual behaviors such as kissing or intercourse disgusting. Sexual fantasies are common, however, and may be a source of guilt. Desired sexual activities are of a nonphysical nature during this period. The early adolescent is most likely to express her sexual urges through dress, body language, and curiosity about sexual acts (Murray & Zentner, 2001).

MIDDLE ADOLESCENCE

The most turbulent stage is age 14 to 16 years or middle adolescence. During this period, the adolescent is becoming psychologically egocentric and is preoccupied with self (Erikson, 1965). Self-esteem is established through recognition of the peer group. Behavior is characterized by rebellion and profound mood swings as the adolescent struggles to establish independence. The middle adolescent begins to use abstract reasoning and introspection to develop a better understanding of herself and others. The middle adolescent often exhibits a feeling of immortality or indestructibility, however, as a result of increasing intellect, physical size, and peer identity. This false sense of security can contribute to impulsive and risk-taking behaviors, with no thought of the danger or the sequelae (Moore, 1996; Wadsworth, 1996).

By middle adolescence, physical maturation is well established and menarche has occurred in the majority of females. Sexual energy is high with an emphasis on physical contact. Sexual behavior, however, is primarily explorative and exploitative in nature. Dating leads to casual relationships with both coital and non-coital contacts. Sexual interests continue to grow and heterosexual relationships become important but are of short duration and erratic. Asynchrony between physical maturity and psychological immaturity in the middle adolescent leads to denial of the potential consequences of sexual behavior. Typically, she believes that the complications of sexual activity, such as sexually transmitted diseases (STDs) or pregnancy, cannot happen to her (Moore, 1996).

Middle adolescence may also mark the adolescent's realization that she is attracted to members of her own gender. The heterosexual orientation of societal expectations can result in confusion and anxiety for the lesbian adolescent (see Chapter 7). The process of establishing a healthy individual identity, or the fusion of emotions and sexuality into a meaningful whole, is an important developmental task (Smith & McClaugherty, 1993).

LATE ADOLESCENCE

Late adolescence, or ages 17 to 21, coincides with full sexual maturity for most individuals. The individual has developed a sense of self and purpose to her life. Sexual behavior is more expressive and less exploitative (Murray & Zentner, 2001). Relationships that are monogamous and intimate are developed. Abstract reasoning skills are fully operational, and the individual is able to interact in the adult world and consider the long-term implications of her actions (Wadsworth, 1996). She also achieves socio-legal maturity during this stage.

HEALTH ISSUES AND RISKS

A major focus of health care for the adolescent is on the physical changes resulting in reproductive maturity and on the psychosocial changes resulting in the establishment of independence. There are a number of other issues and risks that need to be considered in the care of the adolescent, however, to assure adaptive coping and positive growth.

NUTRITION AND EATING DISORDERS

The adolescent's nutritional needs are increased as a result of the increased metabolic processes associated with accelerated growth. The female adolescent between ages 11 and 14 years needs 2,200 kcal/day while the 15- to 18-year-old needs 2,400 kcal/day (Murray & Zentner, 2001). Nutrient intake should include good dietary sources of protein, calcium, and zinc to meet rapid growth and development demands. In addition, the female adolescent requires an adequate intake of iron. Dietary iron is necessary for the increasing blood volume that accompanies growth as well as to replace the iron lost during menstrual bleeding.

Eating disorders during adolescence include compulsive overeating, anorexia nervosa, and bulimia. Overeating resulting in obesity is the most common malnutrition problem among adolescents and is demonstrating a rising incidence. In the early 1970s, 6.1 percent of adolescents were overweight in contrast to 1988–1994 when the percentage rose to 10.5 percent (CDC, 2000). In other words, one out of ten adolescents is considered overweight (CDC, 2000). Female high school students were more than twice as likely as male students to be attempting weight loss (AMA, 2001). Eating disorders can be associated with the individual's anxiety about weight, distortion of body image, and desire to exert control. Therefore, eating disorders are often symptoms of an underlying problem, rather than a primary disease entity. Food has come to be associated with more than a source of nutrition; it is a source of celebration, consolation, punishment, or reward (Murray & Zentner, 2001). Adolescent eating disorders frequently begin subsequent to an emotional trauma and are the manifestation of an overwhelming feeling of helplessness, dissatisfaction, or unattractiveness (Moore, 1996). Feelings of low self-esteem and negative self-image may trigger eating disorders but may also be exacerbated as the eating disorder progresses. Critical to the prevention and resolution of eating disorders is the promotion of self-esteem and a positive self-image. Consequently, the primary goal in managing the adolescent's nutritional well-being is based on understanding the adolescent's perception and the underlying pressures that influence the meaning of food to the adolescent. Establishing a healthy lifestyle, including healthy eating habits and exercise, during the adolescent period can influence the individual's nutritional habits throughout her lifetime (see Chapter 23 for further discussion of eating disorders).

MENSTRUAL DISORDERS

Menstrual complaints of the adolescent are primarily related to abnormal bleeding or painful bleeding. Prior to maturation of the HPG axis, disorders manifested as abnormal menstrual bleeding are usually related to the anovulatory nature of the menstrual cycle in the adolescent (Speroff et al., 1999). Menstrual irregularities in adolescents can also be related to stress, weight changes, change in level of physical activity, pregnancy, and trauma (Furniss, 1996).

Acute adolescent menorrhagia can present as a minor deviation in the amount of blood loss to life-threatening hemorrhage (Maxson & Rosenwaks, 1995). Due to lack of cognitive maturity manifested as embarrassment or fear of being different, the adolescent may attempt to ignore or hide an episode of excessive blood loss. Consequently, menorrhagia can lead to excessive blood loss and a clinical presentation of a pale, anxious girl presenting with heavy bleeding of several days' or weeks' duration. The primary etiology of acute adolescent menorrhagia is an anovulatory menstrual cycle. Pregnancy-related complications also should be explored and ruled out, however. After anovulatory uterine bleeding, pregnancy-related states, such as spontaneous abortion, complications of an elective termination, and ectopic pregnancy are the leading etiologies (Maxson & Rosenwaks, 1995).

Therapy for acute adolescent menorrhagia is focused on controlling bleeding, restoring circulating volume, and preventing recurrence. In anovulatory cycles, the main cause of bleeding is extreme endometrial proliferation secondary to fluctuating estrogen levels and the lack of progesterone secretion. Consequently, a primary component of treatment is exogenous hormones to stabilize circulating levels of estrogen and to stabilize the endometrium with progestogen (Maxson & Rosenwaks, 1995). Long-term follow-up includes surveillance for the spontaneous onset of ovulatory cycles, through measurement of basal body temperature, a difficult monitoring parameter to implement with the adolescent population. Individuals with acute adolescent menorrhagia are at greater risk for chronic anovulation disorders (see Chapter 8).

Dysmenorrhea is one of the most common complaints of adolescent women and accounts for a large number of days lost from work or school. The typical presentation is an adolescent one to three years following menarche, complaining of cramps and lower abdominal pain coinciding with the first day of the menses. Dysmenorrhea may be experienced as an isolated symptom or as a component of premenstrual syndrome (PMS). The onset of pain occurs within one to four hours of the beginning of the menses, lasts for twenty-four to forty-eight hours, and can be mild to severe in intensity (Maxson & Rosenwaks, 1995). The adolescent usually presents with primary or functional dysmenorrhea, that is, painful menstruation with a nonpathological etiology. In the adolescent, dysmenorrhea is usually associated with the onset of ovulatory menses. Ovarian maturation and cyclic progestogen secretions are associated with the myometrial spasms characteristic of dysmenorrhea. The adolescent with severe dysmenorrhea should be thoroughly evaluated, however, to rule out a pathological etiology such as endometriosis. In sexually active adolescents, dysmenorrhea may be symptomatic of pelvic inflammatory disease. Treatment of primary dysmenorrhea is usually symptomatic (see Chapter 8).

SEXUALLY TRANSMITTED DISEASES

Sexually transmitted diseases (STDs) are a significant source of potentially reversible morbidity in the adolescent population. The most common STDs in adolescents ages 15 to 19 years in 1999 were chlamydia at a rate of 1,383 per 100,000 among all teens and 2,359.4 per 100,000 females and gonorrhea at a rate of 534 per 100,000 teens. The infection rate for chlamydia increased in 1999, while the rate for gonorrhea has decreased slightly (CDC, 2000). Data may underestimate the actual prevalence rate in adolescents, however, since the most frequently occurring sexually transmitted infections in this population, chlamydia and HPV infections, are not routinely reportable. The presence of STDs accelerates the risk for HIV infection, and the incidence of HIV is increasing most rapidly among young women age 13 to 24 years (CDC, 2000).

The reasons adolescents engage in sexual activity are varied. The individual's ability to physically engage in sexual activity does not correspond with cognitive or social maturity. This disparity between physiological ability and cognitive understanding is often a contributing factor in unprotected sexual practices. Recently, there has been an upward trend in high school students who report being sexually active. In 1999, 49.9 percent of all high school students reported ever having sexual intercourse. The prevalence rate of sexual activity increases from grade 9 to grade 12: 33 percent of female students and 45 percent of male students in grade 9 compared to 66 percent of female and 64 percent of male students in grade 12 report being sexually active (MacKay, Fingerhut, & Duran, 2000).

The clinical presentation of STDs in the adolescent is essentially the same as in the adult: abnormal vaginal discharge, vulvar irritation, perianal sores, ulceration, dysuria or lower abdominal pain. There are some special considerations in the etiology and the implications of STDs in the adolescent population, however.

Physiologically, two factors, transitional vaginal epithelium and the lack of cervical mucous production, make the adolescent more susceptible to sexually transmitted bacterial and viral organisms. During puberty, the vaginal epithelium is in continual transition. The everted columnar cells on the portico of the cervix are preferentially attached to by organisms such as gonorrhea neisseria, chlamydia, and trachomatis (Furniss, 1996). The metamorphosis of the vaginal mucosa and the establishment of an acidic environment serve as protective mechanisms in the mature female. The second factor is the lack of cervical mucosa production. Cervical mucosa is the result of cyclic progesterone production from the mature ovary. Cervical mucosa forms a protective barrier to exclude pathogens from the internal reproductive structures and has specific protective properties including phagocytic cell production. These protective mechanisms are not functional, however, until after ovarian maturation, establishment of ovulation, and ovarian progesterone secretion. As previously discussed, ovarian maturation usually does not occur until one to two years after menarche.

For many sexually transmitted infections, the time from infection to diagnosis and treatment is influential of the prognosis. The lack of adequate or prompt treatment can result in the development of long-term sequelae. Women are at particular risk for complications from untreated or inadequately treated STDs. The long-term complications include sterility, ectopic pregnancy, fetal or infant death, and chronic pelvic inflammation (Furniss, 1996).

The progressively earlier age of first sexual intercourse is associated with an increased number of lifetime sexual partners and an increased risk of exposure to STDs. In addition, many adolescents become sexually active prior to seeking professional guidance related to safe sexual behaviors. Also, data indicate that while sexual activity increases by grade level, older students are less likely to use condoms: 66.6 percent of ninth graders compared to only 47.9 percent of twelfth graders. Recognizing the significance of the problem and the implications for future well-being, the health care provider has an obligation to screen all adolescents for risk specific behaviors, educate patients about transmission, and counsel adolescents about safe sex practices that reduce their risk for contracting a sexually transmitted disease.

ADOLESCENT PREGNANCY

More than 900,000 adolescents become pregnant each year (AMA, 2001). Adolescent pregnancy has become a major concern for all sectors of society. Adolescents who become parents tend to have less formal education, lower paying jobs, and higher rates of unemployment, as compared with their childless peers. In 1998, the birth rate for teens (15–19 years) was 51.1 per 1,000 births. Fortunately, the U.S. teen birth rate decreased by 22 percent to a record low in 2000 (National Center for Health Statistics, 2001). The *Healthy People 2010* target is 43.0 teen births per 1,000 births (National Center for Health Statistics, 2001). A majority of teen pregnancies are unintentional. Seventy-eight percent of teen pregnancies are unplanned and account for one-quarter of all unintended pregnancies (MacKay et al., 2000). An unintended pregnancy can be a crisis for the adolescent and her family. A minority of adolescent pregnancies are intended. The adolescent's desire to conceive usually emerges from the desire to please her partner or to solidify a relationship, to have someone to love and to take care of, to change her status in the family or to assert her independence, and to establish her fertility. Whether a pregnancy is accidental or intended, the normal process of adolescent maturation is interrupted. In addition, a pregnancy can exacerbate an adolescent's feeling of loss of control.

Presenting symptoms of an adolescent pregnancy—secondary amenorrhea, breast tenderness, morning nausea and weight gain—are typical of any pregnancy. Many adolescents may deny their concern about an unplanned pregnancy, however, by presenting with alternative complaints such as fatigue, weight changes, abdominal pain, or a request for contraception. Consequently, careful history and physical examination by the provider are essential to an accurate diagnosis. As a result of denial, fear, or lack of recognition of existing signs and symptoms, adolescents often present for diagnosis of the pregnancy and initiation of prenatal care after the completion of the first trimester. Late prenatal care limits both the quality and quantity of prenatal care services and may also limit the woman's options related to the disposition of her pregnancy.

Following the confirmation of a pregnancy, the adolescent must make a decision about the disposition of the pregnancy. It is important that the decision is made by the adolescent; the role of the health care provider is to offer supportive counseling and information about all options and resources. Of 893,000 teen pregnancies (ages 15 to 19) in 1996, there were 492,000 live births, 264,000 induced abortions, and 137,000 fetal losses (U.S. Census Bureau, 2001). Ten- to 14-year-olds had 26,000 pregnancies, 11,000 live births, 10,000 induced abortions, and 4,000 fetal losses in that same year. The highest pregnancy rates were in white teens. If abortion is the option of choice, the adolescent not only needs information about the procedure but needs appropriate follow-up care for both physical and emotional adaptation. Another option is adoption. Prior to 1970, the majority of unmarried, white adolescents chose adoption, but since that time the percent of teens choosing adoption is declining. Adoption has never been a highly chosen option by African American teens. The third option is parenthood. When parenthood is chosen, the adolescent needs high-quality prenatal care as well as preparation for the emotional, financial, and physical demands of parenting. Adolescents attempting to establish their own independence and to formulate their personal identity have difficulty balancing their own psychological responses with the demands of an infant.

If the adolescent chooses to continue the pregnancy, she is at greater risk for perinatal complications than the pregnant nonadolescent. Females under age 17 years have a high incidence of pregnancy related iron deficiency anemia, pregnancy-induced hypertension, operative births, preterm delivery, and low birth weight infants. In part, the increase in perinatal complications is related to competition between the adolescent's growth needs and the fetal demands on the maternal system for metabolic support. From a dietary perspective, additional amounts of pro-

tein, iron, and calcium are necessary for individual growth and fetal development. The role of folate in prevention of neural tube defects and promotion of DNA synthesis is becoming widely publicized. Current recommendation is for folic acid supplementation of 800 to 1,000 micrograms daily (Butterworth & Bendich, 1996; Lewis, Crane, Wilson, & Yetley, 1999).

Adolescents who conceive within two years of menarche are at particular risk. Pregnant adolescents of young gynecologic age have not completed their physical growth. Consequently, fetal distress and cephalopelvic disproportion during labor account for an increased risk for cesarean births among young adolescents. In addition, there is an increased incidence of low birth weight among infants born to adolescent mothers, related to competition between mother and fetus for nutritional resources. (National Center for Health Statistics, 2001). Reports indicate that the increased morbidity seen in adolescent pregnancy is related more to socioeconomic factors than the chronologic age at conception, particularly, the lack of early and adequate prenatal care (CDC, 2000). Many adolescents receive late or inadequate care either because the pregnancy was denied or the resources were lacking to access prenatal care. The adolescent's access to prenatal care is further complicated by factors including lack of money, transportation, knowledge, and not valuing prenatal care as contributing to a healthy pregnancy outcome. Adolescents who lack early and adequate obstetrical care have a higher incidence of spontaneous abortions, placental disorders, low birth weight, PIH, and prolonged labor (National Center for Health Statistics, 2001).

Although there are physical risks associated with an adolescent pregnancy, most pregnant adolescents do well physically. The biggest risk to both the adolescent and the infant, however, is the lack of parenting skills. Inadequate parenting skills predispose the adolescent to an increased risk of frustration, feeling of failure and social isolation, and negative self-image. Furthermore, these inadequate skills place the infant at great risk for physical and emotional developmental delay and, in extreme situations, an increased risk of injury or abuse.

SMOKING

Smoking has been listed as the most important source of preventable morbidity and premature death in every report of the surgeon general since 1964 (CDC, 2000). Despite these warnings, data indicate that 6,000 adolescents experiment with smoking and 3,000 teens become daily smokers each day (CDC, 2000). Smoking initiated during the adolescent years is the single most preventable cause of death, including heart disease and cancer. Reasons adolescents begin to smoke include peers and parents or siblings who smoke. Adolescents with high exposure to cigarette advertising and role models are significantly more likely to be smokers than those with low exposure. (National Center for Health Statistics, 2001). One study of smoking behaviors suggested that self-esteem may be a factor in the smoking behavior of female adolescents, but not for males. Therefore, female adolescents may have unique motivations to initiate tobacco use, making them more susceptible to advertising and media portrayals. Adolescents frequently do not enjoy smoking but report doing it to "fit in." (Murray & Zentner, 2001). A study of 155 adolescent smokers found that 95 percent knew the health risks and hazards associated with smoking, but those risks were of little concern to 70 percent of participants. Adolescent smoking has a negative correlation with academic performance and a positive correlation with use of alcohol and illicit drugs (AMA, 2001).

It is estimated that 5.5 minutes of life is lost for each cigarette smoked (Childtrends, 2001). Adolescents also need to be aware of the addictive effects of nicotine, the effects on the cardiovascular and respiratory systems, the alterations of blood coagulation and the use of oral contraceptives, an increased incidence of cervical cancer, as well as the effect of passive smoke on pregnancies, infants, and children. Interventions focused on preventing initiation of smoking or cessation of smoking need to include more than giving the facts. The provider must explore the individual's idea of health and the social dynamics of smoking. Smoking cessation is a loss. The provider needs to aid the individual to recognize what is gained by not maintaining a smoking habit.

SUICIDE

Suicide is the third leading cause of death, after accidents, in 13- to 24-year-olds (CDC, 2000). While male suicides are more successful, females attempt suicide four times more frequently than males (CDC, 2000). Adolescent suicide is often associated with impulsivity and anger. Neinstein, Julian, and Shapiro (1996) have identified a four-step progressive behavioral pattern evident in suicidal adolescents:

- Long-standing problem: lack of social connections or problems that create vulnerabilities.

- Escalation: childhood problems exacerbate during adolescent development.
- Progressive social isolation: failure of available adaptive techniques leading to social isolation and depression.
- Final state: the attempt preceded by increased despair.

In 1999, 28.3 percent of high school students (35.7 percent female and 21.0 percent male) reported feeling so sad or hopeless for a period of at least two weeks duration that they stopped some of their regular activities. While males are more likely to succeed when they attempt suicide (18.5/100,000 males versus 3.3/100,000 females), females (37.7 percent versus 21.0 percent) are more likely to experience feeling of sadness and hopelessness leading to suicidal ideation (CDC, 2000).

Asking adolescents about suicide doesn't give them the idea. Asking key questions as part of health care visits can identify the adolescent in trouble and open the opportunity to secure help and counseling.

CARDIOVASCULAR DISEASE RISK

The pathogenesis of atherosclerosis begins in childhood and results from the interaction of genetic and environmental factors (Childtrends, 2001). Although genetics cannot be altered, environmental factors such as dietary intake of saturated fats and cholesterol, exercise patterns and smoking patterns can be modified during the adolescent years.

The adolescent's blood pressure should be evaluated annually. Hypertension in teens may begin early and is often associated with obesity (USDHHS, 2000). Usual interventions include low-salt diet, weight reduction, exercise, and relaxation as the foundation of a healthy lifestyle.

SEXUAL ASSAULT

Female adolescents are the most likely victims of sexual assault. Approximately 50 percent of rape victims are between 10 and 19 years and the perpetrator is usually a known acquaintance (MacKay et al., 2000). Sexual assault or rape with a known perpetrator can lead to self-blame and guilt.

The adolescent who is assaulted or raped is the object of hostile, dehumanizing attacks that may have long-standing effects on the victim's self-worth and identity. These effects are particularly difficult for the adolescent still dealing with issues of separation, independence, and development of sexual identity. Helton (1986) found that asking two questions about the possibility of abuse increased the opportunity for positive responses and communicated that the provider was concerned and committed. Once abuse is identified, the adolescent needs to hear that she is not alone, it is not her fault, she needs to talk about it, and she needs help and support.

CARING FOR ADOLESCENTS

Providing health care for the adolescent can present complex and difficult situations. Strategies for promoting adolescent health care need to emphasize helping the individual to adapt to the physical and psychological changes, become aware of the risk and negative consequences of behaviors, and help her to engage in responsible decision-making processes. Although many of the physical problems experienced by the adolescent are similar to problems seen in the adult population, the adolescent presents with emotional characteristics that require special attention. The adolescent is often confused and ambivalent about her feelings and may be unable or unwilling to share her concerns, needs, or questions. Therefore, providers need to allot adequate time and use language appropriate to the adolescent's developmental and cultural background.

During adolescence, the individual makes the transition from patterns of child health care to adult health management and care systems. During childhood, health care providers primarily work with parents to make decisions related to health care as well as to educate and counsel parents about the intervention implemented for their child. The child is primarily a passive recipient of health evaluation and management. During adolescence, the emerging woman needs to become an active participant in her health care. The adolescent's activities have consequences that may impact current and future health care status. Thus, she not only becomes an active participant in health care choices but also learns to accept responsibility for the consequences of a choice. The adolescent should perceive that she is in partnership with the health care provider. Empowering the adolescent in the delivery of health care enhances compliance and further open, honest communication between the client and the provider.

Adolescents have reported that they would find it helpful to talk with a health care provider about health-related topics (Public Health Foundation, 1999). Adoles-

cents also report, however, that one of the barriers to communication is failure of the provider to raise a subject or the provider's lack of response when the adolescent asks about a subject. Consequently, the adolescent needs to be seen by a provider who will obtain a thorough assessment of sexual knowledge and behaviors, and who has the time to listen and respond to the adolescent's needs with satisfactory explanations and to answer questions in a manner appropriate to her level of development and comprehension. The interaction between the adolescent and the health care provider provides an opportunity for the adolescent to establish an important relationship outside the family and peer group structure.

SEXUAL BEHAVIOR DECISIONS

Adolescents need to discuss issues of sexuality and their decisions related to sexual activity. Therefore, a sexual history needs to be taken and risk prevention discussed with all adolescents. The sexual history should use language understandable to the adolescent and should progress from least to most intimate areas to establish a sense of respect and trust between the provider and the adolescent. A well-conducted sexual history allows the provider to gather data and to facilitate expression by the adolescent in a direct but nonconfrontational manner. Based on the information obtained in the sexual history, the provider is able to identify areas of counseling, education, prevention, and referral. It is important to acknowledge the adolescent's desire for autonomy and to encourage and support the adolescent's values and choices throughout this process.

Educational and counseling strategies need to focus on safer sexual practices and contraception to prevent sexually acquired diseases and pregnancy. In addition, female adolescents need information focused on decisions regarding becoming sexually active, empowering women to say no, and helping women in abusive or coercive relationships. Strategies and awareness of situational factors leading to sexual violence may foster preparedness in this at-risk population. Childtrends (2001) reports that 2.3 percent of girls between ages 12 and 15 years and 4.8 percent of women between 16 and 19 years of age have been victims of sexual assault, making the female adolescent the most likely victim of sexual violence.

Promotion of school-based clinics, distribution of condoms, and family life programs are efforts to provide education and resources for health enhancing and risk avoiding behaviors. All adolescents have a right to and a need for information about healthy and responsible sexual behavior. Without factual information, the young woman is denied her right to protect herself and to make decisions within the framework of her emerging personal identity. Information and resources should be accessible and provided in an accepting, supportive, and nonjudgmental environment. Providing supportive and honest information and feedback to the adolescent will enhance her development of self-esteem, acceptance of responsibility for her actions, and the establishment of a values system. Support must also exist for the adolescent who chooses virginity or not to become sexually active. The adolescent needs to be reassured about the acceptability of abstinence. Support includes discussion of how to effectively say no and how to interact with pressure from peers or acquaintances who may not understand or want to accept her decision. Respecting and supporting the choice of the adolescent and promoting a healthy adolescence are the interventions that promote the emergence of a healthy adult.

PELVIC EXAMINATION

The first pelvic examination should be approached with care and gentleness. The provider should be aware of the adolescent's developmental level since the internal examination is a source of anxiety for many adolescents. Common concerns include the fear of pain, embarrassment, or discovery of an anomaly as well as inadequate knowledge of the vaginal anatomy and physiology. The impact of the first examination can leave long-term positive or negative effects that can impact the individual's future health care practices. Basically, the indications for a pelvic examination include symptoms specific to the female reproductive system, initiation of sexual activity, or age 18 years, at which time annual examination should commence (Speroff et al., 1999) (see Chapter 4). Virginal females find the gynecologic examination particularly distressing. In nonsexually active, younger adolescents, a recto-vaginal examination is an alternative that may provide information about the status of the external genitalia and may assist in identifying possible abnormalities of the vaginal, uterine, and adnexal structures (Speroff et al., 1999). When an internal examination is necessary, younger adolescents and virginal girls prefer a female family member to be present during the examination, whereas older or sexually active adolescents prefer a female chaperone to be present. Prior to the first examination, the adolescent should receive a thorough explanation and demonstration of what will be done and offered the opportunity to voice questions or concerns. Establishing a good rapport prior

to the examination and maintaining eye contact and a professional but caring relationship during the examination are essential to the adolescent's psychological well-being.

CONFIDENTIALITY AND TRUST

Health care is traditionally provided in an environment of confidentiality and trust. But, when interacting with the adolescent, it is important to be aware of the unique issues of confidentiality and trust inherent in the client/provider relationship. Health issues related to sexuality and sexual activity raise unique dilemmas for the health care provider and can influence the provider's relationship with the client and thereby impact the quality of the care provided.

Most adolescents are minors, that is, under the age of 18. The power to consent to a minor's medical care has belonged traditonally to the parents or the parent's surrogate. The adolescent's status related to ability to seek and consent to health care is based either on the status of the minor or on the type of health care needed. Although there is variation among states, most states have laws that allow the adolescent the right to seek and consent to certain types of health care including the diagnosis and treatment of STDs, provision of contraception, and the diagnosis and treatment of pregnancy (MacKay et al., 2000). In addition, an individual under the age of 18 who has been declared an emancipated minor or meets the criteria for the mature minor rule may seek and consent to medical treatment. An emancipated minor is an individual who has attained a specific status based on marital status, parenthood or pregnancy, military service, or residency and financial independence (English, 1996). Typically, the courts have considered these individuals emancipated from their parents. The status of emancipation, however, is rarely conferred by the court proactively. In fact, in most states, the right to seek emancipation of a minor belongs to the parent, not to the adolescent. Consequently, the designation of emancipation may need to be made by the health care provider within the context of the professional relationship. The mature minor doctrine states that there is "little likelihood that a practitioner will incur liability for failure to obtain parental consent in situations in which the minor is an older adolescent (typically at least age 15) who is capable of giving an informed consent and in which the care is not high risk, is for the minor's benefit, and is within the mainstream of established medical opinion" (English, 1996). Basically, the criteria for determining the adolescent's ability to consent is based in her ability not only to understand the risks, benefits, and alternatives but also to make a voluntary choice. These are the same criteria for informed consent with adult clients.

Issues of confidentiality should be discussed proactively with the adolescent and the parent. The nature of the adolescents seeking health care, however, may not make these types of discussion realistic or desirable. Thus, the health care provider needs to be familiar with state statutes and needs to communicate his or her philosophy to the adolescent at the initiation of the client/provider relationship.

CONCLUSION

Unlike other cultures that celebrate the transition of adolescence, U.S. culture views the adolescent period as a time of anxiety, awkwardness, and turmoil (Childtrends, 2001). Although stereotypical descriptions predominate, adolescence is often a time of positive growth and development, a time for the development of healthy lifestyles, practices, and behaviors. The stage of adolescence includes a rapidly changing body and new expectations, norms, and social roles. Conceptualizations of adolescence need to focus on monitoring the physical changes as well as mastering the psychosocial tasks that allow advancement to higher levels of development. Health care providers must recognize that adolescents are "not just big children or small adults—they have unique problems that demand unique solutions" (Shalala, 1996). A healthy adolescence equates with a successful transition manifested as physical well-being, coping, adaptation, and psychosocial growth. Working with adolescents offers the health care provider a unique opportunity for investing in the health and well-being of future generations.

REFERENCES

Albertsson-Wikland, K., Rosberg, S., Karlberg, J., & Groth, T. (1994). Analysis of the 24 hour growth hormone profiles in healthy boys and girls of normal stature: Relation to puberty. *Journal of Clinical Endocrinology and Metabolism, 78,* 1195–1201.

American Medical Association (AMA). (2001). *Healthy youth 2010.* Chicago: Author.

Baram, D.A. (1996). Sexuality and sexual function. In *Novak's gynecology* (12th ed). Baltimore MD: Williams and Wilkins.

Butterworth, C.E., & Bendich, A. (1996). Folic acid and the prevention of birth defects. *Annual Review of Nutrition, 16,* 73–97.

Centers for Disease Control and Prevention (CDC). (2000). Youth risk behavior surveillance: CDC surveillance summaries, June 9, 2000. *MMNR, 2000, 49* (no SS-5).

Childtrends. (2001). Facts at a glance. Available at: *www.childtrend.org.* Date accessed: 5/30/02.

English, A. (1996). Understanding legal aspects of care. In L.S. Neinstein (Ed.), *Adolescent health care: A practical guide* (3rd ed., pp. 50–163). Baltimore: Williams and Wilkins.

Erikson, E. (1965). *Childhood and society.* New York: Norton.

Furniss, K. (1996). Common clinical problems and issues. In *Current practice issues in adolescent gynecology* (pp. 8–14). Washington, DC: AWHONN and NANPRH.

Hechinger, F.M. (1992). *Fateful choices: Healthy youth for the 21st century.* New York: Carnegie Foundation.

Helton, A. (1986). Battering during pregnancy. *American Journal of Nursing, 86,* 910–913.

Lewis, C.J., Crane, N.T., Wilson, D.B., & Yetley, E.A. (1999). Estimated folate intakes: Data updates to reflect food fortification, increased bioavailability and dietary supplements use. *American Journal of Clinical Nutrition, 70,* 198–207.

MacKay, A.P., Fingerhut, L.A., & Duran, C.R. (2000). *Adolescent health chartbook: Health, United States of America.* Hyattsville, MD: National Center for Health Statistics.

Maxson, W.S., & Rosenwaks, Z. (1995). Dysmenorrhea and premenstrual syndrome. In K.J. Ryan, R.S. Berkowitz, & R.L. Barbiere (Eds.), *Kistner's gynecology* (6th ed.; pp. 168–187). St. Louis: Mosby.

Moore, R. (1996). Overview of developmental and physical milestones and psychosocial issues. In *Current practice issues in adolescent gynecology* (pp. 4–7). Washington, DC: AWHONN and NANPRH.

Murray, R.B., & Zentner, J.P. (2001). *Health promotion strategies through the life span* (7th ed.). Upper Saddle River, NJ: Prentice Hall Health.

National Center for Health Statistics. (2001). *National survey of family growth.* Available at: *www.cdc.gov/nchs/nsfg.htm.* Accessed 5/30/02.

Neinstein, L.S., & Kaufman, F.R. (1996). Normal growth and development. In L.S. Neinstein (ed.), *Adolescent health care: A practical guide* (3rd ed., pp. 3–39). Baltimore: Williams and Wilkins.

Neinstein, L.S., Julian, M.A., & Shapiro, J. (1996). Suicide. In L.S. Neinstein (ed.), *Adolescent health care: A practical guide* (3rd ed., pp. 1116–1123). Baltimore: Williams and Wilkins.

Public Health Foundation. (1999). *Healthy People 2010 toolkit: A field guide to health planning.* Available at: *http://www.health.gov/healthypeople/state/toolkit.* Accessed 5/30/02.

Shalala, D.E. (1996). I believe in angels. *Journal of Adolescent Health, 19,* 195.

Smith, S., & McClaugherty, L.O. (1993). Adolescent homosexuality: A primary care perspective. *American Family Physician, 48,* 33–36.

Speroff, L., Glass, R.H., & Kase, N.G. (1999). *Clinical gynecological endocrinology and infertility.* Baltimore, MD: Williams and Wilkins.

U.S. Census Bureau. (2001). Table No. 86. Numbers and rates of pregnancies, live births, induced abortions, and fetal losses for teenagers by age, race, and Hispanic origin. In *Statistical Abstract of the United States: 2001* (121st ed.). Washington, DC: U.S. Government Printing Office.

U.S. Department of Health and Human Services. (2000). *CDC's guidelines for school and community programs: Promoting lifelong physical activity: An overview* [Online]. Available: *http://www.cdc.gov/nccdphp/dash/phactaag.htm.* Accessed 11/19/02.

Wadsworth, B. (1996). *Piaget's theory of cognitive and affective development* (5th ed.) New York: Longman.

CHAPTER 4

ASSESSING WOMEN'S HEALTH

Ellis Quinn Youngkin ◆ *Marcia Szmania Davis*

Consider any inter-action with a client a therapeutic interven-tion by permitting the free expression of is-sues and concerns.

Highlights

- Mortality, Morbidity, and Risk Factors
- Screening Methods
    Health History
    Special Assessment: Family, Nutrition,
        Stress/Risk, Fitness, Occupation, Sleep
    Physical Examination
- Overview of Commonly Indicated Laboratory Tests
    Cervical Cytology
    HPV DNA Testing
    Gonorrhea and Chlamydia Tests
    Wet Mounts
    Urinalysis
    Herpes Culture and Type-Specific Tests
    Sensitivity, Specificity, and Predictive Value

❖ INTRODUCTION

Women's life span, opportunities and risks, and challenges and stresses are ever increasing. As perhaps the only person a woman sees for health care, the woman's health care provider must approach assessment holistically. Indeed, all factors impinging on the woman's health and well-being must be considered if significant omissions in detecting problems and offering care are to be avoided. Pender (1996), in discussing health and wellness, refers to Dunn's suggestion that optimum health, or high level wellness, only emanates from an environment that is favorable. Thus, the provider must help the woman become more attuned to her body and its cues and use the assessment period as an opportunity for teaching and counseling.

Healthy People 2010 has as its main goal helping Americans live longer with improved quality of life (U.S. Department of Health and Human Services [USDHHS], 2000). One important focus for the provider is assessing the woman's risk factors and working with her to change her behaviors and lifestyle to more healthful ones. Of interest are results of a study that examined the role of cognitive-perceptual factors (control over health, self-efficacy, and health status) in maintenance of health-promoting behavior of over 1,000 women. The investigators found that cognitive-perceptual factors had only small effects on specific health promoting behaviors.

Progress to decrease deaths has been made. From 1998 to 1999, deaths from cancer, stroke, influenza/pneumonia, suicide, homicide, and aortic aneurysm declined (National Center for Health Statistics [NCHS], 2001). However, deaths from septicemia, hypertension, chronic lower respiratory diseases, and diabetes increased. Heart disease, accident, and chronic liver disease deaths—all leading causes of mortality—changed insignificantly. Alzheimer's disease deaths moved from twelveth place to eighth. Decreasing health disparities based on gender, race/ethnicity, income, disability, rural residency, and sexual orientation comprises *Healthy People 2010*'s second goal (USDHHS, 2000). Although women have an overall lower death rate than men, it has risen in the last ten years as men's has declined. Racial disparities are thought to derive from "the complex interaction among genetic variations, environmental factors, and specific health behaviors" (p. 12). Income and education account for most of the morbidity and mortality levels for such diseases as heart disease, obesity, diabetes, and low birth weight infants. Access to medical care, better housing, safer neighborhoods, and a better health promotion lifestyle are all a function of higher education and income.

MORTALITY, MORBIDITY, AND RISK FACTORS IN U.S. WOMEN

LEADING CAUSES OF MORTALITY IN U.S. WOMEN

The average life expectancy for U.S. women has increased from about 50 years in 1900 to 79.4 years in 1999; this is a 0.1 year decline from 1998 (USDHHS, 2000; NCHS, 2001). The discrepancy between white and black women continues to be significant: 79.9 for white women in 1999; 74.5 for black women (National Vital Statistics Report [NVSR], 2002a, b). The causes of death differ significantly for U.S. women, depending on age and race (Tables 4–1, 4–2, 4–3, 4–4, and 4–5). By 1999, heart disease, cancer, and stroke led the way as the top three causes of death, with chronic lower respiratory diseases in fourth place and continuing to increase (Eberhardt, Ingram, Makuc, et al., 2001). Cancer deaths declined six percent between 1990 and 1998, but the number of cases being diagnosed is up and people are living longer (Eberhardt et al., 2001; Youngkin & Davis, 1998). Better screening and diagnostic technologies are partially responsible for this trend. Women's lung cancer deaths since 1950 are up about 600 percent; it is the leading cause of cancer deaths (Kelley, Blair, & Pechacek, 2001). Smoking is a major contributor to cancer deaths and COPD in women. Kidney disease became a top ten cause of death for all U.S. women in 1999 (Eberhardt et al., 2001). HIV infection, although no longer among the top ten causes of death for women, remained the tenth leading cause of death for African American women, in particular for ages 25 to 44 years. For white women, Alzheimer's disease became the sixth leading cause of death, and pneumonia/influenza remained in the top ten (Eberhardt et al.,

TABLE 4–1. Death Rates for U.S. Women by Selected Cause and Age (Per 100,000 Population)

Age	Heart Disease[a]	Cancer[a]	MVRIs[a,b]	Cerebv. Dis.[a,i]	CLRD[a,c]	Pneumonia[d,e]	Suicide[a]	Liver Disease[d]	DM[d]	Homicide[a]
1–14	1.6	5.0	3.7	0.5	0.5	1.3	3.4	[g]	[g]	3.3
15–24	2.2	3.8	16.3	0.5	0.5	0.5	5.6	[g]	[g]	4.4
25–34	5.6	10.7	9.3	1.5	0.9	1.9[f]	4.7	2.9[f]	2.4[f]	4.6
35–44	17.4	41.1	8.9	5.6	2.1		6.3			4.0
45–54	51.8	125.9	8.2	14.0	8.5	8.2[f]	6.6	10.1[f]	20.1[f]	2.4
55–64	167.4	328.7	9.6	35.5	43.6		5.2			1.5
65–74	503.1	676.7	13.4	118.5	151.4	233.6[f]	4.2	[g]	139.1[d]	1.7
75–84	1,562.6	1,067.9	19.5	458.3	328.9		4.7	[g]		2.0
85–	5,913.6	1,448.9	18.7	1,670.2	509.0		4.1	[g]		2.0
Totals for women	220.8	169.9	9.8	60.5	58.1	[g]	4.0	[g]	67[h]	2.9
Totals for men	327.9	251.6	21.8	60.1	38.2	[g]	18.1	[g]	86[h]	9.3

[a]Eberhardt et al., 2001: Tables 37, 38, 39, 42, 45, 46, 47.
[b]Motor vehicle-related injuries
[c]Chronic lower respiratory diseases
[d]U.S. Census Bureau, Statistical Abstract of the United States: 2001. Table No. 108. Deaths by age and leading cause: 1998.
[e]Pneumonia and influenza
[f]Rates for this and next age category combined
[g]Not available
[h]USDHHS, 2000, pp. 5–18.
[i]Cerebrovascular diseases

TABLE 4–2. Death Rates for U.S. Women in 1990 and 1999 from Homicide, Motor Vehicle-Related Injuries, Suicide (Per 100,000 Resident Population)

		Ages 15 to 24 years			Ages 25 to 44 years			Ages 45 and over		
		Homicide	MVRI	Suicide	Homicide	MVRI	Suicide	Homicide	MVRI	Suicide
White	1990	4.0	19.5	4.2	3.8	20.8	6.6	2.2	17.4	6.8
female	1999	3.0	17.3	3.2	3.0	18.2	6.3	1.6	16.7	4.6
Black	1990	18.9	9.9	2.3	21.0	20.5	3.8	9.4	13.5	1.9
female	1999	11.5	12.1	2.0	11.9	18.6	2.5	3.4	13.0	1.5
AI	1990	*	31.4	*	6.9	37.0	*	NA	*	*
female	1999	*	28.6	*	10.2	59.8	8.3	NA	28.0	*
Hispanic	1990	8.1	11.6	3.1	6.1	17.4	3.1	*	14.9	*
female	1999	4.9	11.7	2.0	3.7	14.8	2.5	*	12.9	2.2
White,	1990	3.3	20.4	4.3	3.5	21.0	7.0	2.2	17.5	7.0
NH fem.	1999	2.6	18.2	3.4	2.8	18.5	6.8	1.7	16.8	4.8
Asian	1990	*	11.4	3.9	3.8	14.8	3.8	NA	24.3	8.5
PI female	1999	2.8	8.7	4.4	2.8	9.4	4.0	NA	15.1	6.5

*Based on fewer than 20 deaths
AI—American Indian or Alaska Native female
NH—Non-Hispanic female
PI—Asian or Pacific Islander female
NA—No data available

Source: Eberhardt et al., 2001, Tables 45, 46, 47; Health, United States 2001. Starting with 1999 data, cause of death is coded according to ICD-10.

TABLE 4–3. Differences in Death Rates for U.S. Women by Selected Cause for all Ages and Detailed Race/Hispanic Origin (per 100,000 Population)[1]

Disease/Cause	White females	Black females	Native AI/AN females	Asian/ PI females	Hispanic females	White non-Hispanic females
Heart disease	215.4	290.4	138.3	121.6	146.6	218.0
Cerebrovascular diseases	50.8	78.1	38.3	48.2	36.3	59.6
Malignant neoplasms	168.6	200.0	109.1	104.1	104.1	172.1
Respiratory cancer	41.5	40.5	26.9	19.6	13.1	43.4
Breast cancer	26.4	35.6	15.4	13.1	15.4	26.9
Chronic liver disease	40.2	23.9	27.3	11.9	15.3	41.6
Motor vehicle injuries	9.9	9.2	21.4	7.3	8.1	10.0
Suicide	4.4	1.6	4.7	3.6	1.9	4.7
Homicide	2.2	7.5	5.9	2.3	2.8	2.0
Cancer of cervix[2]	7.4	10.5	NA	9.3	12.0	6.4
Cancer of colon[2]	35.5	45.5	NA	27.8	21.3	36.9
Cancer of uterus[2]	22.7	15.3	NA	15.9	13.7	23.5
Cancer of ovary[2]	14.6	9.8	NA	11.6	10.1	15.2
Chronic lower respiratory disease	40.2	23.9	27.3	12.0	15.3	41.5

AI/AN—American Indian or Alaska Native female

PI—Pacific Island female

[1] Eberhardt et al., 2001. Tables 37, 38, 39, 40, 41, 42, 45, 46, 47, data from 1999.

[2] Eberhardt et al., 2001. Table 55, data from 1997.

2001). Although the twentieth century, by and large, saw declines in infectious diseases, recent increases in mortality raise concerns about prevention and treatment in the future (Armstrong, Conn, & Pinner, 1999).

TABLE 4–4. Death Rates for Human Immunodeficiency Virus (HIV) Infection, According to Sex, Detailed Race, Hispanic Origin, and Age: 1987, 1992, 1994, 1996, 1998, 1999 (per 100,000 Resident Population)

Race and Sex	1987	1992	1994	1996	1998	1999
White male	8.7	19.0	21.2	13.2	4.6	4.9
Black male	26.2	65.5	87.2	71.5	34.0	37.0
Hispanic male	18.8	35.5	42.4	28.2	10.7	11.3
Asian/Pacific Islander male	2.5	4.6	7.0	4.5	1.4	1.4
American Indian/ Alaskan Native male	*	4.9	9.5	7.1	4.0	5.0
Non-Hispanic white male	10.7	16.8	18.7	11.3	3.8	4.0
White female	0.6	1.6	2.3	1.9	0.8	1.0
Black female	4.6	14.8	22.6	21.1	12.2	13.3
Asian/Pacific Islander female	*	0.5	0.7	0.5	*	*
American Indian/ Alaskan Native female	*	*	*	*	*	*
Hispanic female	2.1	5.8	8.1	6.5	2.8	3.1
Non-Hispanic white female	0.5	1.0	1.6	1.3	0.5	0.7

* Age-specific death rate based on fewer than 20 deaths.

Source: Eberhardt et al., 2001, Table 43.

Adolescence to Young Adulthood (Ages 15 to 24)

The number of young people in this country has increased since a decline from 1976 through 1991. By 2020, 43 million teenagers, up from 35 million in 1992, will live in the United States. Adolescent and young adult women are at greatest risk for death from accidents and violence. Most unintentional injuries are from motor vehicle fatalities. In adolescents, alcohol is a major contributing factor (CDC National Center for Chronic Diseases Prevention and Health Promotion [CDCNCCDPHP], 2000). Despite this, alcohol-related traffic deaths decreased by one-third in the 15- to 24-year-old age group (Sells & Blum, 1996). Death by assault is nearly four times higher in 15- to 24-year-old black women as compared with white women (Eberhardt et al., 2001). Interpersonal violence causes significant mortality and morbidity for adolescent girls. Moskowitz, Griffith, Discala, and Sege (2001) found that those girls who were killed or disabled from assault were more likely than adolescent boys to have preexisting impairments, cognitive or psychosocial, and more likely to have been injured at a home or residence. Motor vehicle-related injuries (MVRI) as a cause of death in the 15- to 24-year-old age group increased in 1999 in young black, American Indian and Alaskan Native, and Hispanic females, while deaths from homicide and suicide decreased across all races as compared to 1990 data (Table 4–2). Deaths and death rates for injury by firearms for females declined in 1997, 1998, and

TABLE 4–5. Leading Causes of Death by Rank of 1 through 10 in U.S. Females According to Detailed Race and Hispanic Origin: United States, 1999.

Disease	White	Black	American Indian/ Alaska Native	Asian/ Pacific Islander	Hispanic
Heart disease	1	1	1	2	1
Malignant neoplasms	2	2	2	1	2
Cerebrovascular diseases	3	3	5	3	3
Unintentional injuries	6	5	3	5	5
Pneumonia/influenza	5	9	8	7	7
Diabetes mellitus	8	4	4	4	4
Alzheimer's disease	7				
Chronic lower respiratory diseases	4	7	7	6	6
Perinatal conditions					8
Chronic liver disease			6		9
HIV infection		10			
Nephritis/nephrotic syndrome/nephrosis	9	6	9	8	10
Septicemia	10	8	10	10	
Essential hypertension and hypertensive renal disease				9	

Source: Eberhardt et al., 2001, Table 32; updated October 2001.

1999 (Eberhardt et al., 2001). Suicide rates are highest for Asian/Pacific Islander females in the 15- to 24-year-old age group, the only group in which the rates increased in 1999. Suicide is less likely to be successful in females. The United States has higher homicide and MVRI death rates in age groups 15 to 34 than twenty-three other countries (Heuveline & Slap, 2002). Females have lower rates in both MVRIs and homicides. Fatal risk behaviors increase in teen years, indicating a need to target this group for prevention. 1999 saw a decline in deaths from HIV infection among the 15- to 24-year-old age group. However, African American reproductive-age women continue to be at highest risk, especially those living in the South (Phillips & Sowell, 2000). Black U.S. females have the highest mortality rate from HIV disease of any race with Hispanic females a distant second (Table 4–4). White, black, Hispanic, and white non-Hispanic females all had an increase in mortality from HIV in 1999 from 1998, which may suggest an increased reliance on drug therapies over protective behaviors among women and men.

Young Adulthood to Mid-Adulthood (Ages 25 to 44)

Cancer remained the number one killer for women ages 25 to 44 in 1999 (Table 4–1). MVRI was second and heart diseases third in the 25- to 34-year-olds, but these causes were reversed for women 35 to 44 years. Suicide remained fourth as it was in 1997, when it tied with HIV infection which was not a major cause of death in 1999.

Homicide deaths were fifth and sixth respectively in 1999 for 25- to 34-year-olds and 35- to 44-year-olds. Motor vehicle deaths became significantly increased for American Indian and Native Alaskan women in these age groups.

Mid-Adulthood to Older Adulthood (Ages 45 to 64)

Cancer and heart diseases lead the causes of mortality for this age group. Cerebrovascular and chronic lower respiratory diseases are third and fourth with motor vehicle accidents and pneumonia next. Liver disease, diabetes, suicide, and homicide continue as significant causes of death. Homicide is higher in black and Hispanic females; suicide in white and white non-Hispanic females. Autoimmune diseases are frequent causes of death in women under 65 years (Walsh & Rau, 2000).

Maturity (Ages 65 and Older)

Heart disease increases dramatically with age, as do cancer, cerebrovascular diseases, chronic lower respiratory diseases, pneumonia/influenza, and diabetes. Leading causes of death in a report of 1996 data differed by race with Alzheimer's disease a cause more often in white women, and diabetes, renal diseases, hypertension, and septicemia more common among blacks (Desai, Zhang, & Hennessy, 1999). Falls are a main cause of injury resulting in death after age 75, causing 47 percent of such deaths (Schnitzer & Runyan, 1995). Falls, orthostatic systolic blood pressure, and increased foot reaction time are significant risk factors for motor vehicle crashes and fatality rates in elderly women (Margolis, Kerani, McGovern, et al., 2002). Older women with diabetes die at an excess rate as compared to older women without diabetes (Bertoni, Krop, Anderson, & Brancati, 2002). Stroke and ischemic heart disease are higher complications of diabetes in the elderly.

Differences in Causes of Death for Women by Race

Compared with white women, black women have a higher incidence of death from heart disease; malignant neoplasms including breast, cervical, and colon cancer; cerebrovascular diseases; and homicide (Table 4–3). Deaths from motor vehicle-related injuries are significantly higher among American Indian/Alaskan Native women than any other race/origin (Table 4–2). Deaths from HIV infection are significantly higher in black women with Hispanic women much lower but higher than other races (Table 4–4). Deaths from lung cancer and chronic lower respiratory diseases are highest in white and white non-Hispanic females (Table 4–3). Heart disease and malignant neoplasms are the leading killers of all women regardless of race and Hispanic origin. Although the risk of dying from pregnancy and childbirth-related causes is low in the United States (i.e., 6.1 deaths per 100,000 live births in 1999 as compared to 7.3 in 1992), black women in 1999 had nearly four times the deaths per 100,000 live births than white, Hispanic, and non-Hispanic women (Eberhardt et al., 2001). Leading causes of pregnancy-related deaths include hypertensive disorders, hemorrhage, and embolism (Berg, Atrash, Koonin, & Tucker, 1996). For the period 1979–1992, the pregnancy-related mortality ratio of maternal deaths per 100,000 live births was 10.3 for Hispanic women, 6.0 for non-Hispanic white women, and 25.1 for black women (Hopkins, MacKay, Koonin, Berg, et al., 1999). Puerto Rican women had the highest mortality ratio for Hispanic women at 13.4, with Cuban women at 7.8 and Mexican women at 9.7. Among African American inner-city women, earlier age at first delivery (under 25 years) and having a high school education or higher predicted longevity in one study (Astone, Ensminger, & Juon, 2002).

Cancer

In 1999, cancer was the second leading cause of U.S. deaths (USDHHS, 2000). The most common sites for cancer regardless of gender or race/ethnicity were lung, trachea, and bronchus; prostate; female breast; and colon and rectum. Male lung, female breast, prostate,

and colorectal cancers declined from 1990 to 1996 (USDHHS, 2000). More than half of medical costs for cancer, estimated at $107 billion per year, are for lung, breast, and prostate cancers. Lung cancer deaths, the leading cause of women's cancer deaths, continue to rise; breast cancer is second (USDHHS, 2000). Cancer deaths decreased more in men than women from 1990 to 1996, particularly for lung cancer (Garfinkle & Mushinski, 1999). In 1999, white, non-Hispanic females had the highest death rate from respiratory cancers, with white then black females next (Eberhart et al., 2001, Table 40). African American women in 1999 had the highest breast cancer death rate, with white non-Hispanic then white women following (Table 4–3). Incidence rates in the United States for breast cancer are higher overall in whites, probably due to longer lives, but black women under 40 have the highest incidence rates in that age group (Lacey, Devesa, & Brinton, 2002). Reasons related to reproductive and socioeconomic differences are said to explain a higher mortality rate for breast cancer in women from some areas of the Northeast (Lacey et al., 2002). White women have seen a decline in breast cancer deaths due to better screening (USDHHS, 2000). Hispanic women are experiencing increasing incidences of lung and breast cancer and have the highest rates of cervical cancer (USDHHS, 2000). Colorectal cancer deaths, the third leading overall cancer death cause, are higher in black women, indicating a need for earlier detection. Rates of ovarian cancer deaths are increasing in women 65 and older, but decreasing in younger women, a change thought to be due to oral contraceptive use (Oriel, Hartenbach, & Remington, 1999).

Lung cancer is higher among whites and in the northern states. The highest incidences of selected cancers in women in 1997 were as follows: cervical—blacks and Hispanics; uterine and ovarian—white non-Hispanics and whites; stomach—Asian/Pacific Islanders; pancreatic—blacks; urinary bladder—white non-Hispanics; and non-Hodgkin's lymphoma and leukemia—white non-Hispanics, blacks, and whites (Eberhardt et al., 2001). Endometrial, cervical, and ovarian cancers kill about 25,000 American women annually (Fontaine, 1998).

HIV/AIDS

HIV death rates quadrupled between 1985 and 1994, becoming the sixth leading cause of death for U.S. women (Horton, 1995). However, HIV practically disappeared by 1999 in the top ten causes of death for women, being tenth for black women only (Tables 4–4 and 4–5; Eberhardt et al., 2001). Black women have an HIV death rate more than four times that of the second highest group, Hispanic women. The high disparities in rates of HIV infection among African American and Hispanic populations are related to cultural, socioeconomic, and high-risk behavior factors (USDHHS, 2000). In 1998, women comprised 20 percent of people over 13 living with AIDS, compared to 13 percent in 1992.

Heart Diseases

Heart diseases are the leading causes of death in U.S. women. They rank first for all races and ethnicities except for Asian/Pacific Islanders (National Women's Health Information Center [NWHIC], 2000). Coronary heart disease (CHD) is the major cause of heart disease deaths, and high blood cholesterol, a modifiable feature, is the most significant risk factor (USDHHS, 2000). The other major risk factors are smoking and hypertension, and strangely, though smoking has decreased in men and increased in women over the last three decades and lung cancer has increased in women, a sex difference based on smoking has not been found for CHD (Lawlor, Ebrahim, & Smith, 2001). Cerebrovascular disease, which includes the major type, stroke, is the third leading cause of death in U.S. women (USDHHS, 2000), but in women 85 and older, it is second (Desai, Zhang, & Hennessy, 1999b). Hypertension, one of the main risk factors for stroke, CHD, and heart failure, is often "silent" until too late (USDHHS, 2000). It is suggested that as the number of people live longer and survive a heart attack, atrial fibrillation will become more prominent as a disease. Heart disease is responsible for nearly 25 percent of hospital discharges among older adults (Desai, Zhang, & Hennessy, 1999b). Now it is seen more in elderly women because they live longer, not that there are proportionately more cases in elderly women than men (USDHHS, 2000). African American (AA) women have the greatest cardiovascular risk, two to three times that of Asian/Pacific Island women (Cooper, 2001). A study comparing AA, Asian Indian American (AIA), and Caucasian U.S. women found that AA and AIA women 30 years of age or older had more lifestyle, dietary, hemodynamic, anthropometric, and laboratory identified risk factors than Caucasians, including higher apolipoprotein A-1, lipoprotein (a)(Lp(a)), fibrinogen, and fasting insulin levels in AA women, and higher Lp(a) and fibrinogen levels in AIA women (Palaniappan, Anthony, et al., 2002). Many lifestyle factors were modifiable, such as eating too much fat in the diets and being sedentary. Smoking only four or fewer cigarettes per day increases the risk of myocardial infarction by two times. Better screening for and managing diabetes, hypertension, smoking, overweight, inactivity, and high cholesterol can significantly improve the one in every three women's risk for coronary heart disease (USDHHS, 2000). Obesity is now one of the major preventive health dilemmas in the United States. As obesity and overweight grow as public health problems, efforts to begin in childhood to change the trajectory become critical.

LEADING CAUSES OF MORBIDITY IN U.S. WOMEN

Conditions Requiring Emergency Department (ED) or Hospital Visits

Visits for injuries to hospital emergency departments (ED) increased for all women between 1995–1996 and 1998–1999 (Eberhardt et al., 2001, Table 84). Falls led the list in 1999 as the major cause of unintentional injuries for all ages, except 18- to 24-year-old women, and leaped upward dramatically in the 65 and over age group. Motor vehicle accidents were the major reason for ED visits for those ages 18 to 24 and were the second major reason in all other age groups. Intentional injuries were highest in the 25- to 44-year-old age group. Major diagnoses for hospital stays in 1999 were for pneumonia; injuries and poisoning in females 18 and under; delivery, serious mental illness, and injuries and poisoning for 18- to 44-year-olds; heart disease, cancer, injuries and poisoning, and pneumonia for 45- to 64-year-olds; heart disease, injuries and poisoning, and cancer for women ages 65 to 74. Women 75 and over were discharged primarily with diagnoses of heart disease, injuries and poisonings (fractures predominantly), pneumonia, and cerebrovascular diseases (Eberhardt et al., Table 93).

Chronic Conditions

In women under 45 years old, chronic sinusitis and hay fever and allergic rhinitis without asthma are leading causes of chronic conditions (U.S. Bureau of the Census, 2000b). Women 45 years and older suffer primarily from arthritis and hypertension. By age 65, heart conditions become a cause of major chronic disease, and after 74, hearing and vision impairments are significant problems. Arthritis affects approximately 1.5 million women in the United States, about 71 percent of all those who suffer with this major debilitating disease (NWHIC, 2000). Rheumatoid arthritis, osteoarthritis, osteoporosis, and chronic back conditions "have the greatest impact on public health and quality of life" (USDHHS, 2000). Heart disease is the number one cause of work disability; arthritis is second. However, arthritis involves severe pain that alters the quality of life and mental health. By 2020, it is estimated that 18 percent of all Americans will develop arthritis. It is the leading chronic condition in whites and greatly affects African Americans, Hispanics, American Indians, and Alaskan Natives as a leading cause of activity limitation. After age 50, up to 18 percent of women currently have osteoporosis, with its major complications from fractures, especially of the hip (USDHHS, 2000). Twenty-four percent of persons 50 and older with hip fractures die within the next year. Greater functional disability results from hip fracture than from MI, stroke, and cancer (USDHHS, 2000). African Americans, American Indians, and Alaska Natives have a greater incidence of kidney disease than whites or Asians, with some of the disproportionate effect explained by higher numbers of these races with hypertension and diabetes (USDHHS, 2000). Fewer women than men are affected, but as obesity and diabetes type 2 increase in women, more kidney disease will be seen. Type 2 diabetes, increasing rampantly in the United States, occurs less frequently in women than men. However, any increase leads to more coronary heart disease, blindness, and renal disease (USDHHS, 2000). Those groups most at risk are African Americans, Hispanics, American Indians, and Alaska Natives, Asian/Pacific Islanders, older (over 60), and the poor. The increase of obesity, poor nutrition, and sedentary lifestyle contributes significantly to chronic illness. Other chronic serious diseases that occur most often in women are autoimmune diseases, systemic lupus erythematosus, multiple sclerosis, scleroderma, Hashimoto's thyroiditis, Graves' disease, Alzheimer's disease, urinary incontinence, major depression, dysthymia, and anxiety disorders (NWHIC, 2000). Hypertension increases steadily in U.S. women as they age, and is significantly higher in black and Hispanic women (Eberhardt et al., 2001, Table 67).

LEADING RISK FACTORS FOR WOMEN

An overall evaluation of risk factors should include assessment of the following behaviors.

Unsafe Lifestyle Behaviors

Such behaviors are related to personal choices and are amenable to change in most instances.

- **Cigarette smoking** continues to be the "single most preventable cause of disease and death" in this country (USDHHS, 2000). Smoking is associated with many diseases, including lung cancer and chronic respiratory diseases; heart diseases; cerebrovascular and peripheral vascular diseases; cancers of the cervix, larynx, oral cavity, pharynx and esophagus, bladder, kidney, and pancreas; peptic ulcer disease; increased cataracts; deaths by fire; lowered estrogen levels and early menopause; rapid skin aging and wrinkling; and secondhand smoke risk (USDHHS, 2000). Nonsmokers are at greater risk from secondhand smoke for heart disease than smokers (Glantz & Parmley, 1995). Secondhand smoke causes about 3,000 cancer deaths annually and increases children's risk of serious respiratory and middle ear infections (Rigotti & Polivogianis, 1995). (Also see Exposure to Environmental Hazards: Unsafe home environment.) Although women's rates of smoking have dropped significantly since they peaked in 1965, 21.6 percent of adult women smoked in 1999 (Eberhardt et al., 2001, Table 60). Women ages 35 to 44 had the highest number of smokers, 26.5 percent, with 18- to 24-year-olds close behind at 26.3 percent. Black women 35 to 44 years old and white females 18 to 24 years old had the highest percentage of smokers, and those with a bachelor's degree or higher smoked the least (Eberhardt, et al., 2001, Table 61). Overall, it is estimated that nearly 30 percent of American Indian and Alaska Native women, nearly 24 percent of non-Hispanic white women, 22 percent of non-Hispanic black women, nearly 14 percent of Hispanic women, and about 12 percent of Asian/Pacific Islander women smoke (National Women's Health, 2000). In the 1990s, the number of adolescent women smokers increased to 34.9 percent in 1999; many started to smoke to prevent gaining weight (National Women's Health, 2000). However, 2001 data from the Centers for Disease Control (CDC) showed a significant drop in U.S. high school students who smoked as compared with five years ago (now 28.5%, then 36.4%) (McClam, 2002a). Boys were more likely to smoke as compared to girls, 29.2 percent to 27.7 percent. White and Hispanic students were more likely to smoke. Smoking is associated with premature births, mental retardation, miscarriage, and low birth weight in infants, yet 17 percent of pregnant women 15 to 44 years of age smoke. The number of low birth weight infants was nearly two times higher in smokers than nonsmokers in 1999 (Eberhardt, et al., 2001, Table 12). Factors associated with smoking in women include higher body mass index, longer prior attempts to stop smoking, greater dependence on nicotine, lower education, lower exercise patterns, stress, and depressive symptoms (Borrelli, Hogan, et al., 2002; Ludman, Curry, et al., 2002; Tseng, Yeatts, Millikan, & Newman, 2001). Assessment should include what the woman smokes, the number smoked per day, the number of years she has smoked, ill effects, and others in the household who smoke or are affected.

◆ **Substance use/abuse** includes alcohol, nicotine, caffeine, heroin, cocaine, marijuana, tranquilizers, inhalants, and most recently, a designer drug called Ecstacy. Use of Ecstacy, a hallucinogenic amphetamine, can cause serious acute effects such as seizures and myocardial infarction and long-term destruction of nerve endings that produce serotonin that later regrow abnormally (Hess & DeBoer, 2002). Twenty to 25 percent of patients seen in primary care settings have alcohol-abuse problems. Accompanying diagnoses of sexual abuse, mental health disorders such as phobias, eating disorders, and posttraumatic stress disorder are often seen in women with alcohol use issues (Becker & Walton-Moss, 2001). Women have been found to use alcohol and drugs more than men, but do not receive counseling as often as men (Roeloffs, Fink, et al., 2001). More than 13 million people, 17 percent of those who drink alcohol, are alcohol dependent or abusers (USDHHS, 2000). Those who begin drinking as young adolescents, 14 and under, are at significant risk for alcohol dependency. A family history of alcoholism predisposes to this disease. Breast cancer risk is increased if a woman drinks only two drinks daily, and long-term and/or heavy use increases risks for hypertension, arrhythmias, cardiomyopathy, stroke, cirrhosis, liver disease, and cancer of the esophagus, mouth, throat, and larynx, as well as deaths from homicide, suicide, high-risk sexual behavior, and motor vehicle accidents (USDHHS, 2000). Alcohol is involved in two-thirds of violent situations where the perpetrator is someone intimate to the victim (USDHHS, 2000). It is imperative to screen for alcohol abuse, particularly in women who could bear children, since fetal alcohol syndrome is a leading cause of birth defects (Enoch & Goldman, 2002).

The most commonly used illicit drug is marijuana, and it is associated with illegal and dangerous behaviors by adolescent users (USDHHS, 2000). The most chronically abused drug is cocaine, and relapse into drug use for any chronic drug user is common (USDHHS, 2000). STD and HIV/AIDS, tuberculo-

sis, strokes, heart failure, heart arrhythmias, convulsions, mental health disorders, and memory defects are associated with illicit drug use.

Whites are more likely to use alcohol, tobacco, and illicit drugs that any other race. In adolescents, substance abuse and dependence were associated with a history of physical or sexual assault, witnessing violence, a family history of alcohol or drug use, posttraumatic stress disorder, and Caucasian, Hispanic, or Native American race/ethnicity (Kilpatrick, Acierno, et al., 2000). Women substance abusers are more likely to be successful with treatment if they have personal and social resources such as education, job abilities, and past employment histories (Kelly, Blacksin, & Mason, 2001). The average first age for alcohol use in U.S. women in 1997 was 13.4 years; for marijuana use, 14.0 years (USDHHS, 2000). Half of high school female seniors had used an illicit drug in 1998, and 81 percent had used alcohol. Women, particularly older women, require less alcohol to become intoxicated because they have less body water. Women with disabilities have a higher risk of illicit drug use associated with lower self-esteem, peer pressure, and other factors that influence use (Li & Ford, 1998). Women are treated significantly more often than men with drugs that have abuse potential (Simoni-Wastila, 2000).

◆ **Overuse of any medication or supplement** may occur when clients fail to read warnings or are not cautioned about the excessive use of legal drugs, such as gastric mucosal irritation with non-steroidal anti-inflammatory drugs (NSAID). Neurological abnormalities with excessive vitamin B_6 ingestion is another example. Assess the type of drug or substance, amount used, years of use, and effects.

◆ **Sedentary lifestyle and lack of exercise and personal fitness** are associated with a shorter life span, more dependence on others for activities of daily living, and poorer quality of life (USDHHS, 2000). Diseases/conditions associated with lack of physical activity include hypertension, diabetes, heart disease, colon cancer, lower back problems, breast cancer, osteoporosis, and arthritis. The highest percentages of less or no-leisure activity are found in women, African Americans and Hispanics; the older adult; those with less education and funds; those with disabilities; and people living in the northeastern and southern states. The biggest decrease in physical activity occurs most significantly in girls by grade 12. Girls participate less in team sports but more in dance and aerobics. Self-esteem and strength influence physical activity participation. Only 30 percent of women in the U.S. spent 20 minutes in physical activity three or more days per week in 1997 (USD-HHS, 2000). Data collected from interviews with 68,000 U.S. adults in 1997 and 1998 by the National Center for Health Statistics and published April 7, 2002, found that most adults (7 of 10) do not exercise regularly, 4 of the 7 not at all, and only 3 of 10 adults are physically active for 30 minutes 5 times a week doing moderate exercise, or 20 minutes 3 times a week performing vigorous exercise, either of which is considered being regularly physically active (Mc-Clam, 2002). Factors associated with being more physically active were earning four times the poverty level or more, being better educated, being married, and being white.

◆ **Nutritional excesses and deficits** are associated with many serious and potentially lethal conditions such as obesity, coronary heart disease, some cancers, stroke, type 2 diabetes, and osteoporosis (USD-HHS, 2000). The cost in the U.S. is over $200 billion annually. Eating disorders, such as binging, purging, and anorexia, occur primarily in younger women (American Psychiatric, 2000). Underweight women report having had more stress during mealtime communications with their families, while overweight women report more effects from emphasis by their families on appearance and weight control (Worobey, 2002). Women who have an eating disorder have a significant relationship between thinking that their appearance will help them get dates and their self-esteem as compared to women who do not have an eating disorder (Mendelson, McLaren, Gauvin, & Steiger, 2002). Binging and purging in both male and female adolescents is associated with a significantly higher risk of having been physically or sexually abused (Ackard et al., 2001; Grilo & Masheb, 2001). Mexican American college women from family backgrounds of greater rigidity and who had poor peer socialization were found to be at a greater risk for bulimia and preoccupation with body size and slimness (Kuba & Harris, 2001). Over-concern and eating disturbances partially explain the current increase in depression being seen in adolescent girls (Stice & Bearman, 2001). More Americans than ever are overweight or obese, and these conditions are associated with a greater risk of hypertension, abnormal lipid levels, Type 2 diabetes, cardiovascular and cerebrovascular diseases; cancers of the endometrium, breast, prostate, and colon; gallbladder disease; breathing disorders and sleep disturbances; and arthritis (Field et al., 2001; USDHHS, 2000). Between 1960 and 1994, the incidence of obesity in U.S. women rose from 15.7 percent of the population to 26.0 percent (Eberhardt, Ingram, & Makuc, 2001, Table 69). The greatest rises have been in black, and Hispanic women, with 39.0, and 36.1 percent incidences in their respective populations. Findings from the Nurses Study indicated that significant deaths were associated with being overweight (Mason, Willett, & Stampfer, 1995). Almost a third of cancer deaths were attributed to being overweight. Women of average weight by today's standards and those mildly overweight had death rates higher than lean women. The average American woman was found to be 5 feet 5 inches tall and weighed 150–160 pounds. This weight was found to be about 30 pounds too high and associated with a significant risk of cardiovascular and cancer deaths. Health is associated with eating a balanced diet that provides adequate sources of vitamins and minerals with adequate protein, complex carbohydrates, vegetables, fruits, low fat (especially saturated fat and cholesterol), moderate salt and sugar, and moderate alcohol if it is consumed (USDHHS, 2000; American Dietetic Association, 2001). A study that looked at diet quality using the health eating index (HEI), food consumption patterns, and body mass index (BMI) found that BMIs were lowest among women who ate vegetarian diets or high carbohydrate/low fat diets, and these diets provided the lowest energy intakes (Kennedy et al., 2001). The highest quality diets were high complex carbohydrate. Eating out usually provides diets with higher fat and sodium and lower grains, vegetables, and fruits, at a cost about 40 percent higher than if meals were taken at home (USDHHS, 2000). The American Cancer Society guidelines for diet to decrease cancer morbidity and mortality parallel those of the American Heart Association to prevent heart disease (Byers et al., 2002). One example of how diet influences risk and progression of disease is with osteoarthritis. Not only does diet affect weight, which, if excessive, can significantly increase risk of injury and pain with osteoarthritis, but vitamins C, E, and D have been shown to be beneficial in slowing the progression of this disease (McAlindon, 2000). Childbearing-age women need folic acid and adequate iron, and all women, especially those past menopause, need adequate calcium and vitamin D. The American Dietetic Association emphasizes total diet, not one food or another, the importance of moderation, balance in the diet, to get all needed nutrients from food, and physical activity (Freeland-Graves & Nitzke, 2002). Older U.S. women, in a study to compare diets of healthy seniors living at home with recommended guidelines, ate recommended vegetable and fruit servings more often than men, fewer grain and protein servings than men, fewer vitamins D, E, B9, and calcium from the diet than needed, and less dairy than needed (Foote, Giuliano, & Harris, 2000). It is essential that older women consume foods and/or supplements providing adequate calcium, vitamin D, and protein along with exercise to help prevent osteoporosis or further bone loss if present. Because changing eating habits is tied to so many factors—sociocultural, psychological, environmental, physiological, and genetic—assessment must focus on all these parameters to offer assistance for change to individuals and families (USDHHS, 2000). The change must begin with families and children, and include regular physical activity regimens.

- **Unsafe automobile driving,** inattention to precautions, and lapses in driving safety are associated with a high level of morbidity and mortality for women up to age 64, especially young women. The greatest number of deaths from motor vehicle accidents are in the 15 to 24 and 65 and over age groups respectively (Eberhardt et al., 2001). Older women are more likely to die if injured in a motor vehicle accident than younger women, due to increased vulnerability to serious complications. Substance abuse, nonuse of protective devices (seatbelts), and reckless driving need to be assessed. Safety cautions should be integrated into the history routinely.

- **Violence.** Women are significantly more likely to be the victims of physical assault as well as sexual assault and rape (USDHHS, 2000). The lifetime prevalence for women to be violently attacked is more than four of every ten women; intimate partner violence accounts for 34.6 percent, rape, 20.4 percent, physical assault, 19.1 percent, and child abuse, 17.8 percent (Plichta & Falik, 2001). Up to 30 percent of U.S. women are domestic abuse victims (Moore, Zaccaro, & Parsons, 1998). More than one-third of women seen in emergency rooms of hospitals for violence-related injuries were victims of their intimate

partners. The husband, ex-husband, or boyfriend in 1995 data was the murderer in almost 50 percent of 5,000 cases of murdered women (USDHHS, 2000). Data indicate that rape, attempted rape, and sexual assault are much higher than actually reported (USDHHS, 2000). The National Women's Study estimated that 0.7 percent of adult women had been raped by force in the prior year (Kilpatrick, Edmunds, & Seymour, 1992). African American women age 12 and older are at greatest risk of rape, and Hispanic women 12 and older are at greatest risk of sexual assault. A national study of more than 3,000 women identified risk factors for rape and physical assault separately (Acierno, Resnick, Kilpatrick, Saunders, & Best, 1999). Findings showed that having been a past victim, being young, and current posttraumatic stress disorder were associated with an increased risk to be raped. The increased risk of physical assault was associated with a past history of being a victim, minority status, current active depression, and drug use. A study of 2,109 North Carolina women found that perception of health as fair or poor, past history of ill health or mental health problems in the last month, and a history of poor mental health were associated with sexual assault (Cloutier, Martin, & Poole, 2002). These women were more likely to be cigarette smokers, hypertensive, obese, and have hyperlipidemia. The authors urged screening for sexual assault in all settings to institute interventions to help victims cope. Assessment should include asking about dangerous, conflictual relationships and living conditions such as violent families and neighborhoods.

Date rape and the victimization of young women who are drugged before being assaulted are growing concerns. Teens in one study were more likely than adults to suffer the assault during the day, in a residence, to know the assailant, and to receive medical follow-up; less likely to be injured, to have a weapon used in the assault, and to have rape-centered counseling (Strickland, 2001). In a study of 617 African and Mexican American women who had been sexually abused, a higher risk existed for earlier intercourse, multiple sex partners, recurrent STDs, PID, and delay in health-seeking behaviors (Champion, Piper, et al., 2001). Both heterosexual and lesbian women experience sexual assault, however, one study found that childhood sexual assault was more common in lesbians (Hughes, Johnson, & Wilsnack, 2001).

Alcohol abuse for their entire lives was associated with having been abused sexually as children in both groups of women. Adult sexual assault and adult alcohol abuse were associated in heterosexual women.

Reports of abuse in pregnancy are as high as 60 percent with 25 percent being teens (Anderson, 2002). The most common time for pregnant women to present to the emergency room is between weeks 20 and 40, and nurses are ideally suited to identify these women. Only 23 percent of 77 percent of women who had been abused postpartally had medical care (Martin, Mackie, et al., 2001). Greater incidences of substance abuse and psychological stress are associated with abuse in pregnancy (Curry, 1998).

Pediatric providers are important sources through which to identify abused mothers. Sixteen percent of mothers visiting a pediatric practice had been physically abused by a partner at some time in their lives, and 10 percent reported a gun in the household (Parkerson, Adams, & Emerling, 2001).

The incidence of elder abuse based on substantiated cases in the United States was 2.7 per 1,000 population in a 1996 study (Hajjar & Duthie, 2001). Factors that geriatricians have identified that help in assessing for elder abuse include having a good rapport with the client; evidence that the client is not adhering to the medical regimen or not being involved in social activities; and finding physical evidence, most commonly bruises, traumatic injuries, poor general appearance and hygiene, malnutrition, and dehydration (Harrell, Toronjo, et al., 2002). In older women, sexual assault was associated with an increased risk of arthritis and breast cancer, and a history of multiple sexual assaults increased the risk by two- to threefold (Stein & Barrett-Connor, 2000).

◆ **Exposure to HIV, hepatitis, and sexually transmitted diseases (STDs)** may cause life-threatening, incurable, or disabling conditions (see Chapters 11 and 12). Nearly four million of the estimated 15 million new cases of STDs that occur annually are in teens (USDHHS, 2000). Many of the same characteristics that put women at risk for HIV also put them at risk for non-HIV STDs. A study of sexual behaviors of inner-city adolescent women considered to be at high risk for STDs found that the choice of the partner and the partner's risk behavior were more significant factors for risk to the woman than her own high-risk behavior (Katz, Fortenberry, et al., 2001). In addi-

tion, young women may use fewer protective measures, putting themselves at greater risk for STDs and HIV (Hutchinson, Sosa, & Thompson, 2001). Nonoxynol-9 gel is not recommended as a preventive since it has been found to be associated with a greater risk of some STDs (Richardson, Lavreys, et al., 2001). Less self-efficacy, self-esteem, knowledge about sexual issues, and ability to communicate are associated with higher risk (Raphan, Cohen, & Boyer, 2001). Women who are poor, African American, or Hispanic are at the greatest risk for STDs and HIV infections, supporting the need to expand access to assessment and to education for prevention (Aral, 2001; USDHHS, 2000). Women's complications of STDs—PID, HPV, cervical malignancy, ectopic pregnancy, infertility, chronic pelvic pain—are far more serious than those of men. Women whose only sexual partners are women are still at risk for STDs and should be tested (Bauer & Welles, 2001). Assessment should include questions about the frequency of sexual contacts, the number of partners currently and in the past, the risk status of partners, forms of sexual expression, type of contraception and/or barrier/chemical methods of protection. Perception of risk should be assessed; it may be significantly different from real risk.

◆ **Lack of health-directed behaviors, or poor personal care,** is associated with a substandard health status and inadequate detection and prevention behaviors, such as immunization status, and use of contraception. Personal assessment should include breast self-exam, regular dental and eye exams, general screening physical and diagnostic exams including pelvic and rectal exams, cervical cytology and indicated cultures/tests, occult fecal blood testing, mammography, and vulvar self-exam. Demographic characteristics related to underuse of screening services in one study included such factors as being single, divorced, or widowed; an educational level less than high school; older age (over 65); living in specific parts of the country, for example, women from the Northeast or South were less likely to have had a clinical breast exam in the last year (What's happening, 1996). Providers must ask about health-directed behaviors, including immunizations.

◆ **Inadequate, excessive, or unusual sleep.** About 33 percent of all Americans in a national sleep survey had occasional insomnia, and 9 percent had nightly problems (Ancoli-Israel & Roth, 1999). Most do not seek medical help, and 40 percent self-medicate with alcohol or over-the-counter drugs. Most frequently, people complained of waking tired and drowsy in the morning. Consequences were impaired memory and concentration, decreased enjoyment of interpersonal relationships, as well as inability to complete daily duties (Roth & Ancoli-Israel, 1999). A managed care enrollees survey yielding 3,447 responses found that 46 percent of respondents had either difficulty initiating sleep, maintaining sleep, or daytime dysfunction from lack of sleep (Hatoum, Kania, et al., 1998). Decreased education, less income, increased age, female gender, non-Caucasian race, and many co-morbidities were associated with daytime dysfunction from insomnia. A complaint of insomnia necessitates further assessment for underlying medical and psychiatric disorders as well as sleep disorders (Roth, 2000). Young women attending a rural U.S. college in the south had more sleep problems than the men, and most of the students reported some sleep disturbance (Buboltz, Brown, & Soper, 2001). Sleep disturbances are commonly reported in women going through menopause, after hysterectomy, with aging, and with depression and stress. Assessment should include evaluation of duration and quality of sleep, breathing difficulties, snoring, smoking, neuroses, alcohol use, medication use, estrogen decline, time zone or job shift changes, sleepwalking, stress and depression, heavy exercise near bedtime, environmental conditions for sleep, and dozing off during the day. People who are natural short sleepers do not need catch-up sleep or alarms. A serious concern with chronic insomnia is the increased likelihood of accidents secondary to fatigue.

Exposure to Environmental Hazards

Unsafe conditions may be found in the home or work environment.

- **Unsafe home environment** encompasses falls, exposure to chemical/toxic/radon hazards, fire, excessive heat or cold, unsanitary living conditions, unsafe drinking water, lack of running water, rodent or insect infestation, airborne pollutants, and infections among people living in crowded conditions. People spend 90 percent of their time indoors where higher levels of allergens and pollutants are found (USDHHS, 2000). Dust mites, cockroaches, pets, mold,

and rodents contribute to indoor allergens and the development of respiratory diseases at home and at work. More than 36 million homes in 1998–1999 exceeded the dust mite allergen levels of the government (USDHHS, 2000). In the 65 and older age group, falls account for 87 percent of all fractures and cause spinal cord injury and brain injury second only to motor vehicle accidents (USDHHS, 2000). From 1998 to 1999, there were 672 visits per 10,000 persons to U.S. hospital emergency rooms for this age group as compared to a third or less visits by younger age groups. Risks factors for falls in the homes must be assessed, such as throw rugs, poor lighting, unstable railings, and unsafe tub access.

- **Unsafe occupational situations** are associated with life threatening, damaging, or debilitating conditions (also see unsafe home environment information). Increased fetal risks when the pregnant mother is exposed to pesticides in her job in the agricultural industry are suggested from the literature (Arbuckle & Sever, 1998). Working in adverse conditions (prolonged standing or walking, shift work, heavy lifting) or where one is exposed to hazardous substances (radiation, chemicals, solvents, gases, and antineoplastic drugs) are associated with an increase in spontaneous abortions, preterm births, and low birth weight infants, calling for the provider to take a detailed workplace history (Gabbe & Turner, 1997; Gold & Tomich, 1994). Military women exposed to heavy metals, pesticides, petroleum products, and chemicals have a greater risk of abnormal pregnancy outcomes (Hourani & Hilton, 2000). Job strain (work with high demands and low control) was found to cause lower birth weights, particularly among black women (Oths, Dunn, & Palmer, 2001). Exposure to environmental tobacco smoke is associated with increased risk of hay fever, asthma, hearing loss, cold/flu symptoms, and heart disease in women (Iribarren, Friedman, Klatsky, & Eisner, 2001). As people age, an increased sensitivity to exposure to hazardous substances may put them at greater risk to develop illness than when they were younger (Richardson & Wing, 1998). Assessment should include the individual's type of work, work hazards and conditions, and effects. Biological, chemical, environmental-mechanical, physical, and psychosocial hazards should be assessed (see Screening Methods, Special Assessment Guides in this chapter and Chapters 16 and 17 on pregnancy). Providers should

be familiar with their local, state, and national resources such as the local poison control center hotline and Occupational Safety and Health Administration (OSHA).

Negative Influences on Emotional Health

Such influences vary widely from family crises to unrealistic values of thinness.

- **Stress** is associated with a wide array of physical and
  emotional problems. Women raising children and living in a poor, urban city community described stressors as finances, work, family, safety, police, and
  municipal services; depression was significantly associated with finances, police, and safety stress and
  unfair treatment factors (Schulz, Parker, Israel, &
  Fisher, 2001). Researchers at the University of California found that women do not employ the "fight-
  or-flight" response to stress as would men, but rather,
  "tend-and-befriend" to protect their children, establishing a social support system that may help defend
  them (Taylor, Klein, et al., 2000). Women ages 44 to
  55 years from five ethnic groups were asked about
  physical-functional limitations (Pope, Sowers, Welch,
  & Albrecht, 2001). High levels of stress were associated with such limitations, also seen with older
  women. Older women and blacks used prayer to cope
  with stress more often than whites or men (Dunn &
  Horgas, 2000). Women with metastatic breast cancer
  who reported greater spirituality (attended religious
  services more frequently and reported a greater importance of religious or spiritual expression) had
  greater helper and cytotoxic T-cell counts than those
  with lower levels of spirituality (Sephton, Koopman,
  Schaal, Thoresen, & Spiegel, 2001). Assessment includes stressors related to work, home, family, and
  other relationships. One researcher, Lazarus, has
  more closely linked the effects of hassles (the little
  irritating or distressing occurrences that happen
  daily) rather than major life events to emotional
  health (Lazarus, 1981). Stress can affect the person
  physically (reduced immune responses, increased
  risk of cardiovascular, reproductive, and gastrointestinal conditions) and mentally (posttraumatic
  stress syndrome, neuroses, and transient situational
  disturbances). With the September 11, 2001, act of
  terrorism against the United States, a more global
  stressor is affecting women and children. Effects of
  this ongoing stress will be seen in the months and

years to come and should be considered in assessing
stress factors affecting women.

- **Family crises** mean increased physical and emotional risks for both the individual and the family.
  Assessment includes family health, values, health
  care beliefs, cultural influences, and coping abilities,
  as evidenced by past coping with crises, individual
  and family. Such crises include a wide array of problems such as death, serious illness, divorce, loss of a
  job, loss of a home, moving, or substance abuse of a
  member.
- **A poor or absent support system** is associated with
  feelings of loneliness, helplessness, hopelessness,
  and powerlessness. Social support appears to be related to better health and feelings of well-being (Pender, 1996). Social networks are known to decrease
  health risks associated with occupational stress, cancer, and pregnancy (Auslander, 1988). Assessment of
  supports should include determining recent changes
  in life (e.g., marriage, divorce, birth, change of residence, change of job); distance from friends, relatives, cultural group, health resources; and access to
  support systems, such as church. Race and ethnic
  differences must be considered in evaluating
  women's support systems. (Silverstein & Waite,
  1993). In a study that examined social support as a
  predictor of health-related quality of life in chronic
  heart failure patients, changes in social support significantly predicted changes in health-related quality
  of life (Bennett, Perkins, et al., 2001).
- **Depression and other mood disorders** are common
  psychiatric illnesses in women (see Chapter 23, Depression). One in five U.S. women will be clinically
  depressed at some time in her life (Dietch, 2002), and
  twice as many women as men become depressed
  (Cyranowski, Frank, Young, & Shear, 2000). Depression, the most common U.S. mental illness, causes
  more disability than any other illness and two-thirds
  of suicides (USDHHS, 2000). The National Institute
  of Mental Health has labeled depression "the invisible disease," indicating that providers must be alert
  to recognizing and treating this deadly disease
  (Dietch, 2000). Poor women, women on welfare, minority women, and those who are less educated and
  unemployed have a greater risk for depression (USD-
  HHS, 2000). Eighteen to 44-year-olds are most affected. The childbearing years and the hormone level
  fluctuations are often associated with more stress and
  mental illness than any other period in women's lives

(Dietch, 2002). Depression following childbirth affects one in every ten women (Redmond, 2000). Older adults with medical conditions have higher incidences of depression; rates for nursing home dwellers are 15 to 25 percent (USDHHS, 2000). Women often experience depression during the menopause transition attributed to the interaction between vasomotor symptoms, changing hormone levels, and sleep problems (Avis, Crawford, Stellato, & Longcope, 2001). Assessment requires recognizing that five or more signs and symptoms that cluster and persist daily for prolonged periods—weeks to years—are the red flag (American Psychiatric Association, 2000). These signs include changes in mood, sleep patterns, weight, activity level, energy level; decreased motivation, interest in life, sex drive, concentration and memory, and self-esteem/self-worth; and suicidal ideation (Dietch, 2000). A family history of mental disorders is also a warning sign.

- **Unrealistic values** of youth, beauty, and thinness lead to unhealthy, excessive concerns and behaviors related to appearance. These concerns may also indicate an inability to accept the aging process. Assessment includes appearance, age, weight, height, history of unusual or overuse of plastic/reparative surgery, diet and exercise history, any verbal and nonverbal cues, such as great concern with being overweight when in reality one is underweight (see nutrition excesses and deficits in this chapter and Chapter 23, Eating Disorders). Much of the emphasis on attractiveness, weight loss, and fitness has come from the media, focusing on the positives of being thin to the extent that good nutrition and health may be jeopardized (Guillen & Barr, 1994). Adolescents and young adult women reap the fallout of this negative campaign to make money by the larger business world.

- **Lack of recreational and relaxation activities** can cause stress, overwork, anxiety, and in some instances depression. Assessment includes financial, social, physical, and psychological conditions and barriers. Relaxation takes planning and considered time to break from life's usual pressures and competitions.

Poverty, Insufficient Insurance, and Inadequate Material Resources

Women and children (including adolescents) are the fastest growing segment of those living in poverty. For the year 2000, the poverty line, said to be unrealistically low, was $17,436 for a family of four (KIDS COUNT Census, 2002). Being poor is no longer a problem only for welfare recipients. The consistent decrease in the value of low-skilled labor is inversely related to the increasing number of children in working poor families, according to the survey's executive director. Two factors contribute to the working poor being more disadvantaged than welfare recipients: more working poor are without health insurance and less time can be spent with children by the working poor. Poor people often delay seeking health care when ill, use fewer measures to prevent or alleviate illness, have less accurate information about health, and have fewer choices for access to health care. As significant changes in the welfare system occur, more consequences for the working poor will be seen.

As women age, a greater chance for poverty exists. Lower income is associated with greater risk of heart disease, diabetes, and obesity (USDHHS, 2000). Gains in health that have occurred with those in higher income brackets are not mirrored in lower income groups. Lowest income families have three times the limitation in activities from chronic diseases of higher income people. Women who have children at home have a higher risk for depression if unemployed (Danziger, Carlson, & Henly, 2001). Being without a job or being in a low-paying job is associated with depression and a feeling of hopelessness whether the woman is receiving welfare or not (Petterson & Friel, 2001). Single women who are off welfare, but who have health limitations and are mothers of children with health limitations, have a very high risk of losing their jobs (Earle & Heymann, 2002). U.S. women, their children, and families who are poor are at much greater risk of not receiving adequate health care in the years to come as public services for health care decline and privately funded systems grow (Akukwe, 2000). Disparities in health for minorities is significantly determined by socioeconomic factors as well as medical care, geographical location, culture, and migration (Williams, 2002). African American women are excessively prone to chronic illness and disability, regardless of their socioeconomic status, and the reason is proposed to be early health insults and subsequent deterioration, called "the weathering concept" (Geronimus, 2001). Hispanics, especially if young, uninsured, and with fewer than twelve years of education, are less likely to have a usual source of health care, and Hispanics—especially Mexican Americans—have a particularly high rate of uninsured (USDHHS, 2000). Receiving adequate prenatal care is stratified by race/ethnicity, with Mexican American and African American women at greatest risk for receiving inadequate prenatal care (Frisbie, Echevarria, & Hummer, 2001). Williams and Lawler (2001) found that stress and physical illness are linked in low-income women, but that hardiness and being African American buffered these effects. Divorced women who have not been married at least ten years are predicted to be the most impoverished of all women in this marital category in the future as more women become divorced after shorter marriages (Butrica & Iams, 2000).

Hereditary, Cultural, and Ethnic Influences

Family history and culture impact health.

- **Familial diseases** may be detected by assessing family history. Diabetes, breast cancer, colorectal cancer, ovarian cancer, diabetes, heart disease, asthma, and allergies are examples of disease risks inherited from family members. Significant health problems can be prevented or minimized by careful attention to risk factors and management of lifestyle, environmental, and other conditions.
- **Race** is another consideration. According to *Healthy People 2000,* even though a disparate number of minority people die from disease—and much of this disparity can be attributed to socioeconomic factors—a part of the difference cannot be explained by poverty factors alone (Healthy People, 2000). Race plays a role. Some diseases are more common among people of certain races; for example, osteoporosis is more prevalent in light- or yellow-skinned women; sickle cell disease is found in African Americans; and glucose-6-phosphate dehydrogenase (G-6-PD) deficiency occurs more often in people of Mediterranean descent. In many American Indian tribes, diabetes affects more than 20 percent of the members.
- **Ethnic, cultural, and religious influences** may be associated with unhealthy practices: eating uncooked meat, refusing to see a health care provider, lacking health-directed behaviors, and lacking the understanding or education necessary for good health. As an example, Pender (1996) cites one study of a major source of saturated fat for different groups. Hispanic and black children's intake of whole milk was significantly higher than that of white children based on the parents' beliefs that the whole milk was better for the children than lower fat or skim. In contrast, Asian Americans consume low-fat, high-carbohydrate diets, eating much healthier foods than Americans from European origins. Sensitivity to a client's culture, religion, and ethnic influences is essential in trying to assist her with any health behavior changes, for these variables strongly affect her health beliefs.

Current or Past Medical Problems

Of particular concern are the risks of past and present problems and the potential or real effects of current or past illness on new disease conditions. For example, recent research indicates a past history of smoking, even if the person no longer smokes, increases the risk of multiple myeloma and colon cancer. Multiple drug interactions may cause increased risks and confusing presentations. The use of multiple medications, seen most often in the elderly, is essential to assess as interactions may lead to serious consequences. Past pelvic inflammatory disease increases the risk of ectopic pregnancy or infertility.

SCREENING METHODS

HEALTH HISTORY

Interview and Approach Considerations

Effective interviewing and interpersonal skills are required in order to gather accurate, useful data.

- Consider any interaction with a client a therapeutic intervention by permitting the free expression of issues and concerns. Treat the client with dignity and respect; be nonjudgmental, accepting, supportive, concerned, and an appropriate role model (e.g., do not smoke in a client's presence).
- Use clear language and terminology matched to the client's level of understanding, culture, and background. Consider the client's age, education, response to the interview, and ethical, cultural, and religious taboos. Avoid medical jargon and clarify by restating confusing information. Use an interpreter if necessary.
- Appropriate questioning technique includes using open questions early in the interview to facilitate broad information gathering and to assist with mental status and general survey assessment. Open questions draw forth an overview of the client's problems. Ask the client about her concerns. Avoid interrupting, which may cause valuable data to be lost. Use pointed, directive questions to obtain specific data. Avoid leading questions ("You've never had a sexually transmitted disease, have you?"). Phrase sensitive questions in a nonjudgmental manner ("How

many partners do I need to notify about the risk of AIDS?").

- Be aware of nonverbal cues such as facial expressions, body movements, and signs of anxiety. The client may avoid making eye contact or answering questions. She may be reluctant to give information. Such cues may indicate fears or concerns.
- Help the woman understand the importance of telling you her concerns. If the client is able to talk freely, the interaction becomes healing, and there is the increased probability that something will be said that will help in understanding a problem or in management. Recognize that the client's real concerns may not surface until she feels comfortable with you.

Physical and psychological factors affect interaction.

- Provide a quiet, private place for the interview. Ideally, the interview should not take place in the examination room. Use measures, such as a sign on the door, to discourage others from walking in during the interview.
- Maintain the client's comfort. Permit her to remain dressed during the interview and provide comfortable seating that will allow client and interviewer to be at the same eye level. Never obtain a history with the client in lithotomy position.
- Due to the limited time frames for most visits in primary care today, seek to find out early what the problems that most concern her are. For example, you could say, "Since we have a limited time, could you tell me the most important reason(s) to you for your visit here today?" Keep the interview focused to stay within a reasonable time limit, using more than one session if needed.

Components of Health History

- **Demographic and biographical data, called identifying data (ID),** must be accurate. If someone else has obtained this information, recheck vital numbers such as phone, address, and Social Security Number.
- **Record the chief complaint (CC) or reason for visit (RFV).** Use the client's own words in a brief statement and put into a time frame (e.g., "I've had chest pain for two days," or "I need a Pap test and checkup").
- **Probe the history of present illness (HPI) or current health status (CHS).** An introductory statement for all women is essential: gravidity (G); parity (P); full-term or premature pregnancies; abortions (A),

spontaneous and induced, with reasons and length of gestation; number of living children (LC); dates of last and previous normal menstrual periods based on first day of bleeding (LNMP, PNMP); and methods of contraception used by client and partner, for how long or when stopped. If the woman is older, include date of menopause.

Write the remainder of the paragraph as a narrative, giving the following:

- **Usual state of health.**
- **Clear, chronological development/analysis of complaints:** sequencing (starting with onset), causes or associated phenomena, factors worsening/lessening/relieving/aggravating, quality or character of complaint, quantity of problem, effect on activities, location, radiation, severity (on a scale of 1 to 10), timing, past occurrence, others with problem.
- **Relevant family history.**
- **Degree of disability.**
- **Significant negatives.**

If the visit is related to the menstrual cycle, a complete description of the menstrual cycles is needed, including characteristics before and after the use of hormonal or other contraception that may affect the cycles.

If the visit is for routine health maintenance, elicit information about the client's usual health, last exams or tests and their results, current medications, habits, and significant problems or negatives, such as diabetes mellitus or cardiac disease.

- **Assess and record the past medical history (PMH) or past health status (PHS).**
  - *Childhood Diseases.* Measles, mumps, frequent infections, and so on.
  - *Immunizations and Screening Tests.* Dates of childhood immunizations: hepatitis B, diphtheria, pertussis, tetanus, Hemophilus influenza type B, measles, mumps, rubella, chickenpox, polio vaccines (types); dates of adult immunizations: tetanus toxoid, pneumococcus, influenza, hepatitis B, measles (those born after 1956), rubella (women without immunity), varicella; dates of other vaccinations: tuberculosis, meningococcus, smallpox, typhoid, and other special vaccines for at-risk and older populations; screening tests (HIV, rubella, tuberculosis, sickle cell, G-6-PD). Urge importance of maintaining currency of record. (See Table 4–6 for recommended routine adult immunizations).

TABLE 4–6. Adult and Adolescent Immunizations

Vaccine	Schedule/ Timing	Indications	Comments	Precaution/ Contraindications
Adult tetanus/diphtheria toxoid (Td)	First visit 1 IM dose Second visit 4 to 8 weeks after first dose Third visit 6 to 12 months after second dose Booster q 10 years through life; repeat dose with contaminated wounds if five years post booster	All unimmunized adults	1. Not contraindicated in pregnancy 2. Fully immunized women may not need further boosters > age 50 3. Adolescents ≥ 11 years get Td, not DtaP (pertussis not given after age 6)	Neurologic or immediate hypersensitivity after prior dose; severe local reaction after prior dose
Polio vaccines Live oral polio virus (OPV)[a] Not an alternative for routine IPV. Used if travelling in region with polio.	First dose at first visit Second dose in 2 months Third dose 6–12 months after second	1. Persons at risk for future exposure who previously received 1 or more doses of either oral or inactivated vaccine 2. Incomplete childhood series	1. Can give second dose in month if need to accelerate 2. Immunocompromised persons at higher risk for paralysis; rare in healthy persons; greatest risk for paralysis with first dose	1. Avoid in pregnancy unless immediate protection essential; then use OPV or E-IPV 2. Use E-IPV with immunocompromised persons 3. Do not give OPV to people with immunocompromised family members; hypersensitivity to streptomycin and neomycin (trace amounts are used in preparation of vaccine)
Enhanced-inactivated polio virus (E-IPV)[a] (Routinely given)	First dose SC at first visit Second dose 1 to 2 months after first dose Third dose 8 to 14 months after first dose	1. **Preferred for primary adult vaccinations** 2. Unimmunized or partially immunized with compromised immunity 3. HIV infected—symptomatic or asymptomatic 4. Close contacts of immunodeficient individuals 5. Partially immunized or unimmunized in households where children receive OPV 6. Unimmunized at risk of exposure and has had primary series 7. Partially immunized with IPV or OPV at future risk of exposure 8. At future risk of exposure who have had primary series 9. Those refusing OPV 10. Those traveling outside U.S. 11. Incomplete childhood series	1. E-IPV means has enhanced potency and is equal to OPV in seroconversion rates; is available in U.S. 2. Preferred for primary adult vaccinations 3. For those adults who have completed primary vaccinations, booster can be either E-IPV or OPV	See OPV A hypersensitivity reaction may occur if allergic to streptomycin, polymycin B, neomycin

TABLE 4–6. Adult and Adolescent Immunizations (CONTINUED)

Vaccine	Schedule/Timing	Indications	Comments	Precaution/Contraindications
Measles vaccine	One dose SC; no boosters needed	1. Birthdate prior to 1957 gives immunity 2. No evidence of documented vaccination requires 2 doses 1 month apart 3. If person entering college, health care work, or traveling internationally, give revaccination. 4. Revaccinate if received killed vaccine between 1963 and 1967	1. Vaccine of choice is MMR 2. Is live virus vaccine 3. Second dose needed for college students. Health care workers, international travelers, immunocompromised need 2 doses if only one in past	1. Pregnant women 2. Immunocompromised persons 3. History of anaphylactic reaction after ingesting egg or after receiving neomycin
Mumps vaccine	One dose SC; no boosters needed	1. Travelers without immunity 2. No documentation of disease or live vaccine 3. Elderly age no contraindication	1. Is live virus vaccine 2. MMR is vaccine of choice 3. HIV persons may receive	1. Pregnant women 2. Immunocompromised persons 3. History of anaphylactic reaction after ingesting egg or after receiving neomycin 4. Moderately to severely ill persons 5. Recent receipt of antibody-containing blood products
Rubella vaccine	One dose SC; no boosters needed	1. No documentation of live vaccine or immunity by lab test 2. Childbearing-age women 3. Employment in health care, colleges, military base 4. Travelers with susceptibility	1. Risk theoretically to fetus is considered negligible if given to mother in first trimester 2. If person also susceptible to measles and mumps, MMR is vaccine of choice 3. Breastfeeding is not contraindication 4. HIV persons may receive	1. Pregnant women 2. Immunocompromised persons 3. History of anaphylactic reaction after receiving neomycin 4. Recent receipt of antibody-containing blood products 5. Moderately to severely ill persons
MMR	First dose at first visit Second dose at 11–12 years after first visit If measles vaccine alone given and no past documentation, give 2 doses SC 1 month apart	1. Two doses needed if born >1957 2. Older people usually immune by contracting diseases 3. If entering college, immunize 4. No contraindication to vaccination if already immune	1. Susceptible postpartum women can receive vaccine even if breastfeeding 2. Revaccinate those vaccinated 1963–1967 with killed measles vaccine; also students entering college, health care workers, international travelers 3. Five to 55 percent have some local or systemic reaction	1. Do not administer to people with altered immunity except HIV-infected women who need measles protection (give MMR) 2. Contraindicated in pregnancy (live virus) 3. Postpartum women who received transfusion during peripartum—delay vaccine 3 months 4. History of anaphylactic reaction after ingesting egg or exposure to neomycin 5. Moderately to severely ill persons

TABLE 4–6. Adult and Adolescent Immunizations (CONTINUED)

Vaccine	Schedule/ Timing	Indications	Comments	Precaution/ Contraindications
Influenza (Whole or split-virus)	One dose (whole or split-virus) annually; generally in November, but may be offered as early as September	1. Healthy adults age 65± 2. Nursing home residents 3. Chronic care facility residents 4. All health care workers 5. Teens receiving long-term aspirin therapy 6. Persons with chronic illnesses 7. Immunosuppressed persons 8. International travelers	1. Provides protection against A&B strains 2. Does not cause the flu 3. May cause fever, malaise, myalgia 6–12 hours after given; lasts 1–2 days 4. Considered safe for asthmatics 5. CDC encourages flu shots for children 6–23 months. 6. Healthy adults benefit through less work time lost; less money spent on treatment	1. Acute febrile illness (wait until all symptoms abate) 2. Known hypersensitivity to eggs 3. Delay in pregnancy until after first trimester (not live virus)
Pneumococcal	One dose IM; another dose every 6 years may be considered	1. Adults age 65± 2. Immunocompetent adults with chronic disease 3. Immunocompromised adults 4. HIV-infected adults 5. Those living where increased risk of disease exists 6. All persons with asplenia	1. Vaccinate high-risk women before or after pregnancy 2. Half experience injection site pain, erythema; 1% have fever, myalgias, severe local reaction	1. Contraindicated in pregnant women
Hepatitis A Vaccine	One dose IM; booster at 6–12 months	1. Adults at risk such as international travelers, those with hepatitis C, HIV	1. Inactivated virus 2. Side effects: soreness at site, malaise, headache	1. Use only in pregnancy if risk > without
Hepatitis B vaccine	First visit first dose Second dose in 4 weeks Third dose 5 months after second dose Screen with Hb$_S$Ab before booster given; immunity lasts 7 years	1. All health care workers 2. All who are at increased risk occupationally, socially (includes family exposure)	1. Recombinant vaccine 2. Screening for susceptibility before vaccination variability cost effective 3. No therapeutic or adverse effects seen when given to HBV-infected persons	Not contraindicated in pregnancy Screen pregnant women for Hb$_S$Ag; give to all newborn
Varicella zoster vaccine (VZV; Varivax)	Two doses 4–8 weeks apart; if > 8 weeks apart, may still give second dose	Age 12 months and older who have not had varicella	1. Live, attenuated vaccine 2. Herpes zoster risk ≤ natural disease 3. 25% have erythema/soreness at injection site; 5%—rash	1. Avoid in immuno-compromised, hypersensitive, or neomycin-allergic people 2. Avoid pregnancy for 1 month after vaccine 3. Nursing women at high risk for exposure may take 4. Avoid in moderately to severely ill persons 5. Do not give if recent receipt of antibody-containing blood products

TABLE 4–6. Adult and Adolescent Immunizations (CONTINUED)

Vaccine	Schedule/ Timing	Indications	Comments	Precaution/ Contraindications
Variola (Smallpox vaccine)	Not routinely available; multipuncture technique with application of vaccine	1. Exposure to persons with smallpox	1. "Ring" vaccination method an effective approach for outbreaks	1. Pregnant women 2. Persons allergic to polymycin B, streptomycin, neomycin, tetracycline
Meningoccocal Vaccine (Menomune-A/C/Y/W-135)	One dose provides protection for 3 years.	1. Travelers to areas of endemic disease 2. Adolescents living in college/boarding school dorms.	1. Children need a second dose in 2–3 years	1. Not routine immunization

E-IVP—enhanced-potency inactivated poliovirus vaccine; IM—intramuscular; MMR—measles-mumps-rubella; SC-subcutaneous

[a]For detailed recommendations for poliomyelitis prevention, see Poliomyelitis Prevention in the United States: Introduction of a Sequential Vaccination Schedule of Inactivated Poliovirus Vaccine Followed by Oral Poliovirus Vaccine. (January 24, 1997). Morbidity and Mortality Weekly Report. U.S. Department of Health and Human Services, PHS, CDC. Atlanta, GA.

Sources: Bath et al., 2000; CDC, 2001; Gall, 1995; Hearington, 1999; Johnson, 1996; Watkins, 2002; Zimmerman & Ball, 2001.

- *Hospitalizations, Surgeries, and Serious Illnesses.* Dates, places, health care providers, reasons, courses of recovery, sequelae.
- *Accidents and Injuries.* Type of injury, how it occurred, severity, treatment, where, by whom, sequelae.
- *Obstetric History.* All pregnancies, regardless of outcome; dates and types of deliveries, sex and weights of infants, lengths of gestations; antepartum, intrapartum, and postpartum complications.
- *Contraceptive History.* Types of contraceptives used by client or partner, length of use, complications, side effects, satisfaction with method.
- *Sexual History.* (See Chapter 6.) Assess safer sex methods used and sexual satisfaction.
- *Allergies.* Specific allergens (food, environmental, medication), types of reactions, treatments, and results.
- *Medications.* Prescription, over-the-counter, herbs, supplements, dosages, administration routes, frequencies, reasons for use, side effects.
- *Habits.* Recreational or illicit substance use; tobacco, alcohol, caffeine use; type of substances, frequency, duration of use, effects, routes of administration, risk practices such as needle sharing.
- *Transfusions/Transplants.* Dates, reasons, exposure to HIV, hepatitis b and c.
- **Violence History.** Incidents of assault, incest, rape, other violence; injuries, treatment, counseling, sequelae.
- **Family history (FH)** includes hereditary, communicable, and environmental family diseases; causes of death of maternal and paternal grandparents, parents, siblings, children, partners, aunts, uncles, and cousins (if indicated). A genogram can be visually helpful (see Special Assessment Guides, Family Assessment). Note if family history is unknown or the client is adopted. Of particular importance is a family history of breast, colon, or ovarian cancer in mother or sister, congenital anomalies or retardation, multiple births, CVD, and anemia.
- **Psychosocial history taking (PSH) and personal history taking and assessment require sensitivity.**
  - *Nutrition.* (See Special Assessment Guides, Nutritional Assessment.)
  - *Family Relationships, Friendships, and Support Systems.* Significance and quality of relationships and interactions, areas of concern or conflict, verbal or physical abuse, living arrangements, availability of support systems, club and organization memberships, activities enjoyed with friends and relatives (see Special Assessment Guides, Family Assessment).
  - *Culture/Ethnicity.* Foods, religion, values, and beliefs affecting health.
  - *Occupation.* Full- or part-time employment, length of employment, type of work, hazards, stressors (see Special Assessment Guides, Occupational Assessment).
  - *Education.* Highest level obtained (formal and informal); client's feelings of satisfaction and how she learns best.
  - *Economic Status.* Adequacy of income for basic and recreational needs, monetary concerns, adequacy of insurance.

- *Exercise and Activity.* Current levels and types of activity, length of time spent, frequency, tolerance, safety.
- *Developmental Status.* Current level of task accomplishment according to developmental stage (see Chapters 2 and 3).
- *Self-Concept.* Locus of control, positive and negative feelings about self, satisfaction with self, perceived strengths and weaknesses.
- *Coping Mechanisms.* Stressors and usual methods of coping, perceived effectiveness (see Special Assessment Guides, Stress/Risk Assessment).
- *Patterns and Maintenance of Health Care.* Types, sources, and frequency of health care visits; home/folk remedies; general experiences and attitudes about health and care.
- *Sleep and Wakefulness.* Patterns, effects, problems, dreams, medication used to sleep or to stay awake (see Special Assessment Guides, Sleep Assessment).
- *Recreation/Relaxation.* Hobbies and activities for fun or relaxation; associated patterns, roles, and relationships.
- *Living Environment.* Hazards (real or potential), level of comfort; privacy, space.
- *Religion.* Importance to client, source of strength or stress, level of involvement.
- *Daily Profile.* Description of a typical day for the client.

- ◆ **A review of systems (ROS)** includes a thorough past and present history of each system.

  - *General.* General health, fatigue, exercise tolerance, episodes of unusual weight/height loss or gain, malaise, ability to carry out activities of daily living (ADL).
  - *Skin, Hair, Nails.* Diseases; primary or secondary skin lesions, itching, flaking; changes in texture, moisture, color, skin temperature, amount of hair, care practices.
  - *Head and Neck.* Injuries and their treatments, sequelae; headaches (type); range-of-motion limitations, pain, or stiffness; enlarged nodes; swelling.
  - *Eyes.* Use of corrective lenses, reason for prescription, results of last exam and glaucoma test, diseases or infections, pain, itching, discharge, diplopia, cataracts, blurred vision, spots, halos, flashing lights, blind spots.
  - *Ears.* Hearing acuity, test results and dates, use of aids and their effectiveness, diseases, pain, ringing, vertigo, infection, discharge, care habits.

- *Mouth, Teeth, and Throat.* Diseases; condition of teeth (loose, missing, caries), last exam and results, knowledge of routine care; sore throats, lesions, bleeding, hoarseness, voice changes; chewing, swallowing, or taste problems.
- *Nose and Sinuses.* Diseases; problems with sense of smell; nosebleeds; allergies/seasonal problems, sneezing, congestion, drainage, pain; trauma; breathing difficulties; infections and their treatments.
- *Chest and Lungs.* Diseases; dyspnea, cough, hemoptysis, exertion breathing difficulty, wheezing, asthma, pneumonia, bronchitis, tuberculosis (TB), emphysema, orthopnea, night sweats, smoking; time of last chest x-ray, reason, and results; last TB test and results.
- *Cardiovascular.* Diseases; pain, cyanosis, palpitations, murmurs, bruits, irregular heart rate, mitral valve prolapse, hypertension, edema, varicosities, rheumatic fever; coldness, tingling, color changes, hair loss on extremities; recent cholesterol and lipid screening results.
- *Breasts and Axillae.* Diseases; pain, masses, changes related to menstrual cycle, discharge, color, characteristics; skin, vascular, temperature changes; breast self-exam (when, how); last provider exam; last mammogram results; breast-feeding history.
- *Gastrointestinal.* Diseases; abdominal pain, distention, masses, indigestion, food intolerances, belching, nausea, vomiting (character), reflux, jaundice, ascites, diarrhea, constipation, character of stools; hemorrhoids; use of antacids or laxatives; last hemoccult test, results.
- *Genitourinary*
  REPRODUCTIVE. Onset of puberty, menarche (when, character, regularity of menses), current menstrual pattern (frequency, duration, flow amount); premenstrual syndrome (PMS); dysmenorrhea; tampon or pad use, size, correct use, number per day of flow, saturation; problems related to menses; use of medications or hormones, reasons, problems; last pelvic exam and Pap smear (if abnormal results, follow-up, sequelae); vaginitis, itching, discharge, lesions, diseases, abnormalities; sexually transmitted diseases (STDs), including pain, fever, chills; diethylstilbestrol (DES) exposure; fertility problems; sexual satisfaction, discomfort, problems. (Obstetric, sexual, contraceptive, and menopause history data may go here, or in HPI or

CHS if it relates to the reason for visit; see Chapter 16 for further information about obstetric history.) **URINARY.** Character and regularity of urination/ urine; diseases, infections (cystitis or pyelonephritis); dysuria, polyuria, oliguria, anuria, incontinence, hematuria, nocturia, urgency, stones, flank pain, fever, chills.

- *Musculoskeletal.* Diseases, fractures, or other injuries, cramping, pain, fasciculations, weakness/ strength, range-of-motion/activities of daily living limitations, gait problems, joint complaints (swelling, redness, pain, deformity, crepitus); back discomfort, ache, or deformity; loss of height.
- *Neurological.* Diseases; fainting, loss of consciousness, seizures (and medication for them), sensory problems (numbness, tingling, paresthesia), motor problems (balance, gait, spasm, paralysis), cognitive problems (mood changes, memory loss, disorientation, loss of judgment, hallucinations); sleep disturbances.
- *Blood and Immune.* Diseases; anemias, bleeding tendencies, easy bruising, transfusions, allergies, treatments; unexplained infections or node enlargement; blood type.
- *Endocrine.* Diseases; unusual changes in weight, height, glove, or shoe size; increased thirst, urination, appetite; heat/cold intolerance; weakness/fatigue; changes in skin and hair (loss, excessive growth, hirsute, texture).

SPECIAL ASSESSMENT GUIDES

Family Assessment

Determine who lives in the family, their relationships, cultural origins, religious preferences, health practices; the role of each member (education, occupation), communication among members, material management (home, money), goals of the family, relaxation and recreational family activities; and strengths, weaknesses, conflicts, problems, past resolution methods (Sawin & Harrigan, 1995; Seidel, Ball, Dains, & Benedict, 1999).

- **The McMaster Family Assessment Device (FAD)** looks at six family functioning areas, and assumes that some areas can be healthy functional areas while others are not (Sawin & Harrington, 1995). It is a paper and pencil self-report 60-item tool that takes about 20 minutes to complete. Family members' scores can be compared. The overall measure of a

family's functioning can be measured by the General Functioning Scale. Each of the six areas has optimal and unhealthy functioning well clarified. Problem solving, communication, roles, affective responsiveness, affective involvement, and behavior control are measured.

- **"Family APGAR"** is one quick screening tool for identifying areas of family difficulty (Sawin & Harrigan, 1995). It uses five areas for scoring: *adaptation, partnership, growth, affection,* and *resolve.* Each category receives a score of 0 to 2 points. The provider asks the client to score 2 points for "almost always," 1 point for "some of the time," and 0 points for "hardly ever." The following statements are given to the client for scoring:
  - I am satisfied with the help that I receive from my family* when something is troubling me. (Adaptation)
  - I am satisfied with the way my family* discusses items of common interest and shares problem solving with me. (Partnership)
  - I find that my family* accepts my wishes to take on new activities or make changes in my lifestyle. (Growth)
  - I am satisfied with the way my family* expresses affection and responds to my feelings, such as anger, sorrow, and love. (Affection)
  - I am satisfied with the amount of time my family* and I spend together. (Resolve)

A score of 0 to 3 is associated with a severely dysfunctional family; 4 to 6 with a moderately dysfunctional family; and 7 to 10 with a highly functional family. This tool is easy to use and focuses on perception of satisfaction (Sawin & Harrington, 1995).

- **The *genogram* is** a family tree picture that contains a family's relationships, structure, health, and other important data over three generations (Sawin & Harrington, 1995). It has been evolving since the 1970s. This visual picture may be very helpful in identifying tendencies of conditions within families and, thus, risk factors for individual clients. It is also helpful in providing the elderly client with a framework for looking at life events. Cultural differences are exhibited in genograms, as well as ways to compare heritages. Relationship and emotional behaviors can

---

*Substitute spouse, partner, significant other, parent, or children if necessary.

also be demonstrated with the genogram through use of a key that depicts such terms as "loving," "abusive," "domineering" (Visscher & Clore, 1992). Standardization has not been accomplished yet, but the tool is useful nevertheless.

Nutritional Assessment

Appropriate nutrition with adequate exercise will ensure better health. Assess the client's 24-hour diet recall of food/drink intake for balance and adequacy of nutrients. For nonpregnant, nonlactating women, the table of governmental dietary guidelines gives the daily intake (the lesser amounts for less active or older women) (*Dietary Guidelines,* 2000). See Table 4–7 for examples of servings and foods from the food groups appropriate for the nonpregnant woman 25 and over.

Healthy, active women who are not dieting need about 1,800 to 1,900 calories daily (Gennaro, 2001). These calories should be distributed with carbohydrates comprising 55 percent, protein 15 to 20 percent, and fat no more than 30 percent. No more than 10 percent of fat should come from saturated fats such as animal fat or tropical oils like coconut oil. Trans-fat-free foods are advised to decrease LDL-cholesterol levels also (USDHHS, 2000). Blood lipid levels should be maintained at healthful levels: total cholesterol under 200 mg/dL, HDL cholesterol above 40 mg/dL (ideally for women above 50 mg/dL), and LDL cholesterol under 130 mg/dL (optimum level equal to or under 100 mg/dL). (Expert Panel on, 2001). The triglyceride level is emerging as an independent risk factor for women; it should be under 200 mg/dL (optimum under 150 mg/dL).

Sugar and salt should be used in moderation. The maximum amount of salt daily in foods and added in cooking or at the table should be no more than 2,400 mg. A variety of foods that provide the proper number of food group servings should be eaten daily. Moderate alcohol consumption is advised for the woman who drinks. This equates to less than 1 to 1.5 ounces of 80 proof distilled liquor daily or under 7 ounces per week; 5 ounces of wine or one 12-ounce beer daily (USDA, 2000; Position Statement, 2002).

Eating adequate fruits and vegetables (optimum is 9 servings a day) provides the body with antioxidants (5 or more of vegetables and 4 or more of fruits). Six to 11 servings of grains are needed daily. Fiber-rich foods—such as apples, carrots, whole grains, bran, and legumes—are important for reducing risks of bowel cancer, diabetes, obesity, and decreasing serum cholesterol (ACOG, 1996, May; Tapper-Gardizina, Cotugna, & Vick-

ery, 2002). Adequate fiber intake (25–35 grams daily) is advised. Oat bran, kidney beans, and a pear are examples of 4 grams of soluble fiber per serving. Raisins, prunes, and figs provide insoluble fiber that increases transit time and decreases constipation.

Megadoses of vitamins and minerals are not advised without provider knowledge and management. Folate 400 mcg daily is advised from foods or a multivitamin supplement to reduce the risk of neural tube defects in fetuses of childbearing age women (ACOG, 1996; Hilton, 2002). Fortification is added to most enriched breads, flours, and grain products. Women under age 60 in the Nurses' Health Study who had a daily consumption of 352 mg or more of vitamin C were 57 percent less likely to develop cataracts than if they had less than 140 mg per day (Vitamin C and, 2002). Calcium-rich foods daily are advised, or calcium supplements, if such a diet is not adequate or not tolerated. Adolescents and younger women up to age 24 need 1,000 to 1,500 mg/day (By the way, Doctor, 2002; Curry & Hogstel, 2002; National Academy of Sciences, 1997; *Optimal Daily Calcium,* 1994). Those 24 to 50 years (premenopausal) need 1,000 mg daily. Women 50 to 64 years on hormone replacement therapy need 1,000 mg a day; women 50 to 64 not on hormone replacement therapy and women 65 and over whether on or off HRT need 1,500 mg daily. Pregnant and nursing women need 1,200 to 1,500 mg daily. Foods high in calcium include dairy products, broccoli, kale, turnip greens, some legumes, canned fish, seeds, nuts, and fortified products. Not all calcium supplements are as bioavailable as others. Calcium citrate is one of the better sources providing more bioavailable elemental calcium. Best absorption of supplements is in doses of 500 mg or less taken between meals. Calcium carbonate absorption is impaired without the presence of gastric acid, however, and so should be taken with foods promoting secretion of gastric acid. Calcium citrate is not dependent on gastric acid for absorption. Six to eight glasses of water in addition to other fluids are recommended daily for optimal body functioning.

Determine if the client eats breakfast; skips meals; uses vitamin and mineral supplements and types/amounts; wears dentures; eats snacks (how often and what); drinks caffeinated or carbonated beverages (what and how much); eats more beef than fish and poultry; consumes excessive fat, salt, sugar, or substitutes; eats alone or too quickly; chews adequately; uses alcohol, tobacco, or other substances or medications that could alter nutrient intake; is unable to tolerate some foods, eats charcoal grilled or fried foods; eats what someone else cooks; has wide weight fluctuations; abuses food when stressed; or diets constantly. Be sure that the client knows

TABLE 4–7. Examples of Foods Groups, Foods, Daily Servings Needed, and Serving Sizes for Nonpregnant Women 25 Years and Above

Food Group	Food Examples and Serving Sizes		Number Servings
Fruits/Vegetables			
High in Vitamin A	cantaloupe	1/4 medium	1
	tomato	2 medium	
	papaya	1/2 medium	
	apricot	3 medium	
	carrot, spinach, greens, sweet potato, winter squash	1/2 cup cooked or 1 cup raw	
	chili peppers	2 tbsp. raw/cooked	
High in Vitamin C	juices (orange, grapefruit)	6 ounces (3/4 cup)	1
	cantaloupe, papaya	1/4 medium	
	grapefruit	1/2 medium	
	orange, lemon, kiwi	1 medium	
	tomato	2 medium	
	broccoli, brussel sprouts, strawberries, cauliflower, green pepper, cabbage	1/2 cup cooked or 1 cup raw	
Other	raisin	1/4 cup	3
	grapes/watermelon	1/2 cup	
	apple, banana, peach	1 medium	
	asparagus, green beans, potato, peas, yellow squash, corn	1/2 cup cooked or 1 cup raw	
	lettuce	1 cup raw	
Milk Products	milk, yogurt, custard	1 cup	2
	cheese (cheddar)	1-1/2 ounces	
	cheese (American)	2 ounces	
	frozen yogurt, ice milk, ice cream	1-1/2 cups	
	cottage cheese	2 cups	
Breads/Cereals/Grains	bread	1 slice	5
	tortilla	1 small	
	cereal, cold	3/4 cup	
	cereal, hot	1/2 cup	
	macaroni/noodles/spaghetti, cooked	1/2 cup	
	rice, cooked	1/2 cup	
	hot dog/hamburger bun	1/2	
	biscuit, roll, muffin	1 small	
	pancake	1 medium	
	crackers	8	
Protein Foods	cooked dry beans/peas	1/2 cup	1/2
	peanut butter	2 tbsp.	
	soyburger	2 1/2 ounces	
	nuts/seeds	1/3 cup	2
	meat/poultry/fish (serving size 2–3 ounces)	1 piece	
	eggs	1 substituted for 1 ounce meat/poultry/fish	
	canned tuna/fish	1/4 cup	3
Unsaturated Fats	avocado	1/8 medium	
	margarine, mayonnaise, vegetable oil	1 tsp	
	salad dressing—mayonnaise-based	2 tsp.	
	oil-based	1 tsp.	

Sources: Dietary Guidelines, 2000; Gutierrez, 1994; U.S. Department of Agriculture, 2000.

what is included in a balanced diet. For the elderly woman, it is important to assess for conditions that may interfere with nutritional health. Ask about the effect on her diet of any illness, drug, or problem she may have such as dental or oral problems, if she has enough money for food, if she has someone to eat with or eats alone, how many meals she eats a day, unplanned weight loss, and how she shops and cooks for herself (AAFP, ADA, & NCOA, 1994). The Nursing Nutritional Screening Tool (NNST) is a quick and easy tool that may be used to identify women with actual or potential nutritional lacks (Phaneuf, 1996).

Vegetarians can get all the nutrients needed from a diet comprised mainly of plant foods, such as vegetables, grains, legumes, fruits, seeds and nuts, small amounts (3 servings per day) of low or nonfat dairy foods per day, and 3 to 4 egg yolks a week. Readers are referred to the January 1996 issue of the *Harvard Women's Health Watch* for a readable coverage of a vegetarian diet and nutrients requiring special attention, such as folate, calcium, vitamins B-12 and D, iron, and protein. Vegetarian diets are especially beneficial in providing fiber and antioxidants.

Correlate diet patterns with other history, physical examination, and diagnostic test findings; for example, high fat intake may be correlated with obesity and abnormal lipid levels. (See Chapter 17 for nutritional recommendations during pregnancy.) Data have shown that weight in the upper levels of normal and even moderate weight gains after age 18 increase a woman's risks of coronary heart disease (Willett, Manson, Stampfer, et al., 1995). The Body Mass Index (BMI) is the accepted measure for assessing weight most accurately (Willett et al., 1995). The normal BMI range is 18.5 to 24.9 (Gennaro, 2001). A BMI of 25.0 to 29.9 equates with being overweight; 30.0 to 34.9 with obesity; and 35.0 and over with being extremely obese. If the woman's BMI is under 18.5, she is considered underweight. As body fat increases and lean body mass decreases, the risk for cardiovascular disease increases. Waist/Hip Ratio is another helpful measure for assessing health status related to weight. This ratio is calculated by dividing the waist measurement in inches by the hip measurement in inches. The optimal ratio should be 0.80 or under for women. (Clinical Guidelines, 1995; Gennaro, 2001; Gerchufsky, 1996). In general, the waist size is important alone as a measure (Gennaro, 2001). A waist size greater than 35 inches in women is considered a high risk for health problems. If a woman has both a high BMI (25.0 or greater and a waist size greater than 35 inches, she is at high to extremely high risk (see Tables 4–8 and 4–9). Any ratio above this optimum indicates a tendency for central obesity, a significant risk factor for heart disease.

Stress/Risk Assessment

Assess the amount of healthy stress in the woman's life, and the amount of distress (Pender, 1996). Distress is stress overload; therefore, look at factors such as financial problems; changing situations or relationships with family or significant others; and employment, unemployment, or underemployment problems or concerns (such as lack of control or input into the job situation). In addition, assess personal information (age, hereditary factors such as family history of depression, lifestyle, living conditions, habits), coping strategies, and social support. Stress and ineffective coping are associated with the development of illnesses, such as hypertension, coronary artery disease, headaches, back pain, and GI upsets; decreased immunity; mental health problems such as depression and substance abuse; and domestic violence, to name a few. A study to see if perceived family stress was predictive in forecasting health problems found that people reporting a high level of family stress had more severe illness follow-up visits, referrals, and hospitalizations over an 18-month period than low stress persons (Parkerson, Broadnead, & Tse, 1995). Research has also shown that the small stressors in life (daily hassles) can be important sources of stress, perhaps as much or more than major events (Kanner, Cyne, Schaefer, & Lazarus, 1980). Psychological distress is associated with an increased risk for coronary heart disease (Stansfeld, Fuhrer, Shipley, & Marmot, 2002).

Helpful assessment tools for evaluating stress or anxiety are the Holmes and Rahe Life-Change Index, which measures the degree of change from major life events in one's life to predict the chance of illness (Holmes & Rahe, 1967); the hassles and up-lift scales (Kanner et al., 1980); and Speilberger's State-Trait Anxiety Inventory, (Spielberger, Edwards, Lushene, et al., 1983); which measures the amount of anxiety a person feels at the time of testing. Signs of excessive stress (mood swings, disposition changes, physical signs and symptoms) must be correlated with other assessment findings (sleep, appearance, nutrition, relaxation, recreation, self-concept, social supports, use of medications/substances, or unusual behaviors).

Offering ways for managing stress to decrease the potential adverse effects becomes important as a routine part of women's health care in our society today. Using relaxation techniques is one effective way to inhibit the stress effects on the body. Domar and Dreher (1996) suggest minirelaxation techniques to use quickly and effectively in stressful situations. These involve use of conscious abdominal breathing rather than chest breathing, which is associated with anxiety. Sauro et al. (2001) found that sociotropic cognition, a method to moderate stress, did reduce cardiovascular measures of blood pressure and heart rate in college women during interpersonal stress-induced periods.

TABLE 4–8. Body Mass Index

BMI	19	20	21	22	23	24	25	26	27	28	29	30	31	32	33	34	35
Height (inches)								Body Weight (pounds)									
58	91	96	100	105	110	115	119	124	129	134	138	143	148	153	158	162	167
59	94	99	104	109	114	119	124	128	133	138	143	148	153	158	163	168	173
60	97	102	107	112	118	123	128	133	138	143	148	153	158	163	168	174	179
61	100	106	111	116	122	127	132	137	143	148	153	158	164	169	174	180	185
62	104	109	115	120	126	131	136	142	147	153	158	164	169	175	180	186	191
63	107	113	118	124	130	135	141	146	152	158	163	169	175	180	186	191	197
64	110	116	122	128	134	140	145	151	157	163	169	174	180	186	192	197	204
65	114	120	126	132	138	144	150	156	162	168	174	180	186	192	198	204	210
66	118	124	130	136	142	148	155	161	167	173	179	186	192	198	204	210	216
67	121	127	134	140	146	153	159	166	172	178	185	191	198	204	211	217	223
68	125	131	138	144	151	158	164	171	177	184	190	197	203	210	216	223	230
69	128	135	142	149	155	162	169	176	182	189	196	203	209	216	223	230	236
70	132	139	146	153	160	167	174	181	188	195	202	209	216	222	229	236	243
71	136	143	150	157	165	172	179	186	193	200	208	215	222	229	236	243	250
72	140	147	154	162	169	177	184	191	199	206	213	221	228	235	242	250	258
73	144	151	159	166	174	182	189	197	204	212	219	227	235	242	250	257	265
74	148	155	163	171	179	186	194	202	210	218	225	233	241	249	256	264	272
75	152	160	168	176	184	192	200	208	216	224	232	240	248	256	264	272	279
76	156	164	172	180	189	197	205	213	221	230	238	246	254	263	271	279	287

To use the table, find the appropriate height in the left-hand column labeled Height. Move across to a given weight. The number at the top of the column is the BMI at that height and weight. Pounds have been rounded off.

Source: http://www.nhlbi.nih.gov/guidelines/obesity/bmi_tbl.htm

Fitness Assessment

Assess activities at work, home, or play for aerobic quality, stretching/flexibility movement, strength components, and sufficient intensity to meet therapeutic cardiovascular levels without compromising safety. Determine the duration of the exercise session, frequency per week, and the motivation of the client to exercise. To achieve a realistic assessment, evaluate fitness within a framework of lifestyle, diet, weight, stress, and substance use. *Healthy*

People 2010 objectives aim to increase the proportion of U.S. adults who engage in moderate physical activity for a minimum of 30 minutes daily and of adolescents who do so on 5 days a week to 30 percent (USDHHS, 2000). Vigorous activity three or more times a week for 20 or more minutes is the goal for 30 percent of adults. Adolescents become more sedentary, especially females, indicating a need for early fitness habits in children (Pender, 1996). The Centers for Disease Control and Prevention and the American College of Sports Medicine examined

TABLE 4–9. Classification of Overweight and Obesity by BMI, Waist Circumference, and Associated Disease Risks

	BMI (kg/m²)	Obesity Class	Disease Risk* Relative to Normal Weight and Waist Circumference†	
			Men 102 cm (40 in) or less Women 88 cm (35 in) or less	Men > 102 cm (40 in) Women > 88 cm (35 in)
Underweight	< 18.5		-	-
Normal	18.5–24.9		-	-
Overweight	25.0–29.9		Increased	High
Obesity	30.0–34.9	I	High	Very High
	35.0–39.9	II	Very High	Very High
Extreme Obesity	≥ 40.0	III	Extremely High	Extremely High

* Disease risk for type 2 diabetes, hypertension, and CVD.
† Increased waist circumference can also be a marker for increased risk even in persons of normal weight.

Source: http://www.nhlbi.nih.gov/health/public/heart/obesity/lose_wt/bmi/dis.htm

the research on recommended physical activity levels and concluded that every U.S. adult should "accumulate 30 minutes or more of moderate-intensity physical activity on most, preferably all, days of the week." (Pate, Pratt, Blair, et al., 1995). Previous recommendations had said that each person needed moderate- to high-intensity exercise three times a week for 20 to 60 minutes; however, this recommendation is based on the finding that most health benefits can be attained with moderate-intensity exercise not necessarily found in a formal exercise program. Lifestyle exercise, those activities that cumulatively provide the person with moderate exercise during the day, should be assessed for adequacy in total amount (30 minutes) per day at less than 60 percent of maximum heart rate (Pender, 1996).

Provide the woman with the benefits of exercise, such as the positive effects on blood pressure and cholesterol, the improved immunity effects, the decrease in body fat and improved glucose tolerance, the maintenance of bone density and increased lean muscle mass, and the improved self-concept. A study of the effect of a single walking bout on a treadmill on serum lipids and lipoproteins in groups of premenopausal and postmenopausal women found that in the immediate postexercise period, even a single exercise event lowered the total cholesterol and the low density cholesterol (LDL-C) in the premenopausal women and lowered the LDL-C in the postmenopausal group (Pronk, Crouse, O'Brien, & Rohack, 1995). A favorable pattern of cholesterol and lipid changes in older women was produced by a combination of endurance exercise and hormone replacement therapy (HRT) (Binder, Birge, & Kohrt, 1996). Over eleven months, total cholesterol, LDL-C, and high density lipoprotein cholesterol (HDL-C) all changed positively with the combined regimen (Refer to Chapter 15 for current information related to HRT and risks.) A study of over 7,000 women found that women who were least fit had a 110 percent greater risk of death; women smokers had a 99 percent greater risk of death; nonsmoking women who were moderately fit had 55 percent lower all-cause risk of death than lower-fit women; and fitness appeared to offset some of the effects of smoking as well as impacts of hypertension and high cholesterol (Blair, Kampert, Kohl, et al., 1996).

For any exercise regimen, but especially for a moderate or higher intensity exercise program, teach the value of beginning slowly for short periods of time, then gradually building it, with emphasis on increasing tone, strengthening, reducing stress, enhancing flexibility and coordination, promoting relaxation, preventing injury,

and improving self-concept. For a healthy woman who has no contraindications for exercise, advise building up to 20 to 40 minutes of aerobic activity, with a warm-up of 5 to 10 minutes before the more vigorous activity. Advise her to stretch after warming up and to cool down slowly for 5 to 10 minutes after exercising, monitoring her heartrate.

The intensity of exercise is aimed at safely improving cardiovascular function. Referral to an exercise therapist may be necessary for full assessment and program management. A good guideline is that the client should be able to talk while in the safe target percentage range for the heartbeat, but probably not sing. Activities that the usually sedentary individual can integrate into her life to provide short opportunities for moderate exercise include brisk walking, stair climbing, yard work, play with children, and gardening. (Pender, 1996). Suggestions include taking every opportunity to walk, such as changing channels by walking to the television, parking farther from the destination, and taking the stairs instead of the elevator. The more accessible, safe, and aesthetically pleasing the opportunities for physical activity are, the more likely the person is to participate (Humpel, Owen, & Leslie, 2002). Researchers found that women in the Nurses' Health Study II who were underweight or overweight based on BMI had an increased risk of ovulatory infertility, that vigorous activity of one hour each week reduced the risk, and that each hour of increased activity decreased the risk by 7 percent (Rich-Edwards, Spiegelman, et al., 2002). Another study found that women at risk for type 2 diabetes who had at least a 7 percent weight loss and exercised at least 150 minutes a week decreased their risk of developing disease significantly (Knowler, Barrett-Connor, et al., 2002). A study of African American women found that culturally appropriate interventions are important in success of lifestyle modifications (Young, Gittelsohn, Felix-Aaron, et al., 2001). Resting systolic blood pressure was reduced significantly in a meta-analysis of aerobic activity efficacy with older adults (Kelley & Sharpe-Kelley, 2001). Walking programs of exercise statistically decreased resting systolic and diastolic blood pressure in adults ≥ 18 years old (Kelley, Kelley, & Tran, 2001).

Occupational Assessment

Assess the type of work, amount, duration, physical labor involved, rest breaks, environmental risks, and stress overload. Problem areas include prolonged standing or sitting, heavy lifting, excessive noise, excessive heat or cold, exposure to toxins, exposure to chemicals or radiation, excessive hours on the job, boredom, low pay, low recognition, and little or no control over work. An area of increasing concern is environmental tobacco smoke exposure. A 39 percent excess risk of lung cancer was found with exposure in the workplace in a multicenter study that looked at lifetime lung cancer relative risk associated with environmental exposure (Fontham, Correa, Reynolds, et al., 1994).

Be especially concerned about a pregnant woman (see Chapters 16 and 17); determine if she has been exposed to chemicals, anesthetic gases, radiation, or infections. Consider the influence of multiple variables, such as secondhand smoke, stress, nutrition, lack of sleep, and exposure to hazardous materials. Three questions have been found to be essential for a simple occupational history: (1) What is your job like? Describe it; (2) Have you ever worked with any health hazard, such as asbestos, chemicals, noise, or repetitive motion?; and (3) Do you have any health problems that you believe may be related to your work or home? The chief complaint should always be examined for a relationship with the person's work or home activities or exposures. A more in-depth occupational history as presented by Twinings (1995) is needed if the simple history indicates problems.

Sleep Assessment

Assess the sleep and rest patterns of the woman. Eight hours of sleep each night is recommended by the National Sleep Foundation for adults (Women and sleep, 1999). Women ages 30 to 60 are typically sleep-deprived, averaging 1.5 hours less sleep on weeknights and 1 hour less on weekends. The risk of impaired performance—motor vehicle, home, and occupational accidents—is significant (Elliott, 2001). An elevated risk of type 2 diabetes is associated with snoring in women 40 to 65 years old (Al-Delaimy, Manson, Willett, & Stampfer, 2002), and African American women with diabetes and excessive daytime sleepiness have a significant risk for obstructive sleep apnea (Chasen, Umlauf, Pillion, & Singh, 2000). Women report more insomnia, which, along with poor quality sleep, is associated with a higher risk of depression (Ford & Cooper-Patrick, 2001). Sleep disturbances are common in women who have had a hysterectomy (Kim & Lee, 2001), and lower estradiol levels are an important factor for women 45 to 49 who report poor sleep (Hollander, Freeman, et al., 2001). Sleep is comprised of five stages: Stage 1: NonRapid Eye Movement (NREM) sleep for a few minutes as the person moves in

transitional sleep with dreamlike thoughts; Stage 2: NREM sleep that is deeper with fragmented thoughts for 15 to 20 minutes; Stages 3 and 4: Deeper NREM sleep stages (delta sleep) lasting 40 to 70 minutes; REM Stage: Follows the first four stages and is sleep (dream sleep) that can be considered as restorative, or as calisthenics for the brain. The cycles of sleep stages are repeated through the sleep period with increasingly lengthening REM stages until the person awakens. Many activities can interrupt the normal circadian rhythms, disrupting sleep, and causing distress. Lack of sufficient REM sleep affects memory and learning.

If the woman complains of awakening to go to the bathroom, look further because sleep apnea may be the cause (Pressman, Figueroa, & Kendrick-Mohamed, 1996). Sleep apnea is either central or obstructive and affects 2 percent of women (Hahn, 1996; Strauss, 1999). Cardiopulmonary altered function is common (Strollo & Rogers, 1996). Loud snoring, especially with gasping/choking episodes, indicates apnea. Since obstructive problems decrease oxygen to the brain, the body nearly awakes as a warning. If this pattern is repeated multiple times a night, serious repercussions can occur and the woman needs to be seen by a sleep specialist. A history of accidents on the job, sleeping on the job, and/or personality-cognitive changes should raise suspicions. A referral is also needed for women with narcolepsy (periods of sudden sleeping), which can lead to accidents.

Ask the following questions: Does it take you at least an hour to fall asleep? Do you wake up too early? Does your sleep partner complain that you are restless? Do you worry about getting enough sleep most nights? If you wake up in the night, can you go back to sleep? Do you use aids (pills or alcohol) to get to sleep? Do you feel exhausted from lack of sleep? Do you sleep in on days off or take daytime naps to make up for lack of sleep? Do you need caffeine to stay alert during the day? How much? Does your mind continue to work excessively during times when your body is resting? Any "yes" responses can indicate a problem.

PHYSICAL EXAMINATION

Overview

Accurate inspection, palpation, percussion, and auscultation are critical, as is the precise use of appropriate equipment. Understanding the findings is also essential.

- ◆ In preparation for the exam, explain all procedures to the client. Ensure privacy, draping, and comfort.

Have all necessary equipment available and clean and use good lighting. Ask the client to void before the exam. *Clean hands and the use of universal precautions are essential.*

◆ During the exam, give anticipatory advice and information; for example, teach abdominal breathing to help the client relax. Use the exam as an opportunity to teach. Be gentle, systematic, and sensitive. Avoid facial expressions or utterances indicating disgust. Provide tissues for the client after the pelvic exam. When finished, wash hands and allow the client to dress before reviewing findings.

◆ An abbreviated physical examination of a well woman, as done in some family planning clinics or private offices, includes assessment of blood pressure, height and weight, lymph nodes (head/neck, axillae, groin), thyroid, heart, lungs, breasts, abdomen, extremities, and genitourinary tracts and rectum.

◆ A selective exam related to those systems indicated by the chief complaint is required for episodic visits for problems such as vaginal itching or breast pain. Remember that more than one system may cause the problem.

◆ Refer to any current and complete physical assessment text for information on the correct considerations by system for the physical examination. The following information provides special hints for some select systems.

General Survey

Obtain an overall first impression of the client. Obvious and more subtle clues are obtained primarily by sensory observation and listening with a "sixth sense." Be sure to measure height and weight with clothes on and shoes off; compare findings to standardized charts. Consider racial effects: African Americans tend to be heavier and taller than Caucasians; Asians tend to be slighter and shorter than Caucasians. Consider age and gender effects: Girls tend to reach peak height at puberty; older women tend to lose height after menopause. Note body type and posture, whether the woman is obese, slender, average, or stocky; her fat distribution and any deformities. Consider that an older woman may develop a thoracic hump, especially if she is not on hormone replacement therapy. Observe her ability to stand and to sit straight. Assess developmental changes of the breasts and reproductive system (sexual maturity). (See Physical Examination, Developmental Changes of the Breasts and the Reproductive System.)

Skin, Hair, Nails. Teach the client to evaluate moles for changes. Check piercings and tattoos for infection, keloid scarring. Check for cosmetic surgery since clients often fail to provide this in the history. Observe for hair dye, permanent wave, cosmetic damage. Check nails for infection and damage from artificial nail applications.

Thyroid. Be vigilant in checking for nodules and enlargement and associated signs of disease.

Breasts, Areolae, Nipples and Axillae. Note sexual maturity, size, symmetry, dimpling, retractions, color, edema, thickening, vascular pattern, lesions/rashes/scaling, discharge, masses/nodules, rash, unusual pigmentation, abnormal lymph nodes. Teach breast self-exam.

Abdomen. Observe color of skin, lesions, contour, masses, distention, symmetry, vascularity, peristalsis, pulsations, and the umbilicus. Using percussion and/or palpation, assess pulsations, bowel sounds, bruits, ascites, organomegaly, and masses. Note inguinal node enlargement, tenderness/pain, rebound, and rigidity. Perform iliopsoas and obturator maneuvers with acute-abdomen.

Neurological/Psychological. Case-finding instruments are valuable adjuncts in gathering data to diagnose major depression in primary care settings. (Mulrow, Williams, Gerety, et al., 1995). Several instruments such as the *Beck Depression Inventory,* the *Center for Epidemiologic Studies Depression Screen,* and the *Zung Self-Assessment Depression Scale* can be administered in 2 to 5 minutes, are easy in relation to literacy level, and are depression-specific. About 20 percent of depressed clients can be identified with use of a case-finding instrument, a decided improvement over the 50 percent missed if usual history and physical methods are used without a full diagnostic interview. Depression instruments should not be used to the exclusion of other instruments for case-finding additional disorders, however, such as anxiety or drug/alcohol abuse. Some instruments are multidimensional, such as the *Primary Care Evaluation of Mental Disorders* and the *Symptom Driven Diagnostic System,* and should be considered in gathering data. Additionally, specific examinations and tests are needed to rule out physical pathology of somatic complaints, such as chest pain in the woman with panic disorder or headache associated with depression. The reader is referred to Chapter 23, Psychosocial Health Problems for more indepth assessment information.

Pelvic Examination

Use gloves on both hands; maintain strict medical aseptic technique to prevent spread of organisms. Some clinicians recommend double gloves or special high-risk gloves if the HIV-AIDS/Hepatitis B status is known to be positive.

- *Inspect and palpate* femoral nodes, external genitalia and Bartholin glands, urethra, and Skene's (BUS) glands. This includes, in addition to the Bartholin glands and urethra, the mons pubis, labia minora and majora, clitoris, urethral meatus, and vaginal opening. Assess sexual maturity and check pubic hair for pattern/parasite. Note any swelling, enlargement, inflammation, lesions (e.g., excoriations, leukoplakia, folliculitis from shaving), pigmentation, discharge, relaxation/celes, and tenderness. Teach self-examination of the vulva (STD Quarterly, 1995). The two minutes it takes to provide the woman with a "tour" of her genital area may save her life. The self-exam should be done monthly.
- *The vagina and cervix* are examined with a warmed speculum; lubricate with water only; lubricant may interfere with interpretation of cervical cytology. The cervix may more readily come fully into view if the woman is asked to cough out loud three times with a hand covering the speculum and urethral openings (Clinical pearls, 1996). Inspect the cervix and os: size, shape, color, lesions, discharge/bleeding, and position. Obtain the Pap smear and prepare cultures and wet prep specimens (see Overview of Commonly Indicated Laboratory Tests). Inspect the vagina for color, rugae, lesions (erosions, leukoplakia, masses, ulcerations), inflammation, and discharge. With a cotton-tipped applicator, gently remove any discharge that prevents adequate visualization of surfaces.
- *Assess the uterus and adnexa.* Lubricate index and middle gloved fingers; insert into vagina with other hand on abdomen above pubis. Note vaginal nodules, masses, or tenderness; note cervical size, consistency, nodules or masses, tenderness, pain with movement of the cervix, and closure of the os. Assess the position, size, shape, consistency, mobility, and tenderness of the uterus, adnexal organs, and any masses.
- *The rectovaginal area* is evaluated **after gloves are changed** and fingers lubricated again. Inspect the external anal area and palpate the sphincter, rectal walls, septum, posterior surface of the uterus, and palpable adnexal areas for tumors and tenderness. Retroverted or retroflexed uteri are more accessible by rectal exam. Obese women may be evaluated more fully by the rectovaginal route. The reproductive organs of women who are virgins may be more easily assessed in a tense woman via the rectal exam.

Developmental Changes of the Breasts and the Reproductive System

- *Pubertal changes* include functional maturation of the reproductive organs. The breast bud (thelarche) is usually the first sign of puberty, followed soon afterward with the emergence of pubic hair. Axillary hair generally appears about two years after pubic hair begins; rarely does it precede pubic hair growth. Menarche (median age 12.8 years, range 9 to 17.7 years) occurs after the peak of the growth spurt (median age 11.4 years, range 10 to 14 years). (Gordon & Speroff, 2002). See Chapter 3 for more detail.

As the external genitalia develop into adult proportions, the clitoris becomes more erectile and the labia minora more vascular. The labia majora and mons pubis become more prominent at the same time as the breasts develop. The internal organs, including the uterus, ovaries, and fallopian tubes, increase in size and weight. The endometrial lining becomes thick in preparation for menarche, and vaginal secretions increase. (Seidel et al., 1999; Speroff, Glass, & Kase, 1999).

- *Tanner Staging.* This is widely used to assess adolescent pubertal development. (Hacker & Moore, 1998; Murray, 1996; Speroff, Glass, & Kase, 1999). The sample used to develop these guidelines comprised white, middle-class English girls; therefore, modifications may be needed when applying the parameters to other groups.
  - *Stage I (Prepubertal).* Breasts have elevated papilla only. No pubic hair present.
  - *Stage II.* Breasts and papilla are elevated and appear as a small mound with enlarged areola diameter (median age 9.8 years, range <8 to 13 years). Sparse, long, pigmented hair develops chiefly along the labia majora (median age 10.5 years, range 8 to 13 years).
  - *Stage III.* Further breast enlargement occurs without separation of breast and areola (median age 11.2 years). Dark, coarse, curled pubic hair is sparsely spread over mons (median age 11.4 years).

- *Stage IV.* Secondary mound of areola and papilla develop above the breast (median age 12.1 years). Adult-type pubic hair is abundant but limited to the mons pubis (median age 12 years).
- *Stage V (Final Adult Stage).* Recession of areola occurs (median age 14.6 years, range 12 to 18 years). Pubic hair is of adult type in both quantity and distribution (median age 13.7 years, range 12 to 18 years).
- *Although the normal time frame for sexual development varies greatly, deviations do occur.* Variations from normal development are identified by the terms *precocious* and *delayed.* The health care provider must be aware of these aberrations and must ensure that complete family and medical histories are obtained (see Chapter 8).
- *Precocious Puberty.* Sexual development (see preceding discussion of Tanner staging) that occurs before age 8. Menarche may be the first sign of this early onset. Normal girls can begin to develop pubertal changes before age 8, according to new research. A growth spurt is usually the first sign. The onset is idiopathic in 75 percent of cases, but can be due to pathology, such as a CNS lesion or ovarian cyst, so evaluation is necessary (Gordon & Speroff, 2002).
- *Delayed Puberty.* Menarche is absent at age 18, or breast budding is completely absent at age 13. Delay may be familial, but other causes should be sought, including hyper- or hypogonadotropic hypogonadism, or eugonadism (Gordon & Speroff, 2002; Hacker & Moore, 1998; Murray, 1996).

- The reproductive years (Tanner Stage V) involve additional changes, for example, cyclic changes in the size, nodularity, and tenderness of the breasts, related to hormonal changes in the menstrual cycle. (Gordon & Speroff, 2002). These changes, along with an increase in total breast volume, occur maximally three to four days before the onset of menses and minimally in days four through seven of the menstrual cycle. Structural changes also occur, unrelated to the cycle. (Gordon & Speroff, 2002). Pubic hair may spread onto the inner aspect of the upper thighs. The female hair pattern is triangular, while the male is diamond-shaped, a possible clue that testosterone is too abundant if seen in the female. The labia majora increase in prominence; the labia minora and clitoris enlarge. Increased elasticity of vaginal tissue along with attainment of the mature vagina and ovarian size occurs.
- In older women note profound breast and genitalia effects as ovulation and estrogen production decline.

The perimenopause encompasses a period from about age 44 to 58. The median age of menopause is 51, with a normal range of about 45 to 55. Menopause before 40 is premature, and after 55, late. Ovulation usually continues until one to two years before menopause but declines in frequency from about age 40 until ending altogether. (Gordon & Speroff, 2002; Speroff, Glass, & Kase, 1999; Varner & Younger, 1995).

- *Breasts.* Breasts may begin to sag. Glandular tissue atrophies and is replaced by fat.
- *Hair Patterns.* Pubic hair turns gray and decreases in quantity. Axillary hair may also diminish. Hirsutism may develop, with coarse hair on the lip, chin, chest, abdomen, and back.
- *Genitalia and Reproductive Organs.* As estrogen levels decrease, the vulva appears atrophic and the labia and mons pubis flatten. Any lesion, especially in an older woman, may be cancerous and warrants evaluation. Gradually, the vaginal introitus constricts, the vagina becomes shorter and narrower, and the vaginal epithelium becomes thinner and less vascular, appearing pink, dry, and smooth with fewer rugae. The clitoris, cervix, and uterus become smaller. The uterus, about half the size of a woman's fist postmenopausally, may be difficult to palpate or may even prolapse because the ligaments and connective tissue of the pelvis sometimes lose their elasticity and tone. The ovaries and fallopian tubes also atrophy. Many changes may be less drastic with hormone replacement therapy. If significant stenosis is present vaginally, a one-finger bimanual examination is indicated. One-third of pelvic masses in women over 50 are malignant. (Dumesic, 1996). Uterine fibroids occur in one in five menopausal women, especially in African American women. Any enlarged organ or mass must be evaluated by a gynecologist. The normal ovary in menopause is approximately 2 cm $\times$ 1.5 cm $\times$ 0.5 cm.

Guidelines for Routine Examinations and Screening Tests

After menarche until death, self-examination of the breasts, vulva, and skin is indicated for all women. Signs and symptoms of cancer should be taught (see Table 4–10). Despite recent controversy regarding the value of mammography to prolong life, it offers the best breast screening test available at this date. Self-breast examination is advised monthly.

TABLE 4–10. Guidelines for Selected Screening Examinations and Tests for Healthy Nonpregnant Women

Exam/Test	18–39 years	40–59 years	60–74 years	75+ years
Physical examination[a]	q1y	q1y	q1y	q1y
Height/weight/BMI	q1y	q1y	q1y	q1y
Breast clinical examination	q1y	q1y	q1y	q1y
Pelvic and pap	q1y[c]	q1y	q1y	q1y
Rectal exam	q1y if at risk	q1y	q1y	q1y
Mammography	[b]	q1–2y[h]	q1y	q1y
Hematocrit/hemoglobin	Baseline & q10y or[d]	q10y or[d]	q10y or[d]	q10y or[d]
Blood glucose (fasting)	Baseline & [d]	q2–3y	q2–3y	q2–3y
Cholesterol, lipids (fasting)	Baseline & q5y	q5y	q5y	q5y
Stool for occult blood	[d]	q1y	q1y	q1y
Sigmoidoscopy/colonoscopy	[d]	q3–5y/10y[e]	q3–5y/10y[e]	q3–5y/10y[e]
Blood pressure	q1–2y[f]	q1–2y[f]	q1–2y[f]	q1–2y[f]
Urinalysis	[d]	q5y	q5y	q1y
Skin exam	q1y	q1y	q1y	q1y
Dental exam	q1y	q1y	q1y	q1y
Eye exam and glaucoma test	Baseline & q1–2y or[d]	1–2y or[d]	q1–2y or[d]	q1–2y or[d]
Hearing exam	Baseline @ 40	Repeat @ 50[g]	q1–3y[g]	q1–3y[g]
Endometrial sampling	[d]	[d]	[d]	[d]
Tuberculosis	[d]	[d]	[d]	[d]
Chest x-ray or CT lung scan	[d]	[d]	[d]	[d]
Thyroid testing (TSH)	[d]	Baseline & q3y	q3y	q3y
Bone density screening	[d]	Baseline & [d]	Baseline @ 65 & q3–5 years	

[a] After three consecutive normal physical examinations, clinical discretion advised for need for annual exam.

[b] Ultrasound and/or mammography indicated if clinical or risk factors present. Women on HRT with denser breasts may need to use raloxifene or tibolone or avoid HRT for a period prior to mammography.

[c] If sexually active, begin earlier. STD/HIV screen advised for any client at high risk. *Women with hysterectomies for noncancer reasons do not need annual Pap smears.*

[d] Indicated if risk factors present.

[e] After age 50, should have two consecutive annual negative evaluations before extending years between tests.

[f] Every year if BP is 130–139/85–89mm HG; if higher, repeat within two months and evaluate for hypertension.

[g] Audiogram may be needed as the woman ages.

[h] Researchers at University of Toronto reported no increased survival with early screening (Miller, To, Baines, & Wall, 2002).

Source: AWHONN, 2001; Board of Trustees, 2002; Mammography screening, 2002; Should I still, 2002; Slanetz, 2002; Two for 2002, 2002.

Guidelines for General Education and Anticipatory Guidance

Education and guidance should be targeted for certain age groups. See Table 4–11 for suggestions for targeting health information/guidance to all or specific age groups.

TABLE 4–11. Anticipatory Guidance Needed by Age Group

All age groups	Sun exposure, smoking, alcohol use, prescription/over-the-counter drug and supplement use, nutrition, driving accidents/seat belt use, family/marital/other relationships, school and work safety/stressors, fitness, stress, sleep, breast cancer, dental care, sexuality, sexually transmitted diseases/HIV/AIDS, immunizations, and violence/abuse.
Younger ages	Illicit substance use, parenting, contraception, pregnancy, managing multiple roles
Older ages	Falls and other accidents from changes in sensory and physical health, retirement, sensory deficiencies, self-care needs, bowel/bladder problems, menopause/climacteric transitions, loneliness/grief/loss, end-of-life planning

OVERVIEW OF COMMONLY INDICATED LABORATORY TESTS

CERVICAL CYTOLOGY

Papanicolaou Smear

Purpose. The Papanicolau (Pap) smear is a screening test for abnormal/atypical cells suggesting actual or possible preinvasive cervical neoplastic changes (Solomon, Davey, et al., 2002). Cervical cancer deaths have decreased 70 percent since the Pap smear use began in 1950 (Advisor Forum, 2002). New cases of cervical cancer in U.S. women in 2000 were 12,800; approximately 4,600 women died from this cancer in 2001 (CDC, 2001). The U.S. incidence for cervical cancer in 1997 was highest in Hispanic and black women (Eberhardt et al., 2001, Table 55). It ranks thirty-fifth in causes of deaths in U.S. women and is less common than uterine and ovarian cancer. A NIH Consensus expert panel found that women who are poor, over 65, uninsured, ethnic minorities, and rural dwellers have low screening rates and high cervical cancer rates (National Institutes of Health, 1996). Cervical cancer is a major solid tumor that is virally induced in nearly all cases by human papillomavirus (HPV) DNA. There are more than 100 types of HPV; more than thirty infect the genital area (CDC, 2001). The most common types (16, 18, 31, and 45) account for more than 80 percent of all invasive cancers of the cervix (National Institutes of Health, 1996; Richart, Ferenczy, Trofatter, & Tyring, 1999). Thirteen high risk HPV types, most frequently 16, 18, 31, and 51, were found in one study, and two to five types were present at the same time in 24 percent of samples (Perrons, Kleter, et al., 2002). Preinvasive lesions are categorized in a variety of ways. Squamous intraepithelial lesions (SIL), either low-grade (LSIL) or high-grade (HSIL), encompass terminology of cervical intraepithelial neoplasia (CIN) grades 1, 2, or 3 (more serious with the increasing numeral), and dysplasia (mild, moderate, or severe). This varied terminology can be confusing, but the new 2001 Bethesda System for reporting cervical cytology results is helpful in interpretation (see Table 4–12) (Wright et al., 2002a). (See Chapter 13 for more information on cervical cancer.)

Thirty-three percent of SIL lesions regress; 41 percent stay the same; and 25 percent become more advanced. Ten percent of these latter lesions become carcinoma in situ (CIS); one percent become invasive. Viral transmission is through sexual intercourse, with the prevalence decreasing with age. The peak incidence is between 22 and 25 years. Thus, a host immune response may occur, and this knowledge is fueling efforts to find preventive and curative vaccines (NIH, 1996).

Because it has a long preclinical phase, squamous cervical cancer is ideal for screening. Although the Pap smear can identify some infections of the cervix and vagina, other more definitive tests are needed for diagnosis (see Chapter 11). The Pap smear may be used to evaluate the hormonal status of squamous cells, but modern serum hormone levels are more precise. New research and consensus of experts indicate that routine screening every two years from age 20 until death with both Pap and HPV tests may provide the most savings in lives lost to cervical cancer (Mandelblatt, Lawrence, et al., 2002; Solomon, Schiffman, & Tarone, 2002; Wright et al., 2002a). However, risk factors for an individual woman should dictate the need to continue biennial screening beyond age 65. The combined tests (called "parallel screen-

ing") increase sensitivity without decreasing specificity (Mandelblatt et al, 2002, p. 2378). Pap tests alone carry 25 to 50 percent false-negative rates, have poor reproducibility, and have the potential for misclassification of the results. Pap smear plus HPV testing may be more cost effective since years of life would be saved at an acceptable increase in cost. HPV testing alone may become the future screening method of choice as the cost reaches a threshold of $5 per test since it is less costly than Paps in materials and manpower. Its future use for high-risk populations will be preferred since it has greater sensitivity than Pap smears and the potential for the patient to collect the specimen herself (Mandelblatt et al., 2002). The Hybrid Capture®, one example of a HPV DNA test, was found to be 10 to 15 percent more sensitive than Pap smears in a study of 10,000 women in Costa Rica (Study: New test, 1998).

Technique for Conventional Slide Pap Smear. To obtain the best possible specimen for the conventional Pap test (CPT) or any cervical cytology test, be precise. It is essential to get samples from the transformation zone (the squamocolumnar junction), the usual site of abnormal changes. (Solomon et al., 2002). Sampling error is a major factor in false negative smears. Be sure that the entire cervix is visible. For CPT, use the endocervical cytobrush instead of a cotton-tipped applicator and the plastic spatula instead of a wooden spatula; the cotton-tipped applicator and wooden spatula may hold the best cells in porous material. The endocervical brush increases the endocervical cells obtained by sevenfold. (Taylor, Andersen, Barber, et al., 1987). If a cotton-tipped applicator must be used, wet in normal saline first so that the cells will be released from the fibers onto the slide. The brush may be used for the pregnant woman, but warn her that spotting may occur; in fact, this is true for many nonpregnant women. Do not use the long pointed end of the spatula in pregnancy. Be sure all slides are labeled correctly with name, date, source, and that the slides match the paperwork.

Steps in obtaining the Pap smear sample include the following (ACOG, 1993):

- Collect *before* the bimanual.
- *No* lubricant should be used on the speculum; will interfere with cytology. Water is acceptable.
- Collect the Pap smear *before* other tests, such as GC and chlamydia tests. This order of collection is clearly supported by ACOG; the rationale is to ensure the best sample with suspicious cells for the Pap smear.

TABLE 4-12. Cervical Cytology Results, Interpretation, and Recommended Actions for the Primary Care Provider

Cervical Cytology Results	Interpretation	Recommended Actions
Negative for intraepithelial lesions or malignancy. Optional to report non-neoplastic findings other than organisms. These include but are not limited to reactive cellular changes associated with inflammation (includes typical repair), radiation, IUD, glandular cells post hysterectomy, atrophy. Organisms that may be reported include such organisms as _Trichomonas vaginalis_, fungal organisms consistent with _Candida_ species, shift in flora suggestive of bacterial vaginosis, bacteria morphologically consistent with _Actinomyces_ species, cellular changes consistent with herpes simplex virus	Now includes many former "ASCUS, favor reactive" results that have previously been considered more serious. More serious ones are included in ASC. The interpretation of the optional or organism findings should be interpreted in light of the history, the physical findings, and other appropriate laboratory findings.	Repeat in one year. If the woman has had three or more normal consecutive yearly results and has no known risk factors, testing may be repeated in 2 years. If there is a non-neoplastic finding reported, management should be specific to the cause. Treatment of organisms is dependent upon other findings. The woman should be reexamined and tested for the specific problem and then treated appropriately if indicated.
No endocervical cells The presence or absence of endocervical cells is provided if adequate squamous cells are present. Ten endocervical cells should be present that are well-preserved.	The specimen contained no endocervical cells, hence may have missed the squamocolumnar junction in the transformation zone.	If judged "satisfactory for evaluation," repeat cytology is not necessary for one year if the woman is not at high risk and had negative cytology a year past. If judged "unsatisfactory for evaluation," repeat in 3–4 months. If the woman is at risk for cervical cancer, repeat the cervical cytology in 8–12 weeks.
Atypical squamous cells (ASC) (qualified in two categories as follows:)	The cellular abnormalities are more marked than can be attributed to reactive change, but cannot be definitively called squamous epithelial lesions (SIL). They fall short of being SIL in quantity or quality.	See specific recommendations for ASC-US and ASC-H.
ASC-US (Atypical squamous cells of undetermined significance)	All ASC suggests SIL, and some ASC-US is associated with CIN 2,3, but the risk of invasive cancer is low.	Three options available: 1. Repeat cervical cytology. If positive, refer for colposcopy. If negative, repeat at 4–6 months. If positive, refer for colposcopy. If negative, move to routine screening. If liquid-based cytology used for initial cytology, provides for reflex HPV DNA testing. 2. HPV DNA testing; if positive, refer for colposcopy. If negative, repeat cytology at 12 months. 3. Refer for colposcopy and if no CIN or cancer, test for HPV. If negative or unknown, repeat cytology at 12 months. If CIN or cancer, management follows ASCCP guidelines.[1]

TABLE 4–12. Cervical Cytology Results, Interpretation, and Recommended Actions for the Primary Care Provider

Cervical Cytology Results	Interpretation	Recommended Actions
ASC-US in special circumstances *Postmenopause:*	Ascertain if atrophy present; may be causing the results.	If no contraindications and atrophy present, give course of intravaginal estrogen, then repeat cervical cytology test about one week after completion of therapy. If result negative, repeat at 4–6 months × 2. If negative, return to routine cytology. If a repeat test is ASC, refer for colposcopy.
Pregnancy:		Manage same as ASC-US result for nonpregnant woman.
Immunosuppression:	Includes women with HIV, without consideration of CD4 cell count, HIV viral load, or type of therapy.	Refer for colposcopy.
ASC-H (Atypical squamous cells: cannot exclude high-grade SIL)	5–10% of ASC cases are in this category. It contains a mixture of real HSIL and cells that mimic. It is positively predictive for CIN 2,3 that falls between ASC-US and HSIL.	Refer for colposcopy. If biopsy confirms CIN, managed by ASCCP guidelines. If no CIN found, specimens are reviewed again; management proceeds based on the revised finding.
Atypical glandular cells (AGC) *(includes categories of endocervical, endometrial or glandular cells not otherwise specified; AGC favor neoplasia, and AIS.*	Glandular abnormalities are considered less severe than adenocarcinoma, but associated with a much greater risk for cancer than ASC or LSIL.	See categories for AGC.
AGC, either endocervical, endometeral, or glandular cells not otherwise specified (AGC-NOS)	AGC-NOS women are believed to be at lower risk for neoplasia than AGC women.	All AGC results require colposcopy referral except endometrial atypia, which requires endometrial sampling. With invasive disease, refer to a specialist. With no invasive disease for AGC-NOS, if neoplasia, manage by ASCCP guidelines. If no neoplasia, cytology should be repeated at 4–6 months × 4. If ASC or LSIL, colposcopy needed or referral to expert. If HSIL or ACG, diagnostic excision needed.
AGC, favor neoplasia	This result indicates a higher risk of having high grade CIN lesions upon biopsy.	Requires diagnostic excisional procedure such as cold-knife conization.
AIS (endocervical adenocarcinoma in situ)	AIS result is associated with a very high risk of having AIS or invasive cervical adenocarinoma.	Refer to expert for diagnostic excisional procedure and/or other definitive management.
Low-grade squamous intraepithelial lesions (LSIL)	Squamous cervical abnormalities are considered to be noninvasive; with no lesion or CIN1. However, women with LSIL are considered at higher risk for developing CIN 2,3.	Refer for colposcopy. With satisfactory colposcopy and lesion, endocervical biopsy is considered acceptable. With satisfactory colposcopy and no lesion or unsatisfactory colposcopy, endocervical biopsy is preferred. Management is dependent upon findings.

Low-grade squamous intraepithelial lesions (LSIL) in special circumstances:

Postmenopause: Initial colposcopy is not necessary. Important to evaluate for atrophy and contraindication to vaginal estrogen use.

Repeat cytology at 6 and 12 months. If ASC-US or greater, refer for colposcopy. If negative, repeat cytology at 4–6 months. Alternative to cytology is to perform HPV DNA testing at 12 months after initial LSIL Pap; if positive, refer for colposcopy. If negative, repeat cytology at 12 months. If atrophy present, treat first with course of intravaginal estrogen (assuming no contraindications); refer if repeat cytology 1 week after treatment completed indicates ASC-US or greater result.

Pregnancy:

See HSIL in special circumstances.

Adolescence:

Repeat cytology at 6 and 12 months; refer if ASC for colposcopy; **or** do HPV DNA testing at 12 months after initial SIL Pap; refer for colposcopy if positive for high risk HPV DNA; **or** send for colposcopy initially.

High-grade squamous intraepithelial lesion (HSIL)

Not a common diagnosis. Predicts a 70–75% chance of having CIN 2, 3 (biopsy-confirmed) or a 1–2% chance of invasive cervical cancer.

Refer for colposcopy with endocervical assessment. If colposcopy satisfactory without CIN or with CIN 1, specimen reviewed and management based on revised results. If colposcopy satisfactory with CIN 2,3 confirmed, managed by ASCCP guidelines. If colposcopy unsatisfactory and no lesion, specimen reviewed and management based on revised results. If colposcopy unsatisfactory but biopsy confirms CIN, ASCCP guidelines employed.

High-grade squamous intraepithelial lesion (HSIL) in special circumstances:

Pregnancy:

Colposcopic evaluation indicated by experienced clinicians who are experienced in evaluating pregnancy-induced colposcopic changes. Pregnancy contraindicates endocervical curettage.

If colposcopy unsatisfactory, repeat colposcopy at 6 to 12 weeks recommended. If no invasive cancer, repeat cytology and colposcopy. With invasive cancer, diagnostic excisional biopsy recommended. Otherwise no treatment is recommended.

Reproductive age:

If HSIL on cytology confirmed but no CIN 2,3 confirmed with biopsy, colposcopy and cytology is recommended at 4 to 6 month intervals for 1 year (if colposcopic is satisfactory, endocervical sampling is negative, and woman understands and accepts risks). Any lesion that progresses indicates a need for diagnostic excisional biopsy.

---

[1]ASCCP is the American Society for Colposcopy and Cervical Pathology.

Sources: ACOG, 1995; Solomon et al., 2002; Stoler, 2002; Wright et al., 2002a, 2002b.

- If a wet mount is to be done, collect the specimen from the vaginal fornices before the Pap or any test is done to avoid blood from the Pap.
- Remove large amounts of discharge with a cellulose swab from the portio of the cervix gently before taking smears.
- Do not take the sample if large amounts of menses are present; will obscure cytologic field. A partially obscured specimen means 50 to 75 percent of cells cannot be visualized. An unsatisfactory specimen means that more than 75 percent of cells cannot be visualized (Solomon et al., 2002).
- Obtain portio sample first with the spatula, then the endocervical brush sample since bleeding occurs frequently with the latter. If cervical shape/characteristics are not configured to ease of rotating the spatula, gently scrape it over the surface of the cervix. Remember, you want to get as complete a specimen from the transformation zone as possible.
- Rotate the brush 360° gently to minimize bleeding if possible. Be prepared to apply pressure with a large cotton-tipped applicator should bleeding occur after all specimens are obtained and before removing the speculum.
- Apply smear material evenly on the slide without clumping and fix rapidly (within 10 seconds); drying will significantly alter the sample. If using one slide, material must be collected very quickly to prevent drying effects. Ideally, two slides are desirable.
- Be sure to rotate brush or paint cells with spatula onto a slide with slight pressure.
- The squamocolumnar junction may be out on the ectocervix. If so, use the more rounded end of the spatula to collect cells.
- If the newer, fan-type implement is used to collect the squamocolumnar junction specimen, rotate it several times in the os to get an adequate number of cells.
- Do not repeat a Pap smear in fewer than eight weeks. Follow the Bethesda guidelines for repeat intervals if this method is being used for ASC follow-up.

The transformation zone (TZ) may be quite different in different age groups. The TZ at the squamocolumnar junction (SCJ) where the cells from the ectocervix and endocervix meet is the most vulnerable to HPV DNA effects. It is particularly vulnerable in the adolescent woman whose TZ is further out on the portio of the cervix. Hence, ACOG's recommendation to begin cervical cytology at 18 years or with onset of sexual activity.

In the older woman, the clinician must be sure to seek the specimen higher in the endocervix where the SQJ is likely to be found.

Technique for Liquid-Based Cervical Cell Collection. A number of cytological cell collection systems that use a liquid-based or liquid-fixed method are on the market. Typically, a broom implement is used to sweep the cervix (central portion inserted in the cervical os and rotated, then removed and placed in the provided fixative container). Conventional Pap test (CPT) compared with liquid-based cervical cytology (LBCC) found the percentage of satisfactory Pap tests significantly higher for LBCC and significantly lower for the percentage of unsatisfactory or limited satisfactory tests (Ferris, Heidemann, Litaker, Crosby, & Macfee, 2000). The ThinPrep method, as with other methods, uses an automated processor to prepare a thin-layer slide that is read by computers (Massarani-Wafai, Bakhos, Wojcik, & Selvaggi, 2000). Adding an additional slide to evaluate the cellular residue using the ThinPrep method does not enhance the overall diagnosis. The ThinPrep method using one slide provides a satisfactory diagnostic sample; however, it has been found not to be statistically significantly better than the CPT if the portio of the cervix is not cleared gently of mucus and debris before the sample is taken (Obwegeser & Brack, 2001). Another method of LBCC, SpinThin, provides data that correlates well with conventional smears (Khalbuss, Rudomina, Kauff, Chuang, & Melamed, 2000). There are a number of such systems available and clinicians should examine their effectiveness as compared to the conventional Pap smear technique before adopting. The technique for each should be carefully reviewed and applied. LBCC tends to be more expensive for the client. If the woman is high risk, one of these methods may be useful to provide additional data in assessment for reflex testing for HPV DNA if cervical atypia or abnormality are found. The LBCC specimen may be used for the further testing (Wright et al., 2002a, b).

HPV DNA TESTING

Human papillomavirus (HPV) DNA testing employs "highly sensitive, molecular methods" of screening for cervical abnormality (Wright et al., 2002). Sensitivity for finding CIN 2, 3 confirmed by biopsy in women who have ASC is very high: 0.83 to 1.0. The National Cancer Institute (NCI) conducted a study to compare sensitivity and specificity of methods to detect CIN 3 in ASCUS-diagnosed women (Solomon, Schiffman, & Tarone; ALTS Study Group, 2001). Women were randomized for colposcopy, repeat Pap smear every six months, or HPV testing using Hybrid Capture 2™. HPV testing was 96 percent sensitive in accurately indicating a need for colposcopy as opposed to repeat Pap testing being only 86 percent sensitive (even less so with only one repeat Pap). Other studies have supported similar findings, leading the 2001 Consensus Guidelines group to include HPV testing alone or in combination with a cervical cytology test in its recommendations for ASC results (Wright et al., 2002). Reflex HPV DNA testing is an advantage for women with ASC, eliminating a visit for a return pelvic exam to collect the specimen and sparing the need for colposcopy in 40 to 60 percent (Wright et al., 2002). To obtain the sample, collect the endocervical and ectocervical cells specimen following directions for use of the provided swab or other implement from the laboratory and place in the provided transport medium container. Follow instructions for maintaining until transport.

Interpretation of Results and Action

The 2001 Bethesda System is the test reporting system used nationwide that tells the provider the category of the findings and the recommended action (Wright et al., 2002). The categories have been modified from the original Bethesda system to include atypical squamous cells (ASC) with subcategories (ASC-US and ASC-H) and recommendations, including those for special circumstances such as pregnancy; atypical glandular cells (AGC) with subcategories less severe than adenocarcinoma but including endocervical cancer in-situ (AIS) and recommendations for follow-up; low-grade squamous intraepithelial lesion (LSIL) with recommendations for LSIL with and without cervical lesions and in special circumstances such as postmenopause; and high-grade squamous intraepithelial lesion (HSIL) with recommendations for management with colposcopy and special circumstances (see Table 4–12). The information in this table is selected from the most current management recommendations at the time of this writing (Wright et al., 2002a, b).

GONORRHEA AND CHLAMYDIA TESTS

Purpose

Testing is done most often in women, especially if high risk and/or between 15 and 25 years, to diagnose both gonorrhea (GC) and chlamydia (CT) (see Chapter 11 for further information on these diseases) (Chapin, 1999). In many instances, if chlamydia is present, gonorrhea is also. Screening for CT is recommended for all women aged 25 and younger whether pregnant or non-pregnant (USPSTF, 2002). One study by Turner et al. (2002) found that nearly 8 percent of Baltimore adults ages 18 to 35 had GC or CT that was untreated (Hidden STD, 2002). Cultures were the gold standard for years to diagnose both *Neisseria gonorrhoeae* diplococci and the *Chlamydia trachomatis* intracellular parasite. However, newer screening tests are being used now that do not require the intense care that cultures require to maintain stability and proper transport, as well as costly time and money for evaluation. A RNA hybridization assay probe test, the Gen-Probe DNA test, is available to diagnose GC and CT simultaneously (Chapin, 1999). Target RNA is extracted from the woman's specimen; labeled DNA probe sequences specific for GC and for CT are added to the specimen; if the RNA of the organism is present, a tight helix forms on the probe that is measured by an optical scanner. The test has all the components needed for screening: high sensitivity and specificity, fairly low cost, ease of use, and ease of handling (Chapin, 1999). For screening large numbers of people, Turner et al. (2002) used a nucleic acid amplification test (NAAT) that required urine samples. The researchers suggest that all young adults be tested using NAAT. (See Chapter 11 for more information on diagnosis of GC and CT.)

Technique for Gen-Probe DNA Test

Prepare the woman for an exam requiring a speculum insertion. Collect the specimen after the cervical cytology. Use one of the two sterile swabs to clean off excess mucus from the cervical os and portio around os. Be sure to discard this swab. Insert the second swab 1 to 1.5 cm into endocervical canal, rotate 10 to 30 seconds, withdraw without touching the vaginal walls or any other area, and place in the transport medium. Break the swab shaft where scored and place the cap securely. The specimen may be kept at room temperature or refrigerated for up to seven days (Chapin, 1999).

Results

Results are reported as positive or negative for both GC and CT. A small number of samples do not provide definitive results and retesting is needed (0.5 to 1.0 percent). The lab normally repeats the test, but if it continues to be indefinite, the woman may need to return for another specimen to be collected. If there is excessive gross blood, the specimen may be false-positive. Avoid collecting specimens during menses. It is controversial about the order to take the specimen since the cytobrush for the Pap may cause bleeding. Women at risk for GC or CT are also at risk for HPV. All three have negative consequences. Follow the policy of the site where the client is being seen for guidance. If the woman has recently taken an antibiotic, a false-negative result may occur. For positive results, it is crucial to test and treat the partner. Presumptive treatment may be given if signs and symptoms indicate infection. Retesting is indicated if the woman does not improve with treatment or if an area where resistant GC is known to occur. Three weeks after treatment is completed, a test-of-cure is indicated in women who are pregnant, trying to become pregnant, or of a young age (Chapin, 1999).

WET MOUNTS: NORMAL SALINE AND POTASSIUM HYDROXIDE

Purpose

Wet mounts (or preps) are done primarily to diagnose selected vaginal infections and to assist in determining causes of bleeding. A normal saline wet mount of vaginal secretions from a normal childbearing age nonpregnant woman shows lactobacilli and epithelial cells.

Technique

Wear gloves to collect and while handling specimens. Dip cotton swab into vaginal/cervical discharge pooled under the cervix in the posterior and lateral fornices; place in tube with 1 mL saline; mix; drop one drop on clean slide and cover with coverslip. Dip second swab into discharge; place in tube with 1 mL of 10 percent potassium hydroxide (KOH) and mix; drop one drop on clean slide or same slide at other end; cover. Blue or green food dye may be added to enhance visibility of organisms/cells. Evaluate with low and high power microscope objectives. The value of the specimen is proportional to the effectiveness of the collection techniques and the quality of the provider's interpretation. Vaginal/cervical discharge specimen may also be placed directly on a slide with a drop of solution, rather than placed in a tube, and covered with a coverslip for viewing. KOH is used to disrupt the epithelial cells (though not totally destroyed); gets rid of debris that may obscure hyphae and bacteria that are resistant to KOH and easily seen. Obtaining the specimen(s) prior to

cervical cytology or other tests is advised to avoid red blood cells obscuring the field.

Results

The following may be analyzed from a saline wet mount (Iglesias, Alderman, & Fox, 2000; Monif, 2002):

- Normal squamous epithelial cells—have smooth borders, few bacteria visible inside the cell, single central nuclei
- "Clue cells"—squamous epithelial cells with irregular, obscured border from multiple cocci adhered to outer cell membrane; have stippled appearance; indicative of bacterial vaginosis (BV)
- Lactobacilli—rod-shaped bacteria evidencing acidity of normal vaginal environment; not found or decreased significantly in BV
- Polymorphonuclear leukocytes (PMNs)—in great numbers (more than 10 per high power field) indicates infection, such as GC or CT
- Red blood cells—indicates obvious or microscopic bleeding; may indicate need for diagnosis if cause unknown
- Trichomonads—motile protozoa indicative of trichomoniasis vaginitis
- Spores and/or hyphae—indicate fungal infection, such as with *Candida albicans.*

If the wet mount is prepared with 10 percent KOH, the epithelial cells are lysed, and fungal spores and hyphae are easier to visualize (Iglesias et al., 2000). Management of the findings of any wet mount are dependent on the problem (see Chapter 11 for diagnosis and treatment of selected vaginitis and STDs). Providers who use vaginal microscopy for diagnosis should gain depth in this area through special study and practice.

Taking a vaginal swab and storing it for up to 20 minutes at room temperature in a glass tube allows the swab to be cultured for *T. vaginalis* if a wet mount is negative (Schwebke, 2002). This short period of time does not decrease the culture's sensitivity.

EVALUATING VAGINAL pH

Purpose

A pH level of 3.8 to 4.2 is normal in the vagina and must be maintained to help keep the vaginal environment stable (ACOG Technical Bulletin, 1996, No. 226). Lactobacillus acidophilus bacteria keep the vaginal ecosystem healthy by production of lactic acid that suppresses gram-negative and gram-positive anaerobes. Lactobacilli also produce toxic-to-anaerobes hydrogen peroxide. If the lactobacilli growth is suppressed, pH level rises, hydrogen ion concentration falls, and pathogen growth is favored. Testing pH level helps in determining imbalances.

Technique and Results

Special pH paper is placed on the lateral vaginal wall or in vaginal secretions. If the pH is >4.5, an increase in gram-negative facultative anaerobes and gram-positive and gram-negative obligate anaerobes is the probable cause, as is seen with bacterial vaginosis (ACOG, 1996). Placing a drop of vaginal discharge in a drop of 10 percent potassium hydroxide (KOH) gives off a fishy odor as amines are released. This is called a positive whiff test and indicates possible BV or trichomoniasis.

URINALYSIS

Purpose

A urinalysis provides supportive data in diagnosing urinary complaints; however, it should not be used alone if results are negative but other findings indicate that a problem exists. As many as 30 percent of women with acute lower UTIs have low colony counts of the causative bacteria (Mata, 1998). Urine culture is the gold standard for diagnosing UTI. Dipstick reagent strip findings of nitrites, leukocytes, and blood plus microscopic urinalysis data are usually adequate to indicate need for treatment in simple cystitis. Culture and sensitivity should be used with persistent bacteriuria (Mata, 1998). As few as two bacteria seen in a high-power field when the specimen has been centrifuged has a 90 percent sensitivity and specificity for diagnosing significant bacteriuria.

Technique for Urine Specimen

Instruct the client to wash her hands well and collect a midstream urine specimen. A clean-catch specimen is not necessary. Studies indicate that a midstream collection is adequate. (Leisure, Dudley, & Donowitz, 1993). Use a tampon or cotton ball in the introitus during collection of urine if heavy vaginal discharge or bleeding is present. Test or culture the specimen within a few minutes, or refrigerate it with a tight cover and test within a few hours.

- ◆ If screening for nitrite and normal pH, a dipstick test is done on a first morning urine specimen. Keep dipsticks in cool, dark, tightly closed container. Assess glucose, ketones, blood, leukocytes, protein, and specific gravity.
- ◆ Microscopic examination should be done on centrifuged sediment, or a specimen may be sent out for analysis. Look for white blood cells (WBCs, or leukocytes) red blood cells (RBCs, or erythrocytes), crystals, bacteria, epithelial cells, and casts. Use low light to see casts better.
- ◆ Culture and sensitivity tests are indicated when the number of WBCs is greater than five per high power field or when Microstix indicates infection.

Results

All findings should be within normal limits (see standard laboratory testing text or manual).

HERPES CULTURE AND TYPE-SPECIFIC TESTS

Purpose

Culture is done to definitively diagnose herpes simplex genitalis (ACOG Practice Bulletin, 1999, No. 8) (see Chapter 11 for more information).

Technique

Wear glasses to protect eyes and cover unclothed skin with a mask, gloves, gown, and/or lab coat. Carefully puncture (unroof) intact vesicle with sterile tuberculin needle or rub open lesion vigorously (if vesicle already draining) with saline moistened Dacron tipped or cotton swab to get viral sample (ACOG, 1999). Vesicular fluid is needed for testing; it is high in viral particles. Place specimen in culture medium immediately. Do not swab to dry. If obtaining a cervical culture, the swab is inserted in the endocervix and rotated, then rubbed over the ectocervix. Refrigerate and transport within 12 hours or follow directions for transport and storage. There are a number of type-specific serologic assays based upon gG-1 and gG-2 (the significant amino acid that is different between the two types of herpes simplex) (Schmid, Brown, Nisenbaum, Burke, et al., 1999). Herpes simplex type 1 (HSV-1) and herpes simplex type 2 (HSV-2) can be detected using type-specific serologic assays (Palu, Calestri,

Concellotti, Cusan, et al., 2001). Examples of assays are immudot (POCkit HSV-2), enzyme-linked immunosorbent assay (ELISA), HSV-infected cell-based Western blotting, baculovirus–expressed gG immunoblotting, and immunoblot strip (Palu et al., 2001; Schmid et al., 1999). The most reliable method is the Western blotting of HSV-infected cell lysates because it examines the antibody response to more immunogenic HSV proteins than just gG (Schmid et al., 1999). However, these tests often lack either specificity (POCkit HSV-2) or sensitivity (ELISA) (Palu et al., 2001). Although results can be obtained much more quickly than with the culture, which may be an advantage, until the sensitivity and specificity issues of gG-based serology are controlled, such tests should not be used routinely in place of the culture (Schmid et al., 1999).

Results

Positive culture growth of type 1 or type 2 herpes simplex virus (HSV) takes 2 to 3 days for results, but laboratories wait 7 to 14 days to be sure results are negative.

SENSITIVITY, SPECIFICITY, AND PREDICTIVE VALUE OF TESTS

Clinicians must understand the concepts of sensitivity, specificity, and predictive value to use and interpret test results effectively. The Bluestein and Archer (1991) reference is highly recommended to readers.

Sensitivity is the percentage of people who have a positive test who have the disease or condition. A sensitive test is used when the goal is to detect all people with the disease because undetection consequences can be disastrous. An example is the initial ELISA test for HIV antibodies. The test is to miss the lowest number of those exposed to the virus, though some nonexposed are expected to have a positive test.

Specificity is the percentage of people with no disease who have a negative test. It takes the number of people without disease and a negative test and divides it by the total number of nondiseased people. An example is the Western Blot test, which is very specific for HIV antibodies and is quite unlikely to be positive if HIV antibodies are absent.

Predictive value helps predict disease status. Positive predictive value (PV+) is the probability of disease if a test is positive, and negative predictive value (PV−) is the probability if a test is negative. The predictive value of a test utilizes disease prevalence in a particular site along with sensitivity and specificity. For example, a positive ELISA is more likely to be a false positive result in a setting where prevalence of disease is low.

REFERENCES

AAFP, ADA, & NCOA. (1994). *Incorporating nutrition screening and interventions into medical practice: A monograph for physicians.* Washington, DC: The Nutrition Screening Initiative.

Acierno, R., Resnick, H., Kilpatrick, D. G., Saunders, B., & Best, C. L. (1999). Risk factors for rape, physical assault, and post-traumatic stress disorder in women. *Journal of Anxiety Disorders, 13* (6): 541–563.

Ackard, D., Neumark-Sztainer, D., Hannan, P., French, S., & Story, M. (2001). Binge and purge behavior among adolescents: Associations with sexual and physical abuse in a nationally representative sample: The Commonwealth Fund survey. *Child Abuse and Neglect, 25*(6), 771–785.

ACOG Technical Bulletin. (1993). *Cervical cytology: Evaluation and management of abnormalities.* No. 183. Washington, DC: ACOG.

ACOG Committee Opinion. (1995). *Absences of endocervical cells on a Pap test.* No. 153. Washington, DC: ACOG.

ACOG. (1996, May). FDA orders food fortification with folic acid. *ACOG Newsletter, 46* (5): 1–2.

ACOG Technical Bulletin. (1996). *Vaginitis.* No. 226. Washington, DC: ACOG.

ACOG Practice Bulletin. (1999). *Management of herpes in pregnancy.* No 8. Washington, DC: ACOG.

Advisor Forum. (2002, February). HPV screening vs. Pap smear for cancer detection. *The Clinical Advisor, 57.*

Akukwe, C. (2000). Maternal and child health services in the twenty-first century: Critical issues, challenges, and opportunities. *Health Care for Women International, 21*(7), 641–653.

Al-Delaimy, W., Manson, J., Willett, W., & Stampfer, M. (2002). Snoring as a risk factor for type II diabetes mellitus: A prospective study. *American Journal of Epidemiology, 155*(5), 394–395.

American Dietetic Association. (2001). Position of the American Dietetic Association: Food fortification and dietary supplements. *Journal of the American Dietetic Association, 101*(1), 115–125.

American Psychiatric Association. (2000). *Diagnostic and statistical manual of mental disorders* (4th ed.). Washington, DC: Author.

Ancoli-Israel, S. & Roth, T. (1999). Characteristics of insomnia in the United States: Results of the 1991 National Sleep Foundation Survey I. *Sleep, 22*(Suppl 2), S347–S353.

Anderson, C. (2002). Battered and pregnant: A nursing challenge. *AWHONN Lifelines, 6*(2), 95–99.

Arbuckle, T., & Sever, L. (1998). Pesticide exposures and fetal death: A review of the epidemiologic literature. *Critical Review of Toxicology, 28*(3), 229–270.

Armstrong, G.L., Conn, L.A., & Pinner, R.W. (1999). Trends in infectious disease mortality in the United States during the 20th century. *Journal of the American Medical Association, 281*(1), 61–66.

Aral, S. (2001). Sexually transmitted diseases: Magnitude, determinants and consequences. *International Journal of STD AIDS, 12*(4), 211–215.

Astone, N.M., Ensminger, M., & Juon, H.S. (2002). Early adult characteristics and mortality among inner-city African American women. *American Journal of Public Health, 92*(4), 640.

Auslander, G.K. (1988). Social networks and the functional health status of the poor: A secondary analysis of data from the national survey of personal health practices and consequences. *Journal of Community Health, 13,* 197–209.

Avis, N., Crawford, S., Stellato, R., & Longcope, C. (2001). Longitudinal study of hormone levels and depression among women transitioning through menopause. *Climacteric, 4*(3), 243–249.

AWHONN. (2001). *Every woman: The essential guide for healthy living.* New York: Profile Pursuit.

Bath, S., Singleton, J., Stikas, R., Steveson, J., et al. (2000). Performance of U.S. hospitals on recommended screening and immunization practices for pregnant and postpartum women. *American Journal of Infection Control, 28*(5), 327–332.

Bauer, G., & Welles, S. (2001). Beyond assumptions of negligible risk: Sexually transmitted diseases and women who have sex with women. *American Journal of Public Health, 91*(8), 1282–1286.

Becker, K., & Walton-Moss, B. (2001). Detecting and addressing alcohol abuse in women. *Nurse Practitioner, 26*(10), 13–16, 19–23.

Bennett, S., Perkins, S., Lane, K., Deer, M., Brater, D., & Murray, M. (2001). Social support and health-related quality of life in chronic heart failure patients. *Quality of Life Research, 10*(8), 671–682.

Berg, C.J., Atrash, H.K., Koonin, L.M., & Tucker, M. (1996). Pregnancy-related mortality in the United States, 1987–1990. *Obstetrics and Gynecology, 88*(2), 161–167.

Bertoni, A.G., Krop, J.S., Anderson, G.F., & Brancati, F.L. (2002). Diabetes-related morbidity and mortality in a national sample of U.S. elders. *Diabetes Care, 25*(3), 471–475.

Binder, W., Birge, S., & Kohrt, W. (1996). Effects of endurance exercise and hormonal replacement therapy on serum lipids in older women. *Journal of the American Geriatric Society, 44,* 331–332.

Blair, S., Kampert, J., Kohl II, H., et al. (1996). Influences of cardiopulmonary fitness and other precursors of cardiovascular disease and all-cause mortality in men and women. *JAMA, 276*(3), 205–210.

Bluestein, D., & Archer, L. (1991). The sensitivity, specificity and predictive value of diagnostic information: A guide for clinicians. *Nurse Practitioner, 16*(7), 39–45.

Board of Trustees of The North American Menopause Society. (2002). Management of postmenopausal osteoporosis: Position statement of The North American Menopause Society. *Menopause, 9*(2), 84–101.

Borrelli, B., Hogan, J.W., Bock, B., Pinto, B., Roberts, M., & Marcus, B. (2002). Predictors of quitting and dropout among women in a clinic-based smoking cessation program. *Psychology of Addict Behavior, 16*(1), 22–27.

Buboltz, W., Jr., Brown, F., & Soper, B. (2001). Sleep habits and patterns of college students: A preliminary study. *Journal of American College Health, 50*(3), 131–135.

Butrica, B., & Iams, H. (2000). Divorced women at retirement: Projections of economic well-being in the near future. *Social Security Bulletin, 63*(3), 3–12.

Byers, T., Nestle, M., McTiernan, A., Doyle, C., Currie-Williams, A., Gansler, T., Thun, M., & American Cancer Society 2001 Nutrition and Physical Activity Guidelines Advisory Committee. (2002). American Cancer Society guidelines on nutrition and physical activity for cancer prevention: Reducing the risk of cancer with health food choices and physical activity. *CA Cancer Journal Clin, 52*(20), 92–119.

By the Way, Doctor. (2002). Demystifying calcium. *Harvard Women's Health Watch, IX*(9), 8.

CDC National Center for Chronic Disease Prevention and Health Promotion (CDCNCCDPHP). (2000). Adolescent and School Health. (updated June 08, 2000). *National: These leading causes of death result from these risk behaviors.* Retrieved from www.cdc.gov/nccdphp/dash/yrbs/pies99/natl.htm.

Centers for Disease Control and Prevention (CDC). (2001, May). STD prevention: Genital HPV infection. National Center for HIV, STD and TB Prevention. Retrieved May 29, 2002, from http://www.cdc.gov/std/

Centers for Disease Control and Prevention (CDC) (2002). *Immunization education org.* Retrieved May 17, 2002, from http://www.immunizationed.org

Champion, J., Piper, J., Shain, R., Perdue, S., & Newton, E. (2001). Minority women with sexually transmitted diseases: Sexual abuse and risk for pelvic inflammatory disease. *Research in Nursing & Health, 24*(1), 38–43.

Chapin, K. (1999). Probing the STDs. *American Journal of Nursing, 99*(7), 24–27.

Chasen, E., Umlauf, M., Pillion, D., & Singh, K. (2000). Sleep apnea symptoms, nocturia, and diabetes in African American community dwelling older adults. *Journal of the National Black Nurses Association, 11*(2), 25–33.

Clinical guidelines. (1995). Body measurement. *Nurse Practitioner, 20*(4), 65–66, 69.

Clinical pearls. (1996, June). Easier cervical visualization. *Clinician Reviews,* 49.

Cloutier, S., Martin, S.L., & Poole, C. (2002). Sexual assault among North Carolina women: Prevalence and health risk factors. *Journal of Epidemiology and Community Health, 56*(4), 242–243.

Cooper, R.S. (2001). Social inequality, ethnicity and cardiovascular disease. *International Journal of Epidemiology, 30*(Suppl 1), S48–S52.

Curry, L.C., & Hogstel, M.O. (2002). Osteoporosis. *AJN, 102* (1): 26–30.

Curry, M. (1998). The interrelationships between abuse, substance use, and psychological stress during pregnancy. *Journal of Obstetric Gynecologic Neonatal Nursing, 27*(6), 692–599.

Cyranowski, J., Frank, E., Young, E., & Shear, M. (2000). Adolescent onset of the gender difference in lifetime rates of major depression. *Archives of General Psychiatry, 57,* 21–27.

Danziger, S., Carlson, M., & Henly, J. (2001). Post-welfare employment and psychological well-being. *Women Health, 32*(1–2) 47–78.

Desai, M.M., Zhang, P., & Hennessy, C.H. (1999a). Surveillance for morbidity and mortality among older adults— United States, 1995–1996. *Morbidity and Mortality Weekly Report CDC Surveillance, 48*(8), 7–25.

Desai, M.M., Zhang, P., & Hennessy, C.H. (1999b). Surveillance for morbidity and mortality among older adults— United States, 1995–1996. *Morbidity and Mortality Weekly Report [MMWR].* Retrieved April 17, 2002, from http://www.cdc.gov/mmwr/preview/mmwrhtml/ss4808a2.htm.

Dietary guidelines: Building a healthy base. (2000). Department of Health and Human Services. Retrieved April 17, 2002, from www.health.gov/dietaryguidelines/dga2000/docurr

Dietch, K. (2002). The "silent" disease: Diagnosing and treating depression in women. *AWHONN Lifelines, 6*(2), 140–145.

Domar, A., & Dreher, H. (1996). *Healthy mind, healthy women: Using the mind-body connection to manage stress and take control of your health.* New York: Henry Holt & Co.

Dumesic, D. (1996, January). Pelvic examination: What to focus on in menopausal women. *Consultant,* 39–46.

Dunn, K. & Horgas, A. (2000). The prevalence of prayer as a spiritual self-care modality in elders. *Journal of Holistic Nursing, 18*(4), 337–351.

Earle, A. & Heymann, S. (2002). What causes job loss among former welfare recipients: The role of family health problems. *Journal of the American Medical Women's Association, 57*(1), 5–10.

Eberhardt, M.S., Ingram, D.D., Makuc, D.M., et al. (2001). *Urban and rural health chartbook: Health United States, 2001.* Hyattsville, MD: National Center for Health Statistics.

Table 12. Low birth weight live births, according to mother's detailed race, Hispanic origin, and smoking status: United States, selected years 1970–1999.

Table 32. Leading causes of death and numbers of deaths, according to sex, race, and Hispanic origin: United States, 1980 and 1999.

Table 37. Death rates for diseases of heart, according to sex, race, Hispanic origin, and age: United States, selected years 1950–99.

Table 38. Death rates for cerebrovascular diseases, according to sex, race, Hispanic origin, and age: United States, selected years 1950–99.

Table 39. Death rates for malignant neoplasms, according to sex, race, Hispanic origin, and age: United States, selected years 1950–99.

Table 40. Death rates for malignant neoplasms of trachea, bronchus, and lung, according to sex, race, Hispanic origin, and age: United States, selected years 1950–99.

Table 41. Death rates for malignant neoplasm of the breast for females, according to race, Hispanic origin, and age: United States, selected years 1950–99.

Table 42. Death rates for chronic lower respiratory diseases, according to sex, race, Hispanic origin, and age: United States, selected years 1980–99.

Table 43. Death rates for human immunodeficiency virus (HIV) disease, according to sex, race, Hispanic origin, and age: United States, selected years 1987–99.

Table 44. Maternal mortality for complications of pregnancy, childbirth, and the puerperium, according to race, Hispanic origin, and age: United States, selected years 1950–98.

Table 45. Death rates for motor vehicle-related injuries, according to sex, race, Hispanic origin, and age: United States, selected years 1950–99.

Table 46. Death rates for assault (homicide), according to sex, race, Hispanic origin, and age: United States, selected years 1950–99.

Table 47. Death rates for suicide, according to sex, race, Hispanic origin, and age: United States, selected years 1950–99.

Table 55. Age-adjusted cancer incidence rates for selected cancer sites, according to sex, race, and Hispanic origin: Selected geographic areas, 1990–1997.

Table 60. Current cigarette smoking by persons 18 years of age and over according to sex, race, and age: United States, selected years 1965–99.

Table 61. Age-adjusted prevalence of current cigarette smoking by persons 25 years of age and over, according to sex, race, and education: United States, selected years 1974–99.

Table 67. Hypertension among persons 20 years of age and over, according to sex, age, race, and Hispanic origin: United States, 1960–62, 1971–74, 1976–80, and 1988–1994.

Table 84. Injury-related visits to hospital emergency departments by sex, age, intent and mechanism of injury: United States average annual 1995–96 and 1998–99.

Table 93. Rates of discharges and days of care in non-federal short-stay hospitals, according to sex, age, and selected first-listed diagnoses: United States, selected years 1990–99.

Elliott, A. (2001). Primary care assessment and management of sleep disorders. *Journal of the American Academy of Nurse Practitioner 13*(9), 409–417.

Enoch, M., & Goldman, D. (2002). Problem drinking and alcoholism: Diagnosis and treatment. *American Family Physician, 65*(3), 449–450.

Expert Panel on Detection, Evaluation, and Treatment of High Blood Cholesterol in Adults. (May 2001). Third Report of the National Cholesterol Education Program (NCEP). *National Heart, Lung, and Blood Institute.* NIH Publication 01-3670.

Ferris, D., Heidemann, N., Litaker, M., Crosby, J., & Macfee, M. (2000). The efficacy of liquid-based cervical cytology using direct-to-vial sample collection. *Journal of Family Practice, 49*(11), 1005–1011.

Field, A., Coakley, E., Must, A., Spadano, J., Laird, N., Dietz, W., Rimm, E., & Colditz, G. (2001). Impact of overweight on the risk of developing common chronic diseases during a 10-year period. *Archives of Internal Medicine, 161*(13), 1581–1586.

Foote, J., Giuliano, A., & Harris, R. (2000). Older adults need guidance to meet nutritional recommendations. *Journal of the American College of Nutrition, 19*(5), 628–640.

Fontaine, P. (1998). Endometrial cancer, cervical cancer, and adnexal mass. *Primary Care, 25*(2), 433–457.

Fontham, E., Correa, P., Reynolds, P., et al. (1994). Environmental tobacco smoke and lung cancer in nonsmoking women. *Journal of the American Medical Association, 27*(22), 1752–1759.

Ford, D., & Cooper-Patrick, L. (2001). Sleep disturbances and mood disorders: An epidemiolgic perspective. *Depression & Anxiety, 14*(1), 3–6.

Freeland-Graves, J. & Nitzke, S. (2002). Position of the American Dietetic Association: Total diet approach to communicating food and nutrition information. *Journal of the American Dietetic Association, 102*(1), 100–108.

Frisbie, W., Echevarria, S., & Hummer, R. (2001). Prenatal care utilization among non-Hispanic whites, African Americans, and Mexican Americans. *Maternal Child Health, 5*(1), 21–33.

Gabbe, S., & Turner, L. (1997). Reproductive hazards of the American lifestyle: Work during pregnancy. *American Journal of Obstetrics and Gynecology, 176*(4), 826–832.

Gall, S. (1995). Making immunizations a priority for adults and adolescents. *Contemporary Nurse Practitioner, 1*(6), 17–27.

Garfinkel, L., & Mushinski, M. (1999). U.S. cancer incidence, mortality and survival: 1993–1996. *Statistical Bulletin Metropolitan Insurance Company, 80*(30), 23–32.

Gennaro, S. (2001). Weighty matters. *Every woman: The essential guide for healthy living.* Washington, DC: AWHONN.

Gerchufsky, M. (1996). How much is too much? Weight questions. *Advance for Nurse Practitioners, 4*(1), 17–19, 60.

Geronimus, A. (2001). Understanding and eliminating racial inequalities in women's health in the United States: The role of the weathering conceptual framework. *Journal of the American Medical Women's Association, 56*(4), 133–136, 149–150.

Glantz, S., & Parmley, W. (1995). Passive smoking and heart disease: Mechanisms and risk. *JAMA, 273* (13):1047–1053.

Gold, E., & Tomich, E. (1994). Occupational hazards to fertility and pregnancy outcome. *Occupational Medicine, 9*(3), 435–469.

Gordon, J., & Speroff, L. (2002). *Handbook of clinical gynecologic endocrinology and infertility.* Philadelphia: Lippincott, Williams & Wilkins.

Grillo, C., & Masheb, R. (2001). Childhood psychological, physical, and sexual maltreatments in outpatients with binge eating disorder: Frequency and associations with gender, obesity, and eating-related psychopathology. *Obesity Research, 9*(5), 320–325.

Guillen, E., & Barr, S. (1994). Nutrition, dieting, and fitness messages in a magazine for adolescent women, 1970–1990. *Journal of Adolescent Health, 15,* 464–472.

Gutierrez, Y. (1994). *Nutrition in health maintenance and health promotion for primary care providers.* San Francisco: University of California, School of Nursing.

Hacker, N., & Moore, J. (1998). *Essentials of Obstetrics and Gynecology* (3rd ed.). Philadelphia: W.B. Saunders.

Hahn, M. (1996). Search for Mr. Sandman. *ADVANCE for Nurse Practitioners, 4*(5), 36–42.

Hajjar, I. & Duthie, E., Jr. (2001). Prevalence of elder abuse in the United States: A comparative report between the national and Wisconsin data. *Wisconsin Medical Journal, 100*(6), 22–26.

Harrell, R., Toronjo, C., McLaughlin, J., Pavlik, V., Hyman, D., & Dyer, C. (2002). How geriatricians identify elder abuse and neglect. *American Journal of Medical Science, 323*(1), 34–38.

Hatoum, H., Kania, C., Kong, S., Wong, J., & Mendelson, W. (1998). Prevalence of insomnia: A survey of the enrollees at five managed care organizations. *American Journal of Managed Care, 4*(1), 79–86.

Healthy People 2000: National health promotion and disease prevention objectives. (1990). Washington, DC: U.S. Public Health Service.

Hess, D., & DeBoer, S. (2002). Ecstacy. *American Journal of Nursing, 102*(4), 45–47.

Heuveline, P., & Slap, G.B. (2002). Adolescent and young adult mortality by cause: Age, gender, and country, 1955 to 1994. *Journal of Adolescent Health, 30*(1), 29–34.

Hidden STD epidemic exposed. (2002). *Clinician Reviews, 12*(5), 41–42.

Hilton, J. (2002). Folic acid intake of young women. *JOGNN, 31*(2), 172–177.

Hollander, L., Freeman, E., Sammel, M., Berlin, J., Grisso, J., & Battistini, M. (2001). Sleep quality, estradiol levels, and behavioral factors in late reproductive age women. *Obstetrics and Gynecology, 98*(3), 391–397.

Holmes, T., & Raye, R. (1967). The social readjustment rating scale. *Journal of Psychosomatic Research, 11,* 213.

Hopkins, F.W., MacKay, A.P., Koonin, L.M., Berg, C.J., Irwin, M., & Atrash, H.K. (1999). Pregnancy-related mortality in Hispanic women in the United States. *Obstetrics and Gynecology, 94*(5 Pt 1), 747–752.

Horton, J.A. (1995). *The women's health data book: A profile of women's health in the United States, 1995* (2nd ed.). Washington, DC: Jacob's Institutes for Women's Health.

Hourani, L., & Hilton, S. (2000). Occupational and environmental exposure correlates of adverse live-birth outcomes among 1032 U.S. Navy women. *Journal of Occupational Medicine, 42*(12), 1156–1165.

Hughes, T., Johnson, T., & Wilsnack, S. (2001). Sexual assault and alcohol abuse: A comparison of lesbians and heterosexual women. *Journal of Substance Abuse, 13*(4), 515–532.

Humpel, N., Owen, N., & Leslie, E. (2002). Environmental factors associated with adults' participation in physical activity. A review. *American Journal of Preventive Medicine, 22*(3), 188–199.

Hutchinson, M., Sosa, D., & Thompson, A. (2001). Sexual protective strategies of late adolescent females: More than just condoms. *JOGNN, 30*(4), 429–438.

Iglesias, E., Alderman, E., & Fox, A. (2000). Use of wet smears to screen for sexually transmitted diseases. *Infections in Medicine, 17*(3), 175–185.

Iribarren, C., Friedman, G., Klatsky, A., & Eisner, M. (2001). Exposure to environmental tobacco smoke: Association with personal characteristics and self reported health conditions. *Journal of Epidemiology & Community Health, 55*(10), 721–728.

Johnson, C. (1996). Immunizations for adolescents and adults. In C. Johnson, B. Johnson, J. Murray, & B. Apgar (Eds.), *Women's health handbook.* Philadelphia: Hanley & Belfus; St. Louis: Mosby.

Kanner, A., Cyne, J., Schaefer, C., & Lazarus, R. (1980). Comparison of two modes of stress management: Daily hassles and uplifts versus major life events. *Journal of Behavioral Medicine, 4*(1), 1–35.

Katz, B., Fortenberry, J., Tu, W., Harezlak, J., & Orr, D. (2001). Sexual behavior among adolescent women at high risk for sexually transmitted infections. *Sexually Transmitted Disease, 28*(5), 247–251.

Kelley, A., Blair, N., & Pechacek, T.F. (2001). Women and smoking: Issues and opportunities. *Journal of Women's Health and Gender-Based Medicine, 10*(6), 515–518.

Kelley, G., Kelley, K., & Tran, Z. (2001). Walking and resting blood pressure in adults: A meta-analysis. *Preventive Medicine, 33*(2 Pt 1), 120–127.

Kelley, G., & Sharpe-Kelley, K. (2001). Aerobic exercise and resting blood pressure in older adults: A meta-analytic review of randomized controlled trials. *Journal of Gerontology. Series A. Biological Sciences and Medical Sciences, 56*(5), 298–303.

Kelly, P., Blacksin, B., & Mason, E. (2001). Factors affecting substance abuse treatment completion for women. *Issues in Mental Health Nursing, 22*(3), 287–304.

Kennedy, E., Bowman, S., Spence, J., Freedman, M., & King, J. (2001). Popular diets: Correlation to health, nutrition, and obesity. *Journal of the American Dietetic Association, 101*(4), 411–420.

Khalbuss, W., Rudomina, D., Kauff, N., Chuang, L., & Melamed, M. (2000). SpinThin, a simple, inexpensive technique for preparation of thin-layer cervical cytology from liquid-based specimens: Data on 791 cases. *Cancer, 90*(3), 135–142.

KIDS COUNT Census 2000 Supplementary Survey. (2002, May 17). *Children at risk: Summary and findings.* Baltimore, MD: Annie E. Casey Foundation. Retrieved 5/24/02 from http://www.aecf.org/kidscount/c2ss/summary.htm

Kilpatrick, D., Acierno, R., Saunders, B., Resnick, H., Best, C., & Schnurr, P. (2000). Risk factors for adolescent substance abuse and dependence: Data from a national sample. *Journal of Consulting and Clinical Psychology, 68*(1), 19–30.

Kilpatrick, D., Edmunds, C., & Seymour, A. (1992). *Rape in America: A report to the nation.* In U.S. Department of Health and Human Services (2000), *Healthy people 2010* (Conference Edition, in two volumes). Washington, DC: U.S. Government Printing Office.

Kim, K., & Lee, K. (2001). Symptom experience in women after hysterectomy. *JOGNN, 30*(5), 472–480.

Knowler, W., Barrett-Connor, E., Fowler, S., Hamman, R., Lachin, J., et al. (2002). Reduction in the incidence of type 2 diabetes with lifestyle intervention or metformin. *New England Journal of Medicine, 346*(6), 393–403.

Kuba, S., & Harris, D. (2001). Eating disturbances in women of color: An exploratory study of contextual factors in the development of disordered eating in Mexican American women. *Health Care of Women, 22*(2), 281–298.

Lacey, J.V., Devesa, S.S., & Brinton, L.A. (2002). Recent trends in breast cancer incidence and mortality. *Environmental and Molecular Mutagenesis, 39*(2–3), 82–88.

Lanman, G. (1995). Safety and accident prevention. In Carlson, K., Eisenstat, S., Figoletto, F., & Schiff, I. (Eds.), *Primary care of women.* St. Louis: Mosby.

Lawlor, D.A., Ebrahim, S., & Smith, G.D. (2001, September 8). Sex matters: Secular and geographical trends in sex differences in coronary heart disease mortality. *British Medical Journal, 323,* 541–545.

Lazarus, R.S. (1981, July). Little hassles can be hazardous to health. *Psychology Today,* 59–62.

Leisure, M., Dudley, S., & Donowitz, L. (1993). Does a clean-catch urine sample reduce bacterial contamination? *NEJM, 328*(4), 289–290.

Li, L., & Ford, J. (1998). Illicit drug use by women with disabilities. *American Journal of Drug and Alcohol Abuse, 24*(3), 405–418.

Ludman, E., Curry, S., Grothaus, L., Graham, E., Stout, J., & Lozano, P. (2002). Depressive symptoms, stress, and weight concerns among African American and European American low-income female smokers. *Psychology of Addiction Behavior, 16*(1), 68–71.

Mammography screening revisited. (2002). *Clinician Reviews, 12*(3), 41.

Mandelblatt, J., Lawrence, W., Womack, S., Jacobson, D., Yi, B., Hwang, Y., Gold, K., Barter, J., & Shah, K. (2002). Benefits and costs of using HPV testing to screen for cervical cancer. *JAMA, 287*(18), 2372–2381.

Manson, J., Wilett, W., & Stampfer, M. (1995). Body weight and mortality among women. *New England Journal of Medicine, 333,* 677–685.

Margolis, K.L, Kerani, R.P., McGovern, P., Songer, T., Cauley, J.A., Ensrud, K.E. (2002). Risk factors for motor vehicle crashes in older women. *Journal of Gerontology, Aging, Biological Science and Medical Science, 57*(3), M186–M191.

Martin, S., Mackie, L., Kupper, L., Buescher, P., & Moracco, K. (2001). Physical abuse of women before, during, and after pregnancy. *JAMA 285*(12), 1581–1584.

Massachusetts Medical Society. (2001). Flu vaccine safe for asthmatics. *Journal Watch, 21*(24), 192.

Massarani-Wafai, R., Bakhos, R., Wojcik, E., & Selvaggi, S. (2000). Evaluation of cellular residue in the ThinPrep PreservCyt vial. *Diagnostic Cytopathology, 23*(3), 208–212.

Mata, J. (1998). Bacterial infections of the urinary tract in females. In R.E. Rakel (Ed.). *1998 Conn's current therapy* (pp. 668–670). Philadelphia: W. B. Saunders Co.

McAlindon, T. E. (2000). Can diet affect the risk and progression of osteoarthritis? *Women's Health in Primary Care, 3*(10), 741–747.

McClam, E. (May 17, 2002a). Fewer students take up smoking. *Sun-Sentinel,* 3A.

McClam, E. (April 7, 2002b). Most Americans are couch potatoes, report concludes. *Sun-Sentinel,* 8A.

Mendelson, B., McLaren, L., Gauvin, L., & Steiger, H. (2002). The relationship of self-esteem and body esteem in women with and without eating disorders. *International Journal of Eating Disorders, 31*(3), 318–323.

Miettinen, O., Henschke, C., Pasmantier, M. et al. (2002). Mammographic screening: No reliable supporting evidence? *Lancet, 359,* 404–406.

Miller, A., To, T., Baines, C., & Wall, J. (2002). Mammograms in women age 40 to 49: Results of the Canadian Breast Cancer Screening Study. *Annals of Internal Medicine, 137,* 305–312.

Monif, G. (2002, April 15). Infectious vulvuvaginal disease: Obstacles to performing wet mount exams. *Consultant,* 621–624.

Moore, M., Zaccaro, D., & Parsons, L. (1998). Attitudes and practices of registered nurses toward women who have experienced abuse/domestic violence. *Journal of Obstetric, Gynecologic, and Neonatal Nursing, 27,* 175–181.

Moskowitz, H. Griffith, J.L., DiScala, C., & Sege, R.D. (2001). Serious injuries and deaths of adolescent girls resulting from interpersonal violence: Characteristics and trends from the United States, 1989–1998. *Archives of Pediatric Adolescent Medicine, 155*(8), 903–908.

Mulrow, C., Williams, Jr., J., Gerety, M., et al. (1995). Case-finding instruments for depression in primary care settings. *Annals of Internal Medicine, 122,* 913–921.

Murray, J. (1996). Preadolescent and adolescent health promotion and maintenance. In C. Johnson, B. Johnson, J. Murray, & B. Apgar (Eds.), *Women's health care handbook.* Philadelphia: Hanley & Belfus; St. Louis: Mosby.

National Academy of Sciences. (1997). *Dietary reference intake for calcium,* 4–38.

National Center for Health Statistics. (2001). *New CDC report on U.S. mortality patterns:* September 25, 2001. Retrieved April 17, 2002, from http://www.cdc.gov/nchs/releases/01facts/99mortality.htm.

National Institutes of Health. (1996, April 1–3). Consensus Development Conference Statement: Cervical Cancer. Bethesda, MD: Author.

National Vital Statistics Report. (March 21, 2002a). Table 6. Life table for white females: United States, 1999. *50*(6), 17.

National Vital Statistics Report. (March 21, 2002b). Table 9. Life table for black females: United States, 1999. *50*(6), 23.

National Women's Health Information Center (NWHIC). (2000). Women's health statistical information: Leading causes of death for American Women by racial/ethnic group (2000). Retrieved April 17, 2002, from http://www.4women.gov/media/chart.htm.

Obwegeser, J.H., & Brack, S. (2001). Does liquid-based technology really improve detection of cervical neoplasia? A prospective, randomized trial comparing the thin prep Pap test with the conventional Pap test, including follow-up of HSIL cases. *ActaCytol., 45* (5): 709–714.

Optimal daily calcium intake. (1994). National Institutes of Health Consensus Panel on Optimal Calcium Intake. Bethesda, MD: National Institutes of Health.

Oriel, K.A., Hartenbach, E.M., & Remington, P.L. (1999). Trends in United States ovarian cancer mortality, 1979–1995. *Obstetrics Gynecology, 93*(1), 30–33.

Oths, K., Dunn, L., & Palmer, N. (2001). A prospective study of psychosocial job strain and birth outcomes. *Epidemiology, 12*(6), 744–746.

Palaniappan, L., Anthony, M.N., Mahesh, C., Elliott, M., Killeen, A., Giacherio, D., & Rubenfire, M. (2002). Cardiovascular risk factors in ethnic minority women aged < or = 30 years. *American Journal of Cardiology, 89*(5), 524–529.

Palu, G., Calistic, A., Cancellotti, E., Cusan, M., & Mengoli, C. (2001). Evaluation of a near-patient test and 2 enzyme-linked immunosorbent assay-based assays for detecting anti-herpes simplex virus type - 2 antibodies. *Scandinavise Journal of Infectious Disease, 33*(10), 794–796.

Parkerson, G., Adams, R., & Emerling, F. (2001). Maternal domestic violence screening in an office-based pediatric practice. *Pediatrics, 108*(3), E43, www.pediatrics.org.

Parkerson, G., Broadnead, W., & Tse, C. (1995). Perceived family stress as a predictor of health-related outcomes. *Archives of Family Medicine, 4,* 253–260.

Pate, R., Pratt, M., Blair, S., et al. (1995). Physical activity and public health: A recommendation from the Centers for Disease Control and Prevention and the American College of Sports Medicine. *Journal of the American Medical Association, 273*(5), 402–407.

Pender, N.J. (1996). *Health promotion in nursing practice* (3rd ed). Stamford, CT: Appleton & Lange.

Perrons, C., Kleter, B., Jelley, R., Jalal, H., Qunt, W., & Tedder, R. (2002). Detection and genotyping of human papillomavirus DNS by SPF10 and MY09/11 primers in cervical cells taken from women attending a colposcopy clinic. *Journal of Medical Virology, 67*(2), 246–252.

Petterson, S., & Friel, L. (2001). Psychological distress, hopelessness and welfare. *Women and Health, 32*(1–2), 79–99.

Phaneuf, C. (1996). Screening elders for nutritional deficits. *American Journal of Nursing, 96*(3), 58–60.

Phillips, K.D., & Sowell, R.L. (2000). Hope and coping in HIV-infected African-American women of reproductive age. *Journal of the National Black Nurses Association, 11*(2), 18–24.

Pinkerton, S., & Layde, P. for The NIMH Multisite HIV Prevention Trial Group. (2002). Using sexually transmitted disease incidence as a surrogate marker for HIV incidence in prevention trials: A modeling study. *Sexually Transmitted Disease, 29*(5), 298–307.

Plichta, S., & Falik, M. (2001). Prevalence of violence and its implication for women's health. *Women's Health Issues, 11*(3), 244–258.

Pope, S., Sowers, M., Welch, G., & Albrecht, G. (2001). Functional limitations in women at midlife: The role of health conditions, behavioral and environmental factors. *Women's Health Issues, 11*(6), 494–502.

Position Statement. (2002). Management of postmenopausal osteoporosis: Position statement of the North American Menopause Society. *Menopause, 9*(2), 84–101.

Pressman, M., Figueroa, W., & Kendrick-Mohamed, J. (1996). A rarely recognized symptom of sleep apnea and other occult sleep disorders. *Archives of Internal Medicine, 156,* 545–550.

Pronk, N., Crouse, S., O'Brien, B., & Rohack, J. (1995). Acute effects of walking on serum lipids and lipoproteins in women. *Journal of Sports Medicine and Physical Fitness, 35*(1), 50–57.

Raphan, G., Cohen, S., & Boyer, A. (2001). The female condom, a tool for empowering sexually active urban adolescent women. *Journal of Urban Health, 78*(4), 605–613.

Redmond, G. (2000). The management of postnatal depression. *Drug and Therapeutics Bulletin, 38*(5), 33–37.

Richardson, B., Lavreys, L., Martin, H., Jr., Stevens, C., Ngugi, E., Mandaliya, K., Bwayo, J., Ndinya-Achola, J., & Kreiss, J. (2001). Evaluation of a low-dose nonoxynol-9 gel for the prevention of sexually transmitted diseases: A randomized clinical trial. *Sexually Transmitted Disease, 28*(7), 394–400.

Richardson, D., & Wing, S. (1998). Methods for investigating age differences in the effects of prolonged exposures. *American Journal of Industrial Medicine, 33*(2), 123–130.

Richart, R., Ferenczy, A., Trofatter, K., & Tyring, S. (1999, December). New approaches to management of external genital warts. *A Supplment to Patient Care for the Nurse Practitioner.* National Association of Nurse Practitioners in Women's Health.

Rich-Edwards, J., Spiegelman, D., Garland, M., Hertzmark, E., Hunter, D., Colditz, G., Willett, W., & Manson, J. (2002). Physical activity, body mass index, and ovulatory disorder infertility. *Epidemiology, 13*(2), 184–190.

Rigotti, N., & Polivogianis, L. (1995). In J. Carlson, S. Eisenstat, F. Frigoletto, & I. Schiff (Eds.), *Primary care of women.* St. Louis: Mosby.

Roeloffs, C., Fink, A., Unutzer, J., Tang, L., & Wells, K. (2001). Problematic substance use, depressive symptoms, and gender in primary care. *Psychiatric Service, 52*(9), 1251–1253.

Roth, T. (2000). Diagnosis and management of insomnia. *Clinical Cornerstone, 2*(5), 28–38.

Roth, T., & Ancoli-Israel, S. (1999). Daytime consequences and correlates of insomnia in the United States: Results of the 1991 National Sleep Foundation Survey. II. *Sleep, 22*(Suppl 2), S354–S358.

Sauro, M., Jorgensen, R., Larson, C., Frankowski, J., Ewart, C., & White, J. (2001). Sociotropic cognition moderates stress-induced cardiovascular responsiveness in college women. *Journal of Behavioral Medicine, 24*(5), 423–439.

Sawin, K., & Harrington, M. (1995). *Measures of family functioning for research and practice.* New York: Springer Publishing.

Schmid, D., Brown, D., Nisenbaum, R., Burke, R., et al. (1999). Limits in reliability of glycoprotein G-based type-specific serologic assays for herpes simplex virus types 1 and 2. *Journal of Clinical Microbiology, 37*(2), 376–379.

Schnitzer, P.G., & Runyan, C.W. (1995). Injuries to women in the United States: An overview. *Women and Health, 23* (1): 9–27.

Schulz, A., Parker, E., Israel, D., & Fisher, D. (2001). Social context, stressors, and disparities in women's health. *Journal of the American Medical Women's Association, 56*(4), 143–149.

Schwebke, J.R. (2002). Cost-effective screening for trichomoniasis. *Emerging Infections Disease, 8*(7), 749.

Seidel, H., Ball, J., Dains, J., & Benedict, G. (1999). *Mosby's guide to physical examination* (4th ed.). St. Louis: Mosby.

Sells, C.W. & Blum, R.W. (1996). Morbidity and mortality among U.S. adolescents: An overview of data and trends. *American Journal of Public Health, 86*(4), 513–519.

Sephton, S., Koopman, C., Schaal, M., Thorensen, C., & Spiegel, D. (2001). Spiritual expression and immune status in women with metastatic breast cancer: An exploratory study. *Breast Journal, 7*(5), 345–353.

Should I still get mammograms? (2002). *Harvard Women's Health Watch, IX*(7), 8.

Silverstein, M., & Waite, L. (1993). Are blacks more likely than whites to receive and provide social support in middle and old age? Yes, no, and maybe so. *Journal of Gerontology, 48* (4): 5121–5222.

Simoni-Wastila, L. (2000). The use of abusable prescription drugs: The role of gender. *Journal of Women's Health and Gender Based Medicine, 9*(3), 289–297.

Slanetz, P. (2002). Hormone replacement therapy and breast tissue density on mammography. *Menopause, 9*(2), 82–83.

Solomon, D., Davey, D., Kurman, R., Moriarty, A., O'Connor, D., et al. for the Forum Group Members and the Bethesda 2001 Workshop. (2002). The 2001 Bethesda System: Terminology for reporting results of cervical cytology. *JAMA, 287,* 2114–2119.

Solomon, D., Schiffman, M., & Tarone, R.; ALTS Study Group. (2001). Comparison of three management strategies for patients with atypical squamous cells of undetermined significance: Baseline results from randomized trial. *Journal of the National Institute of Cancer, 93*(4), 293–299.

Speroff, L., Glass, R.H., & Kase, N.G. (1999). *Clinical gynecological endocrinology and infertility.* Baltimore, MD: Williams & Wilkins.

Spielberger, C., Edwards, C., Lushene, R., et al. (1983). *Manual for state-trait anxiety inventory.* Palo Alto, CA: Consulting Psychologists Press.

Stansfeld, S., Fuhrer, R., Shipley, M., & Marmot, M. (2002). Psychological distress as a risk factor for coronary heart disease in the Whitehall II Study. *International Journal of Epidemiology, 31*(1), 248–255.

STD Quarterly. (1995, June). Empower your patients by teaching genital self-exam. *Contraceptive Technology Update,* 73–74.

Stein, M., & Barrett-Connor, E. (2000). Sexual assault and physical health: Findings from a population-based study of older adults. *Psychosomatic Medicine, 62*(6), 838–843.

Stice, E., & Bearman, S. (2001). Body-image and eating disturbances prospectively predict increases in depressive symptoms in adolescent girls: A growth curve analysis. *Developmental Psychology, 37*(5), 597–607.

Stoler, M. (2002). New Bethesda terminology and evidence-based management guidelines for cervical cytology findings. *JAMA, 287*(16), 2140–2141.

Strauss, E. (July 1999). Sleep apnea. *Hippocrates,* 12–13.

Strickland, J. (2001). Adolescent acute sexual assault: Contrasting with adult experiences. *Obstetrics and Gynecology, 97*(4 Suppl 1), S6.

Strollo, P., & Rogers, R. (1996). Obstructive sleep apnea. *New England Journal of Medicine, 334*(2), 99–104.

Study: New test for virus better than Pap. (July 10, 1998). *Reuters Limited.*

Tapper-Gardzina, Y., Cotugna, N., & Vickery, C. (2002). Should you recommend a low-carb, high protein diet? *Nurse Practitioner, 27*(4), 52–59.

Taylor, Jr., P., Andersen, W., Barber, S., et al. (1987) The screening Papanicolaou smear: Contribution of the endocervical brush. *Obstetrics and Gynecology, 70,* 734–738.

Taylor, S., Klein, L., Lewis, L., Gruenewald, T., Gurung, R., & Updegraff, J. (2000). Biobehavioral responses to stress in females: Tend-and-befriend, not fight-or-flight. *Psychology Review, 107*(3), 411–429.

Tseng, M., Yeatts, K., Millikan, R., & Newman, B. (2001). Area-level characteristics and smoking in women. *American Journal of Public Health, 91*(11), 1847–1850.

Turner, C., Rogers, S., Miller, H., et al. (2002). Untreated gonococcal and chlamydial infection in a probability sample of adults. *JAMA, 287,* 726–733.

Twinings, S. (1995). The occupational and environmental health history: Guidelines for the primary care nurse practitioner. *Nurse Practitioner Forum, 6*(2), 64–71.

Two for 2002: Identifying and reducing health risk. (2002). *Harvard Women's Health Watch, IX*(6), 1–3.

U.S. Bureau of the Census. (2000a). Death rates by age and leading cause: 1997. (No. 129). *Statistical Abstracts of the United States, 2000* (120th ed.). Washington, DC: U.S. Government Printing Office.

U.S. Bureau of the Census. (2000b). Prevalence of selected chronic conditions by age and sex: 1996. (No. 220).

Statistical Abstracts of the United States, 2000 (120th ed.). Washington, DC: U.S. Government Printing Office.

U.S. Census Bureau, Statistical Abstract of the United States: 2001. (No 108). Deaths by ages and leading cause: 1998. Washington, DC: U.S. Government Printing Office.

U.S. Department of Agriculture and U.S. Department of Health and Human Services. (2000). *Nutrition and your health: Dietary guidelines for Americans* (5th ed.). Home and Garden Bulletin No. 232. Washington, DC: U.S. Government Printing Office.

U.S. Department of Health and Human Services. (2000). *Healthy people 2010* (Conference Edition, in Two Volumes). Washington, DC: U.S. Government Printing Office.

U.S. Preventive Services Task Force. (2002). Screening for chlamydial infection: Recommendations and rationale. *American Journal for Nurse Practitioners, 6*(13), 13, 19–20, 23–24.

Varner, R., & Younger, J. (1995). Menopause. In V. Seltger & W. Pearse (Eds.), *Women's primary health care.* New York: McGraw-Hill.

Visscher, E., & Clore, E. (1992). The genogram: A strategy for assessment. *Journal of Pediatric Health Care, 6*(6), 361–367.

Vitamin C and cataract risk in women. (2002). *Harvard Women's Health Watch, IX*(9), 1.

Walsh, S.J., & Rau, L.M. (2000). Autoimmune diseases: A leading cause of death among young and middle-aged women in the United States. *American Journal of Public Health, 90*(9), 1463.

Watkins, J. (2002). Smallpox (variola). *The American Journal for Nurse Practitioners, 6*(1), 33–36.

What's happening. (1996). Demographic predictors of clinical breast examination, mammography, and Pap test screening among older women. *Journal Americans Academy of Nurse Practitioners, 8*(5), 231–236.

Willett, W., Manson, J., Stampfer, M., et al. (1995). Weight, weight change, and coronary heart disease in women. *JAMA, 273,* 461–465.

Williams, D. (2002). Racial/ethnic variations in women's health: The social embeddedness of health. *American Journal of Public Health, 92*(4), 588–597.

Williams, D., & Lawler, K. (2001). Stress and illness in low-income women: The roles of hardiness, John Henryism, and race. *Women Health, 32*(4), 61–75.

Women and sleep. (October 1999). *Harvard Women's Health Watch,* 1–3.

Worobey, J. (2002). Early family mealtime experiences and eating attitudes in normal weight, underweight and overweight females. *Eating and Weight Disorders, 7*(1), 39–44.

Wright, Jr., T., Cox, J., Massad, L., Twiggs, L., Wilkinson, E., for the 2001 ASCCP-Sponsored Consensus Conference. (2002a). 2001 Consensus guidelines for the management of women with cervical cytological abnormalities. *JAMA, 287*(16), 2120–2129.

Wright, Jr., T., Cox, J., Massad, L., Twiggs, L., Wilkinson, E., for the 2001 ASCCP-Sponsored Consensus Conference. (2002b). *Algorithms from the consensus guidelines for the management of women with cervical cytological abnormalities.* Hagerstown, MD: American Society for Colposcopy and Cervical Pathology.

Young, D., Gittelsohn, J., Charleston, J., Felix-Aaron, K., & Appel, L. (2001). Motivations for exercise and weight loss among African-American women: Focus group results and their contribution towards program development. *Ethnic Health, 6*(3–4), 227–245.

Youngkin, E., & Davis, M. (1998). Assessing women's health. In E. Youngkin & M. Davis, *Women's health: A primary care clinical guide* (2nd ed.). Stamford, CT: Appleton & Lange.

Zimmerman, R., & Ball, J. (2001). Adult vaccinations. *Primary Care, 28*(4), 763–790.

CHAPTER 5

INTEGRATING WELLNESS: COMPLEMENTARY THERAPIES AND WOMEN'S HEALTH

Jo W. Robins ◆ *Leslie Fehan*

We are holistic beings, greater than the sum of our parts.

Highlights

- Diet and Exercise
- Herbal Medicine
- Mind–Body Medicine
- Energy Medicine
- Complementary Therapies in Pregnancy
  - Herbs
  - Aromatherapy
  - Homeopathy
  - Yoga

❖ INTRODUCTION

An integrative approach to wellness involves combining the best of mainstream and complementary therapies. With the introduction of Cartesian dualism in the 18th century, matters of the mind became the domain of the church and the body became the domain of science (Achterberg, 1990). This split resulted in a mechanistic, disease-focused approach to health. Health is a dynamic, holistic state encompassing mind, body, and spirit dimensions, not simply the absence of disease. Additionally, the body possesses an innate healing ability. "Remembered wellness" refers to the body's ability and desire to remain balanced and healthy if supported in this process (Benson, 1996). Complementary therapies share this holistic view of health and focus on accessing and supporting the body's innate healing ability.

Complementary therapies lack randomized clinical trials; however, research in this field is accumulating rapidly, including a growing number of randomized clinical trials as well as other forms of research, including quasi-experimental and qualitative inquiries. Hopefully, research will guide us in the appropriate use of complementary therapies. However, research is but one of multiple ways of knowing when advising clients about health and wellness. Carper's (1978) theory of the fundamental patterns of knowing included empirical ways such as research but also esthetics and personal and ethical ways of knowing (Table 5–1). Following is a brief overview of integrative approaches for women's wellness, including therapies during pregnancy.

DIET AND EXERCISE

Complementary approaches stress the importance of diet and exercise. Diet improves overall health regardless of the health issue. Focusing on whole foods such as grains and fresh fruits and vegetables while minimizing processed foods, establishing and maintaining adequate hydration, and being aware of potential adverse reactions to food and food additives contributes to wellness. For example, monosodium glutamate (MSG) has been shown to aggravate fibromyalgia (Smith, Terpening, Schmidt, & Gums, 2001); aspartame has been empirically linked to headaches (Van den Eeden et al., 1994) and anecdotally linked to a variety of other symptoms including dizziness, seizures, urticaria, and angioedema in susceptible individuals (Smith et al., 2001). Foods can be used medicinally to treat common women's health problems. For example, a low-fat vegetarian diet, omega-3 fatty acids,

vitamin B_6, and magnesium help improve PMS as well as primary dysmenorrhea (Coco, 1999). Regular exercise decreases symptoms associated with a variety of conditions including premenstrual syndrome (Aganoff & Boyle, 1994), menopausal symptoms (Burghardt, 1999; Ivarsson, Spetz, & Hammar, 1998), and depression (Lane & Lovejoy, 2001) to name a few.

HERBAL MEDICINE

Herbal medicine is likely the most widespread complementary therapy with at least two types: traditional and pharmaceutical. Traditional herbalism has been practiced for thousands of years using single herbs in whole form such as the whole flower or leaf or formulas containing several herbs. These formulas are pharmacologically weaker, working more gradually and causing fewer adverse reactions. Pharmacological herbalism is the more modern, Western approach. Extracts of the active constituent(s) in a plant are concentrated for maximal effect. These preparations tend to work faster but potentially elicit more adverse reactions, including interactions with other pharmaceutical preparations. No legally imposed standards exist for manufacturing herbal products, and many reactions occur not because of the herb but because of contaminants in the manufacturing process. Many herbal manufacturers have voluntarily adopted quality control standards such as those

TABLE 5–1. Patterns of Knowing

Patterns	Action
Empirics: The science of nursing	Research—Include new perspectives: Health is more than the absence of disease.
Esthetics: The art of nursing	Empathy
Personal: Therapeutic use of self	Foster wholeness, integrity in encounters.
Ethics: Moral issues	Nursing standards, codes, and values.

imposed in European countries. To maintain safety, it is important to research manufacturers before recommending products. Starting with herbal teas is generally safe because they are less potent and unlikely to cause serious adverse reactions. Teas can be taken internally or used topically in baths or poultices.

Herbs contain all of the seventeen minerals and seventy trace minerals that our bodies need to work properly (Bunce, 1987). Herbal medicine may be helpful in a variety of disorders including PMS (vitex), perimenopause and menopause (black cohosh), mild depression and anxiety (St. John's wort), insomnia (valerian), and urinary tract infections (uva ursi) (Duke, 1997). Herbal medicine in pregnancy is discussed later in this chapter. For additional information on the safe and effective use of herbal therapies, see Youngkin and Israel (1996).

MIND–BODY MEDICINE

Among the safest and most valuable complementary therapies include meditation, imagery, tai chi, yoga (see Complementary Therapies in Pregnancy), and aromatherapy (see Complementary Therapies in Pregnancy), among others. These therapies share the use of breathing to elicit the relaxation response, a state characterized by decreases in blood pressure and heart and respiratory rates and an increase in alpha wave activity in the brain (Benson, 1975). There is a reversal of the stress-induced fight-or-flight response. This response is very common and leads to overstimulation of the sympathetic nervous system, leading to disorders such as depression, anxiety, and insomnia (Weil, 1999). Shallow breathing increases tension and blocks the ability to relax. Learning breathing techniques and teaching them to clients is an inexpensive, efficient way to enhance well-being.

The transition of menopause often creates a sense of great stress and imbalance in women. Mind–body therapies are an excellent way to help women regain balance. Yoga, for example, has been shown to equalize endocrine production of hormones, improve joint mobility, and potentially help prevent osteoporosis (Sander, 1996).

ENERGY MEDICINE

Energy medicine encompasses a variety of therapies based on the conception of the body as an energetic system and includes homeopathy (see Complementary Therapies in Pregnancy), healing touch, therapeutic touch, re-

flexology, acupuncture, and flower essences, among others. This conceptualization stretches our view of the human body, but is not entirely foreign considering electrocardiograms and electroencephalograms are based on energy. The mechanism of action is believed to be the removal of blockages and restoration of free energy flow to foster health and healing in the human energy field (Brennan, 1988).

Perhaps the least known therapy is based on flower essences such as Bach flower essences. Edward Bach, a physician, studied the effects of plants and flowers on mental and emotional states. Typically, the plant is placed in distilled water and exposed to sunlight then the liquid is used to treat various psychological states. One of the most popular is "Rescue Remedy," which is a combination of five flowers and is safe for adults and children experiencing disorders such as anxiety and insomnia (Bach & Wheeler, 1997). The dosage is 4 drops in 4 to 6 ounces of water.

The majority of research in the field of energy therapies is in therapeutic touch and healing touch, homeopathy (see Complementary Therapies in Pregnancy), and acupuncture. For example, therapeutic touch has been shown to decrease anxiety and depression (Leb, 1998; Olson & Sneed, 1995). Acupuncture may help relieve symptoms related to perimenopause and menopause (Dong et al., 2001).

COMPLEMENTARY THERAPIES IN PREGNANCY

In the absence of chronic disease, pregnancy is a state of wellness, not illness. Pregnancy is a time of great change and transition where a woman's mind-body-spirit connection becomes apparent. It is important to support women during this time to enhance their bodies' own natural abilities to be pregnant and give birth. Integrating complementary therapies can enhance mind–body balance and the experience of pregnancy. Complaints are viewed not in isolation but holistically. For example, a woman with backache can be treated solely for the backache with acetaminophen or physical therapy, but discussing activity level and exercise pattern, educating about pregnancy-related musculoskeletal changes, and incorporating strategies to strengthen and support her body may be more effective.

HERBS

The frequency of herbal use during pregnancy is unknown. A recent review of herbs and pregnancy showed many herbs used during pregnancy are safe, though this is based on limited information and few studies (Scialli & Fugh-Berman, 2001). Many herbs should never be used during pregnancy. Those containing high quantities of volatile oils or alkaloids can be teratogenic and affect the central nervous system. Harsh bitters that strongly stimulate digestion and metabolism should be avoided as well as any strong laxatives. Herbs with strong hormonal properties are not advised. For a list of common herbs to avoid in pregnancy and breastfeeding, see Table 5–2.

It is often recommended to take herbs individually rather than in combination to better assess their effects on the body. However, pregnancy tea is a common tonic that can gently support the body's adaptation to pregnancy. The benefits of teas may come from their high nutrient content. Pregnancy tea traditionally contains red raspberry leaf, oatstraw, alfalfa, and stinging nettle. Red raspberry leaf is nourishing to the uterus. It is the safest, most widely used uterine/pregnancy tonic herb (Fugh-Berman, 2001). It has a normalizing effect on the uterus, increasing tone in lax muscle or relaxing a taut or irritable uterus (Belew, 1999). Nettle leaves contain chlorophyll as well as many vitamins and minerals (Weed, 1986). Nettles are a kidney tonic, enhancing the elimination of waste products (Belew, 1999). Oatstraw is nourishing and strengthens capillaries. Alfalfa contains proteins, vitamins C and K, calcium, iron, phosphorus, and chlorophyll to help prevent anemia as well as hemorrhage during delivery (Romm, 1997b).

Though there is no definitive agreement on dosing, it is usually recommended to mix 1 tablespoon of loose tea per cup, steep at least 10 minutes, covered to keep the nutrients in and drink at least 4 cups per day. If women choose to solely take red raspberry leaf tea, the recommendations are the same. Or, she can take 4–8 grams per day in tablet form.

AROMATHERAPY

Aromatherapy is the use of essential oils to stimulate the sense of smell for balancing mind, body, and spirit. Many cultures worldwide recognize the power of smell in treating a variety of conditions and maintaining health and well-being. Essential oils are derived from plants, flowers, trees, herbs, and shrubs. Essential oils are highly concentrated and are usually diluted before use. They can improve many discomforts of pregnancy including emotional changes (bergamot, ylang ylang), morning sickness (peppermint), constipation (rose), and backaches (lavender, clary sage) (Tisserand, 1988).

Excessive stress-related catecholamines can adversely effect the developing fetus (Hawkins, Chestnut, & Gibbs, 2002). Using bergamot and lavender oils prenatally can decrease stress and aid in relaxation. Bringing these oils into the birthing room can help create a sense of safety and security, which is essential to birthing well. Even during postpartum, oils can help with emotional well-being and healing (Table 5–3). All essential oils have antibacterial properties—using these oils can help reduce environmental bacteria and help the pregnant woman's own immune defenses (Table 5–4). Because of their potential stimulating effects, certain oils should be avoided during pregnancy (Table 5–5).

HOMEOPATHY

Homeopathy is based on the theory of "like treats like." Homeopathy helps to restore the body's natural state of balance. Homeopathic preparations are created through a process of repeated dilutions and succussions (shaking the remedy). When completed, there is often no measurable trace of the active ingredient in the remedy. It is believed that through the series of dilutions and succussions, the active ingredient imprints itself on the water molecules and the effect of the remedy is energetic, not pharmacological. Generally, this makes homeopathic remedies safer than herbs. The advantage of homeopathy over herbs is the wrong remedy will cause no harm, whereas the right remedy will assist the body in healing.

TABLE 5–2. Common Herbs to Avoid during Pregnancy

Aloe vera (oral)—cathartic	Feverfew—emmenagogue
Angelica—emmenagogue*	Goldenseal—uterine stimulant
Birthroot—uterine astringent	Gotu kola—CNS stimulant
Black and blue cohosh— emmenagogues	Juniper berries—possibly teratogenic
Cascara sagrada—laxative	Mugwort—emmenagogue
Coltsfoot—possibly teratogenic	Pennyroyal—emmenagogue
Damiana—CNS/hormonal activity	Sage—emmenagogue (safe in cooking)
Dong quai—hormonal, carcinogenic properties	Sarsaparilla—hormonal activity
	Senna—laxative
Ephedra (ma huang)— cardiac stimulant	Shepherd's purse— hemostatic
	Tansy—emmenagogue
False unicorn root— uterine/hormonal effect	Wormwood—emmenagogue

*Induces menstrual bleeding

TABLE 5–3. Therapeutic Essential Oils to Use in Pregnancy

Chamomile (Roman)—calming	Mandarin—rejuvenating
Clary sage—morale booster, balancing	Peppermint—morning sickness
Geranium—uplifting, calming	Rose bulgar—relaxing
Grapefruit—astringent, energizing	Sandalwood—decreases heartburn
Jasmine—emotional balance	Ylang ylang—uplifting, balancing
Lavender—calming, healing	

TABLE 5–4. Essential Oils for the Puerperium

Clary sage—uplifting, balancing	Jasmine—emotional balance
Cypress—healing (use in Sitz baths)	Rosemary—energizing
Lavender (French)—healing (Sitz baths)	Ylang ylang—uplifting, balancing

Therefore, it is the much-preferred treatment during pregnancy and breastfeeding. There have been many European studies documenting the effectiveness of homeopathy. Homeopathic prescribing is often complex, focusing on individual characteristics and symptomatology in choosing a remedy. However, some remedies are more global in their application, such as arnica for muscle trauma and bruising (Castro, 1993). Additionally, several resources are listed at the end of this chapter to assist practitioners in the use of homeopathic remedies.

YOGA

Yoga enhances the mind–body connection during pregnancy. It is an ideal exercise for pregnant women because it fosters balance, relaxation, flexibility, and strength in a gentle, nonstrenuous way. Yoga encourages good posture to help prevent musculoskeletal problems (Romm, 1997a). The stillness and focus on breathing allows women to become peaceful and more in touch with emotions. Yoga is recommended for fatigue, low back pain, nausea, anxiety, headaches, muscle aches, and most other discomforts of pregnancy (Balaskas, 1994).

CONCLUSION

Integrating wellness in the care of women through the use of complementary therapies enhances awareness of the mind-body-spirit connection, fostering health and well-being. When considering these therapies, safety and efficacy are important. Begin with safety issues. Is there any empirical, theoretical, or intuitive information to suggest the therapy is harmful? If not, look for information regarding efficacy. If the research is inadequate, convey this to your client but do not automatically dismiss the potential benefit of the therapy. We are a complex species. We are holistic beings, greater than the sum of our parts. We require holistic care with attention to body, mind, and spirit in order to achieve maximal health and wellness. Expanding our consciousness by integrating complementary therapies will enable us to provide the best potential for treating, curing, and healing the women entrusted to our care.

REFERENCES

Achterberg, J. (1990). *Woman as healer*. Boston: Shambaba.

Aganoff, J., & Boyle, G. (1994). Aerobic exercise, mood states, and menstrual cycle symptoms. *Journal of Psychosomatic Research, 38(3)*, 183–192.

Bach, E., & Wheeler, F. J. (1997). *The Bach flower remedies*. New Canaan, CT: Keats Publishing.

Balaskas, J. (1994). *Preparing for birth with yoga*. Boston: Element.

Belew, C. (1999). Herbs and the childbearing woman: Guidelines for Midwives. *Journal of Nurse-Midwifery, 44(3)*, 231–251

Benson, H. (1975). *The relaxation response*. New York: Morrow.

Benson, H. (1996). *Timeless healing*. New York: Scribner.

Brennan, B. (1987). *Hands of light: A guide to healing through the human energy field*. New York: Bantam Books.

Brennan, P. (1999). Homeopathic remedies in prenatal care. *Journal of Nurse-Midwifery, 44(3)*, 291–299.

Bunce, K. L. (1987). The use of herbs in midwifery. *Journal of Nurse-Midwifery, 32(4)*, 255–259.

Burghardt, M. (1999). Exercise at menopause: A critical difference. *Medscape Women's Health*, 4(1), 1.

Carper, B. (1978). Fundamental patterns of knowing in nursing. *Advances in Nursing Science, 1*, 13–23.

Castro, M. (1993). *Homeopathy for pregnancy, birth and your baby's first year*. New York: Saint Martin's Press, LLC.

Coco, A. S. (1999). Primary dysmenorrhea. *American Family Physician, 60*, 489–496.

Dong, H., Ludicke, F., Comte, I., Campana, A., Graff, P., Bischof, P. (2001). An exploratory pilot study of acupuncture on the quality of life and reproductive hormone secretion in menopausal women. *Journal of Alternative and Complementary Medicine, (6)*, 651–658.

Duke, J. (1997). *The green pharmacy*. Emmaus, PA: Rodale.

Fugh-Berman, A. (2001). Raspberry leaf and pregnancy. *Alternative Therapies in Women's Health, 3* (4), 25–26.

Hawkins, J. L., Chestnut, C. P., & Gibbs, C. P. (2002). Obstetric anesthesia. In S. G. Gabbe, J. R. Niebyl, & J. L. Simpson

TABLE 5–5. Essential Oils to Avoid during Pregnancy

Aniseed	Clove[*]	Myrrh	Savoury[*]
Basil[*]	Fennel[*]	Nutmeg[*]	Spikenard
Bay[*]	Hops	Oregano[*]	Tarragon[*]
Black pepper[*]	Hyssop	Pennyroyal	Thyme[*]
Cedarwood	Juniper	Rosemary[*]	Valerian
Cinnamon bark	Marjoram[*]	Sage[*]	

[*]Safe for culinary use

(Ed.), *Obstetrics: Normal and problem pregnancies* (p. 433). New York: Churchill Livingstone.

Ivarsson, T., Spetz, A., & Hammar, M. (1998). Physical exercise and vasomotor symptoms in postmenopausal women. *Maturitas, 29*(2), 139–46.

Lane, A., & Lovejoy, D. (2001). The effects of exercise on mood changes: The moderating effect of depressed mood. *Journal of Sports Medicine and Physical Fitness, 41*(4), 539–545.

Leb, C. (1998). The effects of healing touch on depression. *Healing Touch International Survey, 9.*

Olson, M., & Sneed, N. (1995). Anxiety and therapeutic touch. *Issues in Mental Health Nursing, 16,* 97–108.

Romm, A. (1997a, March/April). Gentle expectations. *Herbs for Health,* 25–27.

Romm, A. (1997b). The *natural pregnancy book: Herbs, nutrition and other holistic choices.* Freedom, CA: Crossing Press.

Sander, E. (1996, January/February). Menopause—the yoga way. *Yoga Journal,* 61–69, 141.

Scialli, A. R., & Fugh-Berman, A. (2001). Herbs and pregnancy. *Alternative Therapies in Women's Health, 3*(8), 57–60.

Smith, J., Terpening, C., Schmidt, S., & Gums, J. (2001). Relief of fibromyalgia symptoms following dietary excitotoxins. *Annals of Pharmacotherapy, 35,* 702–706.

Tisserand, M. (1988). *Aromatherapy for women.* Rochester, VT: Healing Arts Press.

Van den Eeden, S. K., Koepsell, T. D., Longstreth, W. T., van Belle, G., Daling, J. R., & McKnight, B. (1994). Aspartame ingestion and headache: A randomized crossover trial. *Neurology, 44,* 1787–1793.

Weed, S. (1986). *Wise woman herbal for the childbearing year.* Woodstock, NY: Ash Tree Publishing.

Weil, A. (1999). *Breathing: The master key to self healing.* Boulder, CO: Sounds True.

Youngkin, E. Q., & Israel, D. S. (1996). A review and critique of common herbal alternative therapies. *Nurse Practitioner, 21,* (10), 39–62.

ADDITIONAL RESOURCES

Borysenko, J. (1996). *A woman's book of life.* New York: Riverhead Books.

Castro, M. (1990). *The complete homeopathy handbook.* New York: St. Martin's Press.

Dossey, B., Keegan, L., Guzzetta, C., & Kolkmeier, L. (1995). *Holistic nursing: A handbook for practice.* Gaithersburg, MD: Aspen Publishers.

Dumoff, A. (1995, June/July). Malpractice liability of alternative/complementary health care providers. *Alternative & Complementary Therapies,* 248–253.

Idarius, B. (1996). *The homeopathic childbirth manual.* Ukiah, CA: Idarius Press.

Northrup, C. (2001). *The wisdom of menopause.* New York: Bantam Books.

Robins, J. (1999). The alchemy of homeopathy. *National Academies of Practice Forum, 1,* 107–113.

Robins, J. (1999). Synthesizing reductionism and holism: Integrative advanced health care practice. *National Academies of Practice Forum, 1,* 197–202.

Spencer, J., & Jacobs, J. (1999). *Complementary/alternative medicine: An evidence-based approach.* St. Louis: Mosby.

Sinatra, S. (2000). *Heart sense for women.* New York: Penguin Group.

Weil, A. (1995). *Natural health, natural medicine.* Boston: Houghton Mifflin Company.

Worwood, V. A. (1991). *The complete book of essential oils and aromatherapy.* San Rafael, CA: New World Library.

INTERNET RESOURCES

HealthWorld Online: www.healthy.net

American Holistic Nurses Association: www.ahna.org

Bach Flower Essences: www.bachcentre.com

Dietsite: www.dietsite.com

DrSinatra.com: An Insider's Guide to Smart Medicine and Longevity: www.drsinatra.com

DrWeil.com: Your Guide to Optimum Health: www.drweil.com

The Holistic Health Center: www.forholistichealth.com

Herbal Medicine and Spirit Healing the Wise Woman Way: www.susanweed.com

Motherlove Herbal Company: www.motherlove.com

National Center for Homeopathy: www.homeopathic.org

CHAPTER 6

WOMEN AND SEXUALITY

Catherine Ingram Fogel

*W*omen have the right to intimate and sexual lives and relationships that are voluntary, pleasurable, wanted, and noncoercive.

Highlights

- Dimensions of Sexuality
- Factors That Affect Sexuality
- Sexual Concerns or Problems
- Sexual Dysfunction
- Sexual Health Care Assessment and History
- Sexual Health Interventions: PLISSIT Model

❖ INTRODUCTION

Sexuality is inextricably woven into the fabric of a woman's life and is an important aspect of her health. It is an integrated, unique expression of self that encompasses physiological and psychosocial processes inherent in sexual development, sexual response, sexual desire, view of self as a female, presentation of self to society as a woman, and sexual orientation (Fogel & Lauver, 1990). Sexuality underlies much of who and what a person is, and it is an inherent, ever-changing aspect of life from birth to death. Women express their sexuality differently at different times—alone, with one partner, or with different partners—and no two women express sexuality in exactly the same way (Bernhard, 1995).

Although experts do not agree on a definition of sexual health or what constitutes normal sexual behavior, the World Health Organization definition provides a starting point: "Sexual health is the integration of somatic, emotional, intellectual, and social aspects of sexual beings in ways that are positively enriching and that enhance personality, communication and love."

(WHO, 1995) Essential elements of this definition include a woman's capacity to live in a manner that is congruent with her personal and social ethic while enjoying and controlling sexual and reproductive behavior; the freedom from psychological factors such as guilt, anxiety, fear, shame, and misconceptions that impair sexual response and hurt sexual relationships; and the absence of disease, illness, organic disorders, or deficiencies that interfere with sexual function. Integral to sexual health is an acceptance of one's self-concept, body image, sexual identity, and sexual orientation.

Sexual health is that emotional and physical state that allows enjoyment and the ability to respond to sexual feelings. In short, sexual health may be considered the physical and emotional state of well-being that enables us to enjoy and act on our sexual feelings (BWHBC, 1998). Promoting sexual health is a legitimate role for health professionals and an essential nursing function. The nurse practitioner or other primary care provider can have a primary role in promoting and maintaining the sexual health of women.

DIMENSIONS OF SEXUALITY

Sexuality is a broad concept that encompasses the dimensions of sexual desire, sexual response, and sexual identity. Sexuality is a unique human quality that is an expression of a person's identity and a reflection of the basic need for emotional and physical closeness with another (MacLauren, 1995). Expressed positively, sexuality can bring much pleasure; however, it also has the potential to cause intense pain. It is not limited by age, attractiveness, sexual orientation, or partner participation (Fogel & Lauver, 1990).

SEXUAL DESIRE

Libido is the innate urge for sexual activity, produced by the activation of a specific system in the brain and experienced as a specific sensation that motivates an individual to seek out or be receptive to sexual experience (Kaplan, 1979). The hormone testosterone increases sexual desire in both males and females; in females, the small, influential amount of testosterone is made in the adrenal gland (Charlton & Quatman, 1997). The amount of sexual desire experienced varies across a woman's life span and from woman to woman. Moreover, sexual desire is a re-

sponse learned through feelings of pleasure, enjoyment, or dissatisfaction during sexual activity. Sexual desire derives from interest in sexual activity, preferred frequency of activity, and gender preference for a sexual partner. Further, desire is influenced by one's health, past experiences, and/or cultural and environmental factors. Sexual desire has been incorporated into official diagnostic descriptions of the sexual response cycle (APA, 1994). (See the following section for discussion).

SEXUAL RESPONSE

Sexual response involves *capacity* (what a woman is capable of experiencing) and *activity* (what she actually experiences) and provides the potential for creating a sense of enjoyment, satisfaction, and intimacy for a woman. In the past three decades, much has been learned about healthy sexual functioning. Nurses caring for women can incorporate the information now available into clinical practice. Central to incorporating sexual health care into one's practice is an understanding that emotion and physiology are interwoven in a woman's sexual response cycle.

The human sexual response cycle was first described by Masters and Johnson (1966) and focused on physiologic responses to stimuli. They identified that the endocrine, neurological, vascular, and muscular systems influence sexual response by influencing the amount of blood delivered and retained in the genitals and stimulating the excitation of rhythmic muscular contractions. The two principal physiologic sexual responses to sexual stimulation were identified as vasocongestion and muscle tension (myotonia).

Although Masters and Johnson began the modern movement toward an understanding of the sexual response cycle, their paradigm focused exclusively on physiologic aspects. Because of this focus on physiologic criteria, the subjective nature of sexual arousal was more or less ignored. Excitement was correlated with maximum physiologic performance and assumed that subjective arousal corresponds with physical arousal in the normal individual. No specific consideration was given to sexual desire; "successful" sex was equated with biologically complete and functional sex, and the motivating force behind sexual interaction was seen as the pleasure of arousal and orgasm (Charlton & Quatman, 1997). This approach does not specifically consider sexual desire, disregards passionate and sexual experiences that do not involve all four stages of physical response, and does not consider intimacy, which can be a powerful motivator or fearful inhibitor.

Later authorities incorporated both biologic and psychological components (APA, 1994; Kaplan, 1979; Schnarch, 1991). These models place more emphasis on the emotional and sociocultural context in which sexual activity occurs and the dynamics of relationships rather than solely on physical performance. This more inclusive model incorporating both physiologic and psychosocial factors includes the element of consent (Table 6–1).

Desire Phase

The first phase of the sexual response cycle is characterized by desire for sexual activity (libido) and sexual fantasy. It involves all of the thoughts, images, wishes, and imaging that are a part of sexual activity. While there are no specific physiologic changes associated with this phase, the phase prepares a woman for sexual stimulation and excitement.

Excitement Phase

The excitement phase consists of physiologic changes of sexual arousal and is characterized by vaginal lubrication, external genitalia swelling, narrowing of lower third of vagina, lengthening of upper two-thirds of vagina, and breast tumescence. The clitoris becomes engorged and highly sensitive. Some women may experience a sexual "flush." Systemic responses during this phase include accelerated heart rate and respiration and increased blood pressure. This phase may be interrupted, prolonged or ended by distracting stimuli (APA, 1994; Masters & Johnson, 1966; Roberts, Fromm, & Bartlik, 1998).

Orgasm

Orgasm is the height of sexual pleasure and experienced by a peaking of sexual pleasure followed by an involuntary release of sexual tension and rhythmic contractions of perineal muscles, uterus, and lower third of vagina. The contractions are especially strong in the muscles surrounding the vagina. In addition, heart rate, respiration, and blood pressure continue to be elevated. Orgasms commonly last between 3 and 60 seconds and may vary with each sexual experience and from woman to woman. Unlike men, women are capable of multiple orgasms during a single sexual encounter (Alexander, 1997). Women can experience single and multiple orgasms with vaginal intercourse, mutual masturbation, and self-pleasuring. Orgasms experienced with sexual intercourse have been reported to be more satisfying and less intense than those experienced with masturbation.

Resolution

With resolution, women experience a sense of general relaxation and well-being. A woman's resolution period occurs more slowly than does a man's and does not include a refractory period. The phase is characterized by a bodily return to the pre-excitement state. With adequate stimulation, women may again begin sexual response before complete resolution.

Women and men tend to report differences in body sensations of sexual pleasure. Women appear to be more total body oriented for sexual touching and experience pleasurable, sexual sensations from their skin, whereas men are conditioned to be more genitally oriented. Women report high degrees of sensitivity from mouth or finger contact, whereas men commonly report intercourse to be the most pleasurable form of sexual stimulation.

Although the physical sensations are common to all women, the sequence of physical and emotional sensations are uniquely experienced by each woman and not every woman experiences each response. A woman may experience different affective and physical responses from cycle to cycle. It is not necessary to progress through each of the phases in order to achieve sexual

TABLE 6–1. Sexual Response Cycle in Women

Phase of the Response Cycle	Physiologic/Psychologic Changes
Desire	Sexual fantasy and thoughts Sexual appetite, desire, motivation Active awareness that sexual stimulation is wanted No physiologic changes
Excitement (several minutes to several hours; intense excitement, 30 seconds to 3 minutes)	Subjective sense of anticipation and pleasure Tumescence and subsequent withdrawal of clitoris; labia redden and enlarge; vaginal lubrication; thickening of vaginal walls; expansion of inner two-thirds of vagina; orgasmic platform of outer one-third of vagina Uterus elevates in pelvis Anus tightens Sexual flush (mottling, reddening of skin) in up to 75 percent of women Nipple erection and enlargement in the breasts Increased heart rate, blood pressure, neuromuscular tension, perspiration, pupillary dilation Uterine contractions just before orgasm
Orgasm (3–60 seconds)	Peak of sexual tension, pleasure; sense of release Vasocongestion and muscle tension peak and release Clitoris remains retracted; vagina and labia majora contract rhythmically (about every 3–4 seconds; 3–15 contractions) Strong uterine contractions from fundus towards lower uterine segment; minimal relaxation of external cervical os External urethral sphincter contracts External rectal sphincter may contract; continued anus tightening Well-developed sexual flush Breasts remain enlarged Hyperventilation (up to 40 breaths/min); tachycardia (up to 180 bpm); increased blood pressure (30 to 80 mm Hg systolic; 20–40 mm Hg diastolic)
Resolution (10–15 minutes; if no orgasm, up to one day)	Subjective sense of relaxation Vasocongestion subsides quickly and body returns to unaroused state Clitoris returns to normal position; orgasmic platform relaxes and shrinks; vagina shortens; labia return to normal Uterus decreases in size and descends; cervix drops into seminal pool Breast size decreases Sexual flush resolves Blood pressure, pulse, respirations return to baseline Light perspiration (30–40% of women)

Sources: Charlton & Quatman, 1997; Lauver & Welch, 1990; Roberts et al., 1998; Schnarch, 1991; Zwelling, 1997.

fulfillment (Roberts et al., 1998). And the sexual response is the same whether the stimulus is self-pleasuring, pleasuring from another woman, from a man, or from intercourse (Woods, 1995).

SEXUAL IDENTITY

Sexual identity includes one's view of self as female, presentation of self as a woman, and sexual orientation. This identity is formed in early childhood and evolves throughout a woman's life as life circumstances continue to shape identity. A woman's view of herself as female includes her gender identity (sense of self as a woman); her sense of having characteristics customarily defined as female, masculine, or both (sex role); and body image (mental picture of one's body and its relationship to the environment). While gender identity is influenced by biological or anatomical sex, an individual's gender identity is not necessarily consistent with her biological sex (Alexander, 1997; Alexander & LaRosa, 1994).

Presentation of self as a woman (gender role or sex role) includes all attitudes and behaviors women use—such as dress, hairstyle, speech patterns, and walk—that are considered normal and appropriate for women in a specific culture. Sex role behaviors are a reflection of a woman's internalization of societal and cultural stereotypes and expectations of what a woman's behavior should be (Alexander & LaRosa, 1994). Sex role proscriptions and expectations shape sexual expression. Beliefs about women and men, and assumptions regarding appropriate behaviors for both, affect sexual behavior, communication patterns, and expectations of sexual relationships.

Sexual orientation refers to the preference an individual develops for a partner or the preference for the gender of the person with whom one has an emotional and physical attraction for and wishes to share sexual intimacy (Fogel & Lauver, 1990). Sexual preferences exist on a continuum ranging from complete orientation to the same sex through bisexuality to complete orientation to the other sex.

Sexual lifestyles provide the pattern and context for one's sexuality. While many options exist for women today, not all are equally accepted by society.

- *Heterosexual Martial Monogamy.* This is the most frequently acknowledged pattern for women, and marriage with monogamous partner is assumed to be most desirable by the majority of society.
- *Serial Heterosexual Monogamy.* This lifestyle consists of an established pattern of having one monogamous relationship followed by another.
- *Nonmonogamous Heterosexual Marriage.* Women who choose this lifestyle may participate in sexual activity with other individuals or couples while married to another.
- *Heterosexual Coupling without Marriage.* Women with this lifestyle have sexual relations with one or more male partners without marriage.
- *Single State.* Women with this sexual lifestyle may be unmarried, divorced, and widowed. This lifestyle is often assumed to be transitional by society.
- *Partnering with Either a Woman or a Man* (Bisexual). A woman's sexual and affectional preferences are directed toward individuals of either sex. Women may be married, have partners of both sexes simultaneously or serially, or have lesbian relationships as well as previous sexual relationships with men.
- *Partnering with a Woman* (Lesbian). A woman's sexual and affectional preferences are directed toward women. A woman may be coupled, or single with one or many partners. The most common pattern is serial monogamy.
- *Celibacy.* This lifestyle involves the conscious choice to abstain from sexual activity. Women may view this choice positively as a means of giving oneself time

and energy to devote total attention to other activities. Celibacy may also be nonvoluntary when a woman is between relationships.

FACTORS THAT AFFECT SEXUALITY

DEVELOPMENTAL FACTORS

Adolescence

The period between childhood and adulthood (ages 12 to 18 years) is a time of rapid physical changes and potentially stressful psychological demands including a time of awareness and change in sexual feelings. The development of adolescent sexuality focuses on five aspects (Zwelling, 1997):

- Physical changes of puberty and their relationship to self-esteem and body image.
- Learning about normal bodily functions and sensual and sexual responses and needs.
- Developing one's sense of self as a woman (gender identity) and comfort with one's sexual orientation.
- Learning about sexual and romantic relationships.
- Developing a personal sexual value system.

Sexuality is often defined through activities such as dating. During this time, one selects companions, tests ideas about oneself, and eventually experiences sexual pleasure as adolescents develop a capacity for sexual intimacy, and sexual curiosity and experimentation are common.

In the United States, the likelihood of teenagers' having intercourse increases steadily with age (AGI, 2002). Most very young teens have not had intercourse; eight in ten girls are sexually inexperienced at age 15. In contrast, about 40 percent of all 15- to 19-year-old women have had sexual intercourse (Singh & Darroch, 1999). Unwanted sexual experiences are common, particularly for adolescent girls; for example, between 25 and 42 percent of teenage women report unwanted sexual experiences (Moore et al., 1998; Wilson & Klein, 2002). The younger women are when they first have intercourse, the more likely they are to have had unwanted or nonvoluntary first coitus. Further, young women who initiate sexual activity early have greater numbers of sexual partners. Adolescents often face peer pressure to be sexually active; an additional motivation for sexual activity for girls may be a desire for sexual intimacy rather than a wish for the physical act of intercourse.

Risks associated with early sexual activity are increased risk for contracting sexually transmitted infections (STIs), including human immunodeficiency virus (HIV) and unintended pregnancies. Teenage women experience higher rates of the most common sexually transmitted diseases (STDs) than do older women, with three million teenage women acquiring an STD every year (AGI, 2002). While the teenage pregnancy rate has been declining, 78 percent of teen pregnancies are unplanned and account for about one-quarter of all accidental pregnancies annually (AGI, 2002; Ventura, Mosher, Curtin, Abma, & Henshaw, 2001).

Adulthood

In *early adulthood,* 20 to 45 years, women achieve maturity in a sexual role and in the relationship tasks started in adolescence, including developing intimacy with another individual and development of long-term commitment to a sexual relationship. Important career and personal decisions are made and increasing responsibilities assumed; balancing relationships, career, and children is often a concern. Women face choices regarding sexual lifestyles and often experience several before settling into one. During these years a woman continues to develop her personal sexual value system and must learn to be tolerant of others' sexual values. At some point during a woman's reproductive years (ages 20 to 45 years), she faces decisions about childbearing. Throughout these years, frequency of sexual activity decreases.

In *midlife,* 45 to 65 years, women's sexuality is as varied as are women. Some women report that sex is very good, possibly the best ever. Others report that sex is not the driving force it once was or that sex is less exciting and gratifying. The physiologic changes associated with menopause, which occurs generally between age 40 and 60, can affect sexual desire, expression, and/or functioning. During the perimenopausal years, many women find that their sex drive decreases for a while (Northrup, 2001). In the perimenopause, fluctuating levels of estrogen and related vasomotor instability can result in sleep disturbances associated with hot flashes; the resulting fatigue can adversely affect sexual desire. In the years immediately before and after menopause, women may report a loss of sexual desire associated with decreased vaginal lubrication, vaginal dryness, dyspareunia, painful spasms of the vaginal muscles, loss of clitorial sensations, fewer orgasms, and/or decreased depth of orgasm (Northrup, 2001). In contrast, other women may report increased sexual desire, increased clitorial sensitivity, increased responsiveness, and/or an increase in orgasms (Northrup, 2001). For some women, lessened concern of becoming pregnant may increase sexual desire and lessen inhibitions. An important point is that there is no reason for a diminished sex drive to become a permanent feature in the life of menopausal women.

During *older adulthood,* after age 65, women continue to be sexual and enjoy sexual activity. Although sexual frequency may decline, sexual enjoyment sometimes increases with age, and patterns of sexual behavior remain similar to those in midlife (Alexander & LaRosa, 1994). The need for excitement, pleasure, and intimacy does not fade with aging. A critical issue for older women's sexual expression and activity is availability of a partner. Another important factor is health since good health is positively associated with sexual interest and activity (B. K. Johnson, 1996).

Postmenopausal are not immune to the stressors that have been shown to decrease libido in younger women. The increased responsibilities of different roles that occur with age can increase marital strain and depression and have a negative impact on libido (Murray, 2000). Satisfaction with one's sexual function is also influenced by self-evaluation within the context of personal desires and expectations. Personal expectations are often based on cultural and social factors as well as past sexual experiences. The prevailing cultural view of older women as asexual beings can negatively affect sexual expression and activity and often becomes a self-fulfilling prophecy. Further, current cultural emphasis on youth, beauty, and thinness also contributes to the societal expectation of asexuality in older women.

The physiological changes associated with urogenital aging (i.e., decreased estrogen supply, decreased tissue elasticity, thinning of vaginal tissues) can cause irritation or discomfort with penetration and contribute to lessened desire and activity. The vascular changes that occur in arousal and the intensity of muscular contractions with orgasm may diminish moderately after age 55 to 60 (Alexander, 1997). Loss of fatty tissue of labia and mons pubis may result in tenderness and easily damaged tissue or abrasions and also decrease sexual libido and functioning. Orgasms may decrease in intensity and, in some women, become painful. Breast size also decreases and breasts may sag. While these changes may alter a woman's sexual view of herself, they do not alter her ability to respond sexually.

Body changes may require that a woman and her partners alter how they engage in sexual activity. With aging, sexual practices may include the use of water-soluble lubricant, increased foreplay for arousal, different sexual positions, and planning intercourse for times when energy levels are highest.

While sexual interest and activity may decrease somewhat with aging, many older women maintain sexual relationships, if a partner is available. Old women with partners may find that opportunities for sexual expression within relationships increase as career and family pressures are reduced and more time is available for sharing with a partner. Many older women become celibate due to lack of a partner; however, their need for touch and closeness continues, and they must be encouraged to seek out opportunities for intimacy with another person.

CHILDBEARING INFLUENCES

Sexuality is a concern for many women and their partners during pregnancy and postpartum. Levels of libido and frequency of sexual activity can vary with the trimester of pregnancy. During the first trimester, desire and functioning may be inhibited by nausea and vomiting, breast tenderness, fatigue, and anxiety about the pregnancy. In the second trimester, women often express heightened desire as they feel better although some may be inhibited by increasing weight and bodily changes. Women may experience diminished sexual desire and activity during the third trimester associated with physical discomfort related to increasing size, especially near term.

The physiologic changes associated with pregnancy can contribute to changes in pregnant women's physical sexual response (Alteneder & Hartzell, 1997). Increased vascularity of the genital area can lead to increased sexual tension. Generalized vasocongestion of the pelvic viscera and increased vaginal lubrication occurs by the end of the first trimester and persists throughout pregnancy; vaginal lubrication develops more rapidly and extensively. Orgasm may be triggered more easily during pregnancy due to increased vascular flow to the genital tissues, particularly clitoral erectile tissues, and muscle tension; some women may experience their first orgasm during pregnancy. In the third trimester, women may experience continuous (tonic) uterine contractions with orgasm rather than the typical rhythmic contractions (Zwelling, 1997). The resolution phase may be longer due to increased pelvic vasocongestion that may not be completely relieved by orgasm.

For some couples, pregnancy is a time during which intercourse is avoided. They report a progressive decline in desire, frequency of intercourse, and response through-

out pregnancy (Heiman & Lentz, 2000). Fears about harming the baby or the woman, female self-perceptions of unattractiveness, and/or sexual restrictions associated with high-risk pregnancy (e.g., preterm labor) may contribute to decline in sexual activity and sexual satisfaction during pregnancy.

During the postpartum, women report lessened sexual desire and decreased sexual activity for up to six months (Byrd, Hyde, DeLamater, & Plant, 1998). Reasons for decreased desire and activity are physical discomfort, lessened physical strength, dissatisfaction with appearance, and fatigue. Early postpartum physical manifestations such as lochia, increased vaginal discharge, and episiotomy pain can contribute to decreased sexual desire or activity. Once the initial vaginal discharge has subsided, women may notice a marked vaginal dryness associated with decreased estrogen and progesterone (Peck, 2001). Although the vaginal dryness may be experienced by all postpartum women, it is most common in breastfeeding women. Women who experience vaginal dryness may require some form of lubrication to prevent dyspareunia. Additionally, motherhood allows little privacy and little rest, both of which are necessary for sexual pleasure. Although little is known about possible partner issues with sexuality after childbirth, partner issues such as fatigue, fear of harming the woman or causing pain with intercourse, cultural or religious issues, or jealousy towards the infant may negatively impact partner participation.

Struggles with infertility and repeated attempts to conceive can negatively impact sexual self-esteem, sexual expression, activity, and desire. Women may find the concepts of woman and infertility to be mutually exclusive (C.L. Johnson, 1996). Fertility and virility seem to be inextricably linked in our society. A diagnosis of infertility may negatively affect a woman's sense of sexuality, her self-image, and even her marriage. For women who desire pregnancy, pressure and need to time intercourse may interfere with pleasure and communication because couples no longer have sex for pleasure but rather only for procreation. Years of attempting to conceive and/or bear a child makes spontaneous sex difficult to maintain. Sexuality is an important source of communication and growth in the development of a couple's relationship. When the desired end result of sexual activity is reproduction, sex can become mechanical or take on a demand type of value. Women may initiate sexual activity around the time of ovulation even if they are experiencing low or decreased desire. Reacting to a feeling of threat or resentful of "sex on demand," men may experience "reactive impotence," or an inability to perform sexually, especially around the time of ovulation. Hopelessness, isolation, and self-blame may accompany miscarriage, stillbirth, and infertility.

SOCIOCULTURAL INFLUENCES

Women's sexuality exists within the context of cultural expectations, individual experiences, and biological potential. Family, culture, law, and religion all shape woman's attitudes and behavior regarding sex (see Family Influence). Society and culture are inextricably interwoven with sexuality and influence it as much as do physiology and psychology. Social influences on sexuality begin first within the structure of the family. Through socialization of the individual, the family conveys its own, as well as societal, sexual attitudes and behaviors and can contribute to later sexual dysfunction.

The larger structure of society and its culture also affect sexuality. Society defines what sexual behavior is and the norms for that behavior that are understood and guide behavior of the individuals in a given culture. Current U.S. cultural values present mixed messages to women: Be sexually responsive but within well-defined boundaries. Today, women are defined as dysfunctional if they are "too promiscuous" or if they are not sexual enough—for example, lack desire for an appropriate partner or do not become aroused/reach orgasm with that partner. A specific behavior may be defined as desirable by one cultural group and evil by another. Different views often exist regarding premarital, extramarital, and marital sex; appropriate sexual positions; accepted foreplay activities; and duration of coitus.

To the extent that sexual activity is a coerced activity, full sexual functioning is unlikely to occur. Coercion exists on a continuum from guilt induced by a partner's hurt feelings if refused to the extreme of rape. Male sexual coercion of females in our society is endemic. In almost all present societies, incest is prohibited. Incest contributes to sexual dysfunction particularly when it involves threat or force, occurs at an older age when guilt is more apt to be present, is associated with strong negative feelings or is repeated over time.

In part, women form their ideas of what is sexually appropriate and desirable from years of cultural scripting. In large part, our notions of sexual appropriateness is influenced by our male-dominated culture with an inherent double standard (Northrup, 2001). Cultural scripts are frequently different for men and women and can be the basis of many of the issues women experience in sexual relationships. The notions that men who are sexually aggressive are "macho" or "studs" and that sexually aggressive women are "whores" and "easy" are examples of such cultural beliefs. Current sex role stereotypes prescribe that men initiate sexual activity while women exercise control. Certainly, cultural practices that physically alter sexual response such as clitorectomy will affect sexuality.

Sexual myths abound in every culture and society, are a source of sexual ignorance and misinformation, and can be related to many sexual problems. Often they interfere with women's reaching full sexual potential and establishing fulfilling sexual relationships. The list of sexual myths is long:

- Women should satisfy men; women's needs are secondary to men. Further, men are oversexed, women are undersexed, men initiate sex, and women receive sex.
- Sexual pleasure is the responsibility of the partner. Related to this is the expectation that a partner should somehow be able to sense what a woman's needs are.
- Large amounts of sexual stimulation are needed to arouse a woman; a woman arouses more slowly than a man.
- Orgasms are different for men and women.
- Women who are raped asked for it; every woman wants to be raped; when a woman says no, she doesn't mean it.
- Little girls should not be told about sex because that will put ideas in their heads.
- Women are not interested in sex; they cannot have multiple orgasms.
- Women only want sex for procreation purposes.
- Women are so sexually aggressive that they can never be satisfied.
- Sex and intercourse are synonymous.
- A woman who initiates sex is immoral.
- A woman cannot enjoy sex unless she has an orgasm.
- A partner will find someone else if a woman doesn't satisfy his/her sexual needs.
- Women are supposed to balance career, family, home, and always be ready for sex.
- There are absolute norms for sexual expression.
- Masturbation is dirty.
- Women can only have an orgasm with intercourse.
- Men are more aroused by pornography and fantasy than women.
- Men and women have different sexual age peaks, or men wear out and women wear well.

- It is dangerous to have sex during menstruation; sex during pregnancy can "mark" a child and should be avoided.
- Menopause or hysterectomy ends a woman's sexual life.
- Oral-genital sex indicates homosexual tendencies.

There are also sexual myths that are specific to elderly women.

- Older women are not interested in/capable of sexual expression.
- Older women cannot make love even if they want to.
- Older women are fragile and might hurt themselves if they do attempt sexual relations.
- Older women are physically unattractive and sexually undesirable.
- Older women who do have sexual relations are shameful/dirty.

Religion also influences sexual attitudes, beliefs, and values and can exert a strong influence throughout a person's life. Religious proscriptions can contribute to sexual concerns or problems. For example, a view that sexual intercourse is acceptable only for procreation may raise concerns when pleasurable sensations are felt. Accepting or rejecting premarital sex, contraception to prevent pregnancy, beliefs about monogamy for men and women, and condoning or rejecting homosexuality are examples of religious influences in a woman's life.

Laws are usually made in a society to regulate and control unacceptable sexual behavior. Often periods of societal change are necessary to alter sociocultural beliefs and change laws. One example of such a period was the 1960s and 1970s when women began to redefine their sexuality for themselves. New definitions that recognized that sexuality is created by individuals, not anatomically given and proscribed, began to be developed. During this time women-centered definitions of sexuality that included sensuality, closeness, mutuality, and relationships emerged (Fogel & Woods, 1995).

SEXUAL CONCERNS OR PROBLEMS

ILLNESS-RELATED ISSUES

A number of health-related factors—including illness, surgery, disability, medications, and chemical dependency—can influence sexuality and sexual performance.

Illness can affect sexuality in a number of ways, and a variety of medical conditions can cause sexual dysfunction in women (Table 6–2). Chronic illness with its associated fatigue, pain, and stress affects sexual desire and arousal more often than it affects orgasm. For example, diabetic women report that difficulties with vaginal lubrication, monilial infections, and genital discomfort negatively influence sexual functioning (Shafer, 2002). Many medications can alter sexual functioning and cause sexual dysfunctions including anorgasmia and inadequate lubrication, most commonly antidepressants, antihypertensives, antihistamines, neuroleptics, and antipsychotics (see Table 6–3). The degree of impairment is often dose

TABLE 6–2. Medical Conditions May Interfere with Sexual Functioning in Women

Neurologic Disorders	Endocrine Disorders
Amyotrophic lateral sclerosis	Acromegaly
Cardiovascular accident	Addison's disease
Central nervous system tumors	Cushing's disease
Head trauma	Diabetes mellitus
Herniated lumbar disc	Hypopituitarism
Hypothalamic lesions	Pituitary tumor
Multiple sclerosis	Prolactin-secreting pituitary
Polio	adenoma
Neoplastic spinal cord disease	Thyroid deficiency
Paraplegia, other spinal cord injuries	
Peripheral neuropathies	
Radical pelvic surgery	
Temporal lobe epilepsy	
Gynecologic Disorders/Surgery	Renal and Urologic Disorders
Endometriosis	Chronic renal failure
Episiotomy	Chronic interstitial cystitis
Oophorectomy	Cystitis
Pelvic inflammatory disease	Dialysis
Sexually transmitted diseases	Nephritis
Uterine myomas	Cystocele
Uterine prolapse	
Cardiovascular and Pulmonary Disorders	Other
Asthma	Anemia
Cardiac disease, including angina	Arthritis
Coronary artery disease	Colostomy
Hypertension	Degenerative diseases
Post-coronary syndrome	Infections
Post-stroke syndrome	Malnutrition
Sickle-cell anemia	Liver disease
	Lower bowel disease
	Malignancies
	Mastectomy
	Musculoskeletal disorder
	Pelvic fracture
	Radiation therapy
	Sjogren's syndrome

Sources: Roberts et al., 1998; Shafer, 2002.

TABLE 6–3. Medications Adversely Affecting Sexual Functioning

Category and Generic Name	Trade Name	Category and Generic Name	Trade Name
Anorectics		Diphenhydramine hydrochloride	Benadryl
Phentermine	Ionamin, Fastin	Pseudoephedrine	Sudafed
Fenfluramine	Pondamin	Antiolytics/tranquilizers	
Phenylpropanolamine	Ma huang, Ephedra, Mormon Tea, Dexatrim, Ayds, Acutrim	Benzodiazepines	
		Antipsychotics/neuroleptics	
Diethylpropion	Tenuate		
Mazindol	Sandrex	Phenothiazines	
		Chloropromazine	Thorazine
Anticancer Drugs		Fluphenazine	Prolixin
Vinblastine	Methotrexate	Perphenazine	Trilafan
5-fluorouracil	Efudex	Thioridazine	Mellaril
Tamoxifen	Nolvadex		
		Other	
Antihypertensives		Haloperidol	Haldol
Reserpine	Serpasil		
Methyldopa	Aldomet	Thiothixine	Navane
Guanethidine	Ismelin	Resperidone	Risperdal
Betablockers			
Propranolol	Inderal	Psychotrophics	
Atenolol	Tenormin	Tricyclic antidepressants	
Metoprolol	Lopressor	Clomipramine	Anafranil
Bisoprolol	Zebeta	Amitriptyline	Elavil
Timolol	Timoptic	Doxepin	Sinequan
Betaxolol	Betoptic	Imipramine	Tofranil
		Nortriptyline	Aventyl
Alpha1 blockers		Desipramine	Nopramin
Prazosin	Minipress	Monoamine oxidase inhibitors (MAO inhibitors)	
Doxazosin	Cardura		
Alpha2 blockers		Isocarboxazid	Marplan
Clonidine	Catapres	Phenelzine	Nardil
Guanfacine	Tenex	Tranylcypromine	Parnate
ACE inhibitors		Serotonin uptake inhibitors	
Captopril	Capoten	Fluoxetine	Prozac
Enalapril	Vasotec	Paroetine	Paxil
Calcium channel blockers		Sertraline	Zoloft
Amlodipine	Norvasc	Fluvoxamine	Luvox
Verapamil	Calan, Isoptin	Venlafaxine	Effexor
Diltiazem	Cardizem	Mood stablizers/anticonvulsants	
		Lithium carbonate	
Antiulcer medications		Valproate	Depakote
Cimetidine	Tagamet	Carbamazepine	Tegretol
Famotidine	Pepcid	Phenytoin	Dilantin
Nixatidine	Axid	Phenobarbitol	Dosette
Cold/allergy medications			
Chlorpheniramine	Chlor-Trimeton		

Sources: Charlton & Quatman, 1997; Roberts et al., 1998; Shafer, 2002.

related. Additionally, depending on the dosage and an individual's mental and physical state, some medications known to inhibit sexual function may also enhance it. Examples of such drugs include the benzodiazephine tranquilizers and chlorpheniramine (Roberts et al., 1998).

All cancers can impact sexuality and intimacy. Treatment that affects the vascular system or causes nerve damage may alter sexual function. A crucial factor in predicting sexual dysfunction in women with breast cancer is

treatment with adjuvant systemic chemotherapy. Fatigue associated with cancer and its treatments may affect sexual desire. Changes in body image and self-concept may have a profound influence on sexuality. For example, in our society where breasts are sexual, a woman with breast cancer may have sexuality concerns; greater sexuality problems may be experienced by women who dislike their breasts, have a negative self-image, have been sexually abused, lack a support system, or are uncomfortable discussing personal or sexual concerns (Bernhard, 1995). Results of studies on the effects of hysterectomy on sexuality vary widely and no longer document negative effects only (Katz, 2002).

Sexually transmitted diseases (STDs), including the human immunodeficiency virus (HIV), which are transmitted within the context of a dyadic, interpersonal relationship, have the potential to affect a woman's sexuality and sexual functioning. There is a profound conditioning in our culture that says sex is love, sex is power, and sex makes a woman important. Women who have been diagnosed with an STD often experience depression, low self-esteem, guilt, lack of trust, and/or anger (Fogel, 1995). The adoption of safer sex practices necessitates altered sexual practices. A fundamental characteristic of sexual risk reduction practices, individuals must give up behavior that is enjoyable, gratifying, highly reinforced, often long-standing, and replace it with alternatives that are almost always less gratifying, more awkward or inconvenient, and harder to do than current behaviors (Kelly & Kalichman, 1995). Women may decide to be celibate to avoid risk, decrease the number of their partners or avoid certain partners, and change or avoid specific sexual activities that increase risk. The risk of sexual coercion may be greater for women in power-imbalanced relationships with men who resist using condoms. Sex roles and sexual double standards may hinder a woman's ability to ask for safer sex practices and contribute to a man's resistance to implement these practices.

Chemical dependency can have an adverse effect on sexual functioning and sexuality. Sexual dysfunctions, especially sexual desire disorders, can occur with the use of substances such as alcohol, amphetamines, cocaine, opiods, sedatives, and tranquilizers (Klein, 1997; Zerbe, 1999). Chemical dependency in women is associated with issues such as incest and childhood sexual abuse experiences, rape, and violent relationships as adults. Women who use illicit drugs have been labeled "crack whores" and described as compulsively exchanging sex for a drug. In reality, contrary to popular folklore that crack is an aphrodisiac, women who use crack cocaine report that the drug has an adverse effect on sexual desire and functioning (Henderson, Boyd, & Whitmarsh, 1995). While crack use reduces sexual desire and the physical ability to be orgasmic, crack use is associated with more frequent sex, trading sex for drugs and money, and having multiple partners.

Disability may affect sexuality in a number of ways. Disabled women often are viewed as less sexual or asexual by health providers and the public alike (Cesario, 2002) and thus are not encouraged to express their sexual feelings or to be sexually active. The attitude that a disability somehow "neuters" a woman interferes with her right to sexual feelings and sexual expression. Often women with disabilities have more difficulty finding partners and establishing intimate relationships than do able-bodied women (Zerbe, 1999). Access to social and interpersonal interactions often is limited; however, greater threats to intimacy related to disability may be feelings of worthlessness and unattractiveness. A critical issue for some women who are disabled is body image—they may view their bodies as a problem and a source of anxiety rather than an instrument for pleasure. The reactions of others may suggest that a woman's body is unacceptable/unattractive. The specific physical effects of a given disability on sexual activity differ with the disability. Women with spinal cord injuries (SCI) commonly report autonomic dysreflexia and bladder incontinence (Jackson & Woodley, 1999). SCI women may experience alterations in desire, establishing adequate vaginal lubrication, ability to reach or feel orgasm, and difficulty finding a comfortable position for intercourse (Cesario, 2002).

LOSS OF A PARTNER

Women may define their identity through relationships, and thus the loss of a partner can be a loss of self. Furthermore, the stereotypical view of a widow is of a sad, grieving woman whose sexual life is over. A woman's sexuality after the loss of a partner may be influenced by her past extramarital sexual experiences, age, and sexual satisfaction in her marriage (Bernhard, 1995). Remarriage is correlated with age; the older a woman, the less likely remarriage.

FAMILY INFLUENCE

Poor parent–child interactions contribute indirectly to sexual problems; such a child may have lower self-esteem or difficulty coping with intimacy. Restrictive family upbringing and the belief that expressions of intimacy or sexuality are shameful or taboo may affect a woman's later ability to express herself sexually. Sexual expression or enjoyment may be inhibited by messages that were taught within a restrictive family—messages such as "Sex is something to be endured" or "Women who enjoy sex are no good."

Sexual abuse with its inevitable negative associations, including the case of threats and force, and feelings of guilt and anxiety contributes to sexual dysfunction.

RELATIONSHIP ISSUES

Discord within a relationship may precipitate sexual dysfunction, so much so that many sex therapists suggest that sexual dysfunction is a symptom of the underlying relationship problem. Open communication of one's sexual preferences, feelings, and desires is essential for sexual satisfaction. Communication problems are exacerbated by distrust, feelings of betrayal, and fear of disease. One or both partners may experience difficulty after the disclosure of sexual encounters out of their relationship. Sexual dysfunction in one's partner may precipitate dysfunction in the other. For example, premature ejaculation is often accompanied by lack of vaginal lubrication, orgasmic difficulties, and impaired sexual desire.

SEXUAL DYSFUNCTION

Altered, impaired, incomplete, or absent expressions of human sexual desires and responses become dysfunctional only when there is distress and discomfort associated with them. Sexual dysfunction may be defined as the persistent impairment of an individual's normal patterns of sexual interest and response. Thus, sexual dysfunction is inherently subjective (Roberts et al., 1998). It is not always easy to distinguish between aberrant or merely unconventional behaviors or between healthy and neurotic behaviors. Questions that the nurse practitioner might ask to assist in drawing these distinctions are the following (MacLauren, 1995):

- How does the woman interpret the behavior?
- Does the behavior enhance or impoverish her sexual life and those with whom she has sexual relations?
- Does society in general tolerate the behavior?
- Is the behavior between two consenting adults?
- Does the behavior cause physical or psychological harm to the woman or her partner?
- Does the behavior involve coercion?

Several factors characterize sexual dysfunction.

- Dysfunction may occur in one or more phases of the sexual response cycle but is less common in the resolution phase.
- Dysfunction may occur during masturbation or, more commonly, during sexual activity with a partner.
- Dysfunction may be lifelong or develop after a period of normal responsiveness; it may occur once or recur.
- Most typically, dysfunction is seen among individuals in their late 20s or early 30s.

The prevalence of sexual dysfunctions in women is not precisely known, as epidemiological studies that include sexual dysfunction, especially in women, are rare. Additionally, clinicians often do not elicit the information when providing health care, and client discomfort in answering questions or reporting problems of a sexual nature contributes to underestimating the prevalence of sexual dysfunctions. It has been suggested that most individuals experience some degree of sexual difficulty at some point in their lives. For example, transient, delayed, or absent sexual response might occur with illness or fatigue, when a woman is preoccupied with life demands or with certain medications, drugs, or alcohol. In contrast to popular belief, satisfaction with marriage does not imply adequate sexual functioning or satisfaction (Heiman, 1995).

CAUSES OF SEXUAL DYSFUNCTION

Pathophysiological causes of sexual dysfunction are more common than those that are psychogenic; however, traumatic sexual experiences, such as incest, rape, and coercive sexual encounters may precipitate dysfunction. Other associated factors may be depression and life stress. Anxieties, including fear of partner rejection, fear of failure, and fear of demand for performance, may also result in dysfunction (Hawkins, Roberto-Nichols & Stanley-Haney, 2000). Poor communication between partners about sexual feelings, needs, and desires often occurs and can perpetuate an unsatisfying sexual pattern or escalate problems by limiting knowledge of each other or restricting standards of acceptable sexual behavior.

TABLE 6–4. Female Sexual Dysfunctions

Sexual Desire Disorders
Hyposexual Sexual Desire (HSD): Persistent lack of desire for sexual activity.
Sexual Aversion Disorder: Aversion to, and avoidance of, genital sexual activites. More severe form of sexual inhibition.

Sexual Arousal Disorder
Inability to attain or maintain physiological sexual arousal

Inhibited Female Orgasm
Inability to experience orgasm following normal sexual excitement phase with sexual activity.

Sexual Pain Disorders
Dyspareunia: Recurrent genital pain before, during, or after vaginal intercourse.
Vaginismus: Involuntary vaginal spasm accompanied by pain interfering with or preventing intercourse.

Source: Ayers, 1995; Heiman, 1995; Morrison, 1995; Roberts et al., 1998.

SEXUAL DYSFUNCTIONS IN WOMEN

Sexual dysfunctions may arise from a disruption in any of the phases of the sexual response, most commonly, desire, excitement, and orgasm. Additionally, sexual pain disorders are considered in this classification (see Table 6–4). Sexual dysfunction also is categorized as lifelong (has occurred throughout a woman's active sexual life) or acquired (there has been a time when a woman did not experience sexual dysfunction) and general (disorder occurs with all partners and in all situations) or situational (occurs only with certain partners or situations).

Sexual Desire Disorders

Hyposexual Sexual Desire (HSD). This disorder is a prevalent sexual problem and one for which women most commonly seek assistance (Roberts et al., 1998). Sexual desire depends on many things including inherent sexual drive, self-esteem, previous sexual satisfaction, an available partner, and a good relationship with one's partner in areas other than sex. Women with HSD have little or no desire for sexual activity, sexual dreams or fantasies, do not become frustrated if sexual activity does not occur, and rarely, if ever, initiate sexual activity. Sexual activity occurs infrequently or only in reluctant compliance with a partner's desire for activity (Ayers, 1995; Heiman, 1995). Although the cause is unknown, the disorder is thought to be associated with depression, anxiety, and high levels of stress. Women with HSD may have deeper and more intense sexual anxieties, greater amounts of hostility and/or resentment in their relationships, and more tenacious defense mechanisms than do clients with arousal or orgasm phase difficulties. Two common etiologies are trauma (sexual abuse, assault, or incest) or relationship issues that have created resentment and hostility. Life events such as job loss or family trauma also may play a role. Psychological response to aging in a society that has strict cultural norms of female attractiveness may be a factor in some women. Physical factors also can be involved, particularly hormonal status, general health status, and use of recreational drugs and alcohol.

Desire disorders are difficult to diagnose and diagnosis is made more difficult because there are no norms for sexual desire across the life span. Generalized lifelong hyposexual desire suggests a need for assessment for endocrine disorders, illness, and long-term medication use. Among the areas to assess during the sexual history include (McCafferty, Barnett, & Thomas, 2001): Does she limit physical contact with her partner fearing that it will lead to sex? Does she become irritated when her sexual partner initiates sex? Or feel that having sex is an imposition? Does she have a negative body image? Treatment depends on the extent of the dysfunction, taking into account factors that affect sexual functioning such as age, occupation, and the context of a woman's life. Underlying physical causes should be treated first because desire often returns when a woman's feelings of well-being are restored. Treatment of a primary sexual dysfunction such as dyspareunia or anorgasmia may also alleviate a lack of desire. Treatment is often difficult and frequently incorporates sensate focus and techniques to improve communication between partners. It is essential that health care providers assisting women with HSD provide a supportive environment and frequent opportunities for expression of feelings. Often a client may require referral to a health care professional with advanced training in sexual counseling and therapy. This should not be done during a crisis period. If an underlying depression is suspected, the nurse practitioner should refer a client to a mental health provider for medication and/or psychotherapy. In some instances, referral for couple therapy will be appropriate.

Sexual Aversion Disorder. Extreme repulsion, loathing, and avoidance of almost all genital sexual contact with a partner is classified as sexual aversion disorder. This disorder, which is far less common than HSD, may be the result of painful intercourse, feelings of guilt, or rape or other sexual trauma occurring in childhood or earlier in a woman's sexual life. Physical factors are not usually involved. These women, who experience intense irrational fear of sexual activity and a compelling desire to avoid sexual situations, should be referred to a trained sex therapist for care. Therapy usually includes cognitive behavioral techniques, desensitization, and, when relevant, working through issues of past abuse.

Sexual Arousal Disorder

Female sexual arousal disorder occurs in as many as one-third of all women (Morrison, 1995). The disorder is characterized by partial or complete failure to attain or maintain vaginal lubrication and swelling. Women also report a lack of sexual excitement or pleasure. A number of biological factors may cause insufficient vaginal lubrication, including medications such as antihistamines and anticholinergics or marijuana use prior to a sexual experience (Ayers, 1995). Postmenopausal women may experience lessened lubrication due to lowered estrogen levels. Chronic yeast infections, acute or chronic bacterial vaginosis, or trichomoniasis also may be associated with inadequate lubrication. Once physical causes have been ruled out or treated, women with this disorder should be referred to a trained sex therapist for care.

Inhibited Female Orgasm

A significant minority of women report having difficulty achieving orgasm at some time in their lives. The inability to experience orgasm is defined as a disorder only if a woman reports receiving sufficient stimulation without orgasm. Women with this dysfunction do experience erotic feelings, genital swelling, and vaginal lubrication.

Rarely is primary (lifelong, generalized) orgasmic disorder caused by a physical factor. Rather, factors such as a restrictive home environment, negative cultural conditioning during childhood, unrealistic expectations about performance, current relationship issues, and lack of knowledge about female anatomy or the sexual response cycle are implicated. Physical causes of inhibited female orgasm include illnesses such as hypothyroidism and diabetes; vaginal damage such as episiotomy scars; any physical cause of dyspareunia; or endometriosis. Medications such as antihypertensives, central nervous system stimulants, serotonin-reuptake inhibitors or tricyclic antidepressants, and monoamine oxidase inhibitors also have been associated with inhibited orgasmic response (Morrison, 1995).

Women whose orgasmic difficulties have a physical basis should be treated for the underlying cause. Once physical causes have been corrected, the most common treatments for this problem are behavioral. For example, the woman is taught to experience orgasm through a series of exercises that increase her awareness of genital sensations and masturbatory techniques. Once she has experienced an orgasm through self-stimulation, she is taught to transfer this knowledge to a partner experience. Women with a partner may be given specific couple exercises to practice. Women with an orgasmic dysfunction may also benefit from information about female anatomy and physiology and the differences between male and female response cycles.

Sexual Pain Disorders

Dyspareunia. Pain experienced in the labia, vagina, or pelvis during or after intercourse is called dyspareunia (Jones, Lehr, & Hewell, 1997; Schnare, 1997). Pain may be experienced prior to, with penetration upon intromission, and/or with thrusting. Even when the actual pain is gone, the memory of the pain may persist and interfere with pleasure. Dyspareunia is both a symptom and a diagnosis (Morrison, 1995). All too often women do not seek care for this problem. The incidence of this problem is unknown; estimates of the prevalence in the general population are about 20 percent with a range of 4 percent to 40 percent. Some authorities suggest that as many as 60 percent of women experience dyspareunia at some time in their lives. Further, the incidence appears to be increasing; however, it is not clear if this is a result of the increasing incidence of sexually transmitted diseases, changes in sexual behavior, or women's increased willingness to talk about sexual matters. As women age, they also report more dyspareunia associated with changes in the urogenital system.

Causes of dyspareunia are many and diverse (see Table 6–5 for etiology of dyspareunia). Physical causes are most common and numerous. They include sexually transmitted disease, bladder disease, diabetes, anatomic defects, and decreased estrogen due to aging. Mechanical causative factors may be excessive douching or the use of irritating soaps or sprays. Dyspareunia may also be caused by psychological factors related to family religious taboos or teachings that the vagina should not be touched; traumatic factors such as rape, incest, or previous painful intercourse; or other factors such as a lack of complete arousal and inadequate vaginal lubrication, personal problems, or negative feelings toward one's partner. (Heiman, 1995; Jones et al., 1997; Schnare, 1997).

Presentation of dyspareunia is diverse, necessitating a careful, logical sequence of history taking, physical examination, laboratory studies, and therapies. In general, the history would include inquiring about the following:

- Sexual response cycle and any alterations in phases of sexual response cycle she has noticed.
- Attempts to conceive, previous high-risk pregnancy, postpartal difficulties, contraceptive choices, and problems associated with them.
- Past and present illness, surgery, and medications.
- Client's self-concept and body image.
- Her view of herself as a sexual being and level of confidence in ability to function sexually.
- Past and current psychiatric problems or illness including anxiety and depression and use of psychotrophic medications.
- Her satisfaction with current relationship.
- Any history of sexual abuse.
- Perceptions of sex appropriate roles for men and women in relationships; perception regarding her ability to fulfill these roles competently.
- Sources of sexual education, when received, and reactions to this information.
- A woman's religious affiliation and beliefs and ethnic and cultural belief system also should be noted.

TABLE 6–5. Possible Causes of Dyspareunia

When Pain Occurs	Where Pain Occurs	Consider	Management
Precoital foreplay	External genitalia	Vulvovaginitis Inept male technique Vulvodynia Arthritis in adjacent structures Associated with abuse	Treat organism Education and communication Treatment Treatment Therapy (individual or group)
As penis enters	Introitus	Lack of lubrication Infection/vaginitis Position/angle of penis Urethritis/cystitis Scar tissue Rigid hymen Postmenopausal changes	Education; water-soluble lubricants Treatment Education and communication Treatment Medical/surgical intervention Education; surgical intervention Education; HRT; water-soluble lubricants
Penis in midvagina	Vaginal canal and adjacent structures	Cystitis Vaginitis Postmenopausal changes Scars Position of penis Anorectal problems	Treatment Treatment Education; HRT; water-soluble lubricants Medical/surgical intervention Education Medical/surgical intervention
Deep penetration with thrusting	Lower back Lower abdomen Deep pelvis	Endometriosis PID-related Position of penis Arthritic/orthopedic problems Post-trauma scars Broad ligament varices	Medical (hormonal); surgical intervention Medical/surgical treatment Education Medical/surgical interventions Medical/surgical interventions Medical/surgical interventions
During orgasm	Lower back Deep in pelvis Lower abdomen	Endometriosis Scars at vaginal vault or abdomen Broad ligament varices	Medical (hormonal); surgical intervention Medical/surgical intervention Medical/surgical intervention
Post coitus	Lower back Lower abdomen Deep in pelvis	Endometriosis Scars at vaginal vault or abdomen Broad ligament varices	Medical (hormonal); surgical intervention Medical/surgical intervention Medical/surgical intervention

Source: Adapted from Ayers, 1995.

The nurse practitioner should assess whether the information received was correct and accurate. A history that is specific for dyspareunia would include information about the pain: quality, quantity, location, duration, and aggravating/relieving factors. In addition, the nurse practitioner would obtain complete medical, surgical, obstetrical, gynecological, and contraceptive histories. Within this context, questions about previous vaginal or pelvic surgeries and pelvic trauma such as rape or sexual abuse should be asked. Finally, women are asked about medications, douching, and the use of perineal products such as sprays, deodorants, and minipads.

Physical examination is essential to determine the cause of dyspareunia. Possible components of the physical exam include vital signs, a general physical examination, and an abdominal examination. A pelvic exam always is performed. Special attention is paid to the external genitalia, observing for irritation, lesions, and discharge. During the bimanual examination, the nurse practitioner would note any tenderness in the introitus, vagina, and pelvis and assess for unstretched or rigid hymen (Ayers, 1995). During the speculum examination, cultures, when indicated, are obtained.

The history and physical examination suggest which diagnostic tests are indicated. There are no tests specific to sexual assessment. Laboratory studies may be indicated when there is evidence of infection, for example, cultures for gonorrhea or chlamydia may be done when there is history of purulent discharge. If a woman complains of dyspareunia and a bladder infection is suspected, the nurse practitioner may elect to obtain a clean catch urine for culture and sensititivities.

Treatment for dyspareunia should address the specific cause of dyspareunia, for example, suggesting a water-soluble vaginal lubricant for the menopausal woman, treating the sexually transmitted disease, or providing information about techniques for sexual arousal. Further, the nurse practitioner may act as a consultant to mental health professionals who are referring a client with dyspareunia for a physical and gynecological examination (Shafer, 2002). (See Chapter 13, Common Gynecologic Pelvic Disorders, for related information on dyspareunia.)

Vaginismus. This disorder involves the involuntary, spasmodic, sometimes painful contractions of the pubococcygeus and other muscles in the lower third of the vagina and the introitus (Shafer 2002). The degree of vaginal spasm may range from partial (penetration is possible but painful) to complete (no penetration is possible) (Shafer, 2002). Vaginismus can occur during any phase of the sexual response cycle when vaginal entry is attempted. Vaginismus can be associated with other sexual dysfunctions, including lack of desire, arousal, or orgasm (Shafer, 2002). Although rare, sex therapists believe vaginismus may be more common than is documented and women do not seek help for it. Often a woman will not seek help until she experiences relationship difficulties or wishes to become pregnant.

Causes of vaginismus are varied and include sexual trauma (rape, incest, or sexual abuse), phobia about sexual response or intercourse, strong conservative religious values in the woman's family of origin, dyspareunia, and hostile feelings toward one's sexual partner (Shafer, 2002). Further, repeated experiences with pain can establish a pain-fear-tension-pain syndrome that becomes self-maintaining. Generally, medical conditions are not a significant cause of vaginismus.

When collecting a history from a woman who presents with symptoms suggestive of vaginismus, specific areas to assess include the degree of vaginal spasm she experiences, presence of desire, arousal, lubrication, and orgasm; history of previous pain related to penetration, fear of penetration or ripping; partner's sensitivity to pain; client's ability to communicate needs to partner; erectile difficulty in partner; use of lubricant; and attempts to penetrate virginal hymen. Vaginismus is diagnosed primarily by pelvic examination. It is important to remember that past or present pelvic exams may be connected to trauma. The nurse practitioner must discuss this possibility with a woman, and the two should work together to make the exam as comfortable as possible. During the examination, the nurse practitioner should assess for involuntary contraction of vaginal muscles upon touching vulva or digitally entering vagina.

Treatment usually involves a desensitization process including insertion of progressively larger dilators into the vagina by the woman and/or her partner. At the same time, she is taught to relax vaginal muscles consciously. Often psychotherapy is needed. Treatment of this sexual dysfunction requires a health professional with advanced training in sexual therapy. Clients should be referred to such an individual.

Secondary/Other Sexual Dysfunctions

The majority of the sexual problems just reviewed (with the possible exception of dyspareunia) usually contain a psychological component, are solely caused by psychological factors, or cannot be accounted for by a general medical condition. There are sexual problems, however, that are the result of a medical condition, such as a woman whose orgasm is inhibited by Cushing's disease or hypoparathyroidism. Further, a number of psychoactive drugs such as cocaine or alcohol may affect the sexual abilities of women. Lack of sensation in the genital area may be a problem for women with neurologic disease or injury.

SEXUAL HEALTH CARE ASSESSMENT AND HISTORY

In order to provide adequate sexual health care, nurse practitioners must be aware of their sexual biases, be comfortable with their sexuality, and have a genuine desire to help the client. MacLauren (1995) suggests that health professionals can become aware of their personal attitudes and values about sex and sexuality by asking themselves the questions such as "My religious beliefs teach me that sex is…" and "In my culture, communicating my sexual needs to my partner is considered…" (MacLauren, 1995, p. 109 for the complete list). When providing sexual health care, it is critical that assumptions not be made about a woman's sexual behavior, feelings, or attitudes. Health care providers should know how various health problems, diseases, and their treatment affect sexuality and sexual functioning.

Sexual assessment includes physiological, psychological, and sociocultural evaluations. Peck (2001) suggests that this is most appropriately introduced during the genitourinary, gynecologic, or obstetrical history review. Data are gathered regarding the client's sexual response cycle and any alterations she has noted in its phases. The woman should be asked about attempts to conceive, any previous high-risk pregnancy, postpartum difficulties, and contraceptive choices and any associated problems. In addition, data about past and present illness, surgery, and medications are obtained.

Components of psychological sexual assessment include the client's self-concept and body image; view of self as a sexual being and level of confidence in ability to function sexually; past and current psychiatric problems or illness including anxiety and depression; use of psychotropic medications, history of sexual abuse, quality of personal relationships; and health of sexual partner.

Sociocultural sexual assessment incorporates information about women's attitudes toward sex and aging; attitudes toward alternative expressions of sexuality; and lifelong beliefs and values related to sexuality (Berg, 2001). Further, the clinician should inquire about the client's perceptions of sex appropriate roles for men and women in relationships and her perception of her ability to fulfill those roles competently. Women should be asked about their sources of sexual education, when they received it, and their reactions to the information. The nurse practitioner/primary care provider should assess whether the information that the client received was accurate. The woman's religious affiliation and beliefs and her ethnic and cultural belief system should be noted.

TECHNIQUES FOR TAKING A SEXUAL HISTORY

The health care provider should take responsibility for introducing the topic of sexual health problems. Choose a private location where the client is comfortable and assure her that the information will be held in strict confidence. It is essential that sufficient time be given to build trust and develop rapport before soliciting information that the client may consider highly personal or intimate. Several meetings may be needed to collect the history, especially if anxiety is high. Continually monitor your own responses to detect negative or embarrassed feelings that may easily be conveyed to the client. Usually, you will obtain more information if you begin with open questions that will permit clients to tell their story on their own terms. Yes or no questions do not facilitate descriptive responses and may prevent complete discussion, especially if the woman is uncomfortable (Peck, 2001). Closed questions generally facilitate gathering specific information, such as medical history, menstrual history, and drug reactions.

From Simple to Complex

History taking should always begin with the least threatening material, for example, obstetric history or childhood sexual education, and progress to more sensitive topics, such as current sexual practices. A general guide is to begin with questions about the individual's sexual learning history, proceed to personal attitudes and beliefs about sexuality, and finally assess actual sexual behaviors. Explain to your clients the purpose of your questions and how the information will be used. You can set limits on the length of responses if excessive or irrelevant information is offered or provide encouragement if progress is slow. Tell your clients if information becomes tangential.

Appropriate Terminology

Avoid using excessive medical terminology during an interview; in other words, make sure that both you and the client know the meaning of the terms used. Avoid euphemisms such as "slept with." Pose only one question at a time and give the client sufficient time to answer it. Questions such as "How many times a week do you have sexual intercourse?" should not be asked because norms vary widely among individuals.

"Universalizing" or prefacing questions with phrases such as "many people" or "the Kinsey Report shows" may make a client feel more comfortable when answering sensitive questions.

SEXUAL HISTORY FORMATS

A sexual history can be incorporated into a total health history (brief sexual history) or it can be more formal and inclusive (sexual problem history).

Brief Sexual History

When the sexual history is incorporated into the total health history, various formats can be used.

- Two questions that elicit sexual concerns are "Are you sexually active?" and "Are you having any sexual difficulties or problems at this time?"
- The three-question format is used to gather information about a client's usual sexual roles, views of self as a sexual being, and sexual functioning. These questions are "Has any [illness, pregnancy, surgery] interfered with your being a [mother, wife, partner]?" "Has any [surgery, medical treatment, illness] changed the way you feel about yourself as a woman?" and "Has any [surgery, disease, medication] altered your ability to function sexually?"

Although sexual histories will vary depending on the woman, four key points are appropriate:

- Concerns relating to sexual functioning.
- Changes that have occurred in sexual function in the past six months/since the last visit.
- Degree of satisfaction with sex life.
- Medications, treatments, health problems or conditions that affect sexual function.

These points are usually understood by all patients and provide a nonthreatening starting point for sexual assessment.

Additional questions that could be asked in any of the above formats are "Is sex pleasurable for you?" (desire), "Are you having any difficulty with lubrication during sex?" (arousal), "Are you able to achieve orgasm?" (orgasm), and "Do you experience any pain or discomfort during sexual activity?" (pain). Two other categories that can be incorporated into assessment that relate specifically to sexual dysfunction are satisfaction: "Are you satisfied with your sexual relationship?" "Do you have other sexual complaints?"

Other elements of a customary well-woman history are also significant for a sexual history. The woman's menstrual history is queried, including her age at menarche and the characteristics of her menstrual cycle (i.e., length, duration of flow, presence or absence of associated premenstrual symptoms, and ovulatory discomfort or dysmenorrhea). Ask your client about the presence of vaginal discharge, discomfort, or itching and about her preferred method of sanitary protection and level of satisfaction with that method. If the woman is beyond her childbearing years, ask when menopause occurred and whether she has experienced any difficulties with sexual functioning, such as vaginal dryness. If problems have occurred, ask her how she dealt with them.

Obstetric history data are significant and include the number of pregnancies, deliveries, and spontaneous and induced abortions. Note any difficulties the client has experienced conceiving and any history of infertility. Questions about her contraceptive history include the methods used, her satisfaction or dissatisfaction and confidence with each, and partner participation. Be sure to record any history of sexually transmitted disease, including pelvic inflammatory disease.

Obtain a brief description of the client's sexual response cycle. It is important to clarify the degree of lubrication that develops during sexual arousal or if pain occurs during sexual intercourse. Ask the client to describe briefly her present relationship and to rate it with respect to communication, affection, sexual needs met, and sexual communication.

Sexual Problem History

A sexual problem history is used to supplement a brief sexual history and is obtained within the context of sexual counseling and therapy. It is intended to collect information so that the provider can define the character, etiology, onset, severity, duration, and psychosocial effect of presenting sexual dysfunction. Formats may vary; however, certain commonalties should be explored.

- Description of the problem in the client's own words.
- Exploration of the onset and course of the problem.
- Determination of the client's assessment of the cause and persistence of the problem.
- A description of any past treatment and its results.
- The client's expectations of current therapy.

An in-depth sexual history generally includes several factors:

- The nature of the presenting distress.
- Information about the client's present relationship, such as duration or other partners.
- Life cycle influences and events in childhood, adolescence, premarital adulthood, and marriage.
- The client's perception of self.
- The client's response to sensory stimuli.

These histories can generate extensive information about experiences, feelings, sexual practices, and perceptions of self-concept. *History taking requires several hours of interviewing and is conducted only by health professionals with extensive training in sexual counseling or therapy.*

PHYSICAL EXAMINATION

A physical examination is done when indicated by history, presenting concern, treatment goals, or need for referral. Components might be determination of vital signs and a general physical examination, especially an abdominal and pelvic exam including external genitalia and internal genitalia (using a speculum and bimanual techniques).

DIAGNOSTIC TESTS/METHODS

Although no tests are specific to determine sexual assessment, laboratory studies may be indicated when infection is evident. For example, cultures may be done for gonorrhea or chlamydia if there is history of purulent discharge. If a woman complains of dyspareunia and a bladder infection is suspected, the nurse practitioner may elect to obtain a clean catch urine specimen for culture and sensitivity.

SEXUAL HEALTH INTERVENTIONS: PLISSIT MODEL

The PLISSIT model (Annon, 1974, 1976) is a schema for ordering levels of intervention for sexual problems and is the approach to sexual counseling most used by nurses. It incorporates four levels of counseling: permission, limited information, specific suggestions, and intensive therapy. As the complexity of intervention levels increases, more knowledge and skills are needed. All nurses should be able to provide permission and limited information related to many sexual concerns. Many nurses and all advanced nurse practitioners should also be able to intervene at the specific suggestion level. Intensive therapy, however, requires that nurses be specially trained in sexuality and sex therapy or that the client be referred to experts in sex therapy.

PERMISSION

The provider gives permission to the client to function sexually as she usually does and to accept herself and her desires. Reassurance is offered that such behaviors are normal. The health care professional may also encourage the woman to talk with her partner. It is important never to give permission for activities that are potentially harmful to a woman.

Permission giving involves answering questions about sexual fantasies, feelings, and dreams. Inquiring about the effect of developmental changes, illness, or lifestyle alterations may give a woman permission to be a sexual being. Permission giving is particularly useful for a client with a nursing diagnosis of anxiety related to sexual adequacy or of sexual dysfunction related to guilt over sexual enjoyment. Examples of interventions at this level include providing permission to be sexually aroused by normal feelings; to engage in safe activities that arouse sexual feelings, such as masturbation and fantasizing; and to have sexual intercourse as often as desired.

LIMITED INFORMATION

Provide the client with specific facts that are directly related to her area of sexual concern, making sure that the information is immediately relevant and limited in scope. Limited information helps to change potentially negative thoughts and attitudes about specific areas of sexuality and to refute sexual myths.

The purpose of providing limited information about sexual matters is to open the topic of sexual health for the client so that she, in turn, can discuss her concerns with the health care provider. This approach is particularly useful when the nursing diagnosis is knowledge deficit related to sexuality or anxiety related to sexual misinformation.

SPECIFIC SUGGESTIONS

The health care provider using the specific suggestions approach gives direct behavioral suggestions to relieve a sexual problem that is limited in scope or of brief duration. The client and the health care provider agree on specific goals, and the provider offers specific behavioral suggestions. These interventions are followed up after a brief period.

Numerous suggestions can be made, but they are always tailored to an individual's needs and particular situation. For example, a woman with a recent mastectomy might be counseled to use a side-lying position for intercourse to avoid putting pressure on her wound. Or the health care provider might suggest that a postmenopausal woman who is experiencing vaginal dryness and dyspareunia use a water-soluble vaginal lubricant prior to penile penetration. Additional examples of specific suggestions include sensate focus exercises (mutual stimulation of erotic areas excluding the genitals); medication specific to the organism causing vaginal infection; and alternative ways of sexual pleasuring (oral-genital contact, mutual masturbation, cuddling, holding, massage).

Specific suggestions are used when the nursing diagnosis is sexual dysfunction related to pain with intercourse secondary to vaginal infection, or pain related to sexual position secondary to pregnancy, surgery, or other interfering factors.

INTENSIVE THERAPY

Intensive therapy is used when a client's problems are not relieved by interventions included in the first three levels (permission giving, limited information, and specific suggestions) or when the problems are personal and emotional difficulties that interfere with sexual expression. Intensive therapy is appropriate for women with a nursing diagnosis of sexual dysfunction related to inhibited female orgasm or to vaginismus. This level of intervention is the most complex and should be undertaken only by professionals with advanced training in sexual counseling and therapy. It is essential that nursing professionals recognize the limits of their own knowledge and refer the client appropriately.

REFERENCES

Alan Guttmacher Institute (AGI). (2002). *Facts in brief.* www.agi-usa.org/pubs/fb_teen_sex_html.

Alexander, B.A. (1997). Women's sexuality: A paradigm shift. In J.A. Rosenfeld (Ed.), *Women's health in primary care.* Baltimore, MD: Williams & Wilkins.

Alexander, L.L., & LaRosa, J.H. (1994). *New dimensions in women's health.* Boston: Jones and Barlett Publishers.

Alteneder, R.R., & Hartzell, D. (1997). Addressing couples' sexuality concerns during the childbearing period: Use of the PLISSIT model. *JOGNN, 26*(6), 651–658.

American Psychiatric Association. (1994). *Diagnostic and statistical manual of mental disorders* (DSM-IV-R; 4th rev. ed.). Washington, DC: American Psychiatric Press.

Annon, J.S. (1974). *The behavioral treatment of sexual problems.* Honolulu: Enabling Systems.

Annon, J.S. (1976). *The behavioral treatment of sexual problems: Brief therapy.* New York: Harper and Row.

Ayers, A. (1995). Sexual dysfunction. In *Women's primary health care: Protocols for practice.* Washington, DC: American Nurses Publishing.

Berg, J.A. (2001). Dimensions of sexuality in the perimenopausal transitions: A model for practice. *JOGNN, 30*(4), 421–428.

Bernhard, L. (1995). Sexuality in women's lives. In C. I. Fogel & N.F. Woods (Eds.), *Women's health care.* Thousand Oaks, CA: Sage Publications.

Boston Women's Health Book Collective. (1998). *Our bodies, ourselves for the new century.* New York: Simon & Schuster.

Byrd, J.E., Hyde, J.S., DeLamater, J.D., & Plant, A. (1998). Sexuality during pregnancy and the year postpartum. *Journal of Family Practice, 47*(4), 305–308.

Cesario, S.K. (2002). Spinal cord injuries and childbearing families. *AWHONN Lifelines, 6*(3), 224–232.

Charlton, R.S., & Quatman, T. (1997). A therapist's guide to the physiology of sexual response. In R.S. Charlton (Ed.), *Treating sexual desire.* San Francisco: Jossey-Bass Publishers.

DeMers, D. T. (2001). Intimacy issues: Sexuality, fertility, and relationships. *Seminars in Oncology Nursing, 17*(4), 255–262.

Fogel, C.I., & Lauver, D. (1990). Sexual health promotion. Philadelphia: Saunders.

Fogel, C.I. & Woods, N.F. (1995). *Women's Health Care.* Thousand Oaks, CA: Sage Publications.

Hawkins, J.W., Roberto-Nichols, D.M., & Stanley-Haney, J.L. (2000). *Protocols for nurse practitioners in gynecologic settings* (7th ed.). New York: Tiresias Press.

Heiman, J.R. (1995). Evaluating sexual dysfunction. In D.P. Lemke, J. Pattison, L.A. Marshall, & D.S. Cowley (Eds.), *Primary care of women.* Norwalk, CT: Appleton & Lange.

Heiman, J.R., & Lentz, G.M. (2000). Sexuality. In V.L. Seltzer & W.H. Pearse (Eds.), *Women's primary health care* (2nd ed.). New York: McGraw Hill.

Henderson, D.J., Boyd, C.J., & Whitmarsh, J. (1995). Women and illicit drugs: Sexuality and crack cocaine. *Health Care for Women International, 16,* 113–124.

Jackson, A., & Woodley, V. (1999). Multicenter study of women's self-reported reproductive health after spinal cord injury. *Archives of Physical Medicine and Rehabilitation, 80*(11), 647–656,

Johnson, B.K. (1996). Older adults and sexuality: A multidimensional perspective. *Journal of Gerontological Nursing, 22*(2), 6–15.

Johnson, C.L. (1996). Regaining self-esteem: Strategies and interventions for the infertile woman. *JOGNN, 25*(4), 291–295.

Jones, K.D., Lehr, S.T., & Hewell, S.W. (1997). Dyspareunia: Three case reports. *JOGNN, 26*(1), 19–23.

Kaplan, H. (1979). *Disorders of sexual desire and other new concepts and techniques in sex therapy.* New York: Brunner/Mazel.

Katz, A. (2002). Sexuality after hysterectomy. *JOGNN, 31*(3), 256–262.

Kelly, J.A. & Kalichman, S.C. (1995). Increased attention to human sexuality can improve HIV-AIDS prevention efforts: Key research issues and directions. *Journal of Consulting and Clinical Psychology, 63(6),* 907–918.

Klein, M. (1997). Disorders of desire. In R.S. Charlton (Ed.), *Treating sexual desire.* San Francisco: Jossey-Bass Publishers.

Longworth, J.C.D. (1997). Sexual assessment and counseling in primary care. *Nurse Practitioner Forum, 8*(4) 166–171.

MacLauren, A. (1995). Comprehensive sexual assessment. *Journal of Nurse-Midwifery, 40*(2), 104–119.

Masters, W., & Johnson, V. (1966). *The human sexual response.* Boston: Little, Brown.

McCafferty, R., Barnett, S., & Thomas, D.J. (2001). Seeking satisfaction. Treating decreased libido in women. *AWHONN Lifelines, 5*(4), 30–35.

Moore, K.A., Dviroff, A.K., & Lindberg, L.D. (1999). *A statistical portrait of adolescent sex, contraception, and childbearing.* Washington, DC: National Campaign to Prevent Teen Pregnancy.

Morrison, J. (1995). *DSM-IV Made Easy.* New York: Guilford Press.

Northrup, C. (2001). *The wisdom of menopause.* New York: Bantam Books.

Peck, S.A. (2001). The importance of the sexual health history in the primary care setting. *JOGNN, 30*(3), 269–274.

Roberts, L.W., Fromm, L.M., & Bartlik, B.D. (1998). Sexuality of women through the life phases. In L.A. Wallis (Ed.), *Textbook of women's health.* Philadelphia: Lippincott-Raven Publishers.

Schnarch, D.M. (1991). *Constructing the sexual crucible. An integration of sexual and marital therapy.* New York: W.W. Norton & Company.

Schnare, S. (1997, Summer). Dyspareunia: Evaluation, treatment and management. *Contemporary Nurse Practitioner,* 4–10.

Shafer, L. (2002). Sexual dysfunction. In K.J. Carlson, S.A. Eisenstat, F.D. Frigoletto, & I. Schiff (Eds.), *Primary care of women.* St. Louis: C.V. Mosby Co.

Singh, S., & Darroch, J.E. (1999). Trends in sexual activity among adolescent American women: 1982–1995. *Family Planning Perspective, 31*(5), 212–219.

Ventura, S., Mosher, W., Curtin, S., Abma, J., & Henshaw, S. (2001). Trends in pregnancy rates for the United States: 1976–1997. *National Vital Statistics Report 2001, 49,* 1–9.

Wilson, K.M., & Klein, J. D. (2002). Health care and contraceptive use among adolescents reporting unwanted sexual intercourse. *Archives of Pediatrics and Adolescent Medicine, 156,* 341–344.

Woods, N.F. (1995). Women's bodies. In C.I. Fogel & N.F. Woods (Eds.), *Women's health care.* Thousand Oaks, CA: Sage Publications.

World Health Organization (WHO). (1975). Education and treatment in human sexuality: The training of health professionals. Report of WHO meeting. *Technical Report Series, 572.*

Zerbe, K.J. (1999). *Women's mental health in primary care.* Philadephia: W.B. Saunders Co.

Zwelling, E. (1997). Sexuality during pregnancy. In F.H. Nichols & E. Zwelling (Eds.) *Maternal-Newborn Nursing Theory and Practice.* Philadelphia: W.B. Saunders.

CHAPTER 7

HEALTH NEEDS
OF LESBIANS

Debera Jane Thomas

*A*lthough the health
care needs of les-
bians are the same as
those of all women in
most instances, les-
bians face additional
unique health problems
to which health care
providers must attend.

Highlights

- Care Barriers for Lesbians
- An Inclusive Approach and Environment for Acceptance
- Assessing the Woman's Coping Status
- Special Groups at Greater Risk
- Health Problems of Lesbians
- Desire to Parent
- Health Resources and Organizations

❖ INTRODUCTION

Generally, women who form sexual and affectional relationships with other women are considered lesbian; however, these women may or may not identify themselves as lesbian. The term *lesbian* is used to describe women who have sex with other women either exclusively or in addition to sex with men (behavior); women who identify themselves as lesbian (identity); or women with a sexual preference for women (desire or attraction) (Institute of Medicine [IOM], 1999). The decision to identify as lesbian is influenced by race, ethnicity, socioeconomic class, cultural values, age, religion, or personal history (Gonser, 2000). Women who self-identify as lesbian may do so in their adolescence, as young adults, in middle age, or late in life. Sexual orientation may be fluid over time, and "women may exhibit differing degrees of same-sex sexual behavior, desire, or identity in combinations that vary from person to person" (IOM, 1999, p 26). As with all homosexuals, sexual preference is only one aspect of why a person considers her- or himself same-sex identified.

Lesbians are as diverse as the population at large, crossing all age, occupation, ethnic/racial, religious, economic, and geographic boundaries. The number of lesbians in the United States by any definition is not known, but is estimated to be between 2 and 10 percent (IOM, 1999), although some suggest that this is an underestimation because many women never declare their sexual preference for fear of stigma (Gentry, 1992). Although the health care needs of lesbians are the same as those of all women in most instances, lesbians can experience some health problems with greater frequency than the average. Further, it is imperative that nurses caring for women be attuned to and respectful of this population and its health care needs and problems.

There has been a dramatic interest in lesbian health research since the Institute of Medicine Committee on Lesbian Health Research Priorities published its report in 1999 and the U.S. Department of Health and Human Services presented the Scientific Workshop on Lesbian Health in 2000 (Bradford, Ryan, Honnold, & Rothblum, 2001).

The increased number of articles discussing special needs and concerns of this population not only in the health professional literature but also in other disciplines and lay publications would seem to indicate a tolerant attitude toward lesbians, but prejudice and ignorance remain. Such bias is not limited to lay persons. A literature review of lesbian health care from 1970 to 1990 found that "prejudice is alive and well in present-day clinical practice and health care provider education. . . . This survey evidence suggests that lesbianism was still considered an affliction by many health care providers" (Stevens, 1992, p. 108). Knowing this prejudice exists often impedes lesbians from seeking care that may result in more debilitating, costlier medical problems. Providers can help to decrease barriers by acknowledging any internalized homophobia of their own and attempting to be as impartial as humanly possible to all their women clients.

The health care provider needs to understand first and foremost that, regardless of age, social status, education, and so on, every woman who becomes woman-identified and eventually self-identifies as a lesbian has generally gone through a period of "coming out"—realizing that her sexual and affectional preference is not the societal norm and, in fact, may be condemned by major religious and political groups. "Coming out" is a distressing period for a lesbian at any age and leads to nondisclosure (Williams-Barnard, Mendoza, & Shippee-Rice, 2001; Wilton & Kaufmann, 2001). Because it requires a shift in core identity as well as a need to understand the pros and cons of disclosure, the person may need positive support and counseling. For the adolescent coping with developmental tasks as well as for the woman who finally begins to acknowledge that the heterosexual way of life is not fulfilling, it can be a time of great emotional distress, with greater risks of depression or suicide. Both families and health care providers need to consider questions about sexual identity as a reason for significant behavioral changes. Until the individual becomes comfortable with her choice, *every* "coming out" is a mine field: Will I be rejected, shunned, mocked? Can I live with that? Eventually, lesbians begin to understand that homophobia is the other person's problem. The hard part is knowing that the other's homophobia—internalized or externalized—can indeed affect the lesbian's life in very real and tangible ways.

Providing a safe, comfortable atmosphere, where truth can be told without repercussion, is the ideal. A client who allows a provider to know she is a lesbian has imparted a gift of self. That information should be handled gently and professionally.

CARE BARRIERS FOR LESBIANS

Lesbians experience the same barriers to care that other women do, such as having no transportation, child care, or leave time from work; inconvenient times/location of clinics/practices; inability to communicate due to language barriers or reading ability; physical barriers, or culture; "ism" barriers (race, sex, class, age, ability); putting others ahead of self for care; avoiding health screening as a way to deny problems or viewing it as a non-necessity; seeking care for serious problems only; history of abuse causing distancing from body; fear of procedures causing pain, embarrassment or fear of the unknown; fear of findings of tests; inability to pay; and/or lack of recommendation for a procedure by a health care provider (Bernhard, 2001; IOM, 1999). In addition, lesbians may also face barriers that are particular to a gay identity/behavior (see Table 7–1).

Most lesbians (75 to 94%) do have regular primary care providers, but more than half seek care only if they have a problem. Of concern is the fact that care is often delayed. Stevens found in a narrative study of 45 lesbians in the San Francisco area that "noncare" was common (Stevens, 1994a, 1994b). "Noncare" was negative care, such as feeling a lack of respect, feeling not safe enough to continue with a particular provider, feeling generally poorly cared for. These results confirm prior studies' findings where providers' negative behaviors included such actions as clipped voice tones, constricted affect, roughness in handling, a hurried pace that frightened or humiliated or hurt, and false endearments.

Other reasons and examples of why lesbians may not seek health care, delay health care, or may not disclose their sexual orientation to health care providers include

TABLE 7–1. Special Barriers to Health Care Experienced by Lesbians

- Homophobia from the health care provider
- Internalized homophobia
- Heterosexist assumptions
- Lack of knowledge about special risks and screening needs of lesbians by lesbians themselves
- Incorrect knowledge about health care needs of lesbians by health care providers
- Belief (false) by lesbians and health care providers that lesbians are immune to STDs, cervical cancer, and HIV
- Preventive care sought less since lesbians need routine contraceptive and prenatal care less often
- Insurance lack and/or lack of access under partner's coverage
- Excluded or believe they are excluded from health promotion campaigns

Sources: Bernhard, 2001; IOM, 1999; Marrazzo, Koutsky, Kiviat, Kuypers, & Stine, 2001; Rankow, 1995a.

the following (Claes & Moore, 2000; Deevey, 1995; IOM, 1999; Stevens, 1994b):

- Prejudicial language. Examples are: When taking a history, do not ask any woman if she is married, ask who her support person is. Do not use the term "homosexual"; rather, use "lesbian," which is thought to have a more positive connotation. Do not ask if she is "having intercourse"; ask if she is "sexually active." Better questions are "Are you single, partnered, or married?" "Who is in your immediate family?" If your client uses the term lesbian about herself and her family, she is probably relatively at ease with herself. The term homosexual generally refers to males in the gay culture.
- Negative behavior changes by the provider upon learning that the patient is lesbian. These can be avoiding touching her, superficial or condescending interaction with her, or outright hostility.
- Isolation from those they love—friends and relatives of choice—when in or visiting the hospital. The "traditional family" may be the only people allowed by the hospital staff to visit and support the client.
- Fear that coming out or disclosure will lead to loss of confidentiality. If the client is "labeled" in the charts or records, it may become public knowledge, leading to personal-social-work losses.
- Fear of substandard care or perhaps hurtful care.
- Fear after prior negative experiences.
- Lack of female provider (MD, NP, PA, CNM).

AN INCLUSIVE APPROACH AND ENVIRONMENT FOR ACCEPTANCE

Interview techniques and written materials that do not make the assumption that the woman is heterosexual and that use inclusive language will give the lesbian the message that disclosing her sexual orientation to the health care provider is safe, thus promoting disclosure of more useful information. It is imperative to establish an open, sensitive, and nonjudgmental climate from the onset, reassuring the woman that everything she discloses will be kept confidential. Beginning the conversation with something like the following may be helpful: "In order for me to provide you with care that is specific for your needs, I need to ask some sensitive questions about your sexual history and your support network."

In addition, a safe environment can be created that facilitates disclosure by using open body language, inviting the woman's partner or friend to participate if she wishes, assuring the confidentiality of medical documentation, and having a posted nondiscrimination policy and diversified reading materials prominently displayed in the waiting room.

Because heterosexuality is the accepted societal norm, too often providers assume that the client is heterosexual. The provider who asks a woman if she is sexually active, learns that she is, and then immediately asks what form of contraception is being used, is both insensitive, judgmental, and exhibiting heterosexism.

Examples of questions that give the woman an opportunity to disclose her relationships include the following: "Are you in a committed relationship or partnership?" "Whom do you rely on for support?" "Who do you consider your family?" "Who are the people most important to you?" "Could you tell me about the people you live with?" "What is your relationship with the person(s) you live with?" "Are you in satisfying relationships with people important to you?" "Do you have any concerns you'd like to talk about?" (Rankow, 1995a.)

Asking "Are you sexually active?" and receiving a "Yes" response should then lead to "Are you sexually active with men, women, or both?" "Have your partners been men, women, or both?" Asking these questions in a matter of fact way allows the client to feel free to be truthful since the provider expects any of the answers. However, questions about sexual relationships need to go further than the sex of partner/s and the number of partners. The provider needs to determine if the relationship is a committed one—one where this partner is the most important support person for the woman. This data is important for future reference in case of illness and hospitalization. Because of possible stigma attached to lesbian sexual orientation and the possibility that this information could negatively influence care, permission to place this information in the medical record should be obtained from the patient.

Though the woman may identify as lesbian, she may be reluctant to disclose that she is bisexual, and the provider may need to ask if there is a need to discuss contraception. If the woman is in a committed, long-term monogamous relationship, there may be no need to discuss issues of safer sex, but if she is in a new relationship, a non-monogamous relationship, or bisexual, then the provider is compelled to discuss the possibility of sexually transmitted diseases. Additionally, the provider should ask the woman if she has any concerns she would like to discuss, thereby opening the door to discussions about domestic violence, stress, and any other health concerns.

ASSESSING THE WOMAN'S COPING STATUS

To best meet the needs of the client, the provider must learn how the woman feels about herself, her level of self-esteem, and her ability to cope internally and externally with her identity (Deevey, 1995). How does she feel about being a lesbian? Does she share information about her sexual orientation with others and, if so, does she feel comfortable about this? How has she been and how is she treated by health care professionals? Has she been treated before by or know of health care providers who are open to caring for lesbians? What health needs and risks does she feel she has? Is she aware of support networks? The answers to these questions will allow the provider to give the client more information to help herself and to uncover areas for care.

Lesbians may, in fact, share little or nothing about their self-identification. By controlling this information, the client may believe her environment is safer (Stevens, 1995). She feels less likely to be mistreated, ignored, or misdiagnosed. This is seen as a survival method. Some women may increase their feelings of safety by bringing a friend who will be a witness if they are mistreated or be an advocate if needed. The provider needs to allow this type of support unless there is concern that the friend is abusive or coercive.

Lesbians—or any women—who have been negatively sensitized from past experiences with the health care system (Stevens, 1994b; 1995) may act hostilely toward the provider from the outset or may be disruptive and dissonant. This kind of situation can make them feel more in control, believing that they will more likely receive needed care by using this behavior.

Our society assumes everyone is heterosexual. This heterosexism is most often unintentional but may be associated with the belief that heterosexuality is the only acceptable form of sexuality (Gruskin, 1999). Homophobia is the fear of same-gendered sexual identity (Gruskin, 1999). While heterosexism is unintentional, homophobia is strong anti-homosexual feelings associated with some form of behavior and is most often intentional. An unrealistic fear of anyone who has a different sexual identity from the socially acceptable "norm" is the basis of homophobia, and anyone raised in the U.S. culture is raised with the unconscious fear of anyone different. Lesbians are no exception. This may lead to issues of low self-esteem, self-hatred, and internalized homophobia leading to depression, substance abuse, or negative behaviors.

SPECIAL GROUPS AT GREATER RISK

CHILDREN AND ADOLESCENTS

The Institute of Medicine report on Lesbian Health (IOM, 1999) notes that very little is known about the specific developmental issues that may exist for lesbian children or adolescents. The report goes on to say that much of the older research may not be relevant today because it was conducted when homosexuality was considered a pathologic behavior. Current contextual changes in society have brought homosexuality to a position of increased visibility and less stigma, as witnessed by the popularity of several gay/lesbian television sitcoms in recent years. However, unless the young lesbian child or adolescent is lucky enough to be part of a family who is able to accept and support her in her development regardless of sexual orientation, she may be vulnerable to psychological trauma in her growth and development. The usual message from families and adults who have contact with children today is still one that promotes the beliefs that lesbianism is a deviant, irreligious, and, perhaps, evil orientation. Thus, young girls who are battling inwardly with their same sex feelings and are being told outwardly that same sex feelings are wrong are subject to poor self-identity development, perhaps becoming runaways, homeless, isolated, depressed, or suicidal; furthermore, they may abuse substances, experience domestic violence, and fail in school or work (American Academy of Pediatrics, 1993). These girls need positive lesbian role models and support in developing self-respect to help decrease the risks of these consequences. A number of larger cities have gay and lesbian adolescent social services organizations to which such clients can be referred. (See addresses for several such organizations at the end of the chapter.)

OLDER LESBIANS

Nursing home personnel should be educated to understand the special needs of all clients, including lesbians. A clearinghouse of information on older lesbians is the National Association for Lesbian and Gay Gerontology in San Francisco. (Other resource centers for older lesbians are listed at the end of the chapter.) Older lesbians have a greater risk for unmet health needs because of their triple minority status: being old, being female, and being lesbian (Deevey, 1990). Additionally, older women may have been too afraid of negative consequences of affirming

publicly their woman-identification and thus may never have come out. Consequently, health care providers may not pick up on clues so that effective assistance can be offered to the older person, especially through support from the significant other (Stevens, 1995). Poverty and increasing health problems of aging add to the significant risks for lesbian elders. Health care providers will need to be particularly aware and sensitive to offer needed assistance (Claes & Moore, 2000).

LESBIANS WITH DISABILITIES

See the special section on this topic provided in Chapter 24 on women with disabilities.

RACIAL AND ETHNIC MINORITY LESBIANS

Not only do lesbians face unique challenges due to sexual orientation, but if they are members of a minority race/ethnic group, they face even greater risks of rejection based on racial or ethnic prejudices. Deevey states that "Lesbians of color report triple jeopardy because of their race, sexual orientation, and gender" (Deevey, 1995, p. 197).

HEALTH PROBLEMS OF LESBIANS

Lesbians seek health care for menstrual problems (painful or irregular periods), vaginal infections and sexually transmitted diseases (primarily vaginal infections and herpes), reproductive problems (pelvic pain, uterine infections, infertility problems, painful coitus or orgasms), urinary tract infections, musculoskeletal problems, and breast problems (IOM, 1999). Many women never seek health interventions for these problems, except for musculoskeletal problems. Unique health concerns of lesbians that may go unaddressed if the provider assumes heterosexuality include appropriate screening for cancer, domestic violence, depression, substance abuse, STDs, HIV, as well as relationship issues, pregnancy, and parenting (IOM, 1999; Rankow, 1995b; White & Levinson, 1995).

In a study comparing lesbian and heterosexual women's lifestyles, Buenting (1992) found no difference between the groups on items of regular exercise, smoking cigarettes, social activities, community service, monthly self-breast exams, spiritual-religious activities, abstinence from alcohol, and drinking alcohol. Lesbians had significantly higher mean scores, however, on use of recreational drugs, alternative diets, and meditation/relaxation techniques. Heterosexual women had significantly higher mean scores on regular Pap smears, use of prescribed medications, and fulfilling family obligations. Other research found that lesbian and bisexual women between the ages of 20 and 34 were at higher risk for cigarette smoking and alcohol use than heterosexual women (Gruskin, Hart, Gordon, & Ackerson, 2001). The IOM (1999) reports that, in general, a greater percentage of lesbians describe themselves as being in recovery from alcohol than do heterosexual women, and the limited research on lesbians and drug use seems to point to a greater use of illegal drugs for lesbians than other women.

PHYSICAL HEALTH PROBLEMS

Menstrual Problems and Pelvic Pain

Dysmenorrhea, often severe, is a common complaint of lesbians (38–54%) (Johnson, Smith, & Guenther, 1987). This complaint may never be acted upon because the woman is hesitant to seek care. Endometriosis is presumed to be high, based on the severe dysmenorrhea rate and the high rate of nulliparity. A reported higher rate of hysterectomy among lesbians than among heterosexual women may result from electing hysterectomies as definitive birth control.

Sexually Transmitted Diseases and Vaginal Infections

The prevalence of STDs among lesbians is reported as low. The problem with the data are that there are no current large-scale contemporary studies and no delineation of women who have never had sex with men, who have sex with men and women, or women who have sex with multiple female partners who may also have sex with men (IOM, 1999). Complicating the issue is the fact that there is little data on the actual sexual practices of lesbians. The data are limited with respect to the prevalence of STDs in women who have had sex only with other women, but classical infections such as syphilis, gonorrhea, and chlamydia are rare because of anatomical transmission inefficiency (IOM, 1999). Routine screening for these infections is not indicated. However, lesbians need to be reminded that oral sex can transmit some infections, such as herpes.

The Institute of Medicine (1999) reported several small studies that indicated that bacterial vaginosis (BV) is higher in lesbians than in heterosexual controls. In one study of 101 lesbians who had not had sex with men in the preceding year, the prevalence of BV was 29 percent; of those, 73 percent had partners with BV (IOM, 1999). Another study reported that 33 percent of lesbians in their sample of 149 had at least one episode of BV, and all of them reported having oral and mutual digital-vaginal sex (Marrazzo et al., 1998).

There are several types of human papillomavirus (HPV) that cause genital warts and cervical neoplasia but are often asymptomatic and go undetected, increasing the risk of transmission and delaying effective treatment (Thomas, 2001). The epidemiology of HPV among lesbians has only recently been explored. In a study of 149 lesbians, the prevalence of HPV was 19 percent in women who had never had sex with men and 30 percent in the entire sample (Marrazzo, 2000). Marrazzo and her colleagues (2001) reviewed data for the previous two decades on the occurrence of HPV in lesbians and validated the possibility of transmission in this population. Health care providers need to educate lesbians about the possibility of HPV infection and stress the importance of routine Papanicolaou (PAP) smears.

Although early studies of HIV in lesbians indicated that HIV infection was rare (Chu, Buehler, Flemming, & Barkelman, 1990; Peterson, Doll, & White, 1992), and many lesbian and bisexual women believed themselves to be at low risk, this may not be assumed today. The IOM stresses that, although the research is limited, some unexpected findings regarding women having sex with women are:

- ◆ Higher HIV seroprevalence rates among women who have sex with both women and men (i.e., behaviorally bisexual women) compared to their exclusively homosexual or heterosexual counterparts.
- ◆ High levels of risk for HIV infection through unprotected sex with men and through injection drug use.
- ◆ Risk for HIV infection of unknown magnitude owing to unprotected sex with women and artificial insemination with unscreened semen. (IOM, 1999, p. 76)

Women, in general, are at increased risk today for HIV infection; thus, safer sex information should be shared with lesbians (Gentry, 1992). Use of dental dams, and latex gloves may offer some protection. More accurate information about increasing sexual safety and appropriate prevention rests in knowing the sexual preference of the client. It shows lack of awareness and insensitivity to ask every woman who walks in what kind of contraception she uses and to advise that her partner use condoms without knowing her sexual preference. Women who have male and female partners need to use condoms and spermicide with male partners and other barriers with female partners. Avoidance of contact with blood and secretions/discharges of any partner is important protection from HIV infection.

Obesity

The preliminary data from the Women's Health Initiative (WHI) and the limited data from other studies indicate that 53.3 percent of the lifetime lesbians have a body mass index (BMI) greater than 27, compared to 45.8 percent for heterosexual women (Aaron, Markovic, Danielson, et al., 2001; Cochran, Mays, Bowen, et al., 2001; Dibble, Roberts, Robertson, & Paul, 2002; IOM, 1999). The most ideal BMI is between 20 and 25. Herzog found that lesbians had a higher weight, preferred a higher ideal body weight, and were less concerned about thinness and appearance than were heterosexual women (Herzog, Newman, Yeh, et al., 1992). Lesbians are less likely to have eating disorders and to be concerned with body attractiveness (Siever, 1994). Whether lesbians have a higher incidence of diseases attributable to obesity is unknown. Health care providers need to consider these general risks, however, in providing preventive care.

Cancer Risks

Research has identified factors that put women at greater risk for certain types of cancer. In addition to advancing age and family history of cancer, certain behavioral factors may increase the risk of cancer, such as smoking, alcohol use, and history of HPV (Cochran et al., 2001; Dibble et al., 2002; Gruskin et al., 2001; IOM, 1999). It has been assumed that additional cancer risk for lesbians is associated with less use of oral contraceptives and less likelihood of bearing children (Rankow, 1995c). Additionally, lesbians are less likely to have regular health screenings for cervical cancer (PAP smears), STDs, physical examinations, or mammograms (Aaron et al., 2001; Cochran et al., 2001; IOM, 1999; Marrazzo et al., 2001).

The risk for cervical cancer is strongly associated with HPV infection, which is, in turn, associated with certain sexual behaviors including multiple male sexual partners or partners who have had multiple male sexual partners, early age at first intercourse, and unprotected sex (Reid, 2001). Considering the high-risk behaviors for HPV, it has been assumed that lesbians are at a lower risk for developing cervical cancer than their heterosexual counterparts. HPV can also be transmitted by oral sex, shared sex toys, and some studies have shown it can also be spread by HPV on fomites on underwear and medical

instruments (Bergeron, Ferenczy, & Richart, 1990). In fact, one study found that the prevalence of HPV in women who reported never having sex with men was 19 percent (Marrazzo, 2000). In this same study, the researchers found that PAP smear screening was less frequent in lesbians but that those tested had a prevalence of SIL of 14 percent (Marrazzo, 2000). This is a clear indication that there should be no difference in screening recommendations for lesbians, and health care providers need to inform their patients of the risk.

In general, the incidence of breast cancer among lesbians is unknown. However, a recent study found that the self-reported history of breast cancer in lesbians was not different than the estimates for the female population in the United States (Cochran et al., 2001). Although there have been reports of lesbians performing self-breast exams and obtaining screening mammograms less often than their heterosexual counterparts (Rankow, 1995c), recent studies indicate that lesbians may have mammograms more often than other women (Aaron et al., 2001). More research needs to be conducted to determine if lesbians are at an increased risk for breast cancer because of a lack of or delayed childbearing or higher alcohol consumption.

The cause of ovarian cancer is not known currently, but some data is available about the risk factors that include a diet low in fruits and vegetables and high in fat or whole milk (McCance & Huether, 2002). Other sources cite nulliparity, smoking, high BMI, and non-use of oral contraceptives as factors that increase the risk of ovarian cancer (Dibble et al., 2002). Conversely, any suppression of ovulation (full-term pregnancy, long-term use of oral contraceptive, or a history of tubal ligation) reduces the risk. None of these factors are present in the lesbian population as a whole. In a recent study comparing the risk factors for developing ovarian cancer in lesbians and heterosexual women, the researcher found that lesbians had a higher BMI while the heterosexual women had a higher rate of protective factors such as pregnancy and oral contraceptive use (Dibble et al., 2002). At this point, not enough data are available to determine if lesbians are at an increased risk, but health care providers need to be aware of the potential increased risk.

Heart Disease and Stroke

Those factors that may increase the risk of colon, breast, and endometrial cancer also may increase the lesbian's risk for heart disease and stroke. It is not known what the actual incidence among this group is for these diseases.

The glaring truth is that for all the cancer and cardio-vascular risk factors, routine screening is one safeguard leading to early detection as well as to health promotion efforts that lesbians are less likely to have due to delayed care and irregular care. Both increase the risk of more serious disease.

MENTAL HEALTH ISSUES

Rates of depression among lesbians are similar to those among heterosexual women, but lesbians use counseling more, probably because it is stressful to live in a society where their identification is not readily accepted (Bradford, Ryan, & Rothblum, 1994). Saunders and Valente found a two and one-half times higher rate of suicide in a study of lesbians as compared with heterosexual women (Saunders & Valente, 1987). Adolescents seemed to be more at risk, accounting for half of the suicides among lesbians (Roberts & Sorensen, 1995). The leading cause of death of gay adolescents is suicide (Nelson, 1997). Suicide is the third leading cause of death of U.S. adolescents, and 30 percent of these are by gay adolescents. Information on other mental health problems on lesbians is limited.

If the provider assesses that depression is a health factor, it is appropriate to ask the client, in the course of narrowing down cause, if she has any problems relating to sexual orientation. Once disclosure has been made, the provider—who can comfortably do so—may then ask some or all of the following questions:

- How do you feel about your sexual orientation?
- When did you first come out to yourself?
- Have you been able to talk about this with your friends or family of origin? How did they respond?
- Have you been discriminated against or been victimized because of your orientation? By whom?
- Do you have a support system who you can turn to? Do you need information on how to find gay organizations in the area?

Providing the client with information about mental health professionals who routinely deal with these issues and/or support groups can be immensely helpful and affirming. Even in these so-called tolerant times, the client experiencing emotions toward someone of the same sex for the first time—or acknowledging it for the first time—may still think she's the only one on earth this has happened to. Being gay is a statement of selfhood and identity. Coming to terms with it can involve depression when too many forget that sexual identity is a spectrum and in fact seems to have a genetic basis.

Drinking alcohol has been reported as higher in lesbians, but the studies have been criticized as not being representative but being opportunistic (Roberts & Sorensen, 1995; White & Levinson, 1995). Some studies have found higher rates of substance abuse, especially alcohol, among lesbians (Finnegan & McNally, 1987; Glaus, 1989; Gruskin et al., 2001; Kus, 1990; Lewis et al., 1982; Nicoloff & Stiglitz, 1987), while others have not (Bloomfield, 1993; McKirnan & Peterson, 1989). The criticism is that the data are biased since much of it was gathered in gay bars where there would be a higher number of women who drink. Some areas of the country have AA meetings that are specifically for women or lesbians or gays.

Lesbian relationships are much the same as heterosexual relationships. Issues that cause conflict center around money, sex, and roles much the same as heterosexual relationships. One difference is that in heterosexual relationships, there are societal role expectations. In a lesbian relationship, roles must be negotiated and renegotiated. This is often a source of conflict. Other relational conflicts may exist when one partner in the relationship wishes to keep her sexuality private and the other wishes to be more public or "out."

Little is reported about the frequency of domestic violence in lesbian relationships. In the most recent study available, between 22 percent and 46 percent of lesbians are being physically abused by their partners, which is comparable to the statistics for heterosexual women (Elliot, 1996). One big difference is that same sex domestic violence remains virtually invisible, while heterosexual domestic violence is very visible in the media and legislation. Heterosexism and homophobia successfully keep same-sex domestic violence invisible. Another factor contributing to the invisibility of this type of domestic violence is the fact that women in general are not seen as violent persons and therefore are not seen as perpetrators of domestic violence.

While domestic violence in general includes physical, sexual, and emotional abuse as well as property damage and economic control, same-sex domestic violence can also include the use of an individual's internalized homophobia and the homophobia of other significant people in the victim's life to exercise control (Gruskin, 1999). For example, the perpetrator may threaten to "out" her partner or expose her sexual identity to family, friends, coworkers, or boss. This could threaten her employment or affect her relationship with her family and friends, possibly losing their love and support. The perpetrator can effectively maintain control, especially if the woman is considering leaving the relationship (Elliot, 1996).

The implications for health care professionals include the creation of an environment where a woman feels comfortable talking about her sexual identity and the abuse she suffers. The health care provider also must be aware of internal and external homophobia and the ways that a perpetrator can use this to control her partner. As with reports of any domestic violence, the health care provider needs to understand the ramifications of the patient's reporting of the violence. Ramifications can include retaliation from the perpetrator, negative reactions from the police when learning of the woman's sexual orientation, and loss of support from the lesbian community. Support groups are available for assistance, including the Lesbian Caucus in Boston.

Other forms of violence are experienced by lesbians just as by heterosexual women. The special acts of violence born of hate, however, often unreported in years past, are being reported more often today. The National Gay and Lesbian Task Force hotline in Washington, DC (202-332-6483) offers a way for lesbians who have received violent threats to seek redress.

DESIRE TO PARENT

The needs of lesbians related to childbearing and child rearing have been in the public eye lately. Health care providers must be aware that many lesbians and couples want to have children (Harvey, Carr, & Bernheine, 1989) and should address this area in the history. Studies indicate that children raised in lesbian and gay families are like children from any other families developmentally, behaviorally, and otherwise (Gentry, 1992; Laird, 1993).

Artificial insemination is the usual choice to become pregnant of lesbian couples, and information about this process is often requested of the health care provider (Gentry, 1992). It is advisable for the sperm to come from a screened donor bank to decrease the possible risk of HIV. Adoption poses problems legally, especially if the legal parent dies or the couple separates. Seeking a male to have intercourse with for insemination purposes is another option for pregnancy. It is advisable for lesbians who wish to become pregnant to first consult a legal practitioner or call the Lesbian Mothers National Defense Fund in Seattle, WA (206-325-2643) for a list of attorneys who specialize in this field (Gentry, 1992).

Increased support may be needed when children from a previous heterosexual relationship or children from the lesbian relationship are involved in custody battles because of the client's sexual orientation. Other common fears relate to telling their children about their orientation and to interacting with the straight community—people in the schools, churches, and health care system.

Lesbians represent a large group of clients with unique medical, psychological, and social needs. Often, providers remain unaware that a woman is lesbian and, therefore, unique and diverse needs may go unrecognized. The opportunity to provide optimal care is missed. Clinicians would benefit from further research on lesbian health issues in order to provide appropriate guidelines for care (White & Levinson, 1995).

HEALTH RESOURCES AND ORGANIZATIONS*

COMMUNITY SERVICES CENTERS

Lesbian and Gay Community Services Center
208 West 13th Street
New York, NY 10011
(212) 620-7310

Los Angeles Lesbian and Gay Community Services Center
1625 N. Schrader Blvd.
Los Angeles, CA 90028–9998
(213) 993-7400; GAYLESBLA@AOL.COM

Gay and Lesbian Community Action Council
310 East 38th Street, Room 204
Minneapolis, MN 55409
(612) 822-0127; (800) 800-0350

YOUTH

National Advocacy Coalition on Youth and Sexual Orientation
1638 R Street NW
Washington, DC 20009
(202) 783-4165; (800) 541-6922

The Hetrick-Martin Institute
2 Astor Place
New York, NY 10003
(212) 674-2400; (212) 674-8695

Gay and Lesbian Adolescent Social Services (GLASS)
8961 Melrose Avenue, # 202
Los Angeles, CA 90069-5613
(310) 358-1751

*Source: Rankow, 1995a

Boston Alliance of Gay and Lesbian Youth (BAGLY)
P. O. Box 814
Boston, MA 02103
(800) 42-BAGLY (24-hour hotline)

Indianapolis Youth Group (IYG)
P. O. Box 20716
Indianapolis, IN 46220-0716
(800) 347-TEEN (national peer help line 7:00–
11:45 P.M., EST), (317) 541-8726

Out Youth Austin
909 E. 49 1/2 Street
Austin, TX 78751
(800) 96-YOUTH (peer hotline 5:30–9:30 P.M. EST);
(512) 419-1233

National Runaway Switchboard
(800) 621-4000 (24-hour hotline)
www.nrscrisisline.org

ELDERS

National Association for Lesbian and Gay Gerontology (NALGG)
1290 Sutter Street, Suite 8
San Francisco, CA 94109

Old Lesbians Organizing for Change (OLOC)
P. O. Box 980422
Houston, TX 77098

Senior Action in a Gay Environment (SAGE)
305 7th Ave.
New York, NY 10001
(212) 741-2247

Gay and Lesbian Outreach to Elders (GLOE)
1853 Market Street
San Francisco, CA 94103
(414) 626-7000; (414) 626-7000

FAMILIES AND FRIENDS

Parents and Friends of Lesbians and Gays (P-FLAG)
1011 14th Street NW, Suite 1030
Washington, DC 20035-6363
(202) 638-4200; (202) 638-3852

VIOLENCE

New York City Gay and Lesbian Anti-Violence Project
240 West 35th Street, Suite 200
New York, NY 10001
(212) 807-0197 (24-hour hotline); (212) 714-1141;
(212) 657-9465 (TDD)

Tucson United Against Domestic Violence/ Brewster Center
2711 E. Broadway
Tucson, AZ 85716
(520) 881-7201

The Lesbian Caucus
107 South Street, Fifth Floor
Boston, MA 02111
(617) 426-8492

OTHER

Sexuality Information and Education Council of the United States (SIECUS)
130 W. 42nd Street, Suite 350
New York, NY 10036-7802
(212) 819-9770
www.siecus.org

National Women's Health Network
514 10th Street NW, Suite 400
Washington, DC 20004
(202) 347-1140 (admin)
(202) 628-7814 (information)

REFERENCES

Aaron, D. J., Markovic, N., Danielson, M. E., Honnold, J. A., Janosky, J. E., & Schmidt, N. J. (2001). Behavioral risk factors for disease and preventive health practices among lesbians. *Am J Public Health*, 91(6), 972–975.

American Academy of Pediatrics. (1993). Committee on Adolescence: Homosexuality and adolescence. *Pediatrics*, 92, 631–634.

Bergerson, C., Ferenczy, A., & Richart, R. (1990). Underwear: Contamination by human papillomaviruses. *Am J Obstetrics and Gynecology*, 162, 25–29.

Bernhard, L. A. (2001). Lesbian health and health care. *Annu Rev Nurs Res*, 19, 145–177.

Bloomfield, K. A. (1993). A comparison of alcohol consumption between lesbians and heterosexual women in an urban population. *Drg Alcohol Depend*, 33, 257–269.

Bradford, J., Ryan, C., Honnold, J., & Rothblum, E. (2001). Expanding the research infrastructure for lesbian health. *Am J Public Health, 91*(7), 1029–1032.

Bradford, J., Ryan, C., & Rothblum, E. (1994). National lesbian health care survey: Implications for mental health care. *J Consult Clin Psychol, 62*(2), 228–242.

Buenting, J. A. (1992). Health life-styles of lesbian and heterosexual women. *Health Care for Women International, 13*, 165–171.

Chu, S. Y., Buehler, J. W., Flemming, P. L., & Barkelman, R. L. (1990). Epidemiology of reported cases of AIDS in lesbians. United States 1980–1989. *AJPH*, 80, 1380–1381.

Claes, J. A., & Moore, W. (2000). Issues confronting lesbian and gay elders: The challenge for health and human services providers. *J Health Hum Serv Adm, 23*(2), 181–202.

Cochran, S. D., Mays, V. M., Bowen, D., Gage, S., Bybee, D., Roberts, S. J., Goldstein, R. S., Robison, A., Rankow, E. J., & White, J. (2001). Cancer-related risk indicators and preventive screening behaviors among lesbian and bisexual women. *Am J Public Health, 91*(4), 591–7.

Deevey, S. (1990). Older lesbians: An invisible minority. *J Gerontological Nursing, 16*(5), 35–39.

Deevey, S. (1995). Lesbian health care. In C. I. Fogel, & N. F. Woods, (Eds.), *Women's health care: A comprehensive handbook*. Thousand Oaks, CA: Sage Publications.

Dibble, S. L., Roberts, S. A., Robertson, P. A., & Paul, S. M. (2002). Risk factors for ovarian cancer: Lesbian and heterosexual women. *Oncol Nurs Forum, 29*(1), E1–7.

Elliot, P. (1996). Shattering illusions: Same-sex domestic violence. In C. M. Renzettie & C. H. Miley (Eds.), *Violence in gay and lesbian domestic partnerships* (pp. 1–8). Binghamton, NY: Harrington Park Press.

Finnegan, D. G., & McNally, E. B. (1987). *Dual identities: Counseling chemically dependent gay men and lesbians*. Center City, MN: Hazelden.

Gentry, S. E. (1992). Caring for lesbians in a homophobic society. *Health Care for Women International*, 13, 173–180.

Glaus, K. O. (1989). Alcoholism, chemical dependency, and the lesbian client. In E. D. Rothbaum & E. Cole (Eds.), *Loving boldly: Issues facing lesbians*. (pp. 131–144). New York: Harrington Park Press.

Gonser, P. A. (2000). Culturally competent care for members of sexual minorities. *J Cult Divers*, 7(3), 72–75.

Gruskin, E. P. (1999). *Treating lesbians and bisexual women: Challenges and strategies for health professionals*. Thousand Oaks, CA: Sage Publications.

Gruskin, E. P., Hart, S., Gordon, N., & Ackerson, L. (2001). Patterns of cigarette smoking and alcohol use among lesbians and bisexual women enrolled in a large health maintenance organization. *Am J Public Health, 91*(6), 976–979.

Harvey, S. M., Carr, C., & Bernheine, S. (1989). Lesbian mothers: Health care experiences. *J Nurse-Midwifery*, 34(3), 115–119.

Herzog, D., Newman, K., Yeh, C., et al. (1992). Body image satisfaction in homosexual and heterosexual women. *Int J Eating Disorders, 11*, 391.

Institute of Medicine (IOM). (1999). *Lesbian health: Current assessment and directions for the future*. Washington, DC: National Academy Press.

Johnson, S. R., Smith, E. M., & Guenther, S. M. (1987). Comparisons of gynecologic health care problems between lesbian and bisexual women: A survey of 2345 women. *Journal of Reproductive Medicine, 32*, 805–811.

Kus, R. J. (1990). Alcoholism in the gay and lesbian communities. In R. J. Kus (Ed.), *Keys to caring: Assisting your lesbian and gay clients* (pp. 66–81). Boston: Alyson.

Laird, J. (1993). Lesbian and gay families. In F. Walsh (Ed.), *Normal family process* (pp. 282–328). New York: Guilford Press.

Lewis, C. E., et al. (1982). Drinking patterns in homosexual and heterosexual women. *J Clin Psychiatry*, 43(7), 277–279.

Marrazzo, J. M. (2000). Genital human papillomavirus infection in women who have sex with women: A concern for patients and providers. *AIDS Patient Care STD, 14*(8), 447–451.

Marrazzo, J. M., Koutsky, L. A., Kiviat, N. B., Kuypers, J. M., & Stine, K. (2001). Papanicolaou test screening and prevalence of genital human papillomavirus in women who have sex with women. *Am J Public Health, 91*(6), 947–52.

Marrazzo, J. M., Koutsky, L. A., Stine, K. L., Kuypers, J. M., Grubert, T. A., Galloway, D. A., Kiviat, N. B., & Handsfield, H. H. (1998). Genital human papillomavirus infection in women who have sex with women. *J Infect Dis*, 178(6), 1604–1609.

McCance, K. L., & Huether, S. E. (2002). *Pathophysiology: The biologic basis for disease in adults and children* (pp. 733–734). St. Louis: Mosby.

McKirnan, D. J., & Peterson, P. C. (1989). Alcohol and drug abuse among homosexual men and women: Epidemiology and population characteristics. *Addictive Behaviors, 14*, 545–553.

Nelson, J. A. (1997). Gay, lesbian, and bisexual adolescents: Providing esteem-enhancing care to a battered population. *NP*, 22(2), 94–109.

Nicoloff, L. K., & Stiglitz, E. A. (1987). Lesbian alcoholism: Etiology, treatment and recovery. In Boston Lesbian Psychologies Collective (Ed.), *Lesbian psychologies* (pp. 283–293). Urbana: University of Illinois Press.

Petersen, L. R., Doll, L., & White, C. (1992). No evidence for female-to-female HIV transmission among 960,000 female blood donors. *J Acquir Immune Defic Syndr*, 5, 853–855.

Rankow, E. J. (1995a). *Women's health issues: Planning for diversity*. Durham, NC: Duke University Medical Center.

Rankow, E. J. (1995b). Lesbian health issues for the primary care provider. *J Fam Pract, 40*(5), 486–492.

Rankow, E. J. (1995c). Breast and cervical cancer among lesbians. *WHI*, 5(3), 123–129.

Roberts, S. J., & Sorensen, L. (1995). Lesbian health care: A review and recommendations for health promotion in primary care settings. *NP, 20*(6), 42–47.

Saunders, J. M., & Valente, S. M. (1987). Suicide risk among gay men and lesbians: A review. *Death Stud, 11*(1), 1–23.

Siever, M. D. (1994). Sexual orientation and gender as factors in socioculturally acquired vulnerability to body dissatisfaction and eating disorders. *J Consult Clini Psychol*, 62, 252–260.

Stevens, P. E. (1992). Lesbian health care research: A review of the literature from 1970–1990. *Health Care for Women International, 13*, 91–120.

Stevens, P. E. (1994a). Lesbians' health-related experiences of care and noncare. *Western J Nursing Research, 16*(6), 639–659.

Stevens, P. E. (1994b). Protective strategies of lesbian clients in health care environments. *Research in Nursing and Health, 17,* 217–229.

Stevens, P. E. (1995). Structural and interpersonal impact of heterosexual assumptions on lesbian health care clients. *Nursing Research, 44*(1), 25–30.

Thomas, D. J. (2001). Sexually transmitted viral infections: Epidemiology and treatment. *JOGNN, 30*(3), 316–323.

Trippet, S. E., & Bain, J. (1993). Physical health problems and concerns of lesbians. *Women and Health, 20*(2), 59–70.

Reid, J. (2001). Women's knowledge of Pap smears, risk factors for cervical cancer, and cervical cancer. *Journal of Obstetrics, Gyneology and Neonatal Nursing, 30*(3), 299–305.

White, J. C., & Levinson, W. (1995). Lesbian health care: What a primary care physician needs to know. *West J Med, 162,* 463–466.

Williams-Barnard, C. L., Mendoza, D. C., & Shippee-Rice, R. V. (2001). The lived experience of college student lesbians' encounters with health care providers. A preliminary investigation. *J Holist Nurs, 19*(2), 127–142.

Wilton, T., & Kaufmann, T. (2001). Lesbian mothers' experiences of maternity care in the UK. *Midwifery, 17*(3), 203–211.

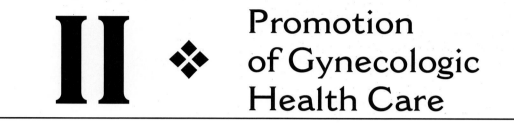

II ❖ Promotion of Gynecologic Health Care

CHAPTER 8

MENSTRUATION AND RELATED PROBLEMS AND CONCERNS

Deborah Griswold

*M*ost women expe-
rience numerous
changes in their men-
strual cycle patterns
during their reproduc-
tive life.

Highlights

- Normal Onset and Occurrence of Menses
- Abnormalities Related to the Menstrual Cycle
    Amenorrhea
    Dysfunctional Uterine Bleeding
    Dysmenorrhea
    Toxic Shock Syndrome
    Premenstrual Syndrome

❖ INTRODUCTION

Menstruation is a normal, cyclically recurring event for most women between the approximate ages of 12 and 50. Like childbirth, it usually occurs without major difficulties and is a universal event for most women. The menstruating woman has been considered unclean or to possess supernatural powers. Some of these powers were regarded as good, while others instilled fear. In some cultures women were isolated during menstruation and only allowed to be in the company of other menstruating women. One theory is that women themselves started the practice of isolation during menstruation to have a time for quiet and reflection and perhaps to provide a time for the older women to impart their knowledge to the younger women (Rome, Reame, & Stanford, 1998).

Historically, menstruation was viewed as a disease rather than a normal condition. Medical treatment during the second half of the 19th century rested on an explicit view of women as fragile and vulnerable, totally dominated by the cyclicity and disability of their reproductive system. This heritage has objectively and subjectively colored society's perceptions of the menstruating woman as weak, suffering, unstable, or physically unable to execute her normal duties competently. There is much argument in the literature about the effect of this conditioning on women's perceptions of menstrual symptoms and events. Feminist literature challenges much of the medical and psychiatric literature on menstrual cycle research as being biased and sexist.

The recent popularity of best sellers on the menstrual changes associated with menopause has opened the way for greater social awareness and knowledge of menstrual norms and changes, made the topic more acceptable for discussion, and continued to alter the attitudes of society toward menstruation. One can hope this trend will help to ameliorate the predominantly negative attitudes about menstruation that past studies have demonstrated. This is important since most women experience numerous changes in their menstrual cycle patterns during their reproductive life. Prevalence rates of primary dysmenorrhea are as high as 90 percent. Menstrual pain is a common cause of absenteeism and decreased quality of life for many females (Coco, 1999). Adequate information about norms, comfort in discussing this body function, and access to reliable health care providers may decrease unnecessary visits, reduce embarrassment and anxiety about common problems, and encourage further studies on women's menstrual experiences.

NORMAL ONSET AND OCCURRENCE OF MENSES

Events preceding the first menses have a characteristic pattern. *Thelarche*, the development of breast buds; *adrenarche*, the appearance of pubic then axillary hair followed by the growth spurt; with culmination in *menarche*. See Chapters 4 and 5 for more details on these developmental milestones.

The menstrual cycle will be repeated 300 to 400 times in the life of the human female. Cycles vary in frequency from 21 to 40 days (regularity is normal), bleeding lasts 3 to 8 days, and blood loss averages 30 to 80 mL (Mitan & Slap, 2002; Speroff, Glass, & Kase, 1999). Small clots are normal; large clots indicate rapid bleeding and inability of fibrinogen to act in the uterus. Only 15 percent of menstrual cycles are the classic 28 days long (Gordon & Speroff, 2002).

ABNORMALITIES RELATED TO THE MENSTRUAL CYCLE

DESCRIPTIVE TERMS

- *Amenorrhea.* Absence of menses.
- *Oligomenorrhea.* Infrequently occurring menses at intervals greater than 35 days.
- *Polymenorrhea.* Menses at intervals of 21 to 24 days or fewer.
- *Hypermenorrhea/Menorrhagia.* Regularly occurring bleeding excessive in duration and flow (greater than 80 mL/cycle or lasting longer than 7 days).
- *Metrorrhagia.* Bleeding occurring irregularly; excessive in flow and length.
- *Menometrorrhagia.* Irregular, heavy bleeding.
- *Hypomenorrhea.* Regular bleeding in less than normal amount.

♦ *Intermenstrual bleeding.* Bleeding at any time between otherwise normal menses (Gordon & Speroff, 2002; Nelson, 1998).

AMENORRHEA

Amenorrhea is a symptom, not a diagnosis, and is categorized as primary or secondary. *Primary amenorrhea* is the absence of menses by age 16 whether normal growth and secondary sexual characteristics are present, or the absence of menses after age 14 when normal growth and signs of secondary sexual characteristics are present. *Secondary amenorrhea* is the absence of menses for three cycles or six months in women who have previously menstruated regularly, or six to twelve months in a woman with a history of irregular periods (Nelson, 1998; Speroff, Glass, & Kase, 1999).

Epidemiology

Etiology. Etiology includes pregnancy, lactation, and age-appropriate menopause, which are by far the most likely causes of amenorrhea and are considered physiological. Among women of reproductive age, amenorrhea that is unrelated to pregnancy may signal stress or a life-threatening disease. Causative factors include anatomic deviations, genetic factors, endocrine abnormalities or imbalances, defective enzyme systems, autoimmune diseases, tumors, eating disorders, excessive exercise, medications, or past surgery (Gordon & Neinstein, 2002).

Incidence. Secondary amenorrhea occurs in 2 to 3 percent of women. Incidences in subgroups such as college students and athletes are higher. Ninety-eight percent of U.S. teenage girls menstruate by age 16 (Minjarez & Carr, 2002).

Subjective Data

The etiology of amenorrhea is revealed in a woman's history most of the time. Questions about each of the following areas should be carefully posed.

♦ Menstrual history includes the following information: age of development of secondary sex characteristics and current status, absence of menarche or age it occurred, date of last menstrual period, symptoms associated with menses, interval between menses, duration and characteristics of flow.
♦ Past illnesses, hospitalizations, and surgeries should be noted. Chronic diseases such as childhood leukemia, thyroid or adrenal dysfunction, and renal or hepatic disease are recorded, along with a description of radiation therapy, chemotherapy, or surgery, particularly a dilation and curettage (D & C), which can affect the menstrual pattern.
♦ Obstetric history records the date and course of any pregnancy. Intrauterine or ectopic pregnancy, abortion, and type of delivery are also noted. Postpartum hemorrhage or infection could be a causative factor of amenorrhea.
♦ Prescription and over-the-counter drugs can affect menstrual function, and a history of oral contraceptives may alter usual patterns. Depot medroxyprogesterone acetate (Depo-Provera) often produces amenorrhea that may persist for a year or more. Illicit drug use, smoking, and alcohol intake also can disturb normal cycles.
♦ Lifestyle evaluation includes eating patterns, weight loss or gain, critical level of body fat, exercise regimens, obesity, anorexia, bulimia, life stressors, and sexual behaviors, including contraception.
♦ History of present illness (HPI) is an assessment of bodily changes or abnormalities, such as nipple discharge, hirsutism, virilization, absense of menses alternating with heavy bleeding cycles, hot flashes, vaginal dryness, insomnia, headaches, or infertility.

Objective Data

Physical Examination

♦ *General appearance and skin.* Observe carefully and note general body habitus, stage of development of secondary sexual characteristics (see Tanner stages, Chapter 5), amount and distribution of hair and fat, and presence of striae.
♦ *Vital signs.* Gather baseline data, height, weight, and blood pressure and compare with norms.
♦ *Head and eyes.* Perform a complete head-to-toe physical, including a visual field exam.
♦ *Neck.* Examine thyroid for nodules or enlargement.
♦ *Breasts.* Observe breasts for discharge, then palpate for masses and attempt to express discharge.
♦ *Abdomen.* Palpate abdomen for masses or hernias.
♦ *Genitalia/reproductive.* Examine genitalia for obstructive problems, such as imperforate hymen. Check for cervical stenosis, vaginal agenesis, transverse vaginal septum, absent uterus, or pregnancy (Gordon & Neinstein, 2002).
♦ *Endocrine.* Assess for signs of androgen excess such as hirsutism, clitoromegaly, or acne. Evaluate hormonal status (estrogen and progesterone) by color of

mucous membranes, presence or absence of rugae, amount and consistency of cervical mucus, and presence of ferning. Vaginal cells may be collected for maturation index.

In the normal woman of reproductive age, mucous membranes are pink and moist; rugae are present; and cervical mucus is clear and ferns if estrogen, without progesterone, is present.

Commonly Recommended Diagnostic Tests and Methods

*   *A pregnancy test should always be done first* to rule out pregnancy or related complications. Immunometric urine pregnancy tests, commonly used in clinic settings, detect hCG levels as low as 5 to 50 mLu/mL (Stewart, 1998). Qualitative (yes/no) beta hCG blood testing is not superior to immunometric urine pregnancy testing used for screening purposes to rule out or confirm pregnancy (Stewart, 1998). Urine pregnancy test results are available within three to five minutes at a lesser cost than blood tests.
*   *Thyroid stimulating hormone (TSH)* and *prolactin hormone* levels are recommended because hypothyroidism and hyperprolactinemia can cause amenorrhea. If the TSH is elevated, indicating hypothyroidism, supplementation may be beneficial. An elevated prolactin level may indicate a pituitary tumor. Appropriate referral to an endocrinologist as well as diagnostic imaging with computerized axial tomography (CT scan) or magnetic resonance imaging (MRI) are essential when the prolactin level is high (Gordon & Speroff, 2002; Nelson, 1998).
*   If tests for pregnancy, hypothyroidism, and pituitary tumor are negative, administer the *progesterone challenge test.* Progesterone in oil 100–200 mg I.M.; or 300 mg oral micronized progesterone; or 5 mg oral medroxyprogesterone acetate (MPA) for seven to ten days; or 10 mg MPA for 5 days is given to test for the presence of estrogen priming and the intactness of the outflow tract (uterus and vagina). If there is no galactorrhea and bleeding occurs in two to seven days after concluding medication, then the cervix is patent, estrogen is being produced, and the endometrium is functional (Gordon & Speroff, 2002; Nelson, 1998).
*   If no bleeding occurs with the progesterone challenge, administer 1.25 mg of *conjugated estrogen* or 2 mg estradiol orally for 21 days to stimulate endometrial proliferation. Add *medroxyprogesterone acetate* 10 mg p.o. for the last five days of estrogen

administration to achieve a withdrawal bleed (Gordon & Speroff, 2002; Nelson, 1998).
*   If no bleeding occurs after the progesterone challenge, measure FSH (follicle stimulating hormone). If the FSH is elevated, ovarian failure (hypergonadotropic hypogonadism) is established (Minjarez & Carr, 2002). If the FSH is normal, an anatomic defect such as Asherman's syndrome may be responsible for the amenorrhea. Asherman's syndrome involves intrauterine adhesions and may occur after a procedure that involves curettage of the uterus. Refer to a gynecologist in this case. The gynecologist may perform sonohysterography (fluid contrast ultrasound), hysterosalpinogram, or hysteroscopy to determine if uterine adhesions are responsible (Minjarez & Carr, 2002).

Ovarian Function Tests

*   Measure serum levels of the gonadotropins FSH and *luteinizing hormone* (LH) and consider *estradiol* level to evaluate the ovaries.
*   An elevated FSH indicates gonadal failure.
*   If the LH and FSH levels are elevated (FSH > 20 IU/L and LH > 40 IU/L) and the estradiol level is low, the woman is menopausal.
*   If the gonadotropins are not elevated, or if the LH is high and the FSH is low or normal, polycystic ovarian syndrome should be considered.
*   If the gonadotropins are low (FSH < 5 IU/L; LH < 5 IU/L), consider prepubertal, hypothalamic, or pituitary dysfunction (Gordon & Speroff, 2002; Nelson, 1998). A normal LH level with a high FSH level indicates impending ovarian failure.
*   *Premature ovarian failure* is defined as amenorrhea with hypoestrogenism and elevated levels of LH and FSH prior to the age of 40 (Minjarez & Carr, 2002). Gonadal dysgenesis is the most common cause of ovarian failure. In gonadal dysgenesis "the germ cells undergo accelerated atresia and the ovary is replaced with a fibrous streak" (Minjarez & Carr, 2002, p. 1074). Genetic aberrations, autoimmune disorders, infections, cancer treatment (radiation and chemotherapy) are among other possible causes of premature ovarian failure. Screening tests for autoimmune disorders may be indicated. Physician referral is recommended for further diagnostic workup.

Ovarian/Adrenal Function Tests

*   Serum total testosterone, dehydroepiandrosterone (DHEA), dehydroepiandrosterone sulfate (DHEA-S), androstenedione, 17-hydroxyprogesterone (17-OHP),

cortisol, TSH, prolactin, and fasting blood glucose are suggested for suspected abnormal androgenic, ovarian, and insulin states. Hyperandrogenism, insulin resistance, and hyperinsulinemia are often associated, as may be seen with polycystic ovarian syndrome (PCOS) and some cases of obesity and non-insulin-dependent diabetes (Gordon & Speroff, 2002).

- Consult with a specialist for tests to order for specific concerns, such as for autoimmune disease (Gordon & Speroff, 2002).

Other. If genetic or chromosomal abnormalities are suspected, consult with a specialist before ordering karotyping. If other disease is a concern, such as anemia or a clotting disorder, specific tests should be ordered.

Differential Medical Diagnoses

Pregnancy Related

- Pregnancy, lactation, or pregnancy complications such as ectopic pregnancy, missed abortion, postpartum hemorrhage, or trophoblastic neoplasm.

Medication Related

- Many medications can cause amenorrhea or oligomenorrhea. Combined or progestin-only contraceptives are frequently the source of diminished or absent menses. Nonhormonal medications may also be responsible for menstrual changes.

Hypothalamic-Pituitary-Ovarian (HPO) Axis Related

- Anovulation secondary to immature HPO axis, obesity, or polycystic ovaries. Polycystic ovarian syndrome (PCOS) is the most common condition associated with chronic anovulation in the presence of estrogen. These women bleed after the progestin challenge. PCOS is associated with hirsutism, elevated body mass index, infertility, amenorrhea, or dysfunctional uterine bleeding (Minjarez & Carr, 2002). Abnormal insulin resistance/activity is associated with PCOS (Gordon & Speroff, 2002).
- Premature ovarian failure secondary to genetic conditions, smoking, autoimmune diseases, infections, chemotherapy, radiation, surgery, ovarian insensitivity to gonadotropins (Savage syndrome), or steroidogenic enzyme defect, 17 α-hydroxylase deficiency.
- Menopause secondary to age appropriate follicular depletion.
- Hyperprolactinemia secondary to pituitary tumor, stress, thyroid disorder, or drug induced.

- Inhibited gonadotropin-releasing hormone (GnRH) secondary to discontinuation of combined contraceptives, use of medications such as danazol or suppression of pulsatile GnRH secretion below its critical range secondary to anorexia or weight loss. Hypogonadotropic hypogonadism involves chronic anovulation without the production of estrogen. In this disorder there is interference in the release of GnRH-gonadotropin releasing hormone or gonadotropin release from the hypothalamic pituitary axis (Minjarez & Carr, 2002). Tumors or other disorders of the hypothalamus and certain syndromes may cause hypogonadotropic hypogonadism. More common causes are eating disorders, weight loss associated with dieting, exercise, and chronic debilitating disease. As many as 55 percent of amenorrheic women may have an eating disorder (Nelson, 1998).

Obstructive Related

- Imperforate hymen.
- Transverse vaginal septum.
- Cervical stenosis following instrumentation or trauma.

Autoimmune Disorders

- See appropriate references.

Asherman's Syndrome. Asherman's syndrome is an acquired anomaly that can occur following vigorous curettage, such as during a D & C or termination of pregnancy. Asherman's syndrome results in intrauterine scarring with destruction of the endometrium (Baase, 2000).

Plan

Psychosocial Interventions. The health care provider must address the diverse causes of amenorrhea, the relationship to sexual identity, perception of normal menstrual function, possible infertility, tumor, or life-threatening disease. Sensitive listening, interviewing, and individualized evaluation are essential. Always consider the possibility of pregnancy and related emergencies, despite the client's history or social situation. All patients diagnosed with ovarian failure prior to age 30 require physician referral for karyotype determination. These tests require sensitive explanations to avoid further emotional trauma.

Medication. The medication prescribed varies with the client situation. Combination oral contraceptives are superior to progesterone-only treatment in a sexually active, nonsmoking client who is younger than 35. Cyclic progesterone may be preferred when estrogen is contraindicated.

Medroxyprogesterone Acetate (MPA)

- Indications are to prevent endometrial hyperplasia in anovulatory clients who do not need contraception (Minjarez & Carr, 2002).
- Administer 5 to 10 mg p.o. the first ten to fourteen days of each month or during cycle days 16 to 26.
- Side effects and adverse reactions most commonly reported include spotting, weight gain, fatigue, depression, or acne.
- Contraindications include pregnancy, thromboembolic disorders, liver dysfunction, known or suspected malignancy of breast or reproductive organs, undiagnosed vaginal bleeding, or missed abortion. The use of medroxyprogesterone acetate (MPA) as a diagnostic test for pregnancy is also contraindicated.
- Anticipated outcome on evaluation is that the client begins cyclic withdrawal spotting or bleeding two to seven days after completing medication.
- Client teaching should include information about the possibility of bleeding's being heavy when medication is completed. Emphasize the importance of taking the medication to prevent endometrial hyperplasia or cancer. Inform the client of side effects and tell her to report any abnormal bleeding or the absence of withdrawal bleeding. Stress the necessity of consistently using reliable birth control measures.

Low Dose Combination Oral Contraceptives

- Indications are to prevent endometrial hyperplasia, to provide contraception for clients with anovulatory cycles (first choice of therapy), and to supplement estrogen for the protection of bone health.
- Administer 21- or 28-day pack cyclic therapy.
- Side effects and adverse reactions most commonly reported include breast tenderness, spotting, scanty menses, and nausea.
- Contraindications are pregnancy, undiagnosed vaginal bleeding, history of breast or reproductive tract cancer, history of thromboembolism, cerebrovascular or coronary heart disease, liver tumor or malignancy, or smoker older than 35, migraine headaches may be preceded by an aura or with neurologic symptoms, lactation, hypertension, complicated prolonged immobilization, or surgery on the legs (Hatcher et al., 2001).
- Anticipated outcomes on evaluation are cyclic withdrawal bleeding, contraception.
- Client teaching and counseling should include information about how to take pills, manage missed pills, and recognize the danger signs (see Chapter 9). Instruct the client to chart dates of menses or spotting.

Hormone Replacement Therapy

- Indications are for hypoestrogenic states secondary to premature or physiological menopause, or in serious exercisers. See Chapter 15 for discussion of the most recent findings related to risks and benefits of hormone replacement therapy. Careful consideration of the individual characteristics of the woman must be considered before use.
- Indicated for women who do not need contraception.
- Implications (see Chapter 9).

Other

- Other medication regimens should be managed by physician referral or with physician consultation because of the complex etiology of amenorrhea.

Surgical Interventions. Usually managed by a gynecologist, endometrial biopsy—curette or flushing of endometrial cells for microscopic examination—may be done to evaluate the uterus for atrophy, phase of endometrium, or abnormalities, although the test is not commonly done unless prior tests and treatments yield no answer to the problem. Destroyed endometrium as a cause of secondary amenorrhea can be determined by hysterogram or hysteroscopy, as an outpatient procedure. Client teaching and counseling include informing the client about the purpose of the biopsy, how the procedure is to be performed, relaxation techniques, follow-up, and the monetary cost.

Follow-Up. Once workup is completed, follow-up is done annually. Prior to refilling medications, evaluate the client's menstrual charts, the client's adherence to the medication schedule, the presence of danger signs or side effects, and the results of the Pap test and breast exam/mammography. Refer all clients with primary amenorrhea for physician evaluation. Reassure young amenorrheic teens and their parents; recommend watchful waiting if results of tests are normal. Refer all clients with secondary amenorrhea caused by central lesions, autoimmune diseases, psychiatric problems, or complex endocrine or metabolic diseases to a physician for evaluation and management.

DYSFUNCTIONAL UTERINE BLEEDING (DUB)

Dysfunctional uterine bleeding (DUB) is prolonged or excessive vaginal bleeding due to endometrial sloughing in the absence of pelvic structural disorder (Mitan &

Slap, 2002). It is frequently associated with anovulatory cycles. Women who ovulate and have abnormal vaginal bleeding are considered to have functional vaginal bleeding, usually a result of a uterine lesion or blood dyscrasia (Fossum, 2002).

Epidemiology

Etiology. The etiology of DUB is usually hormonal disturbance with failure of ovarian follicular maturation resulting in lack of progesterone production, limitation of endometrial growth, and synchronous shedding. Chronic anovulation with continuous estrogen production increases endometrial vascularity and thickness without adequate stromal support for maintenance. Irregular spotting and episodes of profuse and usually painless bleeding result. An atrophic endometrium that bleeds irregularly may be formed by lack of estrogen due to menopause or formed pharmacologically through long-term use of low dose birth control pills or continuous combined hormone replacement therapy (Gordon & Speroff, 2002).

Incidence. Incidence of dysfunctional uterine bleeding is primarily attributed to anovulation and most commonly presents in adolescents and perimenopausal women (Nelson, 1998). Up to 80 percent of menstrual cycles are anovulatory during the first year following menarche and take an average of twenty months to become ovulatory (Mitan & Slap, 2002). One-half of adolescents hospitalized with hemorrhage after menarche have a systemic bleeding disorder (Mitan & Slap, 2002).

Subjective Data

A history of irregular menses is typically exhibited as episodes of heavy painless bleeding alternating with periods of amenorrhea. Subjective reports of excessive bleeding are frequently inaccurate. It is important to take note of any change in bleeding pattern reported by the woman as well as any signs of anemia—including excessive fatigue, headaches, and dizziness. A woman has to experience very significant vaginal bleeding to develop anemia from DUB (Nelson, 1998).

Objective Data

Although no organic problems are associated with DUB, a complete physical examination, including pelvic and rectal exams, is performed to rule out neoplasia. Note passing tissue and test specimens if available and/or suspicious.

Diagnostic tests and methods include a CBC and Pap smear. A pregnancy test should be done with all women of reproductive age who are experiencing abnormal bleeding. Gonorrhea and chlamydia testing should be performed as indicated. Thyroid function tests, especially TSH, are indicated for women who may or may not have signs or symptoms of thyroid dysfunction since menorrhagia has been associated with hypothyroid disease (Gordon & Speroff, 2002; Nelson, 1998). A serum prolactin test may be indicated. In a woman of reproductive age, particularly if unilateral abdominal pain is present, an ultrasound should be done to rule out an ectopic pregnancy. Transvaginal ultrasound may be ordered to measure endometrial thickness. A patient or family history of bleeding disorders mandates coagulation studies. Women with a lifelong history of heavy and prolonged periods should be evaluated for bleeding disorders such as Von Willebrand's disease. Severe DUB with anemia should be discussed with the physician and warrants coagulation studies.

In-Office Endometrial Biopsy

- Evaluation of suspected uterine pathology is usually done by the physician, although some nurse practitioners perform endometrial biopsies. This diagnostic evaluation is done to determine the cytologic status of endometrial tissue. An endometrial biopsy is recommended for women at risk for endometrial hyperplasia and carcinoma (Church, 2000). Endometrial intraepithelial neoplasia (EIN) is of greater concern for cancer than hyperplasia, since cytologic atypia are present (Gordon & Speroff, 2002). Age (over 35 years), obesity, and exposure to unopposed estrogen via medications or intrinsically, as with PCOS, are risk factors for endometrial hyperplasia, EIN, and carcinoma (Gordon & Speroff, 2002; Nelson, 1998).

- Test procedure involves helping the client to assume the lithotomy position. Various devices have been designed for endometrial sampling, which are passed through the cervix to the endometrial cavity in order to obtain a small amount of tissue for examination.

- Nursing implications and client teaching involve informing the client about the purpose of the test, obtaining her signature on the consent form, and explaining the cost of the procedures. Encourage relaxation breathing and convey the progression of each step to the client to alleviate her discomfort and anxiety. Spotting and cramping may occur up to 48 hours following biopsy. NSAIDs can be recommended if there are no contraindications.

Hysteroscopy

- *Hysteroscopy* is visualization of the endometrium through a scope to search for uterine abnormalities. Observation and directed tissue sampling is replacing D & C as the diagnostic procedure of choice. (Minor treatments, such as polyp or septal removal, also can be done through the hysteroscope.)
- The procedure is done in the office or operating room. The hysteroscope is inserted when the cervix is dilated. The uterus is distended with dextran 70, carbon dioxide, or another distention medium to facilitate visualization of the endometrium.
- Nursing implications include teaching the client that some cramps and bleeding are expected following the procedure, and leakage of dextran 70 through the cervix and vagina can be messy. Carbon dioxide distention may cause cramps or shoulder pain. Pain medications should be provided. *Advise the client to report signs of infection, excessive bleeding, or pain—and to report any allergic response that occurs with dextran 70 at once.*

Dilation and Curettage (D & C)

- Dilation of the cervix and curettage (D & C) may be done for diagnostic evaluation. Endometrial D & C is recommended when medical regimens are ineffective, or if polyps, incomplete abortion, or neoplasia is suspected, or if a more complete biopsy sampling of the endometrium may be desired and hysteroscopy is unavailable.

  - The procedure requires that the client be given local or general anesthesia and that specimens be sent to pathology.
  - Nursing implications are to provide appropriate explanations of the procedure, anesthesia, cost, and risks. Postoperative instructions are given, advising the client to report signs of infection, excessive bleeding, and/or pain. Pain medication is also provided.

Differential Medical Diagnoses

- Pregnancy or pregnancy related complications.
- Cervical abnormalities: infection, polyp, carcinoma.
- Uterine abnormalities: fibroids, infection, polyps, endometrial hyperplasia, EIN, carcinoma.
- Medication/herb use: anticoagulants, digitalis, estrogen, phenytoin, ginseng.
- Other diseases: thyroid or adrenal disorders, liver or kidney failure, coagulopathies.

- Other: foreign body, possibly tubal sterilization though data is inconsistent (Gordon & Speroff, 2002; Nelson, 1998).

Plan

Psychosocial Interventions. Educate the client about normal menstrual cycles and possible reasons for her abnormal pattern. Be generous with reassurance. Menstrual calendars are helpful with instruction given about documenting any bleeding or spotting, days and dosages of medications, pad or tampon count, and associated symptoms of dysmenorrhea. By providing information about expected bleeding patterns on discontinuation of medications, you will help the client to avoid fears of recurrence or treatment failure. Because some medications are teratogenic, it is important to address birth control.

Medication

- *Low dose oral contraceptives* are known to control excessive or irregular bleeding and decrease menstrual flow (Gordon & Speroff, 2002; Hillard, 1996). They cycle and suppress the endometrium.
  - Oral contraceptive pills may be started any day of the cycle as long as the woman is not pregnant (Taylor, 2002).
  - Prescribe a pill that contains 35 micrograms or less of estrogen.
  - Side effects may include nausea, breast tenderness, spotting, and scanty menses.
  - Contraindications are pregnancy, undiagnosed vaginal bleeding, history of breast or reproductive tract cancer, history of thromboembolism, cerebrovascular or coronary heart disease, liver tumor or malignancy, or smoker older than 35 (Hatcher et al., 2001).
  - Anticipated outcome on evaluation is that bleeding will abate.
  - *Client teaching and counseling.* If bleeding does not abate, consult a physician. If an anovulatory pattern returns after discontinuing OCs, then resume the low dose combination pills or progesterone therapy described below.
- *Medroxyprogesterone acetate (MPA)* is indicated for clients with anovulatory bleeding in whom estrogen is contraindicated and contraception is not needed. Cyclic oral medroxyprogesterone acetate is used to induce regular withdrawal bleeding (Nelson, 1998).
  - A requirement for beginning therapy is to rule out pregnancy.

- MPA 10 mg is given qd for ten days each month.
- Side effects and adverse reactions most commonly reported include spotting, weight gain, fatigue, depression, or acne.
- Contraindications include pregnancy, thromboembolic disorders, liver dysfunction, known or suspected malignancy of breast or reproductive organs, undiagnosed vaginal bleeding, or missed abortion.
- Anticipated outcome on evaluation is that the first episode of bleeding after progesterone therapy will be heavy.
- Client teaching should include information about the possibility of bleeding being heavy when medication is completed. Emphasize the importance of taking medication to prevent endometrial hyperplasia or cancer. Inform the client of side effects and tell her to report any abnormal bleeding or the absence of withdrawal bleeding.

◆ *Depot medroxyprogesterone acetate (DMPA), Depo-Provera* may be given to suppress the endometrium and provide contraception.

- Rule out pregnancy before providing DMPA. The first dose is usually given during the first five days of the woman's menstrual period; however, if there has been no unprotected intercourse within the previous two weeks and a urine pregnancy test is negative, the injection may be then given regardless of her menstrual period (off label administration). Instruct her to use backup contraception (e.g., condoms) for seven days following the injection (Hatcher et al., 2001).
- Give DMPA 150 mg intramuscularly every twelve weeks (11 to 13 weeks is acceptable).
- DMPA produces amenorrhea in 50 percent of women after the first year of use (Hatcher et al., 2001).
- Side effects include irregular menses, upredictable spotting during the first few months leading to amenorrhea in many users, decreased libido, increased depression or mood changes, weight gain, and acne. Hypoestrogenism is possible due to FSH suppression, leading to hot flashes and decreased bone mineral density (Hatcher et al., 2001). Severe allergic reaction is possible, though rare.
- Many health care providers require the woman to remain for observation 20 minutes following the injection.
- Anticipated outcome is reduced vaginal bleeding, perhaps cessation of menses.

- Contraindications include pregnancy, undiagnosed abnormal vaginal bleeding, history of breast cancer, myocardial infarction, or stroke, current venous thromboembolism, liver dysfunction, or known hypersensitivity to DMPA.
- Client teaching should include the following: Do not massage the injection site, expect irregular bleeding and spotting, which should decrease over time—return to the clinic if it is bothersome. Discuss weight control, watch caloric intake, and exercise at least three times per week. Instruct the woman to be sure she gets adequate calcium for bone health. Women over 25 should take 1,000 mg of calcium per day and women younger than 25 should take 1,300 mg (Hatcher et al., 2001). The woman should be instructed to abstain from intercourse if it has been more than thirteen weeks since her last injection. She should also be advised to seek immediate medical care for severe headaches, heavy bleeding, worsening of depression, or if pus, pain, or bleeding develop at the injection site.

◆ *The Levonorgestrel-20 Intrauterine System, Mirena* was FDA approved in December 2000. It is a T-shaped contraceptive device placed within the uterine cavity that releases 20 micrograms per day of levonorgestrel from its vertical reservoir. Endometrial proliferation is suppressed, which results in reduced bleeding. Menorrhagia generally improves 90 percent, with blood loss decreasing more than 70 percent after three to six months (Hatcher et al., 2001). After twelve months, approximately 20 percent of users have no bleeding (Wysocki, 2002).

- Potential contraindications include pregnancy or suspicion of pregnancy, current cervical or endometrial infection, or uterine anomaly. Candidates are parous women in stable monogamous relationships with low risk of sexually transmitted infections. Testing for infections should be done prior to insertion.
- Side effects may include increase in number of days of bleeding during the first few months, then a decrease in bleeding after three to six months, and possibly cessation of bleeding. Mood changes, acne, headache, and nausea can also occur.
- Anticipated outcome is reduction in vaginal bleeding and menstrual pain, improvement in hemoglobin and hematocrit, and contraceptive protection.
- Client teaching should include checking for the presence of the device strings at the cervical os

monthly. The woman should be told bleeding changes she can expect to occur. She should be advised to return to the clinic if any sign of infection occurs.

♦ *Patients with severe anemia or life-threatening bleeding require immediate physician management.* Intravenous fluids, blood replacement, and conjugated estrogen may be necessary.

♦ *Nonsteroidal anti-inflammatory drugs* (NSAIDs) inhibit the synthesis of prostaglandins and reduce menstrual blood loss (Nelson, 1998), but may cause an alternative response at times with increased bleeding (Gordon & Speroff, 2002). NSAIDs are considered to be a good therapy for initial use (Gordon & Speroff, 2002).

• A requirement for beginning therapy is that pregnancy be ruled out. Prescribe mefenamic acid (Ponstel) 500 mg p.o. t.i.d. for three days *or* naproxen (Naprosyn) 500 mg p.o. b.i.d. *or* ibuprofen 400 mg every 6 hours with food. NSAIDs should be started the first day of menses and continued for three days (Nelson, 1998).

• Side effects and adverse reactions include gastrointestinal upset, rash, and edema.

• Contraindications include pregnancy, peptic ulcers, asthma, sensitivity to aspirin, and inflammatory bowel disease.

• Anticipated outcome on evaluation is reduction in bleeding.

• Client teaching and counseling should include the precaution to take the medication with food. Instruct the client about the dosing regimen and the side effects of the drug.

♦ *Other medical treatments* include estrogen therapy if spotting is due to low stimulation with estrogen; progestin IUD particularly for women with a chronic illness; GnRH agonist Danazol (400 to 600 mg per day) (Gordon & Speroff, 2002, Nelson, 1998). Danazol is an androgenic hormone that blocks gonadotropins and suppresses ovarian estrogen production. The endometrium thins and amenorrhea occurs. Side effects of Danazol limit its use to six to nine months (Nelson, 1998).

Surgical Interventions. Patients should be referred to a gynecologist if large structural lesions are noted on ultrasound or physical exam or if the patients are not responding to treatment. Ablation of the endometrium is an alternative to hysterectomy. A thermal balloon is used to ablate the tissue, and improvement is found in 90 percent

of women (Gordon & Speroff, 2002). It is not used if cancer is suspected. Hysterectomy is a last choice if all else fails. Any surgical procedure and the expected course must be explained fully and follow-up planned.

Follow-Up. Follow-up and referral may include iron therapy; 300 mg ferrous sulfate may be taken by mouth with orange juice 30 minutes after meals in addition to the therapy described above if the hemoglobin level is below 12 g. Anovulatory patterns tend to recur; therefore, clients should have a regular follow-up schedule and keep a menstrual and medication calendar. If more than a year elapses without a health care visit, notify the client. Cancer prevention should be a priority with this population.

DYSMENORRHEA

Dysmenorrhea refers to painful menstruation. It is categorized as primary or secondary. Secondary dysmenorrhea is associated with underlying pelvic pathology; primary is not (Rapkin, 1998).

Epidemiology

Etiology

♦ Primary dysmenorrhea is caused by increased prostaglandin production by the endometrium (Rapkin, 1998). Primary dysmenorrhea generally occurs in women who are ovulatory and produce progesterone in the luteal phase; progesterone stimulates the production of the prostaglandins in the base of the endometrium. Women with primary dysmenorrhea produce excessive amounts of prostaglandins when the endometrium sloughs, which increases the force of myometrial contractions. The contractions increase the pain by reducing blood flow and causing ischemia (Nelson, 1998). Measurements of intrauterine pressure in women with primary dysmenorrhea have shown the pressure similar to the second stage of labor. Uterine contractions cause injection of prostaglandins into the systemic circulation, which can produce nausea, vomiting, diarrhea, and headache (Nelson, 1998).

♦ Secondary dysmenorrhea is painful menstruation due to pelvic or uterine pathology. These women have other complaints such as nonmenstrual pelvic pain or pain with intercourse. The most common causes of secondary dysmenorrhea are endometriosis, adenomyosis, and intrauterine device (Rapkin, 1998). Adenomyosis involves the ingrowth of the endometrium into the uterine musculature, while endometriosis involves ectopic implantation of endometrial tissue in other parts of the pelvis (Rapkin, 1998).

Incidence. Most women experience some degree of dysmenorrhea. Fifteen to 20 percent of women have dysmenorrhea severe enough to interfere with work or school (Kennard, 1998).

Subjective Data

Primary dysmenorrhea typically presents in ovulatory cycles six to twelve months following menarche, and before the age of 20 years. Pain is suprapubic and described as "crampy"; it starts 12 to 24 hours before menses and is intermittent, except in severe cases. Pain is most severe during the first day of menses and disappears in 48 to 72 hours. The lower abdomen is most painful, but frequently pain extends to the back and thighs. About 50 percent experience related symptoms that may include nausea, vomiting, fatigue, dizziness, diarrhea, nervousness, and headache (Braverman & Neinstein, 2002).

Secondary dysmenorrhea typically presents in women with a history of painful menses that are increasingly intense or severe. It occurs most commonly in the third or fourth decades of life. Usually the location or duration of pain changes. Nevertheless, an adolescent should not automatically be assumed to have primary dysmenorrhea (Holmes & Landen, 2002). Endometriosis is the most common cause of secondary dysmenorrhea and is associated with pain beyond menses, dyspareunia, and infertility (Holmes & Landen, 2002). Associated symptoms are frequently dyspareunia with deep penetration, painful defecation, rectal pressure, heavy or irregular bleeding, urinary complaints, diarrhea and/or constipation during menstruation.

Objective Data

Physical Examination. A thorough pelvic exam is mandatory to establish a diagnosis. With primary dysmenorrhea, pelvic findings will be completely within normal limits except a mildly tender uterus on examination. Secondary dysmenorrhea, however, may reveal an assortment of pelvic pathologies, depending on the etiology of the problem:

- Endometriosis may present with a normal pelvic exam, or the examination may reveal nodularity in the cul-de-sac, caused by implants, nonmobile ovaries or uterus due to adhesion formation, and possible adnexal fullness from endometrioma (Holmes & Landen, 2002).

- Adenomyosis will often present in women over the age of 40. The examination will show a diffusely enlarged uterus that is soft and tender with normal mobility (Holmes & Landen, 2002).
- Leiomyoma will present as an irregular or enlarged uterus and may be tender.
- Infection will present with discharge, adnexal tenderness, and/or uterine tenderness. Fever may be present.

Diagnostic Tests and Methods

Variety of Tests

- Diagnostic evaluation to detect specific infection: gonorrhea, chlamydia, herpes; wet mounts for clue cells and/or white blood cells.
- Test procedure (see Chapters 4 and 11).
- Nursing implications are to explain the purpose of the culture or test, the actual procedure, and the cost of specimen collection.

Ultrasound (Vaginal)

- Diagnostic evaluation to diagnose pelvic abnormalities: myomas, ovarian cysts, congenital malformations.
- Nursing implications are to explain the necessary preparation and procedure and to teach the client about ultrasound, its purpose, and its cost.

Laparoscopy

- Diagnostic evaluation to stage and grade endometriosis if treatment fails or fertility workup is desired.
- The procedure is done with the client in lithotomy position in the operating room, using local or general anesthesia. An intrauterine manipulator is used to promote visibility. A small subumbilical incision is made and the laparoscope inserted to visualize the pelvic organs. Carbon dioxide or nitrous oxide is used to insufflate the pelvic region. Some surgery can be performed through the laparoscope.
- Nursing implications are to explain to the client the types of anesthesia, what the procedure entails, the risks, recovery, and the activity schedule that will follow surgery. Obtain the client's written consent for the laparoscopy, and provide pain medication as needed.

Hysterosalpingogram, Hysteroscopy, or D & C

See Dysfunctional Uterine Bleeding (DUB), Objective Data.

Barium Enema

- Diagnostic evaluation done to rule out bowel pathology.
- Test procedure, generally outpatient, begins with barium enema followed by fluoroscopic and radiographic examination of the large intestine.
- Nursing implications and client teaching include explanations of preparation, procedure, follow-up, and test results.

Urinalysis

- Diagnostic evaluation done to rule out bladder pathology.
- Client teaching includes explanations of the procedure and its purpose, the cost, and the results.

Differential Medical Diagnoses

- *Obstructive Defects.* Cervical stenosis; imperforate hymen; congenital disorders of the müllerian tract.
- Endometriosis.
- *Other Differential Diagnoses.* Adenomyosis, pain secondary to an IUD, fibroids, endometrial polyps or carcinoma, pelvic inflammatory disease. Dysmenorrhea refers to pain preceding and during menstruation; pain outside that timeframe requires expanding differential diagnoses to include other causes of pelvic pain (Holmes & Landen, 2002).

Plan

Psychosocial Interventions. Helping the client to understand the normal events surrounding the menstrual cycle and the etiology of the dysmenorrhea is an important part of intervention. In addition, intervention is directed toward pain relief and coping strategies that will promote a productive lifestyle. Explaining the normal menstrual cycle will provide the client with the vocabulary to communicate more accurately about symptoms, and it will help to dispel myths. Give the client charts to record menses, onset of pain, timing of medication, relief afforded by the medication, and relationship of pain to basal body temperature. Charts are a teaching tool; they provide the client with a realistic picture of her pain and an objective record for modifying future therapy.

Carefully explain the nature and severity of the pathology associated with secondary dysmenorrhea. Discuss in detail the rationales for selecting particular tests, treatments, medications, or surgery; this will enhance client understanding and compliance. Be sure to address

the impact that the disease and treatment will have on fertility.

Medication

Prostaglandin Synthetase Inhibitors (PGSIs)

- First choice of therapy for primary dysmenorrhea in clients not needing contraception. Administer these drugs to relieve pain. They prevent the synthesis of prostaglandins, thereby stopping uterine hypercontractility and ischemia and restoring normal function. Commonly prescribed inhibitors include the NSAIDs: ibuprofen (Motrin) 400–800 mg q 4–8 hrs; naproxen (Naprosyn) 250–500 mg q 6–8 hrs; naproxen sodium (Anaprox) 275–500 mg q 8–12 hrs; mefenamic acid (Ponstel) 250–500 mg q 6–8 hrs, rofecoxib (Vioxx) 25–50 mg q 24 hrs. These agents are effective in up to 80 percent of women with primary dysmenorrhea (Holmes & Landen, 2002). Inadequate relief may be improved if NSAIDs are started one to two days before expected menses. These medications should be taken with food.
- Side effects and adverse reactions include gastrointestinal upset, rash, and edema.
- Ibuprofen, naproxen, and naproxen sodium are classified as Pregnancy Category B, and mefenamic acid and rofecoxib are classified as Category C (*Nurse Practitioners' Prescribing Reference*, 2002). Caution should be used if pregnancy is suspected. Also, peptic ulcers, asthma, aspirin sensitivity, and inflammatory bowel disease are contraindications.
- Anticipated outcome on evaluation is relief of pain. The client should use one drug for a minimum of two to four cycles before evaluating effectiveness. If pain is not relieved, choose another NSAID, preferably from a different pharmacological group (e.g., naproxen sodium versus ibuprofen). If no relief occurs after another two to four months, initiate oral contraceptive therapy.
- Client teaching and counseling are the same as for DUB. Tell the client to take the medication with food. Give instructions about the dosing regimen and the side effects of the drug.

Low Dose Combination Oral Contraceptives

- Indication as first choice of therapy is for primary dysmenorrhea in clients who need contraception. Among women who have primary dysmenorrhea, 90 percent are relieved by using an oral contraceptive.

- Administer low dose combination oral contraceptives to reduce pain through the suppression of ovulation and endometrial proliferation. This reduces menstrual fluid volume and prostaglandin production to below normal.
- Low dose monophasic oral contraceptive pills may also be taken following several options for extended OC regimens. Taking active pills on a continuous basis—no placebos—or reducing the pill-free interval can effectively reduce the number of menstrual cycles and the accompanying symptoms (Policar, 2002). There is no clinical evidence that the current regimen of 21 active pills/7 hormone-free days is any safer or healthier than other extended regimens (Policar, 2002). New options include "bicycling," which involves 42 days of active pills, followed by 7 pill-free days; "tricycling," which involves 63 days of active pills, then 7 pill free days; and "quadcycling," which involves 84 days of active pills, followed by 7 pill free days (Policar, 2002). Seasonale (Barr Pharmaceutical), still undergoing trials, is an oral contraceptive pill that delivers pills in the "tricycling" fashion so that the woman gets a period every three months or every season (Policar, 2002). Other options include shortening the pill-free interval (placebo days) from 7 to 5, 4, or 3 days to reduce the number of symptomatic days per menses and probably increase contraceptive efficacy (Policar, 2002).
- Side effects, adverse reactions, and contra-indications are the same as for amenorrhea.
- Anticipated outcome on evaluation is relief of 90 percent of primary dysmenorrhea with oral contraceptives.
- Client teaching and counseling should include information about how to take pills, manage missed pills, and recognize the danger signs (see Chapter 9). Instruct the client to chart dates of menses or spotting.

Depo medroxyprogesterone (DMPA), Depo-Provera

- DMPA is effective in reducing menstrual cramps and decreasing blood loss. Within nine to twelve months of DMPA therapy, 75 percent of women become oligomenorrheic or amenorrheic (Holmes & Landen, 2002).
- DMPA 150 mg is administered intramuscularly every twelve weeks.
- It is essential that the woman understand the bleeding changes that occur with DMPA to improve compliance and patient satisfaction.

If using NSAIDs and/or hormonal contraception does not relieve the pain with primary dysmenorrhea, an evaluation is needed for secondary dysmenorrhea. Referral to a gynecologist is appropriate for a diagnostic workup (Holmes & Landen, 2002).

Lifestyle Changes. Share information about lifestyle factors that can be initiated to restore some sense of control and alleviate the sense of frustration and victimization. For example, exercise increases endorphins, suppresses prostaglandin release, raises the estrone-estradiol ratio that decreases endometrial proliferation, and shunts blood away from the uterus; pelvic congestion and pain are thereby decreased. Menus can be planned to limit salty foods, increase fiber with fresh fruits and vegetables, and increase water to serve as a natural diuretic. Heating pads or warm baths decrease muscle spasms and may increase comfort. Relaxation techniques can supplement medication regimens and enhance the client's ability to deal with pain.

Follow-Up. Follow-up of clients with primary dysmenorrhea can be done on a regular gynecologic exam schedule, once a medical regimen has been found that relieves pain adequately and is well tolerated. Follow clients with secondary dysmenorrhea according to the diagnosis, the type of medication prescribed, and the need for investigative or therapeutic surgery. Explain each procedure carefully and allow adequate time for questioning.

TOXIC SHOCK SYNDROME (TSS)

Toxic shock syndrome (TSS) is a rare but potentially lethal disorder. It has been associated with tampon use and vaginal *Staphylococcus aureus*-produced exotoxins (Hillard, 1998). TSS consists of fever, hypotension, diffuse erythroderma with desquamation of the palms and soles, and the involvement of three or more major organ systems (Hillard, 1998). TSS requires immediate physician referral and hospitalization.

Epidemiology

Etiology. The clinical manifestations of TSS result from the release of various inflammatory mediators in response to a relatively minor infection. TSS is historically associated with tampon use but occurs after surgery, postpartum, with skin or bone infections, burns, dermatologic lesions, and respiratory tract infections, including sinusitis (Davis, 2002).

Incidence. The incidence of TSS peaked in the late 1970s and 1980s, probably as a result of availability of super absorbent tampons. In 1980, approximately 95 percent of reported cases of TSS among women occurred during menstruation. By 1988, that rate dropped to 55 percent. The current overall rate of TSS is 1 to 3 per 100,000 per year. TSS is associated with a 10 percent mortality rate, most often due to adult respiratory distress syndrome (ARDS), intractable hypotension, or kidney failure (Davis, 2002).

Subjective Data

An abrupt onset of symptoms occurs, including high fever, chills, vomiting, watery diarrhea, myalgia, headaches, or abdominal pain in a previously healthy young woman during or shortly after menstruation.

Objective Data

Physical Examination

- Multisystem involvement is typical; hemodynamic instability is prominent. Vital signs include a temperature of 102°F or higher; systolic blood pressure of less than 90 mm Hg. An orthostatic drop in pressure of 15 mm Hg or more may occur when moving from a lying to sitting position.
- The most characteristic symptom is a sunburn-like rash that develops within 24 to 48 hours of onset of symptoms and progresses to desquamation in one to two weeks. Palms and soles are particularly affected.
- Many clients have conjunctival hyperemia, oropharyngeal erythema, strawberry tongue, vaginal hyperemia.
- Nonspecific abdominal tenderness may be found.
- Neurological findings are general confusion and disorientation without focal neurological findings.
- Multisystemic involvement occurs. At least three organ systems must be involved, with no evidence of another cause.

Differential Medical Diagnoses

Rocky Mountain spotted fever, Legionnaires' disease, toxic epidermal necrolysis, rheumatic fever, leptospirosis, rubeola, Lyme disease, Epstein-Barr virus, or disseminated fungal infections (Davis, 2002).

Plan

Organize physician referral quickly. Most clients require intensive care in the hospital.

Follow-Up. Follow-up includes providing the client with information: Inform her that subsequent milder attacks of TSS may develop within two to three months, encourage compliance with antibiotics, and discourage tampon use. If tampons are continued, advise good handwashing with soap prior to insertion or removal of tampons and intermittent use with pads. Advise the the woman to use barrier methods (vaginal sponge, diaphragm, cervical cap) carefully and to adhere to the manufacturer's directions. Advise the woman to seek medical care promptly if she develops any symptoms of TSS, such as fever or rash occuring during the middle or end of a menstrual period (Davis, 2002).

PREMENSTRUAL SYNDROME (PMS)

Premenstrual syndrome consists of a vast array of physical, cognitive, affective, and behavioral symptoms that occur repetitively in a cyclic fashion during the luteal phase of the menstrual cycle and resolve with the onset of menstruation (Braverman & Neinstein, 2002). Over 150 different symptoms are thought to vary with the menstrual cycle (Rebar & Erickson, 2000). *Premenstrual dysphoric disorder (PMDD)* is a similar diagnosis defined by the American Psychological Association that focuses more on affective disorders. PMDD is diagnosed according to criteria in the *Diagnostic and Statistical Manual of Mental Disorders* (4th ed., DSM-IV), whereas PMS is diagnosed according to criteria in the *Tenth Revision of the International Classification of Diseases* (ICD-10) (Dell, Moskowitz, & Sondheimer, 2001). PMS and PMDD are often found blended together in the literature.

Criteria for the diagnosis of PMS or PMDD has been defined by the American Psychological Association and requires that at least five of the following symptoms be present and at least one of the first four symptoms:

- Affective lability—sudden onset of being sad, tearful, irritable, or angry.
- Persistent and marked anger or irritability.
- Anxiety and tension.
- Depressed mood, feelings of hopelessness.
- Decreased interest in usual activities.
- Easily fatigued or marked lack of energy.
- Subjective sense of difficulty concentrating.
- Changes in appetite, overeating, or food cravings.
- Hypersomnia or insomnia.
- Feelings of being overwhelmed or out of control.

◆ Physical symptoms such as breast tenderness, headaches, edema, joint or muscle pain, weight gain (Gordon & Speroff, 2002; Schnare, 2002).

Epidemiology

Etiology. The exact cause of PMS is not known. It is thought to be related to the interaction between hormonal events and neurotransmitter function, specifically serotonin (Linderman, 2000). Not all women respond to serotonin reuptake inhibitors (SSRIs), however, which implies other mechanisms may be involved (Braverman & Neinstein, 2002). Other theories include allergies, endorphin withdrawal, fluid retention, hormonal changes (high estrogen, falling estrogen, changes in estrogen-progesterone ratio, and increased prolactin), prostaglandin effect, increased aldosterone activity, increased renin-angiotensin activity, increased adrenal activity, hypoglycemia, changes in catecholamines, psychological or psychogenic effects, and nutritional deficiencies (Schnare, 2002).

Lifestyle factors have been cited as contributory if not causative; these include increased stress, decreased exercise, poor diet, and increased intake of caffeine, nicotine, alcohol, red meat, and salt. Also implicated are overgrowth of *Candida albicans*, amino acid deficiencies, hyperandrogenism, post-tubal ligation interruption in normal blood supply, sleep deprivation, and altered electroencephalogram (EEG) pattern.

Incidence. It is estimated that up to 85 percent of women have some degree of PMS symptoms (Braverman & Neinstein, 2002). Five to 10 percent of women are thought to experience serious difficulties due to PMS (Rebar & Erickson, 2000). Risk factors include age over 30 years and genetic factors. Studies have shown a higher incidence of PMS symptoms among daughters of mothers who experienced PMS symptoms themselves, as well as higher concordance rates among monozygotic twins than dizygotic twins (Braverman & Neinstein, 2002). Around 60 percent of women who have a diagnosis of an affective disorder also have PMS (Schnare, 2002). The highest incidence of PMS is in the midreproductive years, as is the incidence of depression in women.

Subjective Data

Typically, clients with PMS have a number of physical symptoms, for example, breast tenderness, fluid retention, abdominal bloating, increased appetite and weight gain, craving for salty or sweet foods—chocolate in particular—acne, fatigue, heart palpitations, dizziness, faint-

ness, and/or headaches premenstrually. Usually, several of the following symptoms are present: mood swings, irritability, anxiety, hostility, depression, crying spells, thoughts of suicide, relationship conflict and fear of breakup, guilt over yelling at or battering children, feelings of inadequacy, increased or decreased libido, and inability to cope with the ever recurring symptoms.

Usually, clients delay treatment, deny the syndrome, make and cancel several appointments, and finally see a health care professional as a result of a recent crisis or threat from a significant other. Most women finally seek treatment after experiencing symptoms for ten or more years and report that their symptoms have increased in severity following each successive pregnancy and with advancing age (Rebar & Erickson, 2000). The symptoms, present in the luteal phase, may present in one of four cyclic patterns.

◆ They appear at midcycle, disappear, and reappear the week prior to menstruation.
◆ They begin at midcycle with subtle changes that gradually escalate until menses.
◆ They appear the week prior to menses and intensify until menstruation ensues.
◆ They appear in the first or second luteal weeks and do not disappear until the end of menstruation (Braverman & Neinstein, 2002).

Objective Data

There are no characteristic physical findings associated with PMS, but a complete physical examination should be performed to rule out any other illnesses (Linderman, 2000). No specific laboratory tests are used to diagnose PMS (Braverman & Neinstein, 2002), though a pregnancy test and hormonal assays to rule out menopause, hypothyroidism, and hyperprolactinemia may be of some benefit (Schnare, 2002). Other assays to assess for hyperandrogynism or hypoglycemia may be indicated. Diagnostic tests and methods to rule out other illnesses may include a CBC, Pap smear, and urinalysis.

Differential Medical Diagnoses

Differential diagnoses include psychological or psychiatric disorders such as major depression, panic, dysthymic disorder, or personality disorder (Braverman & Neinstein, 2002), drug addiction, family or social problems, history of rape or molestation, sexual dysfunction, migraine headache, seizure disorder, irritable bowel syndrome, inflammatory bowel disease, chronic fatigue disorders due to anemia or an infectious disease, allergies, idiopathic edema, and endocrine disorders such as hypothyroidism, hyperthyroidism, anorexia/bulimia, adrenal disorders, pheochromocytoma, hyperandrogenism, hyperprolactinemia, panhypopituitarism, and adrenocorticotropic hormone-mediated disorders (Schnare, 2002). Brain, breast, adrenal, or ovarian tumors should also be ruled out.

To diagnose PMS, the symptoms must occur in the luteal phase, they should not be present in the follicular phase, and they should resolve with the onset of menses or soon thereafter (Braverman & Neinstein, 2002). The symptoms must not be caused by other psychological or physical conditions and must be documented over several menstrual cycles and be severe enough to disrupt normal activities (Braverman & Neinstein, 2002).

Plan

Psychosocial Interventions. Assure the client that her symptoms are real, that PMS exists and she is not "crazy." Acceptance and acknowledgment are therapeutic.

Briefly explain PMS. Provide the client with interesting, informative, and accurate articles and books on the topic.

Teach the client the basics of the menstrual cycle and provide a menstrual symptoms chart for her to record and rate symptoms. This will enhance the client's awareness of her problem and the actual timing of PMS, and it will assist in planning and evaluating interventions. Symptoms should be prospectively charted for two to three months.

Focus on stresses contributing to PMS and ways to adjust lifestyle. Encourage the client to talk with family and friends about her needs and symptoms and to ask for nonthreatening types of support. Suggest assertiveness seminars or books about the subject. Role-play new strategies for dealing with troublesome situations that the client presented in her history. Teach her to schedule activities with PMS in mind, namely, not to overschedule when symptoms are worst. Encourage her to get adequate sleep.

Lifestyle changes may include beginning a safe exercise program, preferably outdoors, to increase endorphin production, reduce stress, enhance cardiovascular health, and prevent osteoporosis. Encourage the client to exercise three to five times per week. Exercise may improve the physical complaints and reduce stress, but it does not change the emotional aspects of PMS (Nelson, 1998). Assist the client with planning a balanced diet that avoids

salts and includes a nutritious snack. Previously women were told to resist premenstrual carbohydrate cravings, but now evidence suggests that low-protein, carbohydrate-rich foods consumed during the luteal phase may improve mood swings (Nelson, 1998). Carbohydrates also increase serotonin levels (Schnare, 2002). Many symptoms can be relieved simply by eating a morning meal and avoiding self-induced hypoglycemia. Encourage the client to carry snacks in her purse for times when symptoms such as fatigue, difficulty concentrating, or irritability occur. Advise her to decrease caffeine intake gradually to avoid headaches with the goal of total elimination to reduce irritability and to enhance sleep. Recommend increasing water intake to achieve natural diuresis.

Give the client permission to set aside time for herself. Teach stress reduction techniques, for example, taking long baths and taking time for pleasurable activity, yoga, Lamaze, biofeedback, meditation, or visual imagery—or refer her to a specialist for instruction.

Encourage the client to approach her therapy a little at a time, to seek assistance, and to accept her mistakes. Discourage "all or nothing" thinking patterns.

Review a typical day's communication patterns, sources of conflict, and problematic lifestyle factors. With the client, select one or two realistic goals to begin to pursue right away; accomplishing even small changes enhances self-esteem and the desire to continue making changes. Discourage the client from making too many changes at once.

Stress the importance of *not* smoking because of the overall negative health consequences and toxicity to the ovaries. Encourage limited intake of alcohol or avoiding it. Encourage the client to evaluate her coping styles and discard unhealthy habits, such as alcohol consumption, drug abuse, and smoking, for more functional styles.

Provide information about assertiveness classes, support groups for PMS, Co-Dependency, Al-Anon, Alcoholics Anonymous, counselors, or psychiatrists.

Long-term pharmacological therapy may be needed; therefore, the client should be included in decisions regarding therapy so that concerns about cost and side effects are shared. Therapy should be individualized and tailored to troublesome symptoms determined from menstrual symptom diaries.

Medications

Selective Serotonin Reuptake Inhibitors (SSRIs). Indications for SSRIs are negative emotional symptoms. SSRIs are now frequently used as a first line drug therapy for PMS because of their apparent efficacy and tolerability. Emotional symptoms are decreased more than are physical symptoms, lending support to newer theories that altered serotonergic function is present in women with PMS. Serotonergic agents have been shown to be more effective than placebo in the treatment of PMS. Fluoxetine was approved by the FDA in July 2000 for the treatment of PMS (Dell et al., 2001). SSRIs typically take a month or more to be effective with depression and other disorders, but this is not the case with PMS. SSRIs work immediately and at lower dosages, therefore they can be prescribed intermittently (Dell et al., 2001). Fluoxetine may be prescribed 10 or 20 mg per day for fourteen days premenstrually. Sarafem is fluoxetine marketed for PMS and is available in 10 or 20 mg caps.

Drug interactions with MAO inhibitors and tricyclics may occur. These agents, or combination with other SSRIs, should NOT be prescribed together.

Side effects of dizziness, nausea, headache, and insomnia are common, transient, and usually mild. In contrast to tricyclics, fluoxetine and other SSRIs do not have anticholinergic, hypotensive, or sedative effects. Dependency is not a concern, and they have no particular cardiovascular or serious toxic effects. Patients may have idiosyncratic responses to SSRIs, and their response should be monitored monthly for the first three months. If relief is not obtained, another agent should be chosen.

Advise clients about taking the medication appropriately and that beneficial effects are not immediate but may take as long as two weeks. In PMS, a positive clinical response has been noted to occur more immediately. Fluoxetine is classified as Pregnancy Category C.

Advise clients of common side effects. Encourage them to give the medication at least a two-week trial, since most side effects are temporary. Elicit client's response to SSRI therapy, since the media has given a great deal of coverage to Prozac—both positive and negative. Advise clients that this therapy may well be long-term.

Vitamin and Mineral Supplements

- A good multivitamin supplement can be a benign beginning treatment while the client collects data for charts.
- Vitamins and minerals are commonly indicated for PMS therapy; however, there is no evidence that nutritional deficiencies cause PMS, and their use may be dangerous if taken in inappropriate amounts.

- Pyridoxine (vitamin B_6) has been used in the past for the emotional symptoms of PMS but is now considered of limited benefit and may be potentially harmful in doses above 100 mg per day (Braverman & Neinstein, 2002).
- Overdosage of vitamin A must be avoided because research results have not been definitive on its use as a successful treatment. No more than the recommended daily allowance (5,000 units) should be advised.
- Vitamin E, 400 units per day, has been associated with reduction of negative mood and food cravings, but there is limited evidence of its effectiveness (Braverman & Neinstein, 2002).
- Trials have found that 1,200 mg per day of calcium carbonate significantly decreases symptoms and that 200–400 mg per day of magnesium may also be effective (Evidenced based recommendations, 2000).

Nonsteroidal Anti-Inflammatory Drugs (NSAIDs)

- NSAIDs are useful for the physical symptoms associated with PMS. Indications for these drugs include premenstrual headaches, tension, irritability, depression, abdominal pain, breast tenderness, abdominal bloating, and ankle edema.
- Side effects and contraindications are the same as for dysmenorrhea. Side effects and adverse reactions include gastrointestinal upset, rash, and edema. NSAIDs may be teratogenic; therefore, they are contraindicated in pregnancy. Also peptic ulcers, asthma, aspirin sensitivity, and inflammatory bowel disease are contraindications.
- Client teaching and counseling should begin with a discussion of the client's symptom records. It should include information about taking NSAIDs with meals to avoid gastric upset or ulcer development. The medication should be initiated on the day of the luteal phase when symptoms and signs are perceived, as noted on a previous month's symptom record and limited to somatic symptoms.

Diuretics

- Many women with PMS complain of water retention and bloating. Spironolactone, an aldosterone antagonist, has been shown to be useful for some women. Other diuretics, such as hydrochlorthiazide, should not be used (Nelson, 1998).

- Administer spironolactone during the luteal phase 25 mg two to four times daily for fourteenth days.
- Side effects include gynecomastia, GI upset, drowsiness, headache, rash, mental confusion, irregular menses or amenorrhea, and deepening of the voice.
- Contraindications include hyperkalemia and renal impairment. Precautions include liver disease, hyponatremia, surgery, and pregnancy (*Nurse Practitioners' Prescribing Reference*, 2002).
- Anticipated outcomes on evaluation are decreased bloating, feelings of fullness, and affective/physical symptoms associated with excessive fluid retention.
- Client teaching and counseling should make clear that potassium supplementation in the form of food or medication should NOT be taken with spironolactone. Furthermore, spironolactone should not be taken with other potassium-sparing diuretics. Follow clients with fluid and electrolyte studies to avoid excessive potassium levels. It is better to recommend increasing water intake and reducing sodium rather than to prescribe diuretics.

Oral Micronized Progesterone

- The indication for progesterone supplementation has been suggested since 1938 to relieve a wide variety of PMS symptoms. Controlled clinical trials have failed to demonstrate effectiveness superior to placebo.

Oral Contraceptives

- The indication for oral contraception is elimination of cyclic hormonal fluctuations. Both avoidance and the use of oral contraceptive pills have been recommended. Overall, the efficacy of OCs in the treatment of PMS has not been proven. OCs may be beneficial due to ovulation suppression and may be effective in treating the physical symptoms of PMS, but do not help the mood disorders (Schnare, 2002). Some women have increased breast tenderness, depression, and bloating with OC use (Nelson, 1998).
- Administer low dose, 35 mcg or less, oral contraceptives according to manufacturer's guidelines. (See Chapter 9 for detailed discussion of administration, side effects, and contraindications.) Side effects most commonly include breast tenderness, weight gain, spotting, and scanty menses. Contraindications are pregnancy, undiagnosed vaginal bleeding, history of breast or reproductive tract cancer, history of thromboembolism, cerebrovascular or coronary disease,

liver tumor or malignancy, or smoker older than 35 (Hatcher et al., 2001).
- The anticipated outcome on evaluation is very limited. Little success occurs in reducing symptoms, and oral contraceptives may exacerbate depressive symptoms in some PMS sufferers.
- Advise regarding appropriate use of oral contraceptives (OC), danger signs, and side effects. Advise clients to record their response to OC therapy in order to decide whether the medication should be continued.

Anxiolytics

- The indication for anxiolytics is for the most troublesome emotional symptoms of PMS, notably anxiety, panic, irritability, and depression. Alprazolam (Xanax), a CIV benzodiazepine, is the preferred anxiolytic for women who do not respond to fluoxetine. It is also classified as a smooth muscle relaxant and antidepressant. Many states do not permit nurse practitioners to prescribe controlled drugs such as alprazolam. This medication has the potential for abuse. Alprazolam administration can be limited to the luteal phase. If that is not helpful, it may be given throughout the entire cycle (Schnare, 2002). To avoid withdrawal symptoms, the doses need to be tapered each time alprazolam is used (Nelson, 1998).
- Administer alprazolam 0.25 or 0.5 mg p.o., b.i.d. or t.i.d. during the luteal phase. Prescribe in small amounts and evaluate patient response.
- Side effects include addiction potential, drowsiness, memory impairment, headache, ataxia, tremors, increased salivation, and paradoxical excitement (*Nurse Practitioners' Prescribing Reference*, 2002), and if used with alcohol, a synergistic effect.
- Contraindications include pregnancy, lactation, history of addiction, or acute narrow angle glaucoma. It should not be administered concomitantly with itraconazole or ketoconazole. There may be interactions with many other drugs; potential interactions should be known before prescribing or adding a medication. Use caution with renal, cardiovascular, or hepatic disease.
- The anticipated outcome on evaluation is that the therapy will allow temporary symptom reduction and enable the client to seek problem resolution through counseling or other therapies.
- Client teaching should encourage specialized counseling; therapists may be recommended. Discuss ways to reduce or cope with stress and discuss alternative PMS therapies that may be helpful.

Gonadotropin-Releasing Hormone Agonist (GnRH-a)

- Indications are extremely severe symptoms. GnRH agonists function by suppressing gonadotropin levels at the level of the pituitary and ultimately eliminate ovulation and hormone production (Linderman, 2000). GnRH agonists induce a hypoestrogenic state, are expensive, and should only be used when other measures have failed (Evidence based recommendations, 2000). Estrogen replacement therapy may be needed to prevent bone loss.
- *Administer with physician consultation only.* Requires daily subcutaneous injections (Lupron), intramuscular injection (Depo Lupron), or intranasal sprays (Buserelin).
- Side effects are menopause induced by complete ovulation cessation (see Chapter 15, Hypoestrogenic Changes, for effects of estrogen deficiency).
- The anticipated outcome is consistent elimination of menstrually related disorders through pharmacologic suppression of ovarian steroids.
- Client teaching and counseling require informed consent and in-depth education about the effects of this treatment. Although GnRH can reduce symptoms dramatically, hypoestrogenic effects, and risks of osteoporosis and cardiovascular disease need to be explained.

Surgical Interventions. Oophorectomy is reserved for clients with the most severe cases of PMS and is almost never recommended. To be considered, the following criteria need to be met: no treatment except GnRH agonist was effective, there was complete resolution of symptoms with the GnRH agonist for four to six months, childbearing is complete, and the woman is thought to have at least five more years of menstrual cycles remaining (Evans, 1998).

Hysterectomy has *no* place in the treatment of PMS and will not help the syndrome. Clients should be informed of this.

Follow-Up. Follow-up involves rescheduling the client in one or two months to evaluate her charts and progress and to arrive at a workable diagnosis and plan of care. The first few months involve intense examination of lifestyle, menstrual patterns, and coping strategies. Frequent visits provide time to review and provide more information, reinforce desired changes, give encouragement, assign reading, and discuss referrals. Results of initial lab work can be shared at this time, and continuation of symptom charting is stressed. As the client accrues knowledge and coping techniques and begins to see progress, her visits can be less frequent and shorter.

REFERENCES

Baase, C.A. (2000). Amenorrhea. In R.E. Rakel (Ed.), *Saunders manual of medical practice* (2nd ed.) (pp. 514–516). Philadelphia: W.B. Saunders Company.

Braverman, P.K., & Neinstein, L.S. (2002). Dysmenorrhea and premenstrual syndrome. In L.S. Neinstein (Ed.), *Adolescent health care, a practical guide* (4th ed.; pp. 952–965). Philadelphia: Lippincott Williams & Wilkins.

Church, L. (2003). Dysfunctional uterine bleeding. In R.E. Rakel (Ed.), *Saunders manual of medical practice* (2nd ed.; pp. 554–557). Philadelphia: W.B. Saunders Company.

Coco, A. (1999). Primary dysmenorrhea. *American Family Physician, 60*(20), 489–496.

Davis, D. (2002). Toxic shock syndrome. In R.E. Rakel & E.T. Bope (Eds.), *Conn's current therapy* (pp. 84–86). Philadelphia: W.B. Saunders Company.

Dell, D.L., Moskowitz, D., & Sondheimer, S.J. (2001). PMS and PMDD: Identification and treatment. *Contemporary OB/GYN 2001.* Retrieved March 8, 2002 from http://www.contobgyn.com.

Evans, C.B. (1998). Premenstrual syndrome. In F.P. Zuspan & E.J. Quilligan (Eds.), *Handbook of obstetrics, gynecology, and primary care* (pp. 172–177). St. Louis, MO: Mosby.

Evidence-based recommendations for managing premenstrual syndrome. (2000). *Women's Health in Primary Care, 3*(10), 735–738.

Fossum, G.T. (2002). Abnormal uterine bleeding. In R.E. Rakel & E.T. Bope (Eds.), *Conn's current therapy* (pp. 1070–1072). Philadelphia: W.B. Saunders Company.

Gordon, C., & Neinstein, L. (2002). Amenorrhea. In L.S. Neinstein (Ed.), *Adolescent health care, a practical guide* (4th ed. pp. 973–991). Philadelphia: Lippincott, Williams & Wilkins.

Gordon, J. D., & Speroff, L. (2002). *Handbook for clinical gynecologic endocrinology and infertility.* Philadelphia: Lippincott Williams & Willkins.

Hatcher, R.A., Nelson, A.L., Zieman, M., Darney, P.D., Creinin, M.D., & Stosur, H.R. (2001). *A pocket guide to managing contraception.* Tiger, GA: Bridging the Gap Foundation.

Hillard, P.A. (1998). Benign disease of the female reproductive tract: Symptoms and signs. In J.S. Berek, E.Y. Adashi, & P.A. Hillard (Eds.), *Novak's gynecology* (4th ed.; pp. 331–397). Baltimore, MD: Williams & Wilkins.

Holmes, M., & Landen, C.N. (2002). Dysmenorrhea. In R.E. Rakel & E.T. Bope (Eds.), *Conn's current therapy* (pp. 1076–1078). Philadelphia: W.B. Saunders.

Kennard, E (1998). Dysmenorrhea. In F.P. Zuspan & E.J Quilligan (Eds.), *Handbook of obstetrics, gynecology, and primary care* (pp. 41–44). St. Louis, MO: Mosby.

Kiningham, R., Apgar, B., & Schwenk, T. (1996). Evaluation of amenorrhea. *American Family Physician, 53*(4), 1185–1194.

Linderman, J.C. (2000). Premenstrual syndrome. In R.E. Rakel (Ed.) *Saunders manual of medical practice* (pp. 603–604). Philadelphia: W.B. Saunders.

Minjarez, D.A., & Carr, B.R. (2002). Amenorrhea. In R.E. Rakel & E.T. Bope (Eds.), *Conn's current therapy* (pp. 1072–1075). Philadelphia: W.B. Saunders.

Mitan, L.A.P., & Slap, G.B. (2002). Dysfunctional uterine bleeding. In L.S. Neinstein (Ed.), *Adolescent health care: A practical guide* (4th ed.; pp. 966–972). Philadelphia: Lippincott Williams & Wilkins.

Nelson, A.L. (1998). Menstrual problems and common gynecologic concerns. In R.A. Hatcher, J. Trussel, F. Stewart, S. Cates Jr., G.K. Stewart, F. Guest, & D. Kowal (Eds.) *Contraceptive technology* (17th rev. ed.; pp. 95–140). New York: Ardent Media.

Nurse Practitioner's Prescribing Reference. (2002, Spring), *9*(1).

Policar, M. (2002, March). Extended OC regimens: Practical applications. In *Contraceptive technology*. Conference by Contemporary Forums, Washington, DC.

Rapkin, A.J. (1998). Pelvic pain and dysmenorrhea. J.S., Berek, E.Y. Adashi, & P.A Hillard (Eds.), *Novak's gynecology* (12th ed.; pp. 399–428). Baltimore, MD: Williams & Wilkins.

Rebar, R., & Erickson, G.F. (2000). Menstrual cycle and fertility. In L. Goldman & J.C. Bennett (Eds.), *Cecil textbook of medicine* (21st ed., vol. 2; pp. 1327–1340). Philadelphia: W.B. Saunders.

Rome, E., Reame, N., & Stanford, W. (1998). Understanding our bodies: Sexual anatomy, reproduction, and the menstrual cycle. In Boston Women's Health Book Collective, *Our bodies, ourselves* (pp. 270–287). New York: Simon & Schuster.

Schnare, S. (2002, March). Premenstrual dysphoric disorder (PMDD) also called premenstrual syndrome (PMS). In *Contraceptive technology*. Conference by Contemporary Forums, Washington, DC.

Speroff, L., Glass, R.H., & Kase, N.G. (1999). *Clinical gynecological endocrinology and infertility*. Baltimore, MD: Williams & Wilkins.

Stewart, F. (1998) Pregnancy testing and management of early pregnancy. In R.A. Hatcher, J. Trussell, F. Stewart, W. Cates Jr., G.K. Stewart, F. Guest, & D. Kowal (Eds.), *Contraceptive technology* (17th rev. ed.; pp. 635–652). New York: Ardent Media.

Taylor, M. (2002, March). What's new, what's next in hormonal contraception: Yasmin, Evra Patch, Nuva Ring, Lunelle and more! In *Contraceptive technology*. *Conference by Contemporary Forums*, Washington, DC.

Wysocki, S. (2002, March). Clinical indications for monthly injectable contraception (Lunelle) and the levonorgestrel IUS (Mirena). In *Contraceptive technology*. Conference by Contemporary Forums, Washington, DC.

CHAPTER 9

CONTROLLING FERTILITY

Kathryn A. Caufield

*M*ore contraceptive methods that provide women additional safe, convenient, and effective options are finally being made available to women in the United States. Lowering STD risk remains an essential priority in contraceptive decision making.

Highlights

- Historical and Political Perspectives on Contraception
- Fundamentals
  Principles of Fertility Control
  Issues of Control, Safety, and Choice
  "Safer Sex"
- Methods of Birth Control
  Evaluation of Clients
  Client Education, Informed Consent
  Combined Hormonal Methods: Pills,
   Injection, Patch, Vaginal Ring
  Progestin-Only Methods: Pills, Implants,
   Injections
  Postcoital Emergency Contraception
  Male and Female Condoms
  Spermicides: Foams, Jellies, Creams,
   Suppositories, Vaginal Films
  Barrier Methods: Diaphragms, Cervical Caps,
   Sponge
  Intrauterine Devices
  Sterilization
  Fertility Awareness Methods
  Lactational Amenorrhea Method
  Withdrawal
  Abstinence
- Elective Termination of Pregnancy: Induced Abortion
- Future Methods of Fertility Control

❖ INTRODUCTION

Entering the twenty-first century, more options for controlling fertility are available to women and men in the United States. These methods provide additional safe, effective and convenient choices for couples who wish to prevent or postpone pregnancy. Many available birth control methods also allow women to independently choose and manage their contraceptive needs. Lowering STD risk for individuals and populations, however, remains a priority in contraceptive decision making.

HISTORICAL AND POLITICAL PERSPECTIVES ON CONTRACEPTION

The desire of women and men to control their reproductive destinies has been evident since ancient times. Use of primitive barriers, spermicides, condoms, and withdrawal is documented in the writings of many ancient cultures. Until the mid-nineteenth century, however, few reliable methods to prevent or delay pregnancy were available. Herbal and chemical spermicides, condoms, and coitus interruptus (withdrawal) carried high risks of pregnancy; the latter two also depended on the cooperation of men.

Margaret Sanger (1883–1966), a nurse and feminist and the most important early leader of the U.S. family planning movement, introduced the diaphragm into the United States and fought for women's rights. She founded the American Birth Control League, which later became the Planned Parenthood Federation of America (Lynaugh, 1991). A 1965 U.S. Supreme Court decision in the case of *Estelle T. Griswold and C. Lee Buxton v. State of Connecticut* declared birth control to be a basic right under the Bill of Rights. In the early 1960s, oral contraceptives and intrauterine devices (IUD) became available, beginning the "contraceptive revolution." In the late 1960s, New York, California and other states rewrote their abortion laws culminating in the 1973 U.S. Supreme Court decision of *Roe v. Wade,* which limited the circumstances under which "the right to privacy" could be restricted by local abortion laws. Abortion was thus legalized. The ability to control the timing and circumstances under which they would conceive and give birth bestowed on women a higher degree of personal control, more freedom of choice in many dimensions of their lives, and the self-determination to work toward equality (Boston Women's Health Book Collective, 1998; Fogel & Woods, 1995).

Not coincidentally, the women's movement gained momentum with the introduction of these more "modern" methods of birth control and the right to choose abortion. In turn, the women's movement provided the stimulus to limit family size and to move society toward acceptance of different roles for women. The availability of modern birth control methods has also dramatically reduced maternal and infant mortality.

The national family planning program, Title X of the Public Health Service Act, was established by Congress in 1970. This program provides community based funding/support for comprehensive family planning services (not including abortion) and sexually transmitted disease (STD) care, free or at an affordable cost, based on income. Yearly, over 5 million clients are served by the program nationwide. Additionally, the United States provides support for numerous international family planning programs (again, not including abortion).

Large numbers of women continue to experience unplanned pregnancies, resulting in morbidity, mortality, and social distress. In fact, the United States is far behind other countries in varieties of birth control methods available. Numerous factors contribute to this phenomenon. Issues constraining contraceptive availability and research include product liability lawsuits; antifamily planning activism; pressure from well intended feminist, consumer, political, and religious groups; cautious and lengthy U.S. Food and Drug Administration (FDA) procedural requirements; too little knowledge about reproductive biology, and too little money. Contraceptive technologies, however, are steadily evolving. Research and development underway in many parts of the world should continue to result in a wider array of contraceptive methods, offering advantages over some currently available contraceptive techniques and more choices for consumers.

FUNDAMENTALS

DEFINITION AND PURPOSE

Fertility control may be defined as follows.

1. Purposeful regulation of conception or childbirth.
2. Voluntary avoidance or delay of pregnancy or childbirth.
3. Use of devices, chemicals, abortion, or other techniques to prevent or terminate pregnancy.

Related terms often used interchangeably with fertility control include *birth control, family planning, contraception, pregnancy prevention,* and *planned parenthood.* The reasons for controlling fertility include personal convenience, economics, social values, and lifestyle.

Primary care clinicians are often the main source of accurate information and advice on responsible family planning practices for clients. Family planning services/programs should offer clients a variety of safe, effective, acceptable, affordable contraceptive methods to help them prevent unwanted pregnancies and STDs and to assist families to achieve their childbearing goals.

SELECTING A METHOD OF CONTRACEPTION

A woman's reproductive life spans almost forty years, and throughout those years, a variety of contraceptive methods may be used. Women need assistance in reevaluating contraceptive choices as their needs change over time and in understanding and recognizing the many variables that can influence those choices. Many individual factors may enhance or impair contraceptive behavior and impact the selection of birth control methods. (Barnett, 1995; Forrest, 1993; Hatcher, Trussell, Stewart, Cates, et al., 1998).

- Age and maturity.
- Stage of reproductive life (desire for future fertility).
- Marital status.
- Cultural and religious beliefs.
- Health/medical history.
- Presence of physical or mental limitations.
- Motivation of the woman.
- Degree of cooperation of the male partner.
- Wishes and concerns of the partner.
- Degree of comfort with one's body and one's sexuality.
- Individual locus of control.

- Monogamous versus multiple sexual partners (risk of sexually transmitted diseases).
- Lactation status.
- Cost of methods.
- Previous experience with birth control methods (successes, failures, problems, side effects).
- Frequency of intercourse.
- Other patterns of sexual activity.
- Effectiveness of methods.
- Safety of methods.
- Access to health care.
- Noncontraceptive benefits.
- Short-term versus long-term contraceptive needs.
- Confidence in methods.
- Perceived convenience of methods.

Characteristics that may impact the selection and use of specific contraceptive methods are summarized in Table 9–1.

GENERAL PRINCIPLES OF FERTILITY CONTROL

- When the goal is to prevent pregnancy, any contraceptive method is better than none.
- *All* sexually active women of every age must have access to effective, confidential, and non-punitive contraceptive services.
- Women need to know their options, the risks and benefits, and which methods may be contraindicated for them and why.
- Women are entitled to professional assistance when selecting a method that meets their own needs and circumstances.
- Health professionals are obligated to educate clients, without undue bias, about the range of possible methods so that fully informed choices can be made.
- No birth control method is 100 percent effective in preventing pregnancy.
- Information and counseling about acquired immunodeficiency syndrome (AIDS) and human immunodeficiency virus (HIV) infection, sexually transmitted diseases (STDs), use of latex and non-allergenic protective condoms, and "safer sex" must be provided to individuals seeking family planning services.
- Responsibility for preventing pregnancy should ideally be shared by the man and the woman in a relationship.
- Every woman needs to have knowledge about emergency contraception and how to obtain it.

TABLE 9–1. Importance of Characteristics Impacting Contraceptive Selection and Use According to Method

Contraceptive Method	Cost	Ease of Use	Coitus Linked	Level of Convenience	Effectiveness	Systemic Effects	Level of Safety	Availability
Combined hormonal contraceptives: pills, injection, patch, vaginal ring	Mod to high	Great	No	High	High	Yes	High for nonsmokers	Wide for COCs Mod for others
Progestin-only methods								
Progestin-only pills	Mod	Great	No	High	Mod	Yes	High	Wide
Implants	High	Great	No	High	High	Yes	Mod	Limited
Injections	Mod	Great	No	High	High	Yes	High	Mod
Diaphragms	Mod to high	Mod	Yes	Mod	Mod	No	Mod to high	Mod
Sponge	Mod	Mod	Yes	Mod	Low to Mod	No	High	Low
Cervical caps	Mod to high	Mod	Yes	Mod	Mod	No	Mod to high	Low
Postcoital emergency methods	High	Difficult	No	Low	Mod to High	Yes	High	Mod
Male condoms	Low to mod	Mod	Yes	Mod to low	Mod	No	High	Wide
Female condoms	Mod	Mod	Yes	Low	Mod	No	High	Mod
Vaginal spermicides	Low to mod	Mod	Yes	Low	Low to Mod	No	High	Wide
Intrauterine devices	High	Great	No	High	High	Some	Mod	Limited
Fertility awareness methods	Low	Difficult	Yes	Low	Low	No	Mod	Mod
Lactational amenorrhea method	Low	Mod	No	High	Mod	No	High	Wide
Withdrawal	None	Mod	Yes	Mod	Low	No	Mod	Wide
Female sterilization	High	Great	No	High	High	No	Mod	Mod
Male sterilization	Mod	Great	No	High	High	No	High	Mod

Note: Mod = moderate; STD = sexually transmitted disease; HIV = human immunodeficiency virus.
*Some protection against PID

Sources: Dickey, 2002; Feldblum & Joanis, 1994; Forrest, 1993; Hatcher et al., 1998; Intrauterine devices, 2000; Rawlins & Smith, 2002.

ISSUES OF CONTROL, SAFETY, AND CHOICE

A "perfect" contraceptive would be 100 percent effective in preventing pregnancy, highly acceptable, free from health hazards and side effects, not coitus related, low maintenance, and easily reversible. In addition, it would be relatively inexpensive and offer noncontraceptive benefits such as protection against sexually transmitted diseases (STDs). Currently, however, all available methods for controlling fertility carry some risks to users; therefore, disadvantages and risks must be carefully weighed against benefits. In assisting clients with contraceptive choices, it is often helpful to compare method risks with the risks of full-term delivery. In most cases, the risks associated with pregnancy and delivery are much greater than those associated with contraceptive use.

In an era when many women wish to delay pregnancy and simultaneously face many hazards to future fertility caused by STDs, choices are indeed difficult. Clients need assistance to select contraceptives that will protect them from both pregnancy and STDs. For young, healthy women, the combination of oral contraceptives or one of the newer combined hormonal methods (patch, ring, monthly injection) and condoms is a very sound choice; however, many options are presented in this chapter (Forrest, 1993; Hatcher, Nelson, Zieman, et al., 2001; Hatcher et al., 1998).

CONTRACEPTION AND "SAFER SEX"

Responsibility for Prevention and Protection

When seeking to prevent pregnancy, both men and women bear responsibility. Today, the question of whether the method offers any protection against STDs must be added to other selection considerations such as convenience, effectiveness, failure rate, safety, and noncontraceptive benefits. Abstinence or sexual intercourse with

TABLE 9–1. (CONTINUED)

			Characteristics		
Partner Involvement Required	Protection Against STDs/HIV	Prescription Required	Health Care System Contact Required	Return to Fertility After Discontinued Use	Can Be Used While Lactating
None	None*	Yes	Yes	Delay—possibly 2–3 months	Not recommended
None	None	Yes	Yes	Rapid	Yes
None	None	Yes	Yes	Delayed—possibly 2–3 months	Yes
None	None	Yes	Yes	Delayed, 6–12 months	Yes
None	Mod	Yes	Yes	Immediate	Yes
No	Mod	No	No	Immediate	Yes
None	Mod	Yes	Yes	Immediate	Yes
None	None	Yes	Yes	Rapid	Not recommended
Yes	High	No	No	Immediate	Yes
Some	High	No	No	Immediate	Yes
None	Low	No	No	Immediate	Yes
None	None	Yes	Yes	Rapid	Yes
Yes	None	No	Yes for teaching	Immediate	Not reliable
None	None	No	No	Rapid	—
Yes	Limited	No	No	Immediate	Yes
None	None	No	Yes	Not applicable	Yes
Yes	None	No	Yes	Not applicable	Yes

one mutually faithful, trustworthy, uninfected partner is the only totally effective prevention strategy against STDs. Individuals with multiple sexual partners must make difficult decisions about responsibility and consequences for actions, sexual expression, communication patterns with partners, and the long-term impact of these decisions. All health care professionals must continue to do their part in providing individual and community education that is culturally and gender appropriate, geared toward safer sexual practices and reducing STD risk.

Safer Sex

When the HIV serostatus or STD status of a person is not certain, there is no such entity as "safe sex"—hence the term "safer sex." Though condoms are not 100 percent effective in preventing infections, male and/or female condoms are the best protection available at this time. Principal problems with male and/or female condom use are improper use, difficulty integrating use into sexual activity, and less often, condom breakage and slippage.

Sexual practices considered *safe* involve no exchange of body fluids of any kind and could include sexual fan-

tasies, non-genital physical touch, mutual masturbation, and erotic books, movies, and conversations. *Possibly safe* activities include wet kissing when there are no breaks in the skin, lips, or mouth tissues; use of latex or plastic barriers during all other oral, anal, and genital contact. *Unsafe sexual practices* include any direct contact with blood, semen, and vaginal secretions; any vaginal or anal intercourse without a latex or plastic condom; or sharing of sex toys (Hatcher et al., 1998).

EVALUATION OF CLIENTS REQUESTING FERTILITY CONTROL

Women seeking care or advice about fertility control are usually in a state of physical wellness; however, they may or may not have been successful in their contraceptive efforts. In addition, health care professionals must be aware that certain clients are at high risk for lack of contraceptive services: teenagers, low income women, and women in underserved areas. These women need services low in cost with convenient hours and accessible locations. Other groups with special family planning concerns

TABLE 9–2. Contraceptive Selection in Special Populations and in Women with Medical Conditions

Special Populations or Medical Conditions	Contraceptive Options and/or Guidelines
Adolescence	• Methods not recommended include IUDs, LAM, natural FP, sterilization. • Most other methods may be successfully used, STD protection is important. • Hormonal methods plus condoms may be the best choice. • FP services for teens need to stress sex education at an early age, contraceptive use, prevention of STDs, affordability, teen-friendly approach, and close supervision with follow-up to encourage continuation. • Adolescents need skills and self-confidence to abstain or reduce risks.
Perimenopause	• Long-term contraception is often preferred. • Any IUD, combined hormonal methods (if no contraindications) are good choices. • Progestin-only methods may be used but can accelerate bone loss. • Noncontraceptive benefits, such as cycle control and relief of vasomotor symptoms, may affect decision making. • Sterilization is a good option.
Physically Disabled	• Progestin-only methods—good choices. • Any IUD—good choice. • Combined hormonal methods generally good choices (though not recommended when client is immobile or has impaired circulation. Caregiver or partner assistance may be needed).
Mental Disability and Psychiatric Illnesses	• Long acting progestins—DMPA, implants—good choices. • Combination hormonal methods especially Lunelle injection generally good choices. • Any IUD second choice. Be aware of potential for increased STD risk and ability to communicate if problems arise.
Epilepsy/Seizure Disorders	• Combined hormonal methods, progestin-only methods, IUDs—good choices. • Anticonvulsant medications may increase catabolism of COCs in liver, prompting higher dose COC use. • DMPA may decrease seizure frequency. • Sterilization—generally good choice with precautions.
Systemic Lupus Erythematosus	• Progestin-only methods—good choices—not associated with SLE flares. • Any IUD—generally good choice.
Liver Disease such as active viral hepatitis, cirrhosis, liver tumors	• Copper IUD—good choice. • Combined OCs—contraindicated. • Progestin-only methods—second choice.
Breast Cancer	• Copper IUD—good choice. • Hormonal methods—contraindicated.
Hypertension: Mild or past history of (140–159/90–99 mm Hg)	• Progestin-only methods, any IUD—good choices. • Sterilization (carries increased anesthesia risk)—generally good choice. • COCs and other combined hormonal methods may be chosen with careful monitoring when health benefits would outweigh potential risks.
Hypertension: Moderate (160–179/100–109 mm Hg)	• Progestin-only methods, any IUD—good choices. • Sterilization (carries increased anesthesia risk) generally good choice. • Combined hormonal methods—generally contraindicated.
Severe Hypertension: (180/110 mm Hg or higher) or coronary artery disease or other vascular disease	• Copper IUD—good choice. • Progestin-only methods—generally undesirable. • Combined hormonal method—contraindicated. • Sterilization (carries an increased anesthesia risk) remains a choice.
Diabetes Mellitus: without Vascular Disease	• Progestin-only methods—good choices. • Low-dose COCs—good choices. • All other methods—good choices.
Diabetes Mellitus: with vascular disease or of more than 20 years duration	• Copper IUD—good choice. • POPs, Norplant, LNG-IUS—second choices. • Combined hormonal methods—undesirable. • DMPA—undesirable. • Sterilization—an option with adequate medical support.
Deep Vein Thrombosis or Pulmonary Embolism (history of or current)	• Progestin-only methods and any IUD—good choices. • Combined hormonal methods—contraindicated. • Sterilization—delay until condition is treated or resolved.

TABLE 9–2. (CONTINUED)

Special Populations or Medical Conditions	Contraceptive Options and/or Guidelines
Sickle Cell Disease	• Progestin-only methods, especially DMPA and LNG-IUS—good choices. • Combined hormonal methods and copper IUD—second choices (when benefits outweigh the potential risks)
Migraine Headaches	• Copper IUD, LNG-IUS, sterilization—good choices. • Progestin-only methods—second choice if migraines are pre-existing and do not increase with their use. • Combined hormonal methods should be used with caution especially in women with focal neurological symptoms such as aura. • Cyclical migraines may be allieviated with COCs especially if given continuously without a pill-free interval. • Women who develop recurring headaches or whose headaches worsen while using hormonal contraceptives should stop the method for a while to see if headaches improve.

Sources: Adolescent Pregnancy Fact Sheet, 1996; Best, 1999, 2000; Dickerson, 2001; Grimes, 1999a, 1999b; Kjos, 1999; Rivera, 1999.

include women with chronic illnesses, women who are physically or mentally handicapped, and women approaching midlife. All women need individualized plans of care, but these groups deserve special attention in order to meet their contraceptive needs fully.

For some women in these groups, unintended pregnancy could pose significant health risks. For these women, barrier methods or natural family planning may not provide adequate protection due to their high failure rates in typical use. The contraceptive needs of special populations groups are briefly addressed in Table 9–2. Consider also that some women have more than one chronic condition.

Initial Evaluation

A thorough initial assessment seeks data to identify risk factors and other influences on method selection (as discussed previously), and contraindications to certain methods. Subsequently, a database is established. During the initial evaluation a complete history is taken, including, but not limited to, the following.

- *Medical History.* Smoking, cardiovascular disease (CVD), thromboembolic disorder, reproductive tract cancer, breast cancer, diabetes mellitus (DM), frequent urinary tract infections (UTIs), migraines, seizures, etc.
- *Obstetric and Gynecologic History.* Menstrual, premenstrual syndrome (PMS), contraceptive, STDs, PID, vaginitis, and sexual.
- *Family History.* Especially cancer, CVD, DM, stroke, and other significant problems.
- *Review of Systems.*
- *Personal and Social Data.* Comfort with touching oneself, use of tampons and female hygiene products, desire or plans for childbearing, and partner involvement.

Objective data are obtained from a screening physical examination with special attention to height, weight, blood pressure (BP), and examination of thyroid, breasts, abdomen, and pelvis (noting position of uterus and any anatomic variation), and extremities. Other components of physical examination may also require emphasis, depending on birth control methods being considered.

Diagnostic testing may include the following.

- Cervical cytology (Pap smear).
- Wet mounts (saline and potassium hydroxide [KOH] highly recommended; others as indicated).
- Hematocrit.
- Urinalysis.
- STD (especially gonorrhea and chlamydia).

In addition, consider human papillomavirus (HPV) testing, and blood chemistries, especially lipid profile and blood glucose. In the presence of symptoms, all appropriate examinations/investigations should be carried out.

Clinical breast and pelvic exams, though customarily required, are not essential for prescribing hormonal contraceptives and could hinder some women's access to much-needed birth control. A thorough medical history and blood pressure are essential because they reveal most of the medical conditions known to contraindicate hormonal contraceptive use. A woman should have the option to defer these procedures to a later time and still receive hormonal contraception. This does not apply to women requesting hormone-releasing IUDs (New approach, 2001).

Subsequent Evaluations

All women who are sexually active or using a method of contraception that requires a prescription should be seen annually to evaluate new risk factors, contraindications, side effects, concerns, or new problems associated with the present birth control method and to identify any other reproductive problems.

Subjective data include a review of the client's history, any significant changes in her health status, and her method of birth control (including satisfaction with the method and any problems). Objective data include the client's weight and blood pressure, screening physical, breast, pelvic exam, and Pap smear. Other lab tests are performed as indicated (see previous information). Include a mammogram at the recommended intervals after age 35. (See Chapter 14.)

METHODS OF BIRTH CONTROL

Birth control methods currently available:

- Combined hormonal methods containing estrogen and progestin (pills, injection, patch, vaginal ring).
- Progestin-only methods (pills, implants, injection).
- Postcoital methods (emergency contraception).
- Barriers (male and female condoms, sponges, diaphragms, cervical caps).
- Vaginal spermicides (creams, jellies, suppositories, films).
- Intrauterine devices (IUDs).
- Fertility awareness methods.
- Lactational amenorrhea method.
- Coitus interruptus (withdrawal).
- Abstinence.
- Sterilization.
- Abortion.

MANAGEMENT CONSIDERATIONS, GUIDELINES FOR CLIENT EDUCATION, AND INFORMED CONSENT

- The client must participate in choosing the birth control method; she must be an informed user.
- Always obtain informed consent: Consent should be written for a client choosing an intrauterine device (IUD), implant, abortion, or sterilization. *Informed consent* implies that client makes a knowledgeable, voluntary choice; receives complete counseling about the procedure and its consequences; and is free to change her mind prior to the procedure.
- For a client planning to use any birth control method, carefully screen for contraindications.

- Set aside time for teaching as a routine part of the visit. During the initial visit, assist the client in selecting a birth control method, then use additional counseling after the visit to teach specific information about the method chosen.
- *For certain methods (diaphragms, cervical caps, IUDs, implants, vaginal rings, sterilization), the health provider must receive formal education, training, and practice in fitting, insertion, and other technical aspects.*
- During the visit, the health professional is responsible for providing client education and the opportunity for practice and validation of skills pertaining to selected methods (as applicable).
- Make all presentations, counseling, and educational materials compatible with the language, culture, and education of the client.
- Be aware of local myths and misperceptions about particular methods. Address misconceptions sensitively but directly. For example, douching, or "washing" semen out of the woman's body, will not prevent sperm from entering the uterus. Indeed, douching could theoretically enhance the movement of sperm up the cervical canal by washing them deeper into the vagina toward the cervix or by washing away protective mucus.
- To prevent the omission of important information, use a standard teaching checklist outlining key information that the user should know.
- Instruct about female and male anatomy, using models and illustrations.
- Provide the client with method-specific teaching and counseling, using models, illustrations, and handouts to describe key information.

  - How the methods work.
  - Effectiveness of methods.
  - Advantages and disadvantages of methods.
  - Noncontraceptive benefits.
  - What to expect during the visit.
  - Recommendations concerning follow-up.
  - Descriptions of short- and long-term side effects that can occur and how to deal with them.
  - Danger signs associated with the method selected.

- Explore factors that could place the client at risk for method failure (e.g., frequent intercourse, age, parity, previous failure of method, sexual or lifestyle patterns that make consistent use difficult). Counsel the client regarding these factors.

- If it is determined that the client is at risk for failure with her chosen method, recommend its use in combination with another method.

- Clients who choose a coitus-associated method need accurate understanding of the timing of ovulation and awareness of days with high risk for conception. An additional method may be employed during high risk times.

- Provide both oral and written instructions. Instruct the client to read specific package literature and follow the instructions carefully.

- Inform the client that regardless of the method chosen, she must always keep a second birth control method available and be familiar with its use.

- Advise client to keep sufficient quantities of contraceptive products/supplies available at all times in a convenient location. Counsel her about the importance of budgeting her finances for the purchase of products and supplies and for annual exams.

- Teach the proper care and storage of contraceptive devices and supplies.

- For devices requiring insertion, instruct the client to wash her hands before and after insertion to minimize possible introduction of contaminants into the vagina; also instruct her to wash applicators with soap and water after each use.

- Ask the client to repeat important information.

- Inform all clients about the availability of postcoital protection (emergency contraception) in the event of method failure. All clients should be offered a prescription for emergency contraception.

EFFECTIVENESS

The determination of contraceptive efficacy is indeed, an inexact science, some statistics and trends being more measurable than others. Table 9–3 presents the best information available on the percentage of women in the United States experiencing contraceptive failure during the first year of typical use, and the first year of perfect use, and the percentage of women continuing use of the method at the end of the first year. Typical use reflects how effective methods are for the average person who may not always use the methods correctly or consistently. Perfect use is when the method is used consistently, that is, correct use with every act of intercourse. Use of two contraceptive methods simultaneously dramatically lowers the risk of unintended pregnancy (Hatcher et al., 1998).

TABLE 9–3. Methods of Contraception: Effectiveness Estimates Comparing Perfect Use and Typical Use, Continuation Rates at One Year, and How Obtained by Client[1]

Method	Perfect Use[2]	Typical Use[3]	Continuation at One Year (%)	How Obtained
Nuva-Ring	<1.0	—	—	Rx
Norplant/Norplant-2	0.05	0.05	88	Rx
LNG-IUS IUD	0.1	0.1	81	Rx
Combined OCs	0.1	3.0	71	Rx
Male sterilization	0.1	0.15	100	Sx
Lunelle injection	0.2	1.0	—	Rx
Depo-Provera	0.3	0.3	70	Rx
Ortho-Evra patch	0.5	0.99	—	Rx
Female sterilization	0.5	0.5	100	Sx
Progestin-only OC	0.5	5.0	71	Rx
Copper T 380A IUD	0.6	0.8	78	Rx
Abstinence post-ovulation	1.0	25.0	63	Tx
Progesterone-T IUD	1.5	2.0	81	Rx
Symptothermal ovulation method	2.0	25.0	63	Tx
	3.0	25.0	63	Tx
Male condom	3.0	14.0	61	OTC
Withdrawal	4.0	19.0		Tx
Female condom	5.0	21.0	56	OTC
Diaphragm	6.0	20.0	56	Rx
Spermicides	6.0	26.0	40	OTC
Sponge—nulliparas	9.0	20.0	42	OTC
Cap—nulliparas	9.0	20.0	56	Rx
Calendar abstinence method	9.0	25.0	63	Tx
Sponge—multiparas	20.0	40.0	42	OTC
Cap—multiparas	26.0	40.0	42	Rx
Chance	85.0	85.0	—	—

[1] How obtained: Rx = prescription; Sx = surgical procedure; Tx = teaching; OTC = over-the-counter.

[2] Perfect use is percentage of couples who become pregnant who begin use, use perfectly (consistently and correctly) for first year of use without stopping for any other reason (Hatcher et al., 1998).

[3] Typical use is percentage of couples who become pregnant accidentally who begin use and do not stop use for any other reason (Hatcher et al., 1998).

Sources: Modified from Darney & Speroff, 2001; Gutierrez, 1999; Hatcher et al., 1998; Rawlins & Smith, 2002; Williams, 2002; Wysocki et al., 2001.

COMBINED ORAL CONTRACEPTIVES

Birth control pills (BCPs) or combined oral contraceptives (OCs or COCs), also called "the pill," have been available in the United States for over forty years. It is estimated that about 60 million women worldwide and almost 20 million U.S. women use OCs. Pill use, its effectiveness, risks, benefits, and side effects have been well researched over the past forty years. Low dosages of estrogen and progestin in today's pills make them very safe and effective for most women. Many noncontraceptive benefits have been identified.

Combined OCs contain two primary components, synthetic estrogen and progestin. The two estrogen compounds currently used in oral contraceptives in the United States are ethinyl estradiol or mestranol. Synthetic progestins are all derived from 19-*nortestosterones*. OCs currently available in the United States contain one of several progestins. First generation progestins currently in use include norethindrone, norethindrone acetate, ethynodiol diacetate; second generation progestins are norgestrel and levonorgestrel. OCs containing norethynodrel are no longer marketed in this country. (Dickey, 2002; Hatcher et al., 1998).

New generation progestins derived from levonorgestrel have been developed. These are gestodene, norgestimate, and desogestrel. Combined OCs containing desogestrel and norgestimate are now available in the United States. Gestodene is marketed in Europe and other countries. There appears to be little difference among these newer progestins with regard to clinical efficacy. These newer progestins are very potent in their ability to inhibit ovulation and to transform estrogen primed endometrium into secretory endometrium. Of the three newer agents, it appears that gestodene is most potent with regard to progestational activity. The three newer agents have more specific progestational activity, little estrogenic effect, a longer half-life, and are weak anti-estrogens. They have far less androgenic activity in animal studies in vivo than older progestins. (Dickey, 2002; Hatcher et al., 1998). A new COC known by the brand name *Yasmin* is the first FDA-approved OC containing drospirenone, a progestin and analog of spironolactone and ethinyl estradiol. The 3 mg dose of drospirenone has antimineralocorticoid activity, including a risk of hyperkalemia comparable to that of a 25 mg dose of spironolactone (Kupecz & Berardinelli, 2002).

Several studies have shown a higher risk of venous thromboembolism (VTE) among women using two of these newer progestins, gestodene and desogestrel. As previously stated, of these two, only desogestrel is available in the United States and is contained in three currently marketed formulations, Desogen, Mircette (Organon), and Ortho-Cept (and their generic equivalents). The increase in risk of VTE is from 1 in 10,000 to 2 in 10,000 for the pills containing these progestins (pregnancy is associated with the greatest risk of VTE). This increased risk is for VTE only and not for other cardiovascular events. In fact, studies have suggested a possible protective effect against myocardial infarction (MI) for women using OCs containing desogestrel and gestodene. Family planning providers

TABLE 9–4. Risk Factors for Venous Thromboembolism (VTE)

1. Genetic predisposition, factor V Lieden mutation[a]
2. Acquired predisposition (such as lupus, anticoagulant, malignancy)
3. Increasing age
4. Physiologic factors (such as dehydration)[b]
5. Mechanical factors (such as immobility or trauma)
6. Obesity (defined here as BMI of 30 or over)
7. Varicose veins (the data on the magnitude of risk attributable to varicose veins is conflicting. Extensive varicosities are likely to be a risk factor).
8. Pregnancy

[a] Women with a family history of hereditary thrombophilia in a first degree relative should not be prescribed combined oral contraceptives unless thrombophilia has been ruled out.
[b] May be acute and/or temporary risk factors.
Source: Dickey, 2002; Hatcher et al., 1998; Vandenbroucke et al., 2001

must be aware of the risk factors for VTE (Table 9–4). Implications for practice, considering these studies, are included under Management Considerations later in this section. (Bergett-Hanson, 2001; Pymar & Creinin, 2001).

Estrogen and progestin are combined in fixed dose pills (monophasic) or in variable amounts in relation to one another throughout the pill cycle, as in biphasic or triphasic preparations. Table 9–5 lists the types and dosages of OCs available in the United States and their comparable biologic activity.

Prescription

OCs are available in 21- or 28-day packs. Active pills are taken the first 21 days; 28-day preparations contain 7 "spacer" tablets that are inert (except for some Parke-Davis products that contain ferrous fumarate in the last 7 brown pills of the 28-day pack). Another exception is Mircette (Organon), which contains 21 active pills followed by 2 inert tablets, then 5 tablets of ethinyl estradiol, 10 mcg. These last 5 pills are progestin-free.

Mechanism of Action

Pregnancy is prevented by several effects of estrogen and progestin.

- Gonadotropin-releasing hormone (GnRH) is suppressed, which in turn suppresses follicle-stimulating hormone (FSH) and luteinizing hormone (LH), inhibiting ovulation.
- Ovum/tubal transport is altered.
- Cervical mucus thickens, inhibiting sperm transport.
- Implantation is inhibited by suppression of the endometrium and alteration of uterine secretions.
- Degeneration of the corpus luteum may occur (Bergett-Hanson, 2001; Dickey, 2002; Hatcher et al., 1998).

TABLE 9–5. Oral Contraceptive Types, Dosages, and Physiological Activities

Oral Contraceptive	Progestational Activity	Androgenic Activity	Endometrial Activity
Low Dose Monophasics[1]			
Alesse (Wyeth-Ayerst) 21 or 28 day 　0.10 mg levonorgestrel 　0.02 mg ethinyl estradiol	Low	Low	Low
Brevicon (Watson) 21 or 28 day 　0.5 mg norethindrone 　0.035 mg ethinyl estradiol	Low	Low	Intermediate
Demulen 1/35 (Pharmacia) 21 or 28 day 　1 mg ethynodiol diacetate 　0.035 mg ethinyl estradiol	Intermediate/High	Low	Low
Desogen (Organon) 28 day 　0.15 mg desogestrel 　0.03 mg ethinyl estradiol	Intermediate/High	Low	Low/Intermediate
Genora 1/35 (Rugby) 28 day 　1 mg norethindrone 　0.035 mg ethinyl estradiol	Intermediate	Low/Intermediate	Intermediate
Levlen (Berlex) 21 or 28 day 　0.15 mg levonorgestrel 　0.03 mg ethinyl estradiol	Low/Intermediate	Intermediate	Intermediate
Levlite (Berlex) 21 or 28 day 　0.1 mg levonorgestrel 　0.02 mg ethinyl estradiol	Low	Low	Low
Levora (Watson) 21 or 28 day 　0.15 mg levonorgestrel 　0.03 mg ethinyl estradiol	Low/Intermediate	Intermediate	Intermediate
Loestrin 1/20 (Parke-Davis) 21 or Fe 28 day 　1 mg norethindrone acetate 　0.02 mg ethinyl estradiol 　Fe 28 day contains 7 pills 　75 mg ferrous fumarate	Intermediate	Intermediate/High	Low
Loestrin 1.5/30 (Parke-Davis) 21 or Fe 28 day 　1.5 mg norethindrone acetate 　0.03 mg ethinyl estradiol 　Fe 28 day contains 7 pills 　75 mg ferrous fumarate	Intermediate/High	Intermediate/High	Low
Lo-Ovral (Wyeth-Ayerst) 21 or 28 day 　0.3 mg norgestrel 　0.03 mg ethinyl estradiol	Low/Intermediate	Intermediate	Low/Intermediate
Low-Ogestrel (Watson) 28 day 　0.3 mg norgestrel 　0.03 mg ethinyl estradiol	Low/Intermediate	Intermediate	Low/Intermediate
Modicon (Ortho) 21 or 28 day 　0.5 mg norethindrone 　0.035 mg ethinyl estradiol	Low	Low	Intermediate
Necon (Watson) 21 or 28 day 　1 mg norethindrone 　0.035 mg ethinyl estradiol	Intermediate	Low/Intermediate	Intermediate
Nelova 1/35E (Warner-Chilicott) 　1 mg norethindrone 　0.035 mg ethinyl estradiol	Intermediate	Low/Intermediate	Intermediate

TABLE 9–5. (CONTINUED)

Oral Contraceptive	Progestational Activity	Androgenic Activity	Endometrial Activity
Nelova 0.5/35E (Warner-Chilicott) 0.5 mg norethindrone 0.035 mg ethinyl estradiol	Low	Low	Intermediate
Nordette (Wyeth-Ayerst) 21 or 28 day 0.15 mg levonorgestrel 0.03 mg ethinyl estradiol	Low/Intermediate	Intermediate	Intermediate
Norethin 1/35E (Schiapparelli Searle) 28 day 1 mg norethindrone 0.035 mg ethinyl estradiol	Intermediate	Low/Intermediate	Intermediate
Norinyl 1+35 (Syntex) 21 or 28 day 1 mg norethindrone 0.035 mg ethinyl estradiol	Intermediate	Low/Intermediate	Intermediate
Ortho-Cept (Ortho) 21 or 28 day 0.15 mg desogestrel 0.03 mg ethinyl estradiol	Intermediate/High	Low	Intermediate
Ortho-Cyclen (Ortho) 21 or 28 day 0.25 mg norgestimate 0.035 mg ethinyl estradiol	Low	Low	Low/Intermediate
Ortho-Novum 1/35 (Ortho) 21 or 28 day 1 mg norethindrone 0.035 mg ethinyl estradiol	Intermediate	Low/Intermediate	Intermediate
Ovcon 35 (Mead Johnson) 21 or 28 day 0.4 mg norethindrone 0.035 mg ethinyl estradiol	Low	Low	Intermediate
Yasmin (Berlex) 28 day 3.0 mg drospirenone 0.03 mg ethinyl estradiol	Low/Intermediate	Low	Low/Intermediate
Zovia 1/35E (Watson) 21 or 28 day 1 mg ethynodiol diacetate 0.035 mg ethinyl estradiol	Intermediate/High	Low	Low
Triphasics[2]			
Cyclessa (Organon) 28 day 7 days: 0.1 mg desogestrel 0.025 mg ethinyl estradiol 7 days: 0.125 mg desogestrel 0.025 mg ethinyl estradiol 7 days: 0.15 mg desogestrel 0.025 mg ethinyl estradiol	Intermediate/High	Low	Low/Intermediate
Estrostep (Parke Davis) 21 or Fe 28 day			
Estrostep Fe (Parke Davis) 21 or Fe 28 day 5 days: 1 mg norethindrone acetate 0.02 mg ethinyl estradiol 7 days: 1 mg norethindrone acetate 0.03 mg ethinyl estradiol 9 days: 1 mg norethindrone acetate 0.035 mg ethinyl estradiol 7 days: 75 mg ferrous fulmerate	Intermediate/High	Intermediate/High	Low
Ortho-Novoum 7/7/7 (Ortho) 21 or 28 day 7 days: 0.5 mg norethindrone 0.035 mg ethinyl estradiol 7 days: 0.75 mg norethindrone 0.035 mg ethinyl estradiol 7 days: 1 mg norethindrone 0.035 mg ethinyl estradiol	Low/Intermediate	Low/Intermediate	Intermediate

TABLE 9–5. (CONTINUED)

Oral Contraceptive	Progestational Activity	Androgenic Activity	Endometrial Activity

Tri-Levlen (Berlex) 21 or 28 day
  6 days: 0.05 mg levongorgestrel
       0.03 mg ethinyl estradiol
  5 days: 0.075 mg levonorgestrel
       0.04 mg ethinyl estradiol
 10 days: 0.125 mg levonorgestrel
       0.03 mg ethinyl estradiol
	Low	Low/Intermediate	Intermediate

Tri-Cyclen (Ortho) 21 or 28 day
  7 days: 0.18 mg norgestimate
       0.035 mg ethinyl estradiol
  7 days: 0.215 mg norgestimate
       0.035 mg ethinyl estradiol
  7 days: 0.25 mg norgestimate
       0.035 mg ethinyl estradiol
	Low	Low	Low/Intermediate

Tri-Cyclen Lo (Ortho) 21 or 28 day
  7 days: 0.18 mg norgestimate
       0.025 mg ethinyl estradiol
  7 days: 0.215 mg norgestimate
       0.025 mg ethinyl estradiol
  7 days: 0.25 mg norgestimate
       0.025 mg ethinyl estradiol
	Low	Low	Low

Tri-Norinyl (Watson) 21 or 28 day
  7 days: 0.5 mg norethindrone
       0.035 mg ethinyl estradiol
  9 days: 1 mg norethindrone
       0.035 mg ethinyl estradiol
  5 days: 0.5 mg norethindrone
       0.035 mg ethinyl estradiol
	Low/Intermediate	Low/Intermediate	Intermediate

Triphasil (Wyeth-Ayerst) 21 or 28 day (same as Tri-Levlen)	Low	Low/Intermediate	Intermediate
Trivora (Watson) 21 or 28 day (same as Tri-Levlen)			
Biphasics[3]			

Jenest (Organon) 28 day
  7 days: 0.5 mg norethindrone
       0.035 mg ethinyl estradiol
 14 days: 1 mg norethindrone
       0.035 mg ethinyl estradiol
	Low/Intermediate	Low/Intermediate	Intermediate

Ortho-Novum 10/11 (Ortho) 21 or 28 day
 10 days: 0.5 mg norethindrone
       0.035 mg ethinyl estradiol
 11 days: 1 mg norethindrone
       0.035 mg ethinyl estradiol
	Low/Intermediate	Low/Intermediate	Intermediate

Mircette (Organon) 28 day
 21 days: 0.15 mg desogestrel
       0.02 mg ethinyl estradiol
  2 days: inert
  5 days: 0.01 ethinyl estradiol
	Intermediate/High	Low	Intermediate

Moderate Dose Monophasics			

Demulen 1/50 (Pharmacia) 21 or 28 day
  1 mg ethynodiol diacetate
  0.05 mg ethinyl estradiol
	Intermediate/High	Low	Intermediate

Genora 1/50 (Rugby) 28 day
  1 mg norethindrone
  0.050 mg mestranol
	Intermediate	Low/Intermediate	Intermediate

TABLE 9–5. (CONTINUED)

Oral Contraceptive	Progestational Activity	Androgenic Activity	Endometrial Activity

Norethin 1/50M (Schiapparelli Searle) 28 day
  1 mg norethindrone
  0.050 mg ethinyl estradiol
	Intermediate	Low/Intermediate	Intermediate

Norinyl 1+50 (Watson) 21 or 28 day
  1 mg norethindrone
  0.050 mestranol
	Intermediate	Low/Intermediate	Intermediate

Norlestrin 1/50 (Parke-Davis) 21 day or FE 28 day
  1 mg norethindrone acetate
  0.050 mg ethinyl estradiol
  FE 28 day contains 7 pills
  75 mg ferrous fumerate
	Intermediate	Intermediate	Intermediate

Norlestrin 2.5/50 (Parke-Davis) 21 day or FE 28 day
  2.5 mg norethindrone acetate
  0.050 mg ethinyl estradiol
  FE 28 day contains 7 pills
  75 mg ferrous fumerate
	High	High	High

Ortho-Novum 1/50 (Ortho) 21 or 28 day
  (same as Genera 1/50)
  1 mg norethindrone
  0.050 mg ethinyl estradiol
	Intermediate	Low/Intermediate	Intermediate

Ovcon 50 (Mead Johnson) 21 or 28 day
  1 mg norethindrone
  0.050 mg ethinyl estradiol
	Intermediate	Low/Intermediate	Intermediate

Ovral (Wyeth-Ayerst) 21 or 28 day
  0.5 mg norgtestrel
  0.050 mg ethinyl estradiol
	High	High	Intermediate/High

Zovia 1/50 (Watson) 21 or 28 day
  1 mg ethynodiol diacetate
  0.050 mg ethinyl estradiol
	Intermediate/High	Low	Intermediate

Progestin Only Micronor (Ortho) 28 day 0.35 mg norethindrone	Low	Low	Low
Nor-QD (Watson) 28 day 0.35 mg norethindrone	Low	Low	Low
Ovrette (Wyeth-Ayerst) 28 day 0.075 mg norgestrel	Low	Low	Low

[1]The following new OCs by Barr are 28-day monophasics: Apri (like Alesse); Aviane (like Ortho-Cept); Crysella (like Lo-Ovral); Lessina (like Levlite); Nortrel 1/35 (like Ortho-Novum 1/35); Nortrel 0.5/35 (like Brevicon); Portia (like Nordette and Levlen).

[2]The following new OC by Barr is a 28-day triphasic: Enpresse (like Triphasil and Tri-Levlen).

[3]The following new OC by Barr is a 28-day biphasic: Kariva (like Mircette).

Source: Adapted from Dickey, 2002.

Effectiveness

OCs are considered highly effective in preventing pregnancy (see Table 9–3). Failures are attributed to the following.

- ◆ Method failure, improper use, user error.
- ◆ Discontinuing the pill without immediate use of another method.
- ◆ Drug interactions.

Little difference exists in the failure rates among individual OCs.

Advantages

- ◆ High rate of effectiveness.
- ◆ Use not associated with the act of intercourse.
- ◆ Use controlled by the woman.

- Easy to use, convenient.
- Rapid reversal of effects after discontinuing use.
- Considered safe for most women throughout their reproductive life span when there are no contraindications.
- Multiple noncontraceptive benefits.

Noncontraceptive Benefits

- *Improved Menstrual Characteristics.* OCs minimize dysmenorrhea and usually decrease the amount and duration of bleeding so that periods are regular and predictable. OCs relieve premenstrual syndrome (PMS) in some women, and they lower the incidence of iron deficiency anemia. They can be used to ameliorate amenorrhea and dysfunctional uterine bleeding. OCs also relieve symptoms related to perimenopause and early menopause.
- *Protection against Ovarian and Endometrial Cancer.* Compared with women who never used OCs, users have half the risk of developing these cancers. Protection is noted after a minimum of twelve months of use and persists long after pills are discontinued.
- *Lower Incidence of Ovarian Cysts.* Incidence is reduced by 90 percent, due to the suppression of ovulation.
- *Prevention of Ectopic Pregnancy.* Prevention occurs through the suppression of ovulation.
- *Lower Incidence of Endometriosis.* Incidence is reduced due to the suppression of endometrial growth.
- Also used in treatment. Active pills often are prescribed for 63 or more days consecutively.
- *Treatment for Polycystic Ovarian Syndrome (PCOS).* Used in treatment once a diagnosis is established. Excessive androgen production of ovarian origin may be suppressed with COCs that have high progestational and low androgenic activities.
- *Protection against Loss of Bone Mineral Density.* Because COCs provide a consistent potent estrogen, higher peak bone mass is achieved. Women who have used COCs enter menopause with stronger bones.
- *Some Protection against Pelvic Inflammatory Disease (PID).* Incidence of PID is 20 to 50 percent lower among users of OCs than among those who use no contraceptive method. The greatest protection is against PID caused by gonorrhea.
- *Lower Incidence of Benign Breast Cysts and Fibroadenomas.* As a result, breast biopsy procedures are decreased.

- *Reduction in vasomotor symptoms in perimenopausal women.*
- *Other Benefits.* OCs may reduce acne in some women; may reduce the incidence of rheumatoid arthritis; are used in treatment of hirsutism. Risk of colon cancer may be reduced (Dickey, 2002; Hatcher et al., 1998; Pymar & Creinin, 2001).

Disadvantages

- Affects all body systems.
- User must remember to take pills daily.
- Some users experience undesirable side effects that cause discontinuance of pills.
- Should not be used while lactating.
- Provides no protection against HIV infection and other STDs.
- High cost for some women.
- For some women, slight delay in becoming pregnant after discontinuing (2 to 3 months).
- Prescription needed.
- Access to pharmacy needed.
- User must interact with medical system.
- OCs may interact with other drugs (see Table 9–6).
- Many possible side effects.

Side Effects and Complications

Side effects and complications are caused by systemic effects of OCs, and may be due to estrogenic, progestational, and/or androgenic activities, or their effects on one or more body systems. Pills with the lowest feasible biologic activity in each of these three areas should be chosen, because of potential long-term adverse effects on some body systems, particularly the cardiovascular system. Table 9–7 summarizes most common side effects of OCs based on their relation to excess or deficient hormone activity.

Managing Side Effects

- Allow the client time to adjust to the pills (two or three cycles).
- Determine that she is taking the pills correctly.
- Determine whether any symptom indicates the possible development of a serious health problem or OC-related complication (especially myocardial infarction, stroke, pulmonary embolism, thrombophlebitis, gallbladder or liver problems). Ask specific questions regarding early pill danger signs, remembering the acronym *ACHES*—severe *A*bdominal pain,

TABLE 9–6. Oral Contraceptive Interactions with Other Drugs

Effect	Substances	Comments
Drugs whose effects may be enhanced in combination with oral contraceptives.	Alcohol, tricyclic antidepressants,[a] some benzodiazepines (alprozolam, chlordiazepoxide, clorazepate, diazepam, flurazepam), β-blockers, corticosteroids, theophylline, Troleandomycin (Tao).[b]	Monitor blood levels when available and monitor affected body systems. Use these drugs with caution.
Drugs whose effects may be diminished in combination with oral contraceptives.	Acetaminophen,[b] oral anticoagulants, some benzodiazepines (lorazepam, oxazepam, temazepam), guanethidine,[a] oral hypoglycemic agents (chlorpropamide, glipizide, glyburide, tolazamide, tolbutamide), methyldopa.	Monitor physiological effect of drug, or use alternative drug, or use alternative contraceptive method.
Drugs that may diminish the effectiveness of oral contraceptives.	Any antibiotic (especially ampicillin, penicillin, sulfonamides, tetracyclines), antacids, anticonvulsants (carbamazepine, ethosuximide, phenobarbital, phenytoin, primidone, valproic acid, valproate), barbiturates, griseofulvin, rifampin, clofibrate, benzodiazepines.	Could result in breakthrough bleeding or pregnancy. Use additional birth control method during drug use and for one cycle after drug discontinuation, or use alternative contraceptive method.

Note: Vitamin C, 1 g or more daily, may cause increased serum concentrations of estrogen and possibly increased adverse effects of estrogens.
[a]Clinical significance of this interaction is unknown.
[b]Increased risk of hepatotoxicity with simultaneous use.

Sources: Dickey, 2002; Hatcher et al., 1998.

severe *C*hest pain, severe *H*eadaches, *E*ye-visual changes, *S*hortness of breath. Other danger signs are severe leg pain, loss of coordination, speech problems, and depression.

◆ Determine which hormonal component of the OC is likely to be responsible for the symptom(s) (Table 9–7).

◆ Determine whether the side effect may be due to an excess or deficiency of a hormonal component (see Table 9–7). If it is determined that the side effect is due to a deficiency or excess of a particular hormonal component, switch the client to a different OC product that has greater or lesser activity of the offending hormone (Table 9–5 and 9–8).

Table 9–8 lists common side effects, suggested hormone adjustments, and other management considerations. Table 9–5 includes hormonal activities of low and moderate dose OCs, and may be used when OC dosage and/or potency adjustments are indicated for management of specific side effects.

Effects of COCs on Blood Lipids

Estrogen alone is known to beneficially affect blood lipids by lowering total cholesterol and low density lipoprotein cholesterol (LDLs) and elevating high density lipoprotein cholesterol (HDLs). Estrogen can also elevate triglycerides.

High doses of progestins (19-nortestosterone derivatives) decrease triglyceride levels and HDL cholesterol levels, and elevate LDL cholesterol levels. Low doses, as used in progestin-only contraceptive pills (POPs), show no significant effects, and depot formulations only lower HDL cholesterol levels. When synthetic estrogens and progestins are combined in COCs, their effects on serum lipids seem to depend on the androgenicity of the progestin. Progestins that are more androgenic show the most unfavorable effects—that is, increasing LDLs, increasing triglycerides and decreasing HDLs.

Formulations containing the third generation progestins (desogestrel or gestodene) show favorable effects on LDLs and HDLs, but they also raise triglycerides.

No causal link between OC use and cardiovascular morbidity resulting from blood lipid changes has been noted. Interest, however, has focused on lipoprotein changes that occur, because they are known indicators of increased risk for cardiovascular disease (CVD).

Studies show no increased risk of atherosclerosis in women who use or have used OCs. Data from the Nurses Health Study indicate no increased risk of coronary heart disease, stroke, or other heart disease among former OC users. Lipid values may indeed vary somewhat in OC users,

TABLE 9–7. Hormone Content of Oral Contraceptives and Related Side Effects

Estrogen Excess			Estrogen Deficiency
Reproductive System	*PMS-Type Symptoms*	*Cardiovascular System*	Absence of withdrawal bleeding
Hypermenorrhea, menorrhagia, and clotting	Nausea	Vascular headaches	Spotting and bleeding (day 1 to day 9, or continuously)
Cervical extrophy	Edema, leg cramps	Hypertension	Hypomenorrhea
Dysmenorrhea	Nonvascular headaches	Cerebrovascular accident	Nervousness
Breast enlargement and tenderness	Irritability	Deep vein thrombosis	Atrophic vaginitis
Mucorrhea	Bloating	Thromboembolic disorders	Vasomotor symptoms
Uterine fibroid growth	Dizziness, syncope	Telangiectasias	Pelvic relaxation
Enlargement of uterus	Cyclic weight gain		
Cystic breast changes	*Miscellaneous Symptoms*		
	Chloasma		
	Hayfever & allergic rhinitis		
	Urinary tract infection		
	Upper respiratory disorders		
	Epigastric distress		
Progestin Excess			Progestin Deficiency
Progestational	*Androgenic/Anabolic*	*Cardiovascular System*	Breakthrough bleeding and spotting during late cycle (days 10 to 21)
Reproduction Symptoms:	Increased libido	Hypertension	Delayed withdrawal bleeding
Post-pill amenorrhea	Acne	Dilation of leg veins	Dysmenorrhea
Libido decrease	Hirsutism	Lowered protective forms of high density lipoproteins (HDLs)	Menorrhagia and clotting
Light menses	Oil skin and scalp		
Cervicitis	Cholestatic jaundice		
Monilial vaginitis	Rash		
Miscellaneous Symptoms:	Pruritis		
Increased appetite	Edema		
Fatigue/weakness			
Depression, mood changes			
Noncyclic weight gain			

Sources: Dickey, 2002; Hatcher et al., 1998.

but these variations tend to remain within the normal range. Women with known hyperlipidemia should be monitored while on OCs, especially if they are hypertensive or diabetic (Bergett-Hanson, 2001; Mantel-Teeuwisse, Kloosterman, & Maitland-Van der Zee, 2001; Pymar & Creinin, 2001).

COCs and Cardiovascular Disease

A dose-response relationship between the risk of arterial and venous thrombosis and the amount of estrogen in combined OCs has been well established. Sub-50 mcg estrogen OCs should always be chosen. Smoking and OC use increase the risk of serious cardiovascular side effects, including MI and stroke, this risk greatly increasing after age 35 and/or in the presence of hypertension. Smokers over age 35 should be advised against using OCs. It should be noted that OCs containing 20 mcg of estrogen have little or no effect on clotting parameters. These preparations should be considered for all smokers, for women over age 35, and for women with other CVD

risk factors such as diabetes mellitus, focal migraine headaches and extreme obesity. A few studies have suggested a small increase in risk of VTE with desogestrel or gestodene-containing OCs (see page 174) (Bergett-Hanson, 2001; Mantel-Teeuwisse et al., 2001; Pymar & Creinin, 2001).

COCs and Stroke

A dose-response relationship has also been established between OC estrogen dose and the risk of both hemorrhagic and ischemic (also called thrombotic) stroke. Studies over the last ten years on women using OCs containing less than 50 mcg of estrogen show the incidence of either type of stroke to be low, but not zero. Factors that increase risk of CVA are: (1) increasing estrogen dosage, i.e, lowest risk for progestin-only pills, slightly higher for 20 mcg estrogen pills, higher still for 30 to 40 mcg estrogen pills, etc.; (2) smoking; (3) presence of moderate to severe hypertension; (4) presence of diabetes; (5) obesity

TABLE 9–8. Management of Side Effects of Oral Contraceptives

Sign, Symptom, Side Effect	Estrogen Adjustment	Progestin Adjustment	Comments and Other Considerations
Acne	Increase	*or* Decrease—less androgenic	Hygiene, diet, topical, antibiotic therapy; choose a pill approved for acne treatment
Amenorrhea or light menses	Increase	Decrease	Rule out pregnancy; pill change not necessary; reassure
Anemia	No change	No change or increase	Diet, iron supplements, evaluate anemia
Bloating, fluid retention	Decrease	Decrease	Consider minipill or alternative BC method
Breakthrough bleeding, spotting	Early cycle (days 1 to 14) increase or give estrogen supplement	No change	Review history for misuse; check for infection, cervical changes, pregnancy
	Late cycle (days 15 to 21) No change	Increase or more biologically active	Change to pill with higher endometrial activity
Breast tenderness, fullness	Decrease	No change or decrease	Consider minipill; decrease sodium, caffeine intake; Vitamin E 400 IU b.i.d.
Breast or uterine cancer	Stop	Stop	Refer
Cervical Ectopy and increased mucus	Decrease	No change or decrease	Examine for infection, annual Pap
Chloasma	Decrease or stop	Lower progestational and/or less estrogenic	Consider minipill; avoid excessive sunlight
Contact lens discomfort, refractive changes	Decrease or stop	No change	Consider minipill; have vision correction reevaluated
Cyclic weight gain	Decrease	No change or decrease	
Decreased breast milk in nursing mothers	Stop	No change or decrease	Combined OCs not recommended—consider minipill or other progestin-only method
Depression	Decrease or stop	Decrease or stop	Try vitamin B_6 20–25 mg per day; monitor closely; treat depression and reevaluate frequently
Diplopia, any loss of vision, papilledema	Stop	Stop	Evaluate
Diabetes, worsening of	Decrease or stop	Decrease or stop; or try OC with desogestrel	Monitor closely
Dizziness	Decrease or stop	No change; or if hypoglycemia present, decrease	If hypoglycemia, eat regularly, and avoid simple carbohydrates
Dysmenorrhea	Decrease	Increase—higher progestational and androgenic	Rule out infection, other pathology
Gallbladder disease	Decrease or stop	Decrease or stop	Evaluate and monitor
Increased facial hair, hair changes, thinning scalp hair	Increase	Decrease—less androgenic	Rule out thyroid dysfunction
High-density lipoprotein (HDL) cholesterol, decrease	Decrease or stop	Decrease or stop	Triphasic pill or try pill with third generation progestin
Headache, migraine	Decrease or stop	Decrease or stop	Evaluate headaches, consult physician, see Table 9–2
Hypermenorrhea	Decrease	Increase—higher progestational and androgenic	Rule out pathology first; can combine decreasing estrogen with progestin/androgen change
Hypertension	Decrease or stop	Decrease or stop	Consider minipill, stop smoking, increase exercise, lose weight, reduce stress, see Table 9–2
Hypoglycemia	Same or increase	Decrease—lower progestational and androgenic	Eat regularly, low CHO/high protein diet

TABLE 9–8. (CONTINUED)

Sign, Symptom, Side Effect	Estrogen Adjustment	Progestin Adjustment	Comments and Other Considerations
Increased appetite	No change or decrease	Decrease—less androgenic	Dietary counseling
Increased growth of benign fibroid tumors	Decrease or stop	No change or decrease	Rule out malignancy
Libido decreased	Decrease	Decrease or higher androgenic	Sexual counseling
Liver disease, jaundice, or benign liver tumor	Stop	Stop	Evaluate
Myocardial infarction or stroke	Stop	Stop	Refer
Noncyclic weight gain	No change or decrease	Decrease—less androgenic	Avoid norgestrel and levonorgestrel
Nausea or vomiting	Decrease or change type	No change	Take after full meal; consider minipill or another combined hormonal delivery system
Nervousness	No change	Decrease or stop	Rule out hypoglycemia; try monophasic pill
Ovarian cysts	No change or increase	Increase—moderate to high progestational activity	If on minipill, triphasic or very low dose OC, then switch to 35 μg dose monophasic or higher
Pelvic inflammatory disease (PID)	No change	No change	Evaluate and treat infection; monitor closely
Pulmonary embolism, thromboembolism, thrombophlebitis (or symptoms of)	Stop	Stop	Refer
Rheumatoid arthritis	No change	No change	Treat rheumatoid arthritis adequately
Thyroid function tests changes	No change	No change	Evaluate for thyroid dysfunction
Urinary tract infection	Decrease	No change	Treat infections
Vaginal dryness	Increase	Decrease	Use additional lubrication
Varicose veins	Decrease	No change	Consider minipill or other progestin-only method
Yeast infections	No change	Decrease	Hygiene measures, treat infection

Sources: Blumenthal & Huggins, 1992; Dickey, 2002; Hatcher et al, 1998; Litchman & Papera, 1998.

(linked to greater risk of ischemic stroke); and (6) African American descent. One study showed a higher risk of thrombotic stroke in women who used OCs with second-generation progestins (levonorgestrel or norgestimate) versus third-generation progestins (gestodene or desogestrel), even after correcting for differences in estrogen dose. CVAs are often preceded by persistent headache for weeks or months and/or transient hemiparesis, worsening migraine headaches, or uncontrolled hypertension (Bergett-Hanson, 2001; Lidegaard & Kreiner, 2002; Pymar & Creinan, 2001; Schwartz et al., 1998).

Effects of COCs on Carbohydrate Metabolism

Older high-dose COCs were shown to increase glucose levels, increase plasma insulin levels, and slightly decrease glucose tolerance. These changes rapidly returned to normal after OCs were discontinued. Some studies have also found that progestins and progesterone increase tissue resistance to insulin by decreasing the number of insulin receptors.

More recent studies of lower dose COCs (50 mcg or less) have shown minimal changes in glucose tolerance, plasma insulin levels, or insulin binding to erythrocytes and monocytes. Carbohydrate metabolism seems to be less affected by the progestins desogestrel, gestodene, and norgestimate. Most nondiabetic women will not experience problems with CHO metabolism when using low-dose COCs (Dickey, 2002; Hatcher et al., 1998; Rivera, 1999). Use of a low-dose pill with low progestin and low androgenicity is advised to decrease resistance to insulin and cardiovascular risks (Hatcher et al., 2001).

ACOG (2000) recommends that OCs in diabetic women be used with caution: only in diabetics who are nonsmokers, under age 35, with no evidence of hypertension, nephropathy, retinopathy, or other vascular disease. Studies have not shown that OCs accelerate diabetic vascular disease (The use of hormonal contraception, 2000). Hatcher et al. (2001) advise prescribing with caution for women with complicated or prolonged diabetes for more than 20 years. A method without estrogen is advised.

Effects of COCs on the Risk of Breast Cancer

The relationship between COC use and risk of breast cancer remains controversial. Studies have led to varying conclusions:

- There is a small but significant increased risk of having breast cancer diagnosed while COCs are being taken and for ten years following discontinuation, especially in women under age 35.
- There is no increased excess risk of breast cancer diagnosis ten years or more after COCs are discontinued.
- Cancers diagnosed in women who used COCs were less advanced clinically than cancers diagnosed in women who had never used OCs. This finding applied for up to twenty years after discontinuing OCs.
- Detection bias may cause a slightly higher number of breast cancer diagnoses in OC users. Regular monitoring of all women for breast disease with self breast exams, clinician breast exams and mammography must be maintained (Bergett-Hanson, 2001; Dickey, 2002; Hatcher et al., 2001; Pymar & Creinin, 2001).

When there is an inherited susceptibility to breast cancer—that is, strong family history (mother, sister, daughter)—or carrier of BRCA1 or BRCA2 mutations, studies support an amplified relative risk of developing breast cancer. COCs are not contraindicated in these women, but they must consider this existing risk and be vigilant about breast cancer screening (Grabrick et al., 2000).

Use of OCs before age 30, first use before 1975, and use for 5 years or more is associated with a higher risk of breast cancer diagnosed before age 40 in women who carry the BRCA1 gene mutation (Narod, Dube, Klijn, Lubinski et al., 2002).

Contraindications

Table 9–9 lists absolute and relative contraindications to the use of oral contraceptives.

TABLE 9–9. Contraindications to the Use of Oral Contraceptives

Absolute Contraindications (Refrain from prescribing OCs in presence of these conditions)

Thrombophlebitis or thromboembolic disorder
Family history of hereditary thrombophilia in a first degree relative
Cerebrovascular disease
Coronary artery or ischemic heart disease
Known or suspected breast cancer
Known or suspected estrogen-dependent neoplasia
Known or suspected pregnancy
Benign or malignant liver tumor
Current impaired liver function
Undiagnosed, abnormal vaginal bleeding

Relative Contraindications (Exercise caution if OC use is considered in presence of these conditions)

Vascular or migraine headaches, especially if they began or worsened with the use of combined oral contraceptives
Hypertension
Acute mononucleosis or recent hepatitis
Presence of factors predisposing to thromboembolic disorder, such as illness or surgery requiring immobilization, long leg cast, trauma to lower leg
Cardiac or renal dysfunction (or history of)
Diabetes mellitus
Obesity (of more than 20 percent of ideal body weight)
Lactation
Age over 50
Age over 35 for a smoker (some providers feel that no heavy smoker should take birth control pills)
Psychic depression
History of myocardial infarction in an immediate family member before age 50 (especially a mother or a sister)
Hyperlipidemia
Active gallbladder disease
Sickle cell (SS) or sickle C disease
Completion of a term pregnancy within the past 10 to 14 days
Ulcerative colitis
Asthma

Sources: Dickey, 2002; Hatcher et al., 1998; Pymar & Creinan, 2001.

Management Considerations

Research on U.S. women's attitudes and beliefs about OCs demonstrates a pervasiveness of misperceptions about the effectiveness and safety of OCs, as well as confusion about the health risks and benefits associated with them. Though COCs are the most popular reversible birth control method in the United States, many women are still unsuccessful in their use. A good clinician–client relationship affects successful use. Empowering the woman with the knowledge to make informed choices, clarifying uncertainties and dispelling her fears and concerns will improve outcomes (Peipert, 1999).

- All clients taking OCs should be advised to stop smoking. Nonsmoking, healthy women (without contraindications) older than 35 may take low dose OCs. Strongly consider a 20 mcg estrogen pill for these older women.
- COCs may be started at three weeks postpartum and immediately after first trimester abortion.
- Instruct that OCs do not protect against STDs, including HIV infection. If the client is not in a mutually monogamous relationship, advise that condoms be used in addition to pills.
- Initial pill selection is based on individual client characteristics. New OC users should generally be started on the lowest dose that is still effective: a 35 µg (or less) pill. Since the introduction of triphasic preparations, many practitioners start new users on one of them. The lowest dose monophiasic combined OCs available with 20 mcg estrogen should be considered for older women. Specific client characteristics that may influence initial OC selection include age, personal and family history, relative contraindications, menstrual patterns, and hormone sensitivity.

    Because of the still controversial information regarding OCs containing desogestrel or gestodene, it is advisable not to start new clients on these pills. For established users of OCs containing desogestrel, consider encouraging them to switch to other OCs if feasible. If clients choose to remain on one of these preparations, fully inform them of the risk of VTE. An informed consent document is advised.

    New users should be reevaluated after three cycles of pill use to determine how they are adjusting. Instruct the client to contact the provider sooner if concerns arise. Early intervention and support when a client experiences bothersome side effects may prevent her from discontinuing the pill for nonmedical reasons.
- Instruct the client about how to take combined OCs. When first initiating pill use, one of the following methods is recommended.

- Start pack on first Sunday after menses begins, regardless of whether bleeding is still present (preferred method) *or*
- Start pack on first day of menstrual bleeding *or*
- Start pack on fifth day after menstrual bleeding begins.
- Postpartum women (not lactating) may begin OCs at day 21 postpartum.

- Postabortion or miscarriage may begin immediately (day 1 or 2).
- Less ideally, OCs may be started any day of the cycle with reasonable assurance that the woman is not pregnant. Starting a pack any day after day 5 requires seven days of back-up contraception.

Pill manufacturers often recommend specific routines for initiating use of their products. Instruct the client to swallow one pill daily, at the same time each day, until the pack is finished.

For second and subsequent packs:

- If using 28-day pack, begin new pack immediately. Do not skip any days.
- If using 21-day pack, stop pills for exactly seven days, then start new pack.
- Periods may be very light while on pills. Even slight spotting or bleeding should be considered a period (as long as no pills were missed).

- Instruct the client to use a second birth control method, such as condoms or a diaphragm used with spermicide, until she completes the first seven pills in the first pack. Another method is always kept on hand to use in case of missed pills, when taking another medication that might interfere with pill effectiveness (see Table 9–6), or when vomiting or diarrhea occurs.
- Missed pills are a common problem. Studies have shown that the most risky time to miss pills is at the beginning of the pack, right after the pill free interval (PFI), or during the third week of active pills, immediately prior to the start of the PFI. Preovulatory follicles may be present after seven days without active pills. If the woman misses 1 or more pills close to the time of the PFI, thus extending the number of days without active pills to more than seven, she could ovulate and conceive. Missed pills during week 2 of the pack do not present a major concern. The following instructions apply if one or more pills are missed.

- If one pill is missed, take the missed pill as soon as remembered and the next pill at the usual time. If the missed pill is taken more than 12 hours late, a backup contraceptive method must be used for the next seven days.
- If two or more pills are missed, take two as soon as remembered and discard the remainder of the missed pills. The next day's pill will be the one

normally taken for that day, had no pills been forgotten. Spotting is very likely to occur. Again, use a backup method for the next seven days.

- If one or more pills are missed during week 3 of the pill pack, follow directions previously given, but skip the pill-free interval (spacer pills) and go directly to the first pill in the new pack. Advise the woman that she may not have a period.

- If a period is missed and pills were taken correctly, the client should begin a new pack as usual. Pregnancy is unlikely. If two consecutive periods are missed and pills were taken correctly, a pregnancy test is done. Emergency contraception should be provided.

- If a period is missed and client missed one or more pills, pills are stopped; pregnancy test is done.

- If a decision is made to stop OCs and pregnancy is not desired, begin using another BC method immediately. If pregnancy is desired, use another method for two or three cycles after stopping pills.

- Birth control pills are considered medication. Always tell any health care provider when OCs are being taken.

- The client who seems to consistently miss pills should consider other methods of contraception.

- Please refer to earlier section in this chapter, Management Considerations, Guidelines for Client Education and Informed Consent (Dickey, 2002; Hatcher et al., 1998; Peipert, 1999).

OTHER COMBINED HORMONAL CONTRACEPTIVES: INJECTION, TRANSDERMAL PATCH, VAGINAL RING

Three new methods of combined hormonal contraception (containing both estrogen and progestin components) have been approved by the FDA are now available in the United States, giving women additional safe, convenient, and effective options for controlling fertility. The three methods discussed improve adherence problems often associated with taking a daily pill.

Lunelle Injection

The Lunelle injection (Pharmacia), medroxyprogesterone acetate/estradiol cypionate (MPA/E_2C), is a combined injectable once-a-month contraceptive. Each 0.5 mL dose contains 5 mg of E_2C and 25 mg of MPA and is administered every 28 days (range can be from 23 to a maximum of 33 days, adding flexibility as an advantage). It is available in single dose vials and prefilled syringes for deep intramuscular (IM) injection (deltoid, anterior thigh, or gluteus maximus muscle). The initial injection of Lunelle is administered within the first five days of the onset of menses, within ten days of a first trimester abortion, or between four and six weeks postpartum. If a client is changing contraceptive methods, it may be given at the end of week 3 of a birth control pill pack or when a Depo-Provera shot comes due. Bleeding usually occurs at two to three weeks after the first injection. With subsequent injections, bleeding generally occurs about 22 days after each injection, averaging one bleeding cycle per month lasting five to six days. Amenorrhea is rare with Lunelle (Darney & Speroff, 2001; Hatcher et al., 2001; Rawlins & Smith, 2002; Wysocki et al., 2001).

Ortho Evra, Transdermal Contraceptive System

The transdermal contraceptive system (TCS) Ortho Evra became available in 2002. The TCS consists of a three-layer patch with an area of 20 cm^2. When applied to one of four primary sites (lower abdomen, upper outer arm, buttocks, or upper torso, excluding the breast), it provides continuous, constant circulating levels of two hormones: 150 mcg of norelgestromin and 20 mcg of ethinyl estradiol are delivered to the serum each day. Users may maintain all usual activities including sports, bathing, swimming, and so on. One patch per week is applied for three consecutive weeks, followed by one week without use of a patch to allow scheduled withdrawal bleeding. The patch is changed the same day of each week. Serum hormone levels are maintained in a therapeutic range for up to nine days, providing contraceptive effectiveness if patch replacement were delayed for up to two days. Studies showed a significantly higher rate of breakthrough bleeding and/or spotting only in the first two cycles of use when compared to a COC. After that, the breakthrough bleeding rates were comparable. A withdrawal bleed is usually experienced during the patch-free week. Side effects include a low incidence of application site reactions, breast discomfort, and dysmenorrhea. These decreased after the second cycle of use. Women with a body weight of 198 pounds (90 kg) or greater had a significantly higher pregnancy rate than women with lower body weights (Darney & Speroff, 2001; Rawlins & Smith, 2002).

NuvaRing, Contraceptive Vaginal Ring

A contraceptive vaginal ring, NuvaRing (Organon), was approved by the FDA in 2001 and became available in 2002. It consists of a flexible, soft, transparent ring made of ethylene vinyl acetate copolymer, with a outer diameter of 54 mm, that releases 120 mcg of etono-gestrel (a metabolite of desogestrel) and 15 mcg of ethinyl estradiol per day. Each ring is to be used for one cycle, which consists of a three-week period of continuous ring use followed by a ring-free week to allow withdrawal bleeding. NuvaRing is inserted by the user and is considered fairly easy to master. No fitting is necessary. The woman compresses the ring and inserts it into the vagina, behind the pubic bone, as far back as possible. The hormones are absorbed through the vaginal mucosa. Precise placement is not critical. For first time use of the NovaRing, it must be inserted between the first and fifth day of the menstrual cycle. Additional contraception (such as condom or spermicide) is needed for the first seven days of that cycle. It is left in place for three weeks, removed, and discarded. After seven days without the ring, a new one is inserted, even if bleeding continues. During the three-week wear period, if the ring is removed or expelled for three hours or more, backup contraception is needed for seven days after it is reinserted. Side effects include a low incidence of headache, leukorrhea, and vaginitis (Darney & Speroff, 2001; Rawlins & Smith, 2002).

Mechanisms of Action

These three combined estrogen-progesterone contraceptives vary in their delivery method, blood levels, and duration of action. The mechanisms of action by which pregnancy is prevented, however, are essentially the same, and result from several effects of estrogen and progesterone.

- Gonadotropin-releasing hormone (GnRH) is suppressed, which in turn suppresses follicle-stimulating hormone (FSH) and luteinizing hormone (LH), inhibiting ovulation.
- Ovum/tubal transport is altered.
- Cervical mucus thickens, inhibiting sperm transport.
- Implantation is inhibited by suppression of the endometrium and alteration of uterine secretions.
- Degeneration of the corpus luteum may occur. (Dickey, 2002; Hatcher et al., 1998; Pymar & Creinin, 2001).

Effectiveness

These three methods are highly effective in preventing pregnancy. Failures may be due to method failure, improper use, user error, or failure to use backup contraception when indicated (see Table 9–3).

Advantages

The following advantages are in addition to those listed previously in the section on COCs:

- Elimination of the need for daily pill taking, so consistent use is improved.
- Delivery systems avoid "first-pass" effect on the liver.
- Low incidence of breakthrough bleeding.
- Similar noncontraceptive benefits to COCs.
- No weight restrictions for patch or shot.

Disadvantages

Also see those listed for COCs on page 179.

- Users of Lunelle shot must make arrangements for monthly injection.
- Possible weight gain.
- Decreased effectiveness of Ortho-Evra patch for women weighing over 198 lbs (90 kg).
- Women using the patch must remember to change it weekly.
- Vaginal ring not recommended for women with uterine prolapse, lack of vaginal muscle tone, or chronic constipation.
- Women must learn and be comfortable with insertion and removal of the NuvaRing.
- With NuvaRing, women may experience a foreign body sensation in the vagina, problems with coitus, expulsion, or vaginal discomfort. These were the most common reasons for discontinuation.
- Backup contraception needed for seven days if the ring is removed for three or more hours.
- Potential for side effects and complications are similar to COCs for all three methods.

Contraindications

See Table 9–9.

Management Considerations

- All clients using these methods should be advised to stop smoking. They should not be prescribed for women over 35 who smoke.

- Instruct that these methods provide no protection against STDs including HIV. Advise condom use for clients not in a mutually monogamous relationship.
- Teach proper use of each method, including initiating use and ongoing use.
- Teach insertion and removal of NuvaRing.
- Also refer to management considerations related to use of COCs (page 184).

PROGESTIN-ONLY PILLS (POPs)

Referred to as "minipills," progestin-only pills (POPs) were introduced ten years after combined oral contraceptives (COCs). POPs are taken daily with no pill-free interval. Although much less popular than COCs, POPs are well suited to women who want to take contraceptive pills but have contraindications to COCs (e.g., women with a history of thrombophlebitis or who developed hypertension or severe headaches while taking COCs). Available POPs contain norethindrone or norgestrel; they contain a fixed dose of progestin in 28-day pack (see Table 9–4).

Mechanisms of Action

There are four mechanisms by which POPs may prevent pregnancy.

- Ovulation is suppressed by inhibition of LH release from the anterior pituitary. Ovulation is inhibited in about 40 percent of cycles.
- Cervical mucus maintains a thick consistency, inhibiting sperm penetration.
- The endometrium becomes thin and atrophic.
- Tubal changes occur, including altered tubal transport, contractility, and histology (Bergett-Hanson, 2001; Dickey, 2002; Hatcher et al., 1998).

Effectiveness

POPs are somewhat less effective than combined OCs (see Table 9–3). Efficacy increases significantly in women of older reproductive age and women who are lactating. (Hatcher et al., 1998).

Advantages

- No estrogen-related side effects.
- Overall safer than combined OCs (fewer and less serious complications).
- May be used by lactating women.

- May be used by clients with prior history of thrombophlebitis (no effect on blood clotting) or with history of other estrogen related contraindications to COC use.
- Minimal effect on carbohydrate metabolism; therefore, may be used (with caution) by diabetic women.
- Rapid reversal of effects after stopping.
- Several noncontraceptive benefits.

Noncontraceptive Benefits

Most health benefits are similar to those of combined OCs. Because only a small number of women use POPs, large-scale studies are not available. Menstrual cycle benefits include decreased cramping, lighter bleeding, shorter periods, decreased PMS-type symptoms, and lessened breast tenderness.

Disadvantages

- Must be taken with meticulous accuracy; no more than 27 hours between pills.
- Less effective than combined OCs.
- May cause irregular bleeding with unpredictable patterns (may include spotting, break-through bleeding [BTB], amenorrhea, prolonged bleeding).
- No protection against HIV infection and other STDs.
- Interaction with other drugs can decrease effectiveness (see Table 9–6).
- Higher incidence of functional ovarian cysts.
- Higher incidence of ectopic pregnancy.
- Progestins may theoretically cause adverse effects on blood lipids by decreasing HDLs and increasing LDLs and triglycerides.
- Less widely available than combined OCs. Also refer to the section on combined OCs and to Tables 9–7 and 9–8 to evaluate and manage side effects.

Contraindications/Precautions

According to the FDA, progestin-only pills are required to carry the same contraindications as combined OCs, even though many of these contraindications are related to estrogen content (see Table 9–9). Several relative contraindications to POPs should be emphasized.

- History of functional ovarian cysts.
- History of ectopic pregnancy.
- Inability to take pills consistently.

◆ Undiagnosed abnormal vaginal bleeding during the preceding three months.

◆ Hyperlipidemia.

Management Considerations

◆ All clients taking POPs should be advised to stop smoking. Nonsmoking, healthy women (without contraindications) older than 35 may take POPs. May also be used by women over 35 who smoke.

◆ Instruct that POPs do not protect against STDs, including HIV infection. If the client is not in a mutually monogamous relationship, advise that condoms with spermicide be used in addition to pills.

◆ If decision is made to stop POPs and pregnancy is not desired, begin using another BC method immediately. If pregnancy is desired, use another method for two or three cycles after stopping pills.

◆ Birth control pills are considered medication. Always tell any health care provider when POPs are being taken.

◆ When taking POPs, it is important to keep track of periods. Tell the client that if more than 45 days pass with no bleeding, a health care professional should be contacted for an examination and pregnancy test.

◆ Spotting or bleeding between periods is not unusual for a woman on the minipill, especially during the first few months of use. Furthermore, some bleeding is very likely if one or more pills are missed. Heavy bleeding, pain, or fever is reported to the health care professional.

◆ *Initiating Use.* Pills are started on the first day of the period, or immediately after completing a 21-day pack of combined OC, or after the 21st pill of 28-day pack (discard remaining pills). A second birth control method is kept on hand to use for (a) the first seven days on minipills, (b) times when pills are missed, (c) when on antibiotics, or (d) when experiencing diarrhea or vomiting.

◆ POPs may be started immediately following delivery, abortion, or miscarriage. Six-week delay is recommended if breastfeeding.

◆ One pill is swallowed daily until pack is finished; new pack is started the very next day—a day is never skipped. In addition, minipills must be taken at *exactly* the same time every day.

◆ When minipills are missed or forgotten, instruct the client as follows.

• If pill is taken more than three hours late, use a backup birth control method for the next 48 hours.

• If one pill is missed, take it as soon as remembered. Take the next pill at the regular time, even if this means taking two pills in one day. Use a backup method for the next 48 hours.

• If two pills or more are missed in a row, there is a good chance of pregnancy occurring. Take two pills as soon as remembered and two the next day. Start using a second method of birth control right away. If no period occurs in four to six weeks, a pregnancy test is needed.

• Emergency contraception may be used if pills were missed and client has had intercourse without adequate protection.

OTHER PROGESTIN-ONLY CONTRACEPTIVES: IMPLANTS AND INJECTIONS

The newer long-acting progestin-only methods are ideal for women who desire long-term, continuous contraception and who may desire future pregnancies. Norplant implants and depo-medroxyprogesterone acetate injections are discussed here.

Norplant

Approved for use in the United States in 1990 and marketed by Wyeth-Ayerst (but not available in the United States at this time), Norplant is a timed-release implant of levonorgestrel. Once in place, it provides five years of continuous, highly effective contraception. The system consists of six Silastic capsules, each measuring 2.4 × 34 mm and containing 36 mg of levonorgestrel. Capsules are implanted in a fanlike pattern through a 3–5 mm incision, usually in the medial aspect of the upper arm. The Norplant system releases 85 µg of levonorgestrel per day during the first few weeks after insertion, decreasing over the next eighteen months to a constant rate of approximately 30 µg per day over a five-year period. It is probably effective for up to seven years (Darney, 2001; Hatcher et al., 1998; Norplant effective, 2000).

A two-capsule Norplant system has been approved by the FDA but is not yet available. This will simplify insertion and removal. This system is effective for a three-year period.

Depo-Provera Injection

Depo-Provera is an intramuscular (IM) injection of depo-medroxyprogesterone acetate (DMPA) that provides twelve weeks of protection. It was approved by the FDA for use as a contraceptive in the United States in 1992, after many years of controversy. The standard dosage is DMPA 150 mg IM every twelve weeks.

Mechanisms of Action

Progestin-only systems vary in their delivery method, blood levels, and duration of action. The mechanisms of action by which pregnancy is prevented are the same, however (Dickey, 2002; Hatcher et al., 1998).

- Ovulation is suppressed by inhibition of LH release from the anterior pituitary. Ovulation is inhibited in about 40 percent of cycles.
- Cervical mucus maintains a thick consistency, inhibiting sperm penetration.
- The endometrium becomes thin and atrophic.
- Tubal changes occur, including altered tubal transport, contractility, and histology.
- There is diminished functioning of corpus luteum.
- Progesterone receptor synthesis is inhibited.

Effectiveness

Failure of long-acting progestins is rare when they are properly administered and used no longer than the specified time limits. DMPA must be injected within the first five days of the menstrual cycle; implants are inserted within the first seven days of onset of menses. *It must be determined that the woman is not pregnant.* These methods are considered highly effective (see Table 9–3).

Advantages

- Long duration of action.
- Highly effective.
- Relative low doses of hormone.
- Few systemic complications.
- Reversible.
- Low ectopic pregnancy rates.
- Major complications are rare.
- Effects on blood lipids appear to be minimal (DMPA may lower HDL cholesterol).
- Estrogen free.
- Safe for women over 35.
- Use not associated with coitus.
- Very light menses or amenorrhea.

- May be used while lactating.
- May be used by smokers over 35.
- Receiving the DMPA injection early by up to a week is not harmful. There is a grace period of one week if late receiving DMPA.
- Some noncontraceptive benefits.

Disadvantages

- Most women experience some side effects; most are usually minor and related to menstrual irregularities. If bleeding is heavy, anemia may occur.
- Implants are very expensive.
- Implants may be slightly visible.
- Implants must be inserted and removed by a specially trained clinician.
- Removal of implants may be difficult.
- In rare instances infection can occur at the implant insertion site.
- Return visit needed every twelve weeks for DMPA.
- If the woman is already depressed, signs and symptoms may increase on DMPA.
- No protection against HIV, other STDs.
- Possible weight gain, nausea, headaches.
- Expulsion of the implant system can occur (rare).
- If first DMPA injection is given later than five days after onset of menses, injection may not be effective for two weeks.
- Return to fertility may be delayed six to twelve months after injection of DMPA.

Contraindications

Progestin-only methods must carry the same contraindications as COCs, even though many are related to estrogen content (see Table 9–9). Several relative contraindications to long-acting progestin-only systems should be emphasized.

- Known or suspected pregnancy.
- History of undiagnosed abnormal vaginal bleeding during the three months prior to use of one of these methods.
- Acute liver disease.
- Jaundice.
- Significant concern about weight gain.
- For Depo-Provera injection, when rapid return to fertility is desired.
- Hypercholesterolemia (DMPA).
- Current significant depression (DMPA).
- Women with existing or risk for bone density loss.

Management Considerations

- For non-breastfeeding women, Depo-Provera and Norplant may be initiated at one week postpartum or immediately post-abortion (first trimester). Lactating women should wait until six weeks after delivery.
- The insertion and removal of implant systems must be done by a professional specifically trained in the proper techniques.
- Teaching and counseling must include information about how long the system is effective; what to expect regarding changes in bleeding patterns; and the importance of continuing annual gynecologic care (see Management Considerations, Guidelines for Client Information, and Informed Consent). Careful client selection, appropriate client education and supportive follow-up care can greatly enhance client satisfaction with these methods.
- Danger signs that indicate possible serious problems associated with use of the methods must be taught.

  - Severe abdominal pain.
  - Heavy vaginal bleeding.
  - Frequent urination.
  - Depression.
  - Severe headache.
  - Pus or bleeding at the insertion site.
  - Excessive weight gain.
  - Expulsion of the implant

- For prolonged and/or frequent bleeding (Norplant or Depo-Provera) obtain the following information: history of bleeding pattern, sexual activity pattern, intercurrent illness, unusual stressful events, medications, substance use/abuse.

  Examine for other causes of bleeding such as infection, genital lesions. Perform gonorrhea and chlamydia tests, saline and KOH preps.

  Treatment options:

1. Ibuprofen 800 mg. t.i.d. for five to seven days.
2. Any currently available low-dose COC (50 mcg or lower) for one cycle.
3. Levonorgestrel 37.5 mcg b.i.d. for 20 days (Ovrette) *or* medroxyprogesterone acetate (Provera) 2.5 mg daily for 30 days *or* megestrol acetate (Megace) 40 mg for 30 days.
4. Ethinyl estradial 20 or 50 mcg for 10 days. If bleeding persists, continue for 20 days *or* Premarin 0.625 mg daily for 25 days.
5. If a low-dose estrogen supplement (oral, transdermal or cream) is added to a progestin-only method to reduce a possible risk of lowered bone density, there may be a risk of thinned cervical mucus and unplanned pregnancy. Condoms are advised as long as the client is taking exogenous estrogen in this circumstance, or advise changing to another method of contraception (Advisor Forum). Serum estradiol levels below 20 pg/mL warrant evaluation for use of exogenous estrogen in some women (Hatcher et al, 1998).

For spotting/bleeding with DMPA, provide reassurance that by second or third injection she may be amenorrheic. If frequent or prolonged, work up as for Norplant outlined previously. Try treatment with one cycle of OCs.

- *Amenorrhea (Norplant or DMPA).* Provide reassurance. Obtain pregnancy test if client is worried or if insertion/injection not done at the recommended time (see previous information). No need to induce menses.
- *Norplant insertion and removal.* Remember the Norplant system that is carefully and properly inserted will be easier to remove. Most important is that all six capsules be at a uniform depth and uniform distance from the incision.

  Several techniques for removal have been developed (Baylor College of Medicine, 1994; Darney, 1995). When performing removal, allow 30 to 45 minutes for the procedure, make sure you and client are comfortable, have ample light and all equipment ready. Palpate all six capsules and mark their locations with a surgical marker. Perform preferred removal technique. Show client all capsules at completion of the removal. Note: Some communities have arranged that one or more providers become very proficient in Norplant removal and all removals are referred to them (Archer, 1995; Bergett-Hanson, 2001; Darney, 1994; Hatcher et al., 1998; Kaunitz, 1994).

POSTCOITAL EMERGENCY CONTRACEPTION

Postcoital contraception, also called *emergency contraception* (EC) or the "morning-after pill," refers to intervention taken to prevent pregnancy after a single act of unprotected intercourse. Indications for use include sexual assault, condom breakage, dislodgement of a cervical cap, diaphragm or sponge, missed OC, incorrect method use, or any unexpected event or emotion that leads to unprotected intercourse and the possibility of pregnancy. The treatment is indicated if the woman has had unprotected intercourse within the last 72 hours and does not wish to become pregnant. EC provides a last chance to prevent pregnancy. Care must be taken, however, that she is not already pregnant. ECPs are an ideal backup method of birth control, especially for couples using barrier methods. ECPs can be provided in advance of need, "just in case."

Emergency contraceptives available in the United States include combined oral contraceptive pills, progestin-only pills, and the postcoital insertion of a copper-T IUD. Emergency contraception is under-utilized in the United States primarily because women are not aware that it is available or they do not know how to obtain it. Use, however, is increasing.

Emergency contraception has the potential to reduce the number of unintended pregnancies each year by half, as well as reduce the need for abortion by half. ECPs are highly cost effective. In Washington state, pharmacists are permitted to prescribe and dispense ECPs. The FDA has been petitioned by over sixty medical and women's health organizations to make ECPs available over the counter (Dickey, 2002; Finger, 2001; Trussell & Stewart, 1998).

In 1995, The Reproductive Health Technologies Project and Bridging the Gap Communications initiated the Emergency Contraceptive Hotline, a toll-free service that enables women to access information about emergency contraception and to obtain referrals to clinicians who provide emergency contraception. The service may be accessed 24 hours a day in English and Spanish. Access numbers are 1-800-584-9911, 1-888-NOT-2-LATE or visit www.not-2-late.com.

Mechanisms of Action

Hormonal methods of EC are believed to work by all or some of the following mechanisms:

- Inhibition or delay of ovulation.
- Luteal phase dysfunction.
- Histologic or biochemical alterations in the endometrium, making the endometrium less receptive to implantation.
- Thickening of cervical mucus.
- Alterations in tubal transport of sperm, egg, or embryo.
- Direct inhibition of fertilization.

Emergency contraceptive pills do not interrupt an established pregnancy. IUD insertion alters the en-dometrium, producing an inflammatory response that makes the endometrium unsuitable for implantation; and interferes with fertilization, and transport (Fahey, 1995; Finger, 2001; Trussell & Stewart, 1998). Patients and providers must also be aware that a small risk of ectopic pregnancy exists if emergency contraception fails (Neilson & Miller, 2000).

Effectiveness

Emergency contraceptive pills, including combined OCs and progestin-only pills, reduce the overall chance of pregnancy by 75 percent. However, in studies comparing the combination pill method with the progestin-only pills, the POPs were found to be twice as effective in preventing pregnancy with far fewer side effects of nausea, vomiting, dizziness, and fatigue (ACOG Practice Bulletin, 2001; World Health Organization, 1998). The POP regimen reduces the risk of pregnancy to 1 in 100 versus 2 in 100 for COCs and 8 in 100 with no EC (World Health Organization, 1998).

The sooner ECPs are taken after unprotected intercourse, the more effective they are. Postcoital emergency insertion of a copper-T IUD is even more effective than ECPs (99% effective) (Trussell & Stewart, 1998).

Contraindications

Contraindications to ECPs are few, but they should not be used with a known or suspected pregnancy, hypersensitivity to any component of the product or undiagnosed abnormal genital bleeding. IUDs should be avoided by women at risk for STDs.

Emergency Contraceptive Pills

Combined OCs. The combined oral contraceptive pills that have been studied and are now used for emergency contraception contain estrogen (ethinyl estradiol) and progestin (norgestrel or levonorgestrel). In the United States, these include Ovral, Lo/Ovral, Alesse, Levlite, Levora, Trivora, Nordette, Levlen, Triphasil, Tri-levlen, and other generic equivalents. There is one dedicated ECP consisting of EE and levonorgestrel called Preven. The current treatment is one dose of the combined OC given as soon as possible after unprotected intercourse, but not later than 72 hours after, followed in 12 hours by a second dose. (Recent studies indicate some protection may be provided up to five days.) This method is referred to as the "Yuzpe" method. Until recently, this was the most commonly used EC method, and almost all women can safely use it. Medical experts believe that even women who should not use estrogen on a continuous basis can usually use this method for one-time emergency contraception (see Table 9–10). Menses should begin in two to three weeks; if it does not, a pregnancy test should be performed. Nausea and vomiting are common with these pills. If vomiting occurs within two hours of taking a dose, that dose needs to be repeated. Extra pills should be dispensed in case this occurs. Antinausea medication should also be given (Finger, 2001; Sterilization, 2001; Trussell & Stewart, 1998; World Health Organization, 1998).

Progestin-Only Pills. Progestin-only pills (POPs) for EC are twice as effective as the Yuzpe COC method. POPS for EC are available in a dedicated product known as *Plan B* (levonorgestrel tablets 0.75 mg each), a two-pill regimen, packaged and labeled for emergency contraception. An alternative is the minipill, Ovrette, containing 0.075 mg norgestrel (which is equivalent to 0.0375 mg levonorgestrel). Twenty pills of Ovrette are required for each dose of EC. The same instructions apply as for the COCs; the first dose is taken within 72 hours of unprotected intercourse, the second dose 12 hours later (Finger, 2001; ACOG Practice Bulletin, 2001; Trussell & Stewart, 1998) (see Table 9–10) Considering the greater effectiveness of

TABLE 9–10. Emergency Postcoital Contraceptive Options

Product	Tablets Taken within 72 Hours of Unprotected Intercourse	Repeat Dose Taken 12 Hours Later
Combined oral contraceptives		
Preven	1 tablet	1 tablet
Ovral	2 tablets	2 tablets
Lo-Ovral; Nordette; Levlen; Levlite; Alesse	4 tablets	4 tablets
Triphasil (yellow tablet only); Tri-Levlen (yellow tablet only); Trivora (pink tablet only)	4 tablets	4 tablets
Progestin-only pills		
Plan B	1 tablet	1 tablet
Ovrette	20 tablets	20 tablets
IUD (copper containing such as CU-T 380-A-Paragard)	Insert up to 7 days after unprotected intercourse. May be left in place for long-term contraception.	

For all methods: Review contraindications. Evaluate for pregnancy if no menses by three weeks.

Sources: ACOG Practice Bulletin, 2001; Finger, 2001; Trussell & Stewart, 1998.

the POP regimen, it is generally felt that these should always be chosen.

Postcoital IUD Insertion

Copper-containing IUDs can be inserted up to seven days (10 days in some cases) after unprotected intercourse. This method prevents pregnancy 99 percent of the time when used postcoitally. The same precautions and contraindications apply when an IUD is inserted for this purpose as when used for routine contraception (see Intrauterine Devices, later in this chapter). In addition, the copper-T IUD may be left in place to provide continuous effective contraception for up to ten years. Other IUDs may also be effective but have not been studied (Hatcher et al., 1998; Trussell & Stewart, 1998).

Other Methods of EC

High dose oral estrogens in the forms of ethinyl estradiol (EE), diethylstilbestrol (DES), conjugated estrogen, or estrone have been used in the past for EC. Danazol, a synthetic androgen, has also been studied. These regimens were less effective, and the incidence of side effects was high. Their use is no longer recommended.

The antiprogesterone drug, mifepristone (Mifeprex, RU-486), is used in countries other than the United States as an emergency contraceptive. European studies have shown it to be highly effective when used within three days of unprotected intercourse. Mifepristone produces less nausea and vomiting than some other EC methods (Fahey, 1995; Hatcher et al., 1998).

THE MALE CONDOM

The male condom, also referred to as a rubber, prophylactic, or skin, is a sheath that is worn over the erect penis to contain fluid from ejaculation. Most U.S. condoms are made from latex rubber. About 1 percent of condoms used in the United States are made of processed collagenous tissue from the intestinal caecum of lambs. Condoms are available in many colors, textures, sizes, shapes, and thicknesses. Clients must be sure to purchase condoms that are labeled for use as contraceptives/prophylactics and that bear a disease prevention claim. Novelty condoms do not prevent pregnancy or disease transmission. In 1994, the FDA approved the first polyurethane ("plastic") male condom, even though limited testing had been performed.

A few brands of polyurethane male condoms are now available. The FDA approved these products only for use by people who are allergic to latex. They are approved but not widely available. Clinical trials to evaluate efficacy are ongoing.

Another nonlatex condom has been developed and approved by the FDA. This is a latex-free, natural rubber, nonallergenic product called the Tactylon condom by Sensicon Corp. Tactylon is a synthetic styrene, butylene styrene, the same material used in the FDA-approved nonallergenic examination gloves. It comes in three styles. This is also not widely available (Feldblum & Joanis, 1994; Gebbie, 1995; Gerchufsky, 1996a,b; Hatcher et al., 1998).

Mechanism of Action

A *condom* is a mechanical barrier to prevent sperm from entering the vagina and cervix. Condoms prevent direct contact with semen, penile lesions, discharges, and infected secretions. Latex condoms prevent transmission of most sexually transmitted infections, including HIV. Spermicidal condoms have the additional action of nonoxynol-9 to immobilize and kill sperm after ejaculation (see Spermicides, later in this chapter). Without condoms, infecting organisms can be physically transmitted into the uterus and tubes by sperm.

Effectiveness

Condoms are considered *moderately* effective at preventing accidental pregnancy (see Table 9–3). Failure to prevent pregnancy is most frequently attributed to inconsistent use. Condom breakage can occur, but this is not a major cause of accidental pregnancy. Effectiveness increases significantly, approaching the effectiveness of oral contraceptives or an IUD, when used concurrently with a vaginal spermicide. Effectiveness of the polyurethane and Tactylon condoms has not been determined (Hatcher et al., 1998).

Advantages

- Available without a prescription or examination.
- Relatively inexpensive.
- Widely available.
- Physiologically safe.
- No adverse effect on fertility.
- Easily reversible contraception.

- Few side effects.
- Significant protection against most STDs and their consequences, including HIV disease.
- Possible protection against cancer of the cervix.
- Male participation in contraception is encouraged.
- Only reversible contraceptive available for use by men.
- May delay premature ejaculation in men for whom this is a concern.
- May be used during lactation.
- Lubricated condoms may reduce friction, preventing irritation to either partner.
- Postcoital drainage of semen from the vagina, which some women find objectionable, is eliminated.
- Allergic reactions are prevented for women who are sensitive to partner's semen.
- Polyurethane ("plastic") condom is stronger than latex and thinner. It may improve sensation and pleasure.
- Polyurethane condom can be safely used with oil-based lubricants.

Disadvantages

- Fairly expensive for frequent use.
- Possible decreased sensation for man.
- Interferes with sexual spontaneity (requires forethought and preparedness).
- Necessity to interrupt foreplay to put condom on.
- "Skin" condoms made from animal membranes may not protect against some STDs, including HIV.
- Some women and men experience irritation with the use of particular lubricants or spermicides on condoms.
- Male partner may be unwilling to cooperate with condom use.
- Most condoms are approved by manufacturers for penis/vagina sex only.

Contraindications

- Allergy of the man or woman to the latex in condoms. The incidence of latex allergy in our society is increasing, especially among individuals such as health care workers who have high environmental exposure to latex in the workplace. Individuals with latex allergies may use the nonallergenic, nonlatex condoms described earlier, or they may use a natural skin type condom over the latex condom (or under it, depending which partner has the allergy) (Gerchufsky, 1996).

Management Considerations

The following instructions will be helpful to couples using condoms:

- Store condoms in a cool, dry place. Heat, even body heat, may weaken the rubber. Always keep the condom in its original package until use. Condoms should keep five years when properly stored. Consider using name brands; these may be of more reliable quality. Spermicidal condoms should be used. Check expiration date.
- The condom is placed on the erect penis (either partner can do this) *before* the penis comes in contact with the woman's genital area.
- Roll the condom all the way down to the base of the penis.
- If the condom does not have a built-in reservoir, leave one-half inch of empty space at the end of it to collect ejaculate. This is accomplished by pinching the tip of the condom as it is rolled on. Leave no air in the tip; this could contribute to tearing.
- Be sure that the vagina and/or condom are well lubricated to prevent condom tearing. If additional lubrication is needed, use only water, saliva, water-based jelly, or contraceptive foam, gel, or cream on latex condoms. Other products, especially petroleum based, will cause rapid deterioration and weakening of latex. Other vaginal products that cause latex condom weakening include miconazole nitrate (Monistat), butoconazole nitrate (Femstat), estradiol (Estrace), and conjugated estrogen (Premarin) creams, Vagisil ointment, Rendell's Cone and Ovule Spermicide, and the sexual lubricant called Elbow Grease. These lubricants do not affect the new polyurethane and Tactylon condoms.
- For added protection, use a second method of birth control (diaphragm, spermicidal foam, gel, film, suppository, or hormonal method).
- After intercourse, remove the condom immediately while the penis is still erect, holding on to the base of the condom to prevent spilling. Dispose of properly after use.
- Check the condom for tears, then throw it away. Use each condom only once. If tears are detected, immediately insert spermicidal gel or cream into the vagina.

FEMALE CONDOMS

The first female condom (Reality) was approved by the FDA in 1993 for over-the-counter sale in the United States. The Reality female condom consists of a polyurethane sheath with an outer ring and inner ring. Each condom is prelubricated with silicone, and a container of water-based lubricant is supplied for those who prefer more lubrication. It is inserted vaginally, like a diaphragm, and held in place by the pubic bone. The closed upper tip is anchored near the cervix by a flexible inner ring that holds the device in place, preventing expulsion. The condom covers the surfaces of the vaginal wall, allowing the penis to move freely inside the condom. An external ring at the outer opening of the pouch remains outside the vagina and partially covers the labia. It is used for one act of intercourse only; however, studies are underway to determine whether it may be used more than once. This would help to reduce cost. If used correctly with every sex act, the female condom also helps to prevent the spread of STD. This product is distributed by Wisconsin Pharmacal. It is approved by the FDA for prevention of pregnancy and STDs. Studies are being conducted on possible reuse of the female condom (The female condom, 1995; Female condoms can be reused, 2001; McNamee, 2000; *Reality female condom,* 1994).

Mechanism of Action

This device serves as a mechanical barrier to prevent sperm from entering the vagina or cervix. The polyurethane female condom also has the ability to prevent transmission of most STDs, including HIV.

Effectiveness

The typical failure rate in U.S. studies was similar to that for diaphragm, sponge, and cervical cap during typical use. The female condom is impermeable to various STD organisms and HIV (see Table 9–3). (The female condom, 1995; Farr, Gebelnick, & Sturgen, 1994).

Advantages

- Use controlled by the woman.
- Available without a prescription or examination.
- Easily reversible.
- Considered medically safe.
- Little danger of systemic effects.
- May provide protection against STDs, cervical neoplasia.

- ◆ May be worn prior to intercourse.
- ◆ Not dependent on male arousal.
- ◆ May be used while pregnant or menstruating.
- ◆ May be used during lactation.
- ◆ May be removed immediately after intercourse.
- ◆ Provides improved sensation for man and woman and allows transfer of body heat.
- ◆ Eliminates postcoital drainage of semen.
- ◆ Prevents allergic reactions for women sensitive to partner's semen or to latex.

Disadvantages

- ◆ Expensive for frequent use (about three times the price of the male condom).
- ◆ For single use only.
- ◆ Cumbersome; insertion can be difficult.
- ◆ Can slip or be pushed out of place.
- ◆ May make noise during use.
- ◆ Unsightly ring dangles outside the vagina.
- ◆ Breakage, tearing can occur (though rarely).

Contraindications

- ◆ Allergy of man or woman to polyurethane.
- ◆ Anatomic abnormalities that interfere with proper placement.
- ◆ Inability to master insertion technique.

Management Considerations

The following instructions will be helpful to the client:

- ◆ Practice wearing and inserting the female condom before depending on it for protection.
- ◆ Be careful not to tear the condom with sharp objects such as rings or long fingernails.
- ◆ Extra spermicidal lubricant may be used if desired.
- ◆ Refer to the package inserts for detailed use and insertion instructions.
- ◆ Insert inner ring high in the vagina, against the cervix.
- ◆ Place the outer ring properly outside the vagina.
- ◆ During intercourse, be sure the penis is placed inside the female condom.
- ◆ After intercourse, remove the female condom carefully to avoid spilling semen (Feldblum & Joanis, 1994).

SPERMICIDES

Spermicides are chemical substances that immobilize and kill sperm. The spermicidal agent available in the United States is nonoxynol-9. This is a surfactant that destroys the sperm cell membrane. Other products, octoxynol and benzalkonium chloride (BZK), are available in other countries. Nonoxynol-9 (N-9) formulations, available in creams, jellies, suppositories, and film, are inserted into the vagina prior to intercourse. When used alone, they are inserted vaginally near the cervix, forming a chemical barrier. Spermicides are also essential components of vaginal barrier methods of contraception (diaphragm, cervical cap, and sponge). Surfaces of male condoms may be coated with spermicide to enhance the effectiveness of this method as a contraceptive.

When used alone, all spermicidal products provide protection for up to one hour and for one episode of intercourse only. Additional acts of intercourse, or intercourse occurring more than one hour after insertion, require repeated application of the product.

In the past, spermicides containing nonoxynol-9 (N-9) were considered protective against transmission of HIV, chlamydia, and gonorrhea infections. However, recent studies refute this. Several recent studies have shown the risk of HIV infection to be higher in N-9 users that in placebo groups and N-9 provided no reduction in the incidences of gonorrhea, chlamydia, trichamoniasis, bacterial vaginosis, and candidiasis compared to placebo. One study linked N-9–induced vaginal inflammation to increased HIV transmission (Fichorova, Tucker, & Anderson, 2001; VanDamme, Ramjee, Alary, Vuylsteke, Chandeying et al., 2002; Wilkinson, Tholandi, Ramjee, & Rutherford, 2002). All the spermicide formulations discussed below contain nonoxynol-9.

Foams, Jellies, Creams

These can be used alone or with a condom, diaphragm, or cervical cap. Foams are available in multidose aerosol containers or in small, single use, prefilled cartridges. Creams and jellies come in multidose tubes with reusable applicators. Some jellies are sold in single use packets.

Suppositories

Referred to as *spermicidal vaginal tablets,* the suppositories are a small ovoid shape. They can be used alone or with a condom but must be inserted ten to fifteen minutes before intercourse in order to melt and disperse the spermicide.

Vaginal Contraceptive Film (VCF)

VCF, which can be used alone or with a condom or diaphragm, is a paper-thin sheet of film containing nonoxynol-9, measuring 2×2 in. The sheet is inserted on or near the cervix (or inside a diaphragm) at least five minutes prior to intercourse in order to melt and disperse the spermicide.

New types of vaginal spermicide film are under development. One version, which incorporates benzalkonium chloride instead of nonoxynol-9 as the active agent, has undergone early clinical trials for safety. Other types, which are made of different materials than the film currently available, are being designed to dissolve more rapidly in the body but maintain their stability in tropical climates.

Mechanism of Action

Spermicides contain a chemical surfactant that immobilizes and kills sperm (by destroying sperm cell membrane) and vehicle ingredients to keep the spermicide in place around the cervix. The active ingredient in spermicidal products sold in the United States is nonoxynol-9. Octoxynol is the active agent in other products and is equally effective as a spermicide. It is not sold in the United States.

Effectiveness

Spermicides used alone are low to moderately effective at preventing accidental pregnancy (see Table 9–3). Spermicides are the least effective of modern contraceptives. Failures are most frequently attributed to inconsistent use. Proper use, including placement of the product deep inside the vagina against the cervix, is essential. Efficacy is much greater if used with a condom or diaphragm. Data are not available comparing the efficacies of the various spermicidal products (Best, 2000a; Hatcher et al., 1998).

Advantages

- Widely available without a prescription or examination.
- Relatively inexpensive.
- Medically safe.
- Readily available as a backup method in a variety of circumstances:
  - In the event of condom rupture.
  - To augment other methods during midcycle, when the woman is most fertile.
  - When a woman begins using oral or other hormonal contraceptives.
  - When a woman taking oral contraceptives misses one or more pills.
- Completely reversible.
- No effect on the return to fertility.
- Women can decide independently to use it.

- Can provide lubrication during intercourse.
- Can be used during lactation.
- Convenient, useful method of contraception after delivery and before the first postpartum visit, and when changing from one method to another.

Disadvantages

- May interfere with sexual spontaneity (requires forethought and preparedness).
- Must be on hand at or near the time of intercourse.
- Suppositories and film require time to disperse before intercourse can take place.
- Perceived as messy by some individuals (drainage of the substance from the vagina occurs after intercourse).
- Incomplete dissolution of suppositories can cause an uncomfortable, gritty sensation for either partner and may impair contraceptive effectiveness.
- Some users experience a warm sensation; some feel that the suppository "burns."
- For couples engaging in oral-genital sex, the taste of spermicides is unpleasant. Spermicide may be inserted after this activity, but before penis-vagina contact takes place.
- Skin irritation of the vulva or penis can result from frequent use of spermicides or from allergy or sensitivity to the spermicide or base ingredients. Another product may be tried.
- A few studies in the early 1980s reported possible adverse effects on the fetus if spermicide was used near or at the time of conception. Subsequent, more carefully designed and controlled studies failed to show adverse effects on the fetus.
- Not protective against HIV/AIDS or other STDs.

Contraindications

- Allergy of either partner to spermicide or its other ingredients.
- Inability to "remember" to use the product associated with intercourse.
- Inability to learn the proper insertion technique.
- Anatomic abnormalities of the vagina that might interfere with the correct placement or retention of the spermicide.

Management Considerations

The following instructions will be helpful to couples using a spermicide.

- The spermicide must be used every time intercourse occurs; must be in place prior to penis-vagina contact.

- Store spermicides in a cool, clean, and dry place.
- Wait the specified time after insertion so that the spermicide is adequately dispersed (for film and suppositories).
- One application is good for one hour after insertion and for one act of intercourse only. Additional application is needed if one hour has passed since insertion or before each additional act of intercourse.
- All spermicides must be left in place for at least six hours after the last act of intercourse. Do not douche or rinse the product out for at least six hours.
- Instructions for specific products include the following.
  - *Foam.* Shake vigorously at least 20 times before dispensing. Insert the applicator as far into the vagina as it will go comfortably. Holding the applicator in place, push the plunger to release the product.
  - *Jelly or cream.* Fill applicator by squeezing the tube from the bottom. Insert as for foam (above).
  - *Suppository (vaginal tablet).* Remove the wrapper and insert as far as possible so that the tablet rests on or near cervix. Wait the specified time before intercourse.
  - *Film.* Fingers must be completely dry. Place one sheet of film on a fingertip and slide it along the back wall of the vagina as far as possible, so that the film rests on or near cervix. Wait at least five minutes before intercourse to allow dispersion.
- If burning or irritation occurs, stop use of the product. Changing brands or the form of spermicide may diminish reactions. If a reaction persists, discontinue use.

VAGINAL BARRIER METHODS: DIAPHRAGMS, CERVICAL CAPS, SPONGE

Diaphragm

A *diaphragm* is a dome-shaped cup made of latex rubber with a flexible-spring metal rim. It is inserted vaginally prior to intercourse, so that the posterior rim rests in the posterior fornix and the anterior rim fits snugly behind the pubic bone. Spermicidal cream, jelly, or film is applied inside the dome of the diaphragm and around the rim before insertion. Diaphragms are available in a range of sizes and four general styles. Specified sizes refer to millimeters in diameter across the rim, for example, 65 mm, 70 mm, 75 mm.

- *Coil Spring Rim.* This type has a sturdy rim with firm spring strength, which most women with average vaginal musculature and average pubic arch depth can use comfortably. The diaphragm folds flat for insertion and can be used with a plastic introducer. Specific products include Koromex diaphragm (latex), sizes 50–95; Ortho coil spring diaphragm (latex), sizes 50–95; Ramses flexible cushioned diaphragm (gum rubber), sizes 50–95.
- *Flat Spring Rim.* Having a thin, delicate rim with gentle spring strength, this type of diaphragm can be worn comfortably by nulliparous women with firm vaginal musculature or by women with a shallow notch behind the pubic bone. It folds flat for insertion and can be used with introducer. An example of this product is the Ortho-White diaphragm (latex), sizes 55–95.
- *Arcing Spring Rim.* The sturdy rim of this type of diaphragm imparts firm spring strength. Furthermore, the arcing rim facilitates insertion. Most women can use it comfortably, and it can be retained in the presence of cystocele and/or rectocele or relaxed vaginal muscle tone. Specific products include the Koroflex diaphragm (latex), sizes 60–95; Ortho All-Flex diaphragm (latex), sizes 55–95; Ramses Bendex diaphragm (gum rubber), sizes 65–95.
- *Wide-Seal Rim.* This type has a thin, flexible flange approximately 1.5 cm wide attached to the inner edge of the rim to keep spermicide in place inside the dome and to enhance the seal between the rim and the vaginal wall. It is made in two styles, arcing and coil spring. Specific products include the Milex Wide-Seal arcing diaphragm (latex), sizes 60–95; Milex Wide-Seal Omniflex coil spring diaphragm (latex), sizes 60–95. Milex diaphragms are not available from pharmacies by prescription, but are only distributed to doctors and clinics by the manufacturer (Hatcher et al., 1998; Tagg, 1995).

Vaginal Contraceptive Sponge

The *Today* vaginal contraceptive sponge was introduced in the United States in 1983. It was removed from the market in 1995, but may return soon. While available, this was a popular over-the-counter contraceptive device. Allendale Pharmaceuticals was recently given FDA approval to manufacture the Today sponge again in the United States. It has yet to come to market.

The Today contraceptive sponge is a small, soft, pillow-shaped disposable polyurethane sponge that is impregnated with nonoxynol-9. After it is moistened with water and inserted high into the vagina, the sponge is immediately effective for the next 24 hours, without need to add more spermicide, even for repeated acts of intercourse. The concave dimple on one side fits over the cervix. A woven polyester loop on the other side facilitates removal. The sponge must be left in place for six hours after the last act of intercourse. It may then be removed and discarded. Maximum recommended wear time is 30 hours (Best, 2000c; Hatcher et al., 1998; *Product Information, Today Sponge*, 2000).

The *Protectaid* contraceptive sponge is available in Canada and other countries. It contains three spermicides (N-9, BZK, and sodium cholate). The *Pharmatex* sponge contains BZK. Use of these products is similar to that of the Today sponge (Best, 2000c).

Cervical Cap

The cervical cap is a soft, rubber, cup-shaped device, resembling a small diaphragm with a deep dome (much like a thimble). It fits over the cervix and is held in place by a seal that forms between its flexible rim and the outer surface of cervix. A small amount of spermicide is placed inside the cap, but not on the rim, which would interfere with forming the seal.

The Prentif Cavity Rim Cervical Cap, the only cap currently approved by the FDA for general use in the United States, was first approved for general distribution in 1988 after several years of investigative testing. The Prentif cap is a soft, deep rubber cap with a firm, rounded rim. A groove along the rim's inner circumference enhances the seal that forms between the inner rim and the surface of the cervix. Available in sizes 22–31 mm (inner rim diameter), it is manufactured in England and distributed in the United States by Cervical Cap Ltd., Los Gatos, California.

Other specific products (not generally available in the United States at this time) are the Dumas Cap and the Vimule Cap (Best, 2000c; Hatcher et al., 1998).

Mechanisms of Action

- The contraceptive effect of the diaphragm is related to the barrier effect, which prevents sperm entry into the cervix, and to the sperm-killing action of spermicide used with all diaphragms.
- Similar in action to the diaphragm, the cervical cap serves as a barrier to the cervix and holds spermicide within its dome.

- The sponge has the barrier effect, sperm-killing action of spermicide, and the additional action of trapping and absorbing semen before sperm can enter the cervix.

Effectiveness

Contraceptive efficacy among these methods is comparable (see Table 9–3). Some cervical cap failures are attributed to cap dislodgement during intercourse and to deterioration of rubber after prolonged use and/or storage.

Vaginal barrier methods depend largely on extremely conscientious use, although individual fertility characteristics are probably equally important. These methods must be used correctly and consistently. They are used with more success by women 30 years of age or older, who have intercourse fewer than four times weekly, and who may have slightly lower fertility than their younger counterparts. Many women who experience accidental pregnancy with these methods report misuse (including inconsistent use). Users must be highly motivated to prevent or delay pregnancy. The role of the clinician can be very significant in assisting women to use these products successfully. (Best, 2000c; Boston Women's Health, 1998; Hatcher et al., 1998).

Advantages

- Attractive method for women needing contraception on an irregular basis and whose sexual patterns are fairly predictable.
- Does not require partner involvement.
- Considered medically safe.
- Little danger of systemic effects.
- Easily reversible.
- Provides significant protection against STDs and PID.
- Can be used during lactation.
- Diaphragm may provide some protection against cervical neoplasia.
- Sponge available over the counter; one size fits all.

Disadvantages

- Both the diaphragm and the cervical cap require accurate fitting by a professional clinician, often accompanied by lengthy office visit.
- Properly trained clinicians not widely available, especially for fitting the cervical cap.
- Costs related to use may be high (i.e., professional care, purchase of products).

- May interfere with sexual spontaneity if not readily available.
- Learning insertion and removal techniques may be difficult.
- Perceived as aesthetically objectionable or messy by some individuals.
- Latex, rubber, polyurethane, or spermicide could cause irritation or allergy in either partner.
- Foul odor or vaginal discharge may occur if the product is left in place more than a few days.
- Oil or petroleum products can damage latex.
- Potential for vaginal trauma associated with difficult insertion or removal of the device.
- Increased risk of urinary tract infection (UTI) in diaphragm users (especially arcing spring).
- Potential for toxic shock syndrome (TSS).
- A few studies have reported Pap smear abnormalities with use of the cervical cap.
- Sponge is somewhat less effective in parous women and can fall out with voiding or defecating. To prevent expulsion, a finger may be held against the introitus. Push the sponge back up in place if it is protruding from the vagina.

Contraindications

- Allergy to latex, rubber, polyurethane, or spermicide.
- Vaginal bleeding, even menses (because of possible risk of TSS). However, the diaphragm may be used during menses.
- Delivery in prior six weeks or abortion in prior two weeks (for cap or sponge).
- Anatomic abnormalities that interfere with proper fitting of the cap or diaphragm.
- Inability to master insertion or removal techniques.
- Recurrent UTIs with use of the diaphragm.
- History of TSS.
- History of cervical malignancy or abnormal Pap that has not been evaluated (for cap).

Management Considerations

Fitting the Diaphragm. During the pelvic exam, check for a palpable pubic notch behind the symphysis pubis, as well as anatomic abnormalities. Estimate the diagonal length of the vaginal canal from the posterior vaginal fornix to the symphysis pubis, by inserting the middle and index fingers until the middle finger touches the posterior wall of the vagina. Use thumb of the same hand to mark the point that touches the symphysis pubis and withdraw fingers. Select a diaphragm with a diameter that equals the measurement from the tip of the middle finger to the point just in front of the thumb where symphysis pubis contact was made. Select the largest rim size that is comfortable for client. Insert the diaphragm and check its fit. The diaphragm should fit snugly between the posterior fornix and the symphysis pubis, touching lateral vaginal walls and covering the cervix. Check for displacement when the client bears down. Have her walk around the room, sit, and squat. Check again for displacement and client comfort. If the client feels the diaphragm while walking around, it may be too large. If it is easily displaced with a finger or with moving/walking, it can be displaced during intercourse. If in doubt about fit, try the next larger size. Two or three different sizes should be tried before a final decision is made. Instruct the client to practice removal and insertion three times, while you verify proper placement each time (Hatcher et al., 1998; Tagg, 1995).

Fitting the Cervical Cap. The client must be involved in the fitting process. During speculum examination, assist her to visualize her cervix. *Specific teaching sessions for health care professionals who will be fitting caps are strongly recommended.* Comprehensive training programs for prospective cap providers are available. Information on these programs may be obtained from the National Women's Health Network in Washington, DC.

During the pelvic exam, visualize the cervix to estimate cap size. The bimanual exam will determine the position and size of the cervix. The cervix must be fairly symmetrical, without excessive scarring or laceration that could interfere with complete contact between the cap rim and the cervix around its full circumference. The cervix also must be long enough to accommodate the depth of the cap. A cervix that is too flat cannot be fitted with the Prentif cap. Try two or more caps sizes to determine the best fit.

To insert the cap, pinch the sides of the cap together, compress the cap dome, insert into the vagina, and place over the cervix. As the dome is released, suction should form between the rim of the cap and the cervix. After inserting the cap, use one finger to feel around the entire circumference of the cap to be sure there are no gaps between the cap rim and the cervix. Probe the cap and cervix from various angles with a finger tip to be sure the cap is not easily dislodged. The cervix must be completely covered.

After a minute or two, check for evidence of suction by pinching the dome and tugging gently. The dome should feel collapsed (or dimpled) and the cap should resist the tug and not slide off easily. Finally, try to rotate the cap at the rim. If the cap rotates too easily or falls off, it is too large. If it does not rotate at all, it is too small and could cause trauma to the cervix. To remove the cap, press the index finger against the rim and tip the cap slightly to break the suction. Gently pull out the device. Instruct the client in proper insertion and removal techniques and have her practice three times during the visit, while you verify proper placement each time. (Best, 2000c; Hatcher et al., 1998; Scott, 1996).

Client Teaching and Counseling

A critical aspect of successful use of either the diaphragm or the cervical cap is that sufficient time be offered to the client for teaching and practice at the office visit. The following points should be part of client teaching.

- Devices may be inserted immediately prior to intercourse; however, some experts recommend waiting 30 minutes after cervical cap insertion to be sure that the seal has formed between the rim and the cervix.
- Devices must be left in place for a minimum of six hours after the last act of intercourse.
- Diaphragm may not be reliable if coitus is to take place in water because spermicide could wash away.
- Do not use during menses (potential for TSS). Have an alternative method, such as condoms, available.
- The danger signs of TSS include sudden high fever, vomiting, diarrhea, dizziness, faintness, weakness, sore throat, aching muscles or joints, rash.
- The diaphragm or cap should be inspected prior to insertion for cracks, holes, tears, or drying of rubber or latex.
- After using a cap or diaphragm, wash the device with soap and water, dry thoroughly, and store in its container.
- Bring the cap or diaphragm to yearly gynecologic visit so that fit can be reevaluated.

Specific Instructions for Diaphragm Use

- Place approximately one tablespoon of spermicidal cream or jelly in the dome and around the rim of the diaphragm.
- Insert the diaphragm up to six hours prior to intercourse.
- The diaphragm must remain in place for six to eight hours following each coitus. If coitus does not take place within six hours of insertion, remove the diaphragm and reapply spermicide. For subsequent

acts of coitus, spermicide is added with an inserter, without removing diaphragm.

Specific Instructions for Sponge Use

- Wet the sponge thoroughly with water. Gently squeeze the sponge to produce suds. Fold the sponge with dimple side facing upward and insert deeply into the vagina, sliding it along the posterior wall of the vagina. The dimple should be up against the cervix.
- The sponge may be inserted up to 24 hours prior to intercourse.
- Six hours after the last act of intercourse, the sponge may be removed by inserting a finger into the vagina and reaching up to find the string loop. Hook the finger around the loop and gently pull the sponge from the vagina. Relaxing and bearing down can facilitate removal. Package instructions are well illustrated (*Product Information, Today Sponge,* 2000).

Specific Instructions for Cervical Cap Use

- To use a cervical cap, the woman should be at least six weeks postpartum or two weeks postabortion.
- Fill the dome of the cap to one-third with spermicidal cream or jelly. Do *not* apply spermicide to the rim—this might interfere with the seal that must form around the cervix.
- Cap may be left in place up to 48 hours without regard to frequency of intercourse during that period. It is not necessary to insert additional spermicide.
- After inserting, check that the seal has formed around the cervix.

INTRAUTERINE DEVICES (IUDs)

Intrauterine devices (IUDs) are small objects, usually plastic, that are placed inside the uterus. They may contain substances such as copper, progesterone, or levonorgestrel that enhance effectiveness. One or two strings are attached that protrude into the vagina so that the presence of the device can be checked by the user and removal facilitated. IUDs are packaged in individual sterile units that include the device, insertion barrel, and manufacturer literature. IUDs are visible on x-ray.

Currently in the United States, three IUDs are available, the copper ParaGard-T-380A marketed by Gyno-Pharma; Progestasert, a progesterone-T device, available through Alza Corporation; and the LNG-IUS (brand name, Mirena by Berlex), which releases levonorgestrel (LNG).

By 1986, most U.S. companies had voluntarily withdrawn IUDs from the U.S. market, not for medical or scientific reasons, but primarily because of decreased popularity, negative consumer perception, increasing litigation costs, and subsequent difficulty obtaining liability insurance. The Dalkon Shield, associated with a high rate of pelvic infections and septic abortions, was removed from the U.S. market in 1975. The Lippes Loop was a popular IUD used in the 1970s and early 1980s. The Lippes Loop was designed to be used indefinitely; consequently, some women still have these in place as they approach menopause.

Fears of side effects or complications continue to hamper widespread acceptance of IUDs among potential users, physicians, and other family planning providers. The modern IUDs, however, are safe, highly effective, and convenient for carefully screened potential users. They should be offered to appropriate clients, especially when hormonal contraceptive methods are contraindicated or not desired. IUDs are also an excellent alternative for women considering sterilization who might be at risk for later regret (see section on sterilization). In many countries of the world, IUDs are the most popular reversible method of birth control.

ParaGard-T-380A

Also referred to as the CU-T, this was approved in the United States in 1984. It is a T-shaped polyurethane device with barium sulphate added (for x-ray visibility). A very fine copper wire is wound around a vertical stem and crossbar. A white polyethylene string attached through a hole in the "T" creates a double string effect that, after insertion, protrudes into the vagina. ParaGard-T-380A is approved for ten years of use, and may be effective for twelve or more years (GynoPharma, 1988; Hatcher et al., 1998).

Progesterone-T (Progestasert)

A T-shaped ethylene vinyl acetate copolymer, the vertical stem contains a reservoir holding 38 mg progesterone and barium sulphate in a silicone oil base. This IUD releases 65 mcg progesterone per day. It may stay in place one year, then must be removed and/or replaced. Black double string is attached to the hole in the base of the "T," which, after insertion, protrudes into the vagina. This was ap-

proved in the United States in 1976 (Alza Corp., 1988; Hatcher et al., 1998).

Levonorgestrel Intrauterine System— LNG-IUS (Mirena)

Approved by the FDA for use in the United States in December 2000, the levonorgestrel intrauterine system (LNG-IUS) consists of a T-shaped polyethylene frame with a steroid reservoir that contains LNG. The IUS releases a low dose of LNG, 20 mcg per day, into the uterine cavity for at least five years and may be effective up to seven years. It has a double thread tail. It is distributed in the United States by Berlex Laboratories, Inc. This system has been used by over 2 million women in Europe since the early 1990s. It has a success rate nearly equal to sterilization (Association of Reproductive Health Professionals [ARHP], 2001; Hatcher et al., 1998).

In addition to its effective contraception, this system has several noncontraceptive benefits: prevention of anemia, therapy for menorrhagia and dysmenorrhea. It protects against uterine fibroid development and growth. Ectopic pregnancy is rare. The antiproliferative effect of the LNG-IUS on the endometrium offers therapy against the proliferative action of estrogen during postmenopausal hormone replacement therapy. It is being studied in the treatment of endometriosis, in the protection of the endometrium exposed to tamoxifen during breast cancer treatment, and as an alternative to hysterectomy in women with bleeding problems. Side effects may include acne, oily skin, benign follicular cysts, and mood changes.

Mirena will alter bleeding patterns. During the first three to six weeks of use, the number of bleeding and spotting days may be increased and bleeding patterns may be irregular. Thereafter, the number of bleeding and spotting days usually decreases, but bleeding patterns remain irregular. Within a year, many women experience little or no bleeding. Overall, there is a 90 percent decrease in menstrual blood loss (Andersson, Odlind, & Rybo, 1994; Hubacher & Grimes, 2002; Pakarinen, Toivonen, & Luukkainen, 2001; Ronnerdag & Odlind, 1999).

Mechanisms of Action

IUDs appear to work primarily by preventing sperm from fertilizing ova. There are effects on fertilization, endometrium, and implantation. IUDs are not primarily abortifacient (although this may occur).

When a foreign body is in the uterus, the endometrium reacts by releasing white blood cells, enzymes, and prostoglandins. These endometrial reactions appear to prevent sperm from reaching the fallopian tubes. In addition, copper-bearing IUDs release copper ions into the fluids of the uterus and the fallopian tubes, enhancing the debilitating effects on sperm. Studies have found fertilization to be rare in IUD users. If fertilization does occur, the local foreign body inflammatory response and increased local production of prostoglandins prevent implantation and cause lysis and/or dislodgment of the blastocyte from the endometrium.

The LNG-IUS and the Progestasert also act by thickening the cervical mucus, thus inhibiting sperm motility and function. With long-term use they also produce an atrophic endometrium. These devices may also prevent ovulation in some cycles, especially in the first months of use (ARHP, 2001; Ortiz, Croxatto, & Bardin, 1996).

Effectiveness

IUDs are highly effective in preventing pregnancy, even more effective than OCs. Effectiveness is impacted by IUD characteristics, such as size, shape, expulsion rates, presence of copper or progesterone; and by user characteristics, such as age and parity. Also influential are medical variables, such as experience of the clinician inserting the device, the ease of insertion, placement of the device at the top of the fundus of the uterus, and likelihood that expulsion will be detected (see Table 9–3) (Andersson et al., 1994; Hatcher et al., 1998; Sieven, Stern, Coutinho, Mattos, & Diaz, 1991).

Advantages

- Once inserted, an IUD requires no continuing action, equipment, or motivation on the part of the user. Is immediately effective.
- Highly effective.
- Continuously effective.
- Very safe for carefully selected users.
- Allows for sexual spontaneity.
- Consider for women who have difficulty following directions or remembering to use a contraceptive or to take a pill every day.
- No messy substances needed.
- After initial cost little additional expense.
- Mirena (LNG-IUS) has several noncontraceptive benefits.
- Return to fertility not impaired.

- Progesterone-releasing IUD and the LNG-IUS may decrease menstrual blood flow and dysmenorrhea.
- Can be used during lactation.

Disadvantages

Use of an IUD carries potential for some side effects and several serious complications; however, careful screening and counseling of potential users can prevent many of them. *If a contraindication to use arises, or when in doubt about the significance of a symptom or complaint, the recommended action is to remove the IUD immediately.* Always provide the client an alternate method of contraception. IUDs are best suited for parous women not desiring future pregnancy.

GynoPharma, the manufacturer of ParaGard-T-380A, distributes directly to physicians and clinics, provides detailed guidelines about who should use the product, and recommends it only for women who have had at least one child and are in a stable, monogamous relationship.

- Insertion requires a skilled professional.
- May aggravate or initiate menstrual cramping.
- May increase bleeding patterns.
- User may experience pain or nausea during insertion.
- User must regularly check for presence of the IUD string.
- May increase the risk of pelvic infection, which could affect future fertility (LNG-IUS may lower PID risk).
- Provides no protection against HIV or STDs.
- Device can be expelled without the user's being aware.
- String may be felt by the partner.
- Progestasert effective only one year; ParaGard-T-380A for ten years; Mirena, LNG-IUS for five years.
- User may neglect to see a health care professional for several years.

Contraindications

Carefully screen potential IUD users for contraindications. Include general and focused histories, a physical examination, appropriate current lab work (CBC, Pap smear, STD testing) and other assessments as indicated.

Absolute Contraindications (IUD Not Recommended)

- Current pelvic inflammatory disease (PID) or PID in past 3 months.
- Known or suspected pregnancy.
- Uterine anomaly.

Strong Relative Contraindications (Strongly Encourage Choice of Another Contraceptive Method)

- History of ectopic pregnancy, especially if future pregnancy is desired.
- Undiagnosed, abnormal vaginal bleeding.
- Risk factors for PID: multiple sexual partners; past history of STD, especially gonorrhea or chlamydia; postpartum endometritis; infection following abortion in past three months; purulent cervicitis.
- Unresolved, abnormal Pap smear.
- Difficult access to medical care.
- Impaired ability (physical or mental) to check for IUD string.
- Known or suspected bleeding disorder.
- Valvular heart disease.
- Anatomic variations that make insertion or retention difficult (e.g., DES exposure, fibroids).
- Severe dysmenorrhea, heavy menses, endometriosis (LNG-IUS may decrease pain and bleeding).
- Anemia.
- History of fainting or vasovagal response.
- Allergy to copper.
- History of impaired fertility (in a client desiring future pregnancy).

Managing Problems and Complications

- Spotting or bleeding may occur at the time of insertion or anytime after. Evaluate for anemia (though less likely with Progestasert and LNG-IUS), infection, pregnancy, and other pathology. Treat according to findings. Remove IUD for severe anemia (Hgb < 9 gm) or uterine infection.
- Cramping or pain also may occur at the time of insertion or at any time after. Giving a dose of a NSAID (assuming no allergy) prior to insertion is helpful. If these problems are severe, persistent or intolerable, remove the IUD. Partial expulsion of the IUD, uterine perforation, cervical or pelvic infection, and pregnancy (intrauterine or ectopic) must be ruled out.
- The IUD may be expulsed or partially expulsed. Most often, expulsion occurs during the first few weeks to months after insertion. Correct placement of the device high in the uterine fundus reduces the risk of expulsion. For partial expulsion, remove the IUD. In either case evaluate for uterine perforation, pregnancy, or infection. If no further problems are identified, another IUD may be inserted. A five- to seven-day course of Doxycycline 100 mg b.i.d. is recommended.

- The IUD can become embedded. If it cannot be removed after reasonable attempts, refer the client to a gynecologist.
- The IUD string may become lost. Attempt to determine whether the device has been partially or completely expelled. Again, evaluate for uterine perforation, infection, pregnancy. If the IUD is determined to still be in place (this can be done with ultrasound), the strings are often in the cervical canal. Insertion of a Pap smear cytobrush into the endocervical canal and rotating it while withdrawing the brush will often extract the strings.
- Uterine perforation can occur. Perforation is most common during insertion, but can occur at any time. Suspect perforation if pain is present; if the string is no longer palpable; if the plastic of the device is felt or visible in the cervix. Ultrasound can help to confirm perforation. If perforation is suspected, refer the client to a gynecologist.
- Pregnancy, ectopic pregnancy (low incidence). There is an increased risk of septic abortion if pregnancy occurs. With delayed menses or suspected pregnancy, evaluate for pregnancy and infection. Ectopic pregnancy rates are higher among users of Progestasert than among users of copper IUD. LNG-IUS has the lowest ectopic pregnancy rate of any IUD. Of users who become pregnant with IUD in place:
  - One-half will experience spontaneous abortion.
  - Twenty-five percent will abort if the IUD is removed early in pregnancy.
  - If the IUD is left in place, severe pelvic infection resulting in death could occur.
  - Five percent will have an ectopic pregnancy.

  Inform the client of the above; assist her to determine whether to continue the pregnancy.
- Potential for increased risk of PID. Most reported cases of PID occur during the first three months after IUD insertion. This is believed to be due to introduction of bacteria into the uterus during the insertion procedure. Beyond three months postinsertion, when client selection procedures include diligent screening for women with risk factors for STDs and PID, the incidence of IUD related pelvic infection is low. *Appropriate* IUD users are at no greater risk of developing PID than non-users. PID is a serious complication that can be life threatening. Infection must be promptly and aggressively treated and the IUD removed. Providers and users of IUDs must be alert to the signs and symptoms suggestive of pelvic infection:

- Fever of 101°F or higher.
- Purulent discharge from the vagina/cervix.
- Abdominal/pelvic pain.
- Dyspareunia.
- Cervicitis.
- Suprapubic tenderness or guarding.
- Pain with movement of the cervix on examination.
- Tenderness on bimanual examination.
- Adnexal tenderness or mass.

(Andersson et al., 1994; ARHP, 2001; Intrauterine devices, 2000; Nelson, 1995).

Management Considerations

- ◆ Women planning to use an IUD must be carefully screened for contraindications. The ideal candidate for an IUD is a woman in a mutually monogamous relationship who has had at least one full term pregnancy. Give each IUD user an identification card with the name and a picture of the IUD, the day of insertion, and the recommended removal date printed on it. Written informed consent is needed.
- ◆ If the client is not accustomed to following a calendar, inform her about recommended dates for checkups and IUD removal.
- ◆ Samples of IUDs should be available so that the client can handle and examine them.
- ◆ Insertion may take place at any time during the menstrual cycle (insertion may be more comfortable at midcycle, when the cervix is softer) as long as it is certain that the client is not pregnant. Higher infection and expulsion rates are noted when IUDs are inserted during menses. The IUD may be inserted at 6 weeks postpartum. Studies conducted in other countries have found that an IUD may be safely inserted immediately after delivery of the placenta (within 10 minutes). Expulsion rates are only slightly higher than for some other types of insertions. IUDs may also be placed during cesarean section with even lower expulsion rates. High fundal placement and a provider trained in these specific postpartum insertion techniques are essential. Higher expulsion rates are associated with later postpartum IUD insertions (more than 10 minutes but fewer than 42 days after full-term delivery). Prophylactic antibiotic use at time of insertion is not recommended.
- ◆ Insertions of IUDs require skill and experience on the part of the provider. Practicing insertions with a model and then several supervised insertions are strongly advised.

- ◆ IUD removal may take place at any time during the menstrual cycle, but may be easier at midcycle or at the time of menses.

(Andersson et al., 1994; ARHP, 2001; Intrauterine devices, 2000; Nelson, 1995; Ronnerdag & Odlind, 1999).

Client Teaching and Counseling

Several points are covered during client teaching and counseling.

- ◆ What to expect during and after IUD insertion.
- ◆ How and when to check for the IUD string (frequently during the first few months, then after each period or when abnormal cramping occurs).
- ◆ Likely bleeding patterns.
- ◆ Signs of infection.
- ◆ Importance of keeping track of periods. Teach the client the IUD early danger signs, using *PAINS:*

  *P*eriod late, abnormal spotting or bleeding.
  *A*bdominal pain, pain with intercourse.
  *I*nfection exposure (especially gonorrhea), abnormal discharge.
  *N*ot feeling well, chills, fever.
  *S*tring missing, shorter, or longer.

(ARHP, 2001; Hatcher et al., 1998; Nelson, 1995).

PERMANENT BIRTH CONTROL

Essure, a technologically new, non-incision procedure, is considered a permanent method of birth control that is 99.8% effective in preventing pregnancy after two years of study (Essure, 2002). Data beyond two years are lacking. Micro-inserts of polyester fibers and metals are placed in the fallopian tubes during hysteroscopy in a 35-minute outpatient procedure. Women generally are able to go home 45 minutes after the procedure is completed, and resume normal activities within 1 to 2 days. No general anesthesia is required. A back-up contraceptive method is used for 3 months until the inserts are totally enmeshed with tissue and block the tubes. At that time, a hysterosalpingogram is done to be sure the inserts are properly placed and are totally blocking the tubes. Essure does not protect against STDs, and like any birth control method, does not guarantee contraception 100%. Women who may desire a future pregnancy should not use this method; it is considered irreversible. Surgery would be required to remove the inserts but there is no guarantee of future fertility. For further information, see the Essure web site: www.essure.com.

VOLUNTARY STERILIZATION

Sterilization is the surgical interruption or closure of the pathways for sperm or ova, preventing fertilization. These methods are considered permanent means of contraception, although some surgical procedures to reverse both vasectomies and tubal ligations have been successful. Sterilization is the most popular method of contraception in the United States and worldwide.

Female sterilization is accomplished by bilateral occlusion of the fallopian tubes, commonly referred to as bilateral tubal ligation (BTL). The fallopian tubes are ligated and cut, occluded with clips or rings, electrocoagulated or plugged to prevent the ovum from moving toward the uterus and joining with sperm. Sterilization is considered to be a safe operative procedure. A hysterectomy (removal of the uterus) accomplishes sterilization, but should *never* be performed solely for that purpose.

Male sterilization, or vasectomy, is an operative procedure that blocks the vas deferens to prevent the passage of sperm into ejaculated seminal fluid. Considered a simple procedure, it can be performed quickly, safely, and inexpensively in an office or clinic setting (Hatcher et al., 1998; Sterilization, 1996).

Sterilization Techniques

Sterilization techniques may be performed using general or local anesthesia with sedation. Local anesthesia with light sedation has definite safety advantages over general anesthesia.

Tubal sterilization can be performed postpartum, postabortion, or as an interval procedure (unrelated to pregnancy). Performing sterilization during the follicular phase of the menstrual cycle is desirable to prevent luteal phase pregnancy. Pregnancy testing should be performed and effective contraception used until after the sterilization procedure.

Tubal occlusion methods include unipolar or bipolar electrocoagulation with or without tubal excision, ligation, and excision by various surgical techniques (Pomeroy, Irving, Prichard/Parkland, fibriectomy, Uchida), or use of various rings, bands or clips (Silastic bands or rings, Falope rings, Hulka or Filshie clips) (Hatcher et al., 1998, 2001; Sterilization, 1996; Update on female sterilization, 1996).

Suprapubic Minilaparotomy. Performed at four weeks or more postpartum or four weeks or more postabortion, i.e., interval BTL (when the uterus is fully involuted). Usually it is performed in lithotomy position. The procedure involves a small (2–5 cm) abdominal incision just above the pubic hairline. The uterus is elevated so that the uterus and tubes are close to the incision. The tubes are lifted, identified, and ligated by any of several occlusion techniques; the incision is sutured.

Laparoscopy. Laparascopic BTL is generally used for an interval procedure. A laparoscope consists of a viewing instrument, light source, and operating channel. *Single puncture technique* involves a small subumbilical incision. The abdomen is insufflated with a gaseous combination of nitrous oxide, carbon dioxide, and room air; the laparoscope is inserted, and the tubes are grasped and occluded through the operating channel of the instrument. With *double puncture technique,* a second tiny incision is made in the suprapubic region through which the operating channel is inserted and the procedure performed. Following bilateral tubal occlusion, the organs are inspected, the scope removed, gas gently expelled, and the incisions closed.

Subumbilical Minilaparotomy. Most frequently used during the immediate postpartum/postabortion period, when the uterus and tubes remain high in the abdomen. A small (1.5–3.0 cm) incision is made just below the umbilicus. Oviducts are usually easily reached for the occlusion procedure. Lithotomy position is not needed, and organ manipulation and instrumentation are less extensive, facilitating a rapid recovery.

Bilateral Tubal Ligation by Laparotomy. BTL using an abdominal incision greater than 5 cm, or during cesarean section, is associated with slightly higher morbidity and complication rates. BTLs performed during cesarean section, however, are relatively common.

Vaginal Approach. For interval BTL, direct visualization of the pelvic organs can be accomplished through an incision high in the vagina, posterior to the cervix (called a colpotomy). The tubes can be reached and directly sutured or cut. This method is rarely used, being less safe and less effective than other methods described above. Infection is more common and the technique is difficult to learn and perform.

Nonsurgical Female Sterilization. Nonsurgical sterilization for women is being studied in several countries around the world. It is not available in the United States. The method involves the use of *quinacrine hydrochloride,* a drug long used to prevent and treat malaria and other parasitic diseases. The quinacrine method of nonsurgical female sterilization (QS) involves transcervical uterine insertion of quinacrine pellets with a modified IUD inserter. This is done during the proliferative phase of the menstrual cycle, usually between the sixth and twelfth days of the cycle. A repeat insertion during the next cycle is needed. The drug causes inflammation and fibrosis in the proximal fallopian tubes leading to sterility. Backup contraception needs to be continued for at least twelve weeks. The failure rate is somewhat higher with QS than with all other forms of female surgical sterilization, at 1 to 3 percent. Cost would be substantially lower. To date, more than 100,000 quinacrine pellet sterilizations have been performed worldwide. No deaths attributed to the use of the pellets have been reported. Experts conclude that further research is needed on toxicology, teratogenicity, and potential carcinogenicity of quinacrine. In the meantime, long-term follow-up studies on women who have already received the pellets are ongoing (Barnett, 1994; Sarin, 1999).

Vasectomy (Male Sterilization). Each vas deferens is cut between two ligated sections, preventing sperm from mingling with ejaculate. Local anesthetic (e.g., 1 percent lidocaine without epinephrine) is injected into each side of the scrotum, where a small incision is made to isolate, occlude, and usually resect the vasa. Closure of the incision(s) requires one or two sutures. A no-scalpel technique for performing vasectomies is now widely used throughout the world and United States. This requires an instrument that "punctures" the scrotal skin and vas sheath. Once this is accomplished, the procedures to isolate, occlude, and resect are the same as for the scalpel technique. Little bleeding occurs, and no sutures are required. About twenty ejaculations are required for existing sperm in the vasa deferentia to be cleared. (Hatcher et al., 1998; No-scalpel vasectomy, 1994; Sterilization, 1996).

Effectiveness

Published in 1996, the U.S. Collaborative Review of Sterilization conducted by the Centers for Disease Control (CREST Study) assessed, over a ten-year period, the long-term risks and failure rates of female sterilization. Failure rates for BTL were found to be higher than previously believed. CREST reported an overall failure rate of 1.9 percent, which is more than double the usually reported failure rate of 0.4 percent. The 0.4 percent rate, however, reflects failures that occurred only during the first year after sterilization (Table 9–3), whereas CREST followed women for ten years or longer.

The CREST study found that women sterilized at a young age had a higher risk of method failure. Failure rates also varied by type of procedure. Unipolar coagula-

tion, interval partial salpingectomy, and postpartum partial salpingectomy all provided consistent protection over ten years. On the other hand, silicone band application, spring clip application, and bipolar coagulation provided less protection, with failure rates increasing consistently and substantially over the ten-year period. In addition, a high percentage (33 percent) of pregnancies that occur following BTL run the risk of being ectopic. Any sterilized woman who suspects she might be pregnant should immediately contact her clinician because of the potential serious health risks involved.

Pregnancy rates following vasectomy (not including pregnancies resulting from intercourse before the reproductive tract was cleared of sperm) are less than 1 percent. Failures may result from errors in technique, such as failing to occlude the correct structure or spontaneous recanalization of the vas. Rarely, congenital duplication of the vas may be present and go unnoticed at the time of the procedure (Peterson et al., 1997; Sterilization, 1996).

Advantages

- One-time decision provides permanent sterility.
- Highly effective, convenient.
- Considered safe; low complication and morbidity rates.
- Following procedure and recovery, very few or no systemic side effects occur.
- BTL has some protective effect against ovarian cancer and PID.
- Partner cooperation not required.
- Short recovery time.
- Certain techniques can be performed immediately after childbirth or abortion.
- BTL immediately effective.
- No interference with love-making.
- Low long-term risks.
- Low long-term cost, covered by 85–90 percent of private insurance plans and Medicaid.
- Can be performed while lactating.
- Vasectomy is equally effective, simpler, safer, much less expensive than BTL.

Disadvantages

- Carries risks inherent in any surgical procedure (infection, injury to other organs, hemorrhage, complications of anesthesia).
- Procedures are difficult to reverse.
- Initial cost may be high.

- Some pain/discomfort during and right after procedure.
- Vasectomy is not immediately effective.
- Some states and third party payors require a waiting period between time of counseling/consent and actual procedure.
- Provides no protection against HIV or STDs.
- Chance of regret.
- Uterine perforation is possible.
- Some women report menstrual pattern changes, increased dysmenorrhea, PMS following BTL. Studies have found no evidence of a post-tubal sterilization syndrome causing menstrual-related abnormalities (Peterson et al., 2000; Gentile, Kaufman, & Helbig, 1998).
- If BTL fails, high probability of ectopic pregnancy.
- Studies on the relationship between vasectomy and the development of prostate cancer, testicular cancer, and atherosclerosis have failed to show a correlation (Peterson et al., 1997; Sterilization, 1996).
- Vasectomy complications can occur (infection, bleeding, hematoma formation, congestive epididymitis, sperm granulation).

Contraindications

- Lack of adequately trained personnel to perform the procedure (especially important for laparoscopy techniques).
- Known or suspected pregnancy.
- Existing infection of the reproductive tract.
- Client ambivalence about future pregnancy or sterilization.
- Serious uncontrolled health problems.

Management Considerations

- A high skill level, involving special training and extensive practice, is needed to perform these procedures (especially for laparoscopy procedures).
- The client must provide informed consent prior to the procedure.
- When federal funds, and in some cases state funds, are used to reimburse for sterilization, the client must have signed informed consent at least thirty days prior to the procedure or before delivery or abortion, if sterilization is planned to immediately follow one of these procedures. The client must also be 21 years of age or older and mentally competent.

- Preoperative assessment includes history (with particular attention to the last menstrual period and most recent use of contraception, to be reasonably confident that the woman is not pregnant) and physical examination (with focus on position and mobility of uterus and detection of possible infection). Minimum lab requirements are hemoglobin and urinalysis.
- The client should have someone accompany her or him home following the procedure.
- The client should rest for a few days following the procedure.
- Sexual activity may be resumed after about one week for women and after two to three days for men.
- Men must be reminded that they are not sterile initially. Another method of contraception must be used for several weeks or for at least the next twenty ejaculations. Microscopic examination of semen is the best way to ascertain that sterility has been achieved.

Client Teaching and Counseling

For several reasons, client teaching and counseling are especially important when an individual is considering sterilization. Sterilization is a surgical procedure, thus involving some risk; there are legal implications; and it is meant to be permanent. Postoperative regret about the sterilization decision is a serious concern. Indicators of future regret include young age (under age 34), poverty, having a BTL postpartum or at the time of a cesarean section, change in marital status, decision was made during a time of personal or family crisis, children very young at the time of procedure, or pressure from partner to have the procedure. Reversal procedures often fail and are very costly. In lieu of sterilization or to postpone the decision for women at risk for later regret, women should be informed about and offered long-term reversible contraceptive options such as IUDs, implants, or DMPA. Documentation of adequate teaching/counseling about sterilization is essential. In addition to the points in the counseling process that follow, also refer to the section at the beginning of this chapter on General Management Considerations, Client Education and Informed Consent (*Family planning counseling,* 1992; Hatcher et al., 2001; Peterson et al., 1997; Wilcox, Chu, Eaker, Zeger, & Peterson, 1991).

- Assess client's interest in and readiness for sterilization, especially risk factors for later regret.

- Emphasize permanence, discuss possibility of failure; provide alternative reversible method information.
- Explain procedure using visual aids, discuss risks/benefits.
- Women who undergo sterilization are much less likely to use condoms or other barriers for prevention of STDs and HIV than are nonsterilized women. Men and women should be assessed and counseled about high-risk sexual behaviors and how to adequately protect themselves and their partners.
- Have client read and sign informed consent form.
- Schedule appointment; provide copy of necessary forms.
- Discuss cost and payment.
- Provide pre- and postoperative instructions.
- Schedule postoperative follow-up visit.

FERTILITY AWARENESS METHODS

Fertility awareness methods (FAM)—also referred to as menstrual cycle charting, natural family planning (NFP), or periodic abstinence—involve making observations and charting of scientifically proven fertility signs that determine whether a woman is fertile on any given day. The three primary fertility signs are (1) waking temperature (basal body temperature), (2) cervical mucus/fluid, and (3) cervical position. These are normal physiological changes caused by hormonal fluctuations during the menstrual cycle that can be observed and charted so that fertile and infertile periods can be identified.

Fertility awareness methods (FAM) are used in combination with coital abstinence or barrier methods during fertile days, when the desire is to prevent pregnancy. Fertility awareness also helps a couple understand how to achieve pregnancy, detect probable pregnancy, detect impaired fertility, or manage PMS. The term *natural family planning* implies exclusive use of these methods and that absolute abstinence is maintained during the fertile phase. The charting of observed changes is an important component for successful use of these methods. The techniques of FAM include basal body temperature method, cervical mucus/fluid (Billings or ovulation) method, and symptothermal method. At least two of these techniques should be used simultaneously. Figure 9–1 is an example of a natural family planning chart for recording fertility signs. Clients may design their own charts or adapt the one shown for their own use.

The calendar (rhythm) method is the original method based on periodic abstinence and is still widely used around the world. It is much less reliable than the newer methods listed above, however, because it relies on a statistical prediction based on past cycles to predict fertility in future cycles. With newer, more effective and well researched methods available, the calendar (rhythm) method is no longer recommended.

Modern fertility awareness methods are considered reliable and are acceptable to diverse population groups with varied religious and ethical beliefs and to couples who do not wish to use other methods for medical or personal reasons. (Hatcher et al., 1998; Weschler, 1995)

Mechanism of Action

Pregnancy is prevented by avoidance of unprotected intercourse during times that a woman is determined to be fertile.

Calendar (Rhythm) Method. This involves calculation of a woman's fertile period based on three assumptions:

- Ovulation occurs on the fourteenth day, plus or minus two days, prior to next menses.
- Sperm are viable for three days.
- The ovum is viable for 24 hours.

The client must chart the length of her menstrual cycles for a minimum of eight months. The earliest day in the cycle she is likely to be fertile is determined by subtracting 18 days from the length of the shortest cycle occurring during that eight-month period. The latest day of potential fertility is obtained by subtracting 11 days from the longest cycle. These two numbers represent the beginning and end of the fertile period.

For example, if the client's shortest cycle was 27 days, subtract 18 from 27; on the 9th day (27 minus 18) the client must begin to abstain from sexual intercourse. If her longest cycle was 34 days, on the 23rd day (34 minus 11) abstinence may be ended. She must abstain from day 9 through day 23, a total of 14 days, during each cycle. This technique is most effective when menstrual cycles are regular. With less variable cycles, the period of required abstinence is shorter. The abstinent period cannot be less than seven days.

As noted earlier, the calendar (rhythm) method is not based on tested scientific principles, relying on information from past cycles to predict fertile patterns in future cycles. Couples should instead be encouraged to utilize the more reliable methods to be discussed now (Hatcher et al., 1998; Weschler, 1995).

Basal Body Temperature (BBT) Method. Basal body temperature (waking temperature) refers to the lowest temperature reached by the body of a healthy person,

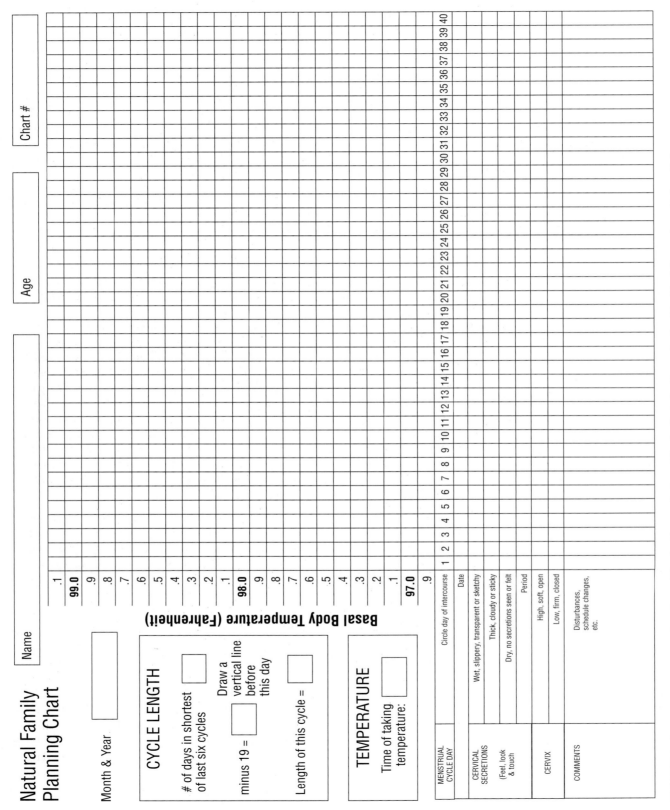

FIGURE 9–1. Natural family planning chart. (*Used with permission of the Institute for Reproductive Health at Georgetown University.*)

taken upon wakening. Generally, a special BBT thermometer should be used (as opposed to a fever thermometer) because the temperatures are shown in increments of 0.1 degrees, and are easier to read and record. The temperature is taken daily after a minimum of three consecutive hours of sleep, before rising, eating, or drinking and is recorded on the chart (see Figure 9–1). The preovulatory temperatures are suppressed by estrogen, whereas postovulatory temperatures are increased by 0.4° to 0.8°F under the influence of heat inducing progesterone. Temperatures typically rise within a day or two *after* ovulation has occurred and remain elevated for 12 to 16 days, until menstruation begins. If the woman were to become pregnant, the temperatures would remain elevated throughout the pregnancy. Some women experience a drop in BBT just prior to ovulation, but this is not a consistent occurrence. Based on the patterns observed, one should be able to predict the end of the fertile phase and the beginning of the safe, luteal phase of the cycle. If using BBT method alone, the client should avoid unprotected intercourse from the beginning of the menstrual cycle (or at least from day 4) until the BBT has been elevated for three days. Using other fertility awareness methods along with BBT should allow for shortening of the abstinent period.

It is important to know that numerous factors can delay or even prevent ovulation, thus prolonging the follicular (estrogenic) phase. These may include stress, travel, illness, medication, strenuous exercise, and sudden weight changes. Once ovulation occurs and the temperature rises, however, it is usually a standard 12 to 16 days until menses. (Hatcher et al., 1998; Kass-Annese & Danzer, 1992; Labbock & Queenan, 1989; Rodrigues-Garcia, 1989; Weschler, 1995).

Cervical Mucus (Billings or Ovulation) Method. This method assesses the character of cervical mucus. The mucus secreted by exocrine glands lining the cervical canal changes in character during the menstrual cycle in response to hormonal levels. The woman is taught to begin checking cervical mucus the first day the period is over and to check it prior to urinating about three times each day. She should first note whether there is a sensation of wetness or dryness in the vaginal area. Then the woman should obtain fluid from the vaginal opening and feel it with her fingers to note changes in the physical properties of the mucus. During a normal menstrual cycle, a woman experiences menses, then a few days of a dry sensation, then early mucus (may be milky white,

translucent, yellow or clear, sticky at first and then smooth). As ovulation approaches, the mucus becomes more abundant, clear, slippery, and smooth. The mucus can be stretched between two fingers without breaking. This is called *spinnbarkeit* and closely resembles egg whites. The vaginal sensation is one of lubrication, being wet and slippery. These characteristics correspond to the peak in estrogen occurring immediately prior to ovulation. This mucus is more permeable to sperm and can prolong the life of sperm. It is now known that sperm can live up to five days in the environment of wet quality cervical mucus. The *peak day* is the last day of egg white-quality cervical mucus, or the lubricative vaginal sensation, or any midcycle spotting.

Before ovulation, the only days that are considered safe are those dry days in which there is no cervical fluid present. Postovulation, the woman is considered infertile the evening of the fourth consecutive day after the peak day. Charting must be done, noting observed cervical mucus characteristics.

Cervical position is an optional fertility sign that can be assessed to augment or confirm the changes in temperature and cervical mucus/fluid. The woman should insert one finger into the vagina and feel the conditions of the cervix, beginning when menses has ended. She palpates the cervix for height in the vagina (low, midway, high), softness (firm, medium, soft), openness (closed, partly open, open), and wetness (nothing, sticky, creamy, egg white). Near ovulation, the cervix feels high/deep in the vagina, soft, open, and wet. These observations should be noted on the chart as well (Hatcher et al., 1998; Katz, 1991; Labbock & Queenan, 1989).

Symptothermal Method. This method merely connotes that at least two indicators are being combined to identify the fertile period. The term *fertility awareness methods* also implies that more than one indicator is used. The symptothermal method usually combines the BBT and cervical mucus methods. It may also incorporate the changes in the cervix (position, texture, openness) described earlier, as well as secondary fertility signs that a woman might observe, such as breast tenderness, libido changes, midcycle pain, spotting, fluid retention, etc.

The Standard Days Method. A new natural family planning method has been developed by the Institute for Reproductive Health at Georgetown University called the Standard Days Method. It is only appropriate for women with menstrual cycles between 26 and 32 days long. For these women, days 8 through 19 of their cycles are the days when pregnancy is likely to occur, so unprotected intercourse is avoided. On all other days, the probability of becoming pregnant is very low. Most women using the Standard Days Method utilize Cycle-Beads, a string of color-coded beads that help her keep track of the fertile and infertile days. No calculations or observation are involved, making it easy for providers to teach and for clients to understand (The Standard Days Method, 2003).

Home Test Kits and Monitors

Home test kits and monitors that predict when ovulation occurs are available from most pharmacies. Most kits/devices measure LH, which can be detected the day before or the day of ovulation. Most were developed to help women achieve conception.

For natural family planning, intercourse should be avoided until four days after ovulation has occurred. Kits and monitors are being developed to help couples who wish to avoid pregnancy by identifying the beginning and the end of the fertile time.

Effectiveness

Fertility awareness methods are considered moderately effective for preventing pregnancy (see Table 9–3). Studies have concluded that when used perfectly, FAMs are very effective in preventing pregnancy with a 3.4 percent failure rate in the first year of correct and consistent use. It is extremely unforgiving, however, of imperfect use. Breaking the rules entails a 27 percent risk of pregnancy per cycle. Effectiveness would be increased if couples limited unprotected intercourse to the postovulatory period only. These techniques require high levels of commitment and participation by both partners. High motivation to prevent pregnancy and ability to learn the necessary concepts are needed. Failures are often related to poor understanding or improper teaching and poor use of methods. Some pregnancies result from couples having trouble coping with periods of abstinence. They may intentionally "break the rules" and take chances. Pregnancy must be an acceptable possible outcome of use of these methods. (Trussell & Grammer-Strawn, 1991; Weschler, 1995).

Advantages

- No damaging side effects.
- No interruption of normal body functions.
- Immediate return to fertility.
- No external or internal devices or chemicals.

- Acceptable to most religious groups.
- Low cost.
- Increases awareness of normal female body processes and fertility.
- Can facilitate diagnosis of gynecologic problems.
- Encourages communication between partners.
- The concepts and charting skills learned can also be applied to planning conception, detecting pregnancy, diagnosis and treatment of fertility problems, and mapping symptoms of PMS.
- Use of Standard Days method with CycleBeads is easily understood by most clients.

Disadvantages

- High failure rate with incorrect use.
- Interferes with sexual spontaneity.
- Requires copious recordkeeping and intensive, ongoing teaching and partner cooperation.
- Couples may have difficulty learning the techniques.
- Periodic abstinence is difficult for some couples.
- Is a less reliable method if infection is present.
- Is a less reliable method if menstrual periods are irregular.
- No identifiable BBT pattern is seen in some women's cycles, even when ovulating.
- Emotional and physiological stress, shift work, and travel can alter the timing of ovulation.
- No protection provided against HIV or STDs.
- Methods are unreliable during lactation and perimenopausal periods.
- If conception occurs, it may involve the fertilization of an "old" or overripe egg and an increased theoretical risk of fetal abnormalities. Convincing studies are unavailable either to support or negate this concern.

Contraindications

There are no absolute contraindications to fertility awareness methods; however, if unplanned pregnancy would be unacceptable or inadvisable for a client or her family, for any reason, a more reliable contraceptive method should be considered. Relative contraindications include the following.

- Irregular menses.
- History of anovulatory cycles.
- Inability to keep careful records.
- Lack of partner cooperation.
- Frequent or persistent vaginal infections.

Management Considerations

Clients must receive intensive and ongoing teaching by a trained fertility awareness counselor usually over several months. They also will need assistance with interpreting charts. It is recommended that health care professionals be familiar with the available community resources for teaching these techniques and with the philosophy and teaching/learning resources used by the counselor. A philosophical "match" between the needs and beliefs of the client and those of the counselor is helpful.

Teaching and counseling involves several aspects.

- Explanation of the normal menstrual cycle.
- Explanation of how the methods work.
- Selection of the methods.
- Techniques involved in the methods selected (e.g., how and when to take BBT, how to evaluate cervical mucus).
- Procedures for charting.
- How to determine fertile periods.
- Alternative sexual activity for fertile periods.

Further information on NFP method research, videos, tools, etc., as well as natural family planning instructor training, may be requested from: Resource Center at the Institute for Reproductive Health at Georgetown University (see Website: www.irh.org).

LACTATIONAL AMENORRHEA METHOD (LAM)

The Lactational Amenorrhea Method (LAM) is a highly effective temporary family planning method for breast-feeding women. LAM is based on the utilization of lactational infertility for protection from pregnancy. LAM can provide women with natural protection against pregnancy for up to six months after a birth, and following the guidelines for this method encourages the timely introduction of complementary methods of birth control while breastfeeding continues beyond six months. Studies have shown that women who meet the criteria for the method have a less than 2 percent pregnancy rate.

According to Hatcher et al. (2001, pp. 40–41), if the woman answers "no" to all the following questions, LAM is a good method for her. If she answers "yes" to even one question, it most likely is not the appropriate method for her. Some method of contraception should be incorporated with LAM for backup while she is breastfeeding, and a method should be provided for use when she starts to give the baby food, other milk supplement, when the

baby is 6 months old, and/or when she has her period for the first time.

- Is the baby 6 months old or more? If "yes," she should choose another method.
- Has she had two consecutive days of menstrual bleeding (not counting bleeding the first eight weeks after the birth)? If "yes," she needs to choose another method.
- Is she breastfeeding less often or supplementing with other than water? If "yes," choose another method.
- Has a nurse, doctor, or other provider told her not to breastfeed? LAM is not appropriate if so. Lactation is contraindicated with certain drugs, such as lithium, ergotamine, antimetabolites, cyclosporine, bromocriptine, tetracycline, heparin, coumadin, radioactive drugs. Also the infant may have a metabolic disorder that contraindicates breastfeeding.
- Does the mother have HIV/AIDS or hepatitis? These viruses can be passed to the infant by breastfeeding.
- How long will you breastfeed before you start giving the baby supplementary foods?

LAM specifies that when any one of these conditions changes, the woman needs to begin to use a complementary family planning method if she desires to continue to have a low pregnancy risk (see Figure 9–2). LAM guidelines are considered extremely safe. The return of menses is the most important indication of the return of fertility (*Are you offering,* 1996; Hatcher et al., 2001; Labbock, Cooney, & Cole, 1994; Labbock, Perez, Valdes, Sevilla, et al., 1994). LAM is less effective for women who are separated from their infants by returning to work, even when they are expressing their milk and exclusively breastfeeding (Valdes, Labbock, Pugin, & Perez, 2000). A 1996 study in the British Medical Journal found LAM to be highly effective for twelve months (a 1 to 3 percent pregnancy rate) for women who remained amenorrheic (LAM effective for 12 months, 1997).

Mechanisms of Action

The physiology of LAM is based on the hypothalamic-pituitary-ovarian feedback system. The hypothalamus reacts to the suckling at the breast by reducing the pulsatile release of gonadotropin releasing hormone (GnRH). This, in turn, changes the pulsatile secretion of prolactin and the gonadotropin hormones, follicle stimulating hormone (FSH), and luteinizing hormone (LH). The result is decreased and disorganized follicular development (Labbock, Cooney, & Cole, 1994; Labbock, Perez, et al., 1994).

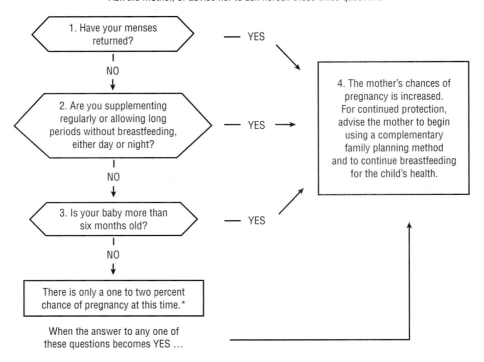

FIGURE 9–2. The Lactational Amenorrhea Method. *(Reproduced, with permission, from the Institute for Reproductive Health, Georgetown University, 1994.)*

Effectiveness

Studies have demonstrated that women who met the LAM criteria had only a 1 to 2 percent chance of pregnancy during the first six months postpartum. The LAM method alone should not extend beyond six months. Research has emphasized the importance of full or nearly full breastfeeding patterns. If the woman is concerned that she is at risk for pregnancy, emergency contraception may be used while breastfeeding. Plan B is advised (Hatcher et al., 2001).

Advantages

- Highly effective (when used perfectly—see criteria).
- No supplies, low cost.
- Not coitus linked.
- Improved infant health through breastfeeding.
- Controlled by the woman.

- Gives women time to choose which complementary family planning method they will use.
- Acceptable to many religious groups.

Disadvantages

- Temporary method, only effective in the postpartum months.
- If mother and baby are separated for extended periods, efficacy as a family planning method decreases.

Contraindications

- Specific infant metabolic disorders.
- Maternal use of mood altering drugs.
- Maternal use of reserpine, ergotamine, anti metabolites, cyclosporine, cortisone, bromocriptine, radioactive drugs, lithium, anticoagulants.

◆ Maternal HIV infection/AIDS.

◆ Active tuberculosis.

Management Considerations

In addition to teaching women the criteria for successful use of the Lactational Amenorrhea Method, several points should be considered in client teaching and counseling.

◆ Emphasize that if there are disruptions in patterns of breastfeeding, resumption of ovulation and fertility cannot be accurately predicted. A woman can become pregnant while breastfeeding and before the first menstrual period occurs.

◆ Women who are uncertain about whether they can continue to meet the specified criteria for LAM, and wish to avoid the risk of pregnancy, should begin using a reliable method of birth control immediately. For some women, this may be at the time of the six-week postpartum examination or even sooner.

◆ If the client wishes to rely on LAM for contraception, she must breastfeed her infant on demand over each 24-hour period, with no formula or food supplementation. When the infant reaches 6 months or menses return, she should begin another method of birth control.

◆ Because U.S. women rarely adhere to such a rigorous breastfeeding pattern, most should be advised not to rely on lactation alone to prevent pregnancy. A complementary method is recommended (Labbock, Perez et al., 1994).

WITHDRAWAL (COITUS INTERRUPTUS)

Coitus interruptus, withdrawal, or "pulling out," involves the man removing his penis from the vagina before ejaculation so that ejaculation occurs away from the vagina and external genitalia. The man must rely on his own sensations to determine when he is about to ejaculate. Though not popular in the United States, withdrawal is one of the most common methods of preventing pregnancy in many countries and cultures of the world. Adolescents frequently use this method. Withdrawal is often used in conjunction with fertility awareness methods.

Mechanism of Action

Coitus interruptus prevents conception when sperm containing ejaculate is deposited away from the woman's genitalia, preventing contact between sperm and ovum. The man must interrupt intercourse and withdraw his penis from his partner's vagina before ejaculation occurs.

Effectiveness

Among typical users, about 19 percent experience method failure in the first year of use (see Table 9–3). Low success rates with this method may be due to the following:

◆ Presence of sperm in the preejaculate fluid that is emitted without sensation to the man.

◆ It is difficult for the man to predict when he will ejaculate.

◆ The required self-control is difficult to achieve. (Boston Women's Health Book Collective, 1998; Hatcher et al., 1998; Lethbridge, 1991).

Advantages

◆ Coitus interruptus involves no artificial devices or chemicals, costs nothing, is always available, and can be used during lactation.

◆ It is a backup method that is always available.

Disadvantages

◆ High failure rate.

◆ Requires considerable self-control by the man.

◆ Can diminish enjoyment for the couple.

◆ Depends solely on the cooperation of the man.

◆ Puts the woman in a dependent role.

◆ Provides no protection against HIV or STDs.

◆ Sexual dysfunction and diminished pleasure could develop, as couples must remain alert, concentrate on timing, and interrupt the excitement or plateau phase of sexual response.

Contraindications

There are no absolute contraindications; however, if unplanned pregnancy is unacceptable or inadvisable, a more reliable method should be used. Relative contraindications include (a) questionable commitment of either partner to the method and (b) lack of effective communication between partners.

Management Considerations

The method should be taught as part of contraceptive counseling, especially for those who tend to use this method (i.e, individuals inexperienced with contraceptive use or those who have exhausted all other contraceptive choices). Counseling and instruction should include several topics.

- Before intercourse, the man should urinate and wipe off any fluid on the tip of the penis; it may contain sperm. This is especially important if the couple intends to have more than one act of intercourse, because semen may be present in clear fluid at the tip of an erect penis.
- When a man feels impending ejaculation, he must immediately remove his penis from the vagina so that ejaculation occurs well away from the vagina and external genitalia.
- Condom use with this method would greatly increase its effectiveness and provide protection against HIV and other STDs.
- A supply of spermicide may be kept on hand in case withdrawal is not accomplished in time. An application could be inserted immediately, although this measure probably would not prevent some sperm from entering the uterus.
- Always advise clients about the availability of emergency contraception.

DOUCHING

"Washing" semen out of the vagina through douching will not prevent sperm from entering the uterus. *Douching is not a contraceptive.* Sperm enter the cervical canal too quickly, as soon as 15 seconds after ejaculation. In fact, douching could theoretically enhance movement of sperm up the cervical canal by washing it deeper into the vagina or by washing away protective mucus. Douching has also been associated with increased risk of pelvic infection and ectopic pregnancy (Hatcher et al., 1998; Rosenberg & Phillips, 1992).

ABSTINENCE

Abstinence refers to refraining from penis-vagina intercourse. It is the most effective form of birth control and may be chosen at any stage of life. Abstinence does not preclude sexual intimacy. Individuals choosing abstinence may decide to engage in activities such as those on p. 169 under *safe* and *possibly safe* practices (that exclude intercourse). Partner cooperation, however, is critical. Health care providers can assist couples in communicating about this choice and in achieving intimacy that is satisfactory to both of them. Be sure the woman is informed about emergency contraception.

ELECTIVE TERMINATION OF PREGNANCY: INDUCED ABORTION

Induced abortions are voluntary interruptions of pregnancy and may be performed as elective or medically therapeutic procedures. Induced abortions involve the expulsion or extraction of the products of conception from the uterus by medical or surgical intervention before the embryo or fetus is capable of independent life. Abortion is the most common surgical procedure performed in the United States, approximately 1.3 million per year, and may be the most common surgical procedure in the world. Excluding miscarriages, about 30 percent of all pregnancies in the United States end in abortions, with most abortions (90 percent) being performed during the first trimester of pregnancy (Gold, 1990; Gordon & Speroff, 2002; Hatcher et al., 1998).

The 1973 U.S. Supreme Court decision *Roe v. Wade* allows women to choose to terminate pregnancy in the first trimester; after that point, individual state laws become effective. In recent years, many states have placed restrictions on access to abortion services in certain circumstances (Boston Women's Health Book Collective, 1998; Hatcher et al., 1998).

Since becoming widely available, controversy about abortion has been commonplace and will continue for the foreseeable future. People who support a woman's reproductive rights must make their opinions known to state and national legislators and at the ballot box. In order to provide health professionals with the information needed to counsel clients in a supportive manner, this section provides a discussion of the health needs of women seeking abortion services and an overview of abortion care.

Death as a result of legal induced abortion is unusual; in fact, maternal mortality associated with carrying a pregnancy to term is sixteen times higher than the risk of death due to abortion. Risk of complications and death from induced abortion vary according to weeks of gestation, method used, and type of anesthesia. Later abortions and general anesthesia are more hazardous. Approximately 99 percent of first trimester abortions in the United States are performed by vacuum aspiration and curettage (Gordon & Speroff, 2002). This is a very safe method of induced abortion. The number of U.S. women reported as dying from abortion declined from nearly 300 deaths in 1961 (mostly illegal abortions), to only 6 in 1987, or 0.4 deaths for every 100,000 legal abortions.

Currently, mortality per 100,000 legal abortions is 0.8 deaths (Gordon & Speroff, 2002). Major and minor complications associated with the procedures do occur. Major complications include retained tissue, sepsis, uterine perforation, hemorrhage, incomplete abortion. Minor complications include mild infection, reaspiration (same day or later), cervical stenosis, cervical tear, underestimated gestation, convulsions/seizure. Major complications are 2.5 times higher for instillation methods than with instrument evacuation procedures in the second trimester. Use of general anesthesia during any abortion procedure carries a significantly higher risk of serious complications and death than use of local anesthesia (Hatcher et al., 1998; Hern, 1990).

Risk of long-term complications after having one or more legal abortions is low. Subsequent problems with fertility, spontaneous abortion, premature delivery, and low birth rate have not been found to be associated with first trimester abortions, or for later abortions when performed by skilled and well-trained abortion providers. Concurrent abortion and sterilization procedures are not recommended due to higher rates of morbidity and mortality.

CLIENT EVALUATION AND PREPARATION COUNSELING

Counseling can assist a woman in decision making and prepare her to give informed consent. When a woman finds out she is pregnant with an undesired conception, it is essential that she (and her partner or other supportive person, if appropriate) has the opportunity to discuss concerns and needs in a nonjudgmental atmosphere. Women seeking abortions may experience feelings of anxiety, conflict, isolation, or fear. If the abortion is sought because of a serious medical condition, loss or sadness may be prominent. Situations involving sexual abuse or rape will require referral for further counseling and support. Abortion counselors should convey the characteristics of empathy, warmth, and genuineness while helping women to resolve confusion, ambivalence, or guilt before the procedure is performed. Sensitivity to cultural differences among clients is essential. In addition, clients must be made to feel safe, considering today's volatile environment related to abortion.

The client should be given the opportunity to discuss her current and future life situations, plans and expectations, and the possible impact of the pregnancy and/or abortion. For women who decide against abortion, referral should be made for prenatal care and information

about adoption. The counselor must be able to provide other referrals that may be indicated such as social services, group or individual support, etc.

It is the responsibility of the counselor to explain—in a kind, thorough and objective manner—all aspects of the procedures, including options, risks, preparations for the procedures, techniques and their effects, pain management, and guidance in what to expect. Postabortion contraceptive options also need to be discussed.

History

The following historical data are needed.

- Menstrual history, especially last and previous menstrual periods.
- Contraceptive history and what methods the client wants to use in the future.
- Obstetric history.
- Reproductive system disease and/or prior surgery.
- Drug/anesthesia allergies.
- Other illnesses affecting health, past or present.
- Current medications.

Physical and Reproductive Examination

The *physical exam* may be brief (heart, lungs, breasts, abdomen, vital signs); however, the *reproductive exam* should be thorough to estimate the size and position of the uterus, to estimate the state of the conceptus, and to determine any abnormality, such as a mass or anatomical variation (Hatcher et al., 1998; Hern, 1990).

Diagnostic Tests

Several diagnostic tests may be done.

- *Pregnancy Test.* A urine test for first screening; if test is negative but pregnancy suspected, a sensitive serum test is done. A wait of one to two weeks may be needed for more definitive test results if the woman is six weeks or less from her last normal menstrual period.
- *Ultrasound Evaluation.* Done for accurate dating when a discrepancy exists between the size of the uterus and gestational age. Ultrasound is routinely performed in the second trimester to ascertain accurate gestational age.
- *Hemoglobin/Hematocrit.*

♦ *Blood type.* Necessary to determine if a woman is Rh negative. Rh negative women will need to receive Rh(D) immunoglobulin (RhoGAM) after the procedure.

♦ *Vaginitis/STD Screening.* Chlamydia, gonorrhea, saline wet mount, and other if indicated.

Reasons for Elective Termination

The decision to have an abortion is rarely simple. A woman may seek to terminate pregnancy for several reasons.

♦ *Elective reasons* do not relate to the health of the mother or fetus. They could be because the pregnancy was a result of rape or incest, but more commonly, because of unreadiness to start or expand one's family, lack of money to support a pregnancy and a child, lack of a supportive relationship, or other personal crisis.

♦ *Maternal indications* are reasons for which the mother's health would be jeopardized if the pregnancy were to continue, such as heart disease, severe depression, or cancer.

♦ *Fetal indications* most commonly are congenital defects, or exposure to a teratogenic agent (Women who have abortions, 1996).

METHODS OF INDUCED ABORTION

Surgical Abortion Methods

Vacuum aspiration or suction curettage is the most commonly used abortion procedure in the United States. It is an ambulatory care procedure and may be done through week 14 of gestation. The procedure is done under local anesthesia or a para-cervical block. Sometimes a mild sedative is also given. Prior to surgery, the cervix is dilated either by graduated instrumentation or by osmotic dilators. The products of conception are removed by suction evacuation. Completion may be confirmed by curettage. The procedure takes about 10 minutes.

Potential complications include incomplete abortion, cervical laceration, seizure, cardiac arrest, allergic reaction, uterine atony, uterine perforation, bleeding, and infection. Advantages of the procedure are that it costs less than procedures performed during later gestation and little time is lost from work. Private physician costs are generally higher. Dilation with a laminaria may be needed prior to the procedure, thus requiring an additional visit to the office. (Hacker & Moore, 1993;

Hatcher et al., 1998, 2001; Hern, 1990; What is surgical abortion?, 1997).

Other surgical methods include dilatation and curettage (D & C), though this is rarely used because of potential complications. Dilatation and evacuation (D & E), also known as dilatation and extraction (D & X), is a commonly used procedure for second trimester abortions, after about 14 weeks. (This is the procedure misleadingly referred to as "partial birth abortion" by those who oppose abortion.) This involves dilatation of the cervix (to about 1.5 to 2 cm) by various possible means, usually with a number of laminaria, and evacuation of the products of conception with specially designed forceps, followed by curettage, then suction. The D & E procedure is considered safer, faster, and less expensive for second trimester abortions than instillation methods (discussion to follow), and can be carried out under local anesthesia. Hysterotomy (essentially a cesarean section) is rarely performed due to high morbidity and mortality. (Hacker & Moore, 1993; Hern, 1990).

Menstrual extraction is a term used to designate the performance of an early abortion before the diagnosis of pregnancy has been made by pregnancy test or examination. It is a simple procedure performed five to six weeks from the LMP, involving a suction device and a small cannula, accomplishing endometrial aspiration (if not pregnant) or an early abortion. It is not without risk, however, and because it is the general consensus of the medical community that potential risks outweigh the possible benefits, it is not recommended (Chalker & Downer, 1992; Hern, 1990).

Medical Abortion Methods

Substances used to induce medical abortion in the second trimester are prostaglandin E_2 suppositories, 12-methyl prostaglandin F_2 intramuscular injection, hypertonic saline intra-amniotic infusion, intra-amniotic prostaglandin infusion, or hypertonic urea intra-amniotic infusion. These are generally referred to as instillation methods of induced abortion. Methods may be combined to ensure evacuation. To ease the procedure, dilation substances such as laminaria, or synthetic osmotic dilators, or prostaglandin suppositories to soften the cervix, are commonly used before the induction is begun. To induce abortion, oxytocin may be given alone intravenously to cause uterine contractions, or it may be given in combination with other substances, such as saline. Infusions are inpatient or outpatient procedures; they become more expensive as a hospital stay lengthens. Moreover, the psychological effects on the client may be traumatic. Only 5 percent of abortions are performed after 15 weeks.

The following two methods of medical abortion are carried out only in early pregnancy. Women choose medical abortion in the first trimester for reasons of greater privacy and autonomy, less invasiveness and a more natural process than surgery. The first to be discussed is the use of methotrexate (first developed as an antineoplastic agent), given intramuscularly at 50 mg per square meter of body surface area, followed by the prostaglandin misoprostol as an 800 mcg vaginal suppository or in oral form three to seven days later. Methotrexate induces abortion because of its toxicity to trophoblastic tissue and is most successful as an abortifacient when used at eight or fewer weeks' gestation. When used in abortion, misoprostol, a prostaglandin, works by causing contractions of the uterus, helping to expel the uterine contents. If abortion does not occur within seven to ten days, a second dose of misoprostol is given. Side effects of methotrexate used in this way are minimal. Misoprostol side effects include diarrhea, nausea, vomiting. This method is 90 to 98 percent successful in accomplishing completed abortion. Incomplete abortions may require a surgical procedure to complete. Follow-up evaluation to be certain abortion is complete is important because of the potential teratogenicity of the drug, should the pregnancy continue. Use of methotrexate for the purpose of inducing abortion is not an FDA-approved indication for this drug (Hatcher et al., 1998; What is medical abortion?, 2000; Wiebe, 1996).

A second method of induced first trimester abortion involves use of mifepristone (Mifeprex, also known as RU-486) followed by administration of the prostaglandin misoprostol (Cytotec). Mifiprex, manufactured by Danco Laboratories LLC, was approved for this use by the FDA in 2000.

Mifepristone is a potent oral antiprogestogen. Mifepristone blocks the action of the natural hormone progesterone, which prepares the lining of the uterus for the fertilized egg and then maintains the pregnancy. Without progesterone, the lining of the uterus softens, breaks down, and bleeding begins. The pregnancy is thus interrupted in its early stages. The actions of misoprostol cause contractions of the uterus and expulsion of uterine contents.

This method of medical abortion is approved for the termination of intrauterine pregnancy with a duration of 49 or fewer days (counting from the last menstrual period). The approved regimen is mifepristone 600 mg on day 1 of the procedure plus misoprostol (Cytotec) 400 mg on day 3. A follow-up visit fourteen days later is required

to determine if termination of pregnancy has occurred. If not complete, vacuum curettage is performed. This method is 95 percent effective. Five percent of women may require surgical completion of the abortion. Clinicians prescribing mifepristone must have a referral plan in place for surgical intervention if necessary. Side effects of the mifepristone are minimal, though some nausea, headache, weakness, and fatigue may occur. The misoprostol has possible side effects of cramping, abdominal pain, nausea, vomiting, diarrhea, and uterine bleeding. Contraindications to mifepristone include confirmed or suspected ectopic pregnancy, adrenal failure, current corticosteroid therapy, allergy to prostoglandins, and bleeding disorders. Mifepristone is also being studied as an emergency contraceptive (Fielding, Lee, & Schaff, 2001; Spitz, Bordin, Benton, & Robbins, 1998).

COMPLICATIONS, SIGNS AND SYMPTOMS, AND PREVENTIVE MEASURES
(Table 9–11)

Postabortion Counseling

Clients who undergo vacuum aspiration or suction curettage need to expect menstrual cramping during and after the procedure and some vaginal bleeding that will taper over the next week. Clients undergoing a D & E in the second trimester can expect to enter the hospital, undergo a thirty-minute procedure to place the laminaria, then allow about six hours or more for the laminaria's effect. Analgesia may be needed after the abortion for cramping and/or breast engorgement.

Infusions later in pregnancy require hospital stays of one to three days; severe cramping, necessitating analgesia, can be expected. Instruct all clients not to put anything in the vagina for seven days after their procedure. They should expect to feel fatigue and breast tenderness for a few days and anticipate feelings of loss, sadness, or relief. Negative feelings are usually short-lived. A return visit should be scheduled for two to four weeks.

Postprocedure Care

Advise clients that fertility can return as soon as ten days following an abortion procedure. Contraceptive options must be discussed and decided on. An IUD may be inserted at the same time as a surgical abortion or otherwise as soon as termination is confirmed (Hacker & Moore, 1993; Henshaw, 1993; Hern, 1990).

TABLE 9–11. Immediate Complications of Induced Medical or Surgical Abortion, Signs and Symptoms, and Preventive Measures

Complication	Signs and Symptoms	Preventive Therapy Measures
Excessive or prolonged bleeding	Occurs during or after procedure. Uterus may be atonic; bleeding may be from trauma (see below).	Local anesthesia, I.V. oxytocin or oral or I.M. ergot, uterine massage. Evacuation of placenta within hour of fetal expulsion. May require transfusion and ergotamine treatment if occurs. Best treatment is aspiration.
Infection	Fever, chills, cramps, foul discharge, backache, abdominal pain, uterine tenderness, muscle aches, tiredness.	Treatment of infections prior to procedure, complete evacuation of products of conception, antibiotic therapy prophylactically. Hospitalization may be indicated for adequate treatment if infection develops.
Intrauterine blood clots/retained products of conception (POC)	Occurs during first 5 days after abortion. Severe pain and cramps; uterus tense, tender, enlarged; no bleeding from cervix. May be accompanied by infection (endometritis). Seen with first trimester abortions.	Vacuum aspiration indicated; oral ergot may decrease occurrence of clots. Complete evacuation of uterus prevents retained POC.
Unsuccessful termination	Pregnancy signs/symptoms continue; products of conception not found; or delay of 6 weeks or more in resuming menses.	Adequate uterine curettage.
Trauma to uterus (perforation) or to cervix (laceration)	Increased risks with younger woman, later gestation, prior delivery.	Preprocedure use of laminaria, osmotic dilators; safe, correct surgical procedure. Experienced practitioner.

Source: *Gordan & Speroff, 2002; Hacker & Moore, 1993; Hatcher et al., 1998; Hern, 1990.*

FUTURE METHODS OF FERTILITY CONTROL

Promising research is being conducted in many parts of the world to discover and test new technologies in contraception targeted for men and women. Methods being investigated for use by men, however, are most likely many years away.

MEN

- *Hormonal.* Administration of testosterone to men signals the pituitary to decrease the levels of testosterone needed for the testes to fully function, thus temporarily suppressing the production of sperm. An important finding from some early studies indicates that total suppression of sperm is not necessary to achieve highly effective contraception. Synthetic forms of testosterone are in varying stages of development, in the forms of injections, implants, transdermal patches or creams; alone or in combination with progestins such as DMPA or levonorgestrel, or in combination with luteinizing hormone releasing hormone (LHRH) antagonists (Amory & Bremner, 2000; Hatcher et al., 1998).
- *Vaccines.* Referred to as immunocontraception, vaccines, now in phase 1 trials, would use the body's immune system to disable sperm. Vaccines under development are LHRH or FSH based and would eliminate sperm production. Future vaccines will focus on interfering with highly specific aspects of spermatogenesis (Comhaire, 1994; Finger, 1995; Hatcher et al., 2001).
- *Sulfasalazine.* An ulcerative colitis drug, sulfasalazine causes decreased sperm counts and impairs sperm motility and function. The effects of this drug are quickly reversed (Finger, 1995).
- *Occlusion of the Vas Deferens.* This is accomplished either by injection of a polymer or with flexible silicone plugs, producing a "reversible sterilization" (Guha, Anand, Ansari, Farrog, & Sharma, 1990; Hatcher et al., 1998).
- *Gossypol.* A natural substance found in cottonseed oil, gossypol suppresses sperm production, is reversible, and has no effect on androgens. Gossypol depletes potassium levels, however, and can lead to dangerous cardiac arrhythmias. Lower, safer doses are being investigated (Finger, 1995; WHO, 1998).
- *Nifedipine.* Routinely used to treat hypertension, nifedipine appears to prevent sperm from fertilizing eggs by entering the membrane of the sperm and preventing it from discharging the enzymes needed to penetrate the protein coating of the egg. This is due

to the blocking of calcium ion channels in the cell membrane. Dosage needs to be established (Finger, 1995; Nowak, 1994).

- *Mifepristone for Men.* Mifepristone and some of its chemical derivatives prevent calcium from penetrating sperm. Calcium is necessary for sperm motility and subsequent fertilization (Finger, 1995; Yang, Serres, & Philbert, et al., 1994).

WOMEN

- *Hormonal.* Newer long-acting progestins are undergoing testing and in some cases are in use in countries other than the United States. They contain levonorgestrel, norethindrone, and other progestins, in the forms of removable and biodegradable implants, injections, and vaginal rings.

  - *Removable implants.* Norplant II, an improved version of Norplant, contains two rods, is as effective and has similar duration of action as Norplant. Implanon is a one-rod implant effective for three years. No incision is required for insertion; it is inserted under the skin, using a large needle. Contains etonogestrel (Darney, 2001).
  - *Biodegradable implants.* Eliminate need for surgical removal of implants. Annuelle consists of pellets the size of rice grains, containing norethindrone fused with cholesterol; effective for two years. Capronor contains levonorgestrel and is effective for up to two years (Darney, 2001; Hatcher et al., 1998).
  - *Injectables.* A long-acting ester, injectable levonorgestrel butanoate, would be an alternative to DMPA.
  - *Vaginal rings.* These may contain only progestin or a combination of estrogen and progestin.

- *Mifepristone* can inhibit ovulation and induce amenorrhea. A small four-month study on 90 women who took a daily dose of mifepristone produced no pregnancies. This may eventually lead to an estrogen and progestin-free oral contraceptive (Brown, Cheng, Lin, & Baird, 2002). Other anti-antiprogestins are being studied (Spitz, Van Look, & Coelingh-Bennink, 2000).

- *Intrauterine devices.* An IUD is being studied that has one end embedded in the fundus. The other end is monitored monthly at the cervical outlet. Called the Gynefix Copper IUD (multiload Copper IUD), it uses six copper sleeves on the string in the uterus. It

offers low failure and expulsion rates (Hatcher et al., 2001).

- *Barriers.* Efforts are underway to improve condoms, diaphragms, caps, and similar devices that provide physical barrier contraception, some of which can reduce exposure to STDs.

  - *Female condoms.* New types of female condoms are being studied.
  - *Sponges.* Protectaid, available in Canada, is made of polyurethane and contains a low dose combination of three spermicides (nonoxynol-9, benzalkonium chloride [BZK], and, sodium cholate). A sponge containing BZK called Pharmatex, is available in Europe. Another N-9-containing sponge called Avert is also being studied.
  - *Diaphragms.* Research is being conducted on the traditional diaphragms to make them easier and more appealing to use. These approaches include wearing the diaphragm for longer periods with and/or without spermicide. The *SILCS intravaginal barrier* is one size and made of silicone rubber. It has a slightly oblong shape and dimpled surface intended to make insertion and removal easier. Studies on acceptability and effectiveness are underway (Best, 2000c).
  - *Lea's Shield.* This is a one-size-fits-all cup shaped barrier that covers the cervix. It is made of silicone rubber and has a valve that allows draining of secretions and menstrual blood; it has a U-shaped loop for removal. It can be worn for 48 hours.

- *Cervical caps.* Femcap is a type of cervical cap, made of silicone rubber, shaped like a hat with a wide upturned brim. It fits over the cervix, may be worn up to 48 hours, and uses a small amount of spermicide. A loop facilitates removal. Fitting is required. Oves Cap is a silicone device that can be left in place for three days. Equipped with a removal loop, it is disposable after one use. Fitting is required (Best, 2000c).

- *Chemical barriers.* Research involving chemical barrier methods (spermicides) is examining these products for their ability to prevent the transmission of STDs, especially HIV, and ways to improve their ability to do so. Spermicides under study include nonoxynol-9, benzalkonium chloride, and menfegol. New delivery systems would enhance ease of use and would increase spreadability and cohesiveness to better protect against pathogens, including HIV, as well as sperm. These may be in the forms of new types of films, slow releasing pellets, gels, and a vaginal ring that would release spermicide for up to 30 days. Substances such as these, which would have spermicidal and microbicidal activity, could provide women with STD protection that would not necessarily require the cooperation of male partners (Barnett, 1996a, 1996b).

♦ *Vaccines.* An antifertility vaccine is being studied that is directed against human chorionic gonadotropin (HCG). HCG is produced by the implanting embryo and is essential for implantation and successful development of early pregnancy. Other vaccines are being developed that act against various targets in the body or at certain stages of embryonic growth. These include vaccines against FSH, LHRH, the zona pellucida, endometrial proteins, inactivation of the secretions of the blastocyte and other points in the processes of fertilization, postfertilization, and implantation (Edwards, 1984; Griffin, 1994; Hatcher et al., 1998).

REFERENCES

ACOG Practice Bulletin. (2001). *Emergency Oral Contraception,* (25), 1–8.

Adolescent Pregnancy Fact Sheet. (1996). *American College of Obstetricians and Gynecologists [ACOG],* 1–8.

Advisor Forum. (2002 May). Depo-Provera and topical estrogen: A risky combination. *The Clinician Advisor,* 98.

Alza Corp. (1988). *Progestasert intrauterine progesterone contraceptive system.* Product information.

Amory, J.K., & Bremner, W.J. (2000). Newer agents for hormonal contraception in the male. *Trends in Endocrinologic Metabolism, 11* (2), 61–66.

Andersson, K., Odlind, V., & Rybo, G. (1994). Levonorgestrel-releasing and copper-releasing IUDs during five years of continuing use: A randomized comparative trial. *Contraception, 49,* 56–72.

Are you offering your clients all the options? (1996). Washington DC: Institute for Reproductive Health, Georgetown University.

Association of Reproductive Health Professionals [ARHP]. (2001). New developments in contraception featuring the levonorgestrel intrauterine system. *ARHP Clinical Proceedings,* 6–16.

Barnett, B. (1994). FHI's role in search for non-surgical sterilization. *Network: FHI, 14* (4), 26–29.

Barnett, B. (1995). Life stages affect method use. *Network: Family Health International, 15*(3), 14–17.

Barnett, B. (1996a). Developing new diaphragms, condoms and similar devices. *Network: Family Health International, 16* (3), 19.

Barnett, B. (1996b). Microbicide research aims to prevent STDs. *Network: FHI, 16*(3), 15–18.

Baylor College of Medicine. (1994). Inserting and removing levonorgestrel subdermal implants: An update. *Contraceptive Reports, 5,* 4–12.

Bergett-Hanson, L. (2001). Oral contraceptives: An update on health benefits and risks. *Journal of the American Pharmaceutical Association, 41*(6), 875–886.

Best, K. (1999). Hypertension raises method choice concerns. *Network: FHI, 19*(2), 8–9.

Best, K. (2000a). How effective are spermicides? *Network: FHI, 20* (2), 11–15.

Best, K. (2000c). New barrier devices may be easier to use. *Network, FHI, 20*(2), 16–17.

Blumenthal, P., & Huggins, G. (1992). A look at the new progestogen oral contraceptives. *Medical Aspects of Human Sexuality, 26* (1), 30–36.

Boston Women's Health Book Collective. (1998). *Our bodies, ourselves for the new century.* New York: Simon & Schuster.

Brown, A., Cheng, L., Lin, S., & Baird, D.T. (2002). Daily low dose mifepristone has contraceptive potential by suppressing ovulation and menstruation: A double blind randomized control trial of 2 and 5 mg. per day for 120 days. *Journal of Endocrinolgic Metabolism, 87* (1), 63–70.

Chalker, R., & Downer, C. (1992). *A woman's book of choices: Abortion, menstrual extraction, RU-486.* New York, London: Four Walls Eight Windows.

Comhaire, F.H. (1994). Male contraception: Hormonal, mechanical and other. *Human Reproduction, 9* (4), 586–590.

Darney, P.D. (1994). Hormonal implants: Contraception for a new century. *American Journal Ob-Gyn, 170,* 1536–1543.

Darney, P.D. (1995). Contraceptive implants: Proper technique for rapid problem-free removal. *Women's Health Reports, 1,* 9–16.

Darney, P.D. (2001). Contraceptive implants update. *Dialogues in Contraception, 7* (3), 4.

Darney, P.D., & Speroff, L. (2001, Winter). New methods. *Dialogues in Contraception,* (3), 4.

Dickerson, V. (2001). Contraception in the perimenopause. *The Female Patient, 26* (3), 12–16.

Dickey, R. (2002). *Managing contraceptive pill patients* (11th ed.). Dallas: EMIS, Inc.

Edwards, R.G. (1994). Implantation, interception, and contraception. *Human Contraception, 9* (6), 985–995.

Essure™ permanent birth control by Conceptus. (2002). Retrieved March 31, 2003, *http://www.essure.com.*

Fahey, M.L. (1995). Pharmacologic update: Emergency postcoital therapies. *Journal of the American Aademy of Nurse Practitioners, 7* (10), 505–508.

Family planning counseling: The international experience. (1992). New York: AVSC International.

Farr, G., Gabelnick, H. & Sturgen, K. (1994). Contraceptive efficacy and acceptability of the female condom. *American Journal of Public Health,* 84, 1960–1964.

Feldblum P., & Joanis, C. (1994). *Barrier methods: Effective contraception and disease prevention.* Research Triangle Park: FHI.

Female condoms can be reused. (2001). *Reproductive Health Matters, 9* (18), 179–180.

The female condom controlled by women. (1995). *Network: FHI, 16* (1), 23–26.

Fichorova, R.N., Tucker, L.D., Anderson, D.J. (2001, August 15). The molecular basis of Nonoxynol-9 induced vaginal inflammation and its possible relevance to human immunodeficiency virus type 1 transmission. *Journal of Infectious Diseases, 184* (4), 418–428.

Fielding, S., Lee, S., & Schaff, E. (2001). Professional considerations for providing mifepristone-induced abortion. *Nurse Practitioner, 26* (11), 44–54.

Finger, W. (1995). Future male methods may include injectables. *Network: FHI, 15* (3), 9–13.

Finger, W. (2000). Female condom reuse examined. *Network: FHI, 20* (2), 20.

Finger, W. (2001). Contraception after intercourse. *Network: FHI, 21* (1), 185.

Fogel, C.I., & Woods, N.F. (1995). *Women's health care: A comprehensive handbook.* Thousand Oaks, CA: Sage Publications.

Forrest, J.D. (1993). Timing of reproductive life stages. *Obstetrics-Gynecology, 82*(1), 105–110.

Gebbie, A. (1995) Barrier methods of contraception. *British Journal of Sexual Medicine,* 12–15.

Gentile, G.P., Kaufman, S.C., & Helbig, D.W. (1998). Is there any evidence of a post-tubal sterilization syndrome? *Fertility-Sterilization, 69* (2), 179–186.

Gerchufsky, M. (1996a). Ending condom confusion. *ADVANCE for Nurse Practitioners, 4* (6), 39–42, 60.

Gerchufsky, M. (1996b). Issues and answers in latex sensitivity. *ADVANCE for Nurse Practitioners, 4* (6), 15–19.

Gold, R.B. (1990). *Abortion and women's health: A turning point for America?* New York: Alan Guttmacher Institute.

Gordon, J.G., & Speroff, L. (2002). *Handbook for clinical gynecologic endocrinology and infertility.* Philadelphia: Lippincott, Williams & Wilkins.

Grabrick, D.M., Hartmann, L.C., Cerhan, J.H., et al. (2000). Risk of breast cancer with oral contraceptive use in women with a family history of breast cancer. *JAMA, 284,* 1791–1798.

Griffin, P.D. (1994). Immunization against HCG. *Human Reproduction, 9* (2), 267–272.

Grimes, D. (1999a). DMPA good choice for women with sickle cell. *Network: FHI, 19* (2), 10–11.

Grimes, D. (1999b). Hormonal methods may affect headaches. *Network: FHI, 19* (2), 11–13.

Guha, S.K., Anand, S., Ansari, S., Farrog, A., & Sharma, D.N. (1990). Time controlled injectable occlusion of the vas deferens. *Contraception, 41,* (3), 323–331.

GynoPharma. (1988). *Paragard-T-280A.* Prescribing Information.

Hacker, N.F., & Moore, J.G. (1993). *Essentials of obstetrics and gynecology.* Philadelphia: Saunders.

Hatcher, R., Nelson, A., Zieman, M., Darney, P., Creinin, M., & Stosur, H. (2001). *A pocket guide to managing contraception: 2001–2002 edition.* Tiger, GA: The Bridging the Gap Foundation.

Hatcher, R., Trussell, J., Stewart, F., Cates, Jr., W., Stewart, G., Guest, F., & Kowal, D. (1998). *Contraceptive technology* (17th revised ed.). New York: Ardent Media.

Henshaw, S.K. (1993). The accessibility of abortion services in the United States. *Family Planning Perspectives, 20* (4), 169–176.

Hern, W. (1990). *Abortion practices.* Philadelphia: J. B. Lippincott Company.

Hubacher, D., & Grimes, D.A. (2002). Non-contraceptive health benefits of intrauterine devices: A systematic review. *Obstetric-Gynecologic Survey, 57* (2), 120–128.

Intrauterine devices. (2000). *Network: FHI, 20* (1), 1–19.

Kass-Annese, B., & Danzer, H. (1992). *The fertility awareness handbook.* Alameda, CA: Hunter House.

Katz, D. (1991). Human cervical mucus: Research update. *American Journal of Obstetrics and Gynecology, 32* (2), 387–402.

Kaunitz, A.M. (1994). Long-acting injectable contraception with DMPA. *American Journal of Obstetrics-Gynecology, 170* (5), 1543–1549.

Kaunitz, A. (2001). Prescribing oral contraceptives for peri-menopause. *Women's Health in Primary Care, 4* (9), 579–591.

Kjos, S.L. (1999). Contraceptive selection in women with medical problems. *Dialogues in Contraception, 5* (7), 1–8.

Kupecz, D., & Berandinelli, C. (2002). Drugs and device approval highlights from 2001. *The Nurse Practitioner, 26* (2), 16.

Labbock, M., Cooney, K., & Cole, S. (1994). *Guidelines: Breastfeeding, family planning and the lactational amenorrhea method.* Washington, DC: Institute for Reproductive Health, Georgetown University.

Labbock, M., Perez, A., Valdes, V., Sevilla, F., et al. (1994). The Lactational Amenorrhea Method (LAM): A postpartum introductory family planning method with policy and program implications. *Advances in Contraception, 10* (2), 93–109.

Labbock, M., & Queenan J. (1989). The use of periodic abstinence for family planning. *Clinical Obstetrics and Gynecology, 32* (2), 387–402.

LAM effective for 12 months. (1997). *Network: FHI, 17* (2), 2.

Lethbridge, D.J. (1991). Coitus Interruptus: Considerations as a birth control method. *JOGN Nursing, 20* (1), 80–85.

Lidegaard, O., & Kreiner, S. (2002). Contraceptives and cerebral thrombosis: A five year national case controlled study. *Contraception, 65* (3), 197–205.

Litchman R., & Papera, S. (1998). *Gynecology: Well woman care.* Stamford, CT: Appleton & Lange.

Lynaugh, J. (1991). The death of Sadie Sachs…Margaret Sanger. *Nursing Research, 40* (2), 124–125.

Mantel-Teeuwisse, A., Kloosterman, J., & Maitland-Van der Zee, A. (2001). Drug induced lipid changes: A review of the unintended effects of some commonly used drugs on serum lipid levels. *Drug Safety, 24,* 443–456.

McNamee, K. (2000). The female condom. *Australian Family Physician, 29* (6), 555–557.

Narod, S.A., Dube, M., Klijn, J., Lubinski, J., et al. (2002). Oral contraceptives and the risk of breast cancer in BRCA1 and BRCA2 mutation carriers. *Journal of the National Cancer Institute, 94*(23), 1773–1779.

Nelson, A. (1995). Patient selection is key to IUD success. *Contemporary Ob-Gyn, Reprint,* 2–8.

Neilson, C., & Miller, L. (2000). Ectopic gestation following emergency contraceptive pill administration. *Contraception, 62,* 275–276.

New approach to prescribing oral contraception. (2001). *Clinical Reviews.* [On-line]. Available: www.Medscape.com/viewarticle/407324.

Norplant effective for seven years. (2000). *Network: FHI, 20* (3), 2.

No-scalpel vasectomy: An illustrated guide for surgeons. New York: AVSC International.

Nowak, R. (1994). Antihypertensive drug may double as male contraceptive. *Journal of NIH Research, 6,* 27–30.

Ortiz, M.E., Croxatto, H.B., & Bardin, C.W. (1996). Mechanisms of action of intrauterine devices. *Obstetric-Gynecologic Survey, 51* (12), S42–S51.

Pakarinen, P., Toivonen, J., & Luukkainen, T. (2001). Therapeutic use of the LNG-IUS and counseling. *Seminars in Reproductive Medicine, 19* (4), 365–372.

Peipert, J.F. (1999, Fall). Women's beliefs concerning oral contraptives. *Dialogues in Contraception, 1,* 4–8.

Peterson, H.B., Jeng, G., Folger, S.G., Hillis, S.A., Marchbanks, P.A., & Wilcox, L.S. (2000). The risk of menstrual abnormalities after tubal sterilization. U.S. Collaborative Review of Sterilization Working Group. *New England Journal of Medicine, 343* (23), 1681–1687.

Peterson, H.B., Xia, Z., Hughes, J.M., Wilcox, L.S., Tyler, L.R., & Trussell, J. (1997). The risk of ectopic pregnancy after tubal sterilization. *New England Journal of Medicine, 336* (23), 1681–1687.

Peterson, H.B., Xia, Z., Hughes, J.M., Wilcox, L.S., Tyler, L.R., & Trussell, J. (1996). The risk of pregnancy after tubal ligation: Findings from the U. S. Collaborative Review of Sterilization. *American Journal of Obstetrics & Gynecology, 174,* 1161–1170.

Product Information, Today Sponge. (2000). Allendale Pharmaceuticals, Inc.

Pymar, H., & Creinin, M. (2001). The risks of oral contraceptive pills. *Seminars in Reproductive Medicine, 19* (4), 305–312.

Rawlins, S.I.C., & Smith D.M. (2002). Innovative contraception: New options in hormonal contraception. *The American Journal of Nurse Practitioners, 6* (1), 20–28.

Reality Female Condom: An alternative for women. (1994). Chicago: The Female Health Company. Division of Wisconsin Pharmacal.

Rivera, R. (1999). Diabetic women need effective contraception. *Network: FHI, 19* (2), 9–10.

Roddy, R., Zekeng, L., Ryan, K., Tamoufe, U., & Tweedy, K. (2002). Effect of nonoxynol-9 gel on urogenital gonorrhea and chlamydial infection: A randomized controlled trial. *JAMA, 287*(9), 1171–1172.

Rodrigues-Garcia, R. (Ed.). (1989). *Natural family planning: A good option.* Washington DC: Institute for Reproductive Health, Georgetown University.

Ronnerdag, M., & Odlind, V. (1999). Health effects of long-term use of the intrauterine levonorgestrel-releasing system: a follow-up study over 12 years of continuous use. *Acta Obstet-Gynecol Scand, 78* (8), 716–721.

Rosenberg, M.J., & Phillips, R.S. (1992). Does douching promote ascending infection? *Journal of Reproductive Medicine, 37* (11), 930–938.

Sarin, A.R. (1999). Quinacrine sterilization: Experienced among women at high risk for surgery. *Advances in Contraception, 15,* 175–178.

Schwartz, S., Petitti, D., Siscovick, D., Longstreth, W.T., Sidney, S., Raghunathan, T.E., Queesenberry, C.P., & Kelaghan, J. (1998). Stroke and use of oral contraceptives in young women: A pooled analysis of two U.S. studies. *Stroke, 29* (11), 2274–2284.

Scott, P.M. (1996). How to fit a cervical cap. *Journal of the American Academy of Physicians Assistants,* 83–88.

Sieven, I., Stern, J., Coutinho, E., Mattos, C.E.R., & Diaz, S. (1991). Prolonged intrauterine contraception: A seven year randomized study of the levonorgestrel 20 mcg/day (LNG20) and the copper T 380A IUDs. *Contraception, 44* (5), 473–480.

Spitz, I.M., Bordin, C.W., Benton, L., & Robbins, A. (1998). Early pregnancy termination with mifepristone and misoprostol in the United States. *New England Journal of Medicine, 338* (18), 1241–1247.

Spitz, I.M., Van Look, P.F., & Coelingh-Bennink, H.J. (2000). The use of progesterone antagonists and progesterone receptor modulators in contraception. *Steroids, 65* (10–11), 817–823.

The Standard Days Method. (2003). *Institute for Reproductive Health, Georgetown University* [On-line]. Retrieved 1/14/03 from *http://www.irh.org.*

Sterilization. (1996). *ACOG Technical Bulletin, 222,* 1–7.

Tagg, P.I. (1995). The diaphragm: Barrier contraception has a new social role. *Nurse Practitioner, 20* (12), 36–42.

Trussell, J., & Grammer-Strawn, L. (1991). Further analysis of contraceptive failure of the ovulation method. *American Journal of Obstetrics-Gynecology, 165* (62), 2054–2059.

Trussell, J., & Stewart, F. (1998). An update on emergency contraception. *Dialogues in Contraception, 5* (6), 1–5.

Update of female sterilization. (1996, September). *The Contraceptive Report, 7* (3), 4–13.

The use of hormonal contraception in women with coexisting medical conditions. (2000). *ACOG Practice Bulletin, 18.* Washington, DC: American College of Obstetricians & Gynecologists.

Valdes, V., Labbock, M., Pugin, E., & Perez, A. (2000). The efficacy of the lactational amenorrhea method (LAM) among working women. *Contraception, 62* (5), 217–219.

Van Damme, L., Ramjee, G., Alary, M., Vuylsteke, B., Chandeying, V., Rees, H., Sirivongrangson, P., Mukenge-Tshibaka, L., Ettiegne-Traore, V., Uaheowitchai, C., Kari, S.S., Masse, B., Perriens, J., & Laga, M. (2002). Effectiveness of COL-1942, a nonoxynol-9 vaginal gel, on HIV-1 transmission in female sex workers, a randomized controlled trial. *Lancet, 360* (9338), 971–977.

Vandenbroucke, J.P., Rosing, J., Bloemenkamp, K.W., Middeldorp, S., Helmorhorst, F.M., Bourma, B.N., & Rosendaal, F.R. (2001). Oral contraceptives and the risk of venous thrombosis. *New England Journal of Medicine, 334* (20), 1527–1535.

Weschler, T. (1995). *Taking charge of your fertility: The definitive guide to natural birth control and pregnancy achievement.* New York: Harper Collins.

What is medical abortion? (2000). Washington, D.C.: National Abortion Federation.

What is surgical abortion? (1997). Washington, D.C.: National Abortion Federation.

Wiebe, E.R. (1996). Abortion induced with methotrexate and misoprostol. *Canadian Medical Association Journal, 154* (2), 165–170.

Wilkinson, D., Tholandi, M., Ramjee, G., & Rutherford, G.W. (2002). Nonoxynol-9 spermicide for prevention of vaginally acquired HIV and other sexually transmitted infections. *Lancet Infectious Diseases, 2* (10), 613–617.

Wilcox, L.S., Chu, S.U., Eaker, E.D., Zeger, S.L., & Peterson, H.B. (1991). Risk factors for regret after tubal sterilization: 5 years of follow-up in a prospective study. *Fertility-Sterilization, 55,* 927–933.

Women who have abortions. (1996). Washington, DC: National Abortion Federation.

World Health Organization Task Force on Postovulatory Methods of Fertility Regulation. (1998). Randomized controlled trial of levonorgestrel versus the Yuzpe regimen of combined oral contraceptives for emergency contraception. *Lancet, 352,* 428–433.

Wysocki, S., Moore, A., Freeman, S., & Sutton, C. (2001). *New options in hormonal contraception: The monthly combination contraceptive injection.* Dayton, NJ: NP Communications, LLC.

Yang, J., Serres, C., Philbert, D., et al. (1994). Progesterone and RU-486: Opposing effects on human sperm. *Proceedings of the National Academy of Sciences, 91,* 529–533.

CHAPTER 10

INFERTILITY

Jennifer R. Gardella

*T*he etiology of infertility can be identified in 85 to 90 percent of couples: 30 percent have male factor infertility, 35 percent have female factor infertility, and 20 percent have a combination of male and female factors.

Highlights

- Factors Affecting Fertility
- Diagnostic Infertility Evaluation
    Semen Analysis
    Assessment of Ovarian Function
    Assessment of Uterine Cavity
      and Endometrium
    Assessment of the Pelvis
- Female Infertility: Causes, Diagnoses, and Interventions
    Ovulatory Dysfunction
    Hypothalamic, Pituitary, and Adrenal
      Disorders
    Uterine Disorders
    Tubal and Peritoneal Disorders
- Recurrent Pregnancy Loss
- Male Infertility: Causes, Diagnoses, and Interventions
    Endocrine Disorders
    Varicocele
    Disorders of Sperm Transport
    Sperm Transport Dysfunction
- Combined Factors of Male and Female Infertility
- Selected Infertility Treatments
    Ovulation Induction
    Artificial Insemination
    Assisted Reproductive Technologies
- Alternative Family Building
    Nontraditional Family Building
    Egg Donation
    Gestational Carrier
    Adoption
    Childfree Living
- Future Trends and Controversies
    Preimplantation Genetic Diagnosis
    Human Cloning

❖ INTRODUCTION

Infertility is generally defined as one year of unprotected, frequent intercourse without attaining conception. Infertility may also result from recurrent miscarriage. Primary infertility, meaning a couple has never conceived, is a potentially more ominous diagnosis than secondary infertility, or difficulty conceiving after any prior conception.

Today, couples are more aware of specific causes of infertility and of the sophisticated treatments available. Consequently, they are increasingly seeking treatment. The number of available infertility services is also increasing, as evidenced by increased membership in the American Society for Reproductive Medicine (formerly the American Fertility Society) and the creation of the subspecialty Reproductive Endocrinology by the American Board of Obstetrics and Gynecology. The National Certification Corporation for the Obstetric, Gynecologic, and Neonatal Nursing Specialties (NCC) offers certification for registered nurses in reproductive endocrinology/infertility. In many cases, however, health care insurance may not share the burden of treatment costs to diagnose or treat infertility.

Infertility is a widespread problem that often is initially identified in the obstetric/gynecologic, or less commonly, the urologic practice. It is imperative that the nurse practitioner recognize infertility and understand its causes and treatment options. Prevention of infertility, through patient education, can also be incorporated into the nurse practitioner's practice. Evaluation and treatment may be initiated in the general practice, with referral to a reproductive endocrinologist when necessary.

The reproductive endocrinologist and nurse practitioner in an infertility practice collaborate as closely as they would in any medical setting. The health care provider's role is multifaceted: to diagnose and treat; to identify multiple impacts on the individual, couple, and significant others; to provide information, support, and counseling; and to refer to specialties of internal medicine, endocrinology, obstetrics, urology, and psychiatry. Other roles include research, community education, and advocacy.

With the advent of in vitro fertilization (IVF) and other assisted reproductive technologies (ART) in the late 1970s, an increase in media attention focused on infertility, increased public awareness of the availability of fertility services, and increased social acceptance of the use of ART, there has also been an increase in the proportion of women over 35 seeking medical attention for infertility. The rate of infertility in the United States, however, has not risen but has decreased slightly over time. The National Survey of Family Growth performed by the National Center for Health Statistics has been performed several times since 1960. In the most recent survey, performed in 1995, it was reported that 10.5 percent of women in the reproductive age group (or 6.1 million women) were infertile in the United States (U.S. Department of Health and Human Services, 1997; Stephen Chandra, 1998). But despite the availability of medical treatment, only 21 percent of childless couples between the ages of 35 and 44 years ever seek infertility services. One out of five U.S. women has her first child after age 35. Yet about one-third of women who defer pregnancy until the mid-to-late 30s will have an infertility problem (Speroff, Glass, & Kase, 1999). In addition, improved contraceptive methods and liberalized abortion have diminished the availability of adoptable babies to infertile couples.

FACTORS AFFECTING FERTILITY

There are multiple known and unknown factors that impact fertility. The most important factors that reflect current research and practice are discussed in this section.

MATERNAL AGE

Maternal age is one of the most important factors to influence a couple's fertility. A woman's fertility generally begins to decline after the age of 27, due to multiple endocrine changes, decline in number of ovarian follicles, decrease in ovarian volume, and decreased oocyte quality (Lass, Silye, Abrams, et al., 1997). Risk of spontaneous abortion increases from 10 percent under age 30, to 18 percent in the late 30s, to 34 percent in the early 40s (Warburton, Kline, Stein, & Strobino, 1986). The frequency of both euploid (chromosomally normal) and aneuploid (chromosomally abnormal) spontaneous abortions increases with age (see Table 10–1). Studies performed on embryos resulting from in vitro fertilization have confirmed an increased incidence of aneuploidy in embryos

TABLE 10–1. Chromosomal Abnormalities in Liveborn Infants and Maternal Age

Maternal Age	Risk for Down Syndrome	Total Risk for Chromosomal Anomalies[†]
20	1/1667	1/526
21	1/1667	1/526
22	1/1429	1/500
23	1/1429	1/500
24	1/1250	1/476
25	1/1250	1/476
26	1/1176	1/476
27	1/1111	1/455
28	1/1053	1/435
29	1/1000	1/417
30	1/952	1/385
31	1/909	1/385
32	1/769	1/322
33	1/602	1/286
34	1/485	1/238
35	1/378	1/192
36	1/289	1/156
37	1/224	1/127
38	1/173	1/102
39	1/136	1/83
40	1/106	1/66
41	1/82	1/53
42	1/63	1/42
43	1/49	1/33
44	1/38	1/26
45	1/30	1/21
46	1/23	1/16
47	1/18	1/13
48	1/14	1/10
49	1/11	1/8

[†] The other chromosomal anomalies that are increased with maternal age in addition to 47,+21 (Down syndrome) are 47,+18; and 47,+13; 47,XYY (Klinefelter's syndrome); 47,XYY and 47,XXX. The incidence of 47,XXX for women between the ages of 20 and 32 years is not available.

Source: Modified from Hook, Cross, & Schreinemachers, 1983; Hook, 1981.

obtained from older women (Munne, Alikani, Tomkin, et al., 1995). The urgency of the fertility evaluation and treatment increases after age 35. Advanced maternal age presents risks to both mother and fetus in pregnancy including gestational diabetes, pregnancy-induced hypertension, and premature labor (Borini, Bafaro, Violini, et al., 1995). Every woman over the age of 42 should undergo a medical evaluation and counseling by an obstetrician prior to undergoing fertility therapies.

BODY WEIGHT

Extremes of body weight are associated with altered ovarian function. A threshold body weight and fat content are necessary to establish and maintain normal ovarian func-

tion. If body weight is reduced below the 10th percentile for a particular height (body mass index [BMI] < 18) or the body fat content is reduced to less than 22 percent, altered menstrual function and ovulatory dysfunction can develop (Speroff et al., 1999). An increased incidence of amenorrhea in some female athletes and in anorexic women has been well described. Increased body weight can also be associated with ovulatory dysfunction. Obesity also increases the risk of complications in pregnancy and delivery. Obesity is responsible for 18 percent of maternal mortalities and 80 percent of anesthesia-related mortalities (Endler, Mariona, Sokol, et al., 1988). The most important endocrine change in obesity is elevation of the basal body insulin level, leading to increased insulin resistance. Insulin resistance, hyperandrogenism, and anovulation are hallmarks of the polycystic ovarian syndrome. Obese women are also at increased risk for miscarriage and experience decreased success with fertility therapies (ASRM, 2000).

SMOKING

Smoking has been shown to be a reproductive toxin in both men and women. Cigarette smoking reduces fertility, increases the rate of spontaneous abortion, and increases the incidence of abruptio placentae, placenta previa, bleeding during pregnancy, and premature rupture of placental membranes (Fielding, 1987). Smoking has clearly been associated with decreased fertility in several large studies (Bolumar, Olsen, & Boldsen, 1996; De Mouzon, Spira, & Schwartz, 1988). Women who smoke generally go through an earlier menopause by one to five years, suggesting that the metabolic products of cigarette smoke may be directly toxic to the ovaries (American College of Obstetricians & Gynecologists, 1997). Men who smoke have a reduction in all semen parameters, including the concentration, motility, and percentage of sperm with normal morphology (Bayer, Alper, & Penzias, 2002).

ALCOHOL

Alcohol is a known human teratogen, resulting in fetal alcohol syndrome (FAS); it is known to be embryotoxic. Alcohol use increases the risk for spontaneous abortion, and any degree of alcohol intake in a woman can decrease her chance for conception. Alcohol consumption was shown to reduce the ability to conceive in a dose-dependent fashion in two large studies (Jensen, Hjollund, Henriksen, et al., 1998; Hakim, Gray, & Zacur, 1998).

Alcohol should be eliminated from the diet in women attempting to achieve pregnancy. Moderate drinking may be associated with an increased risk for spontaneous abortion in the second and third trimesters (see Table 10–2). Alcohol consumption of more than two drinks per day is associated with a risk of spontaneous abortion twice that in non-alcohol-consuming controls (Harlop & Shinono, 1980). There are no published data, however, that suggest that low to moderate alcohol use affects male reproduction.

CAFFEINE

Several reports link a woman's caffeine intake to decreased fertility (Hatch & Bracken, 1993; Bolumar, Olsen, Rebagliato, & Bisanti, 1997). Caffeine may decrease blood flow to the uterus. A dose-dependent relationship has been confirmed showing any amount of caffeine to be detrimental to fertility. Caffeine in excess of 300 mg/day (3 cups of coffee) is also associated with an increase in risk for spontaneous abortion (Gardella & Hill, 2000).

RECREATIONAL DRUG USE

Combined effects of substances of abuse may be additive with those related to alcohol consumption and cigarette smoking (Jacobson, Jacobson, & Sokol, 1994). Cocaine and heroine use may lead to decreased birth weight, decreased head circumference, prematurity, and severe withdrawal reactions in the baby after it is born. Males who use marijuana on a regular basis have lower serum testosterone levels and decreased sperm counts (Bayer et al., 2002).

ENVIRONMENTAL HAZARDS

Many toxins encountered by women in the environment and workplace may affect reproductive health by decreasing fertility, leading to spontaneous abortion, fetal malformation, or developmental abnormalities (including lead, mercury, and organic solvents). Men are also susceptible to environmental toxins since spermatogenesis is an ongoing and dynamic process. DBCP (a pesticide), lead, ethylene glycol ethers, kepone (an insecticide), organic solvents, and other chemicals have been shown to impact on male fertility (Gardella & Hill, 2000).

PSYCHOLOGICAL STRESS

Infertility is associated with an intense psychological component, which can produce feelings of anger, anxiety, guilt, inadequacy, and overt depression. In addition, the experience of infertility can lead to isolation from social support systems. There are no adequate studies indicating that psychological stress actually causes infertility. Nevertheless, the benefits of relaxation techniques in reducing stress has been reported to potentially improve fertility (Domar, Clapp, Slawsby, et al., 2000). Further research is needed to clarify the association of stress and fertility and the benefits of intervention.

Many couples take for granted that they are fertile and hence are not emotionally prepared for the psychological impact of a diagnosis of infertility. Emotional distress may be no less severe for couples who experience secondary infertility. A couple's ability to admit that they may have a fertility problem is an important first step, but they may also feel threatened as potential causes are identified and treatment recommended. The many complex feelings associated with loss and infertility involve self-image, self-esteem, and sexuality (see Table 10–3). Infertility is a couple's problem, not an individual's. Both partners need to be involved in diagnostic and treatment choices and to accompany each other to appointments when possible. The health care provider can assist the couple experiencing grief by giving accurate information; supporting or making referrals for individual, group, or sex therapy; and encouraging couples to use support services. Couples may contact the American Society for Reproductive Medicine in Birmingham, Alabama for information, or Resolve in Somerville, Massachusetts, to become involved in self-help groups on both a local and national level (see Resources). Couples may also need to be given permission to stop treatment.

TABLE 10–2. Alcohol Effects on Fetal Development

Amount of Absolute Alcohol per Day	Fetal Effect
≥ 4 oz	FAS is induced
2–3 oz	Birth weight reduction
1.5 oz	IQ deficits (reduction of 5 to 7 points)
Five drinks/occasion, at least once per week	Memory and attention deficits
Amount necessary to induce spontaneous abortion	Unknown

Source: Gardella & Hill, 2000.

TABLE 10–3. Common Emotional Responses to Infertility (the manifestation of these responses may differ significantly between men and women)

Guilt
One or both partners assume blame for the infertility. Self-reproach increases and self-esteem decreases.

Depression
One or both partners develop a sense of hopelessness, loss and despair, tearfulness, fatigue, anxiety, sleep or eating disturbances, or an inability to concentrate. The onset of menses can often trigger a depression in many infertile couples.

Anger
The infertile couple often feels that life has treated them unfairly. They may feel out-of-control, resentful, and angry with others, including family, friends, and medical personnel.

Isolation
A sense of social separateness of feeling "left out" of the mainstream of life. Emotional and social isolation negatively impacts self-confidence and self-esteem.

Source: Applegarth, L.D. (1995). The psychological aspects of infertility. In W. R. Keye, Jr. R. J. Chang, R. W. Rebar, & M. R. Soules (Eds.), Infertility: Evaluation and treatment. *Philadelphia: W. B. Saunders Company. Used with permission.*

DIAGNOSTIC INFERTILITY EVALUATION

Expedite the evaluation and treatment of a couple in which (1) the female partner is over the age of 35, (2) she has a history of oligo/amenorrhea, (3) she has known or suspected uterine/tubal disease or endometriosis, or (4) the male partner is known to be subfertile (ASRM, 2000). The etiology of infertility is believed to be roughly equally divided between male and female causes, with approximately one-third of affected couples experiencing a combined problem. Multiple factors of infertility are more difficult to overcome. Unfortunately, 10 to 25 percent of infertility remains unexplained, despite a thorough evaluation. (Bayer et al., 2002; Cowan, 2002).

The infertility evaluation must be couple-oriented and evaluation of both partners should begin at the same time (ASRM, 2000) (see Figure 10–1). The evaluation can become an extremely stressful and dehumanizing experience if not performed by a caring and thoughtful clinician. Providing preconception care and counseling is an important part of the assessment and treatment of the infertile couple. The goal of fertility therapy is not only to establish a pregnancy, but to conceive a pregnancy that is uncomplicated and results in the delivery of a healthy baby (see Chapter 16).

TABLE 10–4. Female History: Summary of Pertinent Data

Age of client

Menstrual history (age at menarche, cycle length, duration/amount of flow, onset/severity of dysmenorrhea, other moliminal symptoms. If amenorrhea present, duration)

Obstetric history (gravidity, parity, pregnancy outcome, associated complications, time to conception)

Contraceptive history (current or past oral contraceptive use, IUD use, duration)

Sexual history (coital frequency, sexual dysfunction, number of partners, sexual orientation, history of sexually transmitted diseases and treatment)

Duration of infertility and results of any previous evaluation and treatment

Medical/surgical history (past surgeries, indications and outcomes, previous hospitalizations, serious illnesses or injuries, pelvic inflammatory disease, or exposure to sexually transmitted diseases)

Symptoms of thyroid disease, pelvic or abdominal pain, galactorrhea, hirsutism, and dyspareunia

Previous abnormal pap smears and any subsequent treatment (LEEP, cryotherapy)

Current medications and allergies

Social and occupation history (use of tobacco, alcohol, recreational drug use, caffeine intake, workplace exposures)

Nutrition history (BMI, vitamin supplementation, herbal remedies)

Family history of birth defects, mental retardation, reproductive failure, and other inheritable disorders

Source: Adapted from American Society for Reproductive Medicine. (2000, June). Optimal Evaluation of the Infertile Female. *A Practice Committee Report: A Committee Opinion. Birmingham, AL.*

After an initial consultation with a couple, which includes a complete history of the female and male partners (see Tables 10–4 and 10–5), physical examination of the female partner (see Table 10–6), preconception counseling, and instruction on how timing of intercourse might be optimized, the remainder of the infertility evaluation can usually be completed within two menstrual cycles (ASRM, 2000; Cowan, 2002). Physical examination of the male partner and referral to a urologist is initiated with abnormal semen analyses (see Table 10–7). Depending on the setting and practice protocols, a nurse practitioner may initiate the infertility evaluation, educate and support the couple, prescribe initial interventions, and refer to a specialist.

In the past, the standard infertility evaluation involved the performance of several tests, including the semen analysis, hysterosalpingogram, postcoital test, endometrial biopsy, and a laparoscopy. Studies confirm that the endometrial biopsy and postcoital testing are not always reliable and do not always differentiate between fertile and infertile populations (Bayer et al., 2002). Moreover, often the findings at the time of a laparoscopy, if done as an initial part of the infertility work-up, do not

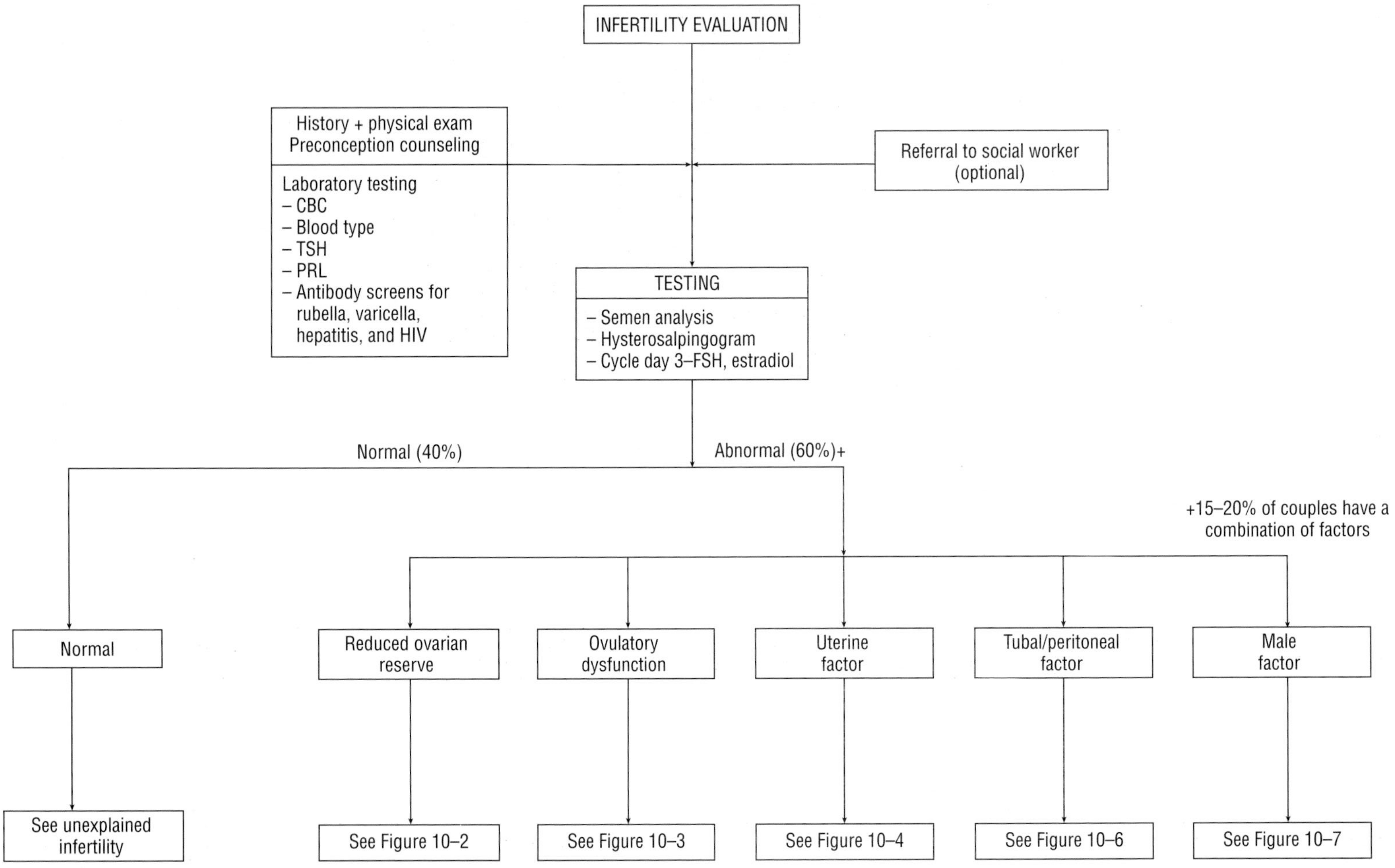

FIGURE 10–1. Infertility evaluation. *Adapted from: Bayer, S. R., Alper M. M., & Penzias, A. S. (2002). Overview of Infertility.* The Boston IVF Handbook of Infertility *(p. 68). New York, NY: Parthenon Publishing Group. Used with permission.*

TABLE 10–5. Male History: Summary of Pertinent Data

Duration of couple's Infertility.

Previous paternities, including time to conceive.

General health, pubescence, disorders of the urogenital tract.

Frequency and timing of coitus, sexual practices.

Contraceptive methods (condoms, vasectomy).

Exposure to toxins, excessive warmth, or irradiation.

Drugs (chemotherapy, anabolic steroids, hypertensive medications, caffeine, nicotine, alcohol, recreational drugs).

Developmental characteristics, e.g., onset of secondary sex characteristics, descent of the testes, and abnormalities of general development. (This may indicate endocrinological causes of reproductive dysfunction.)

Histories of any sexually transmitted diseases, systemic febrile illnesses, or genital infections such as mumps, chickenpox, or other forms of orchitis.

Surgical history, e.g., inguinal herniorrhaphy, injuries to the vas or bladder neck, retroperitoneal node dissection, testicular cancer, or circumcision.

Testicular torsion or general trauma.

Gynecomastia or anosmia.

Source: Adapted from Edwards, R. G. & Brody, S. A. (1995). Principles and practice of assisted human reproduction. Philadelphia: W.B. Saunders Company.

TABLE 10–7. Male Physical Exam: Summary of Pertinent Data

State of virilization (hair pattern, body proportions, muscle development).

Neurological symptoms (libido, headache, visual symptoms, papilledema, olfactory dysfunction).

Thyroid size, consistency, presence of nodules.

Presence of gynecomastia and/or galactorrhea.

Penis, circumcised, Tanner staging.

Testicular location, size, volume, and consistency.

Presence of epididymis and vas deferens.

Varicocele.

Prostate size, consistency.

Sources: Adapted from Sherins, R. J. (1995). How is male infertility defined? How is it diagnosed? Epidemiology, causes, work-up (history, physical, lab tests). In The American Society of Andrology, Handbook of Andrology. Lawrence, KS: Allen Press, Inc. Edwards, R. G., & Brody, S. A. (1995). Principles and practice of assisted human reproduction. Philadelphia: W.B. Saunders Company.

change the recommended course of treatment. Therefore, the infertility evaluation has become more practical, efficient, informative, and cost-effective (see Table 10–8).

SEMEN ANALYSIS (SA)

In 2001, the American Urological Association and the American Society for Reproductive Medicine recommended that the initial screening evaluation of the male partner include, at a minimum, a male reproductive history (see Table 10–5) and two semen analyses. If possible, the two semen analyses should be separated by one month. In practice, if the first semen analysis is normal, many clinicians do not require a second. A full evaluation by a urologist or other specialist in male reproduction should be done if the initial screening evaluation demonstrates an abnormal male reproductive history or an abnormal semen analysis.

Early in a woman's evaluation, her partner, after two to seven (but not more than 10) days of abstinence, collects a semen specimen by means of masturbation or, less commonly, by use of a special condom. The semen is deposited directly into a sterile container and evaluated microscopically within an hour of collection. Semen analyses vary in different labs.

TABLE 10–6. Female Physical Exam: Summary of Pertinent Data

Height, weight, Body Mass Index (BMI)

Thyroid enlargement, nodule, or tenderness

Breast exam (note masses, Tanner stage, any secretions and their character)

Signs of androgen excess (such as hirsutism, cliteromegaly, acanthosis nigricans)

Pelvic exam (note abdominal tenderness, organ enlargement, masses)

Adnexal mass or tenderness

Culdesac mass, tenderness, or nodularity

Uterine size, shape, position, and mobility

Vaginal or cervical lesions, stenosis, secretions, or discharge

Source: Adapted from American Society for Reproductive Medicine (2000, June). Optimal Evaluation of the Infertile Female. A Practice Committee Report: A Committee Opinion. Birmingham, AL.

TABLE 10–8. Past and Present Tests Used for Evaluation of Infertility

Past	Present
Semen analysis	Semen analysis
Endometrial biopsy	Assessment of ovarian function (Cycle day 3 FSH[*]/estradiol or CCCT[**]
Hysterosalpingogram	Hysterosalpingogram
Postcoital test	Laparoscopy (optional)
Laparoscopy	

[*] FSH: follicle stimulating hormone
[**] CCCT: clomiphene citrate challenge test

Source: Bayer, Alper, & Penzias, 2002.

♦ Normal semen analysis per the World Health Organization (WHO) (American Urological Association, 2001):

- *Volume.* 1.5 to 5 mL.
- *Viscosity.* Liquefaction occurs in one hour.
- *pH.* >7.2.
- *Count.* Equal to or greater than 20 million per mL.
- *Motility.* Equal to or greater than 50 percent.
- *Forward Progression.* Greater than 2 (on a 0–4 scale with 0 = no movement, to 4 = excellent forward progression).
- *Morphology.* Greater than 50 percent normal oval heads, midpiece, and tail.
- *Kruger's Strict Criteria.* Greater than 14 percent normal forms. Kruger developed strict criteria for morphology, which have proven to be more predictive of fertilization in in vitro fertilization (IVF) cycles. This system identifies greater than 14 percent normal forms as "normal," 4–14 percent as "good prognosis," and less than 4 percent as "poor prognosis" (Kruger, Acosta, Simmons, Swanson, et al., 1988.)

♦ Abnormal semen analysis requires that the test be repeated in four to six weeks.

♦ If time is not critical, three months should be allowed to complete a sperm cycle if a viral illness, hot bath, or toxicants could have caused poor semen parameters (AUA, 2001).

♦ Some studies suggest that ureaplasma attaches to sperm and reduces motility, so it is reasonable to obtain semen cultures if male factor infertility is present (Speroff et al., 1999). With positive ureaplasma/mycoplasma semen culture, treatment of both partners is indicated: one coated 100 mg doxycycline hyclate pellet (Doryx) daily, p.o., for thirty days, beginning with the first day of the woman's full menstrual flow. It is necessary to prevent pregnancy by protected intercourse or abstinence during the cycle of treatment.

♦ Normal semen parameters indicate no further male evaluation is necessary unless infertility persists (AUA, 2001; Bayer et al., 2002) (see Figure 10–7).

ASSESSMENT OF OVARIAN FUNCTION

Ovulatory dysfunction will be identified in approximately 15 percent of all infertile couples and accounts for up to 40 percent of infertility in women (ASRM, 2000). Ovulatory dysfunction can result in gross menstrual disturbances (oligo/amenorrhea, dysfunctional uterine bleeding), but it is also often more subtle (polymenorrhea, short luteal phase). It is important to discover the underlying cause (e.g., thyroid disease, hyperandrogenism, pituitary tumor, eating disorder, extremes of weight loss or exercise, hyperprolactinemia, obesity) because the correct diagnosis will lead to specific treatment and many conditions have long-term consequences on general health.

Menstrual History

If a woman is having regular menstrual cycles that are 25 to 35 days in length, then she is ovulating. Ovulation is further supported by the presence of moliminal symptoms (fluid retention/bloating, breast tenderness, mood changes).

BBT

A daily record of the basal body temperature (BBT) may provide a simple and inexpensive method for confirming ovulation, with a biphasic pattern characteristic of ovulation. BBT charts, however, can sometimes be difficult to interpret, some ovulatory women exhibit monophasic BBT patterns, and the test cannot reliably define the time of ovulation (see Chapter 9).

Urinary Luteinizing Hormone (LH)

Urinary ovulation predictor kits can identify the midcycle LH surge. These kits can provide reliable, if still indirect, evidence of ovulatory function and can help define the interval in which conception is most likely (intercourse or insemination the day of and the day after the LH surge). Results correlate well with the peak in serum LH.

Assessment of Ovarian Reserve

The maximum number of oocytes during woman's lifetime is present in utero at 20 weeks gestation. There is a developmental and progressive decrease in the number of oocytes from this point forward. Evaluation of the "ovarian reserve" by measurement of cycle day 3 serum FSH and estradiol levels or by the clomiphene citrate challenge test (CCCT) (see Table 10–9) provides an assessment of the number and quality of the remaining oocytes (ASRM, 2000; Bayer et al., 2002). Reduced ovarian reserve is associated with reduced fertility and increased risk of miscarriage (Sharara, Scott, & Seifer, 1998). The routine assessment of ovarian reserve reflects the current practice of most reproductive endocrinologists. Any woman who has evidence of reduced ovarian reserve

DIAGNOSIS:

The diagnosis of reduced ovarian reserve is supported by any of the following:

    1. Cycle day 3 FSH > 10 mIU/ml or estradiol > 50 pg/ml

    2. Abnormal clomiphene citrate challenge test (See Table 10–9)

    3. Documented poor response to aggressive ovulation induction

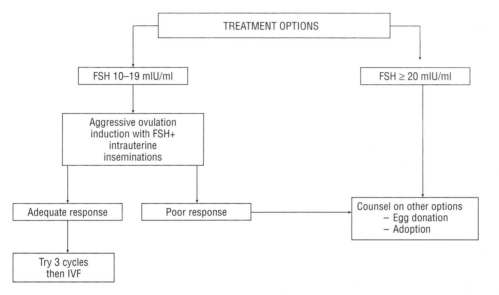

FIGURE 10–2.   Reduced ovarian reserve. *Source: Adapted from Bayer, S. R., Alper M. M., & Penzias, A. S. (2002). Overview of Infertility. The Boston IVF Handbook of Infertility (p. 70). New York: Parthenon Publishing Group. Used with permission.*

should be referred for counseling and offered aggressive treatment (see Figure 10–2).

ASSESSMENT OF UTERINE CAVITY AND ENDOMETRIUM

Hysterosalpingogram (HSG)

An x-ray test is performed by the physician after menses but before ovulation. Radioactive dye is placed in the uterus to outline the uterine cavity and determine the pa-

TABLE 10–9. Clomiphene Citrate Challenge Test (CCCT)

Step 1: Draw serum FSH and estradiol (E2) levels on menstrual cycle day 2, 3, or 4.

Step 2: Administer clomiphene citrate 100 mg (50 mg, 2 tabs po qd) on cycle days 5 through 9.

Step 3: Draw serum FSH level on cycle day 10.

Interpretation: If either of the FSH levels are >10 mIU/ml or the day 3 E2 level is greater than 50 pg/ml, the test confirms reduced ovarian reserve. If either of the FSH levels are greater than 15, the test is considered abnormal. If either (day 3 or day 10) FSH level is ≥ 20, direct the patient toward alternatives such as egg donation or adoption. An FSH level > 40 is menopausal.

tency of the fallopian tubes. Waterbased dye gives a better picture, but oil-based can push mucus out the fallopian tubes, which may have been blocking them. Some physicians will use both to take advantage of the benefits of each type of dye. Cramping can be reduced by having the woman take 600 to 800 mg of ibuprofen one hour prior to the test. The client may have a paracervical block and/or be given a sedative, midazolam HCL/Roche (Versed), which will virtually eliminate discomfort. Advise the client that someone must accompany her home and that she should wear a sanitary pad for fluid leakage and spotting. Prophylactic antibiotic therapy is often given prior to HSG.

Endometrial Biopsy (EMB)

Histologic documentation of secretory endometrial development implies that ovulation has taken place. Some practitioners still assess the functional adequacy of the endometrium with a timed endometrial biopsy. Until recently, luteal phase insufficiency was thought to cause infertility and recurrent miscarriages. Controversies, however, persist regarding the accuracy of the diagnostic criteria, the prevalence, and the clinical relevance of a "luteal phase defect" (ASRM, 2000). Because the chances are small of discovering a significant abnormality, many specialists omit this step, except in patients at high risk of poor response, including women who have received chemotherapy or pelvic radiation or who have a history of severe intrauterine adhesive disease or significant prior uterine surgery (Sauer, 2002). The adequacy of the endometrial response with ovulation induction may be monitored by transvaginal ultrasound. In one series, there were no out-of-phase biopsies when endometrial thickness exceeded 7 mm (Hoffmann, Thie, Scott, & Navot, 1996). Pregnancy rates have also been shown to be stable when embryo transfer is performed in patients with endometrial thickness ≥ 6 mm (Noyes, Hampton, Berkeley, et al., 2001).

If necessary, a late luteal phase endometrial biopsy can be performed two to three days before the onset of menses, with a negative pregnancy test. The nurse practitioner uses a Novak curette or pipelle to take a fundal sample of the endometrium (Winkel, 1995). Discomfort can be reduced by suggesting the client take 600 to 800 mg of ibuprofen one hour prior to the test (see Chapter 8). Histologic dating of the endometrium is correlated with the onset of menses.

ASSESSMENT OF THE PELVIS

Laparoscopy—Diagnostic or Therapeutic

The laparoscopy is performed early in the cycle, after menses, as outpatient surgery, usually under general anesthesia. It is recommended after other tests have been completed, unless the woman is experiencing severe pelvic pain. The laparoscope is inserted through the navel to visualize the pelvis. Laser or cautery can be used to treat endometriosis, pelvic adhesions or scarring, and some tubal diseases at the time of the diagnostic laparoscopy, thereby avoiding the need for major abdominal inpatient surgery. Usually the client can return home in several hours (see Chapter 13).

When uterine anomalies have been identified (abnormal HSG or sonohysterogram), laparoscopy is performed in conjunction with hysteroscopy. Hysteroscopy delineates the internal and external uterine contour, thus differentiating between a bicornate or septate uterus. Laser or cautery can be used at hysteroscopy to lyse adhesions, repair septa, and remove polyps or fibroids.

FEMALE INFERTILITY: CAUSES, DIAGNOSES, AND INTERVENTIONS

Female infertility may be caused by ovulatory dysfunction, uterine factors, and/or tubal or peritoneal factors.

OVULATORY DYSFUNCTION

Ovulatory dysfunction, in which ovulation occurs infrequently (oligo-ovulation) or not at all (anovulation) may be related to normal reproductive development (aging), a variety of endocrine disorders, premature ovarian failure (POF), or gonadal dysgenesis (see Figure 10–3).

HYPOTHALAMIC, PITUITARY, AND ADRENAL DISORDERS

Hyperprolactinemia is a common pituitary disorder; it requires extensive evaluation and referral. Hypogonadotropic hypogonadism and Sheehan's syndrome are rare causes of pituitary disorders (Speroff et al., 1999).

Hyperprolactinemia

Serum prolactin (PRL) levels are greater than 20 ng/mL. Elevated PRL interferes with GnRH release, which in turn results in lowered levels of FSH/LH. Elevated PRL may directly inhibit the gonads (Speroff et al., 1999).

Subjective Data. Take a complete history: infertility; cyclic, irregular menses, or amenorrhea; spontaneous milky breast discharge; headache/visual field disturbances, and stress are commonly reported. Medications such as antipsychotics, antidepressants, clonidine, reserpine, metaclopramide, and cimetidine can cause an elevation in prolactin (Liu, 1995.)

Objective Data

- ◆ *Physical Examination.* This must include a thorough neurological exam. Note any milky breast discharge or abnormal neurological findings, especially visual field disturbances.
- ◆ *Diagnostic Tests and Methods.* The following are indicated:
  - Pregnancy test.
  - PRL level (must be elevated on more than one sample at least several days apart, before a breast

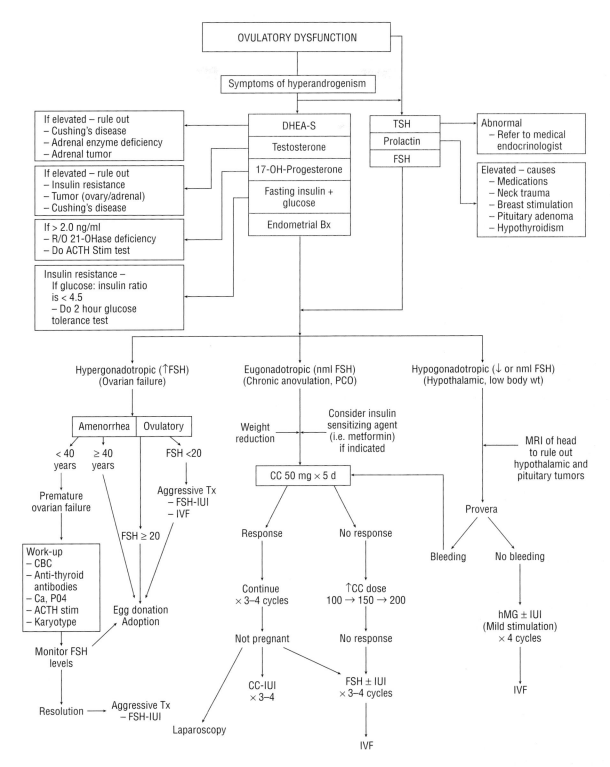

FIGURE 10–3. Ovulatory Dysfunction. *Source: Adapted from Bayer, S. R., Alper, M. M., & Penzias, A. S. (2002). Overview of Infertility.* The Boston IVF Handbook of Infertility *(p. 71). New York: Parthenon Publishing Group. Used with permission.*

exam, or any nipple stimulation, and prior to 11 A.M.).

- TSH and T_3, total T_4, free T_4 to rule out thyroid disease; (see Appendix C for normal values).
- MRI of the sella turcica to rule out pituitary adenoma.

Differential Medical Diagnoses. Galactorrhea, oligomenorrhea/amenorrhea, ovarian dysfunction, hypothalamic lesions, pituitary lesions (tumors, acromegaly, Cushing's disease, empty sella syndrome), hypothyroidism, physiological conditions (pregnancy, breast stimulation), pharmacological effects (reserpine, cimetidine, tricyclic antidepressants, estrogens), idiopathic conditions.

Plan

- Refer the client who desires fertility to a reproductive endocrinologist for continued evaluation and ovulation induction.
- Refer the client to a medical endocrinologist, neurologist, ophthalmologist, or surgeon as indicated.
- Provide the client with information, anticipatory guidance, stress management, and counseling for anxiety and body image disturbance.

Hypogonadotropic Hypogonadism

The hypoestrogenic woman has a negative progesterone withdrawal (i.e., no menstrual bleeding after the administration of progesterone), normal or slightly lower than normal FSH/LH levels, and normal prolactin levels. (Speroff et al., 1999). Amenorrhea can be caused by GnRH pulse suppression, which in turn inhibits pituitary function.

Subjective Data. Obtain an accurate menstrual history and determination of pubertal milestones. Inquire specifically about Crohn's disease, connective tissue disorders, hepatitis, galactorrhea, stress, adequacy of nutrition (take a dietary history to assess for eating disorders), exercise, and medications. Clients commonly report absent menses, monophasic basal body temperatures, history of excessive dieting or exercise, altered eating habits, and/or a stressful lifestyle.

Objective Data

Physical Examination. Assess for low body weight, low fat, little breast tissue, normal secondary sex characteristics, and hair patterns. The vagina may be dry with decreased rugae, and the uterus may be small. If the client has primary amenorrhea, assess the patency of the cervix.

Diagnostic Tests and Methods

Serum pregnancy test (quantitative): Negative

Serum Multiphasic Analysis-12 (SMA-12): Results are evaluated for indications of systemic illnesses that could affect hypothalamic function; may be normal or abnormal.

E2 (estradiol): Low

FSH/LH: Low to normal.

Thyroid studies (TSH, T3, T4, Free T4): May be abnormal

Prolactin (PRL): If elevated, complete work-up of pituitary is required.

Differential Medical Diagnoses. Primary or secondary amenorrhea, anovulation, hyperprolactinemia, psychiatric disorder.

Plan

- Refer the client with primary amenorrhea (see Chapter 8).
- Medical therapy as indicated.
- Refer the client to a reproductive endocrinologist for evaluation and ovulation induction as indicated.
- Ovulation induction in clients with hypothalamic disorders is best managed with the GnRH pump, although clomiphene, menotropin, or urofollitropin are often used. Bromocriptine is used to treat hyperprolactinemia. If no ovulation results, then clomiphene is used. If this does not result in ovulation, menotropin or urofollitropin is used (see Table 10–9).

Androgen Excess

Adrenal gland or ovarian dysfunction may result in androgen excess. Androgen excess is a common cause of ovulatory dysfunction and may also be an indicator of adrenal or ovarian tumor. Careful evaluation and referral are required. The three primary androgens in females are dehydroepiandrosterone sulfate (DHEA-S), androstenedione (A), and testosterone (T). Androgen excess interferes with feedback mechanisms and results in increased FSH/LH levels. Adrenal disorders result in the production of sex steroids which interact with GnRH, FSH/LH, and PRL.

Rapid progression of hirsutism, virilization, and changes in menstrual patterns are suggestive of a tumor. An adrenal tumor is suspected if serum DHEA-S levels are greater than 700 µg/dL (Levy, 1995). Ovarian tumors are suspected if total female serum testosterone is greater than 200 µg/dL (Levy, 1995).

Polycystic Ovarian Syndrome (PCOS)

Women who experience polycystic ovarian syndrome (PCOS) frequently are oligomenorrheic, hirsute, obese, and infertile. The components of PCOS are hyperandrogenism and oligo-ovulation or anovulation in the absence of other hyperandrogenic disorders such as androgen-secreting tumors or nonclassical adrenal hyperplasia. Clinical evidence of hyperandrogenism includes hirsutism and acne. Clinical findings that suggest insulin resistance and hyperinsulinemia are a BMI > 27 kg/m2, waist-to-hip ratio >0.85, waist >100 cm, acanthosis nigricans, and numerous achrochordons (skin tags) (Barbieri, 2000). In a population of women of reproductive age, the prevalence of PCOS is approximately 4 percent. The prevalence of PCOS among anovulatory women is approximately 30 percent (Barbieri, 2000).

PCOS results from an increased resistance to insulin. The compensatory increase in insulin production contributes to excess androgen production and chronic anovulation. In addition to reproductive problems, women with PCOS are predisposed to non-insulin dependent diabetes (NIDDM), hypertension, and heart disease. By the age of 40, up to 40 percent of PCOS patients develop impaired glucose tolerance or clinical diabetes (ASRM, 2001). Given the strong evidence that excess insulin accounts for the symptoms associated with PCOS, current research has shown that by reducing circulating insulin levels, normal reproductive function can be restored (Heard, Pierce, Carson, & Buster, 2002; Nestler, Jakubowicz, Evans, & Pasquali, 1998; Vandermolen, Ratts, Evans, et al., 2001). This is best accomplished through weight loss, improved nutrition, and exercise. Behavioral changes should be the first line of therapy for an overweight woman with PCOS.

Subjective Data. Note BMI, hirsutism, and menstrual history. Ask the client about any use of danazol (Danocrine), progestins, glucocorticoids, anabolic steroids, phenytoin, or minoxidil. The client may reveal concern about a history of excessive body hair, oily skin or acne, being overweight, and having irregular menses.

Objective Data

- *Physical Examination.* A complete physical exam is indicated. Assess the client's face, chin, and abdomen for male hair patterns (fine to coarse); note frontal balding, increased muscle mass, clitoral enlargement, decreased breast size, and voice changes. Also note if obesity is present, and evaluate for ovarian mass.

- *Diagnostic Tests.* Several may be indicated (See Figure 10–3):
  - *FSH.* Low or normal.
  - *LH.* Elevated.
  - LH–FSH ratio greater than 3.
  - *Testosterone.* Free. Normal is 100–200 pg/dL.
  - *DHEA-S.* Normal is 80–350 mcg/mL; normal ranges may decrease with age (Speroff et al., 1999).
  - *17-Hydroxyprogesterone (17 OHP).* Screens for androgen excess due to polycystic ovary syndrome (PCO), enzyme deficiency, or congenital adrenal hyperplasia (normal in follicular phase is 15–70 ng/dL; normal in luteal phase is 35–290 ng/dL). Significant elevation suggests adrenal hyperplasia.
  - *Dexamethasone Suppression.* Dexamethasone 1.0 mg is given orally at 11 P.M. Plasma cortisol is measured at 8 A.M.; if suppressed to less than 5 mcg/mL, Cushing's disease is ruled out (Speroff et al., 1999).
  - *Corticotropin (ACTH) Stimulation Test.* At 8 A.M., an I.V. bolus of synthetic ACTH 0.25 mg is administered; blood samples for 17-OHP and cortisol are obtained prior to the bolus and at 60 minutes (normal random cortisol levels are 5–25 mcg/dL; normal morning levels are 5–25 mcg/dL; normal evening levels are 2–12 mcg/dL). Significant elevation suggests enzyme deficiency or adrenal hyperplasia.
  - *Glucose Tolerance Test:* (3° GTT)
  - *Fasting insulin*
  - *BUN/Creatinine:* Normal renal function is critical to treatment with metformin. Decreased renal blood flow increases metformin toxicity.

Differential Medical Diagnoses. Ovarian disorders (polycystic ovary syndrome, hyperthecosis, androgen producing tumors, virilization of pregnancy). Adrenal disorders (congenital adrenal hyperplasia, androgen producing tumors, Cushing's disease, drug related, obesity, post menopause, incomplete testicular feminization, idiopathic conditions).

Plan

- Weight loss, counseling about improved nutrition and an exercise routine that can be incorporated into a major change in lifestyle.
- Refer the client to an endocrinologist or to a reproductive endocrinologist for evaluation and treatment.

◆ Psychosocial interventions include anticipatory guidance regarding treatment and medication. Offer the client support and referral to a psychologist and referral to a respected weight loss program or nutritionist.

◆ Review risks of endometrial cancer secondary to endometrial hyperplasia resulting from persistent anovulation. Review risks related to overweight such as NIDDM, HTN, and cardiovascular disease.

Metformin (Glucophage) is an antihyperglycemic drug that improves tissue sensitivity to insulin while decreasing insulin levels and inhibiting hepatic glucose production. When used in patients with PCOS, metformin reduces LH, sex hormone-binding globulin, and ovarian androgens and corrects hyperinsulinemia. Metformin also induces the resumption of regular menses and ovulation. Ovulatory response to clomiphene citrate and pregnancy rates can be increased in obese PCOS women when used in conjunction with metformin (Heard et al., 2002; Nestler et al., 1998). Although Metformin is not yet approved by the FDA as a treatment for infertility, of the available options for ovulation induction, metformin may be the most cost-effective intervention with the fewest serious side effects.

Start metformin at 500 mg qhs for one week. Increase the dose to 500 mg bid for one week, then increase the dose to 500 mg tid for one week. Once the client is on a tolerable regimen of metformin 500 mg tid, continue the full dose therapy for five weeks. During the last twenty-one days of therapy, obtain a progesterone level every ten days. If the patient does not ovulate on metformin alone, add clomiphene in a regular regimen. Obtain progesterone levels or other testing to ensure ovulation is occurring. Consider using metformin for up to six months in a solo therapy if it is producing ovulation or in combination with clomiphene. Metformin is a category B drug. The most common side effects are gastrointestinal disturbances, including diarrhea, nausea, vomiting, and abdominal bloating. A gradual increase in the dose over time will minimize GI discomfort. Caution the client to discontinue metformin with severe dehydration of any cause; metformin's toxicity is increased with compromised renal blood flow.

Start folic acid 1 to 4 mg daily. Risk of neural tube defects are increased with obesity.

Premature Ovarian Failure (POF)

In POF, failure of ovarian estrogen production results in elevated FSH levels (greater than 40 mIU/mL) on more than one serum sample (see Figure 10–2). The ovaries do not produce enough estrogen to inhibit hypothalamic release of GnRH. Continued release of GnRH results in elevated FSH/LH levels as ovulation ceases. Failure may occur at any age between menarche and 40 years and requires careful endocrine evaluation. POF can be caused by autoimmune disease (Speroff et al., 1999).

Subjective Data. These include amenorrhea, hot flashes/night sweats, vaginal dryness.

Objective Data. A complete physical examination is indicated; assess for signs of hypoestrogenicity (refer to Table 10–2). Several diagnostic tests are indicated.

◆ Cycle day 3 *FSH/LH* or CCCT (Clomiphene citrate challenge test) (see Figure 10–2) elevated.
◆ *TSH, T_3, T_4, free T_4.* Rule out thyroid disease.
◆ *PRL.* Rule out hyperprolactinemia.

Additional tests to rule out autoimmune disorders include CBC with differential and sedimentation rate, total serum protein, albumin to globulin ratio, rheumatoid factor, antinuclear antibodies (ANA), antithyroid globulin, antimicrosomal antibodies, fasting blood sugar, A.M. cortisol, and serum calcium and phosphorus. If the woman is younger than 30 years, a karyotype is indicated (assessment of normal female versus presence of Y chromosome, which is associated with increased risk of malignant gonadal tumor) (Speroff et al., 1999).

Differential Medical Diagnoses. Chromosome abnormality, autoimmune disease (polyendocrinopathy type I or II, myasthenia gravis, idiopathic thrombocytopenia purpura, hemolytic anemia), thyroid dysfunction (hypoparathyroidism, thyroiditis), adrenal insufficiency/failure, 17-hydroxylase deficiency, gonadal tumor.

Plan

◆ Medical therapy as indicated.
◆ Hormone replacement as necessary.
◆ Refer the client who desires fertility to a reproductive endocrinologist.
◆ Psychosocial interventions involve providing information and anticipatory guidance about the physical and emotional changes that accompany loss of ovarian function, including disturbances in body image, personal identity, self-esteem, the grief process, and sexual dysfunction. The client may need to be referred for individual/marital counseling and possible sex therapy. Review nutrition, including calcium and red meat intake, need for weight-bearing exercise, as

well as the risks of osteoporosis, cardiovascular disease, and endometrial cancer.

- Medication may include estrogen/progesterone replacement, lubricants, estradiol vaginal cream.
- In vitro fertilization (IVF) with donor oocytes.
- Adoption
- Childfree living

Gonadal Dysgenesis (Turner's Syndrome)

Gonadal dysgenesis is a broad term for clients with female genitalia, normal müllerian structures, and streak gonads (Speroff et al., 1999).

Dysgenesis results from the gonads undergoing partial or complete regression, which leads to abnormal sexual development (Nestler & Jakubowicz, 1996). Fibrous gonads caused by complete regression do not produce hormones. This syndrome is associated with a broad range of genetic patterns. Surprisingly, some women with pure gonadal dysgenesis have a normal XX chromosome pattern. A majority of clients with dysgenesis have only one X chromosome; others have multiple cell lines of varying sex chromosome composition (mosaicism) (Speroff et al., 1999). Women with XY chromosome patterns (usually mosaic) are at risk for neoplastic changes in the gonads, thus requiring gonad removal (Speroff et al., 1999).

Turner's syndrome is a gonadal dysgenesis condition in which a woman has only one X chromosome, a structural abnormality in one X chromosome, or mosaicism with an abnormal X. The fetus has a normal complement of ova at 20 weeks' gestation; however, they have totally or partially disappeared by birth. The ovaries appear as streak gonads. The incidence of Turner's syndrome is 1 in 2000 to 5000 liveborn girls (Speroff et al., 1999).

Subjective Data

- *Gonadal Dysgenesis.* Scant or absent pubic or axillary hair; primary or secondary amenorrhea, absent or arrested secondary sexual development.

Objective Data. A complete physical examination is necessary (see Table 10–2).

Gonadal Dysgenesis Clients May Have Any of the Following

- Normal height or short stature.
- Scant or absent pubic/axillary hair.
- Normal appearing female external genitalia.
- Normal or no breast development.

- Ambiguous genitalia (intra-abdominal testes often found in hernia), blind vaginal pouch, and absent or arrested secondary sex characteristics.
- May have no secondary sexual characteristics but normal appearing external female genitalia *or* ambiguous external genitalia.

Turner's Syndrome Clients Classically Have the Following

- Short stature.
- Scant or absent pubic/axillary hair.
- Webbing of the neck.
- Broad shield-type chest with laterally placed nipples.
- Lack of breast development.
- Vagina and uterus present but infantile.
- Ovaries absent.
- Diagnostic Tests.
  - Karyotype—Abnormal chromosome pattern.
  - FSH/LH—Elevated.
  - Testosterone—Normal or elevated.
  - Additional studies to detect cardiac malformations (coarctation of aorta) and renal abnormalities may be indicated in clients with Turner's syndrome.

Differential Medical Diagnoses. Turner's syndrome, testicular feminization, Swyer-James syndrome, coarctation of the aorta, kidney dysfunction.

Plan

- Refer the client to a reproductive endocrinologist and for genetic counseling.
- Medical therapy as indicated.
- During psychosocial interventions, information and anticipatory guidance are provided regarding physical differences and the emotional impacts of body stature, impaired sexual development, and lack of reproductive capacity. Refer the client for individual/marital counseling and, possibly, sex therapy.
- Client teaching is related to estrogen deficiencies: review nutrition, exercise, hormone replacement and risks of osteoporosis, cardiovascular disease, glucose intolerance, and thyroid dysfunction.
- Medication in the management of Turner's syndrome includes oral cyclic administration of estrogen and progesterone. Oral contraceptives are not indicated for this client, as there are only streak gonads and the estrogen dose is not adequate to protect the bones and cardiovascular system.
- IVF with donor eggs is an option for the client with Turner's desiring fertility.

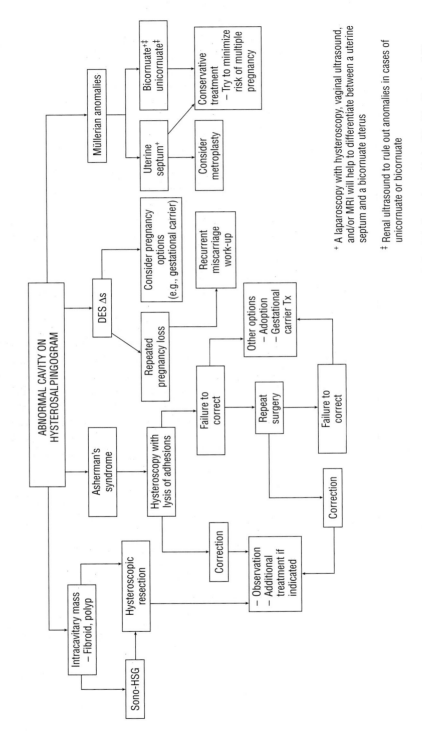

FIGURE 10–4. Uterine disorders. *Adapted from: Bayer, S. R., Alper M. M., & Penzias, A. S. (2002). Overview of Infertility. The Boston IVF Handbook of Infertility (p. 72). New York: Parthenon Publishing Group. Used with permission.*

UTERINE DISORDERS

Uterine causes of infertility are due to anatomic abnormalities or infection (see Figure 10–4). Congenital anomalies result from arrested uterine development, abnormal formation of the uterus, or incomplete fusion of the müllerian ducts, DES exposure, pelvic irradiation, adhesions, infection, fibroids, and polyps can interfere with conception, sperm migration, and implantation.

Müllerian Anomalies

Such abnormalities may result from genetic patterns of inheritance or spontaneous mutations, such as trisomy 13 and 15, which would have been diagnosed as a neonate. Women who are presenting with a history of infertility or recurrent pregnancy loss may be found to have a subtle müllerian anomaly. Fortunately, uterine structural defects, except those caused by DES exposure, are often amenable to surgical correction (see Figure 10–5 and Table 10–10).

Subjective Data. May include a history of infertility and/or pregnancy loss, abnormal uterine bleeding, primary amenorrhea, dysmenorrhea, dyspareunia.

Objective Data

- A physical exam is indicated to assess for abnormal anatomic structures.
- Diagnostic tests and methods including ultrasound, hysterosalpingogram, laparoscopy/hysteroscopy, and/or pelvic MRI are used to detect structural abnormalities. Karyotype is performed to rule out chromosomal abnormalities.

Differential Medical Diagnoses. Congenital anomalies, endometriosis, urinary tract anomalies.

Plan

- Refer the client to a reproductive endocrinologist.
- Psychosocial interventions include providing information, anticipatory guidance, and support.
- If indicated, refer the client to a counselor for individual, group, or sex therapy.
- Laparoscopy/hysteroscopy (metroplasty) is done to correct vaginal and uterine abnormalities and to restore the uterine cavity or endometrium.

Follow-Up. Follow-up depends on the extent of the abnormalities and the procedures needed to correct them.

DES (Diethylstilbestrol) Exposure

Exposure of the female fetus to diethylstilbestrol is associated with uterine cavity abnormalities, including T-shaped uteri, hypoplastic cavities, intrauterine adhesions, and cervical stenosis. In addition, DES exposure in utero is linked with ectopic pregnancy, pregnancy loss, and preterm birth (Speroff, et al., 1999). Later cellular abnormalities (adenosis) in vaginal or ectocervical epithelium are associated with DES exposure during fetal life, result-

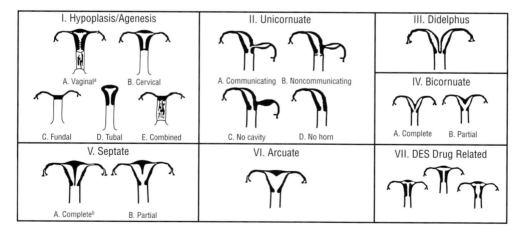

FIGURE 10–5. The American Society for Reproductive Medicine classification of müllerian anomalies. [a]Uterus may be normal or take a variety of abnormal forms. [b]May have two distinct cervices. *(Adapted from The American Society for Reproductive Medicine classifications of adnexal adhesion, distal tubal occlusion secondary to tubal ligation, tubal pregnancies, müllerian anomalies and intrauterine adhesions. Fertil Steril, 49: 6, 1988. Reproduced with permission of The American Society for Reproductive Medicine.)*

TABLE 10–10. Classification of Müllerian Anomalies

Hypoplasia or Agenesis Malformation: Abnormal development of the caudal portion of the uterovaginal primordium. Malformations range from a transverse membrane in the vagina, to vaginal atresia with normal or abnormal uterine shapes, to hypoplasia of the endometrium, to segmental agenesis of the fallopian tubes. Infertility may be the presenting symptom. Obstetrical (OB) complications depend on the anomaly.

Unicornais Uterus: Unilateral abnormality caused by arrested development of one müllerian duct. If implantation occurs in a rudimentary horn pregnancy wastage or tubal pregnancy can be the result. OB complications include malpresentations, intrauterine growth retardation, premature labor, and incompetent cervix.

Uterus Didalphus: The müllerian ducts never fused, so there are two uteri, two cervices, and possibly two vaginas. Outflow from one uterus may be obstructed and cause symptoms. OB complications include malpresentations and premature labor.

Bicornuate Uterus: Partial lack of fusion of the two müllerian ducts produces a single cervix with a varying degree of separation in the two horns. OB complications include early abortions, preterm labor, and breech presentations.

Septate Uterus: Lack of resorption of the midline septum between the two müllerian ducts resulting in defects varying from a slight midline septum to a septum dividing the uterus and vagina. OB complications depend on the severity of the defect, but can include recurrent pregnancy loss, preterm labor, and breech presentations.

Arcrate Uterus: A mild form of septate uterus (heart-shaped cavity) not associated with pregnancy loss.

Diethylstilbestrol (DES) Related Anomaly: Due to in utero DES exposure. T-shaped uterus, small cavity, constriction rings may present in any combination. Cervical defects include anterior cervical ridge, a cervical collar, a hypoplastic cervix, or a pseudopolyp. All may lead to an incompetent cervix.

Source. Sims & Gibbons, 1996; Speroff et al., 1999. Clinical gynecoiodic endocrinology and infertility (6th ed.). Baltimore: Williams and Wilkins; and Sims, J. A. & Gibbons, W. E. (1996). Treatment of human infertility: The cervical and uterine lactors, in E. Y. Adashi, J. A. Rock, & Z. Rosenwaks (Eds.), Reproductive endocrinology, surgery and technology. Philadelphia: Lippincott-Raven.

ing in susceptibility to carcinogenic effects of endogenous estrogens (clear cell adenocarcinomas). (See DES Exposure, Chapter 13.)

DES was synthesized in 1938 and used by several million women from 1945 through 1971 to prevent pregnancy loss, toxemia, stillbirth, and preterm labor (Sims & Gibbons, 1996). Research has documented an increased occurrence of clear cell adenocarcinoma in DES-exposed women between 14 and 22 years of age, with a peak incidence at age 19. It is unknown whether female offspring of DES-exposed offspring will also sustain structural defects (Rock & Markham, 1995).

Subjective Data. Data reveal a history of maternal DES treatment and a client history of menstrual abnormalities,

miscarriage, lower fertility rate, ectopic pregnancy, premature delivery, incompetent cervix, or abnormal Pap smears.

Objective Data. A complete physical examination is indicated to detect abnormalities of anatomic structure. DES-exposed women need to begin having pelvic examinations soon after the onset of menses and to have them at least annually. Common abnormalities include vaginal adenosis (ridge, septum, malformation), cervical adenosis (collar, hood, polyp, malformation, stenosis), and müllerian anomalies.

Diagnostic tests and methods include a Pap smear of the cervix to screen for squamous cell carcinoma, and a colposcopy and biopsy of abnormal vaginal and cervical tissue. Other methods may be indicated to evaluate anatomic abnormalities (ultrasound, hysterosalpingogram, laparoscopy/hysteroscopy, pelvic MRI).

Differential Medical Diagnoses. Congenital anomalies, chromosomal abnormalities.

Plan. Psychosocial interventions include providing information, anticipatory guidance, and support. No medication is recommended. No treatment is indicated unless complications—such as abnormal Pap smears, pregnancy complications, or infertility arise.

Follow-Up. Referrals for individual, group, or sex therapy may be indicated; or an infertility specialist may be indicated if the client is unable to become pregnant or has a history of pregnancy loss. Careful follow-up for clear cell adenocarcinoma and squamous cell carcinoma is required; immediate referral is made if suspicious findings occur.

Intrauterine Adhesions (Asherman's Syndrome)

The syndrome results from damage to the endometrium after excessive curettage, cesarean birth, metroplasty, pelvic irradiation, myomectomy, as well as from infections (Sims & Gibbons, 1996). It interferes with fertility by disrupting sperm migration, mechanically obstructing tubal ostia, and impeding blastocyst implantation. Pregnancy loss may result from decreased size of the uterine cavity or inadequate endometrium (Speroff, et al., 1999).

Subjective Data. The client may report a history of menstrual abnormalities (scant flow, secondary amenorrhea, dysmenorrhea), or normal menses, dyspareunia, uterine infection, pregnancy losses, surgical procedures, cancer therapies.

Objective Data

- A complete physical examination is indicated. Often, findings are normal. Assess for cervical stenosis; cervical discharge; signs of cervical, vaginal or uterine infection; and abnormal uterine contour, firmness, immobility, tenderness.
- Diagnostic tests and methods include endometrial biopsy to diagnose endometritis; hysterosalpingogram to determine abnormalities in uterine contour; laparoscopy and hysteroscopy (when indicated). Repeat hysterosalpingogram may be indicated after surgical correction if conception does not occur. (An endometrial biopsy may diagnose fibrosis, but a normal result does not rule out fibrosis in another area of the uterus.)

Differential Medical Diagnoses. Amenorrhea, dysmenorrhea, cervical stenosis.

Plan

- Provide the client with information, anticipatory guidance, and support.
- Medication may include cyclic high dose estrogen/progesterone replacement to help restore normal endometrium after surgical correction. Postoperative pain is usually managed with acetaminophen or non-steroidal anti-inflammatory agents.
- Laparoscopy and hysteroscopy may be indicated for lysis of adhesions and cervical dilation.
- Following lysis of adhesions, high-dose estrogen therapy is sometimes used to build the endometrium in an attempt to keep the uterine walls from adhering to each other.

Follow-Up. Refer the client to a reproductive endocrinologist and for psychological counseling. Repeat procedures to lyse adhesions are indicated if normal menses is not established.

Endometritis

Endometritis is an endometrial inflammation due to infection caused by pathogens. It may result from ascending infection, use of an intrauterine device (IUD), endometrial trauma, or as a secondary infection associated with cancer. Common pathogens include aerobic/anaerobic bacteria, mycoplasma, chlamydia, gonorrhea, viruses, toxoplasmas, parasites, and rarely mycobacterium tuberculosis. Treatment is controversial when no pathogen is identified because resolution may occur spontaneously. Infertility may be associated with an unfavorable endometrial environment that results from a heightened immune response and interferes with blastocyst implantation (Winkel, 1995).

Tuberculosis (TB) endometritis is rare. Infertility occurs due to extensive tubal scarring and uterine adhesions. Diagnosis is made by curettage and culture of the premenstrual endometrium. Antituberculosis medications are used until repeat curettage is normal.

Subjective Data. The client may report uterine tenderness, dyspareunia, dysmenorrhea, foul odor, or an abnormal vaginal discharge. She may also report a history of D & C or trauma to cervix (decreasing secretion of cervical mucus) (Winkel, 1995). Infertility may be the only sign of chronic endometritis.

Objective Data. Physical examination will reveal tenderness on bimanual examination, especially if it is acute endometritis.

Diagnosis of chronic endometritis is accomplished by follicular phase endometrial biopsy with culture, as well as histologic evaluation of the biopsy tissue (Winkel, 1995). (See Pelvic Inflammatory Disease in Chapter 13 for tests to diagnose acute infection.)

Differential Medical Diagnoses. Urinary tract infection (UTI), acute pyelonephritis, appendicitis, pelvic abscess, thromboembolism, gastrointestinal disease, endometriosis, uterine adhesions.

Plan

- Psychosocial interventions include teaching the client about the causes, treatment, prevention, and effects of infection. Provide support and counseling, and encourage support from significant others.
- Medication specific to the identified organism is prescribed for recurrent endometrial/pelvic infections because the inflammation, abnormal endometrium, and adhesion formation associated with infection decrease fertility (see Chapter 11).
- Endometrial biopsy (follicular phase) is indicated after antibiotic treatment to determine resolution of endometritis.
- Pain management is often indicated.

Follow-Up. Refer the client to a reproductive endocrinologist for continued evaluation and infertility treatment. Diagnostic evaluation and treatment will be affected by a history of recurrent infection and the degree of pelvic and tubal pathology.

♦ Once the infection is resolved, hysterosalpingogram, laparoscopy, laparoscopy/hysteroscopy, and laparotomy for lysis of adhesions and tubal repair may be indicated. After tubal repair, clients are at risk for ectopic pregnancy. IVF may be necessary if other corrective therapies cannot restore normal tubal function. If scarring or adhesions lead to an atrophic endometrium, treatment may involve the use of a gestational carrier.

Uterine Leiomyomata (Fibroids)

Leiomyomata are common tumors occurring in approximately 25 percent of women older than 30 (Propst & Hill, 2000). Fibroids are classified as subserosal, intramural, or submucosal, depending whether they are located just beneath the serosa, within the myometrium, or adjacent to the endometrium, respectively. Depending on the fibroid size, number, and location, if the uterine cavity is partially obliterated or the contour is significantly altered, the fibroid may result in poorly vascularized endometrium and interfere with implantation or otherwise compromise placental development. Submucosal and intramural fibroids affect embryo implantation and development adversely following IVF and embryo transfer, even in the absence of a deformed uterine cavity, compared with women with subserosal or no fibroids (Eldar-Geva, Meagher, Healy, et al., 1998).

Hysteroscopic myomectomy has been shown to improve clinical pregnancy rates and decrease risk of spontaneous abortion. In a large review ($N = 1941$), Buttram and Reiter (1981) reported that in women who underwent an abdominal myomectomy, the subsequent spontaneous abortion rate dropped from 41 percent preoperatively to 19 percent postoperatively. In women with submucous fibroids and either infertility or recurrent pregnancy loss, hysteroscopic myomectomy is recommended because the abdominal approach has been associated with longer anesthesia time, higher blood loss, higher risk for postoperative adhesion formation and infection, and the need for elective cesarean delivery in subsequent pregnancies (Goldenberg, Sivan, Sharabi, et al., 1995).

Subjective Data. The client may report pain (dysmenorrhea or dyspareunia) increased, prolonged, or irregular menstrual flow. Small fibroids may be asymptomatic.

Objective Data. A complete physical exam may reveal an enlarged, irregularly shaped, firm uterus.

♦ Diagnostic tests and methods may include ultrasound, hysterosalpingogram, or hysteroscopy to access the uterine cavity.

Plan

♦ Refer the client to a gynecologist.
♦ *Preoperative Medication.* Surgery may be necessary for a successful pregnancy. Use of Depot Lupron (leuprolide acetate) or other GnRH analogue preoperatively may be indicated with large tumors to impose anovulation and thereby decrease tumor size, the risk of hemorrhage, and trauma to the uterus. Medications such as leuprolide acetate suppress the growth of the fibroid tumor, but as it causes a medical menopause, the risk of osteoporosis increases, and consequently cannot be given on a long-term basis. When the drug is stopped, the tumor starts to grow again, so usually Lupron is used on a short-term (3 to 6 month) basis to shrink the tumor prior to surgery.

- Common transient side effects include hot flashes, night sweats, breakthrough bleeding, vaginal dryness.
- Protected intercourse is indicated during entire course of therapy.

♦ Laparotomy is required to remove large fibroids; small fibroids may be removed with laparoscopy/hysteroscopy.
♦ Pain (dysmenorrhea) management includes acetaminophen and nonsteroidal anti-inflammatory agents.

TUBAL AND PERITONEAL DISORDERS

Sequelae of pelvic inflammatory disease, postoperative adhesions, and endometriosis are involved in the pathogenesis of impaired fertility (see Figure 10–6).

Pelvic Inflammatory Disease (PID)

Every year, one million women are treated for PID (Lewis & Bernstein, 1996). Westrom's classic study demonstrated that the incidence of tubal occlusion after one episode is 11.4 percent, after two episodes, 23.1 percent, and after three or more episodes, 54.3 percent (Westrom, 1980). Early diagnosis of acute PID and aggressive antimicrobial treatment decreases the chances of resulting sequelae (Rogers, 1995).

Tubal pathology is one of the most common causes of infertility in women. Sexually transmitted diseases

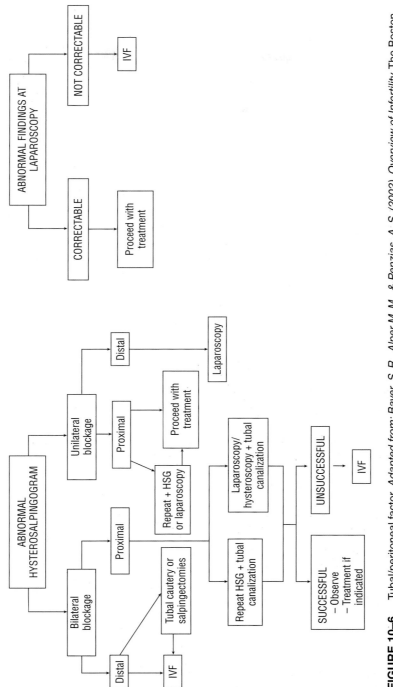

FIGURE 10–6. Tubal/peritoneal factor. *Adapted from: Bayer, S. R., Alper M. M., & Penzias, A. S. (2002). Overview of Infertility. The Boston IVF Handbook of Infertility (p. 73). New York: Parthenon Publishing Group. Used with permission.*

caused by *Neisseria gonorrhoeae* and *Chlamydia trachomatis* are the major source of tubal disease. Other infectious agents include aerobic/anaerobic bacteria, toxoplasmosis, and parasites. Tubal repair may be accomplished by laser or cutting laparoscopy or laparotomy (salpingostomy, fimbrioplasty, reanastomosis). The success of tubal repair depends on the extent of disease and, due to the delicate microsurgery involved, the skill of the surgeon. Further fertility treatment if repair is unsuccessful may include IVF. A repeat surgery usually does not result in functional tubes (see Figure 10–6 and Chapter 13).

Pelvic Adhesions

Pelvic adhesions that interfere with pickup/transport of the oocyte are a major cause of infertility in women. Meticulous surgical technique, minimal tissue handling, stringent hemostasis, constant irrigation, avoidance of abrasion between raw surfaces (adhesion barriers), and microsurgery using unipolar fine wire cautery or laser will reduce adhesion formation and preserve fertility (laparoscopy/laparotomy) (Strickler, 1995).

Subjective Data. The client may report a history of chronic pelvic pain, dyspareunia, menstrual disorders, pelvic surgery. In half of all cases, a history of infertility with no history of antecedent disease is the presentation.

Objective Data. An examination is indicated. Tenderness and a fixed uterus on bimanual examination are common. Diagnostic methods are a hysterosalpingogram and a laparoscopy to diagnose and treat pelvic pathology.

Differential Medical Diagnoses. Chronic salpingitis, residual inflammatory disease, tubal blockage, PID.

Plan

- Psychosocial interventions include providing information and support. Relaxation techniques, biofeedback, and pain management may also be indicated.
- Antibiotic and pain therapy may be used prior to invasive procedures.
- Other possible interventions include laser or cautery laparoscopy for lysis of adhesions; tubal repair (salpingostomy, neosalpingostomy, fimbrioplasty) as indicated; laparotomy to treat severe pelvic disease (adhesion lysis; microscopic tubal or cornual reanastomosis); IVF if indicated.
- Refer the client to a reproductive endocrinologist.

Hydrosalpinges

The presence of large hydrosalpinges has been shown to be associated with decreased clinical pregnancy rates with IVF, decreased implantation rates, increased spontaneous abortions, and increased ectopic pregnancy rates (Cohen, Lindheim, & Sauer, 1999; Nackley & Muasher, 1998). In a large meta-analysis, the effect of salpingectomy was to increase implantation rates, clinical pregnancy rates, livebirth rates with IVF, while decreasing rates of spontaneous abortion and ectopic pregnancies (Johnson, 2002).

Endometriosis

Endometriosis, a major cause of infertility, is a condition in which endometrial tissue, glands, and stroma are located outside of the uterine cavity. The tissue responds to cyclic hormones like the endometrial lining (see Chapter 13). Fertility is impaired by mechanical factors interfering with ovum pickup and tubal transport; by ovulatory dysfunction, and by interference with sperm function, fertilization and implantation. Endometriosis is a chronic disease and can be associated with chronic pelvic pain. (See Resources for the Endometriosis Association.) Treatment depends on the severity of symptoms and the desire for fertility. Infertility management may include both laparoscopy and medical management with GnRH agonists. In mild cases, conservative management (doing nothing), or laser or cautery laparoscopy may be the only treatment needed. Moderate disease may be treated with medication such as Depot Lupron and nafarelin acetate or danazol for six months. These medications suppress estrogen and progesterone production so that atrophy of the endometrial implants occurs. Symptoms often return after the medications are stopped. Severe cases, however, may also require either preoperative or postoperative danazol, Depot Lupron, or nafarelin acetate (Synarel) (Lewis & Bernstein, 1996). Further infertility treatment may include ovulation induction IUI or IVF.

RECURRENT PREGNANCY LOSS

The most common obstetrical complication is spontaneous abortion, which is seen in 15 to 20 percent of all clinically recognized pregnancies. *Recurrent abortion* is defined as three or more consecutive spontaneous pregnancy losses prior to 20 weeks' gestation. This is discouraging for both the couple and the provider. The good news is that almost 70 percent of women will eventually achieve a live birth in subsequent pregnancies without treatment. Treatment is designed to decrease the risk of subsequent pregnancy losses (Cramer & Wise, 2000).

Evaluation of a couple experiencing recurrent abortion should begin after three pregnancy losses, or after two if the woman is over 35 years of age. Pregnancy loss may be caused by anatomic, endocrine, genetic, or immunologic variations; infection; chronic illness; or environmental toxins.

Subjective Data. The client may report a history of recurrent abortion. A detailed history of occupational exposures, cigarette smoking, alcohol consumption, and substances of abuse should be obtained.

Objective Data. A complete physical examination is indicated. During the pelvic examination, special attention is given to detecting anatomic abnormalities, such as fibroids, polyps, hydrosalpinges, and müllerian abnormalities. Diagnostic tests include PRL; TSH, TPO (anti-thyroid antibodies) lupus anticoagulant; anticardiolipin antibodies; antiphosphatidyl serine antibody (IgG, IgM) karyotype (both partners and any products of conception, if possible); chlamydia, ureaplasma, and mycoplasma cultures; endometrial biopsy; hysterosalpingography; ultrasound; laparoscopy/hysteroscopy (Adashi, 2000).

Differential Medical Diagnoses

- *Anatomic Abnormalities (Uterus).* Müllerian defects, fibroids, septum defects, Asherman's syndrome, incompetent cervix.
- *Endocrine Abnormalities.* Thyroid (hypothyroid), hyperprolactinemia, ovulatory dysfunction/LPD.
- *Infection.* Chlamydia, TORCH (T, toxoplasmosis; O, other infections [varicella, listeria, syphilis]; R, rubella; C, cytomegalovirus; H, herpes simplex virus), ureaplasma/mycoplasma.
- *Chronic Illness.* Wilson's disease, heart/renal disease, blood dyscrasias.
- *Genetic Abnormality.* Aneuploidy of products of conception; balanced translocation, sex chromosome mosaicism, chromosome inversions and ring chromosomes of the couple (Adashi, 2000).
- *Immunologic Disorders.* Systemic lupus erythematosus (SLE), parental histocompatibilities.
- *Environmental Toxins.* Radiation, chemotherapy, recreational drugs, smoking, ethyl alcohol abuse, caffeine.

Plan

- Provide the client with information and psychological support; be available for questions and listening.

Evaluate the client's stage of crisis and grief, communication patterns, relationships, coping abilities, and use of support systems.

- Collaborate with medical (reproductive endocrinology) and mental health specialists.
- Medication or surgery is determined by the cause of the recurrent pregnancy loss (Adashi, 2000).

Follow-Up. As appropriate, provide information about Compassionate Friends (see Resources), a support group for individuals and families who have lost pregnancies or children.

MALE INFERTILITY: CAUSES, DIAGNOSES, AND INTERVENTIONS

Male factor infertility is found alone in approximately 30 percent of couples, and is involved in another 20 percent where there is also a female problem. Thus, male factor may be implicated in up to 50 percent of infertile cases. Male factor infertility may result from a variety of causes, such as endocrine disorders, varicocele, antisperm antibodies, occupational and environmental practices, and sexual dysfunction. Evaluation of male fertility should be coordinated with the evaluation of his female partner. Evaluation may be initiated in the general practice or gynecology office (see Figure 10–7). Referral is made to a urologist when abnormalities are identified. Frequently, medical therapies are unsuccessful, but surgery has often been successful in treating post-testicular and ductal disorders.

Subjective Data. A detailed history is essential to identify factors that may affect sperm production (see Table 10–5). For normal spermatogenesis, a delicate balance must exist between the neuroendocrine system and testes (Speroff et al., 1999).

Objective Data

- A thorough physical examination (see Table 10–7) and Doppler evaluation are indicated when sperm parameters are abnormal.
- Diagnostic tests begin with a semen analysis (performed twice) (see Figure 10–7).

Semen culture is obtained if there are five or more white blood cells per high power field or if agglutination of sperm indicates a need for culture. Other tests may include TSH, T_3, T_4, free T_4; FSH (normal is 5–25 mIU/ml); LH (normal is 6–26 mIU/ml); testosterone (normal is

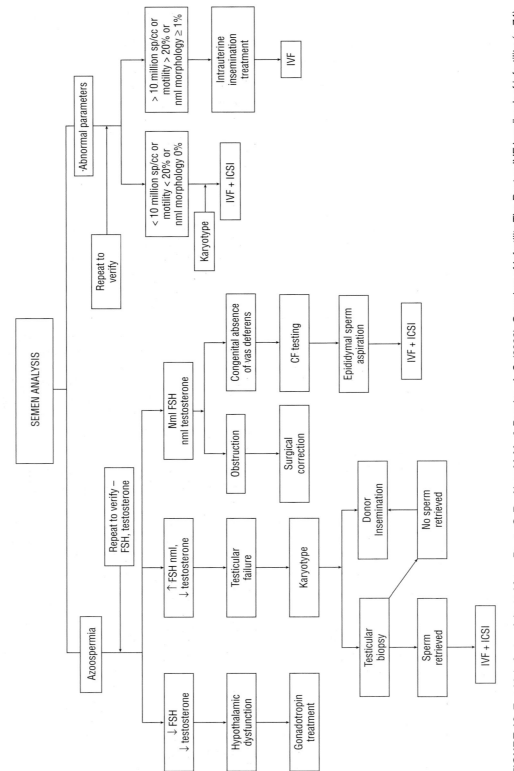

FIGURE 10–7. Male factor. *Adapted from: Bayer, S. R., Alper M. M., & Penzias, A. S. (2002). Overview of Infertility. The Boston IVF handbook of infertility (p. 74). New York: Parthenon Publishing Group. Used with permission.*

250–1200 ng/dL); PRL; CT Scan/MRI of sella turcica; karyotyping. Tests that are rarely used today include anti-sperm antibody testing bovine mucus penetration (because the results would not change the clinical management, which is washed IUI), and the sperm penetration assay (because it does not predict the ability of sperm to bind to or penetrate a human zona pellucida) (AUA, 2001).

ENDOCRINE DISORDERS

Such disorders constitute rare causes of male infertility, and as such endocrine evaluation is indicated when sperm concentration is very low or if there is a clinical suspicion (AUA, 2001). Measurement of TSH, T_3, T_4, free T_4, FSH/LH, PRL, and testosterone may identify abnormalities (Speroff, et al., 1999). Some specific endocrine problems with usual test results are the following.

- Germ cell aplasia; elevated FSH/LH.
- Testicular failure: elevated FSH/LH.
- Pituitary adenoma/impotence: elevated PRL.
- Thyroid dysfunction: elevated or low TSH, T_3, T_4, free T_4.
- Hypogonadotropic hypogonadism (Kallmann's syndrome): low FSH/LH, testosterone (Matsumoto, 1995).

VARICOCELE

This varicosity of the internal spermatic vein is usually on the left side and found in both fertile and infertile men. It impairs infertility by raising testicular temperature, thus killing sperm. Surgical correction is beneficial in some cases (Speroff, et al., 1999).

DISORDERS OF SPERM TRANSPORT

Sperm transport can be caused by congenital disorders, such as absence of major portions of the epididymis, vas deferens and seminal vesicles in males with cystic fibrosis, or acquired disorders due to infections, surgery, or trauma. Such conditions may be surgically corrected.

Functional obstruction occurs in clients with spinal cord injuries, diabetic males with autonomic neuropathy, and with medications such as tranquilizers, antidepressants, and antihypertensives.

SPERM TRANSPORT DYSFUNCTION

Clients with hypospadias, retrograde ejaculation, or sexual dysfunction are unable to deliver sperm to cervical mucus. Sperm collection by means of masturbation for cervical insemination may be indicated. Sperm may also be retrieved from alkalinized urine and prepared for intra-uterine insemination in the client with retrograde ejaculation.

INTERVENTIONS

- Medications. Clomiphene citrate, human menopausal gonadotropins, human chorionic gonadotropin, and the GnRH pump have been used in men to increase sperm count, motility, and to provide normal gonadotropin pulsatility to increase spermatogenesis. Refer to a reproductive endocrinologist or urologist for the above therapies.
- Surgery (varicocelectomy, removal of obstruction, vasectomy reversal).
- Artificial insemination—husband (AIH-cervix).
- Artificial insemination—donor (AID-cervix).
- Ovulation induction IUI—husband or donor.
- Electroejaculation.
- IVF
- Intracytoplasmic sperm injection (ICSI) where one sperm is injected directly into each oocyte with IVF.
- Psychosocial support must be assessed, as self-esteem issues are often dramatic when the diagnosis of male infertility is made. Referral may be indicated for counseling.

COMBINED FACTORS OF MALE AND FEMALE INFERTILITY

Combined factors of male and female infertility may be more difficult to overcome. It is critically important to assess each partner's fertility status before the other undergoes corrective surgery. For example, in vitro fertilization (IVF) may be indicated instead of surgical intervention for couples with tubal pathology and a severe male factor. Individual and couple factors determine the choice of therapy. To maximize chances of conception, evaluation and intervention are coordinated, for example, using varicocele repair and endometriosis surgery.

UNEXPLAINED INFERTILITY

For many infertile couples, no specific cause of infertility can be identified by any of the standard tests. Some couples with unexplained infertility will conceive at an unpredictable time, but many will not. They have multiple needs; although they have the biologic potential to conceive, efforts have been unsuccessful, resulting in frustration for the couple, and there is nothing identified to treat.

Subjective Data. The couple reports a history of infertility.

Objective Data. A complete infertility evaluation is performed resulting in normal findings.

Plan

- Refer the couple to a reproductive endocrinologist.
- Laparoscopy or hysteroscopy may be considered to rule out a tubal or peritoneal factor.
- Psychosocial interventions include providing information and, as treatment becomes more complex, using a variety of educational strategies, such as written information, videotape, demonstration, and individual and group sessions. It is important to be available to answer questions and provide psychosocial support for the individual and couple. Explore all treatment options and allow the couple to regain control by decision making.
- Medication. If the female partner is under 35 years of age and the duration of infertility is less than twelve months, then consider observation alone, or ovulation induction with clomiphene citrate and intercourse for three cycles, or clomiphene citrate and IUI for three cycles. If the female partner is older than 35, consider three cycles of ovulation induction with recombinant FSH and IUI.
- IVF.
- Referral may be made for the individual or couple for counseling for psychological support.

SELECTED INFERTILITY TREATMENTS

OVULATION INDUCTION

This therapy may be used alone with timed intercourse or in combination with inseminations or assisted reproductive technologies. Ovarian response to hMG or rFSH determines dose and duration of therapy.

There is controversy in the field regarding the taking of fertility drugs and the risk of ovarian cancer. Whittemore and colleagues in November 1992 published the findings of a meta-analysis of twelve studies in the *American Journal of Epidemiology.* The study showed a slightly increased risk for ovarian cancer in women with infertility, but no increased risk in women who carried a pregnacy to term.

Another study published in 1994 by Rossing and co-workers found a possible link between the use of clomiphene citrate for twelve or more cycles and ovarian cancer. Today's standard of care with close monitoring makes it highly unusual for a client to have more than six cycles of clomiphene before the recommendation is made to change therapies. To add to the confusion, Rossing and colleagues (1996) published an article that stated the use of clomiphene may reduce the risk of *cervical* neoplasia. Also in 1996, Shushan and others concluded that human menopausal gonadotropin may increase the risk of epithelial ovarian cancer. Mosgaard and co-workers, in a case-control study from Denmark published in 1997, reported that treatment with clomiphene, hMG or hCG did not increase the risk of ovarian cancer, regardless of pregnancy, when compared to nontreated infertile women (Marrs & Hartz, 1993).

The answer to this question is not known. In the first five years of data collection in the NIH supported "Health Surveillance of Women Treated for Infertility by in Vitro Fertilization," no cases of ovarian cancer were reported among approximately 3,100 women (Marrs & Hartz, 1993). This study has been stopped. In addition, there appears to be no increased risk of breast cancer associated with ovarian stimulation with exogenous gonadotropins for IVF (Venn, Watson, Lumley, et al., 1995). A recent statement by the American Society for Reproductive Medicine (Rehan, 2002) concluded that women taking ovulation-inducing drugs face no greater cancer risk than the general population. Clients should be made aware of the potential ramifications of ovulation induction. Since parity is a protective factor, conception and delivery at term may provide protection. Each client must balance the risks, benefits, and her own needs to make a decision.

ARTIFICIAL INSEMINATION

Husband or donor sperm may be used for intracervical (ICI) or intrauterine insemination (IUI). Indications for intracervical insemination include hypospadias, vaginismus, dyspareunia or donor sperm. (see Table 10–11). In a large multicenter randomized, controlled clinical trial, it was shown that ovulation induction and intrauterine insemination (IUI) is three times as likely to result in pregnancy as is intracervical insemination

TABLE 10–11. Indications for IUI

I. Normal Semen Analysis
  A. Anatomic male causes
    1. Retrograde ejaculation
      a. Surgery
      b. Trauma
      c. Systernic disease
      d. Medications
  B. Female causes
    1. Cervical stenosis (conization, cauterization, diethylstilbestrol exposure)
    2. Deficiencies in cervical mucus
    3. Defects in sperm transport or survival
  C. Coital dysfunction
    1. Impotence
    2. Premature ejaculation
    3. Vaginismus
  D. Unexplained infertility

II. Abnormal Semen Analysis
  A. Oligospermia
  B. Asthenospermia
  C. Volume disorders
  D. Immune mediated disorders
  E. Multiple male factor disorders

III. Frozen Sperm
  A. Husband (sperm stored prior to vasectomy, chemotherapy, or radiation)
  B. Donor (azoospermia, genetic disease, Rh incompatibility, single woman)

Source: Byrd, W. (1995). Sperm preparation and homologous insemination. In W. R. Keye, Jr., R. J. Chang, R. W. Rebar, & M. R. Soules (Eds.), Infertility: Evaluation and treatment. Philadelphia: W.B. Saunders Company. Used with permission and adapted from Garner, C. (1995). Infertility. In C. L. Fogel, & N. F. Woods (Eds.). Women's health care: A comprehensive handbook. Thousand Oats, CA: Sage Publications, Inc.

(ICI) and twice as likely to result in pregnancy as is treatment with either ovulation induction and ICI or IUI alone (Guzick, Carson, Coutifaris, et al., 1999). Insemination enables sperm to be deposited closer to the oocyte, which improves the chances of conception. Therapeutic insemination with donor sperm provides hope of parenthood for many single women, lesbian women, and infertile couples.

Procedures

♦ *Artificial Insemination—Husband (AIH).* Requires a fresh specimen for cervical insemination. The partner may assist with insemination. Cervical insemination has a role when due to physical or psychological factors, sperm cannot be deposited in the vagina by intercourse. Otherwise, IUI is the procedure of choice.

♦ *Therapeutic Donor Insemination (TDI).* Must be performed according to The American Society for Reproductive Medicine Guidelines for Gamete and Embryo Donation: 2000–2002. Consent forms are signed and donors selected. Female evaluation includes current history and physical examination, including Pap smear, chlamydia and gonorrhea cultures, rubella titer, cytomegalovirus (CMV) titer, serologic test for syphilis, hepatitis profile, and human immunodeficiency virus (HIV) test. Both partners have blood type and Rh determinations in donor matching. Donors are extensively screened, with cryopreserved specimens guarantined for at least six months, and donors are rescreened for HIV prior to release for use. Laboratory tests include serologic tests for syphilis, hepatitis profile, CMV titer, HIV test, and chlamydia and gonorrhea cultures. Specimens are thawed prior to use.

♦ *Intrauterine Insemination (IUI).* Performed using washed partner's specimen or thawed, cryopreserved sperm. The sperm is separated from the seminal fluid to prevent the proteins, prostaglandins, and bacteria in semen from being deposited in the uterus (Speroff, et al., 1999).

Timing of insemination is determined by using urine luteinizing hormone (LH) ovulation predictor kits or ultrasounds for follicular growth and serum LH or estradiol monitoring. Cervical insemination is performed the day of the LH surge and may be repeated the next day. Unstimulated IUI is performed the day after the LH surge. Stimulated ovulation induction IUIs are performed approximately 18 and 40 hours after ovulation is induced by administration of human chorionic gonadotropin or once at 36 hours after administration of hCG.

If conception with AIH cervical insemination (fresh specimen) does not occur within three to six cycles, then treatment proceeds to unstimulated IUI for three to four cycles, then to stimulated ovulation induction IUI for three to four cycles.

With TDI utilizing thawed specimens, conception should occur no later than twelve cycles. Attempt three to six cycles of stimulated ovulation induction and IUI. If conception does not occur, assisted reproductive technologies are recommended. If the woman is older, it is reasonable to move more quickly to stimulated IUI.

ASSISTED REPRODUCTIVE TECHNOLOGIES

When other treatment options have been exhausted or when other therapies have a poor prognosis, assisted reproductive technologies are used. Options include in vitro fertilization (IVF); gamete intrafallopian transfer (GIFT); embryo cryopreservation, assisted hatching, and intracytoplasmic sperm injection. Assisted reproductive technologies may include the use of donor gametes or donated embryos (see Table 10–12).

Success Rates

Success rates vary from practice to practice. An overall live birth rate of 29.2 percent per egg retrieval and 31.3 percent live birth rate per IVF embryo transfer using

TABLE 10–12. Summary of Procedure and Indications for Assisted Reproductive Technologies

In Vitro Fertilization (IVF)	
Procedure:	**Indications:**
Oocytes are fertilized in the laboratory.	Tubal factor.
Resulting embryos are transferred to the uterus.	Male factor.
	Endometriosis.
	Unexplained infertility.
Gamete Intrafallopian Transfer (GIFT)**	
Procedure:	**Indications:**
Gametes (oocytes and sperm) are transferred to the fallopian tubes.	Religious proscription against IVF.
	Unexplained infertility.
Intracytoplasmic Sperm Injection (ICSI)	
Procedure:	**Indications:**
One sperm is injected directly into the cytoplasm of the oocyte.	Male factor infertility.
Assisted Hatching	
Procedure:	**Indications:**
A hole is made in the zona pellucida with a microinjection needle, laser or acidic Tyrode's solution to enhance embryo hatching.	Failed IVF cycle.
	Woman 35 years or older.
	Frozen embryos.
Donor Oocytes	
Procedure:	**Indications:**
Oocytes are retrieved from a donor, inseminated and resulting embryos are transferred to a recipient in an IVF cycle.	Premature ovarian failure.
	Loss of gonadal function due to surgery, radiation or chemotherapy.
	Congenital absence of ovaries.
	Genetic disorder carrier (X-linked or autosomally dominant).
	Repeated, unexplained pregnancy loss.
	Poor response to gonadotropins.
Gestational Carrier	
Procedure:	**Indications:**
Oocytes are fertilized in the laboratory.	Uterine absence or anomaly (surgical or congenital, distortion of cavity,
Resulting embryos are transferred to the uterus of another woman, who will carry the pregnancy.	trauma, cancer).
	Medical contraindication to pregnancy.
Embryo Cryopreservation	
Procedure:	**Indications:**
Freeze extra embryos from an IVF, GIFT or ZIFT cycle.	To allow for a subsequent attempt at pregnancy without ovarian stimulation or retrieval.
Embryo Donation	
Procedure:	**Indications:**
Previously cryopreserved embryos are transferred to the uterus prepared with estrogen & progesterone.	Infertility (must have an intact uterus).

**Absolute contraindication for GIFT or ZIFT is not having an open fallopian tube.

Source: Adapted from Broer, K. H. & Turanli, I. (Eds.). (1996). New trends in reproductive medicine. Berlin, Germany: Springer.

fresh, nondonor eggs and embryos was reported in 1999 in the United States (the most recent report at the time of this publication). A live birth rate of 41.6 percent per embryo transfer was obtained with fresh donor egg IVF cycles in the same report (CDC, 1999).

High Order Multiple Gestation

A high incidence of multiple births continues to be a major concern in relation to ovulation induction and IVF treatment. In the United States in 1999, of the 20,117 pregnancies conceived through assisted reproductive technologies, 63 percent were singletons, 29 percent twins, 8 percent triplets or greater. Thus, fully 37 percent of all IVF conceived pregnancies were with a multiple gestation (CDC, 1999). Not all of these pregnancies resulted in live births. Many of these spontaneously reduced or the parents decided with the advice of their clinician to opt for a multifetal pregnancy reduction. In a recent review, ovulation induction accounted for 10 to 69 percent of triplet gestations, compared to approximately 30 percent associated with ART and 7 to 18 percent arising spontaneously. Quadruplet and greater multiple gestations were associated with ovulation induction in 50 to 72 percent of cases (ASRM, 2000). The Society for Assisted Reproductive Technology (SART) and the American Society for Reproductive Medicine (ASRM) have jointly published guidelines recommending an optimal number of embryos to transfer based on patient characteristics (ASRM, 2000). In addition, there has been a recent movement to consider transferring only one embryo to a select group of clients, in order to limit risks to mother and fetuses (Hunault, Eijkemans, Pieters, et al., 2002). Clients should be aware of the risks of high order multiple gestation and encouraged to balance these health concerns with their desire for pregnancy.

Stress Management

The complex psychological stressors and emotional impacts of infertility therapies may heighten a couples' feeling of loss of control and intensify over time as the couple undergoes treatment. Stressors are physical, emotional, social, religious, ethical, legal, and financial. Both couples and individuals benefit from counseling, stress management, and assistance with grief resolution (Applegarth, 1995).

Treatment Selection

The risks and benefits of each treatment regimen as well as the couple's prognosis versus their desire of a biologic child need to be carefully weighed before treatment protocols are selected. Treatment choice is often dictated by finances and insurance coverage. Information about clinics in the United States may be obtained from the American Society of Reproductive Medicine (Birmingham, Alabama) at www.asrm.org (see Resources).

ALTERNATIVE FAMILY BUILDING

NONTRADITIONAL FAMILY BUILDING

Lesbian and gay couples experience the same stressors and decision-making difficulties as their heterosexual counterparts, but they also experience additional social (co-parenting), financial (insurance), and legal (adoption-by-partner) concerns (see Chapter 23). In addition, they are coping and must help their children cope with a variety of social stigma that face families with same-sex parents. Family building for lesbian women may require treatment as straightforward as artificial insemination with donor sperm, but becomes increasingly complex if either partner has an additional infertility diagnosis. Gay male couples are parenting through the use of donor eggs and a gestational carrier. Multiple social, financial, and legal obstacles face these couples. As single-parent families are increasingly socially accepted, single women are also increasingly turning to fertility therapies to become pregnant. Currently, few fertility specialists will treat single men desiring children.

EGG DONATION

Oocyte (egg) donation is an increasingly common option offered to couples when the female partner has poor or absent ovarian function. Indications for egg donation are premature ovarian failure (cessation of ovarian function prior to age 40), congenitally or surgically absent ovaries, ovarian failure induced by chemo- or radiation therapy, developmental ovarian failure (menopause), or decreased ovarian function demonstrated by multiple failed IVF or ovulation induction cycles (ASRM, 2002). Many philosophical and legal issues related to egg donation are similar to those of sperm donation, yet there are obvious differences. The technical difficulties related to ovulation induction and egg retrieval in the donor and the difficulty in synchronizing the menstrual cycles of the donor and recipient make the process logistically more complicated. Furthermore, there is no well-developed technology for cryopreserving oocytes as there is for sperm (although intensive research is currently underway). Nonetheless, egg donation in the human has been used quite successfully and has provided many couples with an opportunity to experience pregnancy, childbirth, and breastfeeding who would otherwise not have been able.

Candidates for egg donation must be in good physical health and have a uterus with a normal endometrial cavity. A potential recipient of donated eggs requires medical clearance for estrogen and progesterone replacement and must be considered to be an acceptable risk for carrying a pregnancy. Egg donors should be healthy, ideally between the ages of 21 and 33, and free of infectious disease. There is special concern for the reproductive future of women who have not yet completed their own families. Known egg donors include sisters, relatives, friends, or colleagues. Anonymous egg donors may be recruited by word of mouth, advertising, through recruiting agencies, or over the Internet. Most women who become egg donors express an altruistic desire to help another woman, although financial compensation is an important motivating factor for the majority of anonymous egg donors. Payments for anonymous egg donors can range from $2,500 to over $10,000 per cycle. All egg donors, whether anonymous or known, must be screened to ensure that their motivation appears reasonable and voluntary. Egg donation presents a number of unique legal and emotional issues, which need to be carefully considered. Most egg donation programs require psychological counseling for both recipients and donors, and many programs also recommend legal counsel for both parties and a contract between recipient and donor.

GESTATIONAL CARRIER

Use of a gestational carrier is indicated when the uterus of the female partner is surgically or congenitally absent, when the uterine cavity is distorted by uterine anomalies or trauma, or when the endometrial lining is unreceptive to implantation such as after multiple surgical repairs, Asherman's syndrome, or after chemo- or radiation therapies. Use of a gestational carrier is also indicated if the female partner has a medical contraindication to pregnancy.

Traditional surrogacy implies that a woman is inseminated with the intended father's sperm and at the time of delivery relinquishes her rights to the child. This relationship raises many ethical and legal difficulties. These difficulties can be avoided through the use of a gestational carrier. Utilizing assisted reproductive technologies, embryos created from the gametes of the intended parents, or donor gametes, are transferred to the uterus of another woman, who will carry the pregnancy. Prior to the embryo transfer, extensive psychological counseling of the intended parents and the potential gestational carrier and her spouse is required. In addition, a legal contract between the intended parents and the gestational carrier is critical. A contract establishes intent, so that, at the time of delivery, it is clear who intends to parent the child. Laws regarding this relationship vary tremendously from state to state, and prior to treatment it is important for the couple to seek legal counsel from an expert in reproductive law.

ADOPTION

The decision to adopt may be difficult and is almost always come to gradually. Guide couples toward adoption resources during their infertility treatment if they are interested. Beginning the adoption process does not always resolve a couple's grief over the loss of their own fertility. This process occurs over time with the support of each other, significant others, and professionals (Johnston, 1992). Options for adoption are by means of a private arrangement (parental placement) or through an agency or international organization. Many adoption agencies insist that all infertility treatment be complete and neither partner over 40 years old. Waiting lists may be years long. Adoptive children may have special needs or be an older child. The process can be complicated, time consuming, and costly. Many couples, however, once their child has found their adoptive home, are able to find fulfillment, happiness, and resolution of their desire for biologic children. Adoptive parents often express wonder at how long it took them to take this step and wish that they had begun the process sooner.

CHILDFREE LIVING

Infertile couples are faced with many difficult decisions. They must take into consideration their motivation in pursuing fertility therapies, their energy and resources, and the value of continuing treatment. Choosing to remain without children may be painful, and many couples must come to terms with a tremendous sense of loss. In the end, however, there may be some relief in finding their family complete without children. A couple may no longer feel pressured to perform on demand, put their lives on hold, or conform to medical therapies. They are able to regain privacy, control their lives, and focus their energies on themselves, each other, their relationship, and future life goals (Carter & Carter, 1989; Robertson 1994).

FUTURE TRENDS AND CONTROVERSIES

PREIMPLANTATION GENETIC DIAGNOSIS

Preimplantation genetic diagnosis (PGD) is a technique used during IVF procedures to test embryos for specific genetic disorders and/or chromosomal abnormalities prior to their transfer into the uterus. PGD makes it possible for couples or individuals with serious inherited disorders to decrease the risk of having a child who is affected by the same problem. This technique remains controversial and raises the issues of sex selection and genetic engineering. At present PGD is only available in a few centers, but its use may become more widespread in the near future.

There are over 200 disorders that can potentially be prevented by the gender selection of embryos. Currently, PGD can detect the following single gene disorders and chromosomal abnormalities: alpha-1-antitrypsin deficiency, cystic fibrosis, fragile X syndrome, Lesch-Nyhan syndrome, Charcot-Marie-Tooth disease, Down syndrome, Tay-Sachs disease, Duchenne muscular dystrophy, hemophilia A, retinitis pigmentosa, and Turner syndrome.

PGD is performed during IVF by isolating embryos at the 8-cell stage, when all the cells of the embryo are omnipotent, removing a single blastomere (cell) under microscopic guidance and analyzing the chromosomal material. A diagnosis is obtained within a day of the biopsy, and only the unaffected embryos are transferred to the uterus.

HUMAN CLONING

In a position statement made April 5, 2002, the American Society for Reproductive Medicine (ASRM) states opposition to any attempt at reproductive cloning of a human being. At present, despite claims to the contrary, there is no scientific evidence to justify an attempt to clone a human being. The ASRM urges the media, the public and policy makers to meet such claims with skepticism rather than alarm, unless they are accompanied by peer-reviewed scientific evidence. In addition, the ASRM finds it unconscionable to recruit patients to participate in these efforts. Because infertility can be an emotionally devastating, the ASRM states that any effort that offers false hope to couples with infertility is irresponsible and unethical.

RESOURCES

Adoptive Families of America
2309 Como Avenue
St. Paul, Minnesota 55108
Phone: (800) 372-3300
Fax: (612) 645-0055
www.adoptivefam.org

Network of families built by or interested in adoption. Goals are education, support, and advocacy. Bimonthly magazine available.

The American Society for Reproductive Medicine
1209 Montgomery Highway
Birmingham, Alabama 35216-2809
Phone: (205) 978-5000
Fax: (205) 978-5005
www.asrm.org

Patient education booklets, fact sheets, guidelines available. Nurses' Professional Group of ASRM has developed protocols and procedures to provide nursing care.

The Compassionate Friends
P.O. Box 3696
Oak Brook, IL 60522-3696
Phone: (630) 990-0010
Fax: (630) 990-0246
www.compassionatefriends.org

National self-help group to provide support to families who have experienced the death of a child. National newsletter for parents and grandparents and a newsletter for siblings are available. National and regional conferences are held annually.

Resolve, Inc.
1310 Broadway
Somerville, MA 02144-1731
Helpline: (617) 623-0744
www.resolve.org

National lay organization with local chapters dedicated to providing education, support, and advocacy for couples experiencing infertility. Newsletter and fact sheets available.

American Infertility Association
666 Fifth Ave. Suite 278
New York, NY 10103
Phone: 203-740-7874
www.americaninfertility.org

Endometriosis Association International

8585 North 76th Place

Milwaukee, WI 53223

Phone: 414-355-2200

www.endometriosisassn.org

The endometriosis association is a nonprofit, self-help organization dedicated to providing information and support to women and girls with endometriosis.

Serono Symposia, International

One Technology Place

Rockland, MA 02370

Phone: 781-982-9000 *or* (800) 283-8088

Fax: 781-681-2915

www.seronosymposiausa.org

Has free patient education booklets on various infertility topics. Sponsors professional and lay symposia to provide education in the field of reproductive medicine. Syllabi from various symposia are available free of charge to nonparticipants of the symposia.

REFERENCES

Adashi, E. Y. (2000). Recurrent Pregnancy Loss: State of the Art. *Seminars in Reproductive Medicine, 18,* 327–443.

American College of Obstetricians and Gynecologists. (1997). *Smoking and Women's Health.* Education Bulletin, Number 240.

American Society for Reproductive Medicine (ASRM). (2000, June). *Optimal evaluation of the infertile female.* A Practice Committee Report: A Committee Opinion. Birmingham, AL: Retrieved June 20, 2002 from http://www.asrm.org.

American Society for Reproductive Medicine (ASRM). (2000). A Practice Committee Report, an educational bulletin. *Multiple Pregnancy Associated with Infertility Therapy.* Retrieved January 7, 2002 from http://www.asrm.org.

American Society for Reproductive Medicine (ASRM). (2002). A Practice Committee Report: Guidelines and Minimum Standards. *Guidelines for Gamete and Embryo Donation.* Retrieved December 8, 2002 from http://www.asrm.org.

American Urological Association (AUA). (2001). Infertility: Report on Optimal Evaluation of the Infertile Male: An AUA best practice policy and ASRM practice committee report Vol. 1 (ISBN 0-9649702-7-9).

Applegarth, L. D. (1995). The psychological aspects of infertility. In W. R. Keye, Jr., R. J. Chang, R. W. Rebar, & M. R. Soules (Eds.), *Infertility: Evaluation and treatment* (pp. 19–24). Philadelphia: W. B. Saunders Company.

ASRM Statement on Attempts at Human Cloning, April 5, 2002. Statement Attributable to William Keye, M.D., President, American Society for Reproductive Medicine. Retrieved January 7, 2002 from http://www.asrm.org.

American Society for Reproductive Medicine (ASRM). (2000). *A Practice Committee Report: Use of Insulin Sensitizing Agents in the Treatment of Polycystic Ovarian Syndrome.* Retrieved December 1, 2002 from http://www.asrm.org.

Barbieri, R. (2000). Induction of ovulation in infertile women with hyperandrogenism and insulin resistance: Clinical opinion. *American Journal of Obstetrics and Gynecology, 183,* 1412–1418.

Bayer, S. R., Alper M. M., & Penzias, A. S. (2002). Overview of infertility. In *The Boston IVF handbook of infertility* (pp. 1–23). New York: Parthenon Publishing Group.

Bolumar, F., Olsen, J., & Boldsen, J. (1996). Smoking reduces fecundity: A European multicenter study on infertility and subfecundity. European Study Group on Infertility Subfecundity. *American Journal of Epidemiology, 143,* 578–87.

Bolumar, F., Olsen, J., Rebagaliato M., Bisanti., L. (1997). Caffeine intake and delayed conception: A European multicenter study in infertility and subfecundity. *American Journal of Epidemiology, 145* (14): 324–334.

Borini, A., Bafaro, G, Violini, F., Bianchi, L., Casadio, V., & Flamini, C. (1995). Pregnancies in postmenopausal women over 50 years old in an oocyte donation program. *Fertility & Sterility, 63,* 258.

Buttram, V. C., & Reiter, R. C. (1985). *Surgical Treatment of the Infertile Female.* Baltimore: Williams & Wilkins, p. 149.

Byrd, W. (1995). Sperm preparation and homologous insemination. In W. R. Keye, Jr., R. J. Chang, R. W. Rebar, & M. R. Soules (Eds.), *Infertility: Evaluation and treatment* (pp. 696–711). Philadelphia: W. B. Saunders Company.

Carter, J., & Carter, M. (1989). *Sweet grapes: How to stop being infertile and start living again.* Indianapolis, IN: Perspective Press.

Centres for Disease Control (CDC). (1999). *Assisted reproductive technologies success rates.* www.cdc.gov/ncadphp/drh/art.htm.

Cohen, M. A., Lindheim, S. R., & Sauer, M.V. (1999). Hydrosalpinges adversely affect implantation in donor oocyte cycles. *Human Reproduction, 14,* 1087–1089.

Cowan, B. D. (2002). Evaluation of the female for infertility. In D. B. Seifer, & R. L. Collins (Eds.), *Office-based infertility practice* (pp. 1–9). New York: Springer-Verlag.

Cramer, D. W., & Wise L. A. (2000). The epidemiology of recurrent pregnancy loss. In Adashi, E. Y., Silver R. M., and Hill, J. A. (Eds.), Seminars in Reproductive Medicine. *Recurrent Preganancy Loss: State of the Art, 18*(4), 331.

De Mouzon, J., Spira, A., & Schwartz, D. (1988). A Prospective study of the relation between smoking and fertility. *International Journal of Epidemiology, 17,* 378–384.

Domar, A. D., Clapp, D., Slawsby, E. A., et al. (2000). Impact of group psychological interventions on pregnancy rates in infertile women. *Fertility & Sterility, 73,* 805–811.

Eldar-Geva, T., Meagher, S., Healy, D. L., MacLachlan, V., Breheny S., & Wood C. (1998). Effect of intramural, subserosal, and submucosal uterine fibroids on the outcome of assisted reproductive technology treatment. *Fertility and Sterility, 70,* 687–691.

Endler, G. C., Mariona, F. G., Sokol, R. J., et al. (1988). Anesthesia-related maternal mortality in Michigan, 1972–1984. *American Journal of Obstetrics and Gynecology, 159,* 187–193.

Fielding, J. E. (1987) Smoking and women: Tragedy of the majority. *New England Journal of Medicine, 317,* 1343–1345.

Gardella, J. R., & Hill, J. A. (2000). Environmental toxins associated with recurrent pregnancy loss. In E. Y. Adashi, R. M. Silver, & J. A. Hill (Eds.), Seminars in Reproductive Medicine. *Recurrent Preganancy Loss: State of the Art, 18*(4), 409.

Goldenberg, M., Sivan, E., Sharabi, Z, Bider, D., Rabinovici, J., & Seidman, D.S. (1995). Outcome of hysteroscopic resection of submucous myomas for infertility. *Fertility and Sterility, 64,* 714–716.

Guzick, D. S., Carson, S. A., Coutifaris, C., Overstreet, J. W., Factor-Litcak, P., Steinkampf, M. P., Hill, J. A., Mastroianni, L., Buster, J. E., Nakajima, S. T., Vogel, D. L., & Canfield, R. E. (1999). Efficacy of superovulation and intrauterine insemination in the treatment of infertility. *New England Journal of Medicine, 340*(3), 177–183.

Hakim, R. B., Gray, R. H., & Zacur, H. (1998). Alcohol and caffeine consumption and decreased fertility. *Fertility and Sterility, 70,* 632–637.

Harlep, S., & Shiono, P. H. (1980). Alcohol, smoking, and incidence of spontaneous abortions in the first and second trimester. *Lancet 2:* 173–178.

Hatch, E. E., & Bracken, M. B. (1993). Association of delayed conception with caffeine consumption. *American Journal of Epidemiology, 138*(12): 1082–1092.

Heard, M. J., Pierce, A., Carson, S. A., & Buster, J. E. (2002). Pregnancies following use of metformin for ovulation induction in patients with polycystic ovarian syndrome. *Fertility and Sterility, 77*(4), 669–673.

Hoffmann, G. E., Thie, J., Scott, R. T., & Navot, D. (1996). Endometrial thickness is predictive of histologic endometrial maturation in women undergoing hormone replacement for ovum donation. *Fertility and Sterility, 66,* 380–383.

Hook, D. B., Cross, P. K., & Schreinemachers, D. M. (1983). Chromosomal abnormality rates at amniocentesis and in liveborn infants. *Journal of the American Medical Association, 249,* 2034–2038.

Hook, E. B. (1981). Rates of chromosomal abnormalities at different maternal ages. *Obstetrics–Gynecology, 58,* 282–285.

Hunault, C. C., Marinus, J. C., Eijkemans, M. S., Pieters, M. H., Velde, E. R., Habbema, J. D. Fauser, B. C., & Macklon, N. S. (2002). A prediction model for selecting patients undergoing in vitro fertilization for elective single embryo transfer. *Fertility and Sterility, 77*(4), 725–732.

Jacobson, J. L., Jacobson, S. W., & Sokol, R. J. (1994). Effects of alcohol use, smoking and illicit drug use on fetal growth in black infants. *Journal of Pediatrics, 124,* 757–764.

Jensen, T. K., Hjollund, N. H. I., Henriksen, T. B., et al. (1998). Does moderate alcohol consumption affect fertility? Follow up study among couples planning first pregnancy. *Br Med J, 317,* 505–510.

Johnson, N. P., Mak, W., & Sowter, M. C. (2002). Laparoscopic salpinectomy for women with hydrosalpinges enhances the success of IVF: A Cochrane review. *Human Reproduction, 17* (3): 543–548.

Johnston, P. (1992). *Adopting after infertility.* Indianapolis, IN: Perspective Press.

Kruger, T. F., Acosta, A. A., Simmons, K. F., Swanson, R. J., Matta, J. F., & Oehninger, S. (1988). Predictive value of abnormal sperm morphology in in vitro fertilization. *Fertility and Sterility, 49,* 112–117.

Lass, A., Silye, R., Abrams, D. C., Krausz, T., Hovatta, O., Margara, R., & Winston, R. M. (1997). Follicular density in ovarian biopsy of infertile women: A novel method to assess ovarian reserve. *Human Reproduction, 12,* 1028.

Levy, M. J. (1995). Hirsutism. In W. R. Meyer (Ed.), *Infertility and reproductive medicine clinics of North America, 6*(1), 215–227. Philadelphia: W. B. Saunders Company.

Lewis, J. A., & Bernstein, J. (1996). *Women's health: A relational perspective across the life cycle.* Boston: Jones and Bartlett Publishers.

Liu, J. H. (1995). Hypothalamic-pituitary disorders. In W. R. Keye, Jr., R. J. Chang, R. W. Rebar, & M. R. Soules (Eds.), *Infertility: Evaluation and treatment.* Philadelphia: W. B. Saunders Company.

Marrs, R. P., & Hartz, S. C. (1993, January). Comments on the possible association between ovulation inducing agents and ovarian cancer. Statement from the American Fertility Society to its members.

Matsumoto, A. M. (1995). Pathophysiology of male infertility. In W. R. Keye, Jr., R. J. Chang, R. W. Rebar, & M. R. Soules (Eds.), *Infertility: Evaluation and treatment* (pp. 555–579). Philadelphia: W. B. Saunders Company.

Mosgaard, B. J., Lidegaard, Ø., Kjaer, S. K., Schou, G., & Andersen, A. N. (1997). Infertility, fertility drugs and invasive ovarian cancer: A case-control study. *Fertility and Sterility, 67*(6), 1005–1012.

Munne, S., Alikani, M., Tomkin, G., et al. (1995). Embryo morphology, developmental rates and maternal age are correlated with chromosome abnormalities. *Fertility and Sterility, 64,* 382–391.

Nackley, A. C., & Muasher S. J. (1998). The significance of hydrosalpinx in in vitro fertilization. *Fertility and Sterility, 69,* 373.

Nestler, J. E., & Jakubowicz, D. J. (1996). Decreases in ovarian cytochrome P450c17 activity and serum free testosterone after reduction of insulin secretion in polycystic ovary syndrome. *New England Journal of Medicine, 335,* 617–623.

Nestler, J. E., Jakubowicz, D. J., Evans, M. D., & Pasquali, R. (1998). Effects of metformin on spontaneous and clomiphene-induced ovulation in the polycycstic ovary syndrome. *New England Journal of Medicine, 338*(26), 1876–1880.

Noyes, N., Hampton, B. S., Berkeley A., et al., (2001). Factors useful in predicting the success of oocyte donation: A 3-year retrospective analysis. *Fertility and Sterility, 76,* 92–97.

Propst, A. M., & Hill, J. A. (2000). Anatomic factors associated with recurrent pregnancy loss. In E. Y. Adashi, R. M. Silver, & J. A. Hill (Eds.), Seminars in Reproductive Medicine. *Recurrent Pregnancy Loss: State of the Art, 18*(4), 409.

Rebar, R. (2002). ASRM statement on risk of cancer associated with fertility drugs. Retrieved January 24, 2002, from http://www.asrm.org.

Robertson, J. A. (1994). *Children of choice: Freedom and the new reproductive technologies.* Princeton, NJ: Princeton University Press.

Rock, J. A., & Markham, S. M. (1995). Developmental anomalies of the reproductive tract. In W. R. Keye, Jr., R. J. Chang, R. W. Rebar, & M. R. Soules (Eds.), *Infertility: Evaluation and treatment* (pp. 387–411). Philadelphia: W. B. Saunders.

Rogers, S. F. (1995). Pelvic inflammatory disease: Effects on future fertility. In W. R. Meyer (Ed.), *Infertility and Reproductive Medicine Clinics of North America, 6*(1), 95–101. Philadelphia: W. B. Saunders Company.

Rossing, M. A., Daling, J. R., Weiss, N. S., Moore, D. E., & Self, S. G. (1994). Ovarian tumors in a cohort of infertile women. *New England Journal of Medicine, 331,* 771–776.

Rossing, M. A., Daling, J. R., Weiss, N. S., Moore, D. E., & Self, S. G. (1996). In situ and invasive cervical carcinoma in a cohort of infertile women. *Fertility and Sterility, 65,* 19–22.

Sauer, M. V. (2002). *Milestones in oocyte donation: A 20-year review.* ART of Donor Oocytes and Third Party Reproduction. Fourth annual conference: Charleston, SC.

Sharara, F. I., Scott, R. T., Jr., Seifer, D. B. (1998). The detection of diminished ovarian reserve in infertile women. *American Journal of Obstetrics and Gynecology, 179,* 804–812.

Shushan, A., Paltiel, O., Iscovich, J., Elchalal, U., Peretz, T., & Schenker, J. G. (1996). Human menopausal gonadotropin and the risk of epithelial ovarian cancer. *Fertility and Sterility, 65,* 13–18.

Sims, J. A., & Gibbons, W. E. (1996). Treatment of human infertility: The cervical and uterine factors. In E. Y. Adashi, J. A. Rock, & Z. Rosenwaks (Eds.), *Reproductive endocrinology, surgery, and technology* (pp. 2141–2169). Philadelphia: Lippincott-Raven.

Speroff, L., Glass, R. H., & Kase, N. G. (1999). *Clinical gynecologic endocrinology and infertility* (6th ed.). Baltimore: Lippincott, Williams & Wilkins.

Stephen E. H., & Chandra A. (1998). Updated projections of infertility in the United States: 1995–2025. *Fertility and Sterility, 70*(30).

Strickler, R. C. (1995). Factors influencing fertility. In W. R. Keye, Jr., R. J. Chang, R. W. Rebar, & M. R. Soules (Eds.), *Infertility: Evaluation and treatment* (pp. 8–18). Philadelphia: W. B. Saunders Company.

U.S. Department of Health and Human Services. (1997). *Fertility, family planning, and women's health.* New data from the 1995 National Survey of Family Growth; Centers for Disease Control and Prevention/National Center for Health Statistics. Series 23, No. 19. U.S. Department of Health and Human Services. (www.cdc.gov/nchs/nsfg.htm)

Vandermolen, D. T., Ratts, V. S., Evans, W. S., Stovall, D. W., Kauma, S. W., & Nestler, J. E. (2001). Metformin increases the ovulatory rate and pregnancy rate from clomiphene citrate in patients with polycystic ovary syndrome who are resistant to clomiphene alone. *Fertility and Sterility, 75,* 310–315.

Venn, A., Watson, L., Lumley, J., Giles, G., King, C., & Healy, D. (1995). Breast and ovarian cancer incidence after infertility and in vitro fertilization. *Lancet, 346,* 995–1000.

Warburton, D., Kline, J., Stein, Z., & Strobino, C. (1986). Cytogenetic abnormalities in spontaneous abortions of recognized conceptions, In I. H. Porter (Ed.), *Perinatal genetics: Diagnosis and treatment* (p. 133). New York: Academic Press.

Westrom, L. (1980). Incidence, prevalence, and trends of acute pelvic inflammatory disease and its consequences in industrialized countries. *American Journal of Obstetrics and Gynecology, 138*(7), 880–892.

Whittemore, A. S., Harris, R., Itnyre, J., Halpern, J., & The Collaborative Ovarian Cancer Group. (1992). Characteristics relating to ovarian cancer risk: Collaborative analysis of 12 U.S. case-control studies. *American Journal of Epidemiology, 136,* 1175–1220.

Winkel, C., (1995). Lesions affecting the uterine cavity. In W. R. Keye, Jr., R. J. Chang, R. W. Rebar, & M. R. Soules (Eds.), *Infertility: Evaluation and treatment* (pp. 387–411). Philadelphia: W.B. Saunders Company.

World Health Organization (WHO). (1995). *Physical status: The use and interpretation of anthropometry.* Report of a WHO expert committee. WHO Tech. Rep. Ser. 854. Geneva: Author.

Zuckerman, A. L. (1995). Amenorrhea: Diagnosis, evaluation, and treatment. In W. R. Rebar & M. R. Soules (Eds.), *Infertility and Reproductive Medicine Clinics of North America, 6*(1): 25–36.

CHAPTER 11

VAGINITIS AND SEXUALLY TRANSMITTED DISEASES

Susan D. Schaffer

*F*irst-void urine tests *and self-obtained vaginal swabs have the potential to simplify screening and diagno-sis of many sexually transmitted infections. Outside of life-long monogamy with an un-infected partner, consis-tent latex condom use provides the best risk reduction for STDs. However, appreciable risk remains.*

Highlights

- Sexually Transmitted Diseases and the Centers for Disease Control
- Vaginitis
    Bacterial Vaginosis
    Vulvovaginal Candidiasis
    Trichomoniasis
- Cervicitis
    Chlamydia Trachomatis Infections
    Gonorrhea
    Mucopurulent Cervicitis
- Ulcerative Genital Infections
    Herpes Simplex Virus
    Syphilis
    Chancroid
    Granuloma Inguinale
    Lymphogranuloma Venereum
- Epidermal Diseases
    Human Papillomavirus
    Molluscum Contagiosum
    Pediculosis Pubis
- Hepatitis B

❖   INTRODUCTION

Vaginitis and sexually transmitted diseases (STDs) are frequently occurring problems among women. These conditions occur most often during the reproductive years; in fact, many reach their peak incidence during adolescence and young adulthood.

Women bear the greatest burden of STDs, suffering more frequent and more serious complications than men. Gonorrhea and chlamydia can cause pelvic inflammatory disease, with resultant infertility or ectopic pregnancy. Infection with some types of human papillomavirus (HPV) is associated with cervical cancer. Bacterial vaginosis and herpes virus infections are associated with adverse pregnancy outcomes, and most STDs have been shown to increase the risk of acquiring human immunodeficiency virus (HIV) (Rotchford, Strum, & Wilkinson 2000).

Early diagnosis and appropriate treatment can prevent many adverse STD outcomes. But diagnosis and treatment are not enough. Preventing the spread of STDs requires providers to determine the sexual history of all women in their care and to deliver prevention messages when risky behaviors are identified. Counseling skills such as respect, compassion, and a nonjudgmental attitude are essential to the effective delivery of prevention messages as well as STD care. Prevention messages should include a description of actions to avoid acquiring or transmitting STDs. Consistent condom use provides the best STD risk reduction for women outside of a life-long monogamous relationship with an uninfected partner. Although consistent condom use reduces HIV risk by 85 percent in men and women, studies to date have not demonstrated that condoms consistently protect women from any other STD (NIAID, 2001).

Table 11–1 provides an overview of general information that should be provided to women with vaginitis or a sexually transmitted disease.

SEXUALLY TRANSMITTED DISEASES AND THE CENTERS FOR DISEASE CONTROL

Some STDs, but not all, are reportable by state agencies to the Centers for Disease Control (CDC) in Atlanta, Georgia. The CDC is part of the U.S. Public Health Service and charged with, among other functions, assisting states to identify and control certain diseases. The actual mandate to report specific diseases comes from individual states through their legislative bodies. The CDC can recommend which diseases should be reported; however, the final decision rests with the states. The following STDs are reportable by states to the CDC: AIDS, gonorrhea, hepatitis B, chlamydia, chancroid, and syphilis (CDC, 1999). In addition, some states also require the reporting of HIV infection, herpes simplex, and nonspecific urethritis (Schaffer, Gorzon, Heroux, & Korniewicz, 1996).

Three factors are considered in determining which diseases should be reported.

Ability to Test. If no reasonable test for a condition is readily available (e.g., herpes), then that disease is unlikely to become reportable.

Ability to Cure. Especially important to report are readily curable diseases (e.g., gonorrhea) in order to control epidemics.

Public Awareness. Diseases that gain widespread public attention and represent a public health threat (e.g., AIDS) are usually reportable.

In addition to compiling STD statistics, the CDC recommends treatment for individual diseases. Approximately every four to five years, it publishes STD treatment guidelines. The most recent of these guidelines, published in 2002, are used throughout this chapter when discussing medication, although some newer research based recommendations are also included.

The remainder of this chapter is organized according to clinical syndromes. This facilitates clinical decision making when the clinician is faced with vaginitis or a possible STD. First, the clinician must determine the type of clinical syndrome based on presenting symptoms. Then the possible causes of that syndrome can be considered. Although HIV infection is primarily sexually transmitted, it is discussed in a separate chapter due to the complex psychosocial and medical management required by persons with this infection (see Chapter 12).

TABLE 11–1. General Information Needed in the Care of Women with Vaginitis and Sexually Transmitted Diseases (STD)

Provide both written information and verbal explanations to the client.

Disease Process	Etiology, incubation, risk factors, diagnosis, management, follow-up.
Treatments	Medications and their side effects; signs of allergic response; discomfort; time commitments; simultaneous partner treatment; the need to keep appointments for treatment and thereby control growth and spread of lesions and worsening of disease and symptoms; avoidance of douching and tampon use (unless medically directed) until healing is complete.
Transmission	A description of all possible modes; the need to suspend genital and oral sexual relations, foreign body insertion, and manual manipulation until healing is complete; use of lubricated latex condoms until partners are examined and determined disease-free; the dangers of multiple partners and the principles of "safer sex."
Comfort Measures	Sitz baths and oral analgesics may help some conditions.
Hygiene	The importance of cleanliness and dryness to enhance healing. Use of a hair dryer on low setting to aid drying. Avoidance of powders, douches (especially perfumed or deodorized), perfumed sprays. Discussion of secondary infection and how it may occur. Wearing clean cotton underwear, loose clothing, and fabrics that "breathe"; washing hands thoroughly before and after touching genitalia; not wearing underwear more than one day; not wearing anyone else's underwear; not allowing anyone other than oneself to wear one's underwear or tight fitting trousers; changing out of moist clothing as soon as possible.
Other Prevention	Decreasing smoking in infection with human papillomavirus (HPV); self-monitoring of the vulva (HPV); client examination of partner and asking about past exposure; empowerment of client (through role playing) to be motivated and skillful in talking about sensitive issues with her partner; caution in new sexual liaisons; avoidance of alcohol and drugs that limit inhibitions; an agreement ("contract") with her partner that they have a mutually monogamous relationship; for their mutual safety, an agreement between the two partners in the relationship to tell each other if either one has sexual relations with someone else.

VAGINITIS

Vaginitis occurs when the vaginal ecosystem has been disturbed, either by the introduction of an organism, or by a disturbance that allows the pathogens normally residing in this environment to proliferate. Factors that may alter the vaginal ecosystem include antibiotics, hormones, contraceptive preparations (oral and topical), douches, vaginal medication, sexual intercourse, STDs, stress, and changes in sexual partners. The hallmarks of vaginitis are excessive or malodorous vaginal discharge, pruritus or irritation, and sometimes external dysuria. Diagnosis of vaginitis is made by close inspection of the external genitalia, determination of the pH of the vaginal discharge (normally 3.8–4.2) and microscopic examination of the discharge. Although bacterial vaginosis, vulvovaginal candidiasis, and trichamoniasis are the most common causes of abnormal vaginal discharge, other etiologies such as gonorrhea, chlamydia, herpes virus infection, foreign body, allergies, and hormonal deficiency should also be considered.

BACTERIAL VAGINOSIS (BV)

Bacterial vaginosis (BV) is a clinical syndrome characterized by alterations in vaginal flora. It is the most prevalent form of vaginitis among childbearing women. BV is a syndrome in which normal H_2O_2 producing *Lactobacilli*

in the vagina are replaced with high concentrations of anaerobic bacteria (e.g., *Gardnerella vaginalis, Mobiluncus* species, *Mycoplasma hominis, Ureaplasma uealyticum,* and *Prevotella* species (Koumans & Kendrick, 2001). Research suggests that BV is associated with preterm labor, chorioamnionitis, postpartum endometritis, and PID (CDC, 2002).

BV accounted for 83 percent of attributable risk for preterm birth in one study (Purwar, Ughade, Bhagat, et al., 2001). The CDC (2002) recommends that women with a previous premature birth be screened and treated for BV after the first trimester. However, intervention trials targeting BV to reduce preterm birth have been inconsistent (Koumans & Kendrick, 2001).

Epidemiology

Etiology/Risk Factors. Longitudinal studies suggest that douching and multiple sexual partners are associated with acquisition of BV; however, women without these risk factors also acquire the infection. The presence of vaginal lactobacilli that produce H_2O_2 seems to confer protection (Hilliar, 2002).

Transmission. Research suggests a nonsexual mode of transmission, although BV occurs almost exclusively in sexually active women. The treatment of male partners does not reduce the risk of recurrence; however; condom use does (Weissman, 2001).

Incidence. BV prevalence ranges from 10 to 40 percent, depending on the population of women studied.

Subjective Data

Clients with BV may be asymptomatic or may have malodorous vaginal discharge. Often, clients report foul odor after intercourse. Symptoms such as pruritus, abdominal pain, dyspareunia, and dysuria do not reliably correlate with BV.

Objective Data

Physical Examination. Clinical diagnosis of BV requires that three of the following four criteria be met: thin, white homogeneous malodorous adherent vaginal discharge, pH level above 4.5, positive whiff test, and/or presence of clue cells on wet-mount microscopic examination. Cultures are not recommended (CDC, 2002).

Diagnostic Tests and Methods

- *Saline Wet Mount.* Diagnostic evaluation for clue cells: characteristic epithelial cells with bacteria adherent to the cell wall, giving it a stippled, granular appearance (see Figure 11–1). Cell margins become blurred, and few white blood cells are noted.

   The test procedure is to mix a sample of vaginal secretions (obtained from the vaginal pool or posterior blade of the speculum) with normal saline, place on a slide, and cover with a coverslip. Examine microscopically under low and high power. Explain the

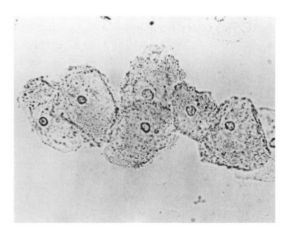

FIGURE 11–1. Saline wet mount of clue cells from *Gardnerella vaginalis* infection. Note the absence of inflammatory cells. *(Reproduced with permission from DeCherney, A. H., & Pernoll, M. L.: Current obstetric and gynecologic diagnosis and treatment, 8th ed. Appleton & Lange, 1994.)*

procedure to the client. Advise her that an immediate diagnosis is possible.

- *"Whiff" Test.* Diagnostic evaluation for a "fishy" amine odor. The test procedure is to mix vaginal secretions with 10 percent potassium hydroxide (KOH); the characteristic odor is readily emitted. Advise the client of the test purpose.
- *Vaginal pH.* Diagnostic evaluation for acidity of vaginal secretions. In BV, pH is greater than or equal to 4.5, but this is not specific for BV alone. The test procedure is to dip appropriate pH paper (pH range 4.0 to 6.0) into vaginal secretions and observe the color change. The sample may be obtained by swabbing the lateral and posterior fornix and applying directly to pH paper, or by dipping pH paper into the posterior blade of the speculum after removal from the vagina. Advise the client of the purpose of the test.

Differential Medical Diagnoses

Trichomonas vaginitis, foreign body vaginitis, monilia.

Plan

Psychosocial Interventions. Because the etiology of BV is uncertain and changing, a client's confusion is understandable. Counsel clients about what is currently known and what is being suggested. Treatment regimens for BV are only 80 percent effective, and up to 20 percent of women will have recurrences within one month of treatment (Koumans & Kendrick, 2001). Recent studies suggest that oral or vaginal *Lactobacilli* capsules can help to restore normal urogenital flora (Reid, Beuerman, Heinemann, & Bruce, 2001; Reid, Bruce, Fraser, et al., 2001). However, the *Lactobacillus* preparations used in the studies are not widely available. Daily ingestion of active culture yogurt has been suggested by some authorities as a treatment adjunct (Ostrzenski, 2002), but has not been rigorously tested.

Medication

Metronidazole Oral Tablets/Metronidazole Vaginal Gel

- *Indications.* Oral metronidazole is recommended for BV (including during pregnancy). Vaginal gel should not be used in pregnancy (CDC, 2002).
- *Administration.* Oral tablets: 500 mg b.i.d. for seven days. The CDC (2002) recommends Metronidazole 250 mg orally t.i.d. in pregnant women. Other authorities recommend the standard dose of 500 mg orally b.i.d. in second trimester pregnant women due

to low efficacy of standard regimens and the association of BV with adverse pregnancy outcomes (Wilson & Henry, 2001; Gilbert, Moellering, & Sande, 2001). Vaginal gel 0.75 percent: one applicator full intravaginally q.d. (CDC, 2002) b.i.d. (Gilbert, Moellering, & Sande, 2001) for five days.

- *Side Effects and Adverse Reactions.* All alcohol products must be avoided with any metronidazole regimen because profuse nausea and vomiting (disulfiram reaction) may occur. Transient nausea and a metallic taste have also been reported. Because metronidazole has a broad antimicrobial spectrum, normal vaginal flora may be suppressed with subsequent monilial infection. Vaginal gel: vaginal candidiasis, occasional genitourinary-perineal itching, irritation, swelling; gastrointestinal complaints.
- *Contraindications.* Known allergy to metronidazole.
- *Anticipated Outcomes on Evaluation.* Symptoms clear rapidly after treatment. A test for cure is not routinely indicated.
- *Client Teaching and Counseling.* Stress the need to avoid alcohol. If symptoms return, reexamination is indicated. Treatment of the sexual partner with recurrent infection is recommended. Sexual abstinence or use of condoms during treatment is recommended. Advise the client about side effects.

Clindamycin

- *Indications.* Alternative treatment of BV; may be useful in recurrent cases and orally during pregnancy.
- *Administration.* Two percent clindamycin cream intravaginally daily (usually at bedtime) for 7 days in nonpregnant women (CDC, 2002). Clindamycin may be used orally 300 mg b.i.d. for seven days, but this is less effective and severe side effects are more common with this regimen (CDC, 2002; Wilson & Henry, 2001).
- *Side Effects and Adverse Reactions.* Colitis may be severe (more common with oral form). Vaginitis from *Candida albicans* is more common with clindamycin use.
- *Contraindications.* Known sensitivity to clindamycin. Do not use condom or diaphragm within 72 hours of cream use.
- *Anticipated Outcome on Evaluation.* Symptoms resolve rapidly. Test for cure is not necessary.
- *Client Teaching and Counseling.* The regimen of medication must be completed.
- *Follow-Up and Referral.* No follow-up is necessary.

VULVOVAGINAL CANDIDIASIS

About 30 percent of women with a healthy vaginal environment harbor *Candida,* usually *Candida albicans.* An upset in the homeostatic balance in the vagina leads to an overgrowth of this organism and symptoms of infection. Vulvovaginal candidiasis (VVC) is a common, irritating, and recurrent cause of vaginitis that is not generally sexually transmitted. Predisposing factors include antibiotic use, obesity, diabetes, HIV infection (or other immunosuppressive conditions), and pregnancy. Other names for the condition are monilia and yeast infection.

Epidemiology

C. albicans is a fungal species that is responsible for 75 to 85 percent of infections. *C. tropicalis* and *C. glabrata* are responsible for the remainder of infections. As many as 75 percent of women will experience at least one episode of VVC during their lifetime; 40 to 50 percent of women will experience two or more infections (CDC, 2002). The organism gains access to the vaginal mucosa primarily from the perianal area.

C. albicans can be transmitted from infected mother to newborn at delivery. Neonates develop an oral infection known as thrush.

Subjective Data

VVC presents with vaginal itching, burning, and irritation. Dysuria (burning when urine hits the involved tissue) is common. Vaginal discharge, which may be scanty or profuse, is white and thick. Symptoms frequently worsen prior to menses. Most clients report an acute onset of symptoms that rapidly clear with treatment. A small subset of women experience persistent chronic infection that does not respond well to classic treatment.

Objective Data

Physical Examination. The vulva may be red and inflamed and edematous or appear normal. Excoriations may be present. Typically, a white discharge with the consistency of cottage cheese is adherent to the vaginal mucosa, which may also be inflamed and edematous. Odor is absent and the pH is normal.

Diagnostic Tests and Methods. Microscopic examination of vaginal solution diluted with saline (wet mount) or 10 percent KOH preparations will demonstrate hyphal forms or budding yeast cells in 50 to 70 percent of infected women (see Figures 11–2 and 11–3). The test procedure involves mixing a sample of vaginal secretions with

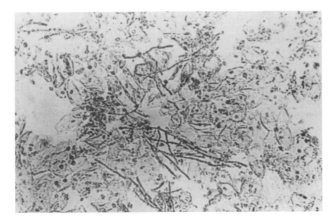

FIGURE 11–2. Saline wet mount demonstrating *Candida albicans. (Reproduced with permission from DeCherney, A. H., & Pernoll, M. L. Current obstetric and gynecologic diagnosis and treatment, 8th ed. Appleton & Lange, 1994.)*

saline, covering with coverslip, and viewing under microscope. A wet mount prepared with 10 percent potassium hydroxide will obliterate cellular material so that yeasts may be seen more easily.

Some cases of VVC are not detected in a wet mount because there are relatively few organisms or because of poor smear technique. Additionally, nonalbicans species tend not to form pseudohyphae.

Focus client teaching on explaining that immediate diagnosis is possible.

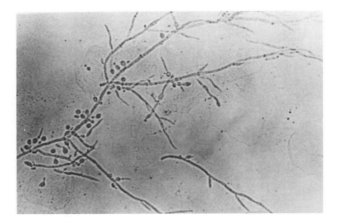

FIGURE 11–3. KOH preparation showing branched and budding *Candida albicans. (Reproduced with permission from DeCherney, A. H., & Pernoll, M. L. Current obstetric and gynecologic diagnosis and treatment, 8th ed. Appleton & Lange, 1994.)*

♦ *Vaginal Culture.* Although routine culture is not cost effective, cultures may be helpful in recurrent VVC. Cultures are prepared by placing a sample of vaginal secretions on Nickerson's medium or Sabouraud's agar. Accurate culture is only possible using the appropriate medium. Advise the client that the yeast culture is the most sensitive test but results take up to 72 hours to obtain.

Differential Medical Diagnoses

Bacterial vaginosis, trichomonas, allergic contact dermatitis, pediculosis pubis.

Plan

Psychosocial Interventions. Advise the client that infection is not sexually transmitted and treatment of her partner is unnecessary unless pruritic balanitis is present in her partner. Rigorous, immediate treatment in pregnancy is recommended to avoid neonatal thrush. Women with chronic moniliasis need intensive counseling to cope with discomfort and long-term medication regimens. Often chronic infection leads to chronic dyspareunia, which can stress relationships. Advise clients to wear cotton underwear, avoid tight fitting nylons and slacks, wipe the perineum from front to back, and use mild soaps. Douching should be avoided. *Clients should be advised that topical vaginal creams or ointments formulated with petrolatum will weaken latex; latex condoms and diaphragms may not be reliable if used within 72 hours of treatment.*

Medication. Many effective topical azole drugs are available over the counter. Self-treatment with OTC medications should be reserved for women who have been previously diagnosed with VVC and experience the same symptoms. Uncomplicated VVC (mild, sporadic symptoms in a normal host) will respond to short-term treatments. Women with severe or recurrent symptoms, women with uncontrolled diabetes, or women who are immunosupressed should be treated for 7 to 14 days (CDC, 2002).

Miconazole (Monistat). 2 percent cream, 100 mg vaginal suppository, 200 mg vaginal suppository. Available over the counter.

♦ *Indications.* Acute and chronic infections. Safe during pregnancy (Category B).
♦ *Administration.* One applicator of 2 percent cream in vagina q.h.s. for seven nights, *or* one 100 mg vaginal suppository q.h.s. for seven nights, *or* one 200 mg suppository q.h.s. for three nights (CDC, 2002).

- *Side Effects and Adverse Reactions.* Few reactions are reported. Occasional burning after application may occur.
- *Contraindications.* Known hypersensitivity to miconazole.
- *Anticipated Outcomes on Evaluation.* Symptoms will rapidly resolve. Routine test for cure (wet mount) is not recommended for acute infection but is advised with chronic recurrent vaginitis.
- *Client Teaching and Counseling.* Advise the client that medication is to be completed as prescribed. Symptoms often will abate before medication is finished, but it must be completed to avoid recurrence. Cream or suppositories should be inserted immediately before retiring or lying down. Some may leak out on arising. Panty liners are helpful during the daytime to prevent moist underwear. Avoid tampon use with cream or suppository because tampons absorb medication, interfering with delivery of the therapeutic dose.

Clotrimazole (Gyne-Lotrimin, Mycelex). 1 percent cream, 100 mg vaginal tablet (over the counter), 500 mg vaginal tablet.

- *Indications.* Acute and chronic infections. Safe during pregnancy (Category B).
- *Administration.* One applicator of 1 percent cream in vagina q.h.s. for seven to fourteen nights, *or* one vaginal tablet q.h.s. for seven nights, *or* two vaginal tablets q.h.s. for three nights, *or* one single 500 mg vaginal suppository once (CDC, 2002).
- *Side Effects and Adverse Reactions.* Same as miconazole.
- *Contraindications.* Known hypersensitivity to miconazole or clotrimazole.
- *Anticipated Outcomes on Evaluation.* Symptoms will rapidly resolve. Routine test for cure (wet mount) is not recommended for acute infection but is advised with chronic recurrent vaginitis.
- *Client Teaching and Counseling.* Same as for miconazole.

Terconazole (Terazol). 0.4 or 0.8 percent vaginal cream; 80 mg vaginal suppository.

- *Indications.* Acute infection; suspected C. tropicalis and C. glabrata may respond better to terconazole than to miconazole or clotrimazole. Not recommended in pregnancy (Category C).
- *Administration.* One applicator of 0.4 percent cream intravaginally q.h.s. for seven days *or* one application of 0.8 percent cream intravaginally q.h.s. for three

days *or* one vaginal suppository q.h.s. for three days (CDC, 2002).
- *Side Effects and Adverse Reactions.* Same as miconazole.
- *Contraindications.* Same as miconazole.
- *Anticipated Outcomes on Evaluation.* Same as miconazole.
- *Client Teaching and Counseling.* Same as miconazole.

Fluconazole (Diflucan). 150 mg oral tablet.

- *Indications.* Acute infection with *Candida* (not recommended for non-*Candidal* species) for clients who prefer not to use topical vaginal medications. Not recommended in pregnancy (pregnancy category C).
- *Administration.* One 150 mg oral tablet.
- *Side Effects and Adverse Reactions.* Most common side effects include headache, nausea, and abdominal pain. Hepatic toxicity has been associated with Fluconazole (not dose related) (Nisson, 2002).
- *Contraindications.* Hypersensitivity to Fluconazole. There is no information related to cross hypersensitivity between Fluconazole and other azoles. Avoid with other hepatoxic drugs.
- *Drug Interactions.* Clinically significant hypoglycemia may be precipitated by the use of Diflucan with oral hypoglycemic agents. Prothrombin time may be increased in patients receiving Fluconazole with coumarin-type anticoagulants. Diflucan increases the plasma levels of Dilantin, cyclosporin, and theophylline. Rifampin enhances the metabolism of Fluconazole (may require increased dose of Diflucan when given with Rifampin). Fluconazole may inhibit the metabolism of ethinyl estradiol and levonorgestrel. The clinical significance of these effects is unknown (Nisson, 2002).
- *Anticipated Outcomes on Evaluation.* Symptoms will improve.
- *Client Teaching and Counseling.* Client should be advised of possible drug interactions.

Ketoconazole (Nizoral). 200 mg oral tablet.

- *Indications.* Should be reserved for long-term suppression of chronic infection with *C. albicans* (resistance, however, has been associated with chronic use).
- *Administration.* Suppressive therapy: one tablet p.o. daily for six months (CDC, 2002).
- *Side Effects and Adverse Reactions.* Hepatotoxic: Monitor hepatic function before and during treatment.

- ◆ *Contraindications.* Known sensitivity to ketoconazole. Hepatic dysfunction. Pregnancy Category C.
- ◆ *Drug interactions:* Potentiates triazolam, midazolam, possibly oral anticoagulants, and oral hypoglycemics. Avoid antacids, anticholinergics, and H2 blockers within two hours of ketoconazole. Avoid rifampin, isoniazid. Monitor digoxin, phenytoin, cyclosporine, and tacrolimus. Caution with other hepatically metabolized drugs (Nisson, 2002).
- ◆ *Anticipated Outcomes on Evaluation.* Symptoms will improve.
- ◆ *Client Teaching and Counseling.* Once long-term therapy is completed, rebound infection may result. Oral absorption may be impaired by antacids, cimetidine, or rifampin.

Other Medications. Other intravaginal formulations that may be used include butoconazole 2 percent cream q.d. for 3 days or tioconazole 6.5 percent ointment once intravaginally in one single dose (now available over-the-counter) (CDC, 2002). Both are pregnancy category C.

Nontraditional Interventions. Boric acid 300 mg in size 0 gelatin capsules inserted into the vagina nightly for fourteen days followed by 300 m.g.s. for five days each month has been reported to be effective for recurrent infections (Guashino et al., 2001). Boric acid has not gained widespread acceptance, perhaps because so many other preparations are readily available. The use of intravaginal yogurt has not been scientifically studied, and reports of its efficacy are only anecdotal; however, a recent study compared the rates of infection among women who ate yogurt containing *Lactobacillus acidophilus* for six months and women who did not. The yogurt group had significantly fewer infections (Hilton et al., 1992).

Follow-Up and Referral

Clients with simple, acute candidiasis do not require a follow-up visit. Those with chronic infection must be seen one to two weeks after treatment. A test for cure, preferably via culture, should be done.

TRICHOMONIASIS

In this common form of vaginitis, women may be markedly symptomatic or asymptomatic. Men are asymptomatic carriers. Although this infection is localized, there is increased incidence of premature delivery and postpartum endometritis in women infected with *Trichomonas vaginalis* (CDC, 2002).

Epidemiology

Trichomonas vaginalis, a flagellated, anaerobic protozoan, is the causative organism. Sexual contact is the primary means of transmission. Although nonsexual transmission via fomites is theoretically possible, clinically it is rare. The organism lives in the vagina, urethra, Bartholin's and Skene's glands in women and in the urethra and prostate gland of men. It is transmitted during vaginal-penile intercourse, and transmission rates are high. There is no finite incubation period. Trichomoniasis occurs in approximately 3 million women annually and is responsible for 15 to 20 percent of vulvovaginitis complaints (Gorroll, 2001a). Prevalence is highest in STD clinics and lowest in the private sector.

Subjective Data

Foul-smelling, yellow-green, frothy vaginal discharge may be profuse or scanty. Vaginal odor is the primary presenting symptom. Infrequently, women report dyspareunia and dysuria. Rarely, men have symptoms of urethritis or prostatitis.

Objective Data

Physical Examination. Infection is often detected on routine examination in the absence of subjective complaints. In addition to discharge as previously described, physical examination reveals vulvar erythema and edema and occasionally petechial lesions on the cervix (sometimes called "strawberry cervix"). The pH will be elevated. Signs and symptoms alone are insufficient to make the diagnosis.

Diagnostic Tests and Methods. A culture is the most sensitive and specific diagnostic method, but it is expensive and not widely available. Wet mount using saline is the most clinically useful test. Diagnosis is made when a motile flagellated trichomonad is visualized (see Figure 11–4). In addition, an increased number of white blood cells may be evident in the wet mount. Pap smear results often include reporting of trichomonads, but the sensitivity of the method is low (65%).

Differential Medical Diagnoses

Bacterial vaginosis, candidiasis, foreign body vaginitis.

Plan

Psychosocial Interventions. The client may experience anxiety and fear with the knowledge that trichomoniasis is sexually transmitted. Reassure her that the infection is

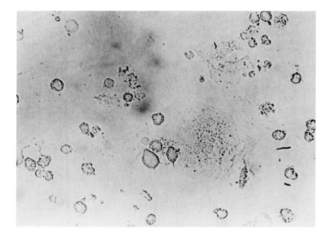

FIGURE 11–4. Saline wet mount with motile trichomonads in the center. (*Reproduced with permission from DeCherney, A. H., & Pernoll, M. L.* Current obstetric and gynecologic diagnosis and treatment, *8th ed. Appleton & Lange, 1994.*)

curable. Counseling should include the need to treat male partners.

Medication

Metronidazole

- *Indications.* Symptomatic and asymptomatic clients and partners; it is the drug of choice for *Trichomonas* infection.
- *Administration.* Metronidazole 2 g p.o., in a single dose for both partners. If treatment fails, nonpregnant clients should be retreated with metronidazole 500 mg b.i.d. for seven days. Symptomatic pregnant women should be treated with 2 grams orally in a single dose (CDC, 2002). Data on the treatment of pregnant women with trichomoniasis who fail on the 2 gram dose is not clearly stated by the CDC. Consultation is advised with a specialist.
- *Side Effects and Adverse Reactions.* Avoid alcohol during and for three days after use. May potentiate oral anticoagulants, phenytoin, and lithium. Antagonized by phenytoin, phenobarbital, and other hepatic enzyme inducers. Potentiated by cimetadine. Use reduced dose in hepatic disease. Rare seizures, peripheral neuropathy, pancreatitis (Nisson, 2002). Transient nausea and a metallic taste have also been reported. Because metronidazole has a broad antimicrobial spectrum, normal vaginal flora may be suppressed with subsequent candidal infection.

- *Contraindications.* Known allergy to metronidazole.
- *Anticipated Outcomes on Evaluation.* Symptoms clear rapidly after treatment. A test for cure is not routinely indicated.
- *Client Teaching and Counseling.* Stress the need to avoid alcohol 24 hours before and 72 hours after treatment. If symptoms return, reexamination is indicated. Routine treatment of the sexual partner is recommended, and the client should be sexually abstinent or use condoms until her partner is treated.

CERVICITIS

Although many sexually transmitted pathogens may gain entry through the vagina, vulva, or cervix, infections characterized by cervicitis primarily use the cervix as a portal of entry. Thus, barrier methods such as condoms and diaphragms are particularly effective in the prevention of cervicitis. Clinical syndromes characterized by cervicitis are considered when mucoid or purulent discharge is observed in the cervical os or when cervical bleeding can be easily induced. Women with cervicitis may have vaginal discharge and dysuria, although many women with cervicitis (perhaps most) are asymptomatic.

CHLAMYDIA TRACHOMATIS INFECTIONS

Chlamydia trachomatis is the most common STD in the United States, with more than 3 million estimated new cases each year (CDC, 2000). Asymptomatic infection is common among both men and women (CDC, 2002). Men primarily develop urethritis. In women, chlamydia is associated with cervicitis, acute urethral syndrome, salpingitis, pelvic inflammatory disease, infertility, and perihepatitis. Some women with apparently uncomplicated cervical infection have been shown to have subclinical upper reproductive tract infection. All women with chlamydia should be tested for gonorrhea before treatment is begun since both are reportable and a specific diagnosis may enhance partner notification and treatment (CDC, 2002).

Newborns delivered to infected mothers may develop conjunctivitis or pneumonitis. In the adult population worldwide, chlamydia is the etiologic agent of trachoma, the leading cause of preventable blindness. Trachoma is not endemic to the United States, however.

Epidemiology

Chlamydia trachomatis is an obligate intracellular parasite that displays some bacterial properties and some viral properties. Unable to produce its own energy, it depends on the host for survival. Risk factors parallel those of gonorrhea. Transmission may be sexual, requiring direct contact with an infected individual, or it may be congenital, acquired at birth when delivery occurs through an infected birth canal. Transplacental transmission does not occur. The incubation period is 10 to 30 days.

The infection is particularly prevalent among adolescents and young adults, so testing sexually active adolescent women should be routine during gynecologic examination. If the availability of chlamydial testing is limited, priority should be given to screening adolescents, high-risk pregnant women, and those with multiple sexual partners. See Chapter 4 for the proper sequencing of the Pap smear and chlamydia/gc tests. Women using oral contraceptives have been found to be at increased risk for Chlamydia, possibly because oral contraceptive induced ectopy exposes more susceptible cells to infection (Baeten et al., 2001).

Incidence ranges from 3 to 5 percent among asymptomatic women and 20 percent among women attending STD clinics.

Subjective Data

Women may be asymptomatic. Subjective symptoms are similar to those seen with gonorrhea and relate to the site of infection. They include vaginal discharge, pelvic pain (dull or severe), fever, dysuria (frequency and urgency). Men may report a penile discharge and burning with urination.

Objective Data

Physical Examination. The physical examination may reveal nothing abnormal, or the cervix may show mucopurulent discharge, hypertrophic ectopy, and friability. There may be mild to severe adnexal tenderness and/or cervical motion tenderness.

Diagnostic Tests and Methods. A wet mount of the discharge may show numerous white blood cells but also may be negative in the presence of infection. Urine culture may be sterile in the presence of urinary symptoms.

Selection of a diagnostic test for chlamydia depends on availability, local expertise, and prevalence of chlamydia in the test population. Nucleic acid detection assays and ligase chain reaction assays are more sensitive than culture or antigen tests (Wilson & Henry, 2001). Testing first-void urine specimens by these techniques has shown

that amplification tests are as sensitive as tests with endocervical swabs (Guaschino & Deseta, 2000). When endocervical swab tests are used, excess secretions should be removed before endocervical sampling to ensure that cellular material is obtained for testing (Loeffelholtz, Jirsa, Teske, & Woods, 2001). Explain to the client the minor discomfort that may occur with endocervical sampling.

Differential Medical Diagnoses

Gonorrhea, mucopurulent cervicitis, salpingitis, pelvic inflammatory disease.

Plan

Psychosocial Interventions. Encourage clients to have chlamydia screening if they are in a risk group. Those with multiple partners or a new sexual partner are especially at risk. Partners of individuals diagnosed with chlamydia should be tested and treated; if testing is unavailable, the partners should be treated presumptively. High risk pregnant women need screening and treatment to prevent congenital transmission. Individuals with chlamydia should be tested for other STDs because of the high rate of concurrent disease. Instruct the client that all medication must be taken. Partners should be treated concurrently and should abstain from intercourse until the treatment is completed.

Medication

Azithromycin

- *Indications.* Treatment of uncomplicated urethral, endocervical, and rectal infections in women and men. Useful if compliance may be a problem. Expense must be considered.
- *Administration.* 1 gm once p.o. (CDC, 2002).
- *Side Effects and Adverse Reactions.* GI side effects, photosensitivity, and overgrowth of vaginal candida are common; hepatic changes (cholestatic jaundice), renal changes, head-ache, dizziness, rash, and angioedema are less common. Caution should be used in patients with impaired hepatic function. Although not reported with Azithromycin, the following reactions/interactions have been observed with other macrolides: ventricular arrhythmias, increased serum levels of theophylline, increased anticoagulant effects with coumarins, elevated digoxin levels, elevated ergot levels, increased pharmacologic effect of Triazolam, and elevated levels of Dilantin, carbamazepine, cyclosporine, and hexobarbital. Because of the long

half-life of azithromycin, allergic reactions may be persistent and should be carefully monitored.

- *Contraindications.* Sensitivity to macrolides. Clinical experience and preliminary data suggest that Azithromycin is "safe and effective," although efficacy and safety data in pregnancy and lactation are not fully established (CDC, 2002, p. 34).
- *Anticipated Outcomes on Evaluation.* Test of cure unnecessary.

Erythromycin

- *Indications.* Chlamydial infection during pregnancy.
- *Administration.* 500 mg p.o., q.i.d. for seven days (CDC, 2002).
- *Side Effects and Adverse Reactions.* Gastrointestinal distress.
- *Contraindications.* Sensitivity to erythromycin.
- *Anticipated Outcomes on Evaluation.* Because experience in treating with erythromycin is limited, a test for cure three weeks after completion of medication is recommended. Retesting should be done at three weeks to allow time for antigen to clear (Gorroll, 2001a).
- *Follow-Up and Referral.* Necessary only if the client was nonresponsive to the medication.

Doxycycline

- *Indications.* Treatment of uncomplicated urethral, endocervical, and rectal infections in women and men.
- *Administration.* Doxycycline 100 mg p.o., b.i.d. for seven days. (CDC, 2002). Avoid antacids during treatment.
- *Side Effects and Adverse Reactions.* Gastrointestinal (GI) upset, rash, photosensitivity. Overgrowth of vaginal candida.
- *Contraindications.* Known pregnancy, sensitivity to tetracyclines. Not for use in children.
- *Anticipated Outcomes on Evaluation.* Antimicrobial resistance to this treatment has not been observed. Provided that treatment is completed, test for cure is not recommended.

Other Medications. Ofloxacin 300 mg p.o., b.i.d. for seven days has been recommended by the CDC, but is expensive and cannot be used in pregnancy or with adolescents age 17 years and under. A recent randomized trial found that Amoxicillin 500 mgs t.i.d. for seven days is equivalent to 1 gram of Azithromycin (Jacobson, Autry, Kirby, Liverman & Motley, 2001).

GONORRHEA

Gonorrhea is a classic bacterial STD that can be symptomatic or asymptomatic in both men and women. In women, gonorrhea primarily infects the cervix and fallopian tubes and is a leading cause of PID. Rectal transmission is common with anal intercourse, and pharyngeal transmission with oral sex is possible but rare. Gonorrhea (GC) can be transmitted during birth and cause conjunctivitis and blindness in neonates. Other rare manifestations of gonorrhea include arthritis, meningitis, perihepatitis, and disseminated gonococcal infection. In pregnancy, gonorrhea has been associated with chorioamnionitis, premature labor, premature rupture of membranes, and postpartum endometritis.

Epidemiology

In 2000, 360,000 new cases of gonorrhea were reported in the United States (CDC, 2001). The causative agent is *Neisseria gonorrhoeae,* a gram-negative intracellular diplococcus. Risk factors include low socioeconomic status, urban residency, nonmarried status, and multiple sexual partners. Infection rates in African Americans and Latins are greater than those in whites. Often, gonorrhea and chlamydia coexist (CDC, 2002).

Direct sexual contact with mucosal surfaces of an infected individual is required for the transmission of gonorrhea. Although the organism has been recovered from inanimate objects artificially inoculated with the bacteria, there is no evidence that natural transmission occurs this way. The incubation period is three to seven days.

Subjective Data

Among women, asymptomatic infection can be present in the urethra, endocervix, rectum, or pharynx. Symptoms may include vaginal discharge, pelvic pain, fever, menstrual irregularities, and dysuria.

Objective Data

Physical Examination. The examination may be normal. Some women exhibit mucopurulent cervicitis, erythema, and friability of the endocervix. Bartholin's abscess is infrequent. Other infections, among them chlamydia, trichomonas, monilia, and herpes, are frequently seen with gonorrhea and may confound the clinical picture.

Diagnostic Tests and Methods. Although gram stains showing intracellular gram-negative diplococci are reliable in males with gonorrhea, gram stains are not reliable in females.

N. gonorrhoeae are readily cultured in a selective growth medium such as Thayer-Martin in a CO_2 rich environment. Rapid antigen tests, enzyme immunoassays, and ligase chain reaction tests are sensitive and specific for urethral, cervical, and urine specimens (Wilson & Henry, 2001).

Differential Medical Diagnoses

Chlamydia trachomatis infection, mucopurulent cervicitis.

Plan

Psychosocial Interventions. Advise the client that persons with untreated gonorrhea risk the development of PID and subsequent infertility. Sexual partners must be treated concurrently and abstain from intercourse during their treatment. With appropriate treatment gonorrhea is curable. Clients must be checked for other STDs before treatment, especially chlamydia and syphilis, as multiple infections are common. Pregnant clients should be screened at the first prenatal visit, and those at high risk should be rescreened late in the third trimester.

Medication

The CDC recommends that persons treated for gonorrhea also be treated routinely with a regimen effective against uncomplicated chlamydia trachomatis if chlamydia has not been ruled out (CDC, 2002). Effective drugs for chlamydia include Doxycycline 100 m.g.s. b.i.d. for 7 days or 1 gram azithromycin orally. In pregnant women Doxycycline may not be used, but Azithromycin 1 gram orally, or Amoxicillin 500 mg p.o. q.i.d. for 7 days may be given (see section on chlamydia).

Ceftriaxone

- *Indications.* This is the treatment of choice for uncomplicated urethral, endocervical, and rectal infection.
- *Administration.* Ceftriaxone 125 mg I.M. once (CDC, 2002). Ceftriaxone is the most effective drug for pharyngeal infection and anal infection in males.
- *Side Effects and Adverse Reactions.* Although usually well tolerated, ceftriaxone has occasionally been associated with pain at injection site, diarrhea, rash, and headache. See discussions of chlamydia for more information about drugs for concurrent treatment of chlamydia.
- *Contraindications.* Known sensitivity to cephalosporins. Patients with a history of IgE-mediated allergic reactions to a penicillin (e.g., anaphylaxis, angioneurotic edema, immediate urticaria) should not receive cephalosporin.
- *Anticipated Outcomes on Evaluation.* Treatment failure is rare. Test for cure with this regimen is not essential.
- *Client Teaching and Counseling.* Advise the client to complete all oral medication and report any drug intolerance. If symptoms recur, retesting is needed. Stress the need for the partner's treatment.

Other Medications. Other recommended regimens for uncomplicated urogenital or rectal gonococcal infections in adults include cefixime 400 mg p.o. in a single dose *or* Ciprofloxacin 500 mg p.o. in a single dose *or* Ofloxacin 400 mg p.o. in a single dose (CDC, 2002). Gonorrhea acquired in Asia, the South Pacific, or Hawaii is likely to be resistant to fluoroquinolones (CDC, 2002). Pregnant women and clients under age 18 may not take Ciprofloxin or Ofloxacin. Pregnant women allergic to cephalosporin antibiotics may be treated with Spectinomycin 2 g I.M. (not effective for pharyngeal gonorrhea) (CDC, 2002). All of these drugs must also be given concurrently with an antibiotic that will cover chlamydia, if chlamydia has not been ruled out.

Recommended regimens for pharyngeal gonorrhea include ceftriaxone 125 mg I.M. in a single dose, or Ciprofloxacin 500 mg p. o. in a single dose. (CDC, 2002).

Recommended treatment schedules for special circumstances and complications are available from the CDC.

MUCOPURULENT CERVICITIS (MPC)

Chlamydia trachomatis and gonorrhea are the most common etiologic agents in women who have mucopurulent cervical discharge. In about half of women with mucopurulent discharge, however, the diagnosis cannot be established. Although *Ureaplasma urealyticum* and *Mycoplasma hominis* testing is not done routinely, these organisms have been recovered in women with nongonococcal/nonchlamydial mucopurulent cervicitis and in women with chronic voiding symptoms (Potts, Ward, & Rackley, 2000; Sendag, Terek, Tuncay, Ozkinay, & Guven, 2000).

Epidemiology

Ureaplasma urealyticum and *Mycoplasma hominis* are bacterial organisms that are sexually transmitted in adults. Colonization in infants may occur through an infected birth canal, although disease rarely results and colonization does not persist. The incidence of genital mycoplasma infections is unknown, but it is believed to be common. Infection is more common among low socioeconomic groups and minorities.

Subjective Data

May be asymptomatic or may present with dysuria, vaginal discharge, abnormal vaginal bleeding and/or abdominal pain. Mycoplasma/ureaplasma infection may also be suspected in women who present with infertility or recurrent miscarriages.

Objective Data

Physical Examination. Mucopurulent cervicitis is characterized by a yellow endocervical exudate visible in the endocervical canal or in an endocervical swab specimen (the yellow color of the exudate is apparent when contrasted with the white swab).

Diagnostic Tests and Methods. Tests for chlamydia, gonorrhea will be negative. Wet prep will contain many white blood cells, but no *Candida* or *Trichomonads*.

Culture. MPC may be treated empirically by many clinicians; however, confirmation of the diagnosis may be made by vaginal culture. Culture is particularly important when the client has infertility or recurrent miscarriage. The test procedure is to do a vaginal culture, which is better than an endocervical culture. An adequate sample from the vagina is necessary to enhance the yield. Obtain the specimens, place them immediately in medium, and transport them to the lab as soon as possible. Keep specimens refrigerated. Explain the procedure to the client.

Differential Medical Diagnoses

Chlamydia trachomatis, gonorrhea.

Plan

Psychosocial Interventions. Explain to the client the widespread nonspecific nature of genital mycoplasmas and the difficulty in establishing a definitive diagnosis. Partners should be treated empirically.

Medication. Consider empiric treatment for gonorrhea *and* chlamydia. Medications effective for chlamydia are also effective for ureaplasma and mycoplasma. Doxycycline 100 mg b.i.d. for seven days (see chlamydia treatment for prescribing details) (CDC, 2002). Azithromycin 1 g orally as a single dose (some ureaplasma strains are resistant to tetracyclines). May be used in pregnancy

(see chlamydia treatment for prescribing cautions). Ofloxacin 300 mg b.i.d. for seven days (expensive, but also effective for resistant strains) (CDC, 2002; Gilbert et al., 2001). Not in pregnancy or with adolescents under age 18.

ULCERATIVE GENITAL INFECTIONS

In the United States, most genital ulcers are caused by herpes simplex infections. Diagnosis based on history and physical alone, however, is often inaccurate. All persons with suspected genital herpes infection should also be tested for syphilis (CDC, 2002). Since syphilis management is very complex, clinicians unfamiliar with diagnostic and treatment protocols should seek consultation for questions related to diagnostic and treatment strategies. Consultation is also recommended if one of the rare bacterial ulcerative diseases is suspected.

HERPES SIMPLEX VIRUS (HSV)

No cure is known for this recurring viral disease. Characteristic painful lesions can occur in the mouth and genitalia of men and women, although virtually any skin or mucous membrane is vulnerable. Neonates who contract the virus congenitally develop infection of the central nervous system (CNS) and eyes. Significant perinatal morbidity and mortality are associated with congenital herpes simplex. Persons who are immunosuppressed are at risk for disseminated HSV, which often presents as meningitis/encephalitis. Once it enters the body, the herpes virus never leaves, although clinical manifestations disappear as the virus becomes dormant in sensory ganglia. When recurrence is triggered, the virus travels from nerve roots to the skin surface, where lesions develop. Reactivation of the virus is triggered by local or systemic stimuli such as trauma, fever, menstruation, ultraviolet light, and emotional stress (McKenzie, 2001). Many episodes of primary and recurrent HSV are asymptomatic (Gorroll, 2001b).

Epidemiology

Herpes simplex virus type 1 (HSV-1) primarily produces oral lesions, and herpes simplex virus type 2 (HSV-2) primarily produces genital lesions. Differentiation of the two types is academic because they are transmitted identically, their symptomatology is the same, and the procedures for diagnosis and treatment are the same.

Herpes simplex virus is transmitted primarily by direct contact with an infected individual who is shedding the virus. Nearly 20 percent of Americans between 14 and 49 years are believed to be infected with HSV-2 (CDC, 2000). Kissing, sexual contact, and vaginal delivery are means of transmission. Prolonged asymptomatic shedding follows in 20 percent of primary type 2 infections and appears to be responsible for transmission. Primary herpes in pregnancy may be passed to the neonate transplacentally or at birth. Autoinoculation is possible.

Most mothers of infants who acquire neonatal herpes do not have clinically evident genital herpes. The risk of vertical transmission is high among women who acquire genital herpes near the time of delivery (30 to 50%) and low among women with histories of recurrent herpes at term or who acquire herpes during the first half of pregnancy (1%) (CDC, 2002). The incubation period of HSV is two to seven days (Wilson & Henry, 2001).

Subjective Data

Primary herpes is a systemic disease characterized by multiple painful vesicular lesions, fever, chills, malaise, and severe dysuria if the lesions are genital. Symptoms peak four to five days after onset and may last two to three weeks. *Recurrent herpes,* on the other hand, is a localized disease characterized by typical HSV lesions at the site of initial viral entry. Recurrent herpes lesions usually are fewer, are less painful, and resolve more rapidly than primary herpes lesions. Recurrent HSV lasts an average of five to seven days, preceded by a prodromal symptom—frequently a burning, itching or swelling sensation. Lesions will appear within 24 hours of prodrome.

Objective Data

Physical Examination. Characteristic lesions are visible on the vulva and/or cervix. They are vesicular, usually multiple, and exquisitely painful to touch. The vesicles will open and weep and finally crust over, dry, and disappear without scar formation. Clients with primary HSV may have low grade fever and tender lymphadenopathy.

Diagnostic Tests and Methods

Viral Culture. Typical HSV lesions may be diagnosed by clinical signs and symptoms, but laboratory confirmation is desirable. Viral culture has a sensitivity of 70 to 80 percent (Emmert, 2000). The culture yield is best if the specimen is taken during the vesicular stage of disease; viral isolation is markedly reduced as lesions resolve. In primary episodes, viral shedding is prolonged and HSV more easily isolated.

Advise the client that obtaining the culture will be painful because vigorous sampling is essential to collect adequate cells.

Serologic Testing for HSV Antibodies. Serologic testing (including recently developed point-of-care testing such as POCkit^tmHSV-2) is sensitive, but not helpful for diagnosis of primary infection because of the delay in antibody development. It may be useful to differentiate seronegative individuals from seropositive individuals and asymptomatic carriers. Many widely used serological assays, however, do not differentiate HSV-1 and HSV-2 anitbodies. Polymerase chain reaction (PCR) tests are sensitive, but expensive.

Differential Medical Diagnoses

Primary syphilis, mucocutaneous manifestations of Crohn's disease, Behçet's syndrome, chancroid, lymphogranuloma venereum (LGV).

Plan

Psychosocial Interventions. Clients diagnosed with herpes require extensive counseling to understand the complex nature of the disease and its ramifications. Support groups may be helpful. Advise clients to abstain from intercourse during the prodrome and when lesions are present in any stage. Consistent condom use may reduce transmission rates. In addition, clients must know to wash their hands after touching lesions to avoid autoinoculation. Risk of acquiring HIV may be enhanced while genital lesions are present. Clients with a history of genital HSV should know to advise their care provider of this history if they become pregnant.

There is no evidence that HSV causes cervical cancer. Annual Pap smears are recommended for women with HSV infection since persons with one STD are at risk for the acquisition of other sexually transmitted infections.

Clients with genital HSV, both primary and recurrent, will benefit from such comfort measures as nonconstricting clothes, lukewarm sitz baths, and air drying of lesions with a handheld hair dryer on medium setting. Clients with severe dysuria may benefit by urinating in water. Extremes of temperature such as ice packs or heating pads should be avoided, as should steroid creams, anesthetic sprays, and any type of lotion or gel (e.g., petroleum jelly).

Management of HSV in Pregnancy. Pregnant women should be asked whether they or their partners have had genital herpes lesions. Suspicious or recurrent lesions should be cultured to document HSV or a type-specific serologic test should be used.

The risk of herpes is high in infants of women who acquire genital HSV in late pregnancy; such women should be managed in consultation with a HSV specialist (CDC, 2002). Routine screening cultures in women with a history of recurrent HSV, however, have not been shown to predict women who will be shedding virus at delivery (CDC, 2002). At onset of labor, women with a history of recurrent HSV should be questioned about symptoms of genital herpes, including prodrome, and all women should be examined carefully for herpetic lesions. Women without symptoms or signs of genital herpes or its prodrome can deliver vaginally (CDC, 2002).

Medication. Note: The dosage of all antiviral drugs should be adjusted in patients with reduced creatinine clearance. When using antivirals for recurrent symptoms, they should be instituted as soon as the client notices prodromal symptoms.

Acyclovir (Zovirax)

- *Indications.* Primary herpes infection and severe recurrent disease. Clients with frequent recurrences (more than six per year) may benefit from daily suppressive therapy. After one year of therapy, medication may be stopped and the client evaluated for recurrences. The safety and effectiveness for up to six years of acyclovir use have been documented.
- *Administration.* For primary HSV: 200 mg p.o., 5 times daily or 400 mg p.o. three times daily for seven to ten days or until symptoms resolve. For recurrent HSV: 200 mg p.o., 5 times daily for five days, *or* 400 mg p.o. three times daily, *or* 800 mg p.o., 2 times daily for five days. Daily suppression: 400 mg p.o. twice daily. Dosage may be individualized (CDC, 2002).
- *Side Effects and Adverse Reactions.* These are minimal, even with long-term use. Nausea, vomiting, and headache have been reported, however. Clients on long-term suppression can expect a rebound recurrence when therapy is stopped.
- *Contraindications.* Known hypersensitivity to acyclovir.
- *Anticipated Outcomes on Evaluation.* Accelerated healing and shortened course of the disease.
- *Client Teaching and Counseling.* Advise the client that short courses of acyclovir neither eradicate HSV

nor have an impact on the subsequent risk and frequency of recurrences. Daily suppressive therapy reduces the frequency and severity of recurrences, but this effect does not persist after medication is discontinued. The extent to which suppressive therapy prevents HSV transmission is unknown (CDC, 2002). Topical therapy with acyclovir ointment is substantially less effective than oral medications (CDC, 2002). The first clinical episode of genital herpes during pregnancy may be treated with oral acyclovir, however, routine administration of acyclovir to pregnant women with a history of recurrent genital herpes is not recommended (CDC, 2002).

Other Medications. Famciclovir tablets (Famvir) are approved for the management of recurrent genital herpes in adults. Famciclovir is dosed 250 mg p.o. three times daily for seven to ten days for primary infection, 125 mg p.o. for five days for recurrent herpes, or 250 mg p.o. twice daily for suppression (CDC, 2002). Side effects and activity are similar to acyclovir.

Valacyclovir HCL caplets (Valtrex) are also approved for the management of primary and recurrent genital herpes in adults. Valacyclovir is dosed 1 gram p.o. twice daily for seven to ten days for primary infection, or 500 mg p.o. twice daily for five days for recurrent infection. For suppression, Valacyclovir may be dosed 500 mg p.o. once daily or 1 g once daily (CDC, 2002). Side effects and activity are similar to acyclovir.

SYPHILIS

Syphilis is a complex sexually transmitted disease that can lead to serious systemic illness and even death if untreated. Infection manifests in distinct stages with diverse clinical manifestations. Its natural history begins with *primary syphilis,* which is characterized by a chancre at the site of bacterial entry. *Secondary syphilis* is recognized by flulike symptoms and a maculopapular rash of the palms and soles. Following secondary syphilis, *latency* occurs. Ultimately *tertiary (late) syphilis* occurs, characterized by irreversible cardiovascular, neurologic, dermatologic, or bony disease.

Clients with any STD or genital ulcer should be evaluated for syphilis. All pregnant women should have a nontreponemal serologic test for syphilis at the first prenatal visit. Women suspected of being at risk for syphilis should have the test repeated during the third trimester and at delivery (CDC, 2002). Clients who have been exposed to syphilis within the preceding three months may be infected but sero-negative and thus should be treated for early syphilis (CDC, 2002). All clients who have syphilis should be offered HIV testing.

Epidemiology

Treponema pallidum, a bacterium in the spirochete family, is the causative organism. Direct sexual contact (or, less frequently, blood contact) with an infected individual transmits the disease. The risk of developing syphilis after one unprotected contact is up to 50 percent (Jacobs, 2001). Because the initial anorectal or vaginal chancres are not likely to be noticed, syphilis is infrequently diagnosed in the primary stage among women or homosexuals. Transplacental transmission of an infected mother to her fetus is also possible and results in about 60 percent fetal loss; up to half of surviving infants have stigmata (Davis & Simon, 2000). Longstanding untreated disease is less contagious than the primary or secondary stage. The incubation period is from 10 to 90 days (3 weeks average).

Rates of syphilis in the United States are currently declining, but remain high among young adult African Americans in urban areas and in the southern states (CDC, 2000).

Subjective Data

- *Primary Syphilis.* Client is an asymptomatic contact or may report a lesion.
- *Secondary Syphilis.* Low-grade fever, headache, sore throat, rash on the palms and soles.
- *Tertiary Syphilis.* Cardiovascular symptoms (chest pain, cough), neurological symptoms (headache, irritability, impaired balance, memory loss, tremor), skeletal symptoms (arthritis, myalgia, myositis), or skin symptoms (multiple nodules or ulcers).
- *Congenital Syphilis.* See Objective Data.

Objective Data

Physical Examination

- *Primary Syphilis.* Classic chancre is a painless, rounded, indurated ulcer with serous exudate (see Figure 11–5). It may be genital or extragenital. Usually a single chancre occurs, but multiple chancres may be present. An extragenital chancre is likely to be atypical in appearance. Lymphadenopathy, which may accompany the chancre, will resolve spontaneously in three to six weeks. Must be distinguished from genital herpes, chancroid, lymphogranuloma, or neoplasm.

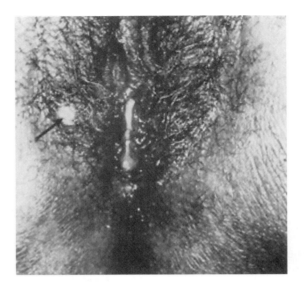

FIGURE 11–5. Chancre of primary syphilis (arrow). *(Reproduced with permission, from DeCherney, A. H., & Pernoll, M. L.* Current obstetric and gynecologic diagnosis and treatment, *8th ed. Appleton & Lange, 1994.)*

- *Secondary Syphilis.* Classic maculopapular rash that gradually covers the body, including the palms and the soles. Less common signs include patchy alopecia, generalized nontender lymphadenopathy, mucosal ulcers, and condyloma lata (flat broad wartlike papules on warm, moist skin surfaces). Spontaneous healing of all secondary manifestations occurs. Must be distinguished from infectious exanthems, pityriasis rosea, and drug eruptions.
- *Tertiary Syphilis.* Manifestations are dependent on whether the client has neurosyphilis, cardiovascular syphilis, or other expressions of the disease. Aortic diastolic murmur, aneurysms, and congestive failure characterize cardiovascular syphilis; meningeal irritation, unequal reflexes, irregular pupils with poor light response, wide-based gait, and personality deterioration characterize neurosyphilis. Must be distinguished from neoplasms of the skin, liver, stomach or brain; other forms of meningitis; and primary neurologic lesions.
- *Congenital Syphilis.* Premature birth, intra-uterine growth retardation, mucocutaneous lesions, snuffles (serous nasal discharge), hepatosplenomegaly, condyloma lata, skeletal lesions, CNS involvement, ocular lesions, and others.

Diagnostic Tests and Methods. Diagnosis is largely dependent on microscopic examination of primary and secondary lesion tissue and serology during latency and late infection. Direct darkfield microscopic examination requires considerable expertise and is unavailable in most offices. However, an immunofluorescent staining technique is available for demonstrating *T. pallidum* in fluid taken from suspicious lesions, spread on slides, fixed appropriately and mailed to a reference lab.

Direct Microscopic Examination. Diagnostic evaluation for definitive identification of *T. pallidum* is possible when lesions (e.g., chancre, rash) are present. If antibiotics have been taken, the test is not useful.

The test procedure is first to cleanse the lesion with sterile saline. Then gently abrade to produce oozing of serous fluid. Avoid active bleeding. Collect serous fluid on a slide and fix as directed by the laboratory. Advise the client that the testing procedure is not uncomfortable, but results will have to be obtained from the laboratory.

Serological Tests, Nontreponemal. Diagnostic evaluation for antilipid antibodies produced by the host exposed to *T. pallidum.* Examples are Venereal Disease Research Laboratory (VDRL) and Rapid Plasma Reagent (RPR). Used for syphilis screening and follow-up after treatment. Twenty-five percent of patients with syphilis develop negative nontreponemal tests in late latent disease; however, treponemal tests will still be positive (Jacobs, 2001).

The test procedure is to collect a blood sample in a dry tube without anticoagulant. Advise the client that venipuncture is required. Results are reported as either reactive (positive) or nonreactive (negative). *Reactive results* are quantitated in the form of a titer. The false positive rate is 1 to 2 percent in the general population, higher in low risk groups. False positive reactions are encountered in connective tissue diseases, mononucleosis, febrile diseases, intravenous drug use, old age, HIV infection, and pregnancy (Jacobs, 2001). False negative results may occur when high antibody levels are present. If syphilis is strongly suspected and the nontreponemal test is negative, the laboratory should be instructed to dilute the specimen to detect a positive reaction.

All reactive results require confirmation by the treponemal test (description follows). Tests become reactive fourteen days after the chancre appears. If results are equivocal, repeat testing is indicated. A rising titer is evidence of primary syphilis. If syphilis is suspected and the initial nontreponemal test is nonreactive, repeat in one week, one month, and three months. *Nonreactive results* after three months exclude the diagnosis of syphilis.

Serological Tests, Treponemal. Diagnostic evaluation to detect *T. pallidum* specific antibodies. This test is designed to confirm the diagnosis of a reactive nontreponemal test. One example is fluorescent treponemal antibody absorption (FTA-ABS). The test procedure is to collect a blood sample in a dry tube without anticoagulant.

The treponemal test should only be used *after* the nontreponemal test is reactive—never as the initial screen. It is also used if symptoms of tertiary syphilis are present. The results are reported as reactive or nonreactive. Although the FTA-ABS test may remain positive after treatment, this is not a reliable marker of previous infection (Jacobs, 2001). Pregnant patients who are allergic to penicillin should be desensitized and treated with penicillin (CDC, 2002). Final decisions about the significance of serologic tests results must be based on a total clinical appraisal of risks.

Plan

Psychosocial Interventions. Extensive counseling and support are needed. Explain the complex nature of the disease and its ramifications. Case finding and treatment of sexual partners are essential to epidemic control but difficult when the relationship is associated with crack or cocaine use. The need must be stressed for follow-up testing to ensure adequate treatment. Explain the meaning of test results, especially rising or falling titers and persistent reactive results. Clients with serological evidence of syphilis in any stage are best treated by practitioners experienced in the management of this complex disease. Suggest HIV counseling and testing.

Medication. Penicillin is the treatment of choice for all clients with syphilis and the only proven therapy for syphilis during pregnancy and for congenital syphilis. Penicillin prevents congenital syphilis in 90 percent of cases, even when given late in pregnancy (Jacobs, 2001).

Benzathine Penicillin G

- ◆ *Indications.* Primary and secondary syphilis and early latent syphilis of less than one year's duration.
- ◆ *Administration.* 2.4 million units I.M. in one dose. Clients with syphilis of greater than a year's duration (latent or tertiary stages) require weekly treatment with 2.4 million units of Benzathine Penicillin G for three weeks. Neurosyphilis (diagnosed by lumbar puncture) requires intravenous treatment (CDC, 2002).
- ◆ *Side Effects and Adverse Reactions.* Penicillin adverse effects include wheezing, weakness, abdominal pain, nausea or vomiting, diarrhea, rash, fever, increased thirst, and seizures. In addition, Jarisch-Herxheimer reaction, an acute febrile illness with

headache and flulike symptoms, may occur a few hours after antibiotic administration. It is probably due to treponemal lysis and subsides within 24 hours. It may be severe. The reaction may be prevented or modified by simultaneous administration of antipyretics or corticosteroids (Jacobs, 2001).

♦ *Contraindications.* A known sensitivity to penicillin.

♦ *Anticipated Outcomes on Evaluation.* Clients treated for syphilis must be followed with a nontreponemal test at three and six months. Titers should fall fourfold by six months in those treated for primary and secondary syphilis, indicating adequate therapy (Jacobs, 2001).

♦ *Client Teaching and Counseling.* Provide the client with information about the possibility of the Jarisch-Herxheimer reaction and its treatment: rest, fluids, and antipyretics. Stress the importance of follow-up testing. Clients allergic to penicillin may be treated with doxycycline/tetracycline/erythromycin/Ceftriaxone (not single dose). Specific protocols are recommended by the Centers for Disease Control (CDC, 2002).

CHANCROID

Chancroid is a sexually transmitted disease characterized by painful genital ulceration. Lesions are usually confined to the genitals and accompanied by inguinal lymphadenopathy. Systemic illness does not occur. Although more common in Africa, the West Indies and Asia, scattered pockets continue to exist in the United States. New York, South Carolina, and Texas accounted for 72 percent of cases reported in 1999 (CDC, 2000). Ten percent of patients with chancroid have co-infection with herpes simplex virus and/or syphilis. An increased rate of HIV infection has also been associated with chancroid, so those with suspected chancroid should be tested for HIV (CDC, 2002).

Epidemiology

Haemophilus ducreyi, a gram-negative bacillus, is the causative agent. The incubation period is three to five days. The condition occurs most commonly in uncircumcised males; incidence among women is low. Transmission is by direct contact with an infected individual. Fomite transmission does not occur.

Subjective Data

The initial lesion is a vesicopapule that breaks down to form a painful soft ulcer. Multiple lesions may develop, spread by autoinoculation. These may rupture sponta-

neously. Fever, malaise, and chills may also develop. Women may have nonspecific symptoms such as dysuria, vaginal discharge, and dyspareunia, or they may be asymptomatic.

Objective Data

Physical Examination. A characteristic ulcerative lesion is seen on the genitalia with a necrotic base and surrounding erythema. In over 50 percent of the cases, a bubo will be present (a greatly enlarged, inflamed lymph node). This unilateral inguinal adenitis is tender and the overlying skin is inflamed. Buboes may spontaneously rupture. One or two lesions are the norm, although more may occur.

Diagnostic Tests and Methods

Culture of Ulcers. Diagnostic evaluation to isolate *H. ducreyi.* The test procedure is to swab the base of the ulcerative lesion with a cotton or calcium alginate swab. Transport the specimen to a laboratory within four hours (refrigerate the swab if transportation time is longer). Do not culture a bubo unless it has ruptured; unruptured bubos are usually sterile.

The laboratory must be informed that chancroid is suspected. The organism is best cultured on chocolate agar with 1 percent Isovitalex and vancomycin 3 mg/ml. Explain to the client that a culture is the best test. (A gram stain may be inaccurate, and newer enzyme immunoassay tests are still being developed.) Culture results take up to one week.

Differential Medical Diagnoses

Genital herpes, syphilis, granuloma inguinale.

Plan

Psychosocial Interventions. Chancroid may in-crease the risk of HIV infection. Advise the client that her sexual partners within the past ten days need examination and treatment. Symptoms improve within three days; ulcers heal within seven days. Bubos resolve more slowly and may require aspiration.

Medication

Azithromycin

♦ *Indications.* Suspected or culture proven chancroid. A presumptive diagnosis is made if the clinical picture is clear. Single dose facilitates compliance; however, treatment failures have been reported with single dose Azithromycin in HIV-positive clients (CDC, 2002).

- *Administration.* One gram orally as a single dose (CDC, 2002).
- *Side Effects and Adverse Reactions.* Gastrointestinal distress, rare angioedema, and cholestatic jaundice. Caution should be used in patients with impaired hepatic function. See also side effects listed under chlamydia.
- *Contraindications.* Known hypersensitivity to any macrolide drug.
- *Anticipated Outcomes on Evaluation.* Ulcerative lesions resolve.

Ceftriaxone

- *Indications.* Suspected or culture proven chancroid. A presumptive diagnosis is made if the clinical picture is clear. Single dose facilitates compliance.
- *Administration.* 250 mg I.M. (CDC, 2002).
- *Side Effects and Adverse Reactions.* Although usually well tolerated, ceftriaxone is occasionally associated with pain at the injection site, diarrhea, rash, and headache.
- *Contraindications.* Known sensitivity to cephalosporins. Use with caution for clients sensitive to penicillin.
- *Anticipated Outcomes on Evaluation.* Treatment failure is rare. Test for cure with this regimen is not essential.

Erythromycin

- *Indications.* Suspected or culture proven chancroid. A presumptive diagnosis is made if the clinical picture is clear.
- *Administration.* 500 mg p.o., q.i.d. for seven days (CDC, 2002).
- *Side Effects and Adverse Reactions.* Gastrointestinal distress. (See Azithromycin under chlamydia treatment for drug reactions/interactions that have been reported with macrolides.)
- *Contraindications.* Known hypersensitivity to erythromycin. Concomitant use of ketaconazole (Nizoral).
- *Anticipated Outcomes on Evaluation.* Ulcerative lesions resolve.

Other Medications. Ciprofloxacin 500 mg p.o., b.i.d. for three days (CDC, 2002). With the exception of ciprofloxacin, which is contraindicated for pregnant and lactating women and children under 17, all of the regimens just listed may be used in pregnancy.

Client Teaching and Counseling. Azithromycin must be taken one hour before or two hours after a meal. It should not be taken with food. If no improvement occurs within two to three days, diagnosis must be reconsidered. Infection with other STDs, including HIV, may also exist. Partners should be treated.

Follow-Up/Referral

Only if nonresponsive to drug treatment.

GRANULOMA INGUINALE

A chronic, progressive bacterial infection of the genitals, granuloma inguinale presents with large, unsightly ulcers of the genitalia, inguinal region, and anus. Other names for the condition are donovanosis and granuloma venereum. Since other sexually transmitted diseases frequently coexist, cultures for these and serological tests for syphilis and HIV must be performed.

Epidemiology

Calymmatobacterium granulomatis, a gram-negative bacterium, is the causative agent. Anal intercourse, often associated with homosexuality, is a particular risk factor. Transmission is by sexual or nonsexual trauma to infected sites, primarily the anus and penis. The disease is mildly contagious; repeated exposures are needed in order for clinical manifestations to develop. The incubation period is seven days to twelve weeks (Chambers, 2001).

Rarely reported in the United States, granuloma inguinale is epidemic in parts of Australia and common in India and many tropical and subtropical environments. Donovan bodies (bacteria encapsulated in mononuclear leukocytes) are found in tissue scrapings that are stained with Wright's stain.

Subjective Data

The disorder often begins as a papule, which then ulcerates, leaving a beefy-red, relatively painless granular area with clean sharp rolled edges. The ulcer is persistent, and satellite ulcers may unite to form a large ulcer. Inguinal swelling is common, with late formation of painful abscesses (buboes). Superinfection of the ulcer with spirochete-fusiform organisms is common; the ulcer then becomes purulent, painful, and foul smelling. Rarely, granuloma inguinale presents with granulomatous cervical lesions which must be distinguished from carcinoma.

Objective Data

Physical Examination. An examination reveals the characteristic lesions, as noted previously.

Diagnostic Tests and Methods. Wright's or Giemsa Stain. Diagnostic evaluation for pathognomonic Donovan bodies (common name for causative organism). The test procedure is to crush/smear a clean piece of granulation tissue on a slide. Air dry, then stain using appropriate Wright's or Giemsa staining technique. Explain to the client that the test procedure is simple and reliable. Must be done by a laboratory familiar with these techniques.

Differential Medical Diagnoses

Chancroid, carcinoma, syphilis, amebiasis.

Plan

Medication. A variety of antibiotics are useful. The first-line treatment is Doxycycline.

Doxycycline

- *Indications.* Positive diagnosis of granuloma inguinale.
- *Administration.* Doxycycline 100 mgs b.i.d. for three to four weeks until lesions have healed (CDC, 2002).
- *Side Effects and Adverse Reactions.* GI upset, rash, photosensitivity. Overgrowth of vaginal candida.
- *Contraindications.* Pregnancy; allergy to tetracyclines.
- *Anticipated Outcomes on Evaluation.* Lesions will heal and Donovan bodies will disappear from the smears.
- *Client Teaching and Counseling.* Advise the client that compliance with treatment is critical. Medication must be continued until all lesions are healed. This may take up to four weeks. Discontinuing therapy early results in high recurrence rates.

Other Medications. Trimethoprim 160 mg/sulfamethoxazole 800 mg (Bactrim DS) tablets b.i.d. for at least 3 weeks or until lesions have healed. Ciprofloxacin 750 mg p.o. daily for three weeks (not in pregnancy). Erythromycin 500 mg q.i.d. for at least three weeks may be used in pregnancy (CDC, 2002).

Follow-Up and Referral

The client should be seen one to two months after the initial diagnosis to ensure resolution. Partners must be treated.

LYMPHOGRANULOMA VENEREUM (LGV)

This chronic bacterial STD initially presents as a vesiculopustular eruption that may go unnoticed. After the genital lesion disappears, the infection spreads to lymph channels and lymph nodes of the genital and rectal areas (in women the genital lymph drainage is to the perirectal glands). This secondary invasion is characterized by painful ulceration, lymphedema and draining abscesses (buboes). Early anorectal manifestations are proctitis with tenesmus and bloody purulent discharge; late rectal manifestations include inflammation, scarring, and stricture of rectal and vaginal tissue. Systemic symptoms (fever, headache, abdominal pain, chills, and arthralgias) may develop.

Epidemiology

The causative organisms are *Chlamydia trachomatis serovars:* L1, L2, and L3. LGV is rare in the United States. LGV is endemic in some tropical and developing areas, such as Papua New Guinea, Australia, and southern Africa (CDC, 2002). Men with the disease outnumber women by 5 to 1. The incubation period is three to twelve days or longer.

Subjective Data

LGV contacts are initially asymptomatic, or may report genital ulcers and painful groin nodes or abscesses. A wide variety of nonspecific symptoms may be present.

Objective Data

Physical Examination. Tender inguinal lymphadenopathy is the most common sign. A spectrum of other clinical symptoms may occur, including papules, ulcers, cervicitis, proctitis, bubo formation (tender abscesses), and genital edema. A hard cutaneous induration may also be present.

Diagnostic Tests and Methods. Serological tests using fixation, neutralizing antibody, or immunofluorescents are available. Because LGV is so rare in the United States, specific information should be obtained from the local laboratory when testing is required.

Differential Medical Diagnoses

Chancroid, genital herpes, syphilis. Lymph node involvement must be distinguished from that due to tularemia, tuberculosis, or neoplasm. Rectal strictures must be distinguished from neoplasm and ulcerative colitis.

Plan

Psychosocial Interventions. Prevention is critical. When LGV is diagnosed, all sexual contacts must be identified and treated to eliminate a reservoir of continued transmission (CDC, 2002). Surgical excision of lesions may be necessary after infection has been halted.

Medication. *Clients should be referred to an infectious disease specialist if LGV is suspected.* Antibiotic therapy is indicated, and adequate treatment and follow-up are essential.

Doxycycline

- ◆ *Administration.* Doxycycline 100 mg p.o., b.i.d. for 21 days (CDC, 2002).
- ◆ *Side Effects and Contraindications.* The same as those discussed in the section on tetracycline therapy for granuloma inguinale.
- ◆ *Anticipated Outcomes on Evaluation.* Resolution of symptoms. Relapse is common.
- ◆ *Client Teaching and Counseling.* Assist the client to complete the medication regimen, which is difficult because it lasts 21 days.

Other Medications. Alternative treatment regimens include erythromycin 500 mg p.o., q.i.d. for 21 days (may be used in pregnancy) (CDC, 2002).

EPIDERMAL DISEASES

Clinical syndromes with epidermal manifestations vary in seriousness, persistence, and treatment approaches. Human papillomavirus infections are unique in that different viral types have different clinical manifestations.

HUMAN PAPILLOMAVIRUS (HPV) INFECTION

Human papilloma virus infection is the most prevalent viral STD in the United States (Carey & Rayburn, 2002). HPV-mediated oncogenesis is responsible for up to 95 percent of cervical squamous cell carcinomas and nearly all preinvasive cervical neoplasms (Morris, 2002). However, prospective studies in young women screened for HPV DNA suggest that HPV is frequently a transient infection, with most initially positive DNA tests becoming negative within one year. As many as 40 percent of women are positive for HPV by polymerase chain reaction testing (Carey & Rayburn, 2002). Clinically evident genital warts are only present in 2 percent of women and men (Sonnex & Lacey 2001). Infection with high-risk HPV types and older age are risk factors for persistent HPV infection that may in turn increase the risk for cervical

squamous intraepithelial lesions (Ho, Bierman, Beardsley, Chang, & Burk, 1998). The outcome of exposure to these viruses depends on multiple factors including HPV type, type of skin infected, host immunity, and smoking status.

Individuals with clinical evidence of HPV in one genital site have a significant risk of other HPV manifestations in another genital site (vulva, vagina, cervix, urethra, perianal skin, and rectum) (Carey & Rayburn, 2002). Unlike the treatment goal for bacterial sexually transmitted infections, the goal of HPV treatment is to remove obvious lesions and prevent the progression of neoplasias, not to eradicate HPV.

HPV infections are classified as clinical, subclinical, or latent. Clinical lesions are fleshy papules. Subclinical lesions are identified as whitened areas visible after application of 5 percent acetic acid and inspection under magnification. Subclinical infection of the cervix is generally diagnosed by typical changes (koilocytosis or neoplasias) diagnosed by Papanicolaou smear. Latent infections have no visible lesions and are evident only by DNA hybridization tests for HPV (Sonnex & Lacey, 2001).

Epidemiology

Human papillomavirus (HPV) is a slow-growing DNA virus of the papovavirus family; more than 100 strains are identified, twenty of which have been associated with genital tract infections (Morris, 2002). Condyloma acuminata and low grade neoplasias are usually associated with human papilloma types 6 and 11. Other HPV types in the anogenital area (16, 18, 31, 45, and 56) are strongly associated with higher grades of genital dysplasia and carcinoma (Morris, 2002). More than one type may be present at one time.

HPV is most commonly spread by means of sexual or other intimate contact. The organism may have limited survival on fomites, but nonsexual transmission is rare and difficult to document. Autoinoculation and mother-child transfer at birth can occur. The incubation period is three weeks to eight months or longer.

Subjective Data

Clinical HPV lesions are papular lesions with a warty, granular surface. They are usually painless; however, malodorous vaginal discharge, pain and burning with urination, pruritus, and bleeding during and after coitus may occur. The lack of visible lesions or complaints is not uncommon, however. A woman may have a history of an infected partner but have no evidence of infection. Lesions may grow so large in pregnancy as to affect urination, defecation, mobility, and descent of the fetus, although rarely is cesarean delivery necessitated (Carey & Rayburn, 2002).

Objective Data

Physical Examination. Genitalia/reproductive tract shows one or more soft, pale, pink or flesh-colored, dry, irregular lesions on the external genitalia, perineum, or anus. The lesions, 1 mm or larger, may be flat, papular, or pedunculated papules on the vulva, introitus, vagina, cervix, perineum, urethra, and/or anus. Small condylomata should not be confused with vulval vestibular papillae that are normally located on the epithelium of both labia minora. In true condyloma acuminata, multiple papilla converge toward a single base, whereas each papillae has its own base in normal vulvar tissue (Ferenczy, 1995). Examination of the vulva after topical application of 3 to 5 percent acetic acid may assist in identification of subclinical lesions. These will be slightly elevated, well demarcated, and aceto-white. Candidiasis, folliculitis, contact dermatitis, and psoriasis may also turn white, however, with acetic acid application (Ferenczy, 1995). Large lesions may be cauliflower-like in appearance, exist in coalesced clusters, and be friable. Areas most often traumatized during coitus are common sites for HPV infection.

Diagnostic Tests and Methods

Pap Smear (Cytology). It is imperative that women with vulvar HPV or partners with HPV have a cervical examination with a Papanicolaou smear. The application of 3 to 5 percent acetic acid to the cervix may identify areas of aceto-whitening that can be targeted by the Pap smear. This screening evaluation will identify squamous intraepithelial lesions on Bethesda System reports. A Pap smear is a screening test and not diagnostic since the sample can miss the lesion. The severity of any cervical lesion reported on a Pap smear can be determined best by HPV molecular testing or colposcopically directed cervical biopsy. (See Chapters 4 and 13 for Pap smear techniques and management of abnormal Pap smears.) It is important to note that any grossly visible suspicious cervical lesion requires biopsy, regardless of the Pap smear findings.

Colposcopy with Directed Biopsy (Histology). Diagnostic evaluation for subclinical lesions, dysplasia, and malignancy, performed by trained, experienced colposcopist using colposcope. The procedure provides a magnified view of direct biopsy sites. An abnormal Pap report, cervical lesions, or extensive external lesions warrant referral for colposcopy and biopsy. Endocervical curettage should not be performed if the client is pregnant.

The test procedure includes the application of 3 to 5 percent acetic acid to the tissue of the vulva or cervix. After several seconds, abnormal areas turn white. The tissue is then examined under magnification with the colposcope. Directed biopsy is done on the most abnormal sites (e.g., aceto-white with punctuation and mosaic pattern).

Explain the procedure to the client: no anesthesia required; lithotomy position; instrument introduced through wide speculum opening; uncomfortable stinging from acetic acid; pinching, cramping sensation when tissue is removed. Tell the client that no excessive bleeding should occur, although a blood-tinged discharge may continue for two to three days; no coitus, douching, tampon use, or putting other objects in the vagina for three days.

DNA Typing (Nucleic Acid Hybridization Tests). Diagnostic evaluation to determine the specific HPV strain; may be useful to discriminate between low-risk and high-risk HPV types when Pap smear reveals ASCUS or LGSIL. If test is positive for high-risk types, the client is referred for colposcopy. If low-risk HPV types are identified, the client can be given the option of colposcopy or serial Pap smears (Bryant-Greenwood, 2002). A specimen for testing can be obtained with a fluid phase collection system such as Thin Prep®.

Explain to the client that HPV typing may identify particularly virulent strains of the virus.

Differential Medical Diagnoses

Condyloma lata, molluscum contagiosum; carcinoma; concomitant sexually transmitted diseases.

Plan

Considerable disagreement exists regarding protocols and recommendations for diagnosis and treatment. There is no consensus on treatment for male partners of women infected with HPV, and there is disagreement on the effectiveness of condoms in preventing transmission or recurrence of HPV (Sonnex & Lacey, 2001). Recurrence rates of 25 to 50 percent are believed to be an evolution from latent to active infection at different sites or reexposure of the healing treated area to the woman's colonized adjacent tissue.

Although treatment of subclinical lesions in monogamous sexual partners is not justified, condom use during treatment of clinical warts may also reduce viral spread in partners who may not yet be infected.

Psychosocial Interventions. Implications for counseling include relationship dissatisfaction, depression, and fear related to the seriousness of the diagnosis (dysplasia or cancer). Referral may be indicated. Discuss treatment options with the client (and partner, if appropriate); fully involve her in the therapy plans.

Emotionally, HPV infection may affect self-esteem, body image, feelings (shame, guilt, or blame), satisfaction with intimate relationships, and overall mental health (Krieger, 1995). Anxiety associated with knowing one has a potentially malignant disease and lack of a definitive cure may necessitate referral for psychological counseling and support. Partners may also be involved in counseling. Through education about HPV, anxiety may be reduced. Involvement in controlling decisions empowers the client by decreasing her dependency.

Medication. Drug therapies may be alternated or combined in some arrangement, such as TCA and liquid nitrogen on alternating weeks. With any topical application, an alternative treatment should be tried if lesions have not resolved in four to five treatments. Clients should be referred for biopsy of any nonresponsive or atypical lesions.

Trichloracetic Acid (TCA) 80 to 90 Percent

- *Indications.* To reduce the size of external genital and vaginal lesions.
- *Administration.* Apply TCA solution sparingly to lesions, using a cotton swab and avoiding the surrounding tissue. Calcium alginate swabs may be preferred since they are smaller and decrease damage to surrounding tissue. Treated areas will turn white. A mixture of baking soda and water may be applied to neutralize the acid after application or to prevent damage from solution inadvertently applied to normal skin. A burning sensation occurs for several minutes following application but may be avoided by pretreatment spraying of topical anesthetic (Sonnex & Lacey, 2001). Applications are repeated once weekly; may be repeated twice weekly if the client can tolerate it.
- *Side Effects and Adverse Reactions.* Burning sensation on application should resolve quickly. There may be erythema, tenderness, swelling, and sloughing of tissue in the area for a few days after application. No systemic effects.
- *Contraindications.* TCA is contraindicated with severely irritated tissues. The medication has been used safely in pregnancy.

- *Anticipated Outcomes on Evaluation.* Lesions will become smaller and finally disappear after a few applications. If no visible improvement occurs after three treatments, use another method. If lesions persist or are multiple or internal, refer the client to a gynecologist.
- *Client Teaching and Counseling.* Tell the client that it is not necessary to wash off the acid. Persistent leukorrhea, increased pain, and redness may indicate infection. Spotting or bleeding may occur if the healing tissue is jarred. In addition, lidocaine (Xylocaine) ointment may be given, or warm sitz baths and a baking soda/water mixture may soothe.

Liquid Nitrogen Cryotherapy

- *Indications.* External warts. For internal lesions, the client is referred to a gynecologist.
- *Administration.* Application may be accomplished with a finely twisted cotton tip, or the wooden end of a cotton tipped applicator, or a special applicator jet. The lesion will turn white. May be followed by application of podophyllin or TCA.
- *Side Effects and Adverse Reactions.* The same as for TCA and podophyllin.
- *Contraindications.* None.
- *Anticipated Outcomes on Evaluation.* The lesions will disappear after one to four weekly treatments.
- *Client Teaching and Counseling.* Inform the client that the application of the drug may burn. For the discomfort, the same teaching and counseling as used for application of TCA or podophyllin are appropriate.

Imiquimod 5% Cream (Aldara)

- *Indications.* Imiquimod is an immune response modifier indicated for external genitalia and perianal warts. Pregnancy category B. Studies suggest that recurrence may be less frequent than with other treatments (Sonnex & Lacey, 2001).
- *Administration.* Clients apply a thin layer to warts and rub in three times weekly at bedtime. May be used for a total of sixteen weeks.
- *Side Effects and Adverse Reactions.* Causes mild to moderate skin erythema and erosion.
- *Contraindications.* Not for urethral, intravaginal, or intra-anal warts.
- *Anticipated Outcomes on Evaluation.* Gradual clearing of warts over the treatment period.
- *Client Teaching and Counseling.* Cream must be washed off with soap and water six to ten hours after

application. Cream is petrolatum based and will cause condoms and diaphragms to deteriorate. Sexual contact should be avoided while cream is on the skin. Avoid eyes.

Podofilox 0.5 Percent. Podofilox 0.5 percent, a self-treatment, may be prescribed. Unlike podophyllin, this is a stable, purified product that does not need to be washed off (Sonnex & Lacey, 2001). Advise the client to apply it twice a day (only to the warts) for three days with a cotton swab followed by four days of no therapy. The treatment may be repeated for a total of four cycles. The health care provider must teach wart identification, proper medicine application, and avoidance of getting any solution on other areas. The total treatment area should be 10 cm^2 or less. No more than 0.5 mL of solution should be used daily. It is contraindicated in pregnancy (Sonnex & Lacey, 2001).

Podophyllin. 10 to 25 percent in tincture of benzoin compound.

- *Indications.* For external lesions only. Because of potential toxicity and variations in potency of this natural plant extract, podophyllin is not recommended as a first line treatment.
- *Administration.* Compound is applied to the lesion using a cotton swab and avoiding normal tissue. Unaffected areas may be protected by applying petroleum or lubricant jelly to them. Podophyllin must be washed off four hours after application. Applications are repeated weekly; more frequent use may result in burning.
- *Side Effects and Adverse Reactions.* Erythema, burning, swelling, tissue damage. Lesions may become tender several days after treatment.
- *Contraindications.* Pregnancy or presence of large warts. Absorption may cause toxicity.
- *Anticipated Outcomes on Evaluation.* The same as for trichloracetic acid (TCA). Do not exceed four applications if no significant improvement results.
- *Client Teaching and Counseling.* Provide the client with information about the signs of toxicity: nausea, vomiting, lethargy, coma, paralysis. Repeated use may be carcinogenic. Instruct the client to wash off podophyllin four hours after application with mild soap and water, sooner if irritation causes discomfort.

Surgery and Other Interventions. Indications are internal lesions, large lesions, or external lesions unresponsive to prior therapy. The client is referred to a trained, experienced specialist.

Laser Carbon Dioxide Vaporization. This outpatient procedure is done with the client under general or regional anesthesia or heavy sedation. A laser beam vaporizes large areas of lesions without scarring. Small lesions are done under local anesthesia. During the procedure, warmth and menstrual-like cramps are felt. Pain after treatment is mild to moderate; profuse, watery discharge occurs for up to two weeks. Healing takes three to four weeks. The secondary infection rate is higher with large treatment areas.

Electrodiathermy Loop Excision Procedure (LEEP). LEEP is increasingly popular as an office procedure for cervical lesions when the entire lesion and entire transformation zone can be visualized by colposcopy, there is no evidence of endocervical involvement, and there is no evidence of invasive disease. LEEP procedures result in less thermal damage compared to cryotherapy and also provide a specimen for histology (Ostrzenski, 2002).

Cryosurgery (Nitrous Oxide). Cryosurgery is performed as an office procedure for cervical disease (dysplasia). Lesions treated by cryosurgery must meet the same criteria as those treated by LEEP. Nitrous oxide is the freezing agent of choice. The cryoprobe is applied to the cervix using a 3–5–3 minute technique. Mild to moderate cramping during the procedure usually subsides once freezing is complete. A profuse, watery, foul-smelling vaginal discharge continues for two to three weeks. Nothing is to be put into the vagina for three weeks. The client may shower or bathe in a clean tub.

Surgical Excision. Performed on an outpatient or inpatient basis, depending on the extent of disease and the location of lesions. Healing varies with the degree of trauma but generally takes two to three weeks for smaller lesions.

Interferon. Interferon is an antiviral agent thought to reduce human papillomavirus (HPV) lesions by improving the immune system. It is injected directly into anal lesions three times per week for one month. Useful for recalcitrant cases or immunosuppressed clients. This expensive treatment is available primarily in medical centers. Side effects include fever, flulike symptoms, and malaise (Ostrzenski, 2002).

5-Fluorouracil. 5 percent cream (Efudex).

- *Indications.* Used by specialists to treat widespread papillary vaginal lesions (not FDA approved for this indication). Flat, keratinized lesions in the vagina do not respond as well as do papillary lesions. It is a cytotoxic agent and not useful for external warts, because side effects are too severe. Because of variable response, treatment must be individualized to prevent chronic vaginal ulcerations.

◆ *Administration.* Treatment protocols vary widely. *Initial treatment:* Use 1/4 applicator inserted deep in the vagina daily at bedtime for one week, then weekly for ten weeks. May also be used twice weekly for ten weeks (Rajavel & Yuk-Kuen Kao, 2001). Monitor weekly for side effects.

◆ *Side Effects and Adverse Reactions.* Erosion of vaginal mucosa.

◆ *Contraindications.* Pregnancy: During pregnancy the drug is teratogenic. No systemic toxicity is usual.

◆ *Anticipated Outcomes on Evaluation.* Vaginal warts will disappear and the Pap smear return to normal. The client should be reevaluated in three months.

◆ *Client Teaching and Counseling.* Include information about inflammation, discharge, and local discomfort caused by 5-fluorouracil. Severe pain and burning are *not* usual. A vaginal tampon may be inserted after application to reduce irritation to other tissues. Effective contraception is essential since this medication is teratogenic (some clinicians will not use in patients who are capable of becoming pregnant).

Long-Term Follow-Up

Women with any history of HPV infection should be evaluated with biannual Pap smears for the first two years after treatment and annually thereafter (NIH, 1996). Self-examination of external genitalia is recommended on a regular basis.

MOLLUSCUM CONTAGIOSUM

This benign, viral, papular infection occurs on the abdomen, thighs, and genitals of adults and on the face, trunk, and extremities of children. Molluscum are common in persons infected with HIV and are difficult to eradicate in these persons. The infection is generally minor and self-limited. Another name for the condition is seed wart.

Epidemiology

Molluscum contagiosum virus (*MCV*), a member of the pox virus family, is the causative organism. In adults, transmission is primarily sexual; in children, it is nonsexual and via fomites. Autoinoculation may also occur. The incubation period ranges from one week to six months (two to three month average).

Subjective Data

The client is generally asymptomatic, and diagnosis is often made when treatment is sought for some other reason.

Objective Data

Physical Examination. A firm, smooth, waxy non-tender dome-shaped papule with a central umbilication is seen (may be single or multiple). Lesions contain a caseous material. Principal sites of involvement include face, upper thighs, lower abdomen, and genitals. In HIV-infected patients, the infection is often generalized (Wilson & Henry, 2001).

Diagnostic Tests and Methods. Diagnosis is made upon sight of a characteristic lesion. Biopsy reveals molluscum bodies.

Differential Medical Diagnoses

Genital warts, genital herpes, dermatologic folliculitis, lichen planus, basal cell epithelioma.

Plan

Psychosocial Interventions. Reassure the client that MCV is benign, self-limiting, and grows slowly. Clients with multiple or persistent lesions, however, should be questioned about risk factors for HIV. Many cases spontaneously resolve over a few months. Bacterial superinfection may require a systemic antibiotic, but such a condition is rare. Clients should avoid sharing razors. Advocate good handwashing.

Surgical Interventions. Unroofing the lesion with a fine gauge needle to remove the central core is effective and practical if there are only a few lesions. Multiple lesions have been successfully treated using cryotherapy with liquid nitrogen; direct destruction is achieved. Electrosurgery with a fine needle may be used.

PEDICULOSIS PUBIS

A species of human lice causes this common sexually transmitted disease. Another name for this condition is pubic lice or crabs. Body and head lice also occur in humans but do not infect the pubic area. Pubic lice, however, have been found in axillae, beards, eyebrows, and eyelashes.

Epidemiology

Phthirius pubis is the crab louse. It requires human blood to survive. Off the host, pubic lice will die within 24 hours. Transmission is through infected humans, clothing, or bedding (Liu & Shellow, 2000). The examination table and toilet used by the client will need to be washed with an appropriate disinfectant, or the rooms may be closed for the life span of the lice (24 hours) if this is feasible. Young adults (15 to 25 years old) have the highest incidence of pubic lice; prevalence declines after age 35.

Subjective Data

Itching is the primary symptom. It leads to scratching, erythema, and skin irritation. The client may be asymptomatic. The underwear of the client with pubic lice may be speckled with blood.

Objective Data

Physical Examination. Adult lice may be viewed moving along pubic hairs. Eggs (nits) appear as minute white dots adherent to pubic hair.

Diagnostic Tests and Methods. Characteristic lice and nits may be observed; microscopic examination confirms. Clients who report pubic lice do not need an office visit to confirm.

Differential Medical Diagnoses

If small white flakes are noted in the pubic hair, seborrheic dermatitis must be considered.

Plan

Psychosocial Interventions. Assist the client to deal with the anxiety and embarrassment that diagnosis causes. Tell her that pubic lice are usually curable and have no long-term consequences. In addition, advise her that contacts need to be checked and treated if they are infected. Clothing and household items require disinfection. Washable items may be laundered in hot water or dry cleaned. Non-washable items can be treated with products that contain pyrethrin (Black Flag or Raid). These products should be used only on inanimate objects.

Medication. A variety of prescription and over-the-counter medications are available. Ideally, medication should be lethal to both adult lice and eggs, however, there is some indication that head lice are developing resistance to usual treatments and this may be seen in the future with pubic lice.

Permethrin. 1 percent liquid (Nix).

- *Indications.* For treatment of pubic lice and eggs. This is an over-the-counter preparation.
- *Administration.* Application is as a shampoo or liquid. Manufacturer's directions for application must

be followed exactly. Repeat application is usually unnecessary but may be done seven to ten days after initial treatment if living lice are seen. Pregnancy category B.

- *Side Effects and Adverse Reactions.* Minimal but minor skin irritation may occur. Avoid contact with mucous membranes.
- *Contraindications.* Sensitivity to pyrethrin or chrysanthemum: for these individuals the solutions should be used with caution.
- *Anticipated Outcomes on Evaluation.* Destruction of pubic lice and eggs. Reexamination is needed one week after initial treatment to confirm positive outcome.
- *Client Teaching and Counseling.* Encourage the client to follow the directions exactly. Instruct her in the use of the fine-tooth comb usually provided with the medication; dead nits are combed out of the pubic hair.

Lindane. 1 percent (Kwell).

- *Indications.* This prescription solution is used in the treatment of pubic lice. It kills both adult lice and eggs. Should be reserved for second-line treatment due to potential neurotoxicity.
- *Administration.* Application is as a shampoo. Apply exactly according to the manufacturer's directions. One application is usually adequate, but the treatment may be repeated in seven days.
- *Side Effects and Adverse Reactions.* May include skin irritation, but it is usually minor. Lindane permeates human skin and has potential central nervous system (CNS) toxicity. Care must be taken to avoid contact with the eyes.
- *Contraindications.* Known seizure disorders and known sensitivity to lindane. Do not use during pregnancy and lactation or on infants/children.
- *Anticipated Outcomes on Evaluation.* The same as that achieved with the use of permethrins.

HEPATITIS B

Hepatitis B, or serum hepatitis, is a viral inflammation of the liver that results in a broad spectrum of disease from mild illness to chronic carrier state with possible cirrhosis, liver cancer, and death secondary to liver failure. Most infected persons never become jaundiced; their illness is mistaken for a nonspecific viral syndrome unless liver biochemical tests are ordered.

Women infected with hepatitis B may transmit the virus to their neonates at the time of delivery; the risk of chronic infection in the infant is as high as 100 percent (Drew, 2001). Testing for hepatitis B is indicated for persons who are jaundiced, who have elevated liver transaminases (ALT and AST), or who are sexual partners of a person diagnosed with hepatitis B. Persons with presumptive hepatitis B should also be tested for hepatitis A, hepatitis C, and hepatitis D. Hepatitis D is caused by a defective RNA virus that requires coinfection with hepatitis B. Further information about hepatitis A and C is beyond the scope of this chapter since their transmission is not primarily sexual (Drew, 2001).

Epidemiology

Hepatitis B virus (HBV) is the causative organism. Those at special risk include intravenous drug users, heterosexuals and homosexuals with multiple partners, sexual partners of HBV carriers, infants of HBV-infected mothers, health workers who have contact with blood, and people born in areas where HBV is endemic. Hepatitis B may occasionally be transmitted to household contacts. Hepatitis B may be transmitted parenterally, sexually, or perinatally. The incubation period ranges from four weeks to six months (average is ten weeks). One to 2 percent of persons with hepatitis B become chronic carriers, remain capable of transmitting the virus, and may progress to cirrhosis or liver failure.

Although up to 300,000 cases and 300 deaths due to fulminant disease have been reported each year in the United States (Drew, 2001), cases are expected to drop with routine immunization of health care workers and infants. The majority of current cases in the United States are adults.

Subjective Data

Many persons have asymptomatic infection and develop lifelong immunity. The symptoms, which may be mild or severe, include fatigue, loss of appetite, dark urine, light-colored bowel movements, nausea/vomiting, diarrhea, malaise, and myalgias. The onset of symptoms is usually gradual, and resolution is slow.

Objective Data

Physical Examination. Examination may reveal jaundice, low grade fever, or the only sign may be mild right upper quadrant pain.

Diagnostic Tests and Methods. Initial diagnostic workup for acute hepatitis should include a urinalysis (for bilirubin), a check of serum transaminases (ALT and AST), hepatitis B surface antigen (HBsAG), antibody to hepatitis B core antibody (Anti-HBc IgM), antibody to hepatitis A (Anti-HAV IgM), and antibody to hepatitis C (Anti-HCV). Antibody to hepatitis D (anti-HDV) should be measured in all persons diagnosed with acute hepatitis B. If hepatitis B is diagnosed, prothrombin time and serum albumin should be measured. The test procedure is to obtain a blood sample. Advise the client that blood testing is highly accurate and can determine active infection.

Differential Medical Diagnoses

Hepatitis A, C, and D.

Plan

Medical Management. Nonphenothiazine anti-emetics (such as Tigan suppositories 200 mg t.i.d.) should be used to control nausea and vomiting since phenothiazines may cause cholestatic jaundice. Clients should be followed weekly in the acute phase to monitor symptom management.

Prothrombin time, serum bilirubin, and aminotransferases should be rechecked weekly if there is suspicion of worsening. At three months, transaminases should be repeated along with serum bilirubin and prothrombin time. HBsAG should be rechecked to determine antigen status. If symptoms and laboratory evidence of activity persist after three months, evaluations should be repeated monthly. If antigen persists six months after acute infection, referral for liver biopsy should be considered (Dienstag, 2000).

Psychosocial Interventions. Advise the client that there is no specific treatment for hepatitis B. Rest and nutritious diet are important. Alcohol should be restricted, but oral contraceptives need not be stopped (Dienstag, 2000). Activity restrictions are based on how the individual feels. Sexual partners and household contacts should be vaccinated. In addition to vaccination, general counseling to prevent transmission of HBV includes information about using latex condoms, and not sharing needles, razors, or toothbrushes.

Medication

Hepatitis B Immune Globulin (HBIG)

- *Indications.* Sexual contacts of clients with acute HBV, those who have sexual contact with HBV carriers, nonimmunized health care workers with needlesticks from patients with hepatitis B, and newborns of mothers with HBV. HBIG should be followed by HBV immunization.

◆ *Administration.* Intramuscular injection, 0.06 mL/kg. In neonates, 0.5 cc I.M. at birth.
◆ *Side Effects and Adverse Reactions.* Minimal, local irritation at the injection site.
◆ *Contraindications.* None known.
◆ *Anticipated Outcomes on Evaluation.* Highly effective, immediate immunity, although temporary.
◆ *Client Teaching and Counseling.* HBIG should be given within fourteen days of HBV exposure. Three dose immunization with hepatitis B vaccine should follow.

Hepatitis B Vaccination

◆ *Indications.* Persons with multiple sexual partners, homosexual/bisexual men, illicit intravenous drug users, prison inmates and other institutionalized individuals, prostitutes, health care workers with exposure to blood products, infants of HBV-infected mothers, clients attending STD clinics, and household or sexual contacts of HBV carriers. Universal vaccination of newborns is now recommended (CDC, 2002).
◆ *Administration.* Requires three intramuscular injections: an initial injection, another one month later, and the third at six months. The deltoid muscle should be used. May give first dose concurrently with HBIG.
◆ *Side Effects and Adverse Reactions.* Minimal, local soreness at injection site.
◆ *Contraindications.* None.
◆ *Anticipated Outcomes on Evaluation.* Active immunity to HBV, lasting five years or longer. Postvaccination testing to confirm immunity is not routinely recommended.
◆ *Client Teaching and Counseling.* Educate the client that prevaccination HBV testing is recommended only for very high risk groups where the presence of HBV antibodies would negate the necessity of vaccination. The cost effectiveness of such testing in moderate risk groups must be considered. HBsAg positive individuals who receive the vaccine are unharmed.

REFERENCES

Baeten, J. M., Nyange, P. M., Richardson, B. A., Lavreys, L., Chohan, B., Martin, H. L., Mandaliya, K., Ndinya-Achola, J. O., Bwayo, J. J., & Kreiss, J. K. (2001). Hormonal contraception and risk of sexually transmitted disease acquisition: Results from a prospective study. *American Journal of Obstetrics and Gynecology, 185* (2), 380–385.

Bryant-Greenwood, P. (2002). Molecular diagnostics in obstetrics and gynecology. In S. B. Ransom, M. P. Dombrowski, M. I. Evans, & K. A. Ginsburg (Eds.), *Contemporary therapy in obstetrics and gynecology* (p. 276). Philadelphia: S. B. Saunders Company.

Carey, J. C., & Rayburn, W. F. (2002). Obstetrics and gynecology (p. 127; 4th ed.). Philadelphia: Lippincott Williams & Wilkins.

Centers for Disease Control and Prevention (CDC). (1999). Summaries of notifiable disease in the United States. *Morbidity and Mortality Weekly Report, 47* (53), 1–116.

Centers for Disease Control and Prevention (CDC). (2000). *Tracking the hidden epidemics: Trends on STDs in the United States 2000.* Atlanta, GA: U. S. Department of Health and Human Services, Centers for Disease Control and Prevention.

Centers for Disease Control and Prevention (CDC). (2001). *Sexually transmitted disease Surveillance, 2000.* Atlanta, GA: U.S. Department of Health and Human Services, Centers for Disease Control and Prevention.

Centers for Disease Control and Prevention (CDC). (2002a). General Recommendations on immunization: Recommendations of the advisory committee on immunization practices and the American Academy of Family Physicians. *MMWR, 51* (RR-2), 1–44.

Centers for Disease Control and Prevention (CDC). (2002b). Sexually transmitted disease guidelines 2002. *MMWR, 51* (RR-6), 1–76.

Chambers, H. F. (2001). Infectious diseases: Bacterial and chlamydial. In L. M. Tierney, S. J. McPhee, & M. A. Papadakis (Eds.), *Current medical diagnosis and treatment 2001.* New York: Lange Medical Books/McGraw Hill.

Davis, B., & Simon, H. B. (2000). Management of syphilis and other sexually transmitted diseases. In A. H. Gorroll & A. G. Mulley (Eds.), *Primary care medicine: Office evaluation and management of the adult patient.* Philadelphia: Williams & Wilkins.

Dienstag, J. L. (2000). Management of hepatitis. In A. H. Gorroll & A. G. Mulley (Eds.), *Primary care medicine (Eds.), Office evaluation and management of the adult patient.* Philadelphia: Williams & Wilkins.

Drew, W. L. (2001). Hepatitis. In W. R. Wilson & M. A. Sande (Eds.), *Current diagnosis and treatment in infectious diseases.* New York: Lange Medical Books/McGraw-Hill.

Emmert, D. H. (2000). Treatment of common cutaneous herpes simplex virus infections. *American Family Physician. 61,* 1697–1704.

Ferenczy, A. (1995). Epidemiology and clinical pathophysiology of condyloma acuminata. *American Journal of Obstetrics and Gynecology, 172* (4), 1331–1339.

Gilbert, D. N., Moellering, R. C., & Sande, M. (2001). *The San-ford guide to antimicrobial therapy* (31st ed.). Hyde Park, VT: Antimicrobial Therapy, Inc.

Gorroll, A. H. (2001a). Approach to the patient with a vaginal discharge. In A. H. Gorroll & A. G. Mulley (Eds.), *Primary care medicine: Office evaluation and management of the adult patient.* Baltimore: Lippincott Williams & Wilkins.

Gorroll, A. H. (2001b). Management of cutaneous and genital herpes simplex. In A. H. Gorroll & A. G. Mulley (Eds.), *Primary care medicine: Office evaluation and management of the adult patient.* Baltimore: Lippincott Williams & Wilkins.

Guaschino, S., & De Seta, F. (2000). Update on chlamydia tra-chomatis. *Annals of the New York Academy of Sciences, 900,* 293–300.

Guaschino, S., De Seta, F., Sartore, A., Ricci, G., De Santo, D., Piccoli, M., & Alberico, S. (2001). Efficacy of maintenance therapy with topical boric acid in comparison with oral itra-conazole in the treatment of recurrent vulvovaginal candidia-sis. *American Journal of Obstetrics and Gynecology, 184,* 598–602.

Hilliar, S. L. (2002). Implications of bacterial vaginosis in ob-stetrics. In S. B. Ransom, M. P. Dombrowski, M. I. Evans, & K. A. Ginsburg (Eds.), *Contemporary therapy in obstetrics and gynecology* (p. 18). Philadelphia: S. B. Saunders Com-pany.

Hilton, E., Isenberg, H., Alperstein, P., France, K., Borenstein, M., et al. (1992). Ingestion of yogurt containing lactobacillus acidophilus as prophylaxis for candidal vaginitis. *Annals of Internal Medicine, 116,* 353–357.

Ho, G. Y. F., Bierman, R., Beardsley, L., Chang, C. J., & Burk, R. D. (1999). Natural history of cervicovaginal papillo-mavirus infection in young women. *New England Journal of Medicine, 338* (7), 423–428.

Jacobs, R. A. (2001). Infectious diseases: Spirochetal. In L. M. Tierney, S. J. McPhee, & M. A. Papadakis (Eds.), *Current medical diagnosis and treatment 2001.* New York: Lange Medical Books/McGraw Hill.

Jacobson, G. F., Autry, A. M., Kirby, R. S., Liverman, E. M., & Motley, R. U. (2001). A randomized controlled trial compar-ing amoxicillin and azithromycin for the treatment of chlamy-dia trachomatis in pregnancy. *American Journal of Obstetrics and Gynecology, 184* (7), 1352–1354.

Koumans, E., & Kendrick, J. S. for the CDC Bacterial Vaginosis Working Group. (2001). Preventing adverse sequelae of bac-terial vaginosis: A public health program and research agenda. *Sexually Transmitted Diseases, 28* (5), 292–297.

Krieger, J. N. (1995). New sexually transmitted disease guide-lines. *The Journal of Urology, 154,* 209–213.

Liu, A. Y., & Shellow, W. V. R. (2000). Management of scabies and pediculosis. In A. H. Gorroll, & A. G. Mulley (Eds.), *Primary care medicine: Office evaluation and management of the adult patient.* Philadelphia: Williams & Wilkins.

Loeffelholz, M. J., Jirsa, S. J., Teske, R. K., & Woods, J. N. (2001). Effect of endocervical specimen adequacy on ligase chain reaction detection of chlamydia trachomatis. *Journal of Clinical Microbiology, 39* (11), 3838–41.

McKenzie, J. (2001). Sexually transmitted diseases. *Emergency Medicine Clinics of North America, 19* (3), 723–743.

Morris, R. T. (2002). Human papillomavirus and genital neopla-sia. In S. B. Ransom, M. P. Dombrowski, M. I. Evans, & K. A. Ginsburg (Eds.) *Contemporary therapy in obstetrics and gynecology.* (p. 481). Philadelphia: W. B. Saunders Company.

National Institute of Allergy and Infectious Diseases (NIAID) National Institutes of Health, Department of Health and Human Services. (2001). *Workshop summary: Scientific evi-dence on condom effectiveness for sexually transmitted dis-ease (STD) prevention.* Washington, DC: Author.

National Institutes of Health (1996). Consensus development conference statement: Cervical Cancer. Washinton, DC: Author.

Nisson, D. (Ed.) (2002). *2002 Mosby's drug consult.* St. Louis: Mosby. [Electronic version]. Retrieved 12/2/2002 from http://online.statref.com

Ostrzenski, A. (2002). *Gynecology integrating conventional, complementary, and natural alternative therapy.* New York: Lippincott Williams & Wilkins.

Potts, J. M., Ward, A. M., & Rackley, R. R. (2000). Association of chronic urinary symptoms in women and ureaplasma ure-alyticum. *Urology, 55,* 486–489.

Purwar, M., Ughade, S., Bhagat, B., Agarwal, V., & Kulkarni, H. (2001). Bacterial vaginosis in early pregnancy and adverse pregnancy outcome. *The Journal of Obstetrics and Gynaecol-ogy Research, 27* (4), 175–81.

Rajavel, S., & Yuk-Kuen Kao, R. (2001). Nephrology and urol-ogy. In M. A. Graber & M. L. Lanternier (Eds.), *The family practice handbook* (4th ed). St. Louis: Mosby.

Reid, G., Beuerman, D., Heinemann, C., & Bruce, A. W. (2001). Probiotic lactobacillus dose required to restore and maintain a normal vaginal flora. *FEMS Immunology and Medical Mi-crobiology, 32* (1), 37–41.

Reid, G., Bruce, A. W. Fraser, N., Heinemann, C., Owen, J., & Henning, B. (2001). Oral probiotics can resolve urogenital in-fections. *FEMS Immunology and Medical Microbiology, 30* (1), 49–52.

Rotchford, K., Strum, A. W., & Wilkinson, D. (2000). Effect of coinfection with STDs and of STD treatment on HIV shed-ding in genital-tract secretions: Systematic review and data synthesis. *Sexually Transmitted Diseases, 27* (5), 243–248.

Schaffer, S., Garzon, L., Heroux, D., & Korniewicz, D. (1996). *Infection prevention and safe practice.* St. Louis: Mosby, Inc.

Sendag, F. Terek, C., Tuncay, G., Ozkinay, E., & Guven, M. (2000). Single dose oral azithromycin versus seven day doxy-cycline in the treatment of non-gonococcal mucopurulent en-docervicitis. *The Australian & New Zealand Journal of Ob-stetrics and Gynecology 40,* 44–47.

Sonnex, C., & Lacey, C. J. N. (2001). The treatment of human papillomavirus lesions of the lower genital tract. *Best Practice & Research Clinical Obstetrics and Gynaecology, 15* (5), 801–116.

Weissman, A. (2001). Gynecology. In M. A. Graber & M. L. Lanternier (Eds.), *The family practice handbook* (p. 512; 4th ed.) St. Louis: Mosby.

Wilson, J. W., & Henry, N. K. (2001). Sexually transmitted diseases. In W. R. Wilson & M. A. Sande (2001). *Current diagnosis and treatment in infectious diseases.* New York: Lange Medical Books/McGraw-Hill.

CHAPTER 12

WOMEN AND HIV

Rachel Effolia Smith ◆ *Susan D. Schaffer*

The growing number of women living with HIV/AIDS is a dominant feature of the evolving epidemic.

Highlights

❖ INTRODUCTION

Acquired immunodeficiency syndrome (AIDS), first identified in 1981, is a viral infection caused by the human immunodeficiency virus (HIV). Although once inevitably fatal, HIV infection is now a highly treatable chronic infection with the advent of highly active antiretroviral therapy (HAART). The spectrum of HIV disease ranges from asymptomatic to full-blown infection (AIDS). Through a loss of cell-mediated immune function and the depletion of T4 lymphocytes, individuals who do not receive antiviral treatment progress from HIV infection to death in about eleven years (Bartlett & Gallant, 2001). The deterioration of the immune system confers susceptibility to rare opportunistic infections and malignant tumors. These phenomena, along with dementia and a wasting syndrome, signal the end stage of HIV infection (AIDS). HIV infection has a profound effect on women both as an illness and as a social and economic challenge. HIV affects women's caregiving role in the family; women must deal with their own life-threatening illness while they also deal with the impact of disease on their families. Women who become pregnant while HIV infected or who contemplate pregnancy while infected need information on risks to the fetus as well as information on caring for themselves. The stigma attached to HIV/AIDS can subject women to discrimination, job loss, social rejection, and other violations of their rights. Although primarily sexually transmitted, AIDS is covered in a separate chapter from other sexually transmitted infections because of the devastating effect HIV/AIDS has on infected women and their families and because of the complex psychosocial and medical management that is required to delay the effects and to promote a high quality of life in infected women.

Since there is no cure for HIV infection, primary prevention remains the most important strategy for primary care providers. Well-known measures that women can take to prevent acquisition of HIV include abstaining from intercourse, selecting low-risk partners, negotiating partner monogamy, and male/female condom use. However, the rising HIV incidence of women in the United States speaks to the prevention barriers women face in heterosexual relationships (Wang & Celum, 2001). Advances in the use of antiviral agents to prevent debilitating opportunistic infection highlight the importance of early diagnosis and treatment. Women with HIV require diagnostic evaluation, periodic physical examinations, monitoring of prognostic markers (CD4 counts and viral load tests), antiviral and prophylactic therapy, therapy for HIV-related complications and supportive counseling. As the disease progresses, women require assistance with pain control and durable power of attorney. Because of the complexity of initiating, maintaining, and adjusting HAART, only a practitioner with a specialty in HIV/AIDS should provide this type of service. Specialty care providers are physicians, nurse practitioners, and physician assistants who have been trained in initiating and monitoring antiretroviral therapy (Bartlett & Gallant, 2001). Strategies to combat HIV infection depend on understanding the epidemiology of the virus.

EPIDEMIOLOGY OF HIV

VIRAL LIFE CYCLE

T lymphocytes play a central part in the immune system by destroying infected cells and helping B cells make antibodies. T4 helper cells (CD4+ cells) are specialized T lymphocytes that do little to repel intruding substances themselves but instead become activated to alert B cells, killer cells, and phagocytes to the presence of a bacterial, fungal, or viral antigens. When the HIV virus is introduced into the bloodstream, the virus joins the host T4 cell's DNA and awaits activation of the cell. Only after the HIV infected T4 cells are activated by some non-HIV antigen do the T4 cells manufacture HIV viral RNA strands, replicating the virus and destroying themselves in the process. Over one billion virons are produced daily. With ongoing destruction and replacement of the T4 cells, the body gradually loses its ability to mount an immune response. It is difficult to eradicate the virus entirely because HIV hides out in places such as the brain, testes, lymph nodes, and retina that are poorly penetrated by drugs (NIAID/NIH, 2002).

INCIDENCE

As of December 2001, 40 million people are estimated to be living with HIV/AIDS worldwide, including 17.6 million women. In the United States, 800,000 to 900,000 people are currently estimated to be living with HIV, and 774,476 have AIDS (134,441 of these are women). Women of color are disproportionately affected by HIV. African American and Hispanic women represent approximately 25 percent of U.S. women and account for 77 percent of AIDS cases. Rates of infection are increasing in women of color (Native Americans, Hispanics, and African Americans) and in women over age 45. AIDS is the third leading cause of death among women 25 to 44 and the leading cause of death among African American women, partly due to difficulty accessing health care (NIAID/NIH, 2001). Race and ethnicity are not risk factors but serve as markers of socioeconomic status and access to medical care.

Unprotected heterosexual intercourse with an HIV-infected partner accounts for 40 percent of new HIV infection in women, and injection drug use accounts for 27 percent. Perinatally acquired HIV is among the ten leading causes of death in infants and young children. However, AZT prophylaxis and cesarean delivery have significantly decreased the rate of perinatal infection (CDC, 2001).

TRANSMISSION

Three main routes of HIV transmission have been documented: (1) sexual contact with infected body fluids; (2) contact with infected blood or blood products via transfusion, organ transplants, shared needles, or accidental needlestick injury (health care workers); and (3) transmission from an infected woman to her infant prenatally, at birth, or during breastfeeding. With 284 cases reported in 2000 compared to 1,098 in 1993, current use of antibody screening for donated blood has greatly diminished the risk of transfusion associated HIV transmission (CDC, 2001). Transmission via casual contacts, fomites, and insect bites does not occur. Transmission via artificial insemination is possible; however, current safeguards make this unlikely. Oral-genital contact is less risky than vaginal or anal sex; however, 8 percent of infected men in a recent study were apparently infected through this route. Gum infection and bleeding increases the risk of acquiring HIV through this route (CDC, 2002). Receptive anal intercourse is especially risky because traumatic lacerations of the delicate rectal mucosa provide direct bloodstream access for the HIV virus.

Women are at far greater risk of contracting HIV during heterosexual intercourse than are men. Semen has greater quantities of lymphocytes that may be infected than does vaginal fluid. Women have a larger mucosal surface area available for HIV penetration (vagina and cervix), but the only exposed mucosal surface in men is the urethra. Vaginal mucosa can suffer microscopic abrasions during intercourse, increasing susceptibility to HIV penetration.

RISK FACTORS

HIV infected individuals may be relatively asymptomatic or asymptomatic for ten years or longer (Greenblatt & Hessol, 2001). Diagnosis while asymptomatic provides optimal opportunities to slow disease progression. Testing for antibodies to HIV is an important first step in establishing a diagnosis. Based on studies documenting the efficacy of zidovudine (ZDV) therapy in reducing the perinatal transmission of HIV (USDHHS, 2002), the Centers for Disease Control and Prevention (CDC) has published guidelines urging routine counseling and voluntary testing for all pregnant women in the United States (Perinatal HIV Guidelines Working Group, 2002). Recommendations for testing of nonpregnant women should be based on risk behaviors and/or symptoms that include the following.

Risk Behaviors

Anal sexual activity, injection drug use, frequent casual unprotected intercourse, intercourse with commercial sex workers, previous treatment for sexually transmitted infections (human papilloma virus, herpes simplex, gonorrhea, syphilis, chlamydia), or sexual activity with partners having any of these characteristics (CDC, 2001).

Symptoms

Flu-like symptoms within one to two months after exposure, unexplained fever or weight loss, severe fatigue, recurrent vaginal candidiasis, oral thrush, pharyngitis, shingles, swollen glands, diarrhea, and other nonspecific but persistent symptoms (NIAID/NIH, 2001).

Signs

Signs that should alert practitioners to possible HIV infection include persistent or recurrent vaginal candidiasis, weight loss, lymphadenopathy, oral candidiasis or oral hairy leukoplakia of the tongue, skin lesions such as varicellazoster, psoriasis, seborrheic dermatitis or folliculitis. Persistent or recurrent genital herpes simplex infection, recurrent cervical neoplasia (despite treatment), and nonspecific genital ulcers may suggest HIV infection. Recurrent (nonpneumocystis) pneumonias, recurrent or particularly severe pelvic inflammatory disease (PID), and persistent urinary tract infections unresponsive to standard treatments may also be markers for early HIV infection. Hepatosplenomegaly and/or mental status changes may also be suspicious.

DIAGNOSTIC TESTING

Except for blood donors, newborns, and military personnel, HIV testing must be performed with voluntary informed consent. HIV antibody usually becomes detectable in the blood between one to three months after exposure. However, incubation periods up to six months are possible (NIAID/NIH, 2001). The enzyme linked immunosorbent assay (ELISA) test detects antibody to HIV antigens and is used as an initial screening test for HIV. The ELISA test is usually performed on venous blood obtained through venipuncture. As with all blood collection, gloves should be worn.

If the ELISA is positive, it is repeated by the reference lab before results are reported. People may test false positive for the ELISA if they have underlying liver disease, have received a blood transfusion or gamma globulin, have lymphoma, are injection drug users, or have received vaccines for influenza or hepatitis B. The confirmatory Western blot test, however, will almost always be negative in these cases. Combined ELISA and Western blot tests, if repeatedly run, have a better than 99 percent overall accuracy rate (Feinberg & Maenza, 2001).

ELISA and Western blot technologies are available for home testing. Home Access Express uses blood obtained with a lancet. Drops of blood are absorbed onto a pad before mailing to a laboratory. OraSure uses saliva obtained with a special absorbent pad. In-office screening tests are available that use urine or vaginal secretions. In-office screening tests should be confirmed with Western blot (Feinberg & Maenza, 2001).

In addition to these antibody tests, quantification of viral burden in persons known to be HIV infected can be performed by polymerase chain reaction (PCR), nucleic acid sequence-based amplification, or branched chain DNA signal amplification. These methods quantify single strands of HIV RNA in plasma.

PRE- AND POST-TEST COUNSELING

It is recommended that all women being tested for HIV receive extensive pretest counseling about viral transmission, implications for pregnancy, modes and prevention of transmission, personal risk, possibility of positive test results, and available support mechanisms. It is generally preferable for all HIV test results to be presented in person.

Persons testing negative for HIV can probably be reassured that they are virus free if it has been six months since their last possible exposure to HIV. Persons testing negative should be counseled about primary prevention strategies, however, and should be encouraged to have the test repeated if they have had more recent possible exposure.

Women testing positive for HIV require extensive counseling. Disclosure should consider social, cultural, and psychological characteristics of the person tested. Immediate interventions should include assessing the woman for the potential for violence to herself or others, ensuring access to a comprehensive medical evaluation, scheduling the next appointment, prevention of further HIV transmission, assessing the availability of key support persons, and providing information on local and national sources of support. Referral should be made for any services not available on site.

Later counseling should also include the natural history of HIV infection and available treatments. Disclosure of HIV status to sexual and needle-sharing partners by the woman should be encouraged so they can be tested. At the same time providers must be aware of the potential for domestic violence that may be triggered by this disclosure. Women should be advised that discrimination based on HIV status or AIDS regarding matters of employment, housing, state programs, or public accommodations is illegal. It should also be recommended that children born after acquisition of maternal infection be tested.

HIV-infected pregnant women should additionally be advised of the risk for perinatal HIV transmission (15 to 25 percent) ways to reduce this risk (including not breastfeeding), and the prognosis for infants who become infected. Breastfeeding increases risk by 16 percent with greatest risk in the first four to six months (Bartlett & Gallant, 2001). They should be given information concerning zidovudine (ZVD) therapy to reduce the risk for perinatal transmission. A three-part regimen of ZVD (orally from fourteen weeks gestation on, intravenously during labor, and to the newborn for the first six weeks of life) is recommended for all HIV-infected pregnant women (Perinatal HIV Guidelines Working Group, 2002). Information about ZVD treatment should include addressing the potential benefit and short-term safety of zidovudine and the uncertainties regarding risks of therapy and effectiveness. A woman's decision not to accept zidovudine treatment should not result in punitive action or denial of care.

INITIAL EVALUATION OF THE WOMAN WITH HIV

SUBJECTIVE DATA

The medical history for all HIV-infected women should include the following: sexual and drug use history and history of exposure to bacterial, viral, parasitic, and fungal infections such as tuberculosis, syphilis, herpes simplex and other STDs, or giardia lamblia. Immunization history should be determined as well as the presence of household pets (cat litter boxes transmit toxoplasmosis and reptiles transmit salmonella). A social history should include family system history, occupational history, socioeconomic needs (insurance, disability benefits, etc.), and psychiatric history (medications and potential for suicide).

OBJECTIVE DATA

A complete physical examination should be done, including weight and nutritional status, blood pressure and temperature, oral cavity and tongue, skin and nails (lesions and clubbing), fundoscopic exam (for exudates associated with CMV retinitis), ears, nose, and sinuses, neurological status (including mental status, cranial nerves, reflexes, gait, and fine motor skills), lymph nodes, heart and lungs, extremities (muscle mass, myositis), and abdominal exam (hepatomegaly, splenomegaly, or tenderness). A breast exam and complete vaginal and perirectal exam should also be done (Feinberg & Maenza, 2001).

Recommended baseline labs include a CD4+ lymphocyte and percentage panel, viral load assay, CBC with differential and platelets, *Toxoplasma gondii* IgG chemistry panel including liver function, lipid profile, serology for syphilis, hepatitis screen (for A, B, and C), and PPD. Simultaneous administration of additional antigens is not recommended. Some authorities recommend PPD retesting following immune reconstitution. (Bartlett & Gallant, 2002). A Pap smear, specimens for gonorrhea and chlamydia, and wet mounts for bacterial vaginosis, trichomonas, white blood cells, and Candida should be obtained at baseline.

MANAGEMENT OF EARLY HIV INFECTION

It has been demonstrated that HIV-infected persons who are followed in a comprehensive program of care survive longer than those who present for care only according to their symptoms. The establishment of trust in a nonjudgmental care provider and sufficient time to express concerns are crucial. Specialty care providers for HIV-infected women should refer them for comprehensive case management services if they are unable to provide such services. Advance directives regarding life-sustaining treatments, durable power of attorney for health care, and guardianship of dependent children should be addressed.

The CD4 cell count is a standard test to stage HIV, determine immune reconstitution, and make decisions regarding antiviral treatment and prophylaxis for opportunistic infections. Viral load is a better predictor of the progression of the disease and the therapeutic effectiveness of antiviral therapy. Current guidelines for HAART should be closely followed and readjusted according to CD4+ T cells and viral load testing (Bartlett & Gallant, 2001).

Women with asymptomatic HIV infection should be followed by a specialty care provider every three to six months as long as their CD4+ counts remain normal. In addition to measuring CD4+ counts and viral load, each visit should include monitoring for mental disorders, alcohol and drug abuse, measurement of weight and temperature, neurological status (including mental status and mood), abdominal examination, assessment of lymph nodes, and assessment of skin, oral cavity, and retina for characteristic lesions. Rescreening for sexually transmitted infection should be based on individual risk assessments. Additional strategies for ongoing care of HIV-infected women follow.

SELF-CARE STRATEGIES

Management of early HIV infection requires extensive teaching in health maintenance and in the avoidance of infectious disease risks. Latex condoms (or latex dental dams) should be encouraged for all vaginal, oral, and anal intercourse for the protection of HIV-infected persons and their partners (SIECUS, 1998). Smoking cessation decreases the risk of oral candidiasis, hairy leukoplakia, and bacteria pneumonia. Women who are abusing drugs or alcohol should be referred to treatment programs. HIV-infected persons experience several unique oral conditions, including frequent oral lesions and rapidly progressive periodontal disease, and should receive twice yearly dental prophylaxis.

HIV-infected persons should avoid pet reptiles who may carry salmonella; they should avoid young animals with diarrhea who may carry enteric pathogens, and they should avoid contact with cat feces that may be infected with *Toxoplasma gondii*. Since *Toxoplasma* may be present in soil, hands should be washed after gardening, and raw fruits and vegetables should be washed before eating. Poultry and meats should be well cooked (> 165 degrees), and uncooked meats should not come into contact with foods that will be eaten raw (CDC, 2002).

HIV-infected persons should be counseled about avoidance of *Cryptosporidium* (transmitted through contact with stools of infected adults and diaper-age children), infected animals, contaminated drinking water, contaminated lake and river water, and uncooked or unwashed foods. Using drinking water purified through reverse osmosis or through distillation may be considered by HIV-infected persons whose municipal water supply is known to be contaminated by *Cryptosporidium.*

IMMUNIZATIONS

The Advisory Committee on Immunizations Practices (ACIP) recommends that no live vaccines be given, with the exception of MMR. However, persons who are severely immunosuppressed should not receive MMR. Inactivated polio vaccine (IPV), pneumococcal, and influenza vaccines should be administered. Pneumococcal vaccine should be readministered every five years and influenza yearly (Atkinson et al., 2002).

GYNECOLOGIC CARE

Cervical dysplasia, vaginal candidiasis, and pelvic inflammatory disease are more common in HIV-infected women and tend to follow more aggressive courses. In the presence of HIV infection, 30 to 60 percent of Pap smears will have cytologic abnormalities and 15 to 40 percent will have evidence of dysplasia. These rates are ten times higher than those observed in HIV-negative women (Maimon, 1998). Women presenting with CIN II and III who are severely immunosuppressed improve to CIN I after undetectable viral loads with HAART are

achieved. Referral for colposcopy and biopsy is recommended for HIV-infected women with atypia or any grade of CIN (Bartlett & Gallant, 2001). Colposcopic evaluation should include the anal canal. Standard excisional or ablative treatment is recommended, although HIV-infected women have a high rate of recurrence (50%). Cryotherapy has the highest recurrence rate and should be avoided if other methods are available (Abularach & Anderson, 2001).

Vaginal candidiasis, although not life threatening, is not a trivial condition in HIV-infected women. Severe pruritus and excoriation can be disabling. Extension of candida to vulvae and thighs is common. Symptoms can often be controlled with topical antifungals, which may be more effective if used for seven days (Abularach & Anderson, 2001). Single-dose Fluconazole 150 mg may be used. Recurrent candidiasis may require maintenance therapy: Fluconazole 100 to 200 mg daily for ten to fourteen days followed by 100 to 200 mg weekly or ketaconazole 100 mg p.o. daily. These regimens should be continued for at least six months. Liver functions should be monitored (Abularach & Anderson, 2001).

Although the bacteriology remains the same, PID is more common in HIV-infected women and is often more severe. Accordingly, inpatient management should be considered. (Abularach & Anderson, 2001).

Genital herpes simplex infections occur more frequently, tend to be more severe, and are more likely to disseminate in immunocompromised hosts. Because of the risk of progressive disease, all herpes simplex should be treated with acyclovir 400 mg, five times a day for seven to ten days, or Famciclovir 200 mg t.i.d. for seven to ten days or valacyclovir 1 gm b.i.d. for seven to ten days (Abularach & Anderson, 2001). Daily suppressive therapy reduces the frequency of recurrences by 75 percent or more in patients who suffer from frequent HSV recurrences (Abularach & Anderson, 2001) (see STD chapter for dosing). Acyclovir-resistant HSV has been demonstrated with low CD4 counts and long-term acyclovir use. Most of these strains are susceptible to foscarnet or cidofovir topical gel (CDC, 1998).

CONTRACEPTION

For HIV positive women, serostatus is one of many factors that influence reproductive decision making. Providers should advise about relative risks and therapeutic options and dangers and refrain from directive counseling where moral judgment is involved. The decision to initiate a pregnancy or to continue a pregnancy must remain a choice of the woman and her partner. The message conveyed to women must be that contraception and protection against STDs are separate issues. Properly and consistently used male and female condoms are the only means to prevent STDs, including HIV (Abularach & Anderson, 2001). Condoms are helpful in protecting uninfected partners and also protect HIV infected women from increased HIV viral load and new viral strains from HIV-positive partners. Polyurethane male condoms or polyurethane female condoms may be recommended for persons who are allergic to latex as laboratory evidence has documented their impermeability to HIV. (Wang & Celum, 2001).

Vaginal spermicides (nonoxynol-9) used with latex condoms enhance prevention of pregnancy as well as STDs such as gonorrhea and chlamydia. However, nonoxynol-9 has been shown to increase the transmission of HIV, possibly due to local irritative effects and ulceration of vaginal mucosa (Wang & Celum, 2001). The use of spermicides alone should be discouraged in women with HIV, and risks of spermicide use with condoms should be discussed.

Hormonal contraceptives are highly effective and should not be denied to women who wish to use them. However, multiple studies report that the use of oral contraceptives and Depo-provera may be associated with a small increased risk of HIV transmission and transmissibility (Baeton et al., 2001; Martin et al., 1998; Wang, 1999). Contraceptive levels may increase or decrease when given in conjunction with protease inhibitors, such as Norvir (ritonavir) and Viracept (nelfinavir), and, thus may be less effective.

Intrauterine devices are not recommended for use in HIV-positive women, since an impaired immune response and increased PID risk are strong relative contraindications (Wang & Celum, 2001). Diaphragms and cervical caps have been associated with microabrasions, and they leave most of the woman's vaginal vault unprotected. They also require use of vaginal spermicides such as nonoxynol-9. These problems make these methods less desirable for HIV-infected women; they should be used only when no other contraceptive option is available.

M. TUBERCULOSIS PREVENTION

Since immunosuppression caused by HIV can cause rapid progression of M. tuberculosis infection to an active state, PPD-positive persons with negative x-rays should receive isoniazid (INH) therapy, usually 300 mg. p.o. daily for nine months. See www.hivatis.org for alternative medications. The addition of 50 mg of pyroxidine (B6) p.o. daily will prevent peripheral neuritis. Since INH is hepatotoxic, persons taking it should be monitored monthly for the development of adverse effects such as nausea, anorexia, fever, rash, visual problems, or jaundice. Monthly hepatic enzymes should be monitored in those over age 35. INH should be avoided in pregnant women (preventive therapy should be deferred until after delivery). A PPD reaction of 5 mm or greater is considered positive in a person with HIV infection (Bartlett & Gallant, 2002). Women should be assessed for health and social conditions (alcoholism, mental illness, or failure to keep appointments) that may affect their ability to complete a course of INH treatment. Case management and directly observed therapy should be used when needed to ensure successful completion of INH treatment (CDC, 1998).

Women presenting with weight loss, hemoptysis, night sweats, or fever should receive an immediate chest x-ray and a sputum smear should be examined. Those who are coughing with symptoms of TB should be placed on respiratory isolation until active TB has been ruled out. Active tuberculosis or infection with possibly drug-resistant organisms should be managed by an infectious disease specialist.

MONITORING IMMUNE STATUS

The assessment of immune status is a key element in the ongoing management of early HIV infection. Measurement of plasma viral load should be used with physical findings and CD4+ cell counts to stage patients and to determine appropriate time for initiating antiretroviral therapy and prophylaxis for P. carinii pneumonia and other opportunistic infections. CD4+ cells and viral load should be measured every six months when the count is greater than 500, and every three months when the CD4+ count is between 200 and 500 cells per microliter (500 to $1400/mm^3$ is normal). If symptomatic and CD4+ is greater than 500, test every six months. If antiviral therapy is readjusted, the CD4+ and viral load should be rechecked in two to four weeks (Bartlett & Gallant, 2002).

MANAGEMENT OF LATE HIV INFECTION (AIDS)

HIV infection is termed AIDS with a CD4+ count of less than $200/mm^3$ (14% lymphocytes) or one or more of the conditions in the 1993 Expanded Surveillance Case Definition for AIDS (See Table 12–1).

TABLE 12–1. 1993 Expanded Surveillance Case Definition for AIDS

HIV Seropositivity *and* CD4+ Count < 200/mm³ *or*
One or More of the Following Conditions:

Candidiasis of bronchi, trachea, esophagus, or lungs, invasive cervical cancer, extrapulmonary coccidioidomycosis (disseminated or extrapulmonary), cryptococcosis, cryptosporidiosis, cytomegalovirus (CMV) disease (other than spleen, liver, and nodes), or CMV retinitis, encephalopathy, herpes simplex virus (chronic ulcers, esophagitis, or bronchitis), histoplasmosis, isosporiasis, Kaposi's sarcoma, lymphoma (Burkitt's, immunoblastic, or primary), mycobacterium tuberculosis (any site) *Mycobacterium avium* complex, *Mycoplasma kansasii* or other species (disseminated or extrapulmonary). *Pneumocystis carinii* pneumonia, any recurrent pneumonia, progressive multifocal leukoencephalopathy, salmonella septicemia (recurrent), toxoplasmosis of brain, or wasting syndrome due to HIV.

Source: Centers for Disease Control (1993). Revised classification system for HIV infection and expanded surveillance case definition for AIDS among adolescents and adults. MMWR 41, 1–19.

Although recurrent vaginal candidiasis, pulmonary tuberculosis, bacterial pneumonia, and persistent generalized lymphadenopathy may occur during early HIV infection, most of the conditions associated with AIDS occur when the CD4+ count falls below 500 cells per microliter according to the CDC (USDHHS, 2002). The distinction between HIV infection and AIDS is important for reporting purposes in some states (see Table 12–2). Persons with AIDS should be managed in conjunction with an infectious disease specialist and may also require referral to oncology or other subspecialty care.

HIGHLY ACTIVE ANTIRETROVIRAL THERAPY (HAART)

The goal of antiretroviral therapy is to maximize suppression of viral load, restore and preserve the immune system (CD4 count), improve the quality of life, and reduce HIV-related morbidity and mortality (USDHHS, 2002).

TABLE 12–2. Reporting Requirements for HIV Infection

By Name	Alabama, Alaska, Arizona, Arkansas, Colorado, Florida, Idaho, Indiana, Iowa, Kansas, Louisiana, Michigan, Minnesota, Mississippi, Missouri, Nebraska, Nevada, New Jersey, New Mexico, New York, North Dakota, North Carolina, Ohio, Oklahoma, South Carolina, South Dakota, Tennessee, Texas, Utah, Virginia, West Virginia, Wisconsin, Wyoming, Virgin Islands
By Unique Identifier	Illinois, Maryland, Massachusetts, Vermont, Puerto Rico
Other	Connecticut, Georgia, Kentucky, Maine, Montana, New Hampshire, Oregon, Rhode Island, Washington

All states require reporting of AIDS cases by name at the state/local level.

Source: Watson & Wasserman (2000).

Antiretroviral drugs do not cure HIV or prevent transmission of HIV. The time for initiating HAART is controversial, but depends on symptoms, cell counts, and patient readiness to adopt a difficult regimen. (USDHHS, 2002). For clients with CD4+ cells above 350 cells/mm³, the risk and toxicities may outweigh the benefits (USDHHS, 2002).

In general, treatment should be offered to all persons with symptoms ascribed to HIV infection, to those with fewer than 350 CD4+ T cells/mm³ and to those with plasma HIV RNA levels exceeding 55,000 copies/ml. Waiting to start antiretroviral therapy until the CD4+ count drops to 200 is a conservative approach that recognizes that immune reconstitution still occurs in patients with CD4+ cell counts in 200 to 350 cells/mm³ range and a viral load of over 30,000 HIV RNA. Delaying treatment minimizes treatment-related drug toxicities and effects of a difficult regimen on quality of life. Delaying treatment may preserve treatment options and delay drug resistance. However, treatment delay risks the possibility that damage to the immune system will be irreversible and suppression of viral replication may be more difficult at a later stage of disease (USDHHS, 2002). Potential benefits of early treatment include preservation of immune function, prolonged disease-free survival, and decrease in viral transmission risk. However, antiretroviral drugs have significant toxicities, complex regimens decrease quality of life, development of drug resistance occurs because of suboptimal adherence, and the durability of effect of current drugs is unknown (USDHHS, 2002).

A high level of adherence is necessary for optimal success of HAART, requiring client understanding and commitment to the treatment plan. Clinicians should inform clients in advance about potential side effects, provide them with treatment for expected side effects, and inform them when to contact the clinician. Daily or weekly pillboxes, timers, pagers, and other devices may be useful along with discussion of compliance at each client encounter (USDHHS, 2002). Results of HAART are evaluated primarily with plasma HIV RNA levels and CD4 cell count (USDHHS, 2002).

There are currently three classifications of antiviral therapy drugs. These are nucleoside reverse transcriptase inhibitors (NRTIs), protease inhibitors (PIs), and non-nucleoside reverse transcriptase inhibitors (NNRTIs) that work on different sites of the virus cell cycle (Table 12–3). Current HAART recommendations are for three to four different drugs to be initiated simultaneously from different classes. Monotherapy should not be used since it rapidly leads to drug resistance. Updated HIV drug man-

TABLE 12–3. Antiretroviral Agents by Class (trade name bolded)

Nucleoside Reverse Transcriptase Inhibitors (NRTIs)	Non-Nucleoside Reverse Transcriptase Inhibitors (NNRTIs)	Protease Inhibitors (PIs)
zidovudine (AZT) **Retrovir**	nevirapine **Viramune**	Indinavir **Crixivan**
didanosine (ddI) **Videx**	delavirdine **Rescriptor**	ritonavir **Norvir**
zalcitabind (ddC) **HIVID**	efavirenz **Sustiva**	nelfinavir **Viracept**
tenofovir disoproxil		saquinavir **Invirase,**
fumerate **Viread**		**Fortovase**
stavudine (d4T) **Epivir**		amprenavir **Agenerase**
abacavir (ABC) **Ziagen**		lopinavir/ritonavir **Kaletra**

agement strategies are provided on the web site maintained by the Panel on Clinical Practices for Treatment of HIV infection convened by the Department of Health and Human Services (DHHS) and the Henry J. Kaiser Family Foundation (*http://www.hivatis.org*). Since developing drug regimens should be left to HIV specialists, drug choices are not discussed further. However, major side effects, adverse reactions, and drug interactions (Table 12–4) are presented for clinicians who provide primary care for women with HIV.

Long-Term HAART-Associated Complications

Changes in body fat distribution (central obesity, peripheral fat wasting, breast enlargement, facial thinning, and dorsocervical fat accumulation) occur in 6 to 80 percent of persons receiving HAART, particularly with PIs and NRTIs. Hyperlipidemia and insulin resistance occur in up to 17 percent and are frequently associated with this lipodystrophy. The effects of lifestyle in reversing these changes is not clear, but exercise and weight maintenance should be encouraged. Concurrent use of statin drugs with PIs must be undertaken with caution, due to the potential for enhanced statin toxicity (see Table 12–5). Oral hypoglycemic agents or insulin may be needed (USD-HHS, 2002).

Potentially severe adverse drug reactions include hypersensitivity reaction (abacavir), severe skin reactions (nevirapine), peripheral neuropathy (zalcitabine), bone marrow suppression, anemia, and neutropenia (zidovudine). Hepatotoxicity (a three- to fivefold elevation in serum transaminases) has been associated with all of the NNRTIs and with PIs. Co-infection with hepatitis C, hepatitis B, alcohol abuse, and other use of other hepatotoxic drugs increases this risk. Close monitoring of clinical symptoms and liver enzymes is required. Although rare, lactic acidosis/hepatic steatosis has been demonstrated with NRTIs and is related to the effect of these drugs on mitochondrial DNA. Risk factors for this adverse effect include female gender, obesity, and prolonged use of NRTIs. Clinical presentation is diarrhea, abdominal pain, vomiting weight loss, dyspnea, respiratory failure, tachypnea, and elevated liver enzymes. Other manifestations of drug-related mitochondrial dysfunction may include pancreatitis, peripheral neuropathy, myopathy, and cardiomyopathy.

Decreased bone density has been demonstrated with more potent antiretroviral therapy. Skin rash is common

TABLE 12–4. Drugs That Should Not Be Used with PI Antiretrovirals

Drug Category	Indinavir	Ritonavir	Saquinavir	Nelfinavir	Aprenavir	Lopinavir + Ritonavir
Ca++channel blocker	(none)	bepridil	(none)	(none)	bepridil	(none)
Cardiac	(none)	amiodarone flecainide propafenone quinidine	(none)	(none)	(none)	flecainide propafenone
Lipid lowering	simvastatin lovastatin	simvastatin lovastatin	simvastatin lovastatin	simvastatin lovastatin	simvastatin lovastatin	simvastatin lovastatin
Anti-mycobacterial	rifampin	(none)	rifampin rifabutin	rifampin	rifampin	rifampin
GI	cisapride	cisapride	cisapride	cisapride	cisapride	cisapride
Neuroleptic	(none)	clozapine pimozide	(none)	(none)	(none)	pimozide
Psychotropic	midazolam triazolam	midazolam triazolam	midazolam triazolam	midazolam triazolam	midazolam triazolam	midazolam triazolam
Ergot alkaloid	all	all	all	all	all	all
Herbs	St. John's wort	St. John's wort	St. John's wort	St. John's wort	St. John's wort	St. John's wort

TABLE 12–5. Drugs That Should Not Be Used with NNRTI Antiretrovirals

Drug Category	Nevirapine	Delavirdine	Efaviren
Ca++channel blocker	(none)	(none)	(none)
Cardiac	(none)	(none)	(none)
Lipid lowering	(none)	simvastatin lovastatin	(none)
Anti-mycobacterial	(none)	rifampin rifabutin	(none)
GI	(none)	cisapride H-2 blockers proton pump inhibitors	cisapride
Neuroleptic	(none)	(none)	(none)
Psychotropic	(none)	midazolam triazolam	midazolam triazolam
Ergot alkaloid	(none)	all	All

Suggested alternatives

simvastatin, lovastatin: atorvastatin, pravastatin, fluvastatin, cerivastatin
rifabutin: clarithromycin, azithromycin, clarithromycin, ethambutol
midazolam, triazolam: temazepam, lorazepam

Source: Adapted from USDDHS, 2002.

with NNRTIs and is seven times more frequent in women (USDHHS, 2002).

FUSION INHIBITORS: A NEW DRUG APPROACH

The FDA has approved Fuzeon (enfuvirtide), a fusion inhibitor medication (FDA, 2003). This drug, which acts by inhibiting viral and cellular membrane fusion, thus interfering with HIV-1 entry into cells, is for use with other anti-HIV medications for advanced HIV-1 infection. A randomized phase 3 study of enfuvirtide found significant antiretroviral and immunologic benefit after 24 weeks of therapy in HIV-1 subjects randomized to the therapy plus three to five antiretroviral drugs or to the antiretroviral drugs alone (Lalezari, Henry, O'Hearn, et al., 2003). This new class of anti-HIV drug offers an additional hope for patients with advanced HIV.

PREVENTING OPPORTUNISTIC INFECTIONS

Life-threatening infection with pathogens that pose little threat to persons with normal immune systems is characteristic of full-blown AIDS. These infections become more evident when the CD4 count drops below 200. Although HAART is effective in preserving and even restoring CD4 cells, some persons are unable or unready to

take HAART, some initiate HAART with CD4 counts below 200, and others have failed antiretroviral treatment. For these persons, medication to prevent opportunistic infections (OIs) remains appropriate. In persons who demonstrate CD4 cell rebound after starting HAART, it may be appropriate to discontinue OI prophylaxis (USPHS/IDSA, 2001).

Pneumocystis Carinii Prophylaxis

Pneumocystis carinii pneumonia (PCP) is the most common opportunistic infection in persons with AIDS. Prophylaxis with the preferred agent trimethoprim/sulfamethoxazole (TMP/SMX), one double strength tablet daily or three times a week, not only prevents this common infection but also prolongs life (USPHS/IDSA, 2001). PCP prophylaxis is recommended for adults and adolescents with a CD4+ count below 200 mm/l^3, a prior episode of PCP, oral candidiasis, or unexplained fever lasting two weeks or more. Because of the importance of TMP/SMX, attempts should be made to continue it even in those who develop the fever and skin rash typical of an allergic reaction, although care must be taken to ensure that life-threatening allergic symptoms do not develop. Women can be referred to an allergist for desensitization, or the dose may be reduced to a daily single strength tablet or a double strength tablet three times a week.

For those unable to tolerate TMP/SMX, Dapsone 50 mg p.o. b.i.d. or 100 mg q.d., or Dapsone 50 mg q.d. plus pyrimethamine 50 mg p.o. weekly, plus leucovorin 25 mg p.o. weekly may be used (USPHS/IDSA, 2001). When TMP/SMX is used, it is necessary to monitor for anemia, neutropenia, and agranulocytosis. Severe dermatologic reactions such as Stevens-Johnson syndrome, erythema nodosum, erythema multiforme, or epidermal necrolysis are possible with TMX/SMX and Dapsone. Agents recommended for prevention of PCP will also prevent toxoplasmosis encephalitis in persons who have a positive titer (USPHS/IDSA, 2001).

When the CD4+ T cell count rises above 200 and has remained stable for three months, prophylaxis maybe discontinued. If prior pneumonia, history of thrush, or wasting syndrome are present, prophylaxis should be continuous (Bartlett & Gallant, 2001).

Mycobacterium Avium Complex

Mycobacterium avium complex (MAC) typically occurs at CD4+ counts below 50/mm^3. Drugs for disseminated MAC prophylaxis are generally started at CD4+ counts of 75 for those with previous infections and at CD4+ counts of less than 50 to 100 for those without previous infections. Prophylaxis for MAC includes clarithromycin 500 mg b.i.d. or azithromycin 1200 mg weekly (Bartlett & Gallant, 2001). Prophylaxis therapy can be discontinued if the CD4+ T cell count remains elevated above 100/mm^3 for three months. However, persons with a prior episode of disseminated MAC should receive prophylaxis indefinitely (USPHS/IDSA, 2001).

Cytomegalovirus Infection

Cytomegalovirus (CMV) retinitis is a common opportunistic infection associated with visual loss in HIV-infected persons. Ganciclovir may be used to delay onset of CMV disease in those with CD4+ counts less than 50. Those with visual symptoms suggestive of CMV retinitis should be referred to an opthamologist for confirmation of diagnosis (USPHS/IDSA, 2001).

REFERENCES

Abularach, S. & Anderson, J. (2001). Gynecologic problems. In R. Anderson (Ed.), *A guide to the clinical care of women with HIV.* [Electronic version]. Washington DC: U.S. Department of Health and Human Services, HIV/AIDS Bureau. Retrieved 12/12/02 from http:/hab.hrsa.gov/publications/womencare.htm

Atkinson, W. L., Pickering, L. K., Schwartz, B., Wenigar, B. G., Iskander, J. K., & Watson, J. C. (2002). General recommendations on immunization: Recommendations of the Advisory Committee on Immunization Practices (ACIP) and the American Academy of Family Physicians (AAFP). *MMWR, 51* (RR-2), 1–36.

Baeton, J. M., Nyange, P. M., Richardson, B. A., Laureys, L., Chohan, B., Martin, H. L., Jr., Mandalya, K., Ndinya-Achola, J. O., Buayo, J. J., & Kreiss, J. K. (2001). Hormonal contraception and risk of sexually transmitted disease acquisition: Results from a prospective study. *American Journal of Obstetrics and Gynecology, 85* (2), 380–385.

Bartlett, J. G., & Gallant, J. E. (2002). The 2002 abbreviated guide to *Medical management of HIV infection.* [Electronic version] Johns Hopkins University School of Medicine. Retrieved 12/12/02 from http://hopkins-aids.edu/publications/abbrevad.html

Centers for Disease Control and Prevention (CDC). (1998). 1998 guidelines for treatment of sexually transmitted diseases. *MMWR, 47* (RR-1), 24.

Centers for Disease Control and Prevention (CDC). (2001). HIV and AIDS—United States, 1981–2000. *MMWR, 50* (21), 430–434.

Centers for Disease Control (CDC), National Center for HIV, STD and TB Prevention: Division of HIV/AIDS Prevention. (2002). *Primary HIV infection associated with oral transmission.* [Brochure, electronic version]. Retrieved March 30, 2002, from http://www.cdc.gov/hiv/pubs/facts/oralsexqa.htm

Feinberg, J., & Maenza, J. (2001). Primary medical care. In R. Anderson, (Ed.), *A guide to the clinical care of women with HIV.* [Electronic version]. Washington DC: U.S. Department of Health and Human Services, HIV/AIDS Bureau. http://hab.hrsa.gov/publications/womencare.htm

Greenblatt, R. M., & Hessol, N. A. (2001). Epidemiology and natural history of HIV infection in women. In R. Anderson (Ed.), *A guide to the clinical care of women with HIV.* Washington, DC: U.S. Department of Health and Human Services, HIV/AIDS Bureau. Retrieved April 26, 2002 from http://hab.hrsa.gov/publications/womencare.htm

Lalezari, J., Henry, K., O'Hearn, M., Montaner, J., et al. (2003). Enfuvirtide, an HIV-1 fusion inhibitor, for drug resistant HIV infection in North and South America. *New England Journal of Medicine.* (Original article retrieved March 19, 2003 from *www.nejm.org*).

Maimon, M. (1998). Management of cervical dysplasia in human immunodeficiency-infected women. *Journal of the National Cancer Institute Monograph, 23,* 954–961.

Martin, H. L., Nyange, P. M., Richardson, B. A., Laureys, L., Mandalya, K., Jackson, D. J., Ndinya-Achola, J. O., & Kreiss, J. (1998). Hormonal contraception, sexually transmitted diseases, and risk of heterosexual transmission of human immunodeficiency virus type 1. *Journal of Infectious Diseases, 178,* 1053–1059.

National Institutes of Allergy and Infectious Disease and National Institutes of Health (NIAID/NIH). (2001). *HIV infection in women.* Bethesda, MD: U.S. Department of Health & Human Services. Retrieved April 24, 2002 from www.niaid.nih.gov/factsheets/womenhiv.htm

National Institutes of Allergy and Infectious Disease and National Institutes of Health (NIAID/NIH). (2002). *HIV infection and AIDS, an overview.* Bethesda, MD: U.S. Department of Health & Human Services. Retrieved 12/12/02 from www.niaid.nih.gov/factsheets/hivinf.htm

Perinatal HIV Guidelines Working Group. (2002). *Recommendations for use of antiretroviral drugs in pregnant HIV-1-infected women for maternal health and interventions to reduce perinatal HIV-1 transmission in the United States.* Public Health Services Task Force. Retrieved April 16, 2002 from www.hivatis.org

Sexuality Information and Educational Council of the United States (SIECUS). (1998) The truth about condoms. *SIECUS Report, 27* (1). Retrieved March 30, 2002 from http://www.siecus.org/pubs/fact/fact0011.html

U.S. Department of Health and Human Services (USDHHS) and Henry J. Kaiser Family Foundation Panel on Clinical Practices for Treatment of HIV Infection. (2002). *Guidelines for the use of antiretroviral drugs in HIV-infected adults and adolescents.* Retrieved March 16, 2002, from www.hivatis.org.

U.S. Food and Drug Administration (FDA). (March 13, 2003). FDA approves first drug in new class of HIV treatments for HIV treatments for HIV-infected adults and children with advanced disease. *FDA News,* 1, 2. Retrieved March 19, 2003 from http://www.fda.gov/bbs/topics/NEWS/2003/NEWoo879 .html

U.S. Public Health Service and Infectious Diseases Society of America (USPHS & IDSA). (2001). *2001 USPHS/IDSA guidelines for the prevention of opportunistic infections in persons infected with Human Immunodeficiency Virus.* Retrieved April 27, 2002 from www.hivatis.org/guidelines

Wang, C., & Celum, C. (2001). Prevention of HIV. In R. Anderson (Ed.), *A guide to the clinical care of women with HIV.* [Electronic version]. Washington, DC: U.S. Department of Health and Human Services, HIV/AIDS Bureau. Retrieved March 6, 2003 from http://hab.hrsa.gov/publications/ womencare.htm

Watson, A., & Wasserman, S. (2000). *HIV reporting in the states.* STATESERV web site. Retrieved April 25, 2002 from www.stateserv.hpts.org/public/pubhome.nsf

Wang, C. O., Reilly, M., & Kreiss, J. K. (1999). Risk of HIV infection in oral contraceptive pill users: A metaanalysis. *Journal of Acquired Immunodeficiency Syndromes, 21* (1), 51–58.

CHAPTER ❖ **13**

COMMON GYNECOLOGIC PELVIC DISORDERS

Donna E. Forrest

*F*rustrating for all health care providers is the client who presents with chronic pelvic pain, because in most cases a specific etiology cannot be determined and care is very difficult.

Highlights

- Endometriosis
- Adenomyosis
- Pelvic Inflammatory Disease
- Adnexal Masses (Ovarian Tumors)
- Dyspareunia
- Nonmalignant Disorders of the Vulva
- Leiomyomas
- Pelvic Relaxation Syndrome
- Chronic Pelvic Pain
- Cervicitis
- Bartholin's Gland Duct Cysts and Bartholinitis
- Cervical Polyps
- Gynecologic Cancers
- Diethylstilbestrol Exposure

❖   INTRODUCTION

The health care provider needs to be familiar with the diagnosis, management, and follow-up of the more common gynecologic pelvic disorders encountered in practice and must recognize when a client should be referred for further evaluation and management. With the changing health care climate where managed care and cost effectiveness are major influences, the practitioner must use sound clinical judgment in gathering pertinent history and physical examination data, selecting cost-efficient diagnostic tests, and implementing medical, nursing, and adjunct therapies. The population of older women is growing rapidly in the United States and quality of life issues are most important and should always be in the forefront of the provider's mind. The provider should be more knowledgeable about those disorders more common in older women, such as genital prolapse, and the importance of screening for gynecologic cancers.

The evaluation of any complaint of pelvic symptoms begins with a thorough client history that includes the following:

- The onset and description of the pelvic symptoms and any associated abdominal symptoms.
- A description of the character, nature, location, and timing of any pain.
- A detailed menstrual and sexual history.
- A history of previous related surgeries or hospitalizations.
- An obstetric history.
- A thorough psychosocial history.

Frustrating for all health care providers, including the gynecologist, is the client who presents with chronic pelvic pain, because in most cases, a specific etiology cannot be determined and care is very difficult. For these clients, a thorough history, physical examination, and diagnostic evaluation are critical. Consultation with a gynecologist is necessary, and in most situations, consultation with a mental health expert, such as an advanced practice nurse specialist in mental health, is beneficial.

Although a goal is to prevent unnecessary medical and surgical intervention, the fact remains that surgical intervention often is necessary to evaluate and manage pelvic disorders. The health care provider has a responsibility to the client to review alternative therapies, to evaluate the severity of her symptoms and their impact on her lifestyle, to discuss the potential benefits of proposed surgery, and to assist the client in seeking consultation with a qualified, reputable surgeon.

In many clinical situations, the provider will find him- or herself in a unique position to thoroughly evaluate a chronic or ongoing problem. In the evaluation, management, and follow-up of nonmalignant vulvar disorders, especially vulvodynia, the provider's most important role is to obtain a complete history, to offer emotional support, and to evaluate therapy.

This section cannot completely address all pelvic/gynecologic disorders. It is intended to be a clinical guideline for current evaluation and management of common, more frequently seen problems. The provider should always be aware of when to seek consultation and/or when to refer. It goes without saying that the provider should stay abreast of ever changing developments in gynecologic health care as she or he continues to gain clinical experience.

ENDOMETRIOSIS

Endometriosis is the presence of endometrial tissue at sites outside the endometrial cavity (Olive & Pritts, 2001; Prentice, 2001). Endometrial tissue responds cyclically to estrogen by swelling and producing local inflammation. The severity of pain appears unrelated to the extent of the disease so that clients with small implants of endometriosis may experience the severest pain (Prentice, 2001). It is generally thought that the extent of the pain is influenced primarily by the location and depth of the endometriotic implant, with deep implants in highly innervated areas most consistently associated with pain.

EPIDEMIOLOGY

A specific etiology for endometriosis is unknown, although several theories have been put forth. Many researchers conclude that endometriosis develops as a result of a combination of factors. Modern explanations of the pathogenesis of endometriosis include the following:

- Sampson's theory of retrograde menstruation describes menstrual or endometrial tissue flowing backward through the fallopian tubes and into the abdominal cavity.
- Lymphatic spread theory describes endometrial tissue spreading to distant sites through the lymphatic system.
- Coelomic metaplasia theory describes the metaplasia of peritoneal mesothelial cells into endometrial epithelium under some unidentified influence, such as repeated inflammation.
- Müllerian cell theory suggests that remnant müllerian cells remain in the pelvic tissue during the development of the müllerian system and later, perhaps under the influence of estrogen, develop into endometrial glands and stroma.
- Recent research suggests that immunologic and genetic factors may have a role in the initiation and progression of endometriosis, including a genetic predisposition that allows retrograde menstrual tissue to implant.

Endometriosis is found equally among caucasian and African Americans, and occurs across all socioeconomic groups. It is more likely to occur and progress in women with early menarche, longer cycle length (greater than thirty days), years of menstruation uninterrupted by pregnancy, and positive family history. There is nearly a 10 fold increased risk of developing endometriosis with an affected first-degree relative (ACOG, 2001, PB 11).

Endometriosis occurs in 7 to 10 percent of women in the general population and in up to 50 percent of premenopausal women. It is prevalent in 38 percent of infertile women and in 71 to 87 percent of women with chronic pelvic pain. The actual prevalence is difficult to determine because of the difficulty of diagnosis (Prentice, 2001). Six million women in the United States report symptoms of endometriosis (Adamson, 2001). Endometriosis should be considered as a potential cause of chronic pain when an adolescent woman presents with this complaint. Early recognition is essential to preserve fertility.

SUBJECTIVE DATA

Dysmenorrhea, pelvic pain, dyspareunia, intermenstrual bleeding, and infertility are the most commonly reported symptoms. The client may also complain of perimenstrual back pain, dyschezia, abdominal pain, urinary symptoms, and/or rectal pain or bleeding. Reported symptoms may be cyclical or constant (ACOG, 2001, PB 11). Because of the strong association of sexual abuse with reported pelvic pain, all clients should be screened for the possibility of past or present physical or emotional abuse (ACOG, 2001, TB 223).

OBJECTIVE DATA

Physical Examination

The genitalia and reproductive tract may appear completely normal if lesions are small and few. In more advanced disease, a speculum exam reveals cervical displacement of 1 cm or more to the left or right of the midline; bimanual exam tenderness and nodularity of the uterosacral ligaments and posterior cul-de-sac are detected. Clinical examination during menstruation may better enable the practitioner to identify tender nodules of endometriosis (Koninckx, Meuleman, Oosterlynck, & Cornillie, 1996). Also seen are fixed retroversion of the uterus and adnexal masses that vary in size, shape, and consistency and may be asymmetric, fixed, cystic, or indurated (ACOG, 2001, PB 11; Keltz & Olive, 1993).

If the history and physical exam suggest endometriosis, especially in the presence of pain and history of infertility, refer the client for gynecologic consultation.

Diagnostic Tests and Methods

CA-125 Assay. Serum cancer antigen is a cell surface antigen found on certain cells derived from embryonic coelomic epithelium (ACOG, 2001, PB 11; Keltz & Olive, 1993). These tissues include the epithelium of the endocervix, endometrium, Fallopian tubes, mesothelial lining of the peritoneum, pleura, pericardium, and fetal müllerian ducts. Used mainly as a marker of response to treatment of ovarian epithelial neoplasms, CA-125 levels are elevated in clients with endometriosis. Levels correlate with severity of the disease and response to treatment. Because elevation of CA-125 levels occurs in several gynecologic and nongynecologic conditions, it is not useful in the diagnosis of endometriosis. Concentrations of CA-125 have been studied as a marker to determine the response to medical therapy for endometriosis. Although CA-125 levels may decrease during treatment, normal values do not confirm the complete absence of endometriosis (ACOG, 2001, PB 11).

The test procedure is to obtain a blood sample and send it to a laboratory with experience in analyzing CA-125.

Tell the client that the assay is very expensive and will most likely not be covered by her insurance. Providing such information will facilitate decisions related to the necessity of the assay. In addition, consult with the physician ordering the assay to ascertain his specific plans for utilizing the test. Assist and educate the client as to its role in her overall plan of care. This assay should be used only in consultation with a physician.

Diagnostic Laparoscopy. Diagnostic evaluation through direct visualization of endometriosis. Procedure of choice for definitive diagnosis of endometriosis (ACOG, 2001, PB 11). Visual inspection and identification of the protean appearances of endometriosis requires an experienced surgeon. Experience is associated with increased diagnostic accuracy. Increased depth of infiltration of endometriosis lesions are associated with an increased level of pain (ACOG, 2001, PB 11; Olive & Pritts, 2001). Gynecologic surgeons employ the American Fertility Society's classification system as a means of communicating and documenting their findings. The severity of endometriosis has been classified by numerous staging systems. The revised classification system of the American Society for Reproductive Medicine was most recently revised in 1996. Unfortunately, there is no true correlation between the stage of endometriosis, the severity of symptoms, and prognosis with treatment (Olive & Pritts, 2001).

The test procedure requires that the client be referred to a gynecologic surgeon with special training and experience using the laparoscope. Laparoscopy is usually performed as an outpatient procedure, with the client under general anesthesia. The laparoscope is inserted through a small incision just above the navel after the abdomen has been inflated with carbon dioxide gas. The surgeon is able to visualize the pelvic organs directly.

Explain the procedure to the client in detail. In addition, discuss the risks. Complications, which are rare, may include bleeding or injuries to nearby organs. Anesthesia complications are rare. Discuss the recovery process. Usually, the client may return home the same day. Common discomforts are neck and shoulder pain from the gas used to inflate the abdomen, mild nausea, pelvic discomfort at the incision site, mild cramps, and mild vaginal discharge. Instruct the client that she may usually shower or bathe in 24 hours and return to normal activities as soon as she feels able. Review the signs and symptoms of infection and explain how to keep the incision site clean and dry. To reinforce this discussion, provide the client with written information about the procedure and recovery.

DIFFERENTIAL MEDICAL DIAGNOSES

Chronic pelvic inflammatory disease, leiomyomata uteri, ovarian cysts, gastrointestinal and urinary tract problems (ACOG, 2001, PB 11).

PLAN

Management of the client with endometriosis should be determined by one or more of the following factors:

- Severity of symptoms.
- Desire for fertility.
- Degree of disease.
- Client's therapeutic goals.

Medical management should be considered initially in clients with mild to moderate symptoms who wish to maintain their fertility potential. Conservative surgery is indicated when medical therapy fails, but fertility is still desired. Medical therapy and conservative surgery can be combined. Those clients who have severe endometriosis with debilitating pain should be counseled to complete their childbearing. Total abdominal hysterectomy and bilateral salpingo-oophorectomy represent definitive treatment of endometriosis.

There are a variety of therapeutic options. Assist the client in determining her desired therapeutic outcome. Monitor side effects of medications and response to therapy. Provide education and emotional support.

Psychosocial Interventions

Encourage active participation by the client and her significant other in treatment decisions. Assess the client's lifestyle and future plans, such as childbearing, marriage, education, and career. Discuss the impact of the disease on her life and which treatment option will best suit her lifestyle. Assess the client for depression, which can be initiated or worsened by chronic pain. Many of the hormonal therapies have side effects such as depression, loss of libido, and/or mood swings. Inform the client of these potential side effects. Sexual therapy should be offered if the disease has significantly impacted sexual relations (Jones, Kennedy, Barnard, Wong, & Jenkinson, 2001; Waller & Shaw, 1995).

Medication

The goal of medication is to interrupt cycles of stimulation and bleeding. The various medications are comparable in their ability to provide relief from dysmenorrhea, dyspareunia, and pelvic pain associated with endometriosis. They are not of proven value in improving fertility. The basis for medical management of endometriosis is to create states of pseudopregnancy, pseudomenopause or chronic anovulation (Olive & Pritts, 2001).

None of the following medications is indicated over any of the others, and the insurance coverage may vary. Recent studies demonstrated that Danazol and Naferelin were equally effective in relieving dysmenorrhea, dyspareunia, and pelvic pain in clients with endometriosis. GnRH analogs continue to be expensive. All have side effects that may be poorly tolerated by the client. Recurrence of endometriosis is common after completion of medical therapies at rates from 20 to 50 percent (Adamson, 2001).

NSAIDs

- *Indications:* First-line treatment in women with pain who have not yet been proven to have the disease. Relief of dysmenorrhea and alleviation of symptoms.
- *Administration:* Initiate NSAIDs immediately upon feeling any premenstrual symptoms and continue medication for three days (Adamson, 2001; Prentice, 2001). Several types of NSAIDs are available, and their dosages vary. The most widely accepted and least expensive are the following:
  - Ibuprofen 600–800 mg., p.o., q.i.d.
  - Naproxen sodium (Naprosyn, Anaprox, Aleve), 550 mg. p.o., b.i.d.
- *Side Effects and Adverse Reactions.* Most often reported is GI irritation. Advise taking with food or after meals.
- *Contraindications.* Previous allergy to NSAIDs and a history of ulcer disease.

Progestogens

- *Indications.* Suppression of the cyclic hormonal response of endometrial implants, and resorption of tissue. Indicated in mild to moderate endometriosis. Progestogens are better tolerated than combination oral contraceptives, having fewer estrogen-related side effects and are less costly than Danazol and GnRH analogs, making them a better initial choice of therapy.
- *Administration.* Medroxyprogesterone acetate (Depo-Provera), 100 mg I.M. every two weeks for four doses, followed by 200 mg I.M. monthly for four additional months, or MPA (Provera), 30 mg p.o. every day for six months.

- *Side Effects and Adverse Reactions.* Breakthrough bleeding, depression, delayed fertility, headache, dizziness, weight gain, nausea, fluid retention, breast tenderness.
- *Contraindications.* Traditionally, contraindications for progestin-only medication have been the same as those for combination oral contraceptives (see Contraindications for Oral Contraceptives, Chapter 8). Progestin-only is also contraindicated for women with undiagnosed abnormal genital bleeding. A relative contraindication is for women who desire fertility immediately after completing therapy.
- *Anticipated Outcomes on Evaluation.* The relief of pain and the resorption of endometrial implants.
- *Client Teaching and Counseling.* Review with the client the instructions for selected regimens, their possible side effects, and the danger signs (see Combined Oral Contraceptives).

Danazol

- *Indications.* Mild to moderate endometriosis in women who desire fertility but not in the immediate future.
- *Administration.* An 800 mg dose is given as two 200 mg tablets p.o. twice daily for six to nine months beginning on the fifth day of menses. Newer studies suggest lower doses may be effective for less severe disease. Therefore, an option is to start at 400 mg daily given as one 200 mg tablet twice daily. If no relief occurs within six weeks, increase the dosage.
- *Side Effects and Adverse Reactions.* Possible weight gain, fluid retention, fatigue, decreased breast size, acne, oily skin, hirsutism, atrophic vaginitis, hot flushes, muscle cramps, emotional lability, voice changes, spotting, and/or decreased HDL cholesterol.
- *Contraindications.* A history of liver disease, hypertension, hyperlipidemia, congestive heart failure, or renal impairment, or pregnancy.
- *Anticipated Outcomes on Evaluation.* The relief of pain, resorption of endometrial implants, return to fertility, and pregnancy if desired; few side effects.
- *Client Teaching and Counseling.* Tell the client about the high cost of Danazol therapy and the length of treatment. Review the side effects and stress the importance of following the administration regimen correctly. Barrier contraception is recommended during therapy with Danazol and during the first menstrual cycle after treatment.

Gestrinone (Ethylnorgestrienone)

- *Indications.* Amenorrhea, suppression of endometrial tissue.
- *Administration.* 2.5 mg. two or three times a week, p.o.
- *Side Effects and Adverse Reactions.* Similar to those of Danazol; mild and transient, less frequent than Danazol. Voice change, hirsutism, and clitoral hypertrophy are sometimes irreversible.
- *Contraindication.* Same as Danazol.
- *Anticipated Outcomes on Evaluation.* The relief of pain, resorption of endometrial implants, return to fertility, and pregnancy if desired; few side effects.
- *Client Teaching.* Tell the client about the possible irreversible side effects.

Combined Oral Contraceptives (OCs)

- *Indications.* Suppression of the cyclic hormonal response of endometrial implants and eventual resorption of the tissue. Oral contraceptives (OCs) induce a "pseudopregnancy." The combination of estrogen and progestin causes endometrial tissue to become decidual and necrotic, leading to resorption. The therapy may be useful for mild to moderate endometriosis associated with clinical symptoms of pain or infertility.
- *Administration.* One pill p.o. daily, of a low dose, monophasic, taken continuously for six to twelve months. May also be administered as continuous active-ingredient tablets for three months, followed by withdrawal, then repetition. Many patients do better with this regimen (Adamson, 2001). Monophasic OCs are superior to triphasic OCs for this indication. Best dosage to begin with is usually 35 mcg of ethinyl estradiol, but this can be decreased if the patient is symptomatic with headaches, or increased in case of breakthrough bleeding. Norethindrone 0.35 to 0.5 mg daily may also be used if this is better tolerated. Treatment lasts three to six months (Adamson, 2001). If breakthrough bleeding occurs, add conjugated estrogen, 1.25 mg per day for one week. Alternatively, the OC dosage may be increased to two tablets or more per day if breakthrough bleeding occurs.
- *Side Effects and Adverse Reactions.* Possible weight gain, breast pain and tenderness, abdominal bloating, nausea, increased appetite, breast secretion, superficial vein varicosities, and increased risk of deep vein thrombosis.
- *Contraindication.* In addition to those usually listed for OCs, other contraindications are known or sus-

pected pregnancy, history of thromboembolic disease, and liver disease (see Chapter 9 and the current *Physicians' Desk Reference*).
- *Anticipated Outcomes on Evaluation.* The relief of pain, resorption of endometrial implants, return to fertility, and pregnancy if desired.
- *Client Teaching and Counseling.* Review with the client the instructions for taking OCs continuously, stressing the importance of not skipping pills. Warn her of the possible side effects and danger signs, for example, abdominal pain, severe headache, and leg pain. Explain the purpose of the therapy.

Gonadotropin-Releasing Hormone Analogues (GnRH-a)

- *Indications.* Suppression of endometriosis by creating a pseudomenopause.
- *Administration.* See Table 13–1, GnRH-Analogue Therapy for Endometriosis. Administered for three to six months; only FDA approved for six months. Studies show that three months of therapy is as effective as six months (Adamson, 2001).
- *Side Effects and Adverse Reactions.* Hot flushes, vaginal dryness, mood swings, depression, weight gain, decreased breast size, decreased libido, fatigue, and insomnia. In addition, GnRH-a may interfere with calcium and bone metabolism. Possible 3 to 8 percent loss of bone density occurring over six months of drug therapy. General consensus is that this is not clinically significant in women with normal bone density (Adamson, 2001).
- *Contradictions.* Known or suspected pregnancy, hypersensitivity to GnRH, undiagnosed abnormal vaginal bleeding, breastfeeding.
- *Anticipated Outcomes on Evaluation.* The relief of pain, resorption of endometrial implants, return to fertility, and pregnancy if desired; few side effects.
- *Client Teaching and Counseling.* Provide instructions for the drug's proper administration, and tell the client that the therapy is costly and will continue for

TABLE 13–1. GnRH-Analogue Therapy for Endometriosis

Drug	Dosage	Route
Lupron (Leuprolide acetate)	3.75 mg IM q 28–33 days	IM sustained release depot
Synarel (Nafarelin acetate)	400–800 mcg (1–2 sprays b.i.d.)	Nasal spray
Zoladex (Goserelin acetate)	3.36 mg implant abdomen q 28 days	Subcutaneous sustained release

Source: Huime & Lambalk, 2001.

three to six months. Review the side effects. Inform client of risk for bone loss. Clients should undergo dual-photon absorptiometry (DPX) and have normal bone density before GnRH agonist retreatment (Adamson, 2001). A calcium supplement may be necessary: 1,000 to 1,500 mg q.d. Barrier contraception is recommended during therapy and for the first menstrual cycle.

Add-Back Therapy

- *Indications.* Relief of side effects, reduction of bone loss induced by GnRH agonists.
- *Administration.* Premarin 0.6 mg daily or norethindrone 2.5 mg daily; *or* Norethindrone 2.5 to 5 mg/day plus alendronate 10 mg/day; plus calcium 1,000 mg/day.
- *Side Effects and Adverse Reactions.* Same as those listed for oral contraceptives. Alendronate may cause severe gastrointestinal distress.
- *Contraindications.* Same as those listed for oral contraceptives.
- *Anticipated Outcomes on Evaluation.* Reduction of bone loss, relief of vasomotor symptoms, continued pain relief from GnRH agonists.
- *Client Teaching and Counseling.* Instruct to take alendronate on empty stomach upon awakening in the morning with a full 8-ounce glass of water. The client should remain upright for 30 minutes after taking the medication. Explain the purpose of add-back therapy and assess client response.

Surgical Interventions

Conservative Surgery. One surgical option is to destroy and dissect endometriomas and endometriotic implants while preserving reproductive function. The procedure may be performed by a specially trained gynecologic surgeon directly after laparoscopic diagnosis, while the client is still under anesthesia. Conservative methods include fulguration, excision and resection, and/or laser vaporization. Conservative surgery is indicated for adnexal masses, symptoms unresponsive to medical therapy, severe endometriosis in a client who desires future fertility, and concomitant conditions such as leiomyomas or adhesions. Some women have been treated with presacral neurectomy and uterosacral ligament ablation for pain if they wish to preserve fertility (ACOG, 2001, PB 11; Adamson, 2001; Olive & Pritts, 2001).

The possible adverse effects are few: a reaction to anesthesia, incisional infection, bleeding, or injury to nearby organs. The anticipated outcomes on evaluation are the relief of pain and return to fertility.

When explaining the procedure to the client, point out that conservative surgery is not curative. Review the postoperative instructions, addressing the client's return to activity, resumption of sexual relations, and signs and symptoms of infection.

Definitive Surgery. Abdominal hysterectomy, with or without bilateral salpingo-oophorectomy, is indicated for clients with severe disease. These are women who either have completed their families, have no desire for future fertility, whose disease has not responded to medical therapy or conservative surgery, or whose disease involves other organs, such as the bowel or bladder. Referral is made to a board-certified gynecologic surgeon. The procedure, performed under general anesthesia, involves removal of the uterus through an abdominal incision. The ovaries and fallopian tubes may or may not be removed; among the determining factors are the age of the client and the extent of endometriosis.

There are possible adverse effects, namely, bleeding, infection, wound infection, or damage to nearby organs. The anticipated outcome on evaluation is complete resolution of the disease, including relief of dysmenorrhea, dyspareunia, dyschezia, and/or dysuria.

Prepare the client by giving her a thorough explanation of the anatomy and physiology, surgical procedure, and risks and benefits. Reassure her that femininity remains unchanged by the surgery. Hormonal replacement therapy may be needed. Full recovery usually takes about six weeks. Review the postoperative instructions, including topics such as the return to activity, the expectation that vaginal bleeding will change to clear discharge, signs of infection, return to sexual activity, and dietary needs.

FOLLOW-UP AND REFERRAL

Endometriosis tends to recur at a rate of 10 to 20 percent per year (Adamson, 2001). Appropriate follow-up intervals depend on the choice of therapy and the client's needs. An initial evaluation, made after six months of therapy, should report the incidence, severity, and cyclicity of pain, dysmenorrhea, and dyspareunia. Review the side effects and their impact on the client. Inquire about the issue of pregnancy and provide emotional support and encouragement. Assess and treat or refer for reactive depression. Encourage the client to adopt healthy lifestyle habits with respect to diet, exercise, sleep, and stress management. Referral sources include: the Endometriosis Association, RESOLVE, and the American Society of

Reproductive Medicine. Personal or group counseling may also be helpful (Adamson, 2001).

ADENOMYOSIS

Adenomyosis occurs when the endometrial glands and stroma within the endometrium grow into the myometrium. The cause is believed to be disruption of the uterine wall during pregnancy, labor, and postpartum involution. It occurs in 5 to 70 percent of multiparous women in their 30s, 40s, and 50s, but it does not occur in postmenopausal women. It is difficult to diagnose and is most commonly identified posthysterectomy (Keckstein, 2000; Seltzer & Pearse, 1995; Siegler & Camilien, 1994).

SUBJECTIVE DATA

Clients most often report severe dysmenorrhea and menorrhagia (Keckstein, 2000).

OBJECTIVE DATA

Physical Examination

Bimanual examination of the genitalia and reproductive organs may reveal a large, symmetrical uterus (Keckstein, 2000).

Diagnostic Tests and Methods

Endometrial Biopsy. Diagnostic evaluation of any abnormal bleeding; requires referral to a gynecologist. Explain the procedure to the client. The test is performed with a biopsy curette, or a suction catheter, or other instrument passed through the cervical canal into the uterus. The client will be an outpatient, and, generally, no anesthesia will be necessary. Obtain the client's menstrual history. Explain that she may return to normal activities immediately.

Ultrasound. Diagnostic evaluation to rule out leiomyomas or other tumors. Transvaginal ultrasound in the hands of a skilled technician can identify the irregular hyperechogenic outlines in the myometrium. (ACOG, 2001, TB 215). The procedure should be performed by a trained professional with expertise in obstetrics and gynecology. The method, performed abdominally or vaginally, employs sound waves to provide detailed images of the pelvic structures.

Explain the procedure to the client and assure her that it is painless. In the *abdominal method*, the lower abdomen is covered with a water soluble gel, a probe is moved slowly across the abdomen, and images are projected onto a video display monitor. In the *vaginal method*, a probe with ultrasound gel is inserted into the vagina. The client remains awake. In order to obtain clearer images, a client may be required to undergo a 24-hour bowel preparation (i.e., laxative, enema, clear liquid diet).

Magnetic Resonance Imaging (MRI). An accurate nonsurgical diagnostic test for adenomyosis, it is indicated preoperatively in symptomatic women who wish to maintain their fertility and who are considering conservative surgery for removal of the adenomyomas. Its usefulness is limited by its cost, and its clinical necessity is best determined by the gynecologic surgeon (Keckstein, 2000).

Hysteroscopy. Operative procedure that allows direct visualization of the endometrial cavity using an optical instrument. Allows the physician to obtain specimens, apply therapies, and perform a wide variety of surgical procedures under direct visualization (ACOG, 2001, TB 191). Usually employed to evaluate abnormal uterine bleeding; can be used to corroborate the diagnosis of adenomyosis (Keckstein, 2000).

Explain the procedure to the client and discuss risks and benefits. Anesthesia is used and the client should be fully informed of the risks of anesthesia.

Contraindications include pregnancy, the presence of a genital tract infection, and medical conditions such as cardiac disease.

Possible complications include fluid overload from direct instillation of electrolyte solutions during the procedure, infection, uterine perforation, bleeding, and/or embolism (ACOG, 2001, TB 191).

The benefit of hysteroscopy in clients with adenomyosis may be the avoidance of hysterectomy (Keckstein, 2000).

DIFFERENTIAL MEDICAL DIAGNOSES

Leiomyomas, endometriosis.

PLAN

Psychosocial Interventions

Discuss the condition with the client and determine the impact of her symptoms. The severity of symptoms will determine therapy, which should be described to the client. Reassure her if necessary.

Medication

No specific medications are given for treatment or resolution of adenomyosis. If symptoms are mild, however, palliative management with non-steroidal anti-inflammatory drugs (NSAIDs) is helpful (see Chronic Pelvic Pain). GnRH-analogues have also proven to effectively reduce symptoms (see Table 13–1).

Surgical Interventions

Hysterectomy is indicated for severe, symptomatic adenomyosis, including severe dysmenorrhea, menorrhagia, or enlarged uterus. (For procedure, see Endometriosis, Definitive Surgery.)

FOLLOW-UP AND REFERRAL

If medical therapy is the initial treatment of choice, then the client is evaluated in three to six months. Increasing pain or bleeding may necessitate referral to a gynecologic surgeon for possible hysterectomy. Sarcoma can be a complication.

PELVIC INFLAMMATORY DISEASE (PID)

In pelvic inflammatory disease (PID), infection and inflammation develop in the pelvic organs—namely the uterus, fallopian tubes, and ovaries. Most often, the condition is localized in the tubes; however, it may occur anywhere in the upper genital tract. Complications include ectopic pregnancy, pelvic abscess, infertility, recurrent or chronic episodes of the disease, chronic abdominal pain, pelvic adhesions, premature hysterectomy, and depression. Because of the seriousness of the potential complications of PID, accurate diagnosis is imperative (Ness, Soper, Holley, Peipert, et al., 2001).

EPIDEMIOLOGY

Neisseria gonorrhoeae and *Chlamydia trachomatis* are the two major causative organisms; however, PID is usually a mixed infection caused by both aerobic and anaerobic organisms. Recent studies demonstrate the presence of bacterial vaginosis in cases of confirmed PID. It is suggested that BV may facilitate the ascent of gonorrhoeae or *C. trachomatis* (Centers for Disease Control, [CDC] 2002; Joessens, Schachter, & Sweet, 1994). Adolescents and young women are three times more likely to develop the infection. Nonwhite women are higher risk. Other risk factors include multiple sex partners (greater than two in the previous thirty to sixty days considered a major risk factor); a history of PID or sexually transmitted disease (STD); intercourse with a partner who has untreated urethritis; recent intrauterine device (IUD) insertion; and nulliparity. Additional risk factors include cigarette smoking, and sex with menses (Joessens et al., 1994). PID is more likely to occur during the first five days of the menstrual cycle.

The causative organisms are transmitted through sexual intercourse with an infected partner. Although accurate estimates of PID are difficult to obtain because of difficulty with accurate diagnosis, it is estimated that 1.5 million new cases of pelvic inflammatory disease are diagnosed annually in the United States. Trends in hospitalized PID have declined steadily during the 1990s, but have remained relatively constant from 1995 through 1999 (CDC, 2002; Rein, Kassler, Irwin, & Rabiee, 2000).

SUBJECTIVE DATA

Because of a wide variety of presenting signs and symptoms in clients with PID, clinical diagnosis can be difficult. A client may report one or all of the following symptoms: pain and tenderness of the lower abdomen, fever, chills, nausea, vomiting, increased vaginal discharge, symptoms of urinary tract infection (UTI), and irregular bleeding. The severity of symptoms may be mild or severe. Recently, experts agree that many cases of PID have gone undiagnosed. Abdominal pain is usually present. If Fitz-Hugh-Curtis syndrome is present, upper abdominal pain will occur due to liver capsule inflammation. A client may also report experiencing any of the aforementioned risk factors. Consultation with a gynecologist is advised due to the seriousness of this condition. The Centers for Disease Control's (CDC) minimum criteria for empiric treatment of PID include all of the following:

- Lower abdominal tenderness.
- Adnexal tenderness.
- Cervical motion tenderness (CDC; Peipert, Ness, Blume, et al., 2001).

OBJECTIVE DATA

Physical Examination

Determination of vital signs may show an elevated body temperature. The abdomen may be distended with rebound tenderness, guarding and hypoactive bowel sounds. The genital and reproductive exam is positive for cervical motion tenderness (pain upon movement of the cervix), purulent cervical discharge, uterine tenderness, adnexal pain and fullness, or the presence of an adnexal mass. The CDC's 2002 *Treatment Guidelines for Sexually Transmitted Diseases* advises that a sexually active young woman should receive empiric antibiotic therapy for PID if all of the minimum criteria for diagnosis are present:

- ◆ Cervical motion tenderness
- ◆ Uterine tenderness
- ◆ Adnexal tenderness
- ◆ WBCs present on saline microscopy of vaginal secretions

Diagnostic Tests and Methods

Complete Blood Count (CBC) and Erythrocyte Sedimentation Rate (ESR). Diagnostic evaluation to detect any inflammatory process. The white blood cell (WBC) count is above 10,000 and erythrocyte sedimentation rate (ESR) is elevated in PID. A venous blood sample is obtained according to laboratory protocol after the procedure and its purpose have been explained to the client.

Pregnancy Test. Diagnostic evaluation (urine or blood level of human chorionic gonadotropin [hCG]) for unsuspected intrauterine pregnancy or suspected ectopic pregnancy. A urine pregnancy test is done, or if ectopic pregnancy is suspected, blood quantitative radioimmunoassay of hCG.

Explain the procedure to the client and determine her last normal menstrual period. If the client is pregnant, ultrasound should be ordered to rule out ectopic pregnancy or missed abortion. Whether a treatment regimen is contraindicated during pregnancy must be determined.

C-Reactive Protein. Diagnostic evaluation to detect inflammation; the test is highly sensitive for detecting PID. A venous blood sample is obtained according to laboratory protocol after the procedure and its purpose have been explained to the client.

Vaginal Smears/Cervical Cultures. Diagnostic evaluation to detect the causative organisms of infection. Wet mount with saline can detect bacterial vaginosis or trichomoniasis. Cervical tests will detect *N. gonorrhoeae* and *C. trachomatis*. PID is usually due to polymicrobial, ascending infection (see Chapter 11 for the test procedures).

Ultrasound. Diagnostic evaluation to identify fluid in the cul-de-sac, distended tubes, masses or a pelvic abscess, and to rule out intrauterine and ectopic pregnancy (see Adenomyosis for a description of the test procedure).

Laparoscopy. Diagnostic evaluation to identify fluid in the cul-de-sac, distended tubes, masses, or pelvic abscess. Indicated if the diagnosis is uncertain, if the client fails to respond to therapy, or if symptoms recur soon after adequate therapy. It may also reveal tubal occlusion and tubal factor infertility associated with PID.

DIFFERENTIAL MEDICAL DIAGNOSES

Ectopic pregnancy, appendicitis, ruptured corpus luteum cyst, septic abortion, torsion of an adnexal mass, pyelonephritis, degeneration of a leiomyoma, endometriosis, endometritis, ulcerative colitis.

PLAN

Psychosocial Interventions

Thoroughly discuss with the client the disease, its implications, and risk factors. If possible, the client's partner should participate. Review the serious sequelae that may occur if the disease is not treated or if the client does not comply with treatment. Refer partners for evaluation and treatment of any sexually transmitted disease that is diagnosed. Discuss the use of condoms, especially if the client has multiple sexual partners. Provide emotional support. Stress the importance of follow-up care and evaluation.

Medication

The client is treated on an ambulatory basis or admitted for hospitalization, and the medication regimen is determined by this choice.

Ambulatory Medication. This regimen is followed when a client with PID can be managed safely on an outpatient basis at home and is based upon the revised 2002 CDC guidelines.

Regimen A:
　　Levofloxacin 500 mg orally b.i.d. for fourteen days
or
　　Ofloxacin 400 mg orally b.i.d. for fourteen days
with or without
　　Metronidazole 500 mg orally b.i.d. for fourteen days
Regimen B:
　　Ceftriaxone 250 mg I.M. once
or
　　Cefoxitin 2 g I.M.

plus

Probenecid 1 g orally in a single dose concurrently once

or

Other parenteral third-generation cephalosporin (e.g., Ceftizoxime or cefotaxime)

plus

Doxycycline 100 mg orally b.i.d. for fourteen days

Stress to the client the importance of taking the complete medication prescription to help prevent complications; review all medication related instructions. *Convey the importance of returning for a follow-up evaluation 48 to 72 hours after the medication is started and again in seven to ten days.* Instruct the client that if symptoms worsen during outpatient treatment, she must call the health professional immediately because hospitalization will probably be necessary. Levofloxacin and ofloxacin should not be used in women 17 years and younger. These drugs are deposited in their cartilage. Both are contraindicated if pregnancy is diagnosed or suspected.

The following factors will contribute to the decision to refer a client to a physician for hospital admission and care.

- Surgical emergencies such as appendicitis cannot be excluded.
- Pregnancy.
- Lack of response clinically to oral antimicrobial therapy.
- Inability to follow or tolerate an outpatient oral regimen.
- Presence of severe illness, nausea and vomiting, or high fever.
- Tubo-ovarian abscess.
- Immunodeficient (i.e., HIV infection with low CD4 counts, taking immunosuppressive therapy, or other disease) (CDC, 2002).

In-Hospital Medication
Regimen A:
Cefotetan 2 grams I.V. every twelve hours

or

Cefoxitin 2 grams I.V. every six hours

plus

Doxycycline 100 mg I.V. or orally every twelve hours

(This regimen should be continued for at least 24 to 48 hours after the client demonstrates substantial clinical improvement, after which oral therapy may be initiated.)

Regimen B:
Clindamycin 900 mg I.V. every eight hours

plus

Gentamicin loading dose I.V. or I.M. (2 mg/kg of body weight), followed by a maintenance dose of (1.5 mg/kg) every eight hours.

(This regimen should be continued for at least 24 to 48 hours after the client demonstrates substantial clinical improvement, then followed with Doxycycline 100 mg orally b.i.d. or clindamycin 450 mg orally q.i.d. to complete a total of fourteen days of therapy.)

Explain to the client the necessity of hospitalization. Make sure that the client understands all discharge instructions and the need to return for evaluation after discharge.

Side Effects and Adverse Reactions

- *Cefoxitan, Cefotetan, Ceftriaxone (Cephalosporins).* Few; most serious is pseudomembranous colitis.
- *Doxycycline.* Gastrointestinal (GI) distress, fetal teeth discoloration if given during pregnancy, photosensitivity.
- *Gentamicin.* Nephrotoxicity, ototoxicity.
- *Clindamycin.* Diarrhea, pseudomembranous enterocolitis.

Contraindications

- *Cefoxitin, Cefotetan, Ceftriaxone (Cephalosporins).* Known allergy to cephalosporins.
- *Doxycycline.* Pregnancy or hypersensivity to tetracyclines.
- *Gentamicin.* Hypersensitivity to aminoglycosides.
- *Clindamycin.* Hypersensitivity to aminoglycosides.

Anticipated outcomes on evaluation are the resolution of symptoms of pelvic inflammatory disease and the prevention of serious sequelae.

Surgical Interventions

Conservative Surgery. This involves removal of grossly abnormal tissue only. The uterus and at least one ovary are preserved to allow for possible later in vitro fertilization. Conservative surgery is indicated when the hospitalized client with acute PID or a pelvic mass does not respond after 72 hours of appropriate therapy or when a ruptured tubo-ovarian abscess is suspected (CDC, 2002). An experienced gynecologic surgeon should perform the surgery.

The potential adverse effects are few: the usual potential anesthesia complications and the risk of excessive bleeding or postoperative infection. The anticipated outcomes on evaluation are the resolution of pelvic infection with the preservation of reproductive capability.

Explain the procedure to the client and inform her that it will be carried out using general anesthesia. Informed consent forms must be signed. Provide postoperative instructions regarding the return to activity, signs and symptoms of infection, and return to sexual activity.

Colpotomy. Colpotomy permits drainage of abscesses located in Douglas' cul-de-sac. It is performed transvaginally by an experienced gynecologic surgeon using direct ultrasonographic or radiographic guidance.

The possible adverse effects include the usual anesthesia complications and the risk of excessive bleeding or postoperative complications. The anticipated outcomes on evaluation are the resolution of the pelvic abscess and the prevention of chronic pelvic infection and chronic pelvic pain.

Explain the procedure to the client and inform her that it will be carried out using general anesthesia. Informed consent forms must be signed. Provide postoperative instructions regarding the return to activity, signs and symptoms of infection, and return to sexual activity.

Unilateral/Bilateral Salpingo-Oophorectomy. One or both fallopian tubes and ovaries are removed, depending on the location and extent of a tubo-ovarian abscess. Indications for the surgery are extensive involvement of the tubes or ovaries by the inflammatory process, including scarring and abscess.

The possible adverse effects are few; the most severe is loss of reproductive capability with a bilateral salpingo-oophorectomy. The usual potential for anesthesia complications and postoperative infection also exists. The anticipated outcomes on evaluation are the complete resolution of infection and symptoms and the prevention of chronic pelvic pain and chronic pelvic infections.

Discuss with the client the impact of the surgery on her reproductive function. Provide emotional support, and refer the client for counseling if her reproductive function is lost.

FOLLOW-UP AND REFERRAL

Any woman with PID who is being treated on an outpatient basis should be seen again in 48 to 72 hours after therapy is initiated. Marked improvement in symptoms should be exhibited by then. If no or less improvement than is deemed acceptable has occurred, the client must be referred to a specialist or hospitalized. If ambulatory care is progressing acceptably, reevaluate again in one week. If tenderness or any mass persists, refer immediately to a specialist. Advise immediate treatment for any sexual partner who has not received evaluation and treatment.

ADNEXAL MASSES (OVARIAN TUMORS)

The word *adnexal* pertains to the appendages of the uterus: the ovaries, fallopian tubes, and ligaments of the uterus. The adnexal masses discussed here are ovarian tumors.

CATEGORIES OF OVARIAN TUMORS

Four major categories of ovarian tumors have been identified: functional, inflammatory, metaplastic, and neoplastic (Hacker & Moore, 1998).

Functional Ovarian Tumors

- *Follicular cyst* is the most common functional cyst. In the normal physiologic course of ovulation, it is caused by the failure of the ovarian follicle to rupture. Follicle cysts may vary in size from 3 to 8 cm and are clinically insignificant. Most disappear spontaneously within sixty days (Callahan, Caughey, & Heffner, 2001).
- *Lutein cyst* forms when the corpus luteum becomes cystic or hemorrhagic and fails to degenerate after fourteen days.
- *Theca-lutein cyst* development is accompanied by abnormally high blood levels of human chorionic gonadotropin (hCG). The cyst occurs in clients with hydatiform mole, or with choriocarcinoma, or who are undergoing ovulation induction with gonadotropins or clomiphene (Callahan et al., 2001).
- *Polycystic ovary syndrome* (Stein-Leventhal syndrome) is characterized by the presence of multiple inactive follicle cysts within the ovary. The syndrome is associated with androgen excess and chronic anovulation (Hacker & Moore, 1998). PCOS is associated with greater LH and GnRH dysfunction with abnormal estradiol levels that fail to stimulate a nor-

mal FSH reaction (Gordon & Speroff, 2002). Obesity often accompanies PCOS; hirsutism occurs in half of patients (DeCherney & Nathan, 2003). PCOS is a complex condition and this text refers the reader to Chapter 8 of this text and Gordon & Speroff (2002) for more detailed information.

Inflammatory Ovarian Tumors

- *Salpingo-oophoritis* is inflammation of a fallopian tube and ovary. (Salpingo-oophorectomy is discussed in the preceding section on pelvic inflammatory disease.)
- *Tubo-ovarian abscess* is the tumor that develops in direct response to acute or chronic salpingo-oophoritis.

Metaplastic Ovarian Tumor

Endometriosis is the presence of endometrial tissue, composed of glands and stroma, at sites outside the endometrial cavity (see Endometriosis, page 304).

Neoplastic Ovarian Tumors

- *Epithelial tumors*, the most common type of tumor, include serous tumors, mucinous tumors, and endometrioid tumors. Epithelial tumors are derived from mesothelial cells lining the peritoneal cavity. They have the highest potential for malignancy (Kenkel, Hricak, Lu, Tsuda, & Filly, 2000).
- *Stromal tumors* are derived from the sex cords and specialized stroma of developing gonads. They include fibromas, granulosa-theca cell tumors, and Sertoli-Leydig cell tumors.
- *Germ cell tumor* is a benign cystic teratoma or dermoid cyst derived from early embryonic germ cells. It may contain calcifications; the majority are benign (Callahan et al., 2001).

EPIDEMIOLOGY

The etiology of adnexal masses is unclear. It is known, however, that the risk of ovarian malignancy increases significantly with age (Rosenfeld, 2001). Benign cystic teratoma (germ cell tumor) is the most common *ovarian* neoplasm; epithelial neoplasm is the most common *malignant* neoplasm. Stromal neoplasms, on the other hand, are uncommon. During the reproductive years, 70 percent of all noninflammatory tumors are functional; 20 percent are neoplastic; 10 percent are endometriomas. After menopause, half of all ovarian tumors are malignant; however, before puberty, only 10 percent are malig-

nant. In prepubertal adolescents, pelvic or ovarian masses are very worrisome and a complete evaluation is necessary (Rosenfeld, 2001; Templeman, Fallat, Blinchevsky, & Hertweck, 2000).

SUBJECTIVE DATA

- *Functional Ovarian Tumors.* A follicular cyst is usually asymptomatic but can cause minor lower abdominal discomfort, pelvic pain, or dyspareunia. A lutein cyst causes pain or signs of peritoneal irritation, delayed menses. The rupture of a cyst may produce acute lower abdominal pain and tenderness.
- *Inflammatory Ovarian Tumors.* A client may report symptoms that are similar to those of pelvic inflammatory disease (discussed earlier in this chapter): pain and tenderness of the lower abdomen, fever, chills, nausea, vomiting, increased vaginal discharge, irregular bleeding patterns.
- *Metaplastic Ovarian Tumors.* A client may report symptoms that are similar to those of endometriosis (discussed earlier in this chapter): dysmenorrhea, dyspareunia, perimenstrual back pain, infertility, dyschezia, abdominal pain, irregular bleeding.
- *Neoplastic Ovarian Tumors.* Subjective data are nonspecific. The client may be asymptomatic unless torsion or rupture occurs. Abdominal enlargement or bloating may occur, usually later in the tumor development. With rupture or torsion of the tumor, mild, intermittent pelvic pain or severe pelvic pain may be reported, as well as peritoneal irritation.

OBJECTIVE DATA

Physical Examination

Bimanual pelvic examination has significant limitations for accurately diagnosing ovarian masses and is influenced by obesity, uterine size, and abdominal scars (Padilla, Radosevich, & Milad, 2000).

Physical examination, including bimanual gynecologic exam, is done to assist in detecting the following.

- Functional ovarian tumor is 4 to 8 cm, noted on bimanual examination. It regresses following the next menstrual cycle, is mobile, unilateral, and may be tender. The normal ovary is 2.5 to 5.0 cm in length, 0.7 to 1.5 cm wide, and 1.5 to 3 cm in span.
- Inflammatory ovarian tumor (see Pelvic Inflammatory Disease).

- Metaplastic ovarian tumor (see Endometriosis).
- Neoplastic ovarian tumor may be palpable by an abdominal exam; percussion may reveal dullness anteriorly with tympany toward the flanks as a result of bowel displacement. Bimanual examination may reveal an adnexal mass, but the clinician should never be reassured by a negative bimanual in the presence of other signs and symptoms, even if vague.

The bimanual pelvic examination should include a rectovaginal examination. Palpate the uterus, adnexae and cervix; repeat with rectovaginal exam. Rectovaginal exam allows detection of lateral and posterior masses. Uterus should be midline. Cervical motion tenderness indicates inflammation versus cyst or tumor. Benign masses are generally cystic, smooth, less than 8 cm and mobile.

Diagnostic Tests and Methods

In some situations, it may be appropriate to begin an initial diagnostic workup, the description of which follows; however, *if the client is premenarcheal or postmenopausal and a palpable adnexal mass is discovered, then refer her immediately to a gynecologist for further evaluation and management* (Rosenfeld, 2001).

Pregnancy Test. Diagnostic evaluation to rule out pregnancy (uterine enlargement may be mistaken for an adnexal mass) and ectopic pregnancy. A urine or blood sample is obtained and measured for quantitative human chorionic gonadotropin (hCG).

Explain the procedure to the client and determine her last normal menstrual period.

Pelvic Ultrasound. Ultrasonography (US) is the primary imaging modality in the evaluation of an ovarian mass and has been made even more accurate with the use of color Doppler flow imaging (Kenkel, et al., 2000; Rosenfeld, 2001). Explain to the client the various aspects of the ultrasound procedure (see Adenomyosis).

Laparotomy/Laparoscopy. Diagnostic evaluation of any adnexal mass larger than 8 cm or any adnexal mass in a premenarcheal or postmenopausal client. (See Endometriosis for the test procedure.)

DIFFERENTIAL MEDICAL DIAGNOSES

Pelvic inflammatory disease (PID), endometriosis, uterine leiomyomas, nongynecologic masses (e.g., neoplastic colon mass), pelvic kidney, pregnancy. If rupture or torsion of the mass occurs and pain is present, rule out ectopic pregnancy and acute PID.

PLAN

If the mass is smaller than 8 cm, unilateral, mobile, smooth, and suspected to be a functional ovarian cyst, then wait and reevaluate the mass after the next menstrual period. If the mass does not meet these criteria or if it does not regress after the next menstrual period, then the health care provider must consult with a gynecologist and refer the client for further evaluation and management. In addition, refer all premenarcheal and postmenopausal clients with a palpable adnexal mass immediately.

Psychosocial Interventions

The client will experience major fear and anxiety with any suspicion of malignancy. Therefore, it is particularly important to provide support, encouragement, and reassurance during any period of observation or evaluation. Stress the importance of compliance with diagnostic testing requirements and of keeping scheduled appointments. Make certain that she understands that early diagnosis and treatment provide the best prognosis.

Medication

An oral contraceptive (OC) is indicated in the management of a functional ovarian cyst. By suppressing gonadotropin levels, the OC increases resolution of the cyst (Rosenfeld, 2001).

Details about OC administration, side effects, and contraindications are discussed in Chapter 9. The anticipated outcome on evaluation is complete resolution of the adnexal mass (functional cyst).

Provide the client with detailed instructions about taking OCs; stress the importance of not skipping any pills. Warn her that pregnancy is possible during the first cycle of pills, and urge use of a barrier method of contraception; and emphasize the importance of returning for the follow-up visit immediately after the first menstrual cycle.

Surgical Interventions

Surgical exploration and management of adnexal masses is headed by a board-certified surgeon specializing in gynecology. The surgical procedure varies with the type of ovarian tumor, but the health care provider should be aware of the possibilities in order to provide counseling and support to the client. Definitive treatment will depend on the client's age and her desire for reproductive capability.

Epithelial ovarian neoplasms may be managed with unilateral salpingo-oophorectomy, including appendectomy. If the client is older than 40, then total abdominal hysterectomy and bilateral salpingo-oophorectomy may be indicated. On the other hand, if the client is young and nulliparous and the ovarian neoplasm is unilocular with no excrescences within the cyst, an ovarian cystectomy that preserves the ovary is performed.

Stromal neoplasms may be managed with unilateral salpingo-oophorectomy and appendectomy. If the client is older than 40, then a total abdominal hysterectomy and bilateral salpingo-oophorectomy may be indicated.

Germ cell tumors are managed with an ovarian cystectomy if future childbearing is desired. If it is not desired, then total abdominal hysterectomy and bilateral salpingo-oophorectomy are indicated (Callahan et al., 2001).

FOLLOW-UP AND REFERRAL

If a functional ovarian mass is suspected, follow-up examination should occur in four to six weeks, or immediately after the next menstrual period. If the mass persists, referral to a gynecologist for further evaluation and management is necessary.

DYSPAREUNIA

Dyspareunia or painful coitus, occurs either on intromission (entry) or on deep penetration of the penis. Pain results from any number of factors, such as infection, inflammation, anatomic abnormalities, pelvic pathology, atrophy or failure of lubrication, or psychological conflicts (Heim, 2001).

EPIDEMIOLOGY

Introital pain may be caused by vulvovaginitis (recurrent and chronic), vulvar vestibulitis (see section on Vulvar Disorders), urethritis/urethral syndrome, interstitial cystitis, cervicitis, lack of lubrication, or levator spasm. Pain on deep penetration may be caused by uterine retroversion, pelvic relaxation, endometriosis, adhesions, adenomyosis, pelvic congestion syndrome or lack of vaginal expansion due to insufficient arousal (Rosenfeld, 2001).

Risk factors for dyspareunia include menopause, psychological factors (including restrictive sexual attitudes), relationship difficulties and history of sexual trauma, history of sexually transmitted disease (STD), recurrent infection (candidiasis), and poor hygiene (Heim, 2001; Marin, King, Sfameni, & Dennerstein, 2000; Rosenfeld, 2001).

The incidence is unclear because clients tend not to report dyspareunia to health professionals. Of the reported cases, the most common cause is vulvo/vaginitis infection. Studies vary in reported incidence of dyspareunia ranging from 8 to 48 percent (Heim, 2001; Rosenfeld, 2001).

SUBJECTIVE DATA

A client's history is crucial to determining if the client has pain and if so, the etiology of dyspareunia. One problem, such as vaginitis, may cause another problem, such as anxiety or fear about pain with intercourse, thus altering sexual response, decreasing lubrication, and increasing pain. Pain may occur on intromission or on deep penetration; it may occur after long pain free intervals or with first intercourse. Vaginal discharge or irritation may be present. There may be a history of chronic pelvic pain. Relationship difficulties may be reported. The client may have been unable to use tampons previously or may have had difficult pelvic exams. Menopausal symptoms may be beginning (ACOG, 2001, TB 211; Heim, 2001; Rosenfeld, 2001).

OBJECTIVE DATA

Physical Examination

Examination includes the genitalia and reproductive tract. The vulvar/vaginal mucosa may reveal irritation, inflammation, lesions, discharge, atrophy, hymenal remnants, Bartholin's cyst/abscess or vestibulitis (focal irritation/inflammation of the vestibular glands, see section on Vulvar Disorders). Involuntary contractions of the perineal muscles (vaginismus) may occur during a speculum or digital exam, prohibiting examination. In this situation, proceed carefully and allow the client control during pelvic exam. Bimanual exam may reveal uterine prolapse, pelvic mass, nodularity of endometriosis, cervical motion tenderness of pelvic inflammatory disease, or loss of pelvic support (cystocele, rectocele) (Heim, 2001).

Diagnostic Tests and Methods

Select tests discriminately as indicated by the findings of the history and physical examination. Review previous test results in order to avoid unnecessary and repetitive diagnostic testing.

Complete Blood Count (CBC) and Erythrocyte Sedimentation Rate (ESR). Diagnostic evaluation to detect any inflammatory process (see Pelvic Inflammatory Disease for test procedure). The white blood cell (WBC) count and ESR are elevated in pelvic inflammatory disease.

Urinalysis. Diagnostic evaluation to identify any urinary tract conditions that might be a source of pain. White blood cells, bacteria, or red blood cells in the urine may indicate chronic or recurrent urinary tract infection (UTI).

To enhance test accuracy, explain to the client how to obtain a clean catch urine sample in a sterile container.

Pregnancy Test (Urine or Blood Level of β-hCG). Diagnostic evaluation to detect unsuspected intrauterine pregnancy or suspected ectopic pregnancy (see Pelvic Inflammatory Disease for procedure).

Vaginal Smears/Cervical Cultures. Diagnostic evaluation to determine whether infection is present. Wet mount with normal saline is used to detect bacterial vaginosis or trichomoniasis; potassium hydroxide (IOH) preparation is used to detect candidiasis; and cervical tests can detect *N. gonorrhoeae* and *C. trachomatis* (see Chapter 11 for the test procedures).

Ultrasound. Diagnostic evaluation using ultrasound may be useful if a bimanual exam is difficult, as with clients who are obese or unable to tolerate the exam. The procedure is most useful in diagnosing acute pelvic pain conditions, such as ruptured ovarian cyst, adnexal masses, or ectopic pregnancy; it should not be performed in clients with a clearly negative pelvic examination (see Adenomyosis for the test procedure).

Diagnostic Laparoscopy. Diagnostic evaluation is accomplished by directly visualizing the pelvic pathology that may be causing dyspareunia (see Endometriosis for the test procedure).

DIFFERENTIAL MEDICAL DIAGNOSES

Vulvovaginitis, atrophic vulvovaginitis, vulvar vestibulitis, urethritis, urethral syndrome, cystitis, cervicitis, muscle spasm, hymenal strands, scar tissue, episiotomy, vaginismus, pelvic relaxation, uterine prolapse, PID, endometriosis, adenomyosis, adhesions, pelvic masses, Bartholin's cyst. Consider possible contributing psychological factors, such as previous sexual trauma, conflictual relationships, stress, or restrictive sexual attitudes.

Also consider inappropriate sexual technique, including lack of foreplay, or low estrogen in the oral contraceptive (ACOG, 2001, TB 211; Heim, 2001).

PLAN

The management of dyspareunia depends on the symptoms and etiology.

Psychosocial Interventions

Refer the client for psychotherapy if her history reveals the possibility of a psychological component to the dyspareunia or if significant discord is present in the couple's relationship. Select a therapist with special training in sexual problems. Discuss fully with the client the findings of the physical examination and diagnostic testing, and include her partner whenever possible. Address and discuss all client fears, concerns, and anxieties. Sexual attitudes may need to be addressed (ACOG, 2001, TB 211; Rosenfeld, 2001).

Medication

The etiology of the dyspareunia determines whether medication is prescribed.

* *Vaginitis/Sexually Transmitted Disease.* See Chapter 11.
* *Atrophic Vaginitis.*
  * Hormonal replacement therapy (HRT) (see Chapter 15). HRT may be the treatment of choice for perimenopausal or menopausal women with atrophic vaginitis. Estrogen revitalizes atrophic tissues.
  * A water-based lubricant (K-Y jelly or Replens) available over the counter or vegetable oil or shortening is indicated for poor vaginal lubrication. The lubricant may be administered prior to or during intercourse to improve vaginal lubrication and enhance foreplay. Do not use latex contraceptives with vegetable-based lubricants. Vaginal suppositories may be inserted three times weekly, without regard to intercourse. Instructing the client in the use of a lubricant is important.
  * Anticipated outcomes on evaluation are improved vaginal lubrication and relief of dyspareunia secondary to vaginal dryness. Local allergic irritation is a potential adverse reaction, however, that would contraindicate lubricant use.
* *Pelvic Inflammatory Disease, Endometriosis, Adnexal Mass, and Leiomyoma.* Medications for these

causes of dyspareunia are described in other sections of this chapter.

Surgical Intervention

The cause of dyspareunia determines whether surgery is necessary. In cases where surgical evaluation is needed, referral should be made to a board-certified gynecologist. For descriptions of specific surgical interventions, see the appropriate section in this chapter: Endometriosis, Pelvic Inflammatory Disease, Adnexal Masses, Leiomyomas, or Pelvic Relaxation Syndrome. Other surgical interventions would depend on the specific cause, such as marsupialization of a Bartholin's cyst.

Progressive Dilation and Muscle Awareness Exercise

This procedure, with appropriate counseling, is indicated for clients with vaginismus, an anatomically narrow introitus, hymenal remnants or scar tissue, or psychogenic factors.

Begin by reviewing the anatomy and physiology of the sexual organs and sexual response, stressing the normalcy of vulvar tissue. Using a mirror, have the client become familiar with her genitalia. Instruct the client on how to perform Kegel's exercises to increase her awareness of the muscles involved. Involve the client's partner whenever possible.

For progressive dilation, the client or health care provider inserts progressively larger objects into the vagina, beginning with a single finger, then a medium Pederson's speculum, two fingers, and finally a medium Graves' speculum. Measured vaginal dilators are also available. Allow the client to stop at any point that pain occurs. Have her bear down on insertion and use water-soluble lubricant to alleviate discomfort.

Progressive digital dilation may be practiced by the client at home in order to familiarize her with her tissue, sensitization, and muscular control. The partner is gradually included in a "bridge-over" manner. Cross-wise intercourse position is suggested to provide the woman with more control over entry and penetration depth (ACOG, 2001, TB 211; Rosenfeld, 2001).

FOLLOW-UP AND REFERRAL

As with the entire evaluation and plan of care for clients with dyspareunia, follow-up will depend on the cause and the therapy selected. Follow-up evaluation is important, especially when dyspareunia is multifactorial. Stress to the client the importance of keeping follow-up appointments. Reassess the client frequently to determine whether psychological intervention is needed.

NONMALIGNANT DISORDERS OF THE VULVA

The client who presents with vulvar symptoms requires conscientious evaluation by the primary care provider/nurse practitioner. Knowledge of the more common nonmalignant disorders of the vulva is important in deciding whether to initiate careful medical therapy or to refer for further evaluation and management, including biopsy and/or surgical therapy. In this section, the more common vulvar conditions are presented. The clinician will most often find her or himself confronted with the client complaining of vulvar burning, itching, and pain. For this reason, vulvar pain/discomfort/irritation will be the primary focus. It is helpful for the practitioner to have available for reference a comprehensive textbook of genital dermatology and/or vulvar disorders.

Most clients who present with either recurrent pain, itching, burning, or irritation are frustrated, desperate for relief, and have previously used a variety of antifungal and/or steroid creams. Many will have already seen a variety of health care providers without resolution of symptoms. Psychological distress, depression, and anxiety may be present as either a risk factor for the current problem or as a result of the chronic discomfort.

The practitioner is in a unique position to obtain a comprehensive, detailed history related to the problem, to identify possible causative factors, to initiate and evaluate therapy, and to provide emotional support. The more experience the clinician gains, the better she or he is able to evaluate and manage vulvar problems. It is most critical to recognize the need for referral to a knowledgeable specialist when necessary.

VULVODYNIA

The International Society for the Study of Vulvar Disease (ISSVD) defines *vulvodynia* as chronic vulvar discomfort characterized by the client's complaint of burning, stinging, irritation, and/or rawness (Kreiter, 2000). Vulvodynia, "burning vulva syndrome" or "vulvar pain syndrome," all terms for the same entity, includes subsets of vulvar disorders. These disorders include the following:

- *Vulvar vestibulitis.* Episodic or continuous stinging or burning accompanied by hyperemia and point tenderness of the vestibule and characterized by dyspareunia.

- *Cyclic vulvovaginitis.* Cyclic burning and/or itching centered around the menses and/or just after intercourse.
- *Vulvar dermatoses.* Characterized by noncyclic pruritus, scratching, dyspareunia and changes in the epithelium, such as in Lichen sclerosus.
- *Vulvar dysesthesia.* Also known as idiopathic vulvodynia, this condition consists of constant severe burning pain of the vulva in the absence of visible pathology (Spadt, 1995).

EPIDEMIOLOGY

The vulvar pain syndrome was recognized and described as early as 1889 by Dr. A.J.C. Skene in his *Treatise on the Diseases of Women*. Many theories exist as to the etiology for vulvodynia. It has been proposed that the syndrome may be precipitated by candidiasis infection, human papilloma virus (HPV), oxalate crystalluria (elevated urinary levels of calcium oxalate), contact dermatitis, allergic response, sexual dysfunction, emotional stress, or hormonal reactions. None of these hypotheses has been proven in the literature and, therefore, a specific etiology is unknown. Most experts agree that the etiology is most likely multifactorial with both pathophysiologic and psychological components (Bornstein, Maman, & Abramovici, 2001).

The exact incidence of vulvodynia is unknown due to the difficulty in making a diagnosis, but current estimates are about 15 percent in the general gynecologic population (Kreiter, 2000).

The client with vulvodynia will usually be white and nulliparous with a wide age range. Mean age range is about 32. The client will most likely have been to multiple clinicians for the condition. Research has shown a high incidence of sexual abuse. The client may have a history of allergies to various substances and/or repeated candida infections. There may be a higher incidence of depression. Sexual history reveals a limited number of sexual partners with a low incidence of history of STDs (Kreiter, 2000).

SUBJECTIVE DATA

Pain is often acute in onset and is described as "burning, stinging, irritation, or rawness." Onset may be associated with recent episodes of vaginitis. Dyspareunia interferes with sexual function. Pain can be mild to severe, interfering with normal activities, and may be continuous or episodic.

Previous treatments have provided either partial or no relief. Clients will report having seen many different clinicians and will generally express frustration and anxiety.

The practitioner can play a major role in evaluating vulvodynia by obtaining a complete history. A comprehensive history for evaluating vulvodynia should include all of the following information (Bergeron, Yitzchak, Khalife, Pagidas, & Glazer, 2001; Kreiter, 2000; Spadt, 1995).

- Description of the client's major symptoms including the duration, quality, cyclicity, and any aggravating or soothing factors.
- Any precipitating event that correlated to the onset of symptoms.
- Complete sexual history including any current or past history of abuse, number of partners, past history of STDs.
- Hygiene habits including use of powders, types of soaps, overbathing, scrubbing, or excessive douching, feminine hygiene sprays.
- Use of personal products such as dryer sheets, types of tampons, chronic use of minipads, contraceptive gels, foams, or suppositories, use of condoms, lubricants.
- Exercise habits such as biking, aerobics, swimming, running, and intensity and frequency of workout sessions.
- Relationship of vulvar symptoms to urinary symptoms.
- History of musculoskeletal trauma, back pain or congenital skeletal abnormalities.
- List of previous treatments used, results of any previous cultures or other diagnostic testing and response to treatments.
- Psychological history including history of traumatic events, marital stress, history of chronic pain, history of depression or anxiety disorder.

OBJECTIVE DATA

Physical Examination

Initial inspection of the vulva generally fails to reveal any obvious abnormality. Closer exam may reveal hyperemia, fine linear excoriations, and/or thickening, atrophy, or whitening of the epithelium in vulvar dermatoses. The vulvar vestibulum consists of the area between the labia minora and hymenal ring, extending upward to the frenulum of the clitoris and posteriorly from the fourchette to the vaginal introitus. The vulvar vestibulum includes the urethra, Skene's glands, Bartholin's glands, and the minor vestibular glands.

Micropapillations are a normal finding of the vulva. Frequently misdiagnosed as HPV, these normal anatomical findings are 1 to 3 mm symmetric papillae that may cover most of the mucosal surface of the labia minora. HPV is more patchy (Black, McKay, & Braude, 1995; Kreiter, 2000; Lynch & Edwards, 1994).

The Q-tip test *may be useful* for assessing vulvar vestibulitis. This test consists of touching the vestibulum lightly with a moist cotton-tipped swab. Ask the client to respond by rating the amount of discomfort she experiences in each area of the vestibulum. Clients with vulvar vestibulitis may experience marked pain at 5 and 7 o'clock between the introitus and posterior fourchette (Bergeron et al., 2001; Black et al., 1995; Lynch & Edwards, 1994).

Although vaginal exam is usually unremarkable in the client with vulvodynia, obtain vaginal secretions for saline and KOH wet mounts. Inspect the vagina for any abnormalities. Use of a Pederson speculum is essential to minimize discomfort.

Screen for any musculoskeletal abnormalities including asymmetry of the spine.

Diagnostic Tests and Methods

Wet Mount and Cultures. Indicated for making a differential diagnosis and for determining any precipitating etiology(ies). Examination of vaginal secretions should include a pH determination and careful microscopic exam for the presence of hyphae, clue cells, trichomonas, lactobacilli, and/or WBCs. The practitioner whenever possible should examine his or her own microscopic slides. Cultures for candidiasis, chlamydia, gonorrhea may be necessary.

- *Vulvar Biopsy*. Indicated for any diagnostically questionable areas or for any suspicion of vulvar intraepithelial neoplasia. Not usually helpful in differentiating vestibulitis. The following are suggested indications for vulvar biopsy.
- Lesions surrounded by either thickened skin or color changes.
- Slightly raised, red, or pigmented lesions.
- Lesions presumed to be genital warts, which do not respond to therapy.
- Chronic dermatoses that do not respond to therapy.
- Any suspicious lesion for neoplasia (Larrabee & Kylander, 2001).

Unless the practitioner has specialized training in vulvar biopsy, referral should be made to either a dermatologist or gynecologist for the procedure. Under local anesthesia, the lesion is biopsied using one of these techniques. The shave biopsy is indicated when the lesion is superficial. A #15 scalpel blade is used to remove a sample of skin well under the lesion but not through to fat. Sutures are not used. Monsel's solution or silver nitrate is used for controlling any bleeding. The punch biopsy is indicated for an ulcer or inflammatory skin condition and removes epidermis, dermis, and some fat. A special punch instrument such as a Keyes biopsy is used, and simple sutures may be necessary.

The biopsy procedure is rapid and can be performed in the office setting, and adverse reactions are rare. Explain to the client the purpose of the procedure and how it will be done. Reassure the client that adverse effects are unusual; rarely, women experience scarring, infection, soreness, bleeding, or bruising. Tissue is sent to a pathologist for diagnostic evaluation.

Aceto-whitening/Colposcopy of the Vulva. Application of acetic acid solution with the use of a specialized microscopic instrument called a colposcope is indicated for directed biopsy and when there is a history of HPV. Colposcopy should also be performed of the vagina and cervix if HPV is found on the vulva. Typically, aceto-white lesions that are diffuse and flat are a result of chronic trauma or inflammation, and those that are raised are typical of HPV infection.

Unless the practitioner has specialized formal training, certification, and experience with colposcopy, referral should be made to the gynecologist for colposcopy.

DIFFERENTIAL MEDICAL DIAGNOSES

Lichen sclerosus, Lichen planus, contact dermatitis, candidiasis, postmenopausal atrophic vaginitis, human papillomavirus infection, herpes simplex infection, pudendal neuralgia, overuse of topical steroids, erythema multiform, Bechet's disease, Reiter's disease, pellagra (Kreiter, 2000; Larrabee & Kylander, 2001).

PLAN

Psychosocial Interventions

The most important intervention in caring for the client with vulvodynia is to validate her feelings. Acknowledge that her pain is real and encourage her to become a partner in her care. Explain the multifactorial nature of the problem and that currently, there is no single known etiology for the condition. Suggest the use of a journal for recording exacerbations and possible related events, foods eaten, stressful events, etc. Request that she not self-medicate and initially, that she be seen for office evaluation during acute episodes. This allows the practitioner to differentiate obvious causes that may confuse the clinical picture such as trichomoniasis, candidiasis, bacterial vaginosis, or urinary tract infection. Include the partner on all discussions to increase his understanding.

Refer for psychiatric evaluation and intervention if there are clinical signs of depression and/or history of sexual abuse. Refer couples for sexual therapy when indicated (Kreiter, 2000).

Medication

Before initiating medical therapy, stop all current topical vulvar medications and review proper vulvar hygiene including the use of cotton underwear, avoidance of constrictive clothing that promotes heat and chafing (pantyhose, jeans, spandex shorts, tights, etc.), use of unscented, hypoallergenic products, avoidance of chemical allergens (hygiene sprays, perfumes, talcum powders, shaving lotions), and use of vaginal lubricants that are nonirritating. Most experts in the area of vulvar disorders recommend the use of Crisco or other vegetable oil as a lubricant for use during intercourse (do not use latex contraceptives with vegetable lubricants). One may also use Vitamin E skin oil (Kreiter, 2000; Spadt, 1995).

Because medical therapy is specific to each subset of vulvodynia, Table 13–2 will be utilized to provide descriptions of the various diagnostic subsets, identifying characteristics and commonly accepted medical therapies. Table 13–3 describes common differential diagnoses, characteristics and treatment.

Medium-Potency Topical Steroids (triamcinolone acetonide 0.1 percent, hydrocortisone valerate 0.2 percent, betamethasone valerate 0.1 percent)

- *Indications*. Prompt improvement of symptoms of Lichen sclerosus.
- *Administration*. Apply thinly b.i.d. to t.i.d.; prescribe in small tubes without refills, ointment base more soothing.
- *Side-Effects and Adverse Reactions*. Super-infection, atrophy, steroid dermatitis, and striae.
- *Contraindications*. Allergy to topical steroids.
- *Anticipated Outcomes on Evaluation*. Relief of symptoms and improvement of the disease process. Noticeable healing of skin, lessening of white lesions.

TABLE 13–2. Evaluation and Management of Common Vulvar Disorders

Disorder	Diagnostic Characteristics		Medical Therapy	Adjunct Therapy
	Subjective	*Objective*		
Vulvar Vestibulitis	Burning, stinging, irritation, rawness, entry dyspareunia	Positive Q-tip test, hyperemia	Topical anesthetics: *2–5 percent topical Xylocaine, alpha-interferon injections,* * *calcium citrate* **	Low-oxalate diet; vestibulectomy*
Dysesthetic Vulvodynia	Constant, severe, burning pain, most common in perimenopausal or menopausal women	Little or no objective findings	Tricyclic antidepressants: *Amitriptyline, 10–75 mg daily*	Psychological counseling; physical therapy; biofeedback
Cyclic Vulvovaginitis	Itching, burning, cyclic, often related to the menses; irritation following coitus; frequent use of antibiotics	Erythema, edema of the vulva with fissure, pustules, scaling, +KOH or yeast culture	Suppressive therapy; 4–6 mos. oral antifungals (*ketodonazole, Diflucan*)	
Lichen Sclerosus	Pruritus, pain, or may be asymptomatic	Well demarcated white plaques of thin, fragile skin; agglutination of labia in advanced cases; may be sores, excoriations	Medium-potent topical steroid, ointment based (*triamcinolone*) or *testosterone cream*, b.i.d. for 4–6 mos., then twice/wk	Monitor annually for malignancy; biopsy as indicated; sleep aids when itching or pain is severe

* Requires physician consultation/referral.
** Theoretical.

Source: Black et al., 1995; Kreiter, 2000; Larrabee & Kylander, 2001; Lynch & Edwards, 1994.

TABLE 13–3. Common Nonmalignant Vulvar Disorders: Differential Diagnoses

| Disorder | Diagnostic Characteristics | | Medical Therapy | Adjunct Therapy |
	Subjective	*Objective*		
Contact/Allergic Dermatitis	Pruritis, burning, stinging; begins 1–2 days after exposure to an irritating agent	Hyperemic, may be vesicular, marked edema, scaling, linear plaques, papules, fissuring, lichenification	Wet prep to r/o yeast; possible biopsy if hx. unclear; low or midpotency steroids; night-time sedation w/antihistamine or tricyclic antidepressant	Avoid all irritants
Seborrheic Dermatitis	More common in men than women; more common in AIDS pts	Erythematous, poorly margined plaques; yellow scale w/greasy texture; lesions occur more in scalp, ears, central face; more severe cases affect genitalia	1 percent hydrocortisone cream; severe cases: oral prednisone, 40 mg 5–10 days	Good hygiene
Hidradenitis	Occurs primarily in the axilla, anogenital areas; occurs after puberty, ages 20–40; higher incidence in African Americans	Red papules, multiform, enlarge to be nodular or cystic; resembles furuncles; draining, scarring, edema may occur; regional lymphadenopathy present	*Tetracycline 500 mg* b.i.d. for several mos; *oral contraceptives* at 50 mcg	Refer for surgery w/severe cases
Furunculosis	Presence of painful boils; fever, malaise may be present	Erythematous nodules that drain	*Dicloxacillin, Cephalexin, Erythromycin*	
Epidermal Cysts	Asymptomatic	White or yellow nodule, firm nontender, varies in size 1mm–several cms.; located near hair follicles		I & D
Lichen Planus	Pain, itching purulent, painful irritating discharge	Well circumscribed flat-topped papules; shiny surface, white, fernlike lesions; ulcers/erosions may be present; may be lesions in the mouth; may be increased vaginal discharge; Vaginal pH > 5.0	Mid- to high-potency topical steroid, b.i.d.	Vulvar biopsy

Source: Black et al., 1995; Lynch & Edwards, 1994.

♦ *Client Teaching and Counseling.* Instruct to apply creams sparingly, in a thin layer and only as often as prescribed. Review the risks of atrophy of the normal skin with overuse.

High-Potency Topical Steroid, Clobetasol Propionate (Temovate)

♦ *Indications.* Improvement of symptoms quickly in more severe, long-standing cases of Lichen sclerosus (Larrabee & Kylander, 2001).

♦ *Administration.* Apply thinly once or twice daily to affected area for about twelve weeks.

♦ *Side Effects, Adverse Reactions, Contraindications, Anticipated Outcomes on Evaluation, Client Teach-*

ing. The same as associated with medium-potency topical steroids.

Testosterone Propionate 2 Percent

♦ *Indications.* Most often used treatment for Lichen sclerosus. Recent research findings, however, indicate that testosterone may have little place in current treatment of Lichen sclerosus (Larrabee & Kylander, 2001).

♦ *Administration.* Must be made up by the pharmacist of 2 percent testosterone propriate in petrolatum. Should be replaced every six months. Apply to affected area twice a day for four to six months. When improvement occurs, taper to twice/week.

- *Side Effects and Adverse Reactions.* Clitoral hypertrophy, increased libido, hirsutism, deepening of the voice. The most common side effect is local irritation and flare up of itching and irritation.
- *Contraindications.* Should not be used in children.
- *Expected Outcomes on Evaluation.* Relief of symptoms. There is generally no improvement in the appearance of the skin.
- *Client Teaching and Counseling.* Discuss possible side effects and advise the client to report changes as soon as possible.
- Testosterone propionate 2 percent and hydrocortisone valerate 0.2 percent, 30 g in a petroleum base; may be ordered from a compounding pharmacy. Women report that this special compounded formulation may be very helpful. Prescribe b.i.d. for two to four weeks, then as needed.

Amitriptyline

- *Indications.* Treatment of essential vulvodynia.
- *Administration.* Initiate at the lowest dose of 10 to 25 mg p.o. in early evening. Gradually increase until relief of symptoms up to 75 mg. Continue at least two months.
- *Side Effects and Adverse Reactions.* Drowsiness, dry mouth, weight gain, tinnitus, palpitations, constipation, loss of balance (especially in the elderly).
- *Contraindications.* Previous hypersensitivity. Should not be given concurrently with monoamine oxidase inhibitors.
- *Expected Outcomes on Evaluation.* Relief of symptoms of burning, pain, and irritation.
- *Client Education and Counseling.* Reassure the client that mitriptyline is commonly used to manage pain syndromes because of its effect on cutaneous nerves and not because they are "crazy" or that the problem is psychosomatic. Discuss common side effects. Advise the client that she will begin with the lowest dosage and will increase the dose by 10 mg every one to two weeks until relief is achieved. If she has difficulty arising in the morning, she may take it at dinnertime.

Antifungals. See Chapter 11.

Topical Anesthetics (Xylocaine Jelly 2 percent or Ointment 5 percent)

- *Indications.* Relief of symptoms of vulvar vestibulitis, may be prescribed for use during sexual activity. First-line therapy for management of vulvar vestibulitis (Kreiter, 2000).

- *Administration.* Apply first in the office setting with a cotton swab to check for burning and local irritation. Then, the client may apply the gel or ointment 15 minutes before anticipated coital activity.
- *Side Effects and Adverse Reactions.* Local irritation.
- *Contraindications.* Should not be used in clients with allergy to benzocaines.
- *Expected Outcomes on Evaluation.* Relief of symptoms, decrease in dyspareunia.
- *Client Teaching and Counseling.* Instruct in proper application. Advise clients to avoid activities that might irritate the affected tissues. Add other lubricants during intercourse.

Interferon

- *Indications.* Last line therapy for vulvar vestibulitis recommended in conjunction with physician consultation. (Black et al., 1995; Lynch & Edwards, 1994; Spadt, 1995).
- *Administration.* Local injections of 1 million units (0.2 mL) intradermally in the vestibule around the circumference on Monday, Wednesday, and Friday for four weeks for a total of twelve injections.
- *Side Effects and Adverse Reactions.* Myalgias, headache, fever and other flulike symptoms; develop about four hours after injection.
- *Contraindications.* Hypersensitivity.
- *Expected Outcomes on Evaluation.* Decrease in symptoms of pain and burning and dyspareunia.
- *Client Teaching and Counseling.* Take 650 mg of acetaminophen prior to the injection and every four to six hours afterward until flulike symptoms resolve. Document thorough informed consent.

Surgical Intervention

Vestibulectomy. Excision of the vestibule to include the hymenal ring. The vagina is undermined and advanced to cover the area. This procedure is indicated when pain and discomfort are severe and interfere with normal daily living and when conservative measures fail. Success rates are reported at 60 to 90 percent. Adverse outcomes include the potential risks involved with anesthesia, postoperative pain, and possible scarring. The anticipated outcomes on evaluation are the complete relief of symptoms with return to normal sexual function.

Discuss with the client the potential risks and the benefits of the surgery. Warn that pain may continue long-term following the surgery. Explain the procedure using anatomical models. The procedure should only be performed by an experienced gynecologic surgeon.

Dietary Interventions

Low-Oxalate Diet. One theory concerning vulvar pain proposes that clients have an elevated urinary level of calcium oxalate, an end product of metabolism. Therefore, it may be beneficial to provide the client with a list of foods that may represent possible dietary irritants and advise her to avoid or limit these particular foods. The following foods are considered to increase calcium oxalate:

- *Beverages*. All teas, coffee, cocoa, and most wines.
- *Fruits and Vegetables*. Beans, beets, berries, celery, cranberries, cranberry juice, eggplant, green peppers, lima beans, plums, prunes, rhubarb, spinach, summer squash, sweet potatoes, tomatoes, vegetable soup, Vitamin C supplement > 250 mg/day.
- *Spices and Condiments*. Black pepper, chiles, dill, mustard, soy sauce, vinegar.
- *Other*. Chocolate, fruit cake, nuts, peanut butter, tofu, wheat germ.

Although a 24-hour urine test for calcium oxalate may help confirm this theory and/or be used to evaluate dietary changes, it is often expensive and may not be covered by insurance. This therapy is best used empirically. Have the client keep a food recall diary and symptom record.

Alternative Therapies

As with any chronic pain syndrome, clients may benefit from biofeedback, massage, acupuncture, acupressure and/or hypnotism. Support the client in pursuing these avenues and evaluate for relief of symptoms.

FOLLOW-UP AND REFERRAL

Continuing, consistent follow-up is extremely important in managing vulvar pain syndromes. Careful observation for visible improvement or worsening of vulvar tissue is crucial. Offer continued emotional support. Clients may need to be seen biweekly when initiating therapy, monthly during active medical therapy, and perhaps every one to two months as improvement occurs.

If improvement does not occur or if the clinician is unsure of the diagnosis, referral to a specialist with knowledge of vulvar disorders is mandatory. Always be aware of the indications for vulvar biopsy (discussed earlier in this section) and refer when indicated. Refer for psychological evaluation and counseling when signs of depression are apparent, when sexual dysfunction is present, or in light of a history of sexual/physical abuse. Re-

ferral sources include the following: the Vulvar Pain Foundation, the National Vulvodynia Association (online at *www.nva.org*) and the Dr. Glazer Vulvodynia Web page (*www.vulvodynia.com*).

LEIOMYOMAS

Leiomyomas are benign smooth muscle tumors of the uterus, commonly called "fibroids." They are classified according to their location within the uterus.

- *Submucous*, protruding into the uterine cavity. Most commonly symptomatic, leading reason for hysterectomy (ACOG, 2001, CO 247).
- *Intramural*, within the myometrial wall.
- *Subserous*, growing toward the serous surface of the uterus.
- *Intraligamentous*, located in the cervix or in between the folds of the broad ligament.

Leiomyomas are estrogen dependent; they rarely occur before menarche or after menopause. Rarely malignant, leiomyomas may be small and asymptomatic or may grow very large and extend up into the abdomen. The two most common reasons for which women seek treatment are pelvic pressure or pain and menorrhagia. Often, menses last seven days or more and cause iron-deficiency anemia. The heavy bleeding may cause significant interruption in a client's normal daily activities. They are the most common indication for hysterectomy and account for an undetermined amount of major and minor conservative surgical procedures, outpatient consultations, and disabilities (ACOG, 2001, CO 247).

ETIOLOGY/EPIDEMIOLOGY

Leiomyomas develop from a single neoplastic smooth muscle cell. Cytogenetic analyses demonstrate abnormalities in chromosomal patterns, but it is still unclear what factors are responsible for the initial neoplastic transformation. Growth of uterine leiomyomata is influenced by steroid hormones including estrogen and progesterone (ACOG, 2001, CO 247; Stewart, 2001).

This condition occurs in 25 to 50 percent of women of reproductive age with a three to nine times higher incidence in African American women (ACOG, 2001, PB 16). Increased risk is also associated with women who are nulliparous, over age 35, obese, sedentary, or who are nonsmokers (Chiaffarino, Parazzini, LaVecchia, Marsico, Surace, & Ricci, 1999). It is no longer accepted that oral contraceptives increase the risk for leiomyomas (Stewart, 2001).

SUBJECTIVE DATA

The majority of clients with uterine leiomyomas are asymptomatic. Symptoms increase as the tumors grow and can be characterized by abnormal uterine bleeding, pelvic pressure and pain, and reproductive dysfunction (ACOG, 2001, CO 247; Stewart, 2001).

OBJECTIVE DATA

Physical Examination

An abdominal exam may reveal a large mass if the leiomyoma has grown larger than a twelve- to fourteen-week pregnant uterus. The absence of ascites and presence of rebound tenderness and normal bowel sounds should be noted.

The genitalia and reproductive tract are also examined. Examine cervix for any extraneous tissue or distortion and examine any bleeding or discharge. Prior to the pelvic exam, ask the client to empty her bladder so that the examiner avoids confusing the tumor with the bladder. A pelvic exam may reveal an enlarged uterus that is firm and irregular but not tender. Usually palpated at midline, a leiomyoma may feel very firm or soft and cystic. If it is situated laterally, it may be mistaken for an adnexal mass. If the mass moves with the cervix, then it is likely to be a leiomyoma. Size should be described in terms of gestational size (ACOG, 2001, CO 247; Stewart, 2001).

Diagnostic Tests and Methods

Hemoglobin or Hematocrit. Diagnostic evaluation to determine whether the client is anemic, especially if she has experienced menometrorrhagia. May usually be obtained by fingerstick and performed via traditional centrifuge or newer instant analyses.

Urinalysis. Diagnostic evaluation to identify urinary tract conditions that might account for any urinary tract symptoms. White blood cells, bacteria, or red blood cells in the urine may indicate chronic or recurrent urinary tract infection (UTI). Hematuria may indicate the presence of renal stone or a tumor of the urinary tract. Further diagnostic testing may be indicated, specifically cystoscopy or intravenous pyelogram.

Explain to the client how to obtain a clean catch urine sample.

Pregnancy Test (Urine or Blood Level of β-hCG). Diagnostic evaluation for unsuspected intrauterine pregnancy (see Pelvic Inflammatory Disease for procedure).

Stool Guiac (Colocare or Hemoccult). Diagnostic evaluation to detect gastrointestinal (GI) pathology that may be the source of a palpable abdominal mass, for example, an inflammatory diverticulum or an intestinal mass. A stool found to be positive for occult blood suggests GI polyps or malignancy, but that result alone is insufficient for a definitive diagnosis. If the test is positive, or if the client's history and physical exam are suggestive, then refer her for gastroenterology consultation and further diagnostic testing, such as upper GI series, barium enema, sigmoidoscopy, and/or colonoscopy.

With the Colocare method, the client floats a special card in the toilet after a bowel movement. A specific color change represents a positive result. The test should be repeated for three bowel movements at home. Alternatively, the older guaiac test (hemoccult) requires the client to smear a stool sample onto a card and return the card to the health care professional, who subsequently applies solution to it; bluish discoloration represents a positive result. This test also should be repeated three times.

Provide instructions that will prepare the client for the test. Tell her that for two days before the test and during the testing period she is not to eat red or rare meats and is not to take vitamin C supplements, laxatives, or medications such as aspirin, corticosteroids, reserpine, indomethacin, or phenylbutazone. A high fiber diet is advised.

Ultrasound. Diagnostic evaluation to identify the leiomyoma and confirm its location. Should identify the uterine volume, number of fibroids, location relative to the endometrial stripe, evaluation of adnexa, and a cursory scan of the kidneys. Ultrasound helps to distinguish between uterine leiomyoma and an adnexal mass, and helps in assessing obese clients or others for whom the exam is not well tolerated (see Adenomyosis for the test procedure).

Sonohysterography. Indicated for the evaluation of abnormal uterine bleeding, identification of intrauterine pathology such as endometrial polyps and submucosal fibroids. Useful in differentiating between fibroids and other etiologies for abdnormal uterine bleeding (Kovacs, 2001). See section on Dysfunctional Uterine Bleeding for description of procedure.

Barium Enema. See Adnexal Masses.

Diagnostic Hysteroscopy. Hysteroscopy employs the use of endoscopic equipment to view the uterine cavity. It enables direct examination of the endocervical canal and lower uterine segment.

The most common indications for hysteroscopy are evaluation of abnormal uterine bleeding and direct observation of uterine fibroids, polyps, adhesions, and location of IUDs. It enables the provider to identify the exact presence, location, size, and number of fibroids and is helpful in treatment planning.

Contraindications to the procedure include a recent or present episode of salpingitis or diagnosed cervical or uterine malignancy. The procedure should be performed with careful consideration in women who are bleeding heavily, pregnant, or have cardiovascular or systemic disease.

Risks are infrequent and include possible cervical trauma, uterine perforation, and infection.

Prior to the procedure, the client is placed in the dorsal lithotomy position and the cervix is cleansed with provodone iodine solution. Paracervical anesthesia may be employed. A light source, camera, carbon dioxide and saline lines are connected, and the hysteroscope is introduced through the cervical canal. The procedure in experienced hands takes about ten minutes.

Counsel the client that she may expect shoulder pain as a result of the CO_2 gas escaping into the abdomen and mild tolerable cramping. She will rest about ten minutes following the procedure and may return home afterward. Advise her to expect possible shoulder pain, cramping, and mild spotting to continue for the next one to three days. She should abstain from intercourse, douching, or use of tampons for two weeks and call if she experiences heavy bleeding, abdominal pain, discharge with odor or fever (Prather, 1995; Siegler, 1995).

DIFFERENTIAL MEDICAL DIAGNOSES

Ovarian neoplasm, tubo-ovarian inflammatory mass, diverticular inflammatory mass, pregnancy, ectopic pregnancy, adenomyosis, pelvic kidney, malignancy, interstitial cystitis, irritable bowel syndrome, obstipation.

PLAN

Psychosocial Interventions

Provide the client with explanations and printed information about leiomyomas (fibroids). Reassure her that leiomyomas occur commonly, that they are rarely malignant, and that if she is asymptomatic or if symptoms are

mild, treatment will be unnecessary. Assess her future reproductive plans and the extent of her symptoms. Stress the importance of regular monitoring and follow-up examinations.

If the client is or becomes pregnant, provide reassurance and support. Reassure her that in most pregnancies, fibroids do not grow enough to cause complication. Advise the client of the signs and symptoms of preterm labor later in the pregnancy.

Medical Management

Expectant Management. Fifty percent of clients with leiomyomata are asymptomatic. In these clients, reassure that no further intervention is necessary. Indications for the treatment of fibroids include menorrhagia, pelvic pressure or pain, infertility or habitual abortion, and compromise of adjacent organs (ACOG, 2001, CO 247).

Medication

The goal of medical therapy is to reduce the symptoms and myoma size.

NSAIDs

- *Indications.* To relieve discomfort and to decrease menorrhagia. Studies show a reduction in menorrhagia by 30 to 50 percent with the use of NSAIDs initiated one to two days prior to the expected menses (Rosenfeld, 2001).
- *Administration.* Several types of NSAIDs are available, and their dosages vary. The most widely accepted and least expensive are the following:
  - Ibuprofen 600 mg, p.o., q.i.d.
  - Naproxen sodium (Naprosyn, Anaprox, Aleve), 550 mg, p.o., b.i.d.
- *Side Effects and Adverse Reactions.* Most often reported is GI irritation. Advise taking with food or after meals.
- *Contraindications.* Previous allergy to NSAIDs and a history of ulcer disease.

Oral Iron Preparation

- *Indications.* The client who is experiencing significant menorrhagia or metrorrhagia and whose hemoglobin and hematocrit are falling below normal levels.
- *Administration.* Select one of many commercially available preparations. Begin with one tablet (300 mg ferrous sulfate or the equivalent) daily; increase to

two daily if hemoglobin falls below 10.0 g/dL. Follow with reticulocyte counts to monitor response to the therapy.

- *Side Effects and Adverse Reactions.* Constipation and other gastrointestinal symptoms, such as indigestion, nausea, loss of appetite.
- *Contraindication.* Known allergy to oral iron preparations.
- *Anticipated Outcome or Evaluation.* Anemia secondary to menometrorrhagia is prevented.
- *Client Teaching and Counseling.* Provide information about foods that are rich in iron (leafy green vegetables, enriched flour products, raisins, prunes, dried apricots). Instruct the client that for better absorption of the iron, she should take the preparation with a citrus juice and avoid eating or drinking dairy products for one hour before and one hour after.

Gonadotropin Releasing Hormone Agonist (GnRHa) (Leuprorelin, Nafarelin, Goserelin).
GnRH analogues bind to GnRH receptors resulting in a decrease in LH and FSH, which produces a hypoestrogenic effect.

- *Indications.* To suppress the growth of leiomyomas and promote possible shrinkage. GnRH-a is useful for reducing the size of the leiomyoma prior to surgery; it may permit vaginal hysterectomy rather than abdominal hysterectomy. It also may prevent the need for surgery in the perimenopausal client (Huime & Lambalk, 2001; Lethaby, Vollenhoven, & Sowter, 2002).
- *Administration. Leuprorelin (Lupron)*, 0.5 mg s.c., q.d. for eight to twelve weeks *or* 3.75–7.5 mg *Depot Luporn* once every twenty-eight days. *Nafarelin (Synarel)*, one spray (200 mg/spray) into one nostril q.a.m. and one spray into the other nostril q.h.s. eight to twelve weeks. *Goserelin (Zoladex)* consists of a small biodegradable cylinder that is inserted subcutaneously monthly.
- *Side Effects and Adverse Reactions.* Hot flashes (75 percent of clients report hot flashes), vaginal dryness, mood swings, depression, weight gain, reduced breast size, decreased libido, fatigue, insomnia, headache, joint and muscle stiffness, and irregular vaginal bleeding.
- *Contraindications.* Known or suspected pregnancy, hypersensitivity to GnRH agonists, undiagnosed abnormal vaginal bleeding, breast-feeding.
- *Anticipated Outcomes on Evaluation.* A reduction in uterine and leiomyoma size.

- *Client Teaching and Counseling.* Instruct the client about proper drug administration and inform her that the GnRH agonists are very expensive. The length of therapy (eight to twelve weeks) needs to be discussed. Review the side effects and the possible need for calcium citrate supplementation. Barrier contraception is recommended during therapy and for the first menstrual cycle. Explain that it is likely that within six months following treatment the leiomyomas will recur.

Add-Back Therapy. See section on Endometriosis.

Surgical Intervention

Myomectomy. This procedure entails the abdominal removal of leiomyomata indicated when the client is symptomatic, the uterus is greater than twelve weeks' size, and conservation of fertility is desired (ACOG, 2001, CO 247; Stewart, 2001). The leiomyoma(s) appears to be either interfering with fertility or causing pregnancy loss.

Refer the client to a board-certified gynecologist. The size and location of the leiomyomas will determine the site of abdominal incision. Some surgeons are skilled at removing small myomas through the laparoscope or hysteroscope. Smaller tumors may be destroyed with the laser. The goal of surgery is to remove all leiomyomas, relieve symptoms, and increase fertility. Adverse effects may develop as a result of a difficult, demanding procedure with the potential for increased blood loss, increased operating time, increased postoperative risks of infection, ileus, anemia, and increased pain. Among women who undergo myomectomy, it is estimated that 51 percent have a recurrence at five years and must have repeated surgery due to recurrence (ACOG, 2001, CO 247). Most myomectomy clients who subsequently become pregnant will require delivery by cesarean section.

Discuss the difficult surgery and its potential complications with the client. Inform her about the high rate of myoma recurrence and the possible later need for a hysterectomy. Warn her not to attempt pregnancy until four to six months after the procedure. Review the postoperative/discharge instruction.

Hysterectomy. This procedure is definitive treatment, indicated when the fibroids become palpable abdominally and are a concern to the client or when menorrhagia occurs or worsens, placing the client at risk for anemia (ACOG, 2001, CO 247; Stewart, 2001). In addition, hysterectomy may be done to resolve any of the following: pelvic pain and secondary dysmenorrhea, urinary symptoms, or uterine growth after menopause. The surgery is indicated if the client has completed childbearing or if the health care provider is unable to evaluate the adnexa because the uterus has become an abdominal organ. The route of hysterectomy depends on the size of the leiomyoma—if less than twelve weeks' size, vaginal hysterectomy is possible.

Surgery should accomplish complete relief of symptoms. Few adverse effects occur; however, bleeding, infection, and damage to nearby organs are possible. After the surgery, the client is at risk for depression and sexual dysfunction.

Client teaching and counseling include discussion of the alternatives to hysterectomy, especially if there is indecision regarding future childbearing. Provide the client with a thorough explanation of hysterectomy, including descriptions of anatomy, physiology, and the surgical procedure, its risks and benefits. Reassure the client that femininity remains unchanged. Hormonal replacement therapy may need to be initiated if salpingo-oophorectomy is done. Full recovery usually occurs within six weeks. Review the postoperative instructions, including the return to activity, expectation that vaginal bleeding will change to clear discharge, signs of infection, resumption of sexual activity when bleeding ceases (usually in about fourteen days), and dietary counseling (including information about preventing constipation and weight gain).

Uterine Artery Embolization. This new radiologic technique provides an alternative to surgery. As of this writing, the number of women treated has been relatively small, the follow-up periods have been relatively short, and the safety of this procedure desiring pregnancy has not been fully demonstrated (ACOG, 2001, CO 247). The procedure involves partial blockage of the uterine arteries, and thus, decreased blood flow to the leiomyomatous uterus. Performed by a specially trained radiologist, an angiographic catheter is placed in the femoral artery and advanced over the aortic bifurcation to the contralateral internal iliac artery, and digital angiography is performed to identify the origin of the uterine artery. Once the microcatheter is deep within the uterine artery, the vessel is embolized with a special solution.

Uterine artery embolization might result in severe pelvic pain as viable uterine tissue becomes ischemic or infarcted. Most patients experience "postembolization syndrome," which may include pelvic pain, fever, malaise, nausea, and vomiting. Most patients are hospitalized overnight. Complications include infection, bleeding, pul-

monary embolus, and death, although thus far the incidence of these problems have been rare.

Current contraindications include pregnancy, infertility, future desire for pregnancy, uterus greater than twenty-four weeks' size.

Client teaching and counseling should include careful explanation of all alternatives for therapy, both medical and surgical. Referral should be made to a board-certified gynecologist with knowledge of this procedure and a radiologist with special training *and* significant experience with the procedure. Informed consent should include all possible complications of the procedure and the fact that the patient population and long-term studies are limited. Positive outcomes should be complete relief of pain, pressure, and bleeding without long-term recurrence (Klein & Schwartz, 2001; Spies, Ascher, Roth, Kim, Levy, & Gomez-Jorge, 2001).

FOLLOW-UP AND REFERRAL

For the client who is asymptomatic or has mild symptoms, the treatment of choice is expectant management (ACOG, 2001, CO 247; Stewart, 2001). During pregnancy, rest and analgesics are appropriate if pain is present. Stress the importance of keeping appointments for close follow-up. If expectant management, medical therapy, or myomectomy is chosen as a treatment option, the client should be reexamined at three- to six-month intervals. It is generally accepted that cancer does not develop from leiomyomata. The client may be monitored without risk of the development of cancer. Rapid increase in uterine size raises the question of malignancy (Stewart, 2001). Uterine size and the leiomyoma should be evaluated carefully by pelvic exam and, if necessary, ultrasound should be used. Discuss with the client any new or worsening symptomology. Alter the plan of care as necessary. Monitor hemoglobin and hematocrit frequently if menorrhagia or metrorrhagia is present. Refer for physician consultation if there is rapid increase in size, increase in menorrhagia or development, or increase in pain/pressure.

PELVIC RELAXATION SYNDROME

Pelvic relaxation syndrome is the failure of the pelvic musculature to maintain support and position of the pelvic organs. When supporting pelvic ligaments, muscles, and fascia can no longer withstand constant increased intra-abdominal pressure, such as that which occurs with obstetric damage, chronic coughing or straining, surgery, or aging, the vaginal wall weakens, descends, and the pelvic organs protrude into the vaginal canal. Five major types of genital prolapse may occur; cystocele, urethrocele, rectocele, enterocele, and uterine prolapse (ACOG, 2001, TB 214; Callahan et al., 2001). The vagina can also prolapse to or beyond the introitus but this generally occurs only when the uterus has been removed.

Types of Genital Prolapse

- *Cystocele*. Prolapse of the posterior bladder wall through the anterior vaginal wall.
- *Urethrocele*. Bulging of the urethra through the anterior vaginal wall; usually not a single entity, occurs with cystocele.
- *Rectocele*. Bulging of the bowel through the posterior vaginal wall; involves loss of support of the fascia and levator ani muscles.
- *Enterocele*. Bulging of the bowel through the posterior cul-de-sac and vaginal wall; may be part of a high rectocele.
- *Uterine Prolapse*. Descent of the uterus through the pelvic floor and into the vaginal canal (see Figure 13–1).

The extent of genital organ prolapse is described in terms of degree: first degree, prolapse of an organ into the vaginal canal; second degree, presence of an organ at the hymenal ring; third degree, presence of an organ beyond the hymenal ring; and fourth degree, organ is fully outside the hymenal ring (ACOG, 2001, TB 214).

EPIDEMIOLOGY

- Weakening of the pelvic support through the stretching and trauma of childbirth.
- Increased intra-abdominal pressure secondary to chronic respiratory problems, heavy lifting, ascites, obesity, and habitual straining due to constipation.
- Normal downward pressure because the human posture is erect.
- Atrophy of the supporting tissues with aging, especially after menopause.
- Congenital weakness.

Risk factors include obesity, caucasian race, multiparity, and menopause with lack of estrogen replacement (Callahan et al., 2001).

Pelvic relaxation occurs with increasing frequency during the postreproductive years; in fact, the majority of parous women show some evidence of pelvic relaxation.

There are nine million women in the United States over the age of 75 (Luber, Boero, & Choe, 2001). With the increase in the aging population, quality of life concerns are increasingly important when caring for this group of women. Factors related to prolapse of the pelvic organs will take a greater portion of the practitioner's time. A study by Luber et al. (2001) found that the median age of women seeking care for pelvic floor disorders was 61 years; however, half of the women seeking care were aged 30 to 60 years. With the population of the United States between the ages of 30 to 89 years expected to grow by 22 percent over the next thirty years, the practitioner should be prepared to deal with this common problem.

SUBJECTIVE DATA

Clients frequently state, "Something feels as if it is falling out." Other symptoms include backache, pelvic pressure or heaviness; bearing-down sensation; urinary frequency, urgency, or incontinence; dyspareunia; discomfort walking or sitting; difficult defecation; or protrusion of an organ through the introitus (ACOG, 2001, TB 214; Heit, Culligan, Rosenquist, & Shott, 2002).

OBJECTIVE DATA

Physical Examination

Physical examination, including complete gynecologic inspection, is the most important step in diagnosing pelvic relaxation.

During the physical examination, the practitioner should be assessing for any of the common complications of prolapse, such as mucosal hypertrophy, irritative bleeding, chronic excoriation, ulceration, and urinary retention (ACOG, 2001, TB 214; Callahan et al., 2001; Davila, 1996).

Examine the external genitalia for atrophy and any obvious protrusion of the uterus, bladder, urethra, or vaginal wall. Use lithotomy position and Sim's speculum (Graves' speculum may be used if the anterior blade is removed). Ask the client to perform the Valsalva maneuver; note which organ prolapses first and the degree to which it occurs.

Systematically examine the anterior and posterior walls of the vagina. Ask the client to contract the pubococcygeal muscles (Kegel's exercise); with two fingers in the vagina, note the strength and symmetry of the contraction. Note any ulcerations of the cervix and uterus if third degree prolapse is present. Note bladder leakage during the exam.

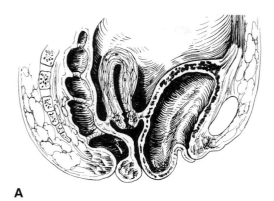

A

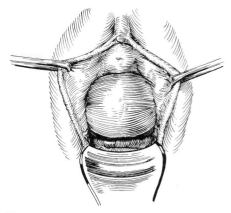

B

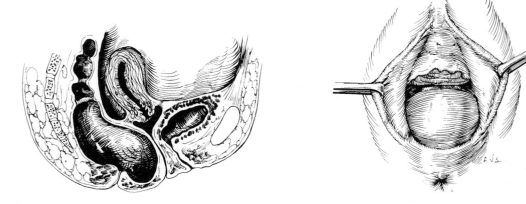

C

D

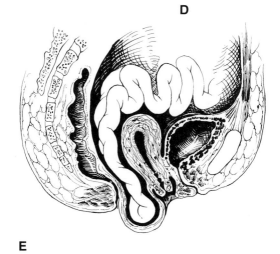

E

FIGURE 13–1. Common Types of Pelvic Floor Relaxation. Diagrammatic representation of cystocele (A & B), rectocele (C & D), and enterocele and prolapsed uterus (E). *(Source: DeCherney, A. H. & Pernoll, M. L. (1994). Current Obstetric & Gynecologic Diagnostics & Treatment. Norwalk, CT: Appleton & Lange.)*

Perform a rectal exam; observe any bleeding, and determine muscle tone and the presence of any rectocele. The client should also be asked to stand and be assessed for prolapse of the vaginal walls or uterus.

The Q-tip test is used by some to assess the degree of descent of the bladder neck. A sterile lubricated tip applicator is placed in the urethra of the urethrovesical junction. It should be at zero degrees in the dorsal-lithotomy position and should only change minimally when the client is asked to strain. If the support of the bladder neck is lax, the applicator will move upward more than than 30 degrees (Davila, 1996; Hacker & Moore, 1998).

Since genital organ prolapse can cause urinary symptoms, such as incontinence or retention, bladder function must be assessed. Determine postvoid residual with catheterization. Retention is present if residual is more than 60 to 100 mL. The client should be referred for further urodynamic evaluation and testing if she is older than 65, has indications for surgery, has had previous unsuccessful anti-incontinence surgery, has serious medical problems, has possible intrinsic sphincter damage or other unexplained urinary symptoms (Davila, 1996).

DIFFERENTIAL MEDICAL DIAGNOSES

Pelvic or abdominal tumors, tumors of the rectovaginal septum, cervical hypertrophy, Gartner's cyst, urethral diverticulum.

PLAN

Psychosocial Interventions

Describe the normal anatomy and the etiologies for pelvic prolapse to the client. If possible, show the client illustrations of normal anatomy and different types of pelvic floor defects. There are many large charts and printed illustrations available. Determine the impact of the prolapse on the client's daily functioning and ask whether she has future reproductive desires. Reassure the client that she can achieve relief of symptoms, restoration or partial restoration of anatomy, and return to normal functioning.

Medication

Estrogen Replacement Therapy. Indicated to improve tone and vascularity of the supporting tissue in perimenopausal and menopausal women.

Nonnarcotic Analgesics. Indicated for temporary relief of associated discomfort, especially back pain. The desired outcome of treatment is partial or complete pain relief. Over-the-counter analgesics, such as acetaminophen, should be tried first, but more potent nonsteroidal anti-inflammatory drugs (NSAIDs) may be needed.

- *Administration.* Continuous use is most effective. Several types of NSAIDs are available, and their dosages vary.
  - Ibuprofen (Motrin), 400 to 800 mg. p.o. q.i.d.
  - Naproxen (Naprosyn, Anaprox, Aleve), 200 mg. p.o. t.i.d. to 550 mg. p.o. b.i.d.
  - Ketoprofen (Orudis), 50 to 100 mg. p.o. b.i.d.
  - New NSAIDs have entered and are continually coming on the market. It is imperative that the clinician remains current on the dosages, benefits, risks, and side effects. It is probably best to select one or two that are inexpensive, low in side effects, and simple to dose and use these interchangeably. See Chapter 22, section on low back pain for additional drug information.
- *Side Effects and Adverse Reactions.* Most often reported is GI irritation. If GI irritation occurs, sucralfate (a GI antiulcerative) may be added to the regimen. Sucralfate dosage is one 1 g tablet p.o. 1 hour before or 2 hours after meals and at bedtime.
- *Contraindications.* Previous allergy to NSAIDs and a history of ulcer disease.
- *Client Teaching and Counseling.* Stress the need to follow the NSAID regimen carefully and to take the drug with food. Counsel the client to report immediately any signs of indigestion, epigastric pain, or hematochezia.

Dietary Interventions

Dietary habits can exacerbate the prolapse by causing constipation and consequently chronic straining. Dietary modifications will help to establish regular bowel movements without discomfort and eliminate excessive gas or bloating.

Teach the client about increasing dietary fiber and fluids to prevent constipation. Explain how constipation can contribute to straining and pelvic prolapse. Provide the client with instruction, materials, and support.

Respiratory Interventions

Correction or improvement of respiratory problems that cause chronic cough will decrease intra-abdominal pressure and thereby prevent worsening of pelvic prolapse. Intervention is indicated for clients who smoke, have asthma, or have chronic bronchitis. Anticipated outcomes on evaluation are that the client has stopped smoking, coughs less, and has less shortness of breath.

Counseling of a client who is not receiving care for a respiratory problem should include referral for evaluation and management. Encourage her to follow prescribed regimens, to stop smoking, and, if possible, to join a support group. Discuss with the client how reducing respiratory symptoms will help improve the symptoms of prolapse and prevent them from worsening. Reinforce the discussion by providing written information.

Surgery

Surgical treatment of genital organ prolapse is designed to correct specific defects, with the goals being restoration of normal anatomy and preservation of function. Procedures that are frequently done include the following (ACOG, 2001, TB 214; Hacker & Moore, 1998):

- *Anterior colporrhaphy* (plication of the pubocervical fascia) to correct cystocele/urethrocele.
- *Posterior colporrhaphy* (midline approximation of the endopelvic fascia and perineal muscles) to correct rectocele/enterocele.
- *Enterocele repair* (approximation of the uterosacral ligaments and levator ani muscles after reduction of the bowel).
- *Manchester operation* (involves anterior colporrhaphy, posterior colporrhaphy, amputation of the cervix, and suturing of the cardinal ligaments in front of the stump) to preserve, support, and antevert the uterus.
- *Vaginal hysterectomy,* done for any degree of uterine prolapse.
- *LeFort's partial colpocleisis* (suturing of the anterior and posterior vaginal walls so that the uterus is supported above), performed in elderly clients with substantial prolapse.

Indications for surgery are when childbearing is completed and/or symptoms begin to interfere with the client's daily living patterns and do not respond to nonsurgical treatment. The procedure chosen depends on the type and severity of pelvic prolapse. The client is referred to a board-certified gynecologic surgeon for evaluation.

Potential adverse effects depend on the surgical procedure performed. For example, with preservation of the uterus and closure of the vaginal canal, abnormal uterine bleeding could occur undetected. Coitus is also affected. A major adverse effect is recurrence of the prolapse; other effects include urinary retention, chronic urinary tract infection (UTI), incontinence, and difficult defecation.

Anticipated outcomes on evaluation are a return to optimal function, cessation or significantly fewer and less severe symptoms, restoration of satisfactory coital function, normal patterns of elimination, and prevention of prolapse of other organs and of recurrence of the prolapse that was repaired.

Provide in-depth discussions of the procedure to be performed, emphasizing anatomy and postoperative instructions. Allow the client to express her fears and anxieties. Stress that femininity will be preserved; however, discuss how sexual function may be altered (Weber, Walters, Schover, et al., 1995).

Pessaries

A *pessary* is a hard rubber or plastic ring used to maintain the normal position of the uterus or bladder by exerting pressure and providing support. It is placed in the vagina behind the pubic arch and the posterior fornix. An indication for pessary use is uterine prolapse or cystocele, especially among elderly clients for whom surgery is contraindicated (ACOG, 2001, TB 214; Callahan et al., 2001; Cundiff, Weidner, Visco, Bump, & Addison, 2000; Hacker & Moore, 1998).

The best type of pessary depends on the individual client's anatomy and symptoms. Clients with uterine prolapse without incontinence require only a space-occupying type (doughnut, inflatable). Clients with urinary incontinence benefit from a Smith-Hodge pessary.

Types of pessaries include the following:

- *Smith-Hodge pessaries* elevate the bladder neck and support it in a retropubic position.
- *Ring pessaries* are similar to diaphragms and are easily accepted by most clients. Inserted similarly to a diaphragm.
- *Cube pessaries* remain in place by adhering to the vaginal side walls. The incidence of mucosal inflammation and ulceration is high with this type, especially in the presence of atrophic vaginitis.
- *Gellhorn pessaries* are the best choice for large prolapse of the anterior vaginal wall.
- *Inflatable pessaries* are inserted and then inflated with a bulb.
- *Doughnut pessaries* are indicated for severe prolapse, may be difficult for the elderly client to insert and remove (see Figure 13–2).

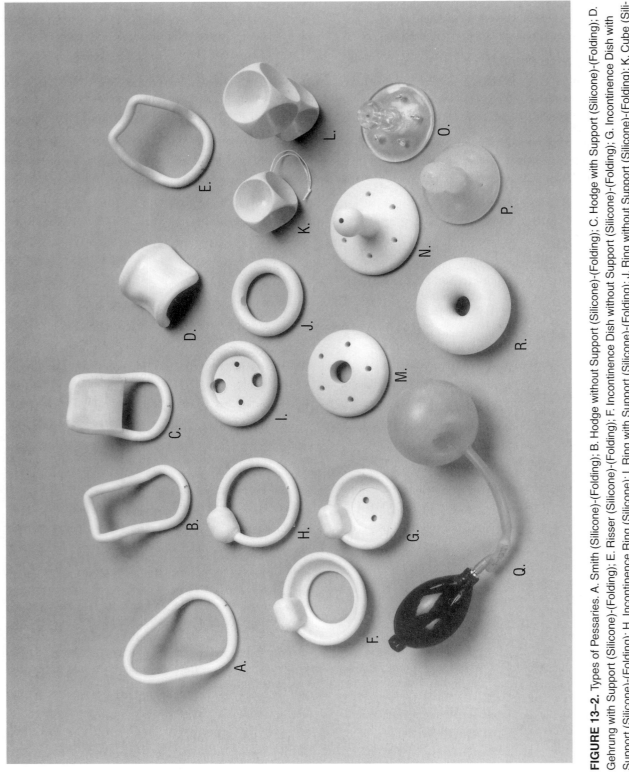

FIGURE 13–2. Types of Pessaries. A. Smith (Silicone)-(Folding); B. Hodge without Support (Silicone)-(Folding); C. Hodge with Support (Silicone)-(Folding); D. Gehrung with Support (Silicone)-(Folding); E. Risser (Silicone)-(Folding); F. Incontinence Dish without Support (Silicone)-(Folding); G. Incontinence Dish with Support (Silicone)-(Folding); H. Incontinence Ring (Silicone); I. Ring with Support (Silicone)-(Folding); J. Ring without Support (Silicone)-(Folding); K. Cube (Silicone)-(Flexible); L. Tandem-Cube (Silicone)-(Flexible); M. Shaatz (Silicone)-(Folding); N. Gellhorn (Flexible)-(Multi-Drain); O. Gellhorn (Acrylic)-(Rigid)-(Multi-Drain); P. Gellhorn (95% Rigid Silicone)-(Multi-Drain); Q. Inflatoball (Latex); R. Donut (Silicone).

Select the largest pessary that can be comfortably admitted through the vaginal orifice. Vaginal estrogen should be used twice weekly (1 gram). The most common recommendations for pessary care include removing the pessary twice weekly and cleansing with soap and water; using lubrication upon insertion, and having regular follow-up exams every six to twelve months after an initial period of adjustment.

Adverse effects include chronic vaginal infection and UTI. Vaginal erosion may occur. Anticipated outcomes on evaluation are that the uterus and bladder are supported, symptoms are decreased, and no interference occurs with intercourse. Client teaching must include instruction for removing and cleaning the pessary. Review the untoward symptoms/signs associated with pessary use; leukorrhea; vaginal burning or itching; loss of pessary; urinary retention; frequency, urgency, and dysuria. Instruct the client to report any symptoms.

Kegel's Exercises

The exercises strengthen pelvic muscles, which prevents further prolapse. They can be performed at any time and are very easy to learn. They have no adverse effect. If the prolapse extends to or beyond the vaginal introitus, however, Kegel's exercises are no longer useful (Davila, 1996).

Help the client to identify the pubococcygeus muscle by having her stop and start her urinary flow. Have her tighten the muscle for a count of 3, then relax it. The client should repeat the exercise ten times. Then instruct the client to contract and relax the muscle rapidly ten times. In addition, have her try to bring up the entire pelvic floor and bear down ten times. This movement may be repeated five times daily.

Lifestyle Changes

Several changes in lifestyle may help to prevent pelvic relaxation. For example, the client should attempt to achieve her ideal weight; wear a girdle or abdominal support; avoid or reduce heavy lifting; avoid high impact aerobics and jogging; and quit smoking.

FOLLOW-UP AND REFERRAL

Emphasize to all clients that worsening or recurrence of any symptoms should be reported immediately. If nonsurgical therapies are employed, regular follow-up visits at least every six months are necessary to assess the degree of prolapse and any worsening symptomatology. If a pessary is used, the client should be seen every two to six months to remove the device for inspection and cleaning. After surgery, the client should be seen at least annually to assess any recurrent prolapse.

CHRONIC PELVIC PAIN

Chronic pain persists for longer than six months and significantly impacts a woman's daily functioning and relationships. It can be *episodic* (i.e., cyclic, recurrent pain that is interspersed with pain free intervals) or *continuous* (i.e., noncyclic pain). Chronic pelvic pain frustrates both the client and her health care providers. Many times an etiology for chronic pain cannot be found or treatment of the presumed etiology fails; hence, pain becomes the illness.

EPIDEMIOLOGY

A significant number of clients with chronic pelvic pain have no obvious pelvic pathology (Gelbaya & El-Halwagy, 2001). Since the 1920s researchers have attempted to discover etiologies for chronic pelvic pain syndrome. At various times, different theories gained popularity, but the studies on which they were based were problematic (e.g., small samples, observer bias). Among the more popular theories that lack definite diagnostic criteria and management protocol are Allen-Masters syndrome (universal joint syndrome), pelvic congestion syndrome, and retrodisplacement of the uterus (Perry, 2001). The more common etiologies of chronic pelvic pain are as follows.

- *Episodic.* Dyspareunia, midcycle pelvic pain (mittelschmerz), dysmenorrhea.
- *Continuous.* Endometriosis, adenomyosis, chronic salpingitis, adhesions, loss of pelvic support.

In clients under 30, the cause of pelvic pain is more likely to be endometriosis or chronic pelvic inflammatory disease. Laparoscopy has revealed that up to 80 percent of women with chronic pelvic pain have endometriosis (Carter & Soper, 2001). In clients who are older, the causes are more likely to be one of the following: leiomyoma; adenomyosis; pelvic relaxation (Mathias, Kupperman, Liberman, et al., 1996).

Risk factors include the following:

- History of childhood or adult sexual abuse or trauma.
- Previous pelvic surgery.
- Personal or family history of depression.
- History of other chronic pain syndromes.

- History of alcohol and drug abuse.
- Tendency toward somatization.
- Dysfunctional family and marital relationships (Lampe, Solder, Ennemoser, Schubert, et al., 2000).

Chronic pelvic pain comprises up to 10 percent of outpatient gynecologic visits and is the reason for 40 percent of laparoscopies and 10 to 15 percent of hysterectomies. Approximately 65,000 to 104,000 hysterectomies are performed annually because of chronic pelvic pain (Winkel, 2001). Recent cost estimates are $1.2 to $2.8 billion annually for physician and mental health visits. Additionally, women who report chronic pelvic pain admit to significantly poorer general health (Mathias et al, 1996; Perry, 2001).

SUBJECTIVE DATA

The major goals in the evaluation of chronic pelvic pain are as follows:

- To identify any treatable sources of pain, either GYN or non-GYN.
- To rule out any potentially life-threatening pathologies.
- To identify associated problems such as depression.

Because the evaluation of chronic pelvic pain can be complicated, a consistent approach to history taking and physical examination is essential. Inquiry about the presence of pelvic pain should be a routine part of health care for women (Carter & Soper, 2001; Gelbaya & El-Halwagy, 2001).

The history should include these essential components:

- Detailed description of the onset, location, nature, character, and timing of the pain.
- Description of any associated symptoms such as nausea, vomiting, fever, urinary symptoms, constipation, diarrhea, bloating, vaginal discharge, dyspareunia.
- Detailed menstrual history including last menstrual period, bleeding patterns, dysmenorrhea, menarche, menopause.
- Reproductive history including pregnancies, births, miscarriages, elective terminations, ectopics, infertility.
- Sexual history including the number of sex partners, use of contraception, history of PID, STDs.
- Psychosocial history with careful attention to any past or present physical or sexual abuse; how the pain has impacted the client's lifestyle (work, sick days, relationships, normal activities, recreation).

- Past medical history and review of systems is pertinent to establishing differential diagnoses and should include past surgeries, previous therapies for the pain, use of pain medications, other providers seen, history of gastrointestinal problems, genitourinary problems, and musculoskeletal problems.

The client may report pain duration of six months or longer; incomplete relief by most previous treatments, including surgery and nonnarcotic analgesics; significantly impaired functioning at home or work; signs of depression such as early morning awakening, weight loss, and anorexia; pain out of proportion to pathology; and altered family roles. The client may also have a history of childhood abuse, incest, rape or other sexual trauma, substance abuse, or current sexual dysfunction. A client usually reports previous consultation with one or more health care providers and dissatisfaction with their management of her condition (Jamieson & Steege, 1996).

OBJECTIVE DATA

Physical Examination

Perform a systematic physical examination of the abdominal, pelvic, and rectal areas, focusing on the location and intensity of the pain. Attempt to reproduce the pain. The use of relaxation/breathing techniques will facilitate examination for both client and health professional (ACOG, 2001, TB 223; Jamieson & Steege, 1996). *Check the client's vital signs; fever indicates an acute process.*

Note the client's general appearance, demeanor, and gait; these may suggest the severity of pain and possible neuromuscular etiology. Vomiting may indicate an acute process.

Abdominal symptoms of a more acute process are rebound tenderness (peritoneal irritation) and decreased abdominal pain on palpation with tension of the rectus muscles. Ask the client to perform a straight leg raise; with the client's legs slightly raised and rectus muscles taut, pain on deep palpation will decrease if it is of pelvic origin and increase if it is of abdominal wall or myofascial origin. Inspect and note any well-healed scars. Palpate scars for incisional hernias, and palpate for any unsuspected masses. To help identify femoral or inguinal hernias, palpate the groin while the client performs the Valsalva maneuver.

During the speculum exam, note any cervicitis, which may be a source of parametrial irritation. With bimanual/rectal exam, a tender pelvic or adnexal mass, abnormal bleeding, tender uterine fundus, or cervical motion tenderness may indicate an acute process, such as pelvic inflammatory disease (PID), ectopic pregnancy, or a ruptured ovarian cyst.

Nonmobility of the uterus may indicate the presence of pelvic adhesions. Note existence of any adnexal mass, fullness, or tenderness. Cul-de-sac nodularities are palpable with endometriosis. Identify any areas that reproduce deep dyspareunia.

Palpate the coccyx, both internally and externally, for tenderness of coccydynia.

Musculoskeletal exam should be performed. View the spine while client is sitting, standing and walking. Observe gait, leg length, and range of motion. Have the client bend at the waist to assess for scoliosis (ACOG, 2001, TB 223; Carter & Soper, 2001; Reiter, 1990).

Diagnostic Tests and Methods

Diagnostic tests should be selected discriminately as indicated by the findings of the history and physical examination. Review previous test results in order to avoid unnecessary and repetitive diagnostic testing.

Complete Blood Count (CBC) and Erythrocyte Sedimentation Rate (ESR). See Pelvic Inflammatory Disease.

Urinalysis. Diagnostic evaluation to identify any urinary tract conditions that might represent the source of pain. White blood cells, bacteria, or red blood cells may indicate either chronic or recurrent urinary tract infections (UTI). Hematuria may indicate renal stones or a tumor of the urinary tract. Further diagnostic testing, specifically cystoscopy or intravenous pyelogram, may be indicated.

Teach the client how to obtain a clean catch urine sample in a sterile container.

Pregnancy Test (Urine or Blood Level of hCG). See Pelvic Inflammatory Disease.

Vaginal Smears/Cervical Cultures. Diagnostic evaluation to detect existing pelvic infection as the etiology of acute or chronic pelvic pain. Wet mount with saline can detect bacterial vaginosis or trichomoniasis. Cervical tests can detect *N. gonorrhoeae and C. trachomatis* (see Chapter 11 for the test procedures).

Stool Guaiac (Colocare or Hemoccult). Diagnostic evaluation to detect gastrointestinal (GI) pathology as a possible source of pain (see Leiomyomas for the test procedure). The stool may be positive for occult blood in cases of ulcerative colitis, irritable bowel syndrome, GI polyps, or malignancy, although this test is not definitive. If the result is positive or if history and physical exam suggest, then refer the client for gastroenterology consultation and

further diagnostic testing, such as upper GI series, barium enema, sigmoidoscopy, and/or colonoscopy.

Ultrasound. Diagnostic evaluation to identify and locate potential causes of pelvic pain (see Adenomyosis for the test procedure).

Laparoscopy. Diagnostic evaluation accomplished by direct visualization, performed when pelvic pathology is not detectable by pelvic exam or other diagnostic testing (see Endometriosis for the test procedure). Laparoscopy is useful in the diagnosis of acute or chronic salpingitis, ectopic pregnancy, hydrosalpinx, endometriosis, ovarian tumors and cysts, torsion, appendicitis, and adhesions. Clients may experience less anxiety about their symptoms when no serious pathology is found. Researchers have been unable to demonstrate a direct correlation between laparoscopic findings and the severity of pelvic pain (Winkel, 2001).

DIFFERENTIAL MEDICAL DIAGNOSES

The evaluation of pelvic pain must differentiate between acute and chronic etiologies and gynecologic and nongynecologic. Table 13–4 summarizes common causes of pelvic pain.

Common medical conditions that are not gynecologic but may present as chronic pelvic pain include GI

TABLE 13–4. Common Causes of Acute and Chronic Pelvic Pain

Common GYN Causes of Acute Pelvic Pain	Common GYN Causes of Chronic Pelvic Pain
Ectopic pregnancy	Endometriosis
Salpingitis	Adenomyosis
Abortion	Uterine fibroids
Ruptured ovarian cyst	Chronic salpingitis
Adnexal torsion	Adhesions
Endometriosis	Dysmenorrhea
Menstruation	Dyspareunia
Ovulation pain	Pelvic relaxation
	Psychopathology/Enigmatic (30–50 percent)

Common NonGYN Causes of Acute Pelvic Pain	Common NonGYN Causes of Chronic Pelvic Pain
Appendicitis	Chronic appendicitis
Cystitis	Irritable bowel syndrome
Diverticulitis	Ulcerative colitis
Ureteral calculus	Diverticulosis
Gastroenteritis/Spastic colon	Urinary tract disease
Trauma	Neuromuscular disorders

Source: ACOG, 2001, TB 223; Carter & Soper, 2001.

conditions, such as irritable bowel syndrome, ulcerative colitis, and diverticulosis; urinary tract disease; and neuromuscular/musculoskeletal disorders, such as disc problems and fibromyalgia (Carter & Soper, 2001; Gelbaya & El-Halwagy, 2001; Zondervan, Yudkin, Vessey, Jenkinson, & Dawes, 2001).

PLAN

Specific management of a client with chronic pelvic pain depends on the pain's etiology. Therefore, careful physical, psychosocial, and diagnostic evaluations represent the most important steps in providing care for these clients. Many clients, however, either fail to respond to therapy or do not demonstrate any known pathology.

The goal of care is to alleviate pain so that the client is able to maintain optimal daily functioning. The emotional, psychological, and physical aspects of the pain should be managed simultaneously.

The most recent research proposes an empiric approach to the treatment of chronic pelvic pain. The American College of Obstetricians and Gynecologists supports this approach, which is as follows:

> Therapy with a GnRH agonist is an appropriate approach to the management of women with chronic pelvic pain, even in the absence of surgical confirmation, provided that a detailed initial evaluation fails to demonstrate some other cause of pelvic pain (ACOG, 2001, PB 11).

Psychosocial Interventions

Listen carefully and demonstrate an attitude of caring and concern. Validate the fact that the client's symptoms are real. If she has one or more of the following indications, then refer her for skilled psychological evaluation and therapy.

- No apparent etiology for pain found during a thorough evaluation, including diagnostic laparoscopy.
- History of psychosexual trauma.
- History of consultation and therapy for multiple unrelated somatic symptoms.
- Symptoms of depression.

Review all findings with the client and involve her in decisions about care. If appropriate, involve the client's partner in planning care. Set realistic goals for evaluating therapy, stressing that a "cure" may not be possible. Refer the client for sexual counseling and therapy if indicated. Encourage her to keep a diary of the timing, location, and severity of the pain and the significant circumstance surrounding it (Carter & Soper, 2001; Gelbaya & El-Halwagy, 2001).

Medication

The goal of treatment with medication is to ameliorate pain, not eliminate it. Long-term narcotic use has been proved ineffective in the management of chronic pelvic pain and may lead to abuse and dependency behaviors (ACOG, 2001, PB 11).

Nonsteroidal Anti-Inflammatory Drugs (NSAIDs). See section on Pelvic Organ Prolapse.

Antidepressants. Antidepressants are used to enhance the effectiveness of NSAIDs, manage simultaneous depression, and improve sleep patterns. Many different types are available, with varying side effects and actions. Tricyclic antidepressants have been most commonly used in the past. The Serotonin-reuptake inhibitors, for example, Prozac and Zoloft are increasingly used. See Chapter 23, Tables 23–1 and 23–2 for a comprehensive list with side effects and dosages.

The anticipated outcomes on evaluation are perception of decreased pain and less interference with the activities of daily living. Instruct the client to monitor her response to the drug and its side effects. Help ensure that the client takes the proper dose and understands the possible side effects.

Oral Contraceptives. Indicated for the management of cyclic, chronic pain, specifically that associated with dysmenorrhea, mild endometriosis, and recurrent functional ovarian cysts (see Endometriosis and Chapter 8, Dysmenorrhea).

GnRH Analogues. Indicated for the management of chronic pain associated with endometriosis and/or uterine fibroids (see sections on Endometriosis and Leiomyomas). Recent studies suggest that a trial of GnRH analogues as a diagnostic/therapeutic modality may be more cost effective than laparoscopy, saving one half the cost of treatment of endometriosis. (Gelbaya & El-Halwagy, 2001; Winkel, 2001).

Dietary Interventions

Modifications in diet may be indicated when the client is experiencing constipation, bloating, edema, excessive fatigue, irritability, or lethargy, or is overweight. Dietary habits may contribute to the pain pattern, although not directly cause it.

Anticipated outcomes on evaluation are regular bowel movements without discomfort; decreased gas, bloating, and edema; improved energy level and stability of mood; and attainment and maintenance of ideal body weight.

Provide the client with information about the need for a high fiber diet and increased fluids to prevent constipation; explain how constipation can contribute to the pain pattern. In addition, less sodium, caffeine, and carbonated beverages reduce edema and abdominal bloating. Discuss with the client alternative cooking and seasoning methods, explain pertinent information on food labels, and suggest alternatives to soft drinks, coffee, and tea in order to limit intake of caffeine and carbonated beverages. Instruction may also include information about achieving stable blood sugar levels and weight loss by reducing refined carbohydrates and sugar in the diet and by eating low fat foods with fewer calories. Reinforce the information with printed materials.

Surgical Interventions

Surgery becomes necessary when anatomic diagnoses are confirmed or when various medical therapies have failed. The client should then be referred by surgical consult. (Carter & Soper, 2001; Winkel, 2001).

Laparoscopy. Indications are for the therapeutic as well as diagnostic purposes. Therapeutically, laparoscopy may be used for lysis of pelvic adhesions and ablation of endometrial implants.

Hysterectomy. This type of surgery is indicated when a known pathology is suspected to represent the source of pain, for example, leiomyomas, endometriosis, chronic PID, adenomyosis, or suspected malignancy. Pain that does not have a known or suspected etiology is not an indication for a hysterectomy; however, chronic pelvic pain is listed as the indication for 10 to 15 percent of the hysterectomies performed in the United States (Reiter, 1990; Winkel, 2001). In a recent study, hysterectomy proved effective in ameliorating pain; however, 25 percent of the hysterectomy clients reported persistent pain one year after surgery (Winkel, 2001).

Alternative Interventions

Other interventions for the management of chronic pelvic pain include biofeedback, stress management techniques, self-hypnosis, relaxation therapy, transcutaneous nerve stimulation (TNS), trigger-point injections, spinal anesthesia, and nerve blocks. For many of these alternative interventions, referral to a chronic pelvic pain clinic is recommended (ACOG, 2001, PB 11; Carter & Soper, 2001).

FOLLOW-UP AND REFERRAL

Regularly scheduled client appointments are crucial to the management of chronic pelvic pain. Visits are scheduled at intervals unrelated to specific pain episodes. Maintain consistent communication with the client, coordinate results of other providers' evaluations and therapies, and review this information with the client (Carter & Soper, 2001).

CERVICITIS

Cervicitis is inflammation or ectopy of the cervix as evidenced by visual presence of yellow endocervical exudate, quantification of leukocytes in cervical exudate or histologic examination of the cervix. Cervical ectopy (ectopia, ectropion, eversion, erosion) refers to the extension of the columnar epithelium from the endocervix outward over the ectocervix, joining the squamous epithelium at the transformation zone, or squamocolumnar junction. Cervical ectopy without the presence of infection is a normal finding in most female adolescents and in women on oral contraceptives (Critchlow, Wolner-Hanssen, Eschenbach, et al., 1995).

EPIDEMIOLOGY

Neisseria gonorrhoeae and *Chlamydia trachomatis* are the two most common organisms that cause cervicitis and the only organisms shown to cause mucopurulent cervicitis (Callahan et al., 2001). Herpes simplex virus (HSV) and human papillomavirus are also common causes of cervicitis, with HPV playing a significant role in the development of cervical cancer (Callahan et al., 2001).

Acute or chronic infectious cervicitis is one of the most common gynecologic disorders affecting more than 50 percent of all women at some time during their adult life. Risk factors for the increased incidence of cervicitis include young age, early age of first intercourse, the presence of *C. trachomatis*; use of oral contraceptives, and sexual contact with men who have nongonococcal urethritis.

SUBJECTIVE DATA

Clients report purulent discharge, postcoital or post-douche vaginal spotting or bleeding.

OBJECTIVE DATA

Physical Examination

Red, edematous, often friable cervix, with the presence of tenacious, yellowish-white discharge. With trichomoniasis, the characteristic "strawberry" cervix is seen with grayish-green discharge.

Diagnostic Tests and Methods

Wet Mount. Microscopic examination of vaginal and cervical discharge for leukocytes, trichomoniasis, candida. See Chapter 4 on Assessment and Chapter 11 on Vaginitis and STDs.

Cultures. Obtain specific cultures for *C. trachomatis, N. gonorrhoeae, Herpes*. See Chapter 4 on Assessment and Chapter 11 on Vaginitis and STDs.

Pap Smear. Indicated to rule out early cervical neoplasia. See Chapter 4 on Assessment and this chapter on Screening for Gynecologic Cancers.

Colposcopy. Indicated if Pap smear shows atypia after repeated dysplasia or if cervicitis is persistent and/or unresponsive to medical therapy. If the practitioner has experience with colposcopic examination, he or she may proceed with evaluation, including biopsy. Otherwise, refer to a gynecologist.

DIFFERENTIAL MEDICAL DIAGNOSES

Ovulation (mucus of ovulation is clear with scant leukocytes); pelvic abscess or mass above the cervix; early neoplasia; syphilis; chronic granulomatous ulcerations of tuberculosis and granuloma inguinale.

PLAN

Psychosocial

Discuss the disease process with the client, reviewing the anatomy and physiology of the vagina, cervix, and uterus. If there is abnormal bleeding, show the client where the bleeding is originating on the cervix, and reassure her that this does not represent an *abnormal period*. Discuss the purpose and importance of the Pap smear in the evaluation of cervicitis. Review the common causes of cervicitis and discuss how high risk sexual behaviors can contribute to the transmission of infection. Encourage the use of condoms. Provide the client with written information. Include the partner when possible and encourage him to be evaluated for the presence of any sexually transmitted diseases.

Medication

Antibiotic therapy should be based upon the specific etiology. See Chapter 11 for specific treatments. Discuss with the client the importance of taking prescribed medications correctly and of completing therapy.

Surgery

Surgical measures in the treatment of cervicitis are indicated for chronic cervicitis that is unresponsive to medical therapy and especially when accompanied by ectopy. Before any procedure is begun, colposcopic examination and biopsy, if indicated, should be performed to rule out cervical neoplasia. Common methods include the following:

◆ *Cryosurgery*. Destroys tissue by freezing with liquid CO_2, nitrogen, freon, or nitrous oxide. A probe is placed directly on the cervical os. Advantages include lack of discomfort, less postoperative bleeding, and less incidence of cervical stenosis. Adverse effects include heavy vaginal discharge for two to three weeks after the procedure.

◆ *Electrocauterization/Loop electrosurgical excision procedure (LEEP)*. Employs the use of heat using a thin wire to incise and destroy diseased tissue. Advantages include good control of tissue destruction, and ability to perform in the office without the use of anesthesia. Adverse effects include postoperative bleeding and cervical stenosis.

◆ *Laser*. Use of directed laser to destroy diseased tissue. Advantages include lack of sloughing of tissue and no resulting leukorrhea, lack of scarring, and control of degree of cellular destruction.

Outcomes on evaluation include destruction of infected tissues with subsequent healing by fibroplastic proliferation and reepitheliazation. Counsel the client about the procedure to be utilized and possible adverse effects. Explain that complete healing may take up to six weeks.

FOLLOW-UP AND REFERRAL

Complications of untreated cervicitis include leukorrhea, cervical stenosis, salpingitis, chronic infection of the urinary tract, and chronic cervicitis. Once treatment is initiated, have the client return in two weeks, and four to eight weeks thereafter until resolved. Refer for further evaluation if the cervicitis does not resolve or if Pap smear reveals cervical intraepithelial neoplasia.

BARTHOLIN'S GLAND DUCT CYSTS AND BARTHOLINITIS

The Bartholin's glands are two pea-sized glands located bilaterally beneath the vaginal vestibule. They are considered major mucous secreting glands, helping to lubricate the vestibule (Black et al., 1995; Lynch & Edwards, 1994).

A Bartholin's gland duct cyst results from obstruction of the gland leading to dilatation of the duct. Bartholinitis is the inflammation of one or both of the Bartholin's glands (Callahan et al., 2001).

EPIDEMIOLOGY

Obstruction of the duct may occur as a result of infection, inspissated mucous, or trauma. Secondary infection is commonly caused by *N. gonorrhoeae, Staphylococcus, Streptococcus, Escherichia coli, Trichomoniasis,* and bacteroides. *Gonococcus* is implicated about 20 to 30 percent of the time (Rosenfeld, 2001).

SUBJECTIVE DATA

May be asymptomatic; however, when size increases, inflammation develops, and clients report unilateral swelling of the labia; extreme tenderness, pain, and throbbing; dyspareunia; and pain when walking or sitting. The client may have a history of recurrent abscess.

OBJECTIVE DATA

Examination of the genitalia/reproductive tract may reveal erythema, acute tenderness, edema, a fluctuant mass located laterally to the vestibule, purulent drainage, tender and enlarged inguinal nodes.

A culture and sensitivity test is done to identify the source of infection, especially with recurrent infection. Drainage from the gland is collected on a sterile swab. If gonorrhea is suspected, the appropriate testing is needed (see Chapters 4 & 11 for more information). Explain the procedure to the client (Callahan et al., 2001).

DIFFERENTIAL MEDICAL DIAGNOSES

Inclusion cyst, sebaceous cyst, primary cancer of Bartholin's gland or duct (especially among women older than 40), secondary metastatic malignancy, lipoma, fibroma, hernia, hydrocele.

PLAN

Psychosocial Interventions

Describe for the client how the infection occurs, and explain the treatment in detail. Allow time for questions and concerns to be expressed.

Medication

Broad Spectrum Antibiotics (Erythromycin, Doxycycline, Cephalosporins). Indicated when gonorrhea is suspected or identified (see Chapter 11).

A side effect is GI upset: Contraindications include previous sensitivity to any of the aforementioned antibiotics. Doxycycline/tetracycline is contraindicated during pregnancy.

Anticipated outcomes on evaluation are relief of symptoms and resolution of infection/abscess. Instruct the client to take the medication with food (meal or snack) but not with milk, to complete the entire course of medication, and if taking doxycycline, to stay out of the sun or use sunscreen.

Analgesics. Used to relieve pain.

Surgical Interventions

Incision and Drainage/Insertion of Word Catheter. This procedure is done by a gynecologist in cases of abscess formation and when response to antibiotic therapy is inadequate. If a practitioner has specialized skills training and experience, he or she may place a word catheter. The procedure involves cleansing the area with povidone iodine (Betadine) and using local anesthetic, such as lidocaine (1 percent). A small incision is made approximately at the opening of the duct, and as much purulent drainage as possible is expressed. The cavity is explored for other pockets of infection. Finally, a word catheter (a bulb-tipped inflatable catheter that remains in the cyst) is inserted and 2 to 4 mL of sterile water is injected to hold the catheter in place for four to six weeks. The plugged end of the catheter is tucked into the vagina.

An adverse effect of overinflation of the bulb is pressure necrosis of the cyst wall with chronic defect.

The anticipated outcome on evaluation is complete resolution of the abscess and infection.

Provide the client with instructions to follow during the four to six weeks that the catheter is in place. The catheter is checked weekly and deflated as the abscess becomes smaller and drainage slows. The client may take sitz baths and warm soaks for comfort. Sexual intercourse is permitted as soon as tenderness subsides; care must be taken not to dislodge the catheter (Callahan et al., 2001; Hacker & Moore, 1998).

Marsupialization. Creation of a pouch is performed in cases of recurrent abscess formation. Referral is made to a gynecologic surgeon, who performs the procedure on an outpatient basis using local, regional, or general anesthesia. After an incision is made over the cyst, exploration and drainage is performed if necessary, and the wall of the cyst is everted and fixed to the surrounding skin. Adverse effects, although rare, may include postoperative infection and pain.

The anticipated outcomes on evaluation are permanent drainage and no further cyst/abscess recurrences (Callahan et al., 2001; Hacker & Moore, 1998).

Alternative Intervention

Rest, heat, and sitz baths may also be used to treat bartholinitis.

FOLLOW-UP AND REFERRAL

Follow-up for conservative treatment (antibiotics, rest, heat) should occur seven to ten days after the treatment is begun. Swelling, pain, erythema, and tenderness or throbbing should be resolved or resolving. If a word catheter is inserted, follow up weekly. A four- to six-week follow-up is appropriate for marsupialization.

CERVICAL POLYPS

Cervical polyps are benign, pedunculated growths of varying size that extend from the ectocervix or endocervical canal. Polyps may occur singularly or they may be multiple (Callahan et al., 2001; Hacker & Moore, 1998).

EPIDEMIOLOGY

The etiology is unknown. Polyps are believed to result from chronic inflammation, however; they may be associated with hyperestrogen states; and they are found commonly with endometrial hyperplasia. Polyps are most common among multiparous women in their 30s and 40s.

SUBJECTIVE DATA

The client is usually asymptomatic, although thick leukorrhea, postcoital bleeding, intermenstrual bleeding, menorrhagia, postmenopausal bleeding, or mucopurulent or blood-tinged vaginal discharge may occur.

OBJECTIVE DATA

Physical Examination

Single or multiple pear-shaped growths may protrude from the cervix into the vaginal canal. They are usually smooth, soft, reddish-purple to cherry red, and readily bleed when touched. They may be small or very large.

Diagnostic Tests and Methods

Pathology. A diagnostic microscopic evaluation of all polyps should be done by a pathologist; diagnosis is confirmed during evaluation. This requires collection of a specimen to be labeled and sent in preservative medium to a pathology laboratory. (See Surgical Interventions, following, for a description of the procedure.)

Explain the procedure to the client and tell her when she can expect test results. Reassure her that the majority of polyps are benign.

Papanicolaou (Pap) Smear. See Chapter 4.

DIFFERENTIAL MEDICAL DIAGNOSES

Endometrial polyps, small prolapsed myomas, cervical malignancy.

PLAN

Psychosocial Interventions

Explain to the client what polyps are and that they are usually benign; encourage her to express her concerns.

Surgical Interventions

Cervical polyps should be removed and sent to a pathology laboratory. The procedure can be performed in an office without anesthesia by any appropriately trained health care provider. Paint the cervix with povidone-iodine (Betadine); using ring forceps, grasp and twist the polyp at the base. Apply silver nitrate or Monsel's solution to the site of removal to control bleeding. Excessive bleeding is a potential adverse effect.

Client teaching includes the need for pelvic rest for 24 hours to ensure that bleeding does not occur at the removal site. If excessive bleeding or excessive vaginal discharge does occur, the client must return for evaluation and possible endometrial sampling.

Treatment of Vaginal Infections

Accompanying vaginal infections must be treated appropriately (see Chapter 11).

FOLLOW-UP AND REFERRAL

Regular Pap smears and gynecologic exams are important, and this needs to be stressed to the client.

GYNECOLOGIC CANCERS: SCREENING AND REFERRAL

CIN AND CERVICAL CANCER

Despite great strides in the reduction of cervical cancer's incidence and mortality in the United States with the widespread use of the Pap smear, the number of cases that are diagnosed yearly has remained fairly constant over the last ten years (Anderson & Runowicz, 2002). The incidence in Caucasian women younger than 50 may be increasing. Approximately 50 percent of reported cases of cervical cancer occur in women who have never had a Pap test (Paley, 2001). It is important that the practitioner be aware of the most common risk factors for CIN and cervical cancer, currently recommended screening protocols, and appropriate follow-up.

Cervical intrapepithelial neoplasia (CIN) is defined as "the spectrum of intraepithelial changes beginning as with a well-differentiated neoplasm, traditionally classified as mild dysplasia, and ending with invasive carcinoma" (Morris, Tortolero-Luna, Malpica, et al., 1996, p. 347).

Cervical cancer (CIS) occurs when malignant cells penetrate the underlying basement membrane of the epithelium and infiltrate the stroma, now considered invasive cervical cancer.

Epidemiology

Each year in the United States there are about 13,000 new cases of cervical cancer, and more than 4,000 women die of the disease (Anderson & Runowicz, 2002). Recent data reveal that the incidence of cervical cancer in the United States is about 8 to 9 percent, with higher rates reported in Native Americans, Hispanics, African Americans, and Filipinos. The lowest rates occur in Japanese women. African American women have about twice the age adjusted incidence rate per 100,000 women compared with white women. Cervical cancer is the third most common cancer among women in the United States and is the second most common worldwide (Morris et al., 1996).

Human papillomavirus infection is highly prevalent, detected in one-third of U.S. female college students and is associated with cervical cancer. HPV types 16 and 18 are the most prevalent types.

Risk Factors

- Early age at first intercourse.
- Multiple sexual partners.
- Immunocompromised state.
- First child prior to age 20.
- Lower socioeconomic status.
- History of sexually transmitted diseases (STDs, especially HPV).
- Exposure to diethylstilbestrol (DES) in utero.
- Cigarette smoking (Morris et al., 1996; Paley, 2001; Rollins, 2000).

Screening. Screening for cervical cancer is very effective because of the presence of a precursor lesion, cervical intraepithelial neoplasm (CIN). Lesions start as dysplasia and progress to carcinoma in situ and finally to invasive cancer. The newly revised 2001 Bethesda System, a standardized description of diagnostic terminology, is discussed in Chapter 4 with the recommendations for management of report results. Abnormalities are categorized into two atypical squamous cell (ASC) groups: *ASC-US* (undetermined significance) and *ASC-H* (cannot exclude high-grade squamous intraepithelial lesions) (Wright et al., 2002). ASC-US cannot exclude that there might be lesions higher than low grade lesions (LSIL), but considers that LSIL represents more transient infection with HPV (Solomon et al., 2002; Wright et al., 2002). ASC-H includes approximately 5 to 10 percent of all the ASC cases and is considered to predict CIN 2 or 3 that may fall between ASC-US and HSIL. Thus, it is believed that women with higher risk lesions are less likely to be missed with the new categorizations and recommendations for management (see Chapter 4). The goal of screening is to identify the precursor lesions at an early stage before progression to malignancy. Fortunately, these precursor lesions appear to have a long latent phase in most cases.

In the United States, widespread use of the Papanicolaou test has decreased the incidence and mortality rates of cervical cancer by 40 percent since 1973. However, recent studies suggest that the rate of false-negative results using the Pap smear alone may be as high as 50 percent. Thus, many new technologies are being studied and introduced clinically (Rollins, 2000; Solomon et al., 2002; Wright et al., 2002). See Chapter 4 for additional information.

- *Automated slide thin-layer preparation (Thin-Prep™)*. Approved by the FDA in 1996, this method is one of several accepted by most major insurance carriers and is increasingly replacing the traditional glass smear. It is a liquid-based cervical cytology (LBCC) technique. A specimen is collected from the cervix using a broomlike device or an endocervical brush and plastic spatula and placed in a vial of fixative solution, which suspends the cells. In the laboratory, the solution is agitated to break up the cellular clumps; disperse blood, inflammatory cells, and debris; and mix the cellular sample. A predetermined number of cells are drawn onto a filter membrane, applied to a glass slide and evaluated by the cytopathologist. A major advantage of this method is improvement of the detection rate of LGSIL and HGSIL (Anderson & Runowicz, 2002).
- *Computer-Assisted Automated Pap Test Rescreening (Autopap™)*. An algorithm-based decision-making technology; identifies slides that should be rescreened by pathologists by determining which samples exceed a certain threshold for the likelihood of abnormal cells. Approved by the FDA, this method is superior to conventional Pap test screening in identifying ASCUS, LGSIL, and HGSIL (Anderson & Runowicz, 2002; Rollins, 2000).
- *HPV-DNA Typing*. The association between certain types of HPV (16, 18, 31, 33, 35, 45, 51, 52, 56) and the development of CIN and invasive cervical cancer is well established. Approved by the FDA in 1995, the *Hybrid Capture™* system can identify high-risk HPV types and holds promise for improving detection and management of cervical disease (Anderson & Runowicz, 2002; Rollins, 2000).
- *Other methods currently under investigation or approved by the FDA*. Computer assisted technology (Cytyc CDS-1000™, AutoCyte™, AcCell™), optical and photographic screening tests such as cervicography and speculoscopy, and acetic acid washing. The practitioner should monitor carefully the continued research of these methods for future use.

Although many professional medical organizations differ in their consensus of opinions as to the frequency of screening for cervical cancer, *the American College of Obstetricians and Gynecologists and the American Cancer Society recommend that annual screening commence when women become sexually active or reach the age of 18 years. If three or more consecutive annual examinations have been normal in a low risk client, then Pap tests may be performed less frequently at the practitioner's discretion*. It is appropriate to continue to perform annual Pap tests in women considered to be at high risk for cervical cancer on the basis of the known risk factors (ACOG, 2001, CO 247; Paley, 2001; Zoorob, Anderson, Cefalu, & Sidani, 2001).

Management of Abnormal Results. Using the 2001 Bethesda system, the currently accepted method of reporting Pap smear results (see Chapter 4), the following are accepted guidelines. (Wright et al., 2002).

- With normal findings, repeat screening every year (see ACOG and American Cancer Society guidelines above).
- *ASC-US:* Repeat either conventional or liquid-based testing at four- to six-month intervals until there are two consecutive negative results for intraepithelial lesion or malignancy, after which the woman may be screened routinely. Colposcopy is recommended for any repeat ASC-US result. If colposcopy does not find CIN, the woman should have a repeat cytological test in twelve months. If colposcopy identifies CIN, management should be according to the 2001 Consensus Guidelines for such abnormalities (Wright et al., 2002). See Chapter 4 for additional management of results.
- *ASC-H:* Refer any woman with ASC-H for colposcopy. If no CIN is found, a review of technique results is advised and a revised interpretation should dictate management. If CIN is found, cytology at six to twelve months or HPV DNA testing at twelve months is advised. Finding ASC or a high-risk type of HPV DNA requires colposcopy (Wright et al., 2002).
- *Atypical glandular cells (AGC) and adenocarcinoma in situ (AIS):* See Chapter 4 for recommended management. The AGC category is significantly associated with a higher risk of cervical cancer (Wright et al., 2002). AGC requires a coloposcopy though it may miss lesions. Follow-up is based upon the subclassification of AGC or the finding of AIS. An excisional biopsy is the recommended approach by many physicians.

Treatment Modalities. The practitioner should be aware of current treatment modalities for CIN:

♦ *Cryosurgery.* Destroys tissue by freezing with liquid CO_2, nitrogen, freon, or nitrous oxide. A probe is placed directly on the cervical os. Studies show a 90 percent cure rate. Advantages include lack of discomfort, less postoperative bleeding, and less incidence of cervical stenosis. Adverse effects include heavy vaginal discharge for two to three weeks after the procedure.

♦ *Loop Electrosurgical Excision Procedure (LEEP).* Employs the use of heat using a thin wire to incise and destroy diseased tissue. Studies show a 95 percent cure rate, slightly better than the rate of cryosurgery or laser. Advantages include good control of tissue destruction and ability to perform in the office without the use of anesthesia. Adverse effects include postoperative bleeding and cervical stenosis (Ferenczy, Choukroun, & Arseneau, 1996). LEEP can also be used to both biopsy and treat within the same procedure. According to Wright et al. (2002), LEEP or any other excisional procedure should be used only with biopsy-confirmed CIN in women with ASC.

♦ *Laser.* Use of directed laser to destroy diseased tissue. Advantages include lack of sloughing of tissue and no resulting leukorrhea; lack of scarring and control of degree of cellular destruction.

♦ *Cone Biopsies.* Removal of a cone shaped section of cervical tissue, including a portion of the endocervix indicated in higher grade or invasive lesions. Can be performed using LEEP, laser, or cold knife conization.

Prevention and Education

♦ Encourage clients to recognize their personal risk factors and to obtain annual screening.
♦ Encourage prevention of STDs and reduction of risk factors.
♦ Advocate postponing sexual activity when counseling adolescents.
♦ Encourage the use of barrier methods of contraception.
♦ Encourage smoking cessation.

UTERINE CANCER

Endometrial or uterine cancer is the most common gynecologic malignancy in women ages 45 years and older (Paley, 2001). It may occur with exposure of the endometrium to high levels of exogenous and/or endogenous estrogen.

Epidemiology

An estimated 36,100 new cases of cancer of the corpus uteri and 6,500 deaths from this cancer were reported by ACOG in 2000 (ACOG, 2001, CO 247). It is the seventh most common malignancy in women. Its incident rate in the United States is about 20 percent. It occurs more frequently in Caucasian and Hawaiian women, moderately in African Americans, Japanese, and Chinese women, and less frequently in Filipino, Korean, and Native American women. It has one of the highest survival rates of all cancers (Paley, 2001).

Risk Factors

♦ Unopposed estrogen replacement.
♦ Hormone replacement therapy, especially unopposed estrogen.
♦ Obesity.
♦ Nulliparity or low parity.
♦ History of diabetes.
♦ History of hypertension.
♦ Menopause.
♦ Chronic anovulation.
♦ Tamoxifen use (Rosenfeld, 2001).

Screening. The incidence of uterine cancer in women younger than 40 is low; hence routine screening of these women is not recommended. Screening of all women over age 40 is neither practical nor cost effective. The criteria used in performing endometrial sampling include the following:

♦ Any unexplained peri- or postmenopausal bleeding (includes light staining or spotting).
♦ Premenopausal clients with polycystic ovarian syndrome.
♦ Premenopausal clients taking unopposed exogenous estrogen.
♦ Obese, nulliparous clients with diabetes or hypertension.
♦ Tamoxifen therapy (baseline, then annually).

Techniques for endometrial sampling vary. Screening is performed by an experienced gynecologist, usually in an office without anesthesia. Fractional dilation and curettage (D & C) with hysteroscopy in a surgical center may be required in some circumstances.

The most commonly used and easiest technique is the pipelle biopsy. It can be performed by the nurse practitioner if he or she has experience and training in the appropriate setting. It employs the use of a slender suction catheter to obtain a small amount of tissue for pathology.

Transvaginal ultrasonography for measuring the endometrial lining is used to detect possible endometrial hyperplasia. If the endometrial lining measures less than 4 mm, then the client is at lower risk (Paley, 2001; Rosenfeld, 2001). US may indicate the need for D & C with hysteroscopy.

Follow-Up and Referral

Any high-risk client (see criteria for endometrial sampling) should be followed with regular biopsies. Positive findings warrant immediate referral to an experienced gynecologist.

Prevention and Education. Prevention should be aimed at weight management and control of obesity, the use of a progestin in hormone replacement therapy, and the early evaluation of any abnormal bleeding.

OVARIAN CANCER

Epidemiology

Ovarian cancer is the fifth leading cancer that is diagnosed in U.S. women and is the leading cause of death from gynecological malignancy (Walker, Schlesselman, & Ness, 2002). ACOG reported 23,100 new cases of ovarian cancer with 14,000 deaths in 2000 (ACOG, 2001, CP 247). Seventy-five percent of women with ovarian cancer are diagnosed with advanced stage disease and the five-year survival rate is poor at 28 percent (Paley, 2001). The rate of ovarian cancer in Native Americans at 17.5 per 100,000 is higher than that of the white population at 15.8/100,000 (Rosenfeld, 2001).

Risk Factors

- Advancing age.
- Family history of ovarian cancer.
- Nulliparity.
- Early menarche and late menopause.
- Personal or family history of breast or colon cancer (ACOG, 2001, EB 250; Rosenfeld, 2001; Walker et al., 2002).

Screening. No effective method of mass screening has yet been developed. Publicity has increased the public's awareness of the difficulty of early detection. Clients may ask about routine ultrasound and CA-125, although neither method is currently recommended for routine screening due to expense and poor sensitivity and reliability. It may be used in women with a first degree relative with ovarian cancer or with a combination of the above risk factors (ACOG, 2001, EB 250; Paley, 2001; Rollins, 2000). An annual bi-

manual examination is currently recommended. Symptoms of ovarian cancer include the following: unusual bloating, fullness and pressure, abdominal or back pain, lack of energy, and urinary symptoms. It has commonly been taught that these symptoms are too vague to assist in making an early diagnosis of ovarian cancer, but more recent studies demonstrate that practitioner and patient awareness of these symptoms may lead to an earlier diagnosis, thereby improving mortality rates (Goff, Mandel, Muntz, & Melancon, 2000; Olson, Mignone, Nakraseive, et al., 2001).

Follow-Up and Referral

Any postmenopausal client with a palpable ovary or mass should be referred for laparoscopic evaluation. Any woman who has completed childbearing and who has two or more first-degree relatives with epithelial ovarian cancer, multiple relatives with colon, endometrial, breast, and ovarian cancer should be considered for a prophylactic bilateral oophorectomy (Rosenfeld, 2001).

Prevention and Education. Pregnancy and oral contraceptives both lower the total number of ovulatory cycles in a woman's lifetime and decrease the risk of ovarian cancer (Walker et al., 2002). In a recent study, physical activity has been shown to reduce the risk of ovarian cancer by 27 percent (Cottreau, Ness, & Kriska, 2000). Discuss the known risk factors with the client. Emphasize the lack of good screening methods and encourage compliance with the annual gynecologic exam. Maintain a healthy weight and low fat diet.

VULVAR INTRAEPITHELIAL NEOPLASIA AND VULVAR CANCER

Vulvar intraepithelial neoplasia (VIN) is a cancer precursor that is often associated with human papillomavirus (Callahan et al., 2001). It is classified just as cervical intraepithelial neoplasia as VIN 1–3, based upon the grade of undifferentiated cells. Invasive vulvar cancer is the presence of a lesion that breaks through the basement membrane (Edwards, Tortolero-Luna, Linares, et al., 1996). During the past two decades, the incidence of carcinoma in situ of the vulva has increased with younger patients being affected—the mean age being approximately 45 years (Joura, Losch, Haider-Ageler, Breiteneclar, & Leodolter, 2000).

Epidemiology

The incidence of VIN in the United States has increased from 1.2 to 2.1 per 100,000 women in the last twenty years (Edwards et al., 1996). The American Cancer Society's 2002 statistics estimate 3,800 new cases of vulvar cancer and 800 deaths for the year 2002. It has increased significantly in Caucasian women under age 35 years. Vulvar cancer is responsible for 1 percent of all malignancies in women and 5 percent of all female genital cancers. It is the fourth most common gynecologic cancer after endometrial, ovarian, and cervical cancers (Ghurani & Penalver, 2001).

Vulvar cancer is predominately found in older women, increasing to more than 50 percent of cases in women age 70 years and older (Edwards et al., 1996).

Risk Factors (Ghurani & Penalver, 2001)

- Granulomatous infection.
- Herpes simplex virus.
- Human papillomavirus.
- Chronic immunosuppression.
- Hypertension.
- Diabetes.
- Obesity.

Screening. The diagnosis of vulvar carcinoma is almost always delayed because symptoms are similar to other conditions. Vulvar pruritis is the most consistent complaint, and women will self-treat with over-the-counter vaginal preparations. Other symptoms include a visible or palpable mass, pain, bleeding, ulceration, dysuria, and vaginal discharge (Ghurani & Penalver, 2001).

Simple inspection of the vulva with biopsy of suspicious lesions is the only available screening method. Careful inspection of the vulva should be an essential part of any physical examination, especially in high-risk clients. Physical examination may reveal some of the various lesions.

Paget disease presents with extreme pruritis and soreness, usually of long duration. Red or bright pink, desquamated, eczematoid areas among scattered, raised, white patches of hyperkeratosis. The borders are well-demarcated and raised.

Basal cell carcinoma is very rare and is associated with a long history of pruritis. The carcinoma occurs over the anterior two-thirds of the labia majora, with slightly elevated margins.

Verrucous carcinoma appears as condyloma, but does not respond to treatment. Invasive squamous cell carcinoma occurs when a woman is in her 60s and 70s. It presents with ulceration, friability, or induration of surrounding tissues.

A melanoma of the vulva involves the labia minora and clitoris. It is a darkly pigmented lesion, rare among African American women. Any recent growths, changes in appear-

ance of existing moles, or bleeding of growths should be investigated. Sarcoma occurs in women of all ages. The vulvar sarcoma is a rapidly expanding, painful mass.

Follow-Up and Referral

Any client with a persistent lesion of the vulva should be referred to a gynecologist for colposcopy, biopsy, and further evaluation and treatment.

Prevention and Education. Teach clients self-examination and advise them to seek evaluation of any persistent itching or unusual lesions. Encourage smoking cessation. Advise clients to avoid constricting undergarments and perfumes and dyes in the vulvar region. Advocate condom use and prevention of STDs. Perform or refer for biopsy for any suspicious lesions (Edwards et al., 1996).

DIETHYLSTILBESTROL (DES) EXPOSURE

DES was used extensively in the United States during the 1940s and early 1950s to treat pregnancy complications, including bleeding, premature labor, diabetes, and preeclampsia. Although studies during the late 1950s proved its ineffectiveness, DES use continued through 1971. An estimated 5 to 10 million were prescribed DES during pregnancy or were exposed to the drug in utero (Palmer, Anderson, Helmrich, & Herbst, 2000). These women exposed to DES are now on average 45 years old (Kaufman, Adam, Hatch, et al., 2000).

DES EXPOSURE SEQUELAE

Women exposed to DES may exhibit one or more of the following sequelae:

- Structural changes including transverse vaginal and cervical ridges (cocks combs, collars, and pseudopolyps), abnormally shaped uterine cavity, uterine hypoplasia.
- Vaginal adenosis with columnar epithelium on or beneath the vaginal muscosa; it is self-limiting and gradually disappears.
- Clear-cell adenocarcinoma of the cervix or vagina (incidence rises at age 15 and median age at diagnosis is 19 years).
- Increased incidences of spontaneous abortion, ectopic pregnancy, premature cervical dilation, and premature rupture of membranes.
- Increased incidence of breast cancer.

Risk

Women who were born in the United States between 1945 and 1971 to mothers who had complicated pregnancies and received DES (Kaufman et al., 2000).

Screening

All women born between 1940 and 1971 should be questioned about possible exposure to DES. If history suggests exposure, the following screening techniques may be employed.

- An initial examination is recommended following menarche or at age 14 if no menarche; routine examination is every six to twelve months thereafter and includes inspection, palpation, and cytology.
- Cytology requires vaginal scrapings taken from all four quadrants of the fornix and fixed on slides for cytological review.
- Careful inspection of the cervix and vagina using one-half strength Lugol's solution and palpation of the entire vaginal wall.
- Colposcopy is performed by an experienced colposcopist if the Pap smear is abnormal. Appropriate biopsies are done for evaluation (Hacker & Moore, 1998).
- DES daughters should be followed as high-risk obstetric patients because of the increased risk of spontaneous abortion, ectopic pregnancy, early cervical effacement, and premature labor (Kaufman et al., 2000). However, recent studies seem to demonstrate an absence of abnormalities in the lower genital tract in third generation offspring of DES daughters (Kaufman & Adam, 2002).

FOLLOW-UP AND REFERRAL

Any abnormal cytology or undiagnosed lesion requires referral to a gynecologist.

Provide the client with information about DES and its possible effects. Stress the importance of having a regular examination and cytology. Allow time for the client to express her concerns. In addition, stress that DES exposure is not known to interfere with fertility, although there may be some risk of premature delivery. Practitioners are encouraged to refer women with known in utero exposure to centers that have focused on the follow-up, treatment, and education of these women. There are no known contraindications to oral contraceptive use.

REFERENCES

Adamson, D. (2001). Endometriosis: Traditional perspectives, current evidence and future possibilities. *International Journal of Fertility and Women's Medicine, 46*, 151–168.

American College of Obstetricians and Gynecologists (ACOG). (2001). *Compendium of Selected Publications*. Washington, DC: Author.

Practice Bulletins (PB)

11. Medical management of endometriosis. (1999). Pages 978–990.

16. Surgical alternatives to hysterectomy in the management of leiomyomas. (2000), Pages 1062–1068.

Technical Bulletins (TB)

191. Hysteroscopy. (1994). Pages 541–545.

211. Sexual dysfunction. (1995). Pages 778–784.

214. Pelvic organ prolapse. (1995). Pages 686–693.

215. Gynecologic ultrasonography. (1995). Pages 479–487.

223. Chronic pelvic pain. (1996). Pages 371–377.

Committee Opinion (CO)

247. Routine cancer screening. (2000). Pages 233–237.

Educational Bulletin (EB)

250. Ovarian cancer. (1998). Pages 671–679.

Anderson, P.S., & Runowicz, C.D. (2002). Beyond the Pap test: New techniques for cervical cancer screening. *Women's Health, 2*, 37–43.

Bergerson, S., Yitzchak, M.B., Khalife, S., Pagidos, K., & Glazer, H.I. (2001). Vulvar vestibulitis syndrome: Reliability of diagnosis and evaluation of current diagnostic criteria. *Obstetrics and Gynecology, 98*, 45–51.

Black, M.M., McKay, M., & Braude, P.R. (1995). *Obstetric and gynecologic dermatology*. Philadelphia, PA: Mosby-Wolfe.

Bornstein, J., Maman, M., & Abramovici, H. (2001). "Primary" versus "secondary" vulvar vestibulitis: One disease, two variants. *American Journal of Obstetrics and Gynecology, 184*, 28–31.

Callahan, T.L., Caughey, A.B., & Heffner, L.J. (2001). *Blueprints in obstetrics and gynecology* (2nd ed.). Boston: Blackwell Sciences.

Carmina, E., & Lobo, R.A. (2001). Polycystic ovaries in hirsute women with normal menses. *The American Journal of Medicine, 111*, 602–606.

Carter, J.F., & Soper, D.E. (2001). Diagnosing and treating nongynecologic chronic pelvic pain; musculoskeletal causes, surgery, and "psychology." *Women's Health, Gynecology Edition, 1*, 166–174.

Centers for Disease Control and Prevention (CDC). (2002). Sexually transmitted disease guidelines 2002. *MMWR Morbidity and Mortality Weekly Report 51* (No. RR-6), 1–76.

Chiaffarino, F., Parazzini, F., LaVecchia, C., Marsico, S., Surace, M., & Ricci, E. (1999). Use of oral contraceptives and uterine fibroids. *British Journal of Obstetrics and Gynecology, 106,* 857–860.

Cottreau, C.M., Ness, R.B., & Kriska A.M. (2000). Physical activity and reduced risk of ovarian cancer. *Obstetrics and Gynecology, 96,* 609–614.

Critchlow, C.W., Wolner-Hanssen, P., Eschenbach, D.A., et al. (1995). Determinants of cervical ectopia and of cervicitis: Age, oral contraception, specific cervical infection, smoking, and douching. *American Journal of Obstetrics and Gynecology, 173,* 534–543.

Cundiff, G.W., Weidner, A.C., Visco, A.G., Bump, R.C., & Addison, W.A. (2000). A survey of pessary use by members of the American Urogynecologic Society. *Obstetrics and Gynecology, 95,* 931–935.

Davila, G.W. (1996). Vaginal prolapse, management with nonsurgical techniques. *Postgraduate Medicine, 99,* 171–185.

DeCherney, A.H., & Nathan, L. (2003). Current obstetric & gynecologic diagnosis & treatment, 9th ed. New York, NY: Lange Medical Books/McGraw-Hill.

Edwards, C.L., Tortolero-Luna, G., Linares, A.C., et al. (1996). Vulvar intraepithelial neoplasia and vulvar cancer. *Obstetrics and Gynecology Clinics of North America, 23,* 259–345.

Ferenczy, A., Choukeroun, D., & Arseneau, J. (1996). Loop electrosurgical excision procedure for squamous intraepithelial lesions of the cervix: Advantages and potential pitfalls. *Obstetrics and Gynecology, 87,* 332–337.

Gelbaya, T.A., & El-Halwagy, H.E. (2001). Focus on primary care: Chronic pelvic pain in women. *Obstetrical and Gynecologic Survey, 56,* 757–764.

Ghurai, G.B., & Penalver, MA. (2001). An update on vulvar cancer. *American Journal of Obstetrics and Gynecology, 185,* 294–299.

Goff, B.A., Mandel, L., Muntz, H.G., & Melancon, C.H. (2000). Ovarian carcinoma diagnosis. *Cancer, 89,* 2068–2075.

Gordon, J.D., & Speroff, L., (2002). *Handbook for clinical gynecologic endocrinology and infertility.* Philadelphia: Lippincott, Williams & Wilkins.

Hacker, N.F., & Moore, J.G. (1998). *Essentials of obstetrics and gynecology* (3rd ed.). Philadelphia: W.B. Saunders & Co.

Heim, L.J. (2001). Evaluation and differential diagnosis of dyspareunia. *American Family Physician, 63,* 1535–1544.

Heit, M., Culligan, P., Rosenquist, C., & Shott, S. (2002). Is pelvic organ prolapse a cause of pelvic or low back pain? *Obstetrics and Gynecology, 99,* 23–28.

Huirne, J.A.F., & Lambalk, C.B. (2001). Gonadotropin-releasing-hormone-receptor antagonists. *Lancet, 358,* 1793–1803.

Jamieson, D.J., & Steege, J.F. (1996). The prevalence of dysmenorrhea, dyspareunia, pelvic pain and irritable bowel syndrome in primary care practices. *Obstetrics and Gynecology, 87,* 55–58.

Joessens, M.R., Schacter, J., & Sweet, R.L. (1994). Risk factors associated with pelvic inflammatory disease of differing microbial etiology. *Obstetrics and Gynecology, 83,* 989–997.

Jones, G., Kennedy, S., Barnard, A., & Jenkinson, C. (2001). Development of an endometriosis quality-of-life instrument: The endometriosis health profile-30. *Obstetrics and Gynecology, 98,* 258–264.

Joura, E.A., Losch, A., Haider-Ageler, M.G., Breiteneclar, G., & Leodolter, S. (2000). Trends in vulvar neoplasia: Increasing incidence of vulvar intraepithelial neoplasia and squamous cell carcinoma of the vulva in young women. *Reproductive Medicine, 45,* 613–660.

Kaufman, R.H., & Adam, E. (2002). Findings in female offspring of women exposed in utero to Diethylstilbestrol. *Obstetrics and Gynecology, 99,* 197–200.

Kaufman, R.H., Adam, E., Hatch, E.E., Noller, K., Herbst, A.L., & Palmer, J.R. (2000). Continued follow-up of pregnancy outcomes in diethylstilestrol-exposed offspring. *Obstetrics and Gynecology, 96,* 483–489.

Keckstein, J. (2000). Hysteroscopy and adenomyosis. *Contributions to Gynecology and Obstetrics, 20,* 41–50.

Kenkel, K., Hricak, H., Lu, Y., Tsuda, K., & Filly, R.A. (2000). Ultrasound characterization of ovarian masses: A meta-analysis. *Radiology, 217,* 803–811.

Klein, A., & Schwartz, M.L. (2001). Uterine artery embolization for the treatment of uterine fibroids: an outpatient procedure. *American Journal of Obstetrics & Gynecology, 184,* 1556–1560.

Koninckx, P., Meuleman, C., Oosterlynck, D., & Cornillie, F. (1996). Diagnosis of deep endometriosis by clinical examination during menstruation and plasma CA-125 concentration. *Fertility and Sterility, 65*(2), 280–287.

Kovacs, P. (2001). Transvaginal ultrasonography, sonohysterography, and operative hysteroscopy for the evaluation of abnormal uterine bleeding. *Medscape Women's Health, 6,* 2.

Kreiter, C.R. (2000). Vulvar vestibulitis. *Advance for Nurse Practitioners, 8,* 67–69.

Lampe, A., Solder, E., Ennemoser, A., Schubert, C., Rumplod, G., & Soliner, W. (2000). Chronic pelvic pain and previous sexual abuse. *Obstetrics and Gynecology, 96,* 929–933.

Larrabee, R., & Kylander, D.J. (2001). Benign vulvar disorders. *Postgraduate Medicine, 109,* 151–164.

Lethaby, A., Vollenhaven, B., & Sowter, M. (2002). Pre-operative GnRH analogue therapy before hysterectomy or myomectomy for uterine fibroids. *Cochrane Review,* 1.

Luber, J.M., Boero, M.D., & Choe, J.Y. (2001). The demographics of pelvic floor disorders: Current observations and future projections. *American Journal of Obstetrics and Gynecology, 184,* 1496–1501.

Lynch, P.J., & Edwards, L. (1994). *Genital dermatology.* New York: Churchill Livingstone, Inc.

Marin, M.G., King, R., Sfamini, S., & Dennerstein, G. (2000). Adverse behavioral and sexual factors in chronic vulvar disease. *American Journal of Obstetrics and Gynecology, 183,* 34–38.

Mathias, S.D., Kupperman, M., Liberman, R.F., et al. (1996). Chronic pelvic pain, prevailing health-related quality of life, and economic correlates. *Obstetrics and Gynecology, 87,* 321–32.

Morphis, L.O., & Steadman, M.S. (1999). Gynecologic disorders and female sexual function. In E. Youngkin, K. Sawin, J. Kissinger, & D. Israel (Eds.), *Pharmacotherapeutics: A primary care clinical guide* (pp. 835–862). Stamford, CT: Appleton & Lange.

Morris, M., Tortolero-Luna, G., Malpica, A., et al. (1996). Cervical intraepithelial neoplasia and cervical cancer. *Obstetrics and Gynecology Clinics of North America, 23,* 347–410.

Ness, R.B., Soper, D.E., Holley, R.L., Peipert, J., Randall, H., & Sweet, R.L. (2001). Hormonal and barrier contraception and risk of upper genital tract disease in the PID Evaluation and Clinical Health (PEACH) study. *American Journal of Obstetrics and Gynecology, 185,* 121–127.

Olive, D.L., & Pritts, E.A. (2001). Treatment of endometriosis. *New England Journal of Medicine, 345,* 266–275.

Olson, S.H., Mignone, L., Nakraseive, C., Caputo, T.A., Barakat, R.R., & Harlap, S. (2001). Symptoms of ovarian cancer. *Obstetrics and Gynecology, 98,* 212–217.

Padilla, L., Radosevich, D., & Milad, M. (2000). Accuracy of the pelvic examination in detecting adnexal masses. *Obstetrics and Gynecology, 96,* 593–598.

Paley, P.J. (2001). Screening for the major malignancies affecting women. *American Journal of Obstetrics and Gynecology, 184,* 1021–1030.

Palmer, J.R., Anderson, D., Helmrich, S.P., & Herbst, A.L. (2000). Risk factors for Diethylstilbestrol-associated clear cell adenocarcinoma. *Obstetrics and Gynecology, 95,* 814–820.

Peipert, J.F., Ness, R.B., Blume, J., Soper, D.E., Holley, R., & Randall, H. (2001). Clinical predictors of endometritis in women with symptoms and signs of pelvic inflammatory disease. *American Journal of Obstetrics and Gynecology, 184,* 856–863.

Perry, C.P. (2001). Current concepts of pelvic congestion and chronic pelvic pain. *Journal of the Society of Laparoendoscopic Surgeons, 5,* 105–110.

Prather, C. (1995). Hysteroscopy: The nurse's role in office hysteroscopy. *Journal of Obstetric, Gynecologic, and Neonatal Nursing, 24,* 813–816.

Prentice, A. (2001). Endometriosis. *The British Medical Journal, 323,* 93–95.

Rein, D.B., Kassler, W.J., Irwin, K.L., & Rabiee, L. (2000). Direct medical costs of pelvic inflammatory disease and its sequelae: Decreasing, but still substantial. *Obstetrics and Gynecology, 95,* 397–402.

Reiter, R.C. (1990). A profile of women with chronic pelvic pain. *Clinical Obstetrics and Gynecology, 33,* 130–136.

Rollins, G. (2000). Developments in cervical and ovarian cancer screening: Implications for current practice. *Annals of Internal Medicine, 133,* 1021–1024.

Rosenfeld, J. (2001). *Handbook of women's health: An evidence-based approach.* New York: Cambridge University Press.

Seltzer, V.L., & Pearse, W.H. (1995). *Women's primary health care.* New York: McGraw-Hill.

Siegler, A.M. (1995). Office hysteroscopy. *Obstetric and Gynecology Clinics of North America, 22,* 457–471.

Siegler, A.M., & Camilien, L. (1994). Adenomyosis. *The Journal of Reproductive Medicine, 39,* 841–853.

Solomon, D., Davey, D., Kurman, R., Moriarty, A., O'Connor, D., et al. for the Forum Group Members and the Bethesda 2001 Workshop. (2002). The 2001 Bethesda System: Terminology for reporting results of cervical cytology. *Journal of the American Medical Association, 287,* 2114–2119.

Spadt, S.K. (1995). Suffering in silence: Managing vulvar pain patients. *Contemporary Nurse Practitioner, 1,* 32–38.

Spies, J.B., Ascher, S.A., Roth, A.R., Kim, J., Levy, E.B., & Gomez-Jorge, J. (2001). Uterine artery embolization for leiomyomata. *Obstetrics and Gynecology, 9,* 29–34.

Stewart, E.A. (2001). Uterine fibroids. *Lancet, 37,* 293–298.

Templeman, C., Fallat, M.E., Blinchevshy, A., & Hertweck, S.P. (2000). Noninflammatory ovarian masses in girls and young women. *Obstetrics and Gynecology, 96,* 229–233.

Walker, G.R., Schlesselman, J.J., & Ness, R.B. (2002). Family history of cancer, oral contraceptive use, and ovarian cancer risk. *American Journal of Obstetrics and Gynecology, 186,* 8–14.

Waller, J.G., & Shaw, R.W. (1995). Endometriosis, pelvic pain, and psychological functioning. *Fertility and Sterility, 63,* 796–800.

Weber, A.M., Walters, M.D., Schover, L.R., et al. (1995). Sexual functioning in women with uterovaginal prolapse and urinary incontinence. *Obstetrics and Gynecology, 85,* 483–487.

Winkel, C.A. (2001). Role of a symptom-based alogorithmic approach to chronic pelvic pain. *International Journal of Gynaecology and Obstetrics, 74,* 15–20.

Wright, Jr., T., Cox, J., Massad, L., Twiggs, L., Wilkinson, E., for the 2001 ASCCP-Sponsored Consensus Conference. (2002). 2001 Consensus guidelines for the management of women with cervical cytological abnormalities. *Journal of the American Medical Association, 287*(16), 2120–2129.

Zondervan, K.T., Yudkin, P.L., Vessey, M.P., Jenkinson, C.P., & Dawes, M.G. (2001). Chronic pelvic pain in the community-symptoms, investigations, and diagnoses. *American Journal of Obstetrics and Gynecology, 184,* 1149–1155.

Zoorob, R., Anderson, R. Cefalu, C., & Sidani, M. (2001). Cancer screening guidelines. *American Family Physician, 63,* 1101–1112.

CHAPTER 14

BREAST HEALTH

Lynette Galloway Branch

*T*horough breast as-
sessment, including
history taking for risk
factors and education
regarding breast self-
exams, should be stan-
dard protocol for the
health provider during
a client's annual exam.

Highlights

- Breast Examination: Professional, Self-Exam, and Mammography
- Benign Breast Disorders
    Fibrocystic Changes
    Fibroadenoma
    Nipple Discharge
- Malignant Neoplasms
- Breast Reconstruction
    Tissue Transfer
    Augmentation Mammoplasty
    Mastopexy
    Breast Reduction

❖ INTRODUCTION

The female breast is closely linked with womanhood in the American culture. The more amply endowed the female bosom, the "sexier" and more womanly one is perceived. Although the primary function of the breasts is lactation, breasts are perceived as erotic. They are attractive and alluring to men and a source of sensual pleasure for women as well. Thus, the loss or injury of these important anatomic structures is potentially psychologically devastating to both sexes.

For women in their childbearing years, breast injury or loss threatens the ability to nourish and nurture offspring by means of breastfeeding. This intimate, interactional process may be perceived as the ultimate way of connecting and communicating with a newborn. Middle-aged women, who have begun to observe the effects of aging on their bodies, may perceive breast loss or injury as an additional change to their once youthful-appearing bodies. Elderly women, who are living longer, desire to maintain their fitness, which entails keeping their bodies healthy and intact. Hence, maintaining breast health is conducive to maintaining optimal physical and psychological health.

Concerns about breasts and breast symptoms are among the most common complaints of women who seek medical attention. Although most concerns have no disease or have benign changes as their underlying condition, the fear of cancer causes great anxiety and stress for most women who have any breast symptoms. This anxiety is indeed warranted since a woman has a one in three chance of developing breast cancer in her lifetime, with the risk increasing substantially with age (American Cancer Society [ACS], 2002a).

Since concerns about breast health are common in primary care settings and since the primary care provider is most often the first point of contact in today's health delivery system, it is important that health care providers have substantial knowledge about breast related disorders and diseases. A basic understanding of the most severe form of breast disease—cancer—is paramount so that immediate referral can be made and mortality reduced.

BREAST EXAMINATION AND ASSESSMENT

Breast examination has a pivotal role in the early detection of breast cancer and diseases. This examination may be carried out by a health professional, the client herself, or by means of mammography. Breast self-examination (BSE) is practiced today by many women and should be taught to adolescents at menarche so that a pattern of breast examination and cancer detection begin early. Breast cancer patients who regularly perform this examination present to their health care providers with lesions that they have discovered (Coates et al., 2001). Yet, many more women fail to carry out this valuable monthly exercise. Why is not clear. It is speculated, however, that motivating factors are health beliefs, fear and anxiety of discovering a lump, hence, a cancer; lack of knowledge or self-confidence regarding the technique of BSE; denial; discomfort with body manipulation; lack of perceived susceptibility to or risk of breast cancer; lack of perceived benefits; and apathy (Adams, Becker, & Colbert, 2001). If this ten-minute routine is not incorporated into a woman's lifestyle, breast cancer may not be detected early and the risk of death due to breast cancer may increase.

The American Cancer Society (2002a, 2000b) recommends the following examination schedule to detect breast cancer in asymptomatic women:

- ◆ *Age 20–39:* Monthly BSE, clinical breast exam every three years.
- ◆ *Age 40 and over:* Monthly BSE, annual clinical breast exam, annual mammography.

The National Cancer Institute (NCI), noting a recent challenge of the effectiveness of screening mammography in saving lives (Olsen & Gotzsche, 2001), and while not offering suggestions regarding breast self-examination and clinical breast exam, differs in its recommendations regarding mammography screening (NCI, 2002). They recommend that:

- ◆ Women in their 40s be screened every one to two years with mammography.
- ◆ Women aged 50 and older should be screened every year.

◆ Women who are at higher than average risk of breast cancer should seek expert medical advice about whether they should begin screening before age 40 and the frequency of screening.

MAMMOGRAPHY SCREENING AND COSTS

Although the American Cancer Society and the National Cancer Institute provide mammography screening guidelines, the health care provider should consider the cost of mammograms for women who do not have coverage by third party payers. Often the cost of the procedure and radiologic interpretation are prohibitive. Some patients may choose to forgo this important screening procedure if they are unable to afford the cost (Adams et al., 2001). Thus, careful investigation should be performed to discover agencies in the community or region who will provide quality mammograms for low or no cost.

TECHNIQUE FOR BREAST SELF-EXAMINATION (BSE)

BSE follows a specific technique (see Figure 14–1). The exam should be done each month, after the menstrual period: Day 4, 5, 6, or 7 is optimal. Menopausal and pregnant women should perform the exam on the first day of each month. For menstruating women, a note placed on a box of feminine hygiene pads or tampons, or on a personal calendar may serve as a reminder to perform BSE.

The Sensor Pad, designed to help women to examine their breasts, has been approved by the Food and Drug Administration. This pad has two layers, is ten inches in diameter, and is filled with a small amount of silicon lubricant. The silicon lubricant is designed to help the fingers to glide easily over the breasts as they do when the breasts are lathered with soap. This pad, used after instruction, not only may help to detect breast lumps but may also serve as a reminder to perform breast exam. Currently, the pad is available by prescription for patients who are interested. Patients who are not interested in using the pad or who find the cost of the pad prohibitive can be encouraged to examine their breasts while bathing.

Breast self-examination proceeds in the following manner:

1. While standing in front of a mirror, observe both breasts for symmetry, dimpling, scaling, redness, bruising, and nipple irritation, discharge, or retraction (Figure 14–1A).

2. Continue observations with hands elevated above the head (Figure 14–1B).

3. Continue observations with hands placed firmly on the hips and body bowed slightly forward (Figure 14–1C).

4. Place one arm above the head and palpate the breast closest to that arm for lumps, masses, and tenderness. Use the fingers (not fingertips) of the opposite hand to glide over the breast in a circular fashion, starting in the upper outer quadrant of the breast and continuing until the entire breast, including the areola and nipple, has been examined (Figure 14–1D). Observe the nipple for discharge during this examination. Next, thoroughly palpate the axillary region for enlarged or tender nodes. Repeat the procedure for the other breast. (*Note:* Right hand examines the left breast, and left hand examines the right breast.)

5. Finally, lie supine with a pillow or towel behind one shoulder and examine the breast as in step 4 (Figure 14–1E). Move the pillow or towel to the opposite shoulder and repeat the procedure for the other breast.

BREAST ASSESSMENT BY THE HEALTH CARE PROVIDER

Despite the advances in breast imaging, a hands-on, clinical examination is vitally important. A thorough breast assessment, including history taking for risk factors and education regarding BSE, should be standard protocol for the health provider during a client's annual exam. To omit breast evaluation from routine examinations may result in missed opportunities for early detection of breast cancer (DiSaia & Creasman, 2002).

History

Obtain the client's history and her family history of breast disease, breast symptoms, and breast cancer. Special attention should be given to breast diseases in the maternal family, especially the mother, siblings, or daughter, since breast cancer in a first-degree relative increases the client's risk of cancer (ACS, 2002a). Also inquire about the client's menstrual and reproductive history, including information about menarche, onset of menopause, number of pregnancies and deliveries and age at both, as well as lactation or breastfeeding history. Ask the client about her current medication usage—specifically, antidepressive or psychotropic drugs, antihypertensives, hormonal therapy (estrogen, progesterone), and oral contraceptives,

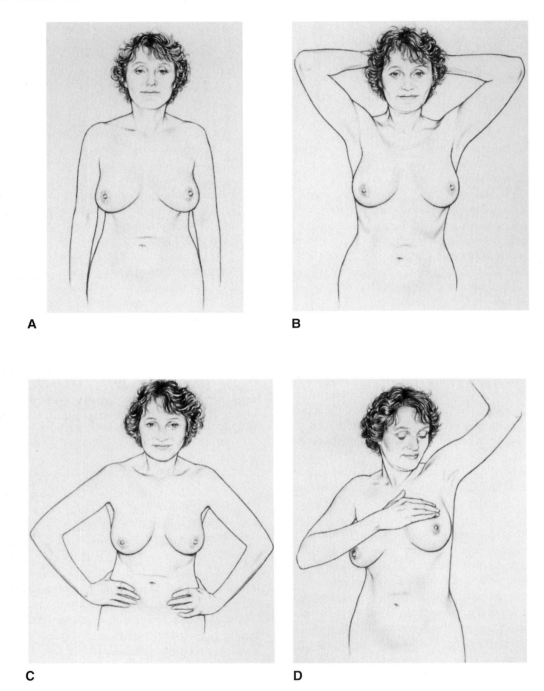

FIGURE 14–1. Breast self-examination (BSE) (perform procedure each month). See page 353. *(From National Cancer Institute (March, 1984). Breast Exams—What You Should Know. (NIH pub. no. 84–2000.) Bethesda, MD: National Institutes of Health.)*

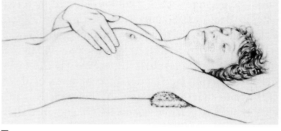

E

FIGURE 14–1 (*cont.*)

which could induce breast changes. Also inquire about her dietary habits, including caffeine intake, frequency of BSE, clinical examination, and mammography.

Breast Examination

Freund (2000) notes that the main goal of the clinical breast examination is to differentiate normal physiologic nodularity from a discrete breast mass.

The health care provider should therefore devote ample time to examining the breasts, teaching the proper technique for BSE, and encouraging monthly BSE. The client should be provided the opportunity and encouraged to demonstrate BSE. Breast models that allow clients to practice on normal and abnormal breasts often help to increase client confidence in BSE. The breast exam by the health care provider should be systematic:

1. Observe the client while she is sitting with her hands resting in her lap, with hands overhead and chest wall forward, and with her hands placed firmly on her hips (which contracts the pectoral muscles). Observe the breasts for dimpling, retraction, color changes, skin thickening, spontaneous nipple discharge, and asymmetry. (*Note:* Some asymmetry is normal, i.e., one breast may be slightly larger or smaller than the other. It is important to ask the client if the asymmetry had been previously observed.)

2. If the client has large, pendulous breasts, ask her to lean over while placing her hands on your shoulders. In this position, observe the breasts for symmetry, retraction, and dimpling.

3. Allow the client's arm to rest diagonally on your arm (positioned from the client's right to your right) as you palpate the axillary nodes. Repeat this procedure for the opposite axilla. Then palpate the supraclavicular and infraclavicular lymph nodes. Since lymph node enlargement or firmness may indicate the

spread of breast cancer, axillary and clavicular lymph nodes should be examined with care (Hindle & Gonzalez, 2001). Next, palpation of the breasts with the patient in the upright position may allow the detection of subtle lesions that would be more difficult to palpate with the patient in the supine position (DiSaia & Creasman, 2002). If the breasts are pendulous, palpate them while the client is seated.

4. Ask the client to lie supine and extend the arm on the side of the breast to be examined overhead. Place a pillow beneath the same shoulder.

5. Then palpate the client's breast from the upper outer quadrant to the nipple in a circular fashion, taking care to cover each breast quadrant. Give careful attention to the Tail of Spence.

6. Observe the nipple for discharge.

7. Perform steps 3 through 6 on the opposite breast.

BENIGN BREAST CONDITIONS

Benign breast conditions account for most breast symptoms and complaints seen in the primary care setting (Hamed & Fentiman, 2001). Frequently, a significant amount of time must be spent reassuring the client that the lesion is indeed benign, thus patience and support are essential.

FIBROCYSTIC CHANGES

Fibrocystic changes of the breast are diverse and are the most frequently encountered benign breast condition seen in the primary practice. The term includes a broad grouping of lesions, including cystic mastitis, large and small cyst formation, epithelial hyperplasia, apocrine metaplasia, fibrosis metaplasia, and sclerosing adenosis (Hindle & Gonzalez, 2001; Hughes, Mansel, & Webster, 2000; Schnett & Connelly, 2000). Breast thickness, lumpiness and/or palpable nodularity is present. Pain is almost always present and is the most common sign and symptom of fibrocystic change. (Hindle & Gonzalez, 2001, Padden, 2000).

Epidemiology

The exact etiology of fibrocystic breast changes is unknown, but several theories exist. The development of mastalgia and tender nodularity is thought to represent a physiological response to hormonal outflow (Hughes et al., 2000). It is thought that an imbalance between estrogen and progestin produces excessive ductal stimulation and proliferation, which produces these symptoms. Pain is also thought to be due to stromal edema. Nodularity and tenderness may be physiological and due to hormone stimulation, or they may be secondary to estrogen excess.

Hyperprolactinemia has been considered a cause of fibrocystic changes. Prolactin levels are elevated in one-third of women with fibrocystic breast changes (Hughes et al., 2000). The hyperprolactinemia is thought to be related to the increased levels of estrogen noticed in some patients. It has not been found to be a consistent causative factor in fibrocystic changes of the breasts; thus, it does not apply to all cases.

Fibrocystic changes are found in all women of reproductive years (Hindle & Gonzalez, 2001).

Subjective Data

The client reports bilateral or unilateral breast pain and tenderness (the symptom is usually bilateral) (Hindle & Gonzalez, 2001). The pain is cyclic and frequently begins seven to fourteen days prior to the menses and resolves sometime after the onset of menses. Sometimes, however, pain is present at all times. Breast lumpiness and nodularity is also noted and may be localized, especially in the upper outer quadrants of the breasts (Hindle & Gonzalez, 2001). The client may also report that the breasts are engorged and occasionally a spontaneous nipple discharge is seen.

Objective Data

Physical Examination. Examination of the breasts reveals thickening and lumpiness (usually bilateral), which is palpated primarily in the outer quadrants. Lymphatic examination reveals tender palpable axillary lymph nodes in some women. No clavicular nodal enlargement is palpable. In older or postmenopausal women, a ridge of nodularity may be found along the inframammary margin, particularly in the lower quadrant of the breast.

Diagnostic Tests and Methods

Mammography. Mammography remains the most widely used imaging modality available today. It is the only technique with proven efficacy for breast cancer screening (Kopans, 2000). It does not detect all cancers early enough to prevent death but can reduce the death rate by 30 percent (Kopans, 2000). Mammography is performed to identify and characterize a breast mass and to detect an early malignancy. It can detect lesions as small as 0.5 cm in size (Willison, 2001), which is commendable consider-

ing that the average size of a tumor detected by a female practicing BSE occasionally is approximately 2.5 cm in size. Occult lesions detected by mammography are eight years old; thus mammography is incapable of detecting a lesion at the cellular level (Willison, 2001). The test procedure involves taking radiographic pictures of the bare breasts while they are compressed between two plastic plates. Generally, cranial-caudal (CC) and mediolateral oblique (MLO) views of the compressed breasts are taken because they provide best coverage of the breast tissue (Willison, 2001). Other images, however, may be taken during diagnostic studies to help to predict the origin of a lesion.

Mammography is not appropriate for all females. It is not usually recommended in women under the age of 30 (Andolina, 2001). Younger women have dense and more radiosensitive breasts. A white-on-white image of a younger women's mostly glandular breasts accounts for more inaccuracy (Andolina, 2001). The decreased incidence of breast cancer in this group also makes screening less cost effective; thus, although a mammogram may detect cancer in younger women, it should not be a standard method of evaluation.

Most women find the ten-minute procedure temporarily uncomfortable but not painful. Inform the client that the tenderness that may be caused by breast compression may be relieved by acetaminophen, ibuprofen, or aspirin. To decrease discomfort, the procedure may be scheduled for a time of the menstrual cycle when breasts are less tender. Deodorant and powder containing aluminum, calcium, or zinc products can cause shadows to appear on the x-rays, making them more difficult to read (Andolina, 2001; Lillé, 2001). They should therefore be removed with soap and water before x-ray or they should be avoided on the day of the exam.

Help the client to choose a mammography facility that is accredited by the American College of Radiology (ACR) and ascertain that machines are designed specifically for mammography. Try to ensure that the mammogram is performed by a registered technologist and that the radiologist is trained to read mammography. The radiology facility may not reveal the results of the x-ray to the client; therefore, it is important that a follow-up visit be scheduled as soon as possible to discuss the mammographic findings or that a note detailing the findings be mailed to the client.

Ultrasound. Sonography is a useful problem-solving tool and is an excellent adjunct to mammography for breast evaluation. The procedure helps to differentiate a cystic mass from a solid one (Hindle & Gonzalez, 2001). Ultrasound is usually performed after mammography in the patient older than 30 years of age and may be the only modality employed in women younger than age 30 (Kossoff, 2000; Sakorafas, 2001). Images of the breasts are produced via sound waves that travel through a gel medium that is applied to the breasts.

Explain the procedure to the client and offer support. The test must be performed by a qualified radiologist. It is not contraindicated in pregnancy.

Fine-Needle Aspiration. Diagnostic evaluation using fine-needle aspiration is done to identify a solid tumor, cyst, or malignancy. The procedure should be done by a trained health care provider, usually an obstetrics/gynecology specialist or a surgeon.

Using universal precautions, the test procedure involves first cleaning the breast with an antiseptic solution (usually alcohol). Then the mass is stabilized between the fingers of the nondominant hand and compressed downward. It should be pushed up and over a rib for stabilization when possible. A 22-gauge needle attached to a 5 cc or 10 cc syringe is inserted into the mass (Kline, Kline, & Howell, 1999). A finer gauge needle may be chosen, but withdrawal of fluid tissue will occur more slowly, which may result in more anxiety for the patient. As the needle is moved around in the mass, suction is applied to remove the contents. The needle is gently withdrawn, and pressure is applied to the puncture site. The specimen should then be placed on a clean glass slide. Gently spread at a 10-degree angle and fix the slide with alcohol or spray fixative (Kline et al., 1999) Prepare a second slide and allow it to air dry. Send both slides to a cytology lab. If straw-colored fluid is withdrawn, the diagnosis is usually benign; in this case the fluid may be discarded. However, if there is doubt, send the remaining fluid to the lab in a sterile glass tube. Absence of fluid may indicate a solid mass, which is suspicious of malignancy, necessitating open biopsy. It is thought that the injection of air post aspiration of a cystic structure will prevent recurrence of that lesion (Gizienski, Harvey, & Sobel, 2002).

Differential Medical Diagnoses

Malignant breast mass; physiological nodularity (when nodularity varies with the menstrual cycle). Pain may be due to cervical (neck) radiculopathy, costochondritis, respiratory infection, rib fracture, peptic ulcer disease, or hiatal hernia (Hindle & Gonzalez, 2001).

Plan

Psychosocial Intervention. Spend significant time performing a thorough breast exam that might assure the client that her complaint is taken seriously. If symptoms are minimal, i.e., occurring two to three days prior to menses, reassurance may be sufficient (Hamed & Fentiman, 2001). Focus on helping to alleviate anxiety by informing the client of the frequency and generally benign nature of the breast changes. Have literature available that provides information in a simplistic manner. Also provide reference books for those who might be interested.

Medication

Oral Contraceptives (OCs)

- *Indications.* Oral contraceptives prevent or slow the development of new fibrocystic changes and minimize symptoms of existing changes. (Hindle & Gonzalez, 2001). Symptoms are suppressed in 88 percent of clients with fibrocystic changes. An OC tends to be very helpful when pain is cyclic and is especially appropriate if the client needs a birth control method and OC use is not contraindicated. The effectiveness of oral contraceptives is based on the reduction of ovarian estradiol production and on the modulation of breast estrogen receptors by progestin.

- *Administration.* Low dose estrogen (e.g., ethinyl estradiol, 0.02 mg) and relatively high dose progesterone (e.g., norethindrone, 1.0 mg) pill daily for 3–6 months or longer. Frequently, symptoms improve drastically after 1 year and maximally after 2 years. If contraception is needed, 0.030 to 0.035 mg of ethinyl estradiol with progestin is used.

- *Side Effects and Adverse Reactions.* Possible water retention, weight gain, hypertension, cardiovascular changes, and breakthrough bleeding (see Chapter 9). Initiation of estrogen replacement may also produce dose-related mastalgia in the higher doses of OCs.

- *Contraindications.* See Chapter 9.

- *Anticipated Outcomes on Evaluation.* A decrease in symptoms associated with fibrocystic changes. If improvement is noted, oral contraceptives are continued. Symptoms will probably recur when therapy is discontinued.

- *Client Teaching and Counseling.* Explain to the client that her menstrual cycle may change and that breakthrough bleeding is possible when the pill is not taken as prescribed. Counsel her about the side effects and danger signs associated with pill use (see Chapter 9). Caution the client about expecting immediate results;

some breast symptoms may improve immediately; however, more severe symptoms require more time. Have the client keep a record of the effectiveness (or lack of) of the medication. Daily recording of symptoms may be extremely beneficial immediately after initiating OCs. Advise the client that symptoms may return when therapy is discontinued. The wearing of a supportive brassiere is essential.

Danazol

- *Indications.* Danazol, a steroid, reduces pain, tenderness and nodularity caused by fibrocystic changes. It is the primary drug of preference for the treatment of severe symptomatology of fibrocystic changes and is the only FDA-approved pharmaceutical treatment for mastalgia (Hindle & Gonzalez, 2001). It has been shown to prevent the midcycle luteinizing hormone surge, find and translocate androgen receptors and inhibit several enzymes involved in ovarian steroidogenesis (DiSaia & Creasman, 2002). Danazol creates a postmenopausal hormonal environment that reduces estrogen production and concentration in breast tissue, thereby reducing symptoms. It should be noted that as Danazol reduces the nodularity of small fibrocystic lesions, large cysts may appear to be more prominent and may require aspiration.
- *Administration.* The usual dose of Danazol is 200 mg per day in divided doses (Hindle & Gonzalez, 2001). Start with Danazol 200 mg per day beginning on menstrual cycle day two. Therapy may be tried for two months (Hughes et al., 2000). If symptomatic relief is maintained, the drug may be reduced to 100 mg every other day (Hindle & Gonzalez, 2001). Therapy should begin during menstruation or after a negative pregnancy test. Three to four months may pass before improvement in symptoms is observed; however, breast pain and tenderness may be significantly relieved in the first month and eliminated in two to three months. The elimination of nodularity usually requires four to six months of uninterrupted therapy.
- *Side Effects and Adverse Reactions.* Weight gain, menstrual irregularity (including amenorrhea), acne, increased cholesterol levels, decreased breast size, oily skin, growth of facial hair, hair loss, deepening voice (which may continue after therapy is terminated), sore throat, hoarseness, liver dysfunction, nervousness, depression, vaginitis. (Faiz & Fentiman, 2000).

- *Contraindications.* Undiagnosed abnormal genital bleeding; markedly impaired hepatic, renal, or cardiac function; pregnancy; breastfeeding; and clients whose symptoms occur only during the premenstrual period or who experience mild fibrocystic changes.
- *Anticipated Outcomes on Evaluation.* A decrease in breast tenderness and nodularity, and a decrease in the size of the breast cyst(s) if present.
- *Client Teaching and Counseling.* Advise the client that improvement normally occurs within the first month of therapy but may require four to six months. Also inform her that 50 to 65 percent of clients notice the return of some symptoms when Danazol is discontinued (Hughes et al., 2000). High cholesterol foods should be decreased in the diet, and a lipid profile and liver function tests should be drawn three months after therapy is initiated. The wearing of a supportive brassiere should be encouraged. A daily diary reflecting the effectiveness of Danazol therapy should be maintained throughout the use of the drug.

Tamoxifen

- *Indications.* Tamoxifen, known more for its use in breast cancer, reduces pain, tenderness, and nodularity caused by fibrocystic changes. It is an estrogen agonist that binds to the estrogen receptor and competes with estradiol for receptors of estrogen located in the breasts, thus decreasing pain. Reduction of symptoms, especially pain, is improved in 70 percent of patients (Hindle & Gonzalez, 2001). Some consider Tamoxifen the most effective treatment for severe *chronic* breast pain (Faiz & Fentiman, 2000).
- *Administration.* Tamoxifen 20 mg per day will normally decrease symptoms after two to three months (Hindle & Gonzalez, 2001). The dosage, however, must be tailored to the individual patient's requirement and symptom control balanced against troublesome side effects (Faiz & Fentiman, 2000). A dosage of 10 mg per day may be effective for some patients (Hughes et al., 2000).
- *Side Effects.* Nausea, vomiting, vaginal discharge, vaginal bleeding, malaise, urticaria, alopecia, weight gain, depression and hot flashes may occur. An increased risk for endometrial cancer also exists (DiSaia & Creasman, 2002, Hughes et al., 2000).
- *Contraindications.* Pregnancy.
- *Anticipated Outcomes.* A decrease in breast tenderness and nodularity.

◆ *Client Teaching.* After assuring that the client is not pregnant by performing a serum pregnancy test, advise the client to avoid pregnancy by consistent use of a barrier method of contraception. Also inform her that breast tenderness may actually increase during the first one to four weeks of therapy but should resolve after that time. Discuss all possible side effects of Tamoxifen. Strongly encourage regular Pap smears and endometrial surveillance. Discuss risk of endometrial cancer. As with other therapies, use of a supportive brassiere should be advocated and a daily diary of breast symptoms should be maintained.

Bromocriptine

◆ *Indications.* This dopamine receptor agonist may reduce the pain and nodularity of fibrocystic changes. (Hindle & Gonzalez, 2001). Because of the possible role of prolactin in the cause of breast pain, bromocriptine will decrease serum prolactin levels (Hughes et al., 2000). Its use, though controversial, has been found to reduce pain and nodularity in some patients. Bromocriptine should not be used frequently and should be restricted to very select patients who may not have had success with other therapies.

◆ *Administration.* Bromocriptine is given at 5 mg per day in two divided doses throughout therapy. Doses may start at 1.25 mg at bedtime, increasing by 1.25 mg every three to four days until the aforementioned dosage is reached.

◆ *Side Effects and Adverse Reactions.* Nausea, vomiting, alopecia, dizziness, edema, headache, and abdominal cramping. (Hindle & Gonzalez, 2001). Side effects are frequently experienced.

◆ *Contraindications.* Clients receiving diuretics and antihypertensives as well as those who are sensitive to ergot alkaloids.

◆ *Anticipated Outcomes on Evaluation.* A decrease in pain and breast nodularity.

◆ *Client Teaching and Counseling.* Inform the client of the possible side effects of this drug. Advise her to avoid pregnancy through the consistent use of a barrier form of birth control. Encourage the use of a supportive brassiere. A daily record of symptoms should be maintained throughout therapy to determine the effectiveness of this drug.

Dietary Intervention

Caffeine. Consumption should be reduced, as this may alleviate breast tenderness and reduce nodularity. This treatment, the effectiveness of which is controversial (Hindle & Gonzalez, 2001), may be tried in conjunction with other treatment modalities. Other nonprescriptive or lifestyle interventions that may help reduce fibrocystic discomfort include low salt diet, warm compresses, a supportive brassiere (even for sleep), and mild analgesics (Hindle & Gonzalez, 2001). The anticipated outcomes on evaluation by the client include decreased breast pain, tenderness, and nodularity.

Advise the client to decrease her intake of coffee, tea, cola drinks, chocolate, and drugs containing caffeine. Explain that three to six months may be required for symptoms to improve. Encourage perseverance, as many clients find it difficult to eliminate such foods as cola, coffee, and chocolate from their diet. Caffeine should be gradually reduced to prevent withdrawal symptoms.

Vitamin E (Effectiveness Controversial)

◆ *Indications.* Vitamin E (alphatocopherol) often decreases pain and tenderness associated with fibrocystic change. Its method of action is unknown, although an alteration in serum gonadatropins and adrenal tropines has been shown in patients taking high doses of vitamin E, which may account for the reduction in breast tenderness (DiSaia & Creasman, 2002). It also decreases the proliferation of breast tissue. Even though the use of vitamin E is controversial, it has been proven effective in relieving the symptoms of fibrocystic changes in some women, with its effectiveness thought to be due to altered lipid metabolism.

◆ *Administration.* Oral vitamin E, 150 to 600 IU daily.

◆ *Side Effects and Adverse Reactions.* Vitamin E's fat solubility and slow excretion may cause it to build up to a toxic level. Blood vessels may become constricted; therefore, the vitamin should be used cautiously in individuals with hypertension, diabetes mellitus, or cardiovascular disease.

◆ *Contraindications.* Hypertension, diabetes mellitus, or cardiovascular disease.

◆ *Anticipated Outcomes on Evaluation.* Decrease in pain, lumpiness, and thickness.

◆ *Client Teaching and Counseling.* Explain that vitamin E is given on a trial basis and should be discontinued in two to three months if no improvement occurs. Caution the client about the dangers of overusing this fat soluble vitamin since vitamin toxicity may result.

Evening Primrose Oil

♦ *Indications.* This homeopathic herb is frequently used in Europe as an initial attempt to control cyclic breast pain (Hindle & Gonzalez, 2001). Its effectiveness is variable (Hughes et al., 2000). The exact mechanism of action of evening primrose oil is unknown; however, it has been found to normalize the ratio of essential fatty acids to saturated fatty acids in some women with cyclic mastalgia. Primrose oil, since its origin is from nature, may be especially useful in young women who require long-term treatment as well as those who desire to avoid hormonal manipulation.

♦ *Administration.* Two 500 mg capsules should be taken three times per day for a minimum of three to four months (Hindle & Gonzalez, 2001).

♦ *Side Effects and Adverse Reactions.* Side effects are few and usually include bloating and nausea.

♦ *Contraindications.* None, however, conflicting reports regarding its efficacy require that the provider be familiar with this herb. In addition, herbal medications are not regulated by the Food and Drug Administration, and sufficient information regarding its interaction with other medications may not be known.

♦ *Anticipated Outcome.* Reduction of breast pain.

♦ *Client Teaching and Counseling.* Inform the client that a minimum trial of three to four months may be required to determine the effectiveness of this therapy. Also describe that side effects are possible with this oil. Advise her that primrose oil may be purchased in health food stores and that no prescription is required.

Practical Interventions. Active breast movement caused by weakened suspensory ligaments may significantly contribute to breast pain. A sports brassiere that provides increased breast support may provide particular comfort for women experiencing mastalgia (Hadi, 2000).

Surgical Intervention

Prophylactic Bilateral Total Mastectomy (see Breast Cancer). Indications for the surgery are to decrease the likelihood of developing cancer in clients who have a strong family history of cancer (Anderson, 2001). The procedure is usually considered too aggressive an approach in treating precancerous changes or as a request from women who are tired of the pain caused by fibrocystic changes. All breast tissue is removed, including the nipple-areolar complex and some axillary nodes. A subcutaneous mastectomy in which the nipple remains attached to the skin envelope and the nipple-areola complex remains intact may be performed. Possible adverse effects include mild lymphedema, disfigurement, and anesthesia reactions.

The anticipated outcomes on evaluation include decreased anxiety related to developing cancer.

When counseling the client, carefully convey the risks and advantages of the voluntary procedure. If breast cancer is of concern, advise the client that breast cancer may not be prevented, even if mastectomy is performed; however, the risk should be decreased. Suggest that testing for the BRCA1/2 gene be done (see Breast Cancer). Professional counseling is strongly advised prior to this extreme surgery. The client should be advised to include significant others of choice in the decision-making process. Refer the client to at least three qualified surgeons for their opinions about the surgery.

Follow-Up

Clients who receive oral contraceptives for fibrocystic breast changes should have a physical examination and evaluation every 3 months for the first 6 months of therapy, followed by a breast exam 6 months later. Clinical breast exam should take place annually thereafter (see Chapter 9).

Clients who receive Danazol will require a lipid profile and liver function tests after 3 months of therapy as well as at the termination of therapy. Normally symptoms associated with fibrocystic breast changes resolve in 3 to 6 months, and Danazol can be terminated, though symptoms may recur.

Endometrial surveillance should be provided for women receiving Tamoxifen. Though controversy exists regarding the most appropriate manner to rule out the presence of endometrial cancer in these women, the American College of Obstetricians and Gynecologists (ACOG, 1996) recommends that all women with breast cancer who take Tamoxifen undergo annual gynecologic evaluation including pelvic examination and cervical cytology. They also advocate the performance of endometrial biopsy in any of these women who complain of vaginal bleeding. ACOG further recommends that screening procedures should be left to the discrimination of the health care provider.

Transvaginal ultrasound is a very sensitive test used for endometrial surveillance and is often performed as a first-line screening test (Renard, Vosse, Scagnol, & Verhest, 2002). Endometrial thickness as evidenced by the ultrasound is an indicator of the presence of cancer, though the exact amount of thickness needed to determine endometrial cancer is debatable (Love et al., 1999; Mourits et al., 1999; Ozsener, Ozaran, Itil, & Dikmen, 1998).

Sonohysterography is useful as an adjunct to transvaginal ultrasound when the endometrial lining is thickened or asymmetric (Cardosi & Fiorica, 2000).

Any unsatisfactory diagnosis or diagnostic test should be evaluated with hysteroscopy, D & C, or even hysterectomy if necessary (Cardosi & Fiorica, 2000). Bromocriptine should be used infrequently and clients who receive bromocriptine should be followed monthly.

Clients who have surgery should be followed per the recommendations of the surgeon.

Advise all clients to try caffeine reduction for three to six months to ascertain if pain and nodularity decrease. Continue reduced intake indefinitely if improvements are noticed.

Evening primrose oil may be tried by all clients as well. The oil may be used indefinitely if effective.

It is important that the health care provider exhibit openness to alternative therapies for those clients who choose such methods as hypnosis. A follow-up should be planned four to six weeks after the initiation of hypnotherapy to assess its effectiveness. All clients should be reminded to wear well-fitted supportive brassieres and to continue to practice monthly BSE.

FIBROADENOMA

A fibroadenoma is the most common benign solid breast tumor (Hamed & Fentiman, 2001) and accounts for the majority of breast biopsies performed (Amshel & Sibley, 2001). It is a discrete, smooth, solid, firm, or rubbery, well defined mobile mass that is usually painless (Clare & Morrow, 2000; Hindle & Gonzalez, 2001). It may be stony hard when calcified. The mass is usually found unilaterally as a single breast mass but may be multiple and bilateral in 14 to 25 percent of women (DiSaia & Creasman, 2002; Kline et al., 1999).

Epidemiology

A fibroadenoma is thought to be hormonal. The mass, considered a disorder of normal breast development—not a neoplasm—presumably arises from the lobules and terminal ducts of the breast (Hughes et al., 2000). It is basically an overgrowth of elements thought to be found in these ducts and is composed of stromal and epithelial cells. Usually a mass will grow to 2 to 4 cm in diameter and remain that size. A small number, however, grow to

be larger than 5 cm; these are called giant fibroadenoma. A fibroadenoma is usually hormonally responsive (Hughes et al., 2000; Kline et al., 1999) and may increase in size toward the end of each menstrual cycle. They do not undergo malignant change.

The occurrence of a unilateral discrete breast mass is most common after puberty and before age 30. It usually appears in young women age 15 to 25 or 30 (Hamed & Fentiman, 2001; Hughes et al., 2000). The young age group is expected because of the lobular origin of the lesion since the time of greatest lobular development is the first years after menarche (Hughes et al., 2000). Often a mass may be detected in postmenopausal women, but it is most likely in these cases that the fibroadenoma developed prior to menopause and became clinically apparent during the involution of surrounding breast tissue (Hughes et al., 2000). Growth of these tumors often occurs during pregnancy, and sometimes the growth during pregnancy may be rapid because of the excess hormone levels associated with pregnancy. The tumor may show involution after parturition (Hughes et al., 2000). Though a fibroadenoma is normally a single, unilateral lesion, it may be multiple and found in both breasts. The risk of developing fibroadenoma is *not* increased by age, weight, parity, age at first pregnancy, socioeconomic status, or a family history of breast cancer.

Subjective Data

The client reports a "seed-like" or "marble-like," discrete, mobile, painless lump in one breast. Less often, she will find a lump in both breasts. It may be observed in any area of the breast, but is most frequently found in the upper outer quadrant. No nipple discharge or retraction, dimpling, or other breast symptoms are reported.

Objective Data

Physical Examination. A physical examination of the breasts reveals a firm, well-delineated, freely mobile, nontender mass, best palpated with the client in the dorsal recumbent position with hand behind her head. Usually the mass is palpable unilaterally, but it also may be bilateral. The lesion may be somewhat less discrete or less mobile in the older patient because involution and fibrotic changes decrease its mobility (Hughes et al., 2000).

Diagnostic Tests and Methods

Fine-Needle Aspiration. (See Benign Breast Conditions, Fibrocystic Changes.) Fine-needle aspiration, if deemed necessary, is cytologically diagnostic if there are abundant sheets of benign ductal epithelial cells, benign stroma, and abundant bipolar bare, benign nuclei. Provide the client with an explanation of fine-needle aspiration and a rationale for it. If referral is necessary, allow the client to participate in the selection of the care provider. If the client wishes to have the mass removed, refer her to a surgeon for excisional biopsy. Encourage her to continue BSE.

Mammography. (See Benign Breast Conditions, Fibrocystic Changes.) A mammogram may be used to evaluate any mass. Fibroadenoma are most common in young adult women who have dense breast tissue, and fibroadenoma may not be visualized accurately via mammography in this age group. Mammography usually shows a circumscribed mass with clear borders and intermediate density. A well-defined mass may show a halo effect from compression of the surrounding breast tissue (Hughes et al., 2000; Kline et al., 1999). In the postmenopausal woman, mammography may reveal atypical, stippled (popcorn) calcifications (Hindle & Gonzalez, 2001).

Ultrasound. (See Benign Breast Conditions, Fibrocystic Changes.) Sonography will differentiate a cystic mass from a solid mass. A fibroadenoma is shown as a circumscribed or lobulated mass with distinct borders and weak internal echoes. The well differentiated, low-level echoes are homogeneous throughout (Clare & Morrow, 2000).

Differential Medical Diagnosis

Breast macrocyst, cystosarcoma phyllodes, tubular adenoma, and mucinous carcinoma.

Plan

Psychological Interventions. Psychological interventions include helping the client to alleviate anxiety by informing her of the usual benign status of this mass. In addition, literature should be provided about common benign breast lesions. Assure her that a fibroadenoma should not impair her ability to breastfeed in the future.

Medication is not indicated.

Surgical Intervention

Excisional (Open) Biopsy. This procedure is done to remove and diagnose a breast lesion. It is performed especially if the lesion persists after repeated aspiration, when a suspicious mass persists beyond menses, if the fluid in a cyst is bloody, if nipple discharge is serous or sero-

sanguineous with no mass but a trigger point is present, or when a suspicious mammogram occurs without clinical findings. Excising the lesion provides the advantage of obtaining a definitive diagnosis and relieving anxiety (Clare & Morrow, 2000). It has also been advised that these lesions be removed before a client decides to become pregnant (even in adolescence) since pregnancy frequently causes the lesions to grow. The lesion may later infarct causing significant increase in size and pain. Removal of a larger lesion causes more unsightly cosmetic changes.

The fibroadenoma is surgically excised under local anesthesia, and adhesive strips are used to close the excision. The fibroadenoma may be excised with a small rim of breast tissue (Clare & Morrow, 2000). Adverse effects are virtually nonexistent. The client, however, may react to the local anesthesia, and bleeding and infection are possible with virtually any surgical procedure.

The anticipated outcomes on evaluation include reduced anxiety because the lesion has been removed. Greater accuracy is achieved in diagnosis because the lesion is sent to a pathology lab.

Explain to the client that the surgery may be done in an ambulatory setting under local anesthesia. A small dressing will be required. The pain is usually mild, but over-the-counter analgesics may be used if needed. Time lost from work is usually minimal. No heavy lifting or strenuous work should be done until the site is healed.

Conservative Treatment. Since fibroadenoma do not undergo malignant change, nonsurgical management may be considered in women who are younger than 30 years of age. The choice to engage this conservative treatment should be made by a surgeon and should take place only after a confident diagnosis of fibroadenoma is made via clinical examination, cytologic evaluation, and breast imaging (Hindle & Gonzalez, 2001). Women should be advised to be reevaluated in six months, perform monthly BSE, and return annually for a clinical breast exam. The client should be encouraged to return if she has any anxiety regarding the presence of the lesion or if the fibroadenoma increases in size. If the tumor enlarges, surgical excision is indicated (Hindle & Gonzales, 2001).

Follow-Up

After fine-needle aspiration and surgery, follow-up should be done at the physician's discretion, but usually in two to four weeks. Routine clinical breast exams should be done every year by a health professional, and breast self-examination (BSE) should be carried out monthly.

NIPPLE DISCHARGE

Fluid emission from the mammary nipple is a common complaint by women seen by health care providers. Nipple discharge is commonly treated in the office or clinic, because many types of discharge can be treated medically and do not require surgery. Concern for an underlying carcinoma may trigger the visit and dictates that the health care provider rule out all pathology (Sakorafas, 2001). Nipple discharge is more commonly associated with benign rather than malignant conditions (DiSaia & Creasman, 2002). Spontaneous nipple discharge is suspicious for pathology (Hindle & Gonzalez, 2001). Discharge may be caused by factors outside the breasts, primarily neuroendocrine or drug induced, by pathology of the ductal system, or by disease of the nipple.

At least seven types of nipple discharge have been identified: serous (yellow), sero-sanguineous, bloody, clear (watery), milky, purulent, and multicolored. (DiSaia & Creasman, 2002). Bloody nipple discharge must always be evaluated to rule out pathology (Hindle & Gonzalez, 2001).

NIPPLE DISCHARGE CAUSED BY FACTORS OUTSIDE THE BREASTS

Galactorrhea

Galactorrhea is a spontaneous milky nipple discharge that is non-puerperal or unrelated to lactation (Dixon & Bundred, 2000; Hindle & Gonzalez, 2001). The condition is usually idiopathic but can be found after discontinuation of oral contraceptive pills or as a persistent discharge after pregnancy (DiSaia & Creasman, 2002). It occurs in 20 to 25 percent of women (Pena & Rosenfeld, 2001) and is usually bilateral, comes from multiple ducts, and is most often found in women of childbearing age.

Epidemiology. Galactorrhea, normally caused by hyperprolactinemia, may have a pharmacologic etiology. For example, it can be induced by oral contraceptives (OCs), antihypertensive medications (e.g., reserpine, methyldopa, and verapamil), or antipsychotic medications (Maguire, 2002) and medications used for antidepression (Peterson, 2001). Estrogen in oral contraceptives causes an increase in prolactin-producing cells of the pituitary (Hughes et al., 2000). Oral contraceptives also stimulate the breasts and prepare them for lactation; estrogen stimulates the ductal system while progesterone stimulates the alveolar system. Antihypertensive medications like reserpine and methyldopa inhibit the synthesis of dopamine, while opiates sup-

press dopamine and stimulate prolactin release, thereby causing hyperprolactinemia. Prolactinomas, tumors of the pituitary gland, frequently produce galactorrhea (Whitman-Elia & Windham, 2000). Galactorrhea can also be due to Forbes-Albright Syndrome, hypothyroidism, chest lesions, renal disease, nonpituitary prolactin producing tumors (such as of the lung or kidney), and dysfunction of the hypothalamus and pituitary tumors. (Brandle & Schmid, 2000). In addition, prolonged stimulation of the nipples and breasts can substantially increase prolactin to high levels and cause galactorrhea. Galactorrhea is often associated with menstrual abnormalities. Details about the incidence of galactorrhea are unknown.

Subjective Data. The client reports an unelicited milky white discharge from both nipples and says that she is not pregnant or lactating. She also indicates that she neither has experienced trauma nor has pain. She may, however, acknowledge amenorrhea or irregular menses. Visual complaints of spots, whiteness, glowing, or progressive blurring may be given by a client suspected of having a pituitary tumor.

Objective Data

Physical Examination. Physical examination of the breasts reveals a milky nipple discharge that occurs spontaneously and with manual stimulation. It is not expressed from any particular areolar quadrant or duct. No redness or tenderness is visible. Fundoscopic examination of the eye may be normal.

Diagnostic Tests and Methods

PREGNANCY TEST. The absence of a pregnancy should be confirmed by performing a pregnancy test. A sensitive urine or blood pregnancy test that measures human chorionic gonadotropin should be performed in the office or sent to a laboratory.

SERUM PROLACTIN TEST. This diagnostic evaluation is performed to identify elevated prolactin, which may be indicative of a pituitary tumor or thyroid disorder (Biller, 1999a). Values greater than 20 ng/mL are considered abnormal. A level of 20 to 100 ng/mL usually represents a tumor or functional hyperprolactenemia. A level between 100 and 200 ng/mL is very suggestive of a tumor. When values of 200 to 300 ng/mL are found, a tumor is present 90 percent of the time. Values greater than 300 ng/mL are essentially diagnostic of a prolactin-secreting tumor. If the blood level is elevated, the test may be repeated to ensure accuracy.

The test procedure is to draw 3 to 5 mL of blood in a red-top tube and send it to a lab for evaluation. Use universal precautions when performing venipuncture. The test is best done in the morning, and manual stimulation of the breast, including breast examination, should be avoided prior to performing the test to avoid abnormally elevated results.

Explain to the client the rationale for the laboratory test and help to allay her anxiety about the diagnosis.

THYROID FUNCTION TEST. This diagnostic test may identify an elevated level of thyrotropin (TSH), which may be indicative of thyroid disease (hypothyroidism). Thyroid-stimulating hormone releasing hormone of the hypothalamus that releases TSH also releases prolactin. (Brandle & Schmid, 2000). If primary hypothyroidism is present, the thyrotropin-releasing hormone increases, which releases TSH and prolactin causing galactorrhea. This test should also be done if the serum prolactin test results show an elevated prolactin level.

The test procedure is to draw 5 mL of blood in a red-top tube and send it to a lab for evaluation. Use universal precautions when drawing blood.

Explain the rationale for the laboratory test and help to allay any anxiety.

SERUM CREATININE/BLOOD UREA NITROGEN. This diagnostic test identifies abnormality in renal function and should be done to rule out a kidney disorder.

Blood (5 mL) should be collected in a red-top tube and sent to the laboratory for evaluation. Universal precautions should be observed.

Rationale for the test should be provided to the patient. An expected date that the test results will be available should be indicated.

COMPUTED AXIAL TOMOGRAPHIC SCAN (CT) SCAN OF THE PITUITARY FOSSA. A CT scan is done to identify pituitary tumors and is performed if the client has hyperprolactinemia.

The test procedure involves the use of narrow x-ray beams to reveal the differences in radiation absorption among different kinds of tissue. Intravenous dye (usually Renografin) is used to enhance the x-ray contrast of vascular lesions. Axial tomography scans 1 mm slices of the pituitary gland and hypothalamus in the coronal plane after 200 cc of iodinated contrast medium is administered. The coronal plane is selected because prolactinomas are usually located in the lateral wing of the anterior pituitary.

Explain to the client the rationale for the test and refer her for financial screening if the test is not covered by medical insurance. Determine if the client is allergic to dyes. Support the client and help to allay any anxiety. Explain that the test is painless, but the client may be required to remain still for long periods during testing.

MAGNETIC RESONANCE IMAGING (MRI). Magnetic resonance imaging is a noninvasive diagnostic tool that differentiates disease or dying tissue from normal healthy tissue (Kline et al., 1999). This test, like the CT scan, will diagnose a pituitary tumor; however, MRI can provide resolution to 1 mm without radiation. The key components in an MRI system are a powerful magnet, a receiving coil, and a radio frequency. Hydrogen nuclei in static magnetic fields, exposed to radiowaves of specific frequency, resonate and depict tissue hydrogen density. This test should also be performed if the prolactin level is elevated.

The procedure requires that the client be placed inside of a large donut-shaped magnet. The magnet creates a magnetic field that aligns all protons inside the patient in a north/south orientation (Kline et al., 1999). A powerful radio frequency signal, which disrupts the magnetic pull, is then sent down the tunnel at a 90-degree angle, causing the protons to spin. The spin-time data is processed and presents an image of the tissue visualized. Normal healthy tissue has a longer spin-time than diseased tissue (Kline et al., 1999).

Explain the test to the client and provide literature if possible. Advise of the expense of testing and suggest financial screening at the local imaging center if available. Inform that she may have to remain immobile for a long period of time during the test. Offer medication to relax if needed.

VISUAL FIELDS MEASUREMENT. This diagnostic evaluation is performed to determine visual field defects caused by a pituitary tumor or mass. It is performed if the CT scan result is abnormal or if the client has visual complaints. Referral to an ophthalmologist is warranted for precise testing to evaluate peripheral vision; gross screening and a fundoscopic exam should be performed by the primary care provider.

Explain the reason for referral and the rationale for the exam. Involve the client in the selection of an ophthalmologist.

CHEST RADIOGRAPH (X-RAY). Radiology of the chest identifies anomalies and lesions of the chest cavity, including the lungs and ribs. Frequently, a cardiac silhouette can also be visualized.

Radiation is used in this brief examination that normally takes fewer than five minutes.

Although most clients are familiar with this exam, an explanation should be offered. Provide test results as soon as possible.

MAMMOGRAPHY. (See Benign Breast Disorders, Fibrocystic Changes.)

Differential Medical Diagnoses. Drug induced galactorrhea, pituitary tumor, prolactinoma, hypothyroidism, chest lesion, renal disease, non-pituitary prolactin-producing tumor, and Forbes-Albright syndrome.

Plan

Psychosocial Interventions. Help to allay the client's anxiety through teaching and providing literature about galactorrhea. Assure the client that galactorrhea is rarely associated with breast cancer. Encourage significant persons in the client's life to be supportive. Discuss sexuality and body image issues as appropriate. (*Note:* Close consultation with the physician is essential while managing a client with galactorrhea.)

Medication

BROMOCRIPTINE

- *Indications.* Bromocriptine is used when an elevated prolactin level is present. Dopamine receptor agonists are the mainstay of therapy for hyperprolactinemia since they rapidly lower serum prolactin and cause tumor shrinkage (Tansey & Schlechte, 2001). Bromocriptine, the primary drug of choice in the treatment of galactorrhea, activates dopamine receptors, acting like long-acting dopamine. It is used to lower prolactin levels, end galactorrhea, and restore the menses to normal if they have been irregular. Bromocriptine may even be used when a tumor is identified, since surgery frequently yields fair to poor results (Zacur, 1999).
- *Administration.* Start with 1.5 to 2.5 mg of bromocriptine daily, with the evening meal, for one week. The dosage is then increased to 1.25 to 2.25 mg twice daily. If necessary, doses of 1.25 to 2.25 mg three times a day may be prescribed. Bromocriptine may also be given vaginally and is as effective as the oral dose when administered by this route. There are practically no gastrointestinal effects when used intravaginally because the metabolism is slower and the liver is bypassed. The daily dosage is a 2.5 mg tablet placed in the fornix of the vagina daily.
- *Side Effects and Adverse Reactions.* Nausea, vomiting, dizziness, fatigue, headache, abdominal cramps, diarrhea, constipation, nasal congestion, and drowsiness (Orrego, Chandler, & Barkan, 2000). Side effects are experienced by a majority of women.

- *Contraindications.* Clients receiving antihypertensives and diuretics and those who are sensitive to ergot alkaloids.
- *Anticipated Outcome on Evaluation.* Cessation of nipple discharge.
- *Client Teaching and Counseling.* Advise the client to practice safe, effective birth control (barrier method) to avoid pregnancy while taking bromocriptine and to notify her care provider of any side effects.

Surgical Intervention

TRANSSPHENOIDAL EXCISION OF PITUITARY TUMOR. Referral for surgical evaluation of prolactinomas should be reserved for patients with neuro defects, such as visual field impairments, or if not improved with medication (Zacur, 1999). This surgery may especially be necessary if the client has a large lesion that is jeopardizing the optic chasm (Biller, 1999b). The purpose of this surgery is to remove the causative pathology and consequently abate the symptom. The tumor is excised through the nasal cavity. Tumor recurrence is possible. Results with surgery depend on the tumor size and prolactin level.

The anticipated outcome on evaluation is cessation of nipple discharge without other adverse health conditions.

Refer the client to a qualified surgeon, encouraging client participation in the selection of a surgeon.

Follow-Up. Consultation with a physician is strongly recommended. If the galactorrhea is being managed with bromocriptine, the client should be evaluated every month. The medication may be discontinued if the symptom resolves in two to three months; thereafter, the client may be evaluated in six months and yearly. If, however, the symptom does not abate in two to three months, bromocriptine may be continued and the client evaluated one month later. If at that time galactorrhea is unresolved, the client should be referred to a physician or managed with frequent consultation with a physician. Bromocriptine should be discontinued temporarily every two years and a prolactin level should be measured six weeks later.

If hypothyroidism is the cause of galactorrhea, then the disorder may be managed with thyroid hormone. The client may be referred to an internist or endocrinologist for management if desired. Evaluate the client every six months once hypothyroidism is stabilized.

If surgery is required for tumor removal, then follow-up is per the surgeon's recommendations.

NIPPLE DISCHARGE CAUSED BY DUCTAL SYSTEM DISORDERS

Intraductal Papilloma

The intraductal papilloma is a small, usually nonpalpable, benign tumor located in the mammary duct that produces a spontaneous serous, sero-sanguineous, or watery nipple discharge (DiSaia & Creasman, 2002; Hindle & Gonzalez, 2001). The tumor is usually solitary and affects only one duct, but occasionally it affects multiple ducts (see Figure 14–2).

Epidemiology. It is thought that intraductal papilloma is caused by a proliferation and overgrowth of ductal epithelial tissue. On rare occasions the papilloma may be intracystic rather than intraductal; however, in these cases, discharge will occur only if the cyst communes with a duct. An intraductal papilloma is generally less than 1 cm in diameter and may be nonpalpable (DiSaia & Creasman, 2002). This lesion, however, may be as large as 4 to 5 cm in size. Sometimes a mass may be palpable near the nipple.

Multiple papilloma may exist, especially in younger women, and are frequently bilateral and located in the periphery of the breasts (Dixon & Bundred, 2000). Multiple lesions have been associated with carcinoma (Schnitt & Connolly, 2000).

Intraductal papilloma occurs most frequently among women in their late menstrual years. Usually the tumor occurs just prior to menopause, but it may occur at any time from adolescence to old age.

Subjective Data. The client reports yellow or bloody discharge on her clothing. The discharge may occur spontaneously or with nipple stimulation. If the papilloma is large, the client may be able to observe a nonpainful, mobile mass usually in the areola. On rare occasions, the client may be able only to palpate the mass. She may complain of an associated feeling of fullness or pain beneath the areola.

Objective Data

Physical Examination. A physical examination of the breasts reveals serous, sero-sanguineous, or watery discharge, which is expressed manually from the affected duct when the nipple is systematically massaged in quadrants. The tumor, if palpable, may be a 1 to 3 cm mass, soft and poorly delineated, and felt in the nipple area (Hindle & Gonzalez, 2001). When multiple lesions are present, they are normally palpated in the periphery

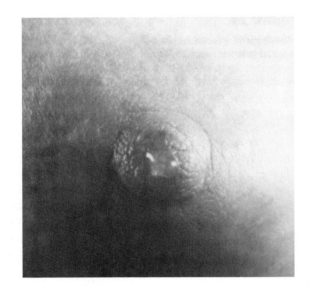

FIGURE 14–2. *Single duct nipple discharge.* Whether the discharge is clear or contains blood is not as useful a diagnostic sign as is often quoted. It is more important to discover whether a palpable or mammagraphic abnormality is present. If cytology of the discharge is carried out and obvious cancer cells are found, clearly an underlying breast cancer is indicated. However, suspicious cells found in nipple discharge are often merely degenerate duct cells.

(Schnitt & Connolly, 2000). Occasionally, skin dimpling is observed.

Diagnostic Tests and Methods

TEST FOR OCCULT BLOOD IN BREAST FLUIDS. This diagnostic evaluation identifies the presence of blood in nipple discharge. The procedure involves placing a small amount of nipple discharge on the designated area of a Hemoccult™ card (front side). Use a gloved finger to transfer the specimen from the nipple (use universal precautions). Apply 2 drops of developer on the designated area on the reverse side of the card. Blue coloration indicates the presence of blood.

Explain the purpose of the test to the client.

CYTOLOGY OF BREAST FLUID (PAPANICOLAOU SMEAR). Cytological evaluation of breast fluid in intraductal papilloma, which screens for cancerous cells, is controversial at best. A negative cytology exam does not exclude cancer, and a positive result cannot distinguish intraductal versus invasive carcinoma (Dixon & Bundred, 2000).

Thus, a cytology exam is considered to be of little value in determining whether duct excision should be performed (Hindle & Gonzalez, 2001). Usually, on microscopic examination, an intraductal papilloma shows scattered macrophages and tight clusters of epithelial cells with minimal atypia.

The test procedure requires that a drop of breast fluid be expressed onto a clean glass slide. The glass slide is held at the opening of the duct and the nipple discharge is expressed directly from the nipple onto the slide. Then the slide is fixed with 95 percent ethanol or commercial spray immediately (Kline et al., 1999). It should be labeled to indicate which breast the sample was taken from and sent to a lab. Immediate fixing is vital to avoid any drying artifact. A small specimen bottle of alcohol preservative works well because the patient may hold the bottle while the nipple discharge is obtained, or the bottle may be placed close to the procedure site. Cell loss, however, is diminished when a fixative spray is used.

Because the discharge is more cellular in the last drops of secretions, it is recommended that several slides be obtained.

Explain the procedure and its purpose to the client; caution that the results are inconclusive.

MAMMOGRAPHY. (See Benign Breast Conditions, Fibrocystic Changes.) Mammography may reveal dilated ducts near the nipple. When a mass is seen, it appears as a smoothly outlined, lobulated lesion about the same density as surrounding glandular tissue (Willison, 2001). A mass may have a raspberry-like configuration.

ULTRASOUND. (See Benign Breast Conditions, Fibrocystic Changes.) Sonogram may reveal dilated ducts, but rarely identifies a lesion. Low level of internal echoes are present when lesions are seen.

DUCTOGRAPHY. Ductography of the breast is an underused procedure that often helps define the cause of unilateral, single-pore spontaneous nipple discharge (Slawson & Johnson, 2001). This diagnostic evaluation identifies, by means of radiography, the ductal orifice that drains the pathological ductal system. Ductography outlines the ductal system, provides information on the reasons for production of nipple discharge, and locates the site within the duct where discharge is produced (Andolina, 2001). It also offers better visualization of small intraductal papillomas. Ductography will not differentiate benign lesions from malignant lesions; thus, surgery may ultimately be required. The test is considered unnecessary by some because the affected ductal quadrant can be identified by manual examination of the nipple and surgery is required whether this radiological procedure is done. Some specialists, however, find the test valuable for a more precise diagnosis and as a guide for surgical intervention (Yamamoto et al., 2001). Ductography is not indicated in patients with bilateral nipple discharge (Andolina, 2001).

The test procedure requires introducing radiographic dye through a cannulated duct, followed by x-rays (Andolina, 2001). Discuss the pros and cons of this procedure with the client and assist her in choosing a qualified radiologist. Intraductal papilloma appears as a smooth, lobulated intraluminal filling defect or a solitary obstructed duct on ductography (Chow, Smith, Kaelen, & Meyer, 2001).

Differential Medical Diagnoses. Intraductal carcinoma, multiple papillomatosis.

Plan

Psychosocial Interventions. Counsel the client regarding the benign etiology of this diagnosis. Encourage her to verbalize her feelings and emotions. Discuss sexuality issues as appropriate.

Medication. Not given for intraductal papilloma.

Surgical Intervention

WEDGE EXCISION. Wedge excision of the affected duct is the removal of the pathological ductal system and papilloma. This is the only method of differentiating this benign lesion from papillary carcinoma (Hindle & Gonzalez, 2001). Also, the nipple discharge will continue if the diseased duct is not removed. Local anesthesia is used. The excised papilloma and duct are sent to a pathology lab to rule out cancer.

Adverse effects may include a reaction to the anesthetic or possibly infection. The anticipated outcomes on evaluation include cessation of the discharge. In addition, anxiety is relieved if pathology results show a benign lesion.

Client counseling includes information that the procedure can be performed in an outpatient surgical setting under local or general anesthesia. Tell the client that usually only a small areolar incision is required; thus, major alteration in the cosmetics of the breast is averted. Only a small surgical dressing is necessary. More extensive surgery is required if the lesion is hard to access. Referral to a surgeon who specializes in the treatment of the breast is required; and client participation in the selection of a surgeon is appropriate.

Encourage the client to follow through with recommendations since surgery is the only method to determine if cancer is present. Advise the client to continue with annual breast exams performed by the health care provider and monthly breast self-examination (BSE).

Duct Ectasia

Duct ectasia is dilation and inflammation of the major mammary ducts, resulting in noncyclic breast pain and pasty nipple discharge that may be straw-colored, cream-colored, green, brown, yellow, gray, or reddish-brown (Hughes et al., 2000).

Epidemiology. The etiology of duct ectasia is unclear; however, ductal inflammation is thought to be present. The evolution of the condition is thought to be periductal inflammation, leading to periductal fibrosis, resulting in ductal dilatation (DiSaia & Creasman, 2002). Squamous metaplasia of the terminal duct epithelium may be an etiological factor in some cases with periductal fibrosis as a common outcome. Duct ectasia increases with age and is more common in perimenopausal women (Dixon & Bundred, 2000; Hindle & Gonzalez, 2001).

Subjective Data. Clients report a bilateral, pasty discharge that may be green, cream, brown, or straw-colored. In addition, dull nipple pain, a "drawing" sensation, subareolar swelling, and burning and nipple itching frequently occur. When the condition is advanced, the client may report an inflammatory breast mass that may resemble a locally advanced Stage III carcinoma (DiSaia & Creasman, 2002).

Objective Data

Physical Examination. Physical examination of the breasts may reveal subareolar redness and swelling. Tortuous tubular swellings are frequently palpated beneath the areola. Nipple retraction and dimpling may also be present (Dixon & Bundred, 2000). There is often mild to moderate tenderness on palpation. Nipple discharge, manually expressed, is green, brown, straw-colored, or cream-colored with the consistency of toothpaste (Hughes et al., 2000). Discharge is usually observed from one ductal quadrant of the nipple when the breast is palpated in a systematic fashion. In advanced cases, a round, firm, and somewhat fixed tumor may be palpable. Also in advanced cases, axillary lymphadenopathy may be observed.

Diagnostic Tests and Methods

TEST FOR OCCULT BLOOD IN BREAST FLUID. (See Benign Breast Conditions, Intraductal Papilloma, p. 367.) In addition to testing for the presence of blood by using a Hemocult™ card, placing a sample of the nipple discharge on a small white gauze pad will frequently reveal the presence of blood in the nipple discharge. The color of the stain usually reflects the true color of the discharge.

MAMMOGRAPHY. (Performed most often for clients with a palpable mass; see p. 356). Mammography may show tubular dilated ducts radiating from the nipple. An abundance of dense tissue may also appear behind the nipple.

ULTRASOUND. (See pp. 356–357). Well-differentiated dilated ducts may be visualized when viewed longitudinally, and lesions that appear to be cysts may be observed when viewed cross sectionally.

CYTOLOGY. (See pp. 366–367). Cytologic exam normally shows acellular material with debris and desquamated epithelium.

DUCTOGRAPHY. (See p. 367).

Differential Medical Diagnoses. Intraductal carcinoma.

Plan

Psychosocial Interventions. Provide information on the benign status of the disease to help alleviate the client's anxiety. Use the opportunity to promote breast self-examination (BSE). Encourage support by significant others in the client's life and encourage the client to express her feelings and emotions. Discuss sexuality issues if problematic and refer the client for professional counseling if indicated.

Surgical Intervention

WEDGE EXCISION. The affected duct, including any mass that is present, is surgically removed by wedge excision and sent to pathology for evaluation. This is the only procedure that may eliminate the symptom (DiSaia & Creasman, 2002).

Follow-Up. If a mass is present or an abscess occurs, it is recommended that wedge excision be performed. If surgery is performed, follow-up care is directed by the surgeon. If symptoms recur, an ice pack may be used for inflammation and nonsteroidal anti-inflammatory drugs (NSAIDs) may be used for pain until a health care provider can be consulted. The usual routine of clinical breast exam should be carried out by the primary care provider, and monthly BSE is done by the client.

Galactocele

A galactocele is a discrete, milk-filled, cystic or firm mass in the breast of a lactating or recently lactating woman. It may or may not be painful.

Epidemiology. The galactocele is thought to arise from dilation and obstruction of the lactiferous duct with retained milk and desquamated epithelial cells. It is most often found in the upper quadrants beyond the areolar border and may be singular or multiple.This lesion normally develops a few weeks to several months after discontinuing lactation (Hughes et al., 2000).

Subjective Data. The client may report a lump, knot, or cyst in her breast that may or may not be painful. Usually no bloody or purulent nipple discharge is reported, but occasionally pain may be described. She may note that the lesion was discovered after lactation was terminated.

Objective Data

Physical Examination. Physical examination usually reveals a visible, palpable, firm, round mass in one or both breasts. Milk may be manually expressed from the nipple and pain may be elicited upon palpation.

Diagnostic Tests and Methods

FINE-NEEDLE ASPIRATION. (See Benign Breast Conditions, Fibrocystic Breast Changes) This test is performed to identify and eradicate the lesion (see page 357 for the procedure). If the fluid is milky, it may be discarded and cytology is not required; however, if doubt exists, the fluid may be sent for cytologic examination. Most often, no further treatment is needed if the mass disappears with aspiration, as aspiration is often curative. If the fluid is other than milky or if the galactocele does not disappear with aspiration, an excisional biopsy is indicated.

MAMMOGRAPHY. (Described on p. 356.) The mammogram usually reveals a well-circumscribed radiolucent mass with clean margins.

ULTRASOUND. (See p. 356–357.) Sonography frequently shows a well-delineated mass with thin echogenic walls (Sahney et al., 2002).

Differential Medical Diagnosis. Microcyst, fibroadenoma.

Plan

Psychosocial Interventions. Once a definitive diagnosis is made, reassure the client that galactocele is a benign condition that rarely interferes with current or future lactation. In addition, discuss issues related to self-concept or sexuality. Encourage the client to express her feelings and concerns. Referral to a breastfeeding support group—for example, La Leche League—may be beneficial.

Surgical Intervention

EXCISION OF THE AFFECTED DUCT. This surgery is often considered inappropriate as the treatment of a galactocele (Marrow, 2000). An incision is made in the quadrant of the areola where the affected duct is located. The duct is then removed and sent to a pathology lab. (Hughes et al., 2000). (More often than surgery, a repeat aspiration is needed.)

Adverse effects, or complications of surgery, may include infection and a possible reaction to the local anesthetic. The anticipated outcome on evaluation is total obliteration of the mass.

Discuss controversies of this treatment methodology. If client insists, help her to choose a surgeon with expertise in this type of breast surgery who will also discuss the pros and cons of this surgical procedure. In addition, explain that the procedure is most often performed in ambulatory surgery under local anesthesia. Inform the client that a periareolar incision is usually made and only a small bandage is required. A minor cosmetic change may result. Mild to moderate pain is associated with the procedure, but there are virtually no complications.

Follow-up visits should be made to the surgeon as directed. Routine breast exams should be continued by the health care provider and a monthly BSE is advocated for the client during and following lactation.

MALIGNANT BREAST NEOPLASMS (BREAST CANCER)

Breast cancer, an overgrowth of neoplastic cells of the breast, is a life-threatening, and when diagnosed, a life-altering, disease. Now that women are living longer, the threat of breast cancer is increasing.

Epidemiology

Breast cancer is the most common cancer among women, excluding nonmelanoma skin cancers (ACS, 2002a). It is estimated that approximately 203,500 new cases of invasive breast cancer will be diagnosed in women in the United States in 2002. In addition, in situ breast cancer accounts for 54,300 new cases annually (ACS, 2002a). Unfortunately, approximately 40,000 deaths from breast cancer are projected in 2002. Only lung cancer causes more deaths in women than breast cancer (ACS, 2002a).

The precise etiology of breast cancer is unknown; however, the disease is thought to develop in response to a number of related factors: increasing age, positive family history, previous breast cancer, late menopause, hormonal factors, and nulliparity (ACS, 2002b, DiSaia & Creasman, 2002).

Age is probably the most important risk factor other than gender with 99 percent of all breast cancer found in women. Early menarche or menarche before age 13 increases risk (DiSaia & Creasman, 2002). If ovulatory cycles begin before age 13, there may be nearly a fourfold increase in risk. Conversely, the later a woman begins menopause, the higher the risk of breast cancer.

Breast cancer is more common following menopause, though women in their third and fourth decades of life have breast cancer. Breast cancer plateaus at approximately 50 years of age and rises thereafter (DiSaia & Creasman, 2002). Approximately 77 percent of women with breast cancer are over age 50 (ACS, 2002a). Women younger than 30 years account for only 0.3 percent of breast cancer cases. Women in their 30s account for about 3.5 percent.

The age at first-term pregnancy appears to be an important risk factor. If a first-term birth occurs before age 19, there is a 50 percent reduction in the risk of breast cancer in comparison with nulliparous women (DiSaia & Creasman, 2002).

Breast cancer is higher among women whose close blood relatives have the disease. Having a mother, sister, or daughter (first-degree relative) with breast cancer approximately doubles a woman's risk, and having two first-degree relatives increases her risk fivefold (ACS, 2002b). There is a fourfold increased risk of breast cancer in the daughters of premenopausal women with breast cancer, but there is no increased risk in daughters of women who developed breast cancer after menopause.

Atypical hyperplasia found on breast biopsy increases the risk for breast cancer. Also, women whose breast biopsies show proliferative changes without atypia or usual hyperplasia are at a somewhat increased risk for breast cancer (ACS, 2002b). The risk is 1.5 to 2 times greater than for other women. A previous breast biopsy result of atypical hyperplasia increases a woman's breast cancer by four to five times.

Women who have had chest area radiation therapy as a young woman or as a child are at significantly increased

risk for breast cancer (ACS, 2002b). Also, a personal history of cancer in one breast has a three- to fourfold increase of developing a new cancer in the contralateral breast or in another part of the same breast (ACS, 2002b).

There is still controversy regarding a relationship between hormone replacement therapy and breast cancer. Some researchers believe that significant evidence to link these two does not exists (DiSaia & Creasman, 2002). Others indicate a slight increase in risk after long-term use (five or more years) following menopause (ACS, 2002b).

The impact of oral contraceptive pill use on breast cancer is also unclear. It appears that women who stopped using oral contraceptive pills more than ten years ago do not have any increased risk for breast cancer (ACS, 2002b) (see Chapter 15 for the latest information on HRT and breast cancer).

Caucasian women are more likely to develop breast cancer than African American women. An estimated 19,300 new cases of breast cancer was expected in African American women in 2001 (ACS, 2000). It is the most common cancer among African American women, though the incidence of newly diagnosed cases is about 13 percent lower than in white women. An estimated 5,800 deaths from breast cancer were expected in African American women in 2001. The death rate of 31 per 100,000 is still approximately 28 percent higher than among white women (ACS, 2000). This may be related to later stage at diagnosis or the greater likelihood of being diagnosed with an estrogen receptor negative tumor or more aggressive tumors, which are more difficult to treat (Adams et al., 2001; Husani et al., 2001; Joslyn & West, 2000; Reis et al., 2000; Underwood, 1999). The five-year survival rate for African American women is 71 percent, compared to 86 percent among white women.

Based on breast cancer incidence rates from the California Cancer Registry, Hispanic women who were 50 years of age had a 0.8 percent (1 in 133) chance of developing breast cancer in five years, 1.6 percent (1 in 63) chance in ten years, and 3.7 percent (1 in 27) in twenty years (Morris, Wright, Schlag, 2001). Risks were lower in Asian/Pacific Islanders with results of 2 percent (1 in 51) in ten years and 3.9 percent (1 in 26) in twenty years. Rates for both groups were 8 to 20 percent higher when in situ tumors were included in the calculations.

Even when all risk factors are accounted for, 75 percent of all women with newly diagnosed breast cancer have no known risk factors (DiSaia & Creasman, 2002).

BRCA1/BRCA2 Genes. Two breast cancer susceptibility genes BRCA1 (Breast Cancer 1) and BRCA2 (Breast Cancer 2) have been identified, and germline mutations of these genes are thought to account for 5 and 10 percent of all breast cancer cases (Martin & Weber, 2000). A woman with an inherited alteration in one of these genes has an increased risk of developing breast cancer at a young age (before menopause) and often has multiple close family members with the disease (NCI, 2002). The likelihood that breast cancer and ovarian cancer are associated with the BRCA1 and BRCA2 genes is highest in families with a history of multiple cases of breast cancer and ovarian cancer, cases of both breast and ovarian cancer, one or more family members with two primary cancers, or an Ashkenazi (Eastern European) Jewish background (NCI, 2002). Fortunately, not every woman in such families carries these altered genes, and not every cancer in these families is linked to these genes.

Thirty-six to 38 percent of women with an altered BRCA1 or BRCA2 gene will develop breast cancer. They are three to seven times more likely to develop breast cancer than the general population (NCI, 2002). Altered BRCA1 and BRCA2 genes are found in 2.3 percent (23 of 1,000) women of Ashkenazi Jewish descent. The frequency of the gene in this ethnic group is about five times higher than the regular population. All women of Jewish ancestry should be tested for this gene.

If someone in a family has a known mutation in BRCA1 or BRCA2, testing other family members for that specific gene alteration can provide information about their cancer risk. In this instance, if a family member tests negative for the known mutation in that family, it is highly unlikely that they have an inherited susceptibility to breast cancer (NCI, 2002). Their risk of cancer is the same as the general population. Positive test results for the BRCA1 and BRCA2 genes provide data regarding a person's risk for developing breast cancer but cannot tell whether a person will actually develop breast cancer (NCI, 2002).

Tumor Marker CA27.29. This test measures CA27.29, a tumor marker found in the blood of patients with breast cancer and other types of cancer (ACS, 2002b). Normally, as breast cancer progresses, the level of CA27.29 antigen in the blood rises. The test is not intended as the sole basis for the diagnosis of cancer, which can be made only after the results are verified by other procedures such as biopsy; however, it provides health care providers with an additional tool to help to detect the recurrence of breast cancer in the earliest stages.

Her2/Neu Oncogene. Her2/Neu is an oncogene whose protein is often elevated in tumors of patients with metastases. About one-third of breast cancers have too much of this protein and too many replications of the gene that instructs the cells to produce Her2/Neu (ACS, 2002b). Amplification of this gene is observed in 20 to 30 percent of invasive breast cancers (Schnitt, 2000). Cancers containing Her2/Neu tend to grow and spread more aggressively than other breast cancers and are reported to be associated with poor clinical outcome (Pegram & O'Callaghan, 2001; Tsutsui, Ohno, Murakami, Hachitanda, & Oda, 2002).

Trastuzumab (Herceptin), an antimonoclonal antibody that attaches to Her2/Neu can shrink some breast cancer metastases that return postchemotherapy or continue to grow during chemotherapy, thereby prolonging the lives of women (ACS, 2002c). Herceptin is generally started after hormonal therapy and chemotherapy are no longer effective. Recent testing demonstrates a 20 percent reduction in relative risk of death and an increase in median survival from 20.3 to 25.1 months when Trastuzumab is used in combination with chemotherapy (Pegram & O'Callaghan, 2001). The side effects of Trastuzumab are fever, chills, weakness, nausea, vomiting, cough, diarrhea, and headache. Cardiotoxicity exists when this drug is used in combination with doxorubicin.

CHK2 Gene. Checkpoint kinase 2, the CHK2 or CHEK-2 gene, when mutated, can lead to a modestly elevated risk of breast cancer (Heijers-Heijboer, et al., 2002). Checkpoint genes that are activated in response to DNA damage and other stresses are frequently targeted for alteration in cancer (Miller et al., 2002). About 1 percent of the population carries a mutated form of this gene. An alteration in this gene can double a woman's risk of breast cancer (ACS, 2002b). Defects in the CHK2 gene contribute to the development of hereditary and sporadic cancers and earmark this gene as a candidate tumor suppressor and a target for drug discovery (Bartek, Falck, & Lukas, 2001).

Profile of Specific Malignant Tumors

Intraductal Carcinoma. This is the most common type of noninvasive breast cancer. The cancer cells reside in the ducts but have not spread through the walls of the duct into the fatty breast tissue. This cancer can be cured in almost 100 percent of women when diagnosed at an early stage (ACS, 2002b).

Lobular Carcinoma in Situ. Though not a true cancer, this disease is sometimes classified as a type of noninvasive cancer. It begins in the lobules of the breast but does not penetrate the walls of the lobule. Women with this condition have a higher risk of developing an invasive breast cancer in the same or contralateral breast (Miller et al., 2001).

Invasive Ductal Carcinoma. This cancer, which peaks in the sixth decade, (Kline et al., 1999), represents about 80 percent of all breast cancers. It can spread rapidly to axillary and other lymph nodes even while small. Breast hardness, dimpling, and nipple retraction develops. Lesions appear more lobulated as they enlarge. This most common type of breast cancer starts in the ducts, breaks through the duct wall, and invades fatty breast tissue.

Medullary Carcinoma. Representing 5 percent of breast cancers, this cancer is most often found among women younger than 50 years. It is a rounded, somewhat soft tumor that characteristically grows rapidly. In this infiltrating breast cancer, the tumor appears well defined with obvious boundaries between the tumor and normal tissue. Necrosis in this lesion is common, which may result in liquefaction and cyst formation. There is a better than average prognosis since they are slow to metastasize. Signs include a large palpable tumor that is fixed to the chest wall or skin and ulceration.

Comedocarcinoma. This cancer originates in the lining of the mammary duct, and as it grows, it fills the duct. Cancer cells undergo necrosis and slough into the lumen of the duct, forming a large quantity of necrotic debris. The tumor is sometimes large but is not likely to spread beyond the breast or into the skin. The prognosis is usually good (ACS, 2002b).

Mucinous Carcinoma. This a ductal cancer that accounts for about 2 percent of breast cancers usually grows slowly and rarely spreads to the nodes. There is characteristically an abundance of extracellular mucin around the tumor cell that is produced by the cancer cells. Mucinous carcinoma may have sharp borders and may be confused with a fibroadenoma. It usually presents as a mass but may be accompanied by nipple discharge, fixation, and skin ulceration. Less often, it is associated with metastasis; thus prognosis is usually good.

Tubular Ductal Carcinoma. Accounting for 29 percent of all breast cancers, this is the best differentiated of the ductal carcinomas and the type with the best prognosis. It is an invasive cancer whose cells are arranged in regular, well-defined tubules typically lined by one epithelial layer and accompanied by fibrous stroma. Axillary metastases are uncommon. The presenting symptom, a palpable mass, is occasionally accompanied by skin retraction or fixation. The prognosis is better than for invasive carcinoma.

Invasive Lobular Carcinoma. This cancer arises in the milk-producing lobules of the breasts, then breaks through the lobular wall. It then spreads invasively elsewhere throughout the breasts. It usually presents as a nondescript skin thickening. Axillary node involvement is common, and this cancer usually metastasizes to sites in the lung, breast, and liver. The presenting tumor is frequently located in the upper-outer breast quadrant. Skin retraction and fixation accompany large lesions. The prognosis is poor in this cancer that accounts for 10 to 15 percent of all cases of breast cancer.

Paget's Disease. This cancer of the nipple is almost always associated with an underlying intraductal carcinoma and frequently with a long history of eczema of the nipple with itching, burning, oozing, erythema, crusting or bleeding. There is frequently a unilateral lesion (see Figure 14–3).

Subjective Data (see prior descriptions)

A client may report one or more of the following conditions.

- A fixed, poorly defined lump or mass may be noted in one breast. Rarely is it painful. The lump is usually located in the upper, outer quadrant of the breast. (*Note:* A lump can be palpated when it reaches a size of approximately 1 cm; it has possibly been present for seven to eight years when palpable at that size.)
- Spontaneous nipple discharge that is clear, yellow, or bloody may appear unilaterally.
- Persistent nipple irritation is reported.
- Dimpling or redness of the skin, nipple retraction, change in breast contour, inflammation, swelling and peau d'orange skin (advanced malignancy) may occur. (These are characteristics of what is called inflammatory breast cancer, which is not a distinct cancer, but represents an extension of the tumor into the intradermal lymphatics.)
- Axillary adenopathy, or supraclavicular/intraclavicular adenopathy (advanced malignancy) is described.

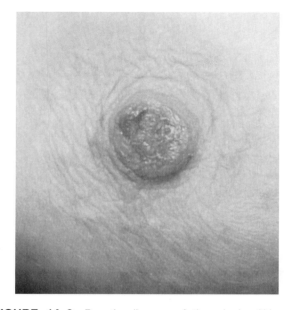

FIGURE 14–3. *Paget's disease of the nipple.* Although there is only a small area of excoriation, biopsy showed this to be Paget's disease of the nipple. Any area of eczematous change of the nipple should be biopsied. Paget's disease of the nipple may heal between episodes of excoriation and a recent history of excoriation is also an indication for biopsy.

Objective Data

Physical Examination. Physical examination should be performed in a slow and meticulous manner. Examination of the breast requires observation for and palpation of the subjective symptoms. Peau d'orange skin of the breast may also be observed, and in advanced malignancies, a mass fixed to the chest wall may be palpated.

Careful lymphatic palpation is performed to determine supraclavicular, infraclavicular, and axillary nodal involvement.

Diagnostic Tests and Methods

Mammography. (See p. 356.)

Ultrasound. (See p. 356–357.)

Fine-Needle Aspiration. (See p. 357.) The procedure for fine-needle aspiration is altered for a solid mass in that several passes are made through the mass while aspirating (Kline et al., 1999). The aspiration continues until aspirate is visualized in the hub of the needle. Aspiration is then stopped and the needle is removed cleanly. The spec-imen is generally confined to the needle. The specimen should be sent to the lab preserved in alcohol.

Stereotactic Core Biopsy. This computerized mammographic biopsy provides a three-dimensional view of a breast abnormality (Willison, 2001). Computerized mammography triangulates the location of the breast lesion to within 1 mm. An automated, large-bore needle (14 gauge), biopsy gun, or vacuum-assisted biopsy device is normally used to obtain multiple samples of the breast lesion (Venta, 2000; Willison, 2001). The samples are sent to the lab for histologic diagnosis. When done well, stereotactic core biopsy has a 98 percent sensitivity that is similar to that of needle-localized excisional biopsy.

Correct needle localization is critical—thus clients who are unable to lie prone, or those who experience severe coughing spells, may not be able to tolerate this procedure (Venta, 2000). It may also be difficult to perform stereotactic biopsy on lesions that are close to the nipple or lie near the chest wall. This procedure can be done with a local anesthetic, may be painful, and normally causes little or no scarring of the breast. The client can usually resume routine activities in 24 hours.

Needle Localization Biopsy. This is a very significant methodology to use with lesions that are detected by mammography but are not palpable (Stomper, 2000). Mammography is used to provide guidance for surgical biopsy of the lesion—in fact, the mammographer's goal is to place the needle close to the lesion so that the surgeon can maximize the size of the biopsy.

A thin guide wire is placed through a percutaneous needle. The wire has a hooked tip that is anchored within the lesion. Mediolateral and craniocaudal views are obtained with the needle and wire in place. Dye may be injected near the lesion as an alternative to the needle, or both may be used. A more precise identification of the lesion is provided with needle localization, and less normal tissue is removed with the biopsy. Less than 5 percent of needle localized biopsies do not contain the lesion.

Local anesthesia is often used and the procedure can be performed on the client as an out-patient. If the lesion is close to the chest wall or deeply situated in large breasts, a more than allowable dose of local anesthetic may be required. General anesthesia may be best suited in these cases.

Excisional Biopsy. (See p. 362.) Excisional biopsy is the complete removal of a lesion with or without a rim of normal surrounding tissue (Foster, 2000). It is usually the definitive treatment for benign lesions but may not be so for cancerous lesions. Excisional biopsy is optimal for removing small lesions of the breast, since the entire mass is often removed with this technique. The procedure requires cleansing the breast with an antiseptic solution. The mass is then surgically excised under local anesthesia, and the biopsied lesion is sent to the pathology lab. When a deeper lesion is present, a combination of intravenous and local anesthetic is very effective. The incision is sutured or held together with adhesive strips.

Explain the procedure to the client and refer her to a qualified surgeon. The client should participate in selecting the surgeon. Review the possible complications of the procedure: hematoma, stitch abscess, malignant tumor remaining partially intact, reaction to local anesthetic, and infection. Provide client support.

Incisional Biopsy. This procedure is usually performed for diagnostic purposes (Foster, 2000). This diagnostic evaluation is done to provide a quick determination of malignancy, especially prior to surgery. It can confirm the diagnosis of advanced cancer.

The procedure requires skin preparation with an antiseptic solution. Under local anesthesia, a small wedge of tissue is excised with sharp dissection from the diseased area. The incision is then closed. Adhesive strips may be used to close the wound. The specimen is submitted to the pathology lab for histologic evaluation.

Explain the procedure to the client and be supportive. Teach her about possible complications: bleeding, infection, reaction to local anesthetic. In explaining, reinforce for the client that only a small wedge of the lesion will be taken and that the remaining, possibly malignant, tumor will be left intact. Thus, it should not be considered a treatment or cure. Referral to a qualified surgeon is required. Encourage the client to participate in selecting a surgeon.

Hormone Receptor Assays. This procedure is done to determine a tumor's dependency on estrogen or progesterone, to determine the likelihood of a tumor's response to endocrine therapy, and to a lesser degree to help assess patient prognosis (Schnitt, 2000). Estrogen appears to stimulate normal ductal growth, while progesterone is responsible for lobular-alveolar development (Hayes, 2000). Tumors with high estrogen receptor (ER) or progesterone receptor (PR) content are better differentiated, and patients with these tumors have a better prognosis (Hayes, 2000). If the estrogen receptor is positive, the client is likely to respond to hormonal therapy in the

treatment of breast cancer. In contrast, if the estrogen receptor (ER) is negative, the client is less likely to benefit from hormonal therapy. Immunohistochemical assays versus biochemical essays are most frequently used because they permit direct visualization of the cells being analyzed. This type of assay can also be performed on very small specimens including core needle biopsies, fine-needle aspirates, and effusions.

Differential Medical Diagnoses

Fibroadenoma, intraductal papilloma, eczema.

Plan

Psychosocial Interventions. Help the client to cope with her fear, anxiety, and impaired self-image, if present, and encourage family support. Referral to a support group, for example, Reach to Recovery, or to a counselor or minister may be appropriate. Remember to provide culturally sensitive counseling. (The client's family usually needs support as well and an appropriate referral should be made.) A cooperative/interactive team approach with this client is vital.

If surgery is performed, explain to the client that the absence of breasts or breast function may not decrease her female sexual response. Orgasm should still be possible, if not directly tied to nipple manipulation and stimulation, since clitoral function is primary to the female sexual response and is still possible. Also, advise the client and her family that the diagnosis of cancer neither equates to imminent death, decrease in attractiveness, nor diminished sexual appetite. Assure her that past misdeeds, family sins, nor improper health caused her to develop breast cancer; however, be mindful that women of some cultures may continue to hold this belief.

Medication

Adjuvant Therapy. Adjuvant therapy, usually chemotherapy or hormonal therapy postsurgery, is most often a preventive measure but actually represents an attempt to ablate micrometastatic disease that may lead to tumor recurrence (Hayes, 2000). This therapy is often used when clients have been determined to be free of disease, post breast cancer treatment, but at great risk for recurrence. Patients are treated with potentially dangerous drugs in hopes of delaying or avoiding recurrence and prolonging life.

Chemotherapy. Chemotherapeutic agents interfere with essential cell processes, leading to cell death (Hayes, 2000). Some agents work by disrupting DNA replication, thereby thwarting the growth of cancer cells. Other agents disrupt the integrity of the cell membrane preventing normal cellular homeostasis (Hayes, 2000). The most active and commonly used chemotherapeutic drugs for breast cancer include alkylating agents, anthracyclines, antimetabolites, and vinca alkaloids.

Any of fifty or more chemotherapy agents may be used to treat breast cancer; however, a combination drug approach versus single drug treatment appears to be more effective. (ACS, 2002b). The drug combinations that are used most frequently are:

Cyclophosphamide, methotrexate, fluorouracil (CMF).

Cyclophosphamide, doxorubicin, fluorouracil (CAF).

Doxorubicin, cyclophosphamide (AC).

Doxorubibin, cyclophosphamide, paclitaxel.

Doxorubicin, followed by CMF.

Cyclophosphamide, epirubicin, fluorouracil (ACS, 2002b; DiSaia & Creasman, 2002; Osborne & Ravdin, 2000).

- *Administration.* Administration of the therapy depends on the agent, the disease stage (Table 14–1), and the site of metastasis if present. It is given intravenously, orally, or possibly intrathecally.
- *Side Effects.* Side effects include nausea, vomiting, alopecia, stomatitis, leukopenia, destruction of healthy cells, cardiotoxicity, early menopause, and infertility (Osborne & Ravdin, 2000).

TABLE 14–1. Staging of Breast Cancer

Stage	Characteristics
0	The earliest type of breast cancer, the disease is in situ.
I	The tumor is less than 1 inch in diameter and has not spread beyond the breast.
II	The tumor is about 1 to 2 inches in diameter and/or has spread to axillary lymph nodes.
III	The tumor is about 2 inches or larger and may have spread to the axillary nodes and/or to other lymph nodes, or to other tissues near the breast.
IV	The cancer has metastasized to other body organs.

Source: American Cancer Society. (2002). Cancer Reference Information. Accessed April 1, 2002, from http://www.cancer.org.

- *Anticipated Outcomes on Evaluation.* Regression in the dissemination of cancer, ablation of micrometastatic disease, and improvement in survivability.
- *Client Teaching and Counseling.* Refer the client to a qualified oncologist for treatment, and advise her to consult with more than one. Provide literature about chemotherapeutic drugs. Discuss possible adverse reactions to the drugs and other possible drug effects on body image, self-perception, or self-esteem. Inform the client that medications may be prescribed to treat some symptoms and that a cap is available to help reduce hair loss. Refer her to a local support group such as Reach to Recovery.

Hormonal Therapy

- *Indications.* Hormone therapy is given to promote tumor regression and to delay recurrence, postmastectomy, among women who have cancer that is sensitive to estrogen. Estrogen plays a central role in the pathogenesis of cancer and treatment with estrogen deprivation has proven to be effective (Dickler & Norton, 2001). The basis of hormonal therapy is to block or counter the effect of estrogen. Selective Estrogen Receptor Modulators (SERM), antiestrogenic agents, are indicated when the cancerous tumor shows estrogen receptors (ER positive). Tamoxifen, the pioneering and most widely used SERM, has been used to treat breast cancer and to reduce the risk of breast cancer in high-risk women (Dickler & Norton, 2001; Jordan, 2000b; Jordan, Gapstur, & Morrow, 2001). Five years of Tamoxifen administration after the diagnosis of breast cancer resulted in a 50 percent reduction in the incidence of cancer in the contralateral breast (Jordan, 2000a). Though its effects are antiestrogenic in the breasts, it produces beneficial effects on bones and lowers circulating cholesterol levels (O'Regan & Jordan, 2001; Jordan 2001). Its use does not come without risks as endometrial cancer, thromboses, cataracts, and possibly diminished quality of life in postmenopausal women can occur (Vogel, 2001). Hormonal therapy was used extensively in the National Surgical Adjuvant Breast and Bowel Project (NSABP), which began in 1992. Most oncologists prescribe tamoxifen therapy for five years, though the duration of therapy is controversial.
- *Administration.* Tamoxifen, one to two 10-mg tablets, p.o., b.i.d.

- *Side Effects and Adverse Reactions.* Hot flashes, nausea, depression, vomiting, vaginal bleeding and discharge, unintended pregnancy, menstrual irregularities, and bone pain. More serious side effects are endometrial cancer, liver cancer, thromboembolitic disease, and retinopathy.
- *Contraindications.* None are known.
- *Anticipated Outcomes on Evaluation.* Tumor regression and increased likelihood of survival. An additional benefit of reduction in cardiovascular death is anticipated because tamoxifen lowers the cholesterol level. This effect occurs within the first three to six months and is sustained during the treatment.
- *Client Teaching and Counseling.* Refer the client to a qualified oncologist; the client should consult with more than one oncologist. Inform the client that therapy is most effective in cancers sensitive to estrogen. Discuss the side effects/risk factors in detail. Discuss data related to the Tamoxifen trials. Advise endometrial evaluation to rule out cancer and recommend close follow-up with the oncologist.
- *Raloxifene.* Raloxifene, a second-generation SERM, is also being evaluated for hormonal therapy. It, like Tamoxifen, blocks the effect of estrogen on breast tissue. It is currently being tested in the STAR trial (Study of Tamoxifen and Raloxifene) (NCI, 2000). Raloxifene is currently used to treat and prevent osteoporosis (Bentrem & Jordan, 2002). Unlike Tamoxifen, Raloxifene does not appear to cause endometrial cancer and when used would be a safer alternative (Dickler & Norton, 2001).

Aromatase Inhibitors. Aromatase inhibitors and inactivators are being evaluated in the adjuvant setting and may have a potential use in breast cancer prevention (Lonning, 2002). Aromatase is the cytochrome P450 enzyme responsible for the last step of estrogen biosynthesis, and aromatase inhibitors constitute an important class of drugs in clinical use for the treatment of breast cancer (Recanatini, Cavali, & Valenti, 2002). Some of these drugs have been found to be superior to Tamoxifen in patients with metastatic breast cancer (Jones, 2002). Trials using these drugs may determine whether aromatase inhibitors show improved tolerability, whether combination therapy is more effective than monotherapy (Jones, 2002), or whether these drugs will eclipse Tamoxifen as the drug of choice for breast cancer prevention.

Radiation Therapy. Radiation therapy is used in conjunction with breast conservation surgery to eradicate residual, subclinical disease (Recht, 2000) and offers a small but important survival advantage. The use of radiation following chemotherapy in women at substantial risk for metastasis is said to improve control of distant disease and survival without compromising the control of local disease. Radiation therapy may also be used postoperatively following mastectomy. It clearly decreases the risk of local-regional recurrence (Recht, 2000).

External radiation (x-rays) is directed to the breast and possibly the axillary lymph nodes (ACS, 2002b). It is uncertain whether the entire breast or a more limited area surrounding the breast should be treated (Recht, 2000). Most radiologists, however, treat the entire breast. The effectiveness of booster doses to the primary site are also controversial (Recht, 2000).

- *Adverse Effects.* Fatigue, temporary discoloration of the skin, itching or peeling, leukopenia, retraction of the breast, breast fibrosis, cancer secondary to radiation therapy, and pleural effusion (ACS, 2002b).
- *Anticipated Outcomes on Evaluation.* Eradication of the pathology, maintenance of breast integrity, and improved chances for survival.
- *Client Teaching and Counseling.* Provide the client with information about the course of radiation therapy, noting that it usually requires five to six weeks of daily trips to the treatment site, where a qualified radiologist administers therapy. Advise the client that she may feel fatigued and that the skin directly exposed to radiation may look or feel as though it has been sunburned. Assure her that the skin should return to normal in one or more months after therapy has been completed and that the use of a sunscreen and protective clothing should help to prevent further irritation. She may also ask the radiologist about specific creams that may be used for irritated skin. Refer her to a support group, such as Reach to Recovery. Discuss the need for annual mammography.

Surgical Interventions. Surgery for breast cancer involves removal of the tumor, with or without complete mastectomy or axillary node dissection and subsequent breast reconstruction if desired. Breast conservation therapy, which includes lumpectomy and partial mastectomy, and modified radical mastectomy or radical mastectomy are performed.

Breast Conservation Therapy/Surgery. Lumpectomy removes only the breast lump and a surrounding margin of tissue (ACS, 2002b). Partial mastectomy, segmental mastectomy, or quadrantectomy removes up to one-quarter or more of the breast along with wide margins of surrounding tissue (ACS 2002b). These procedures are normally followed by a six-week course of radiation therapy. This surgical option is often chosen to maintain the cosmetic and aesthetic appearance of the breast. Breast-conserving therapy usually provides a central incision, limits the volume of breast tissue removed, limits the amount of skin excised, ensures good homeostasis, avoids drains in the breasts, and uses separate breast and axillary incisions (Eberlein & Tsangaris, 2000).

Treatment with conservation therapy for carefully selected patients with invasive breast cancer yields a survival rate equal to that of mastectomy (Recht, 2000). Breast conservation therapy is not an option for women who:

- Have already had radiation therapy to the affected breast.
- Have two or more areas of cancer in the same breast that are too far apart to be removed by one excision.
- Have not experienced complete removal of cancer with previous lumpectomy.
- Have connective tissue/collagen vascular diseases like scleroderma that may cause more sensitivity to radiation and poor cosmesis.
- Are pregnant and will require radiation therapy.
- Have a cancerous lesion that is larger than 5 cm.
- Have a cancer that is large in comparison to the small size of the breast.
- Have infiltrating or invasive tumors without clear margins (ACS, 2002b; Hayes, 2000; Recht, 2000).

This conservative approach is being used more often in the presence of in situ cancer.

Lesions that are removed from the periphery of the breast normally provide a more aesthetically pleasing outcome than tumors that are removed from central locations that include the nipple-areola complex. This should not necessarily deter breast conservation therapy if the client chooses it with full knowledge of the potential cosmetic impairment.

The specific type of breast cancer is not usually considered a strong determinant of the feasibility of breast conservation surgery. In the presence of invasive lobular cancer, with its wide diffuse and vague margins, complete mastectomy might provide a safer choice for the patient.

There is no age limit for breast conservation surgery; however, breast cancer may recur after lumpectomy, and

young women who may live longer can be more at risk for cancer recurrence. Risks include infection, bleeding, scarring, and deformity of the breasts (Eberlein & Tsangaris, 2000).

Clients who have anxiety regarding cancer recurrence following breast conservation surgery may choose to have a complete mastectomy. On the other hand, some clients are more concerned about their physical appearance and may consider breast conservation surgery the only desired option. The anticipated outcomes on evaluation are removal of pathology, preservation of the breast, and improved chances for survival.

Patients who choose breast conservation therapy must have access to a radiation facility and must be followed closely. They must clearly understand that cancer recurrence is a possibility.

TOTAL MASTECTOMY. This surgery is indicated for women with carcinoma in situ (ductal or lobular) with no suspicious axillary involvement or in women whose tumor recurred after partial mastectomy and axillary dissection. The surgery involves removal of the breast and pectoralis major muscle fascia.

Adverse effects may arise if the axillary chain is left intact and not evaluated for cancer. Nodal involvement may be microscopic and nonpalpable. If cancer is later detected in the lymph chain, further surgery, radiation, or other adjuvant therapy may be required. Postoperative infection is possible.

The anticipated outcomes on evaluation are removal of the pathology and improved survival.

In client teaching, contrast and compare total and modified radical mastectomy. Include a discussion of reconstructive surgery. Inform the client that breast prostheses are available. Radiation therapy will frequently be recommended and requires discussion. Refer the client to a support group such as Reach to Recovery for preoperative and postoperative support. Reinforce the practice of BSE.

MODIFIED RADICAL MASTECTOMY. Modified radical mastectomy is indicated when tumors are not large or bulky, when axillary adenopathy is not bulky, and when interpectoral nodes are not grossly involved. The surgery involves removal of the breast, axillary nodes, but not the pectoralis major; thus avoiding a concave anterior chest (DiSaia & Creasman, 2002). All or part of the pectoralis minor may be removed. Modified radical mastectomy is the most commonly performed surgery in patients with invasive breast cancer (Morrow, 2000). Adverse effects include lymphedema, infection, and hematoma.

The anticipated outcomes on evaluation are removal of the pathology and improved chances of survival.

Provide the client with information about the procedure (e.g, surgeon qualifications, anesthesia, and possible complications of surgery). Referral to physical and occupational therapy is imperative. Counsel the client about breast reconstruction and inform her that breast prostheses are available. Refer her to a support group for preoperative and postoperative support. In addition, a professional counselor may be needed. A team approach is necessary for the client's rehabilitation. Reinforce the practice of BSE, advising the client to pay close attention to the contralateral breast.

RADICAL MASTECTOMY. Radical mastectomy is indicated for the removal of cancers with large bulky tumors involving the pectoralis major or fascia, bulky axillary lymph involvement, or grossly involved interpectoral nodes. With improvements in early detection, radical mastectomy is rarely indicated today (Morrow, 2000). The surgery involves removal of the breast, pectoralis major and pectoralis minor muscles, skin overlying the tumor, and all axillary nodes (ACS, 2002b). Adverse effects include extensive scarring, hollow chest, lymphedema, infection, skin necrosis, hematoma, and disfigurement. Breast reconstruction is difficult, if possible at all.

The anticipated outcomes on evaluation are the removal of the pathology and improved chances for survival.

Center client teaching on the procedure and its possible adverse effects. Hospitalization and general anesthesia are required. In addition to a qualified surgeon, a physical and/or occupational therapist will be needed. A team approach is preferable for rehabilitation. Discuss the difficulty of breast reconstruction, and inform the client that breast prostheses are available. A visit by a specialist in fitting breast forms or foundations may be arranged. The management of lymphedema and other side effects must also be taught, and exercises to reduce lymphedema or arm stiffness should begin 24 hours after surgery. Encourage ROM exercises and encourage the client to avoid restrictive clothing such as tight sleeves. The client should also avoid underarm creams, depilatories, and deodorants. Reinforce the importance of BSE and refer the client to a support group such as Reach to Recovery for preoperative and postoperative support. If indicated, suggest professional counseling.

SENTINEL NODE BIOPSY. Historically, as many lymph nodes as possible were removed in the presence of breast cancer to reduce the spread of cancer to other body systems (ACS, 2002b; Eberlein & Tsangaris, 2000). This led to lymphadenopathy and breast edema, which occurs in approximately 10 to 20 percent of women postaxillary dissection (ACS, 2002b; Eberlein & Tsagaris, 2000). The use of the sentinel node as a means of evaluating lymph node status and as an alternative to axillary dissection is becoming more prominent (Beitsch, Clifford, Whitworth, & Abarea, 2001; Leong, Morita, Treseler, & Wong, 2000; Schnitt, 2000). Sentinel node mapping identifies the first lymph node or nodes that drain the breast (Eberlein & Tsangaris, 2000). Theoretically, if the sentinel node is negative, it is unlikely that subsequent nodes in the chain are positive (Ishikawa, Sato, & Mochizuki, 2002).

The procedure involves the injection of blue dye around the periphery of the tumor or at the edge of the biopsy cavity (Morrow & Harris, 2000). An incision is made in the inferior margin of the axilla and a careful search is made for a blue lymphatic channel leading to the blue-stained sentinel lymph node. The node is then harvested and taken for laboratory analysis. Care must be taken to accurately identify the sentinel node so that a false negative report is not provided (Birdwell et al., 2001; McMasters et al., 2001; Morrow & Harris, 2000).

Contraindications to sentinel node biopsy are:

- Suspicious palpable axillary adenopathy.
- Tumor greater than 5 cm in size or locally advanced.
- Use of preoperative chemotherapy.
- Large biopsy cavity.
- Multicentric carcinoma.
- Prior axillary surgery.
- Pregnant or lactating patient (Morrow & Harris, 2000).

AUTOLOGOUS BONE MARROW TRANSPLANT. Transplanted bone marrow is indicated for the treatment of extremely aggressive breast cancer or cancers that have metastasized. Bone marrow is withdrawn from the client to protect it. It is cleaned, treated, and stored. Extremely high doses of chemotherapy are then administered to the client to destroy cancerous cells. Bone marrow is also destroyed, which robs the body of its natural ability to fight infection. Next, the bone marrow is reinjected or transplanted after chemotherapeutic agents have been absorbed. Adverse effects include nausea, vomiting, alopecia, leukopenia, and fatigue. The anticipated outcome on evaluation is regression of the spread of cancer and improved survivability. Clients who are in complete or partial remission prior to transplantation often have a higher response rate.

Advise the client that several weeks of hospitalization will be required. A hospital with the facilities and staff capable of performing transplant will need to be selected. Advise the client that some insurance companies do not cover the cost of this high-risk therapy (Mello & Brennan, 2001).

Follow-Up

The follow-up of clients who have had chemotherapy is variable and depends on their response to the drugs and the oncologist's recommendations. Clients may receive Tamoxifen for two to five years, with follow-up every six months or per the oncologist's preference.

Clients who receive Tamoxifen should have an annual physical examination with endometrial evaluation performed routinely. Annual mammography should occur unless otherwise indicated.

Breast conservation clients who are asymptomatic are often requested to have annual mammography post radiation therapy (Rubin, 2002).

Clients who undergo a mastectomy are evaluated postoperatively at the discretion of the surgeon. Complications, if encountered, may require more frequent evaluation or may necessitate rehospitalization. Clients undergoing autologous bone marrow transplants are followed closely by the oncologist and may require weekly visits after leaving the hospital.

BREAST RECONSTRUCTION

Breast reconstruction, a voluntary procedure, is available to many women who have undergone mastectomy. In addition to being an option following mastectomy, breast reconstruction and augmentation may also be chosen for cosmetic reasons that are unrelated to cancer surgery. Immediate reconstruction postmastectomy has gone from a small minority to a majority in most practices (Fine, Mustoe, & Fenner, 2000). All women would virtually be candidates for this procedure if postoperative adjunctive therapy and surveillance are not delayed.

The need for breast irradiation may be the most commonly cited reason for delaying reconstruction (Fine et al., 2000). An expander may be used during this time to prepare the breast for reconstruction following radiation therapy.

The process of breast reconstruction surgery changed dramatically in 1992 when the Food and Drug Administration (FDA) restricted the use of silicone implants, the

most common breast implant used in the United States. (Reynolds, 1995; Stracner & Bohan, 1995). Silicone breast implants had been used for reconstruction and cosmetic enhancement of the breasts since the early 1960s (Fine et al., 2002). Multiple complaints of rheumatic conditions, including fibromyalgia, systemic lupus erythematosus, polymyositis and Raynaud's phenomenon were reported and associated with silicone implants, which caused the utilization of this long used implant to cease (Stracner & Bohan, 1995). Though the use of these implants was terminated in strictly cosmetic surgeries, the FDA later (1992) approved the use of silicone implants in patients undergoing breast reconstruction surgery, following mastectomy, who were involved in clinical trials. Saline breast implants are now used most often today. The shell of the saline implant is made of a silicon polymer in solid form. This ruling stands today. Saline breast implants are now the only implant available for elective cosmetic breast augmentation that is unrelated to breast cancer.

Some studies show that patients with silicone breast implants are no more likely to get symptoms of connective tissue diseases than are other patients. Still, in 1994 a settlement fund was established by Dow Corning and other manufacturers of silicone gel implants that provided more than $4.2 billion to pay compensation for recipients of these implants who had experienced certain rheumatologic and/or neurologic conditions.

A new implant consisting of a silicone elastomer bag filled with soybean oil is currently being investigated.

TISSUE TRANSFER (TRAM): RECTUS ABDOMINIS MYOCUTANEOUS FLAP

Tissue transfer is recommended when the client chooses to have breast reconstruction while avoiding the possible side effects of breast implants. The procedure gives a superb appearance and a natural feel to reconstructed breast (Eberlein & Tsangaris, 2000). It offers the potential for soft, naturally appearing breast mounds without the associated risks of implanting foreign/manufactured materials. A similar procedure, the latissimus dorsi musculocutaneous flap, may be performed as well when the client has small or moderate-sized breasts. This procedure will leave a scar on the back where it is less visible (Fine et al., 2000).

The rectus abdominis muscle is transferred from the abdomen via a tunnel under the skin and extended through a new incision in the breast area. Artery and blood supply are maintained. The flap is sutured into position and, along with fat, is contoured to form a breast. Sufficient abdominal girth is required to perform the procedure, which can be very painful and may require six to eight weeks for recuperation (Eberlein & Tsangaris, 2000). Untoward responses to anesthesia and postoperative infection and bleeding are possible. Complications of the procedure include vessel thrombosis, partial or total flap loss, mastectomy skin flap necrosis, delayed wound healing, fat necrosis, volume loss, and flap contracture (Tran, Chang, Gupta, Kroll, & Robb, 2001). Initially, sensitivity in the reconstructed breast(s) may be decreased; however, it may later return. Choice of the Free TRAM flap procedure, which avoids use of a pedicle, uses deep inferior epigastric vessels as the primary source of blood supply (Fine et al., 2000). The Free TRAM limits the potential for flap loss, minimizes fat necrosis, and provides up to 100 percent of flap volume for use in women with large breasts. This procedure may be used in women who smoke.

The anticipated outcome on evaluation is a favorable body image and the avoidance of the implantation of foreign substances in the body.

Explain to the client that the recovery period required is often long and that appropriate pain management will be necessary. Inform her that tissue transfer is not recommended for women who smoke or who have chronic disease. In addition, further surgery will be necessary for nipple formation.

AUGMENTATION MAMMOPLASTY (BREAST ENLARGEMENT)

Augmentation mammoplasty is performed to improve the cosmetic appearance of the breast by increasing its size. Many women choose to undergo this procedure to attain a well-proportioned figure or a figure that complies with their and/or society's ideal (Antoniuk, 2002). When this procedure is performed following mastectomy, it is given the term reconstructive breast surgery.

The surgical procedure involves placing an implant behind the breast through an inframammary, periareolar, or transaxillary incision (Sohn, Chung, Kim, & Yoon, 2000). The inframammary placement is preferred by some surgeons because it allows complete visualization of the pockets, which enhances symmetry and allows better hemostasis prior to placement of the implants.

Periareolar incisions introduce the implant in a submuscular or subglandular position. Submuscular placement is often chosen over subglandular placement because there are fewer complications such as hematoma,

infection, and nipple desensitization (Sohn et al., 2000). It is also perceived as safe, versatile, and less painful. Placement of the implants behind the muscle is frequent postmastectomy (Eberlein & Tsangaris, 2000).

The transaxillary approach produces a remote scar that is well hidden in the axilla. Pockets are dissected deep into the pectoralis major muscle, providing less exposure of implants to bacteria from ducts. Care must be given to attain symmetry.

A common complication of silicone gel and saline implants is the formation of a fibrous capsule or capsular contracture around the implant, which causes a firm rigidity of the breast (Eberlein & Tsangaris, 2000; Fagrell, Berggren, & Tarpila, 2001; Rout-Worley, 2001; Sohn et al., 2000). This fibrous capsule forms as a part of the body's normal response to a foreign body. The capsule may contract and become constrictive. This converts the normally disc-shaped implants to appear as a sphere. Some cases may cause disfigurement. Grading of the capsular contracture occurs during physical examination (see Table 14–2).

Treatment of capsular contracture is normally considered ineffective since it probably will recur (Hughes et al., 2000).

Implant rupture may occur spontaneously or after trauma and may cause nodules, decreased breast size, asymmetry, and pain.

Possible side effects of breast enlargement surgery are delayed wound healing, infection, hematoma, changes in breast/nipple sensation, gel bleed, wrinkling, shifting and extrusion of the implant, asymmetry mammography distortion, or inaccuracies and dissatisfaction with cosmetic results (Rout-Worley, 2001). Untoward reactions to general anesthesia may occur. Deflamation, rippling,

TABLE 14–2. Grading of a Capsular Contraction

Grade	Features
Grade 1	The augmented breast is as soft as an unoperated breast; no palpable firmness.
Grade 2	The breast has minimal firmness; is less soft; the implant can be palpated with no visible abnormalities.
Grade 3	The breast is moderately firm; the implant is easily palpated; implant or distortion caused by it is visible.
Grade 4	Severe contracture with tender, painful, cold breast; marked distortion exists.

Source: Howrigan, P. J. (1994). Reduction and augmentation mammoplasty. Obstet Clin North Am. 21:539–549.

Baker, J. T. Jr. (1978). Augmentation mammoplasty. In Ownsley, J. Q. (Ed) Symposium in aesthetic surgery of the breast. St. Louis, MO: Mosby.

wrinkling, sloshing, and encapsulation diminish client's satisfaction with saline implants (Hughes et al, 2000).

Breastfeeding with the presence of breast implants should be possible and should not present problems for the nursing infants or mothers.

Screening for breast cancer and for implant integrity may be difficult since breast implants obscure breast tissue. There are, however, special mammographic procedures used to image the breasts of women with implants (Willison, 2001).

Ultrasound is a very useful tool for the evaluation of the integrity of implants. There is no ionizing radiation, the interior of the implant can be visualized and areas that are difficult or impossible to image with mammography can be seen. The disadvantages of using sonography are that it is very time consuming and requires a highly skilled operator who will scan the breasts meticulously.

Magnetic resonance imaging (MRI) offers an excellent option in the evaluation of the breasts with implants (Willison, 2001). Its major advantage is its ability to distinguish silicone from normal tissues within the breast. Intracapsular ruptures can be diagnosed. The disadvantage is the cost of the test, especially for women who lack insurance coverage. Also many, if not most, insurances might refuse to cover the cost of this test because it is not routinely used.

The anticipated outcomes upon completion of breast augmentation surgery are improved self-esteem and a favorable body image.

Inform the client of the controversies surrounding breast implants and the possible complications of implants and augmentation surgery. Discuss the possibility of decreased sexual pleasure associated with nipple numbness and breast firmness. Clients with a history of or a propensity for keloid formation (common among African Americans) should consider the possibility of unsightly keloid scarring. Encourage the client to continue BSE and provide her with the instruction she needs (see Figure 14–1). Inform her about the American Cancer Society guidelines for mammography screening. Discuss the difficulties associated with imaging breast tissue when breast implants are present and help the client to find a mammography facility that uses specialized techniques for women with breast implants.

MASTOPEXY (CORRECTION OF PTOSIS)

Mastopexy is performed to improve the appearance of sagging breasts, which may be caused by gravity, hormone regression (postpartum, menopausal) or weight loss

(Hughes et al., 2000). Surgical resection of the breasts is done, with elevation of the breast mount, areola, and nipple to a new (usually higher) location.

Markings for breast location following surgery are performed with the client in an upright position, and new sites for the nipple-areola complex are chosen.

General anesthesia is used, and infection, hematoma, nipple numbness (sometimes temporary), asymmetry, and scarring of the breast may develop postoperatively. A reaction to the anesthesia is possible.

The anticipated outcomes on evaluation are a favorable body image and improved self-esteem.

Encourage the client to weigh very carefully the risks and advantages of the procedure. Clients with a history of or a propensity to develop keloids (particularly common in African Americans) should consider possible formation of unsightly keloid scarring. Inform the client that breast ptosis may recur and that sensation in the breast and nipple may be lost, which may decrease sexual gratification. If desired by the client, include significant others in decision making and advise them to seek the opinions of at least two surgeons. Encourage BSE and mammography if age appropriate.

BREAST REDUCTION

The goal of breast reduction surgery is to alleviate the physical symptoms associated with large breasts and to create a breast size and shape that is appropriate for the client's age, body habitus, or desire (Hughes et al., 2000). Breast reduction surgery is performed to reduce breast size and relieve back and shoulder pain caused by heavy pendulous breasts. Many women with large breasts or macromastia complain of neck strain, occipital headache, shoulder pain, disfigurement caused by brassiere straps that burrow into the skin, low back pain, anterior chest discomfort, and paresthesia of the little fingers. Often clients with macromastia find participation in exercise and sports activities difficult because of discomfort or self-consciousness (Hughes et al., 2000). Frequently, unsolicited sexual advances occur, which might be troubling for young adolescents and women who are establishing a sexual identity.

Reduction surgery, which makes breasts smaller, helps to relieve these symptoms and may resolve them totally (scarring and deep shoulder grooves caused by brassiere straps may not resolve). Neck and back pain are frequently relieved. Smaller breasts may also help those who feel embarrassed about their large breasts to improve their self-image and self-esteem.

During breast reduction surgery, the breasts are surgically restructured and made smaller. Preoperative markings are performed as with mastopexy. In some cases the nipple-areola complex requires resection as a full thickness skin graft and is transplanted to the appropriate position on the breast mound. The grafted nipple-areola complex will not have normal sensation and may have irregular pigmentation.

The potential adverse effects and complications are asymmetry, infection, hematoma, nipple numbness, extensive scarring, fat necrosis, and nipple inversion (Hughes et al., 2000).

The anticipated outcomes on evaluation are reduced back and shoulder pain, reduced pressure on skin and irritation from brassiere straps, and improved self-esteem. Some patients find the surgery to be an incentive for total body weight reduction.

Encourage the client to weigh the advantages and risks of this elective surgical procedure. Clients with a history of or propensity to develop keloid (common among African Americans) should consider the possibility of extensive and unsightly keloid scarring. Include significant others of the client's choosing in decision making. Discuss the possible relationship between nipple numbness and decreased sexual gratification. Encourage BSE and mammography if appropriate. Advise the client to seek the opinions of at least two surgeons. Inform her that the procedure generally is covered by insurance because it is not performed for cosmetic reasons alone. The client, however, should consult with her insurance company.

Clients should follow the postoperative care guidelines provided by the surgeon. Immediate evaluation is especially important if signs or symptoms of infection occur in a client who has had the TRAM flap procedure, because abdominal and chest wounds are present. When possible, refer the client to women who have had breast reconstruction and augmentation surgery who are willing to discuss their experiences.

Routine screening mammography should be continued, and annual clinician exam as well as monthly BSE should continue. Mammography should not be performed sooner than 6 months after surgery has been completed.

REFERENCES

Adams, M.L., Becker, H., & Colbert, A. (2001). African-American women's perceptions of mammography screening. *Journal of the National Black Nurses Association, 12*(2), 44–48.

American Cancer Society (ACS). (2002a). *Cancer facts and figures 2002.* Atlanta, GA: Author.

American Cancer Society (ACS). (2000b). *Cancer facts and figures for African Americans 2000–2001.* Atlanta GA: Author.

American Cancer Society (ACS). (2002c). *Cancer reference information.* Accessed April 1, 2002 from http://www.cancer.org.

American College of Obstetricians and Gynecologists (ACOG). (1996, February) *ACOG committee opinion: Tamoxifen and endometrial cancer.* No. 169.

Amshel, C.E., & Sibley, E. (2001). Multiple unilateral fibroadenomas. *The Breast Journal, 7*(3), 189–191.

Anderson, B.O. (2001). Prophylactic surgery to reduce breast cancer risk: A brief literature review. *The Breast Journal, 7*(5), 321–330.

Andolina, V.F. (Ed.). (2001). *Patient considerations: Mammographic imaging.* Baltimore, MD: Lippincott Williams & Wilkins.

Antoniuk, P. (2002). Breast augmentation and breast reduction. *Obstetric and Gynecology Clinics of North America, 29*(1) 103–115.

Bartek, J., Falck, J., & Lukus, J. (2001). CHK2 kinase. *Nature Review: Molecular and Cell Biology, 2*(12), 877–886.

Beitsch, P.D., Clifford, E., Whitworth, P., & Abarea, A. (2001). Improved lymphatic mapping technique for breast cancer. *The Breast Journal, 7*(4), 219–23.

Bell, M.C., & Patride, E.E. (1995, December). Early breast carcinoma: Risk factors, screening, and treatment. *Contemporary OB/GYN, 31–32,* 36, 40 passim.

Bentrem, D.J., & Jordan, V.C. (1999). Targeted antiestrogen for the prevention of breast cancer. *Oncology Research, 11*(9), 401–407.

Biller, B.M. (1999a). Diagnostic evaluation of hyperprolactinemia. *Journal of Reproductive Medicine, 44*(12 Supplement), 1095–1099.

Biller, B.M. (1999b). Hyperprolactinemia. *International Journal of Fertility Women's Medicine, 44*(2), 74–77.

Birdwell, R.L., Smith, K.L., Betts, B.J., Ikeda, D.M., Strauss, H.W., & Jeffrey, S.S. (2001). Breast cancer: Variables affecting sentinel lymph node visualization at preoperative lymphoscintigraphy. *Radiology, 220*(1), 47–53.

Brandle, M., & Schmid, C. (2000). Galactorrhea and pituitary mass: A typical prolactinoma? *Postgraduate Medicine, 76*(894), 232–234.

Cardosi, R., & Fiorica, J. (2000). Surveillance of the endometrium in tamoxifen treated women. *Current Opinion in Obstetrics and Gynecology, 12*(1), 27–31.

Chow, J.S., Smith, D.N., Kaelin, C.M., & Meyer, J.E. (2001). Case report: Galactography-guided wire localization of an intraductal papilloma. *Clinical Radiology, 56*(1), 72–73.

Clare, S.E., & Morrow, M. (2000). Management of the palpable breast mass. In J.R. Harris (Ed.), *Diseases of the breast.* Philadelphia, PA: Lippincott Williams & Wilkins.

Coates, R.J., Uhler, R.J., Brogan, D.J., Gammon, M.D., Malone, K.E., Swanson, C.A., Flagg, E.W., & Brinton, L.A. (2001). Patterns and predictors of the breast cancer detection methods in women under 45 years of age (United States). *Cancer Causes and Control, 12*(5), 431–442.

Dickler, M.N., & Norton, L. (2001). The MORE trial: Multiple outcomes for raloxifene evaluation-breast cancer as a secondary end point: Implications for prevention. *Annals of the New York Academy of Sciences, 949,* 134–142.

DiSaia, P.J., & Creasman, W.T. (2002). *Clinical gynecologic oncology* (Rev. ed.) St. Louis, MO: Mosby.

Dixon, J.M., & Bundred, N.J. (2000). Management of disorders of the ductal system and infections. In J.R. Harris (Ed.), *Diseases of the breast.* Philadelphia, PA: Lippincott Williams & Wilkins.

Eberlein, T.J., & Tsangaris, T.N. (2000). Breast cancer surgery. In D.E. Hayes (Ed.) *Atlas of breast cancer* (Rev. ed.). New York: Mosby.

Fagrell, D, Berggren, A., & Tarpita, E. (2001). Capsular contracture around saline-filled fine textured and smooth mammary implants: A prospective 7.5 year follow-up. *Plastic and Reconstructive Surgery, 108*(7), 2108–2112.

Faiz, O., & Fentiman, I.S. (2000). Management of breast pain. *International Journal of Clinical Practice, 54*(4), 228–232.

Fine, N.A., Mustoe, T.A., & Fenner, G. (2000). Breast reconstruction. In J.R. Harris (Ed.), *Diseases of the breast.* Philadelphia, PA: Lippincott Williams & Wilkins.

Foster, R.J. (2000). Techniques of diagnosis of palpable breast masses. In J.R. Harris (Ed.), *Diseases of the breast.* Philadelphia, PA: Lippincott Williams & Wilkins.

Freund, K.M. (2000). Rationale and technique of clinical breast examination. *Medscape Women's Health, 5*(6), E2.

Gizienski, T.A., Harvey, J.A., & Sobel, A.H. (2002). Breast cyst recurrence after postaspiration of air. *Breast Journal, 8*(1), 34–37.

Hadi, M.S. (2000). Sports brassiere: Is it a solution for mastalgia? *Breast Journal, 6*(6), 407–409.

Hamed, H., & Fentiman, I.S. (2001). Benign breast disease. *International Journal of Clinical Practice, 55*(7), 461–464.

Hayes, D.F. (Ed.). (2000). *Atlas of breast cancer* (Rev. ed.), New York: Mosby.

Hindle, W.H., & Gonzalez, S. (2001). Breast disease: What to do when it's not cancer. *Women's Health in Primary Care, 4*(1), 21–34.

Hindle, W.H., & Gonzalez, S. (2002). Breast cancer: Helping your patients weigh the treatment options. *Women's Health in Primary Care, 5*(4), 225–236.

Hughes, L.E., Mansel, R.E., & Webster, D.J.T. (2000). Benign disorders and diseases of the breast. London, England: W.B. Saunders.

Husani, B.A., Sherkat, D.E., Bragg, R., Levine, R., Emerson, J.S., Mentes, C.M., & Cain, V.A. (2001). Predictors of breast cancer screening in a panel study of African American women. *Women's Health in Primary Care, 34*(3), 35–51.

Ishikawa, H., Sato, K., & Mochizuki, H. (2002). Optimal sentinel node examination and a new strategy for axillary control in breast cancer. *Breast Journal, 8*(1), 10–14.

Jones, S. (2002). Antiaromatase agents: Evolving role in adjuvant therapy. *Clinical Breast Cancer, 3*(1) 33–42.

Jordan, V.C. (2000a). Antiestrogens: Clinical applications of pharmacology. *Journal of the Society for Gynecologic Investigation, 7*(1) Suppl. 47–48.

Jordan, V.C. (2000b). Tamoxifen: A personal perspective. *Lancet Oncology, 1*(1), 43–49.

Jordan, V.C. (2001). The past, present and future of selective estrogen receptor modulation. *Annals of the New York Academy of Sciences, 949,* 72–79.

Jordan, V.C., Gapstur, S., & Morrow, M. (2001). Selective estrogen receptor modulation and reduction in risk of breast cancer, osteoporosis, and coronary heart disease. *Journal of the National Cancer Institute, 93*(19), 1229–1457.

Joslyn, S.A., & West, M.M. (2000). Racial differences in breast carcinoma survival. *Cancer, 88*(1), 114–123.

Kline, T.S., Kline, I.K., & Howell, L.P. (Eds.). (1999). Guides to clinical aspiration biopsy breast. Baltimore, MD: Lippincott Williams & Wilkins.

Kopans, D.B. (2000). Imaging analysis of breast lesions. In J.R. Harris (Ed.), *Diseases of the breast.* Philadelphia, PA: Lippincott Williams & Wilkins.

Kosoff, M.B. (2000). Ultrasound of the breast. *World Journal of Surgery, 24*(2), 143–157.

Leong, S.P., Morita, E.T., Treseler, P.A., & Wong, J.H. (2000). Multidisciplinary approach to selective sentinel lymph node mapping in breast cancer. *Breast Cancer, 7*(2), 105–113.

Lillé, S. (2001). History of mammography. In V.F. Andolina (Ed.), *Mammographic imaging.* Baltimore, MD: Lippincott Williams & Wilkins.

Lonning, P. (2002). Aromatase inhibitors and inactivators for breast cancer therapy. *Drugs and Aging, 19*(4) 277–298.

Love, C., Muir, B., Scrimgeor, J., Leonard, R., Dillon, P., & Dixon, J. (1999). Investigation of endometrial abnormalities in asymptomatic women treated with tamoxifen. *Journal of Clinical Oncology, 17*(7), 2050–2054.

Maguire, G.A. (2002). Prolactin elevation with antipsychotic medications: Mechanism of action and clinical consequences. *Journal of Clinical Psychiatry, 63*(4), 56–62.

Martin, A.M., Weber, B.L. (2000). Genetic and hormonal risk factors in breast cancer. *Journal of the National Cancer Institute, 92*(14), 1126–1135.

McMasters, K.M., Wong, S.L., Chao, C., Woo, C., Tuttle, T.M., Noyes, R.D., Carlson, D.J., Laidley, A.L., McGlothin, T.Q., Ley, P.B., Brown, C.M., Glaser, R.L., Pennington, R.E., Turk, P.S., Simpson, D., & Edwards, M.J. (2001). Defining the optimal surgeon experience for breast cancer sentinel lymph node biopsy: A model for implementation of new surgical techniques. *Annals of Surgery, 234*(3), 292–299.

Meijers-Heijboer, E.J., Verhogg, L.C., Brekelmans, C.T., Seynaeve, C., Tilanus-Linthorst, M.M., Wagner, A., Duke, L., Devilee, P., van den Ouweland, A.M., van Geel, A.N., & Klijn, J.G. (2000). Presymptomatic DNA testing and prophylactic surgery in families with a BRCA1 or BRCA2 mutation. *Lancet, 355* (9220), 2015–2020.

Meijers-Heijboer H., Van Den Ouweland, A., Klijn, J., Wasielewski, M., et al. (2002). Low-penetrance susceptibility to breast cancer due to CHEK 2 (*)1100delC in noncarriers of BRCA1 or BRCA2 mutations. *Nature Genetics, 31*(1) 55–59.

Mello, M.M., & Brennan, T.A. (2001). The controversy over high-dose chemotherapy with autologous bone marrow transplant for breast cancer. *Health Affairs, 20*(5), 107–117.

Miller, C.W., Ikezoe, T., Krug, U., Hoffman, W.K., Tavor, S., Vegesna, V., Tsukasaki, S., & Koeffler, H.P. (2002). Mutations of the CHK2 gene are found in some osteosarcomas, but are rare in breast, lung, and ovarian tumors. *Genes, Chromosomes and Cancer, 33*(1), 17–21.

Miller, N.A., Chapman, J.A., Fish, E.B., Link, M.A., Fishell, E., Wright, B., Lickley, H.L., McCreedy, D.R., & Hanna, W.M. (2001). In situ duct carcinoma of the breast: Clinical and histopathologic factors and association with recurrent sarcoma. *Breast Journal, 7*(5), 292–302.

Morris, C.R., Wright, W.E., Schlag, R.D. (2001). The risk of developing breast cancer within the next 5, 10, or 20 years of a women's life. *American Journal of Preventive Medicine, 20*(3), 214–218.

Morrow, M. (2000). The evaluation of common breast problems. *American Family Physician, 61*(8) 2371–2385.

Morrow, M., & Harris, J. (2000). Local management of invasive breast cancer. In J. R. Harris (Ed) *Diseases of the breast.* Philadelphia, PA: Lippincott Williams & Wilkins.

Mourits, M., Van der Zee, A., Willemse, P., Ten Hoor, K., Holleman, H., & De Vries, E. (1999). Discrepancy between ultrasonography and hysteroscopy and histology of endometrium in postmenopausal breast cancer patients using tamoxifen. *Gynecological Oncology, 73*(1), 21–26.

National Cancer Institute (NCI). (2002). NCI statement on mammography screening. Retrieved April 1, 2002 from http://www.newscenter.cancer.gov.

Olsen, O., & Gotzsche, P.C. (2001). Cochrane review on screening for breast cancer with mammography. *Lancet, 358,* 1340–1342.

O'Regan, R.M., & Jordan, V.C. (2001). Tamoxifen to raloxifene and beyond. *Seminal Oncology, 28*(3), 260–273.

Orrego, J.J., Chandler, W.F., & Barkan, A.L. (2000). Pergolide as primary therapy for microprolactinomas. *Pituitary, 3*(4), 251–256.

Osborne, C.R., & Ravdin, P.M. (2000). Adjuvant systemic therapy of primary breast cancer. In J.R. Harris (Ed.), *Diseases of the breast.* Philadelphia, PA: Lippincott Williams & Wilkins.

Ozsener, S., Ozaran, A., Itil, I., & Dikmen, Y. (1998). Endometrial pathology of 104 postmenopausal breast cancer patients treated with tamoxifen. *European Journal of Gynecological Oncology, 19*(6), 580–583.

Padden, D.L. (2000). Mastalgia: Evaluation and management. *Nurse Practitioner Forum, 11*(4), 213–218.

Pegram, M.D., & O'Callaghan, C. (2001). Combining the anti-her2 antibody trastuzamab with taxanes in breast cancer: Results and trial considerations. *Clinical Breast Cancer, 2* (Supplement 1), 15–19.

Pena, K.S., & Rosenfeld, J.A. (2001). Evaluation of galactorrhea. *American Family Physician, 63*(9), 1763–1770.

Peterson, M.C. (2001). Reversible galactorrhea and prolactin elevation related to fluoxetine use. *Mayo Clinic Proceedings, 76*(2), 215–216.

Recanatini, M., Cavali, A., & Valenti, P. (2002). Nonsteroidal aromatase inhibitors: Recent advances. *Medical Research Reviews, 22*(3), 282–304.

Recht, A. (2000). Breast cancer radiotherapy. In D.F. Hayes (Ed.), *Atlas of breast cancer* (Rev. ed.). New York: Mosby.

Reis, L., Eisner, M., Kosary, C., Hankey, B., Miller, B., & Edwards, B. (Eds.). (2000). *SEER cancer statistics review,* 1973–1997. Bethesda, MD: National Cancer Institute.

Renard, F., Vosse, M., Scagnol, I., & Verhest, A. (2002). Aggressive endometrial carcinoma in a breast cancer patient treated with tamoxifen with normal transvaginal ultrasonography. Case report. *European Journal of Gynaecological Oncology, 23*(1), 25–28.

Reynolds, H.E. (1995). Evaluation of the augmented breast. *Radiological Clinics of North America, 33,* 1131–1145.

Rout-Worley, J. (2001). Augmentation mammoplasty: Implications for the primary care provider. *Journal of the American Academy of Nurse Practitioners, 13*(7), 304–309.

Rubin, N. (2002). What's the "Take Home"? *Consultant, 42*(5), 639–640.

Sakorafas, G.H. (2001). Nipple discharge: Current diagnostic and therapeutic approaches. *Cancer Treatment Reviews, 27*(5), 275–282.

Sahney, S., Petkovska, L., Ramadan, S., Al-Muhtaseb, S., Jain, R., & Sheikh, M. (2002). Sonographic appearance of galactoceles. *Journal of Clinical Ultrasound, 30*(1), 18–22.

Schnitt, S.J. (2000). Processing of breast biopsies. In D.F. Hayes (Ed.), *Atlas of breast cancer* (Rev. ed.). New York: Mosby.

Schnitt, S.J., & Connolly, J.L. (2000). Pathology of benign disorders of the breast. In J.R. Harris (Ed.), *Diseases of the breast.* Philadelphia, PA: Lippincott Williams & Wilkins.

Slawson, S.H, Johnson, B.A. (2001). Ductography: how to and what if? *Radiographics* 21(1), 133–150.

Sohn, B., Chung, Y., Kim, G., & Yoon, W. (2000). Submuscular periareolar approach to augmentation mammoplasy in korean women. *Aesthetic Plastic Surgery, 24*(6), 455–460.

Stomper, P.C. (2000). Breast imaging. In D.F. Hayes (Ed.), *Atlas of breast cancer* (Rev. ed.). New York: Mosby.

Stracner, J., & Bohan, A. (1995). Silicon breast implants: Understanding the current controversies. *Clinician Reviews, 5,* 55–57, 60, 62, passim.

Tansey, M.J., & Schlechte, J.A. (2001). Pituitary production of prolactin and prolactin-suppressing drugs. *Lupus, 10*(10), 660–664.

Tran, N.V., Chang, D.W., Gupta, A., Kroll, S.S., & Robb, G.L. (2001). Comparison of immediate and delayed free TRAM flap breast reconstruction in patients receiving postmastectomy radiation therapy. *Plastic and Reconstructive Surgery, 108*(1), 78–82.

Tsutsui, S., Ohno, S., Murakami, S., Hachitanda, Y., & Oda, S. (2002). Prognostic value of c-erbB2 expression in breast cancer. *Journal of Surgical Oncology, 79*(1), 216–23.

Underwood, S.M. (1999). Breast cancer screening among African American women: Addressing the needs of the African American women with known and no known risk factors. *Journal of the National Black Nurses Association, 10*(1), 46–55.

Venta, L. (2000). Image-guided biopsy of nonpalpable breast lesions. In J.R. Harris (Ed.), *Diseases of the breast.* Philadelphia, PA: Lippincott Williams & Wilkins.

Whitman-Elia, G.F., & Windham, N.Q. (2000). Galactorrhea may be clue to serious problems. Patients deserve a thorough workup. *Postgraduate Medicine, 107*(7), 165–168, 171.

Willison, K.M. (2001a). Mammographic positioning. In V.F. Andolina (Ed.), *Mammographic imaging* (Rev. ed.). Baltimore, MD: Lippincott Williams and Wilkins.

Willison, K. (2001b). Practical applications in problem solving. In V.F. Andolina (Ed.), *Mammographic imaging* (Rev. ed.). Baltimore, MD: Lippincott Williams & Wilkins.

Willison, K.M. (2001c). Thinking in three dimensions. In V.F. Andolina (Ed.), *Mammographic imaging* (Rev. ed.). Baltimore, MD: Lippincott Williams & Wilkins.

Yamamoto, D., Shoji, T., Kanishi, H., Nakagawa, H., Haijima, H., Gondo, H., & Tanaka, K. (2001). A utility of ductography and fiber optic ductoscopy for patients with nipple discharge. *Breast Cancer Research and Treatment, 70*(2), 103–108.

Zacur, H.A. (1999). Indications for surgery in the treatment of hyperprolactinemia. *Journal of Reproductive Medicine, 44*(12 Supplement), 1127–1131.

CHAPTER 15

THE CLIMACTERIC, MENOPAUSE, AND THE PROCESS OF AGING

Valerie T. Cotter ◆ *Ellis Quinn Youngkin*

*W*omen today can expect to live one-third of their lives after their reproductive years.

Highlights

- The Physiology of Menopause
- The Physical Changes of Aging
- Sexuality and Aging
- Hypoestrogenic Changes
    Vasomotor Instability
    Vaginal Changes
    Urinary Tract Changes
    Menstrual Irregularity
- Overview of Current Hormone Replacement Therapy Research and Implications for Practice
- Alterations in Mood
- Cognitive Function/Memory Loss/Alzheimer's Disease
- Sleep Disorders
- Hormone Replacement Therapy: Specific Information
    Client Education and Counseling
    Required Assessment
    Treatment Considerations
- Women's Midlife and Late Life Health Care Program
- Osteoporosis
- Hirsutism/Virilism
- Nonreproductive Health Concerns of Aging Women
    Health Insurance and Income
    Social Support
    Elder Mistreatment
    Chronic Illness
    Functional Status
    Depression and Suicide Risk
    Polypharmacy
    Injury Prevention
    Limited Access to Care

❖   INTRODUCTION

In 1900, the average life expectancy was 48.7 years for white American women and 33.5 years for African American women. By 1999, however, average life expectancy was higher for women (79.4 years) than for men (73.8 years) generally. Today, a woman in the United States who reaches age 65 can expect to live to be 84.9 (National Vital Statistics, 1999).

The elderly population has grown substantially in this century and will continue to grow into the 21st century. In 1997, 13 percent of the U.S. population was 65 years of age and over (USDHHS, 1999). According to the Census Bureau's projections, 20 percent of the population will be 65 years of age and over in 2030 (USDHHS, 1999). The elderly population is becoming more racially and ethnically diverse. In 1994, one in ten elderly were a race other than white. In 2000, 8.8 percent of the U.S. population 65 years and over was black women and 15.8 percent was Hispanic women (U.S. Census Bureau, 2000).

Only recently, then, has society been faced with the issues of aging beyond menopause. Research is now focusing on factors that positively impact physical and psychological aging. Women today can expect to live one-third of their lives after their reproductive years, or one-half of their adult life, and preventive health care and healthy lifestyle habits can greatly improve the quality of life in those later years.

As women age they face numerous transitions that require adaptation. During the middle years, the twenty-year span of time between 50 and 70, a woman refines and integrates the emotional growth that she underwent during the previous twenty or so years and assumes primary responsibility for the continued survival and enhancement of the nation (Stevenson, 1977). During late adulthood, the years between 70 and death, a woman experiences a continuing process of maturation and assumes responsibility for sharing the wisdom of age, reviewing life, and putting affairs in order (Stevenson, 1977).

Developmental Tasks for Age 50–70 Years

- Maintaining flexible views in occupational, civic, political, religious, and social positions.
- Keeping current on relevant scientific, political, and cultural changes.

- Developing mutually supportive (interdependent) relationships with grown offspring and other members of the younger generation.
- Reevaluating and enhancing the relationship with spouse or most significant other or adjusting to her or his loss.
- Helping aged parents or other relatives progress through the last stage of life.
- Deriving satisfaction from increased availability of leisure time.
- Preparing for retirement and planning another career when feasible.
- Adapting self and behavior to signals of accelerated aging processes (Stevenson, 1977).

Developmental Tasks of Late Adulthood

- Pursuing a second or third career, new interest, hobbies, and/or community activities that fulfill some untapped inner resource or otherwise enhance the self-image and maintain worth in society.
- Learning new skills that are well removed from prior learnings or at least do not produce cognitive dissonance with prior learnings.
- Sharing wisdom accrued from the past with individuals, groups, communities, and nations.
- Evaluating the totality of past life and putting successes and failures into perspective.
- Progressing through the stages of grief, death, and dying with significant others and with oneself (Stevenson, 1977).

The Climacteric and Menopause

Menopause is often defined as the permanent cessation of menstruation resulting from loss of ovarian follicular activity and the absence of menses for one year. It is possible to induce menopause surgically by bilateral oophorectomy. The *climacteric* or *perimenopause* refers to the two to seven years prior to menopause and to the subsequent one year of amenorrhea following menopause. The Greek *climacteric* means "rungs on a ladder"—a rather appropriate and positive way to view maturation. The postmenopause is defined as the time after menopause.

The average age of menopause in the United States is 51 years. Despite consistent lowering of the age of puberty, the age of natural menopause has remained consistent. Ovarian failure prior to 30 is premature and requires chromosomal analysis to rule out gonadal dysgenesis. Menopause between ages 31 and 40 is considered early and, because of the increased incidence of autoimmune disorders, requires referral for medical endocrine evaluation. Menopause after age 40 is considered normal. The only consistent predisposing factors for earlier menopause, typically one to two years earlier, are cigarette smoking and nulliparity (Jacobs Institute of Women's Health, 2000).

THE PHYSIOLOGY OF MENOPAUSE

Menopause results from a series of changes initiated in the ovary. General atresia of ovarian follicles begins with the onset of puberty and becomes more significant after age 35 when the ovary contains fewer follicles that are responsive to FSH. Eventually, the atresia leads to a decline in ovarian production of estrogen and progesterone.

LOSS OF ESTROGEN FEEDBACK

In the normal menstrual cycle, rising levels of FSH stimulate the developing dominant follicle to secrete increasing amounts of estradiol. The increasing level of estradiol as well as inhibin from the granulosa cells exert a negative feedback on the hypothalamus and result in decreasing FSH. After menopause, there is an increase in FSH because of the reduction in pituitary gonadotropin inhibition of estrogen and progesterone. This change in ovarian steroid production is often gradual, resulting in anovulatory bleeding patterns. Eventually, the ovaries are completely unable to respond to FSH and LH, and the level of gonadotropin hyperactivity stabilizes. Gonadotropin levels never return to premenopausal levels.

DIAGNOSIS OF MENOPAUSE

- If on no hormonal medication (e.g., HRT, ERT, oral contraceptives), a rise in FSH to 40 mIU/mL is diagnostic (AACE, 1999; NAMS, 2000).
- There is ongoing debate about the best time to switch from OCS to HRT. One suggestion is at age 50, do annual FSH on day 5, 6, or 7 of placebo-pill week; FSH will rise during this week if woman is menopausal. By mid-50s, testing is not necessary—the assumption is that menopause has occurred.
- If on progestin-only contraception or therapy, FSH levels are not affected and can be measured at any time.

POSTMENOPAUSAL ESTROGEN SOURCES

The major source of estradiol prior to menopause is the ovarian follicle. Estradiol is produced cyclically, and the ovary accounts for over 90 percent of total body production. Relatively constant production of estrone by adrenal glandular secretion and peripheral conversion of androstenedione, the major circulating androgen in women, also occur. Postmenopause, little estradiol is produced in the ovarian follicles. Ovarian stroma, under stimulation by LH, continues to produce androstenedione and testosterone, which along with androstenedione produced by adrenal glands, are converted to estrone in peripheral adipose tissue. Thus, the body weight of the woman contributes to her overall postmenopausal level of circulating estrogen. Initially, both the ovary and the adrenal glands are major sources of androstenedione. With advanced age, however, the ovarian stroma ceases production of androstenedione and is unable to maintain sufficient estrone production. Specific target deficiencies may then be noted. The degree of deficiency will vary with the individual woman. During the climacteric, ovarian secretion of androgens decreases markedly; androgens, especially testosterone, may play a role in the maintenance of sexual desire (see Hirsutism).

THE PHYSICAL CHANGES OF AGING

The changes that occur as a woman ages are the culmination of heredity, the effects of living and lifestyle, and hormonal changes.

DERMAL CHANGES

With aging, the skin undergoes progressive changes: The epidermis becomes thinner and flatter, the density of scalp and body hair follicles decreases, and the sebaceous glands and sweat glands have reduced function and become less responsive to stimuli (Blair, 1990). The dermis becomes less elastic, collagen is lost, and a wrinkling of the epidermis results. Decreases in resilience, protection, and moisture occur. The incidence of skin cancer increases markedly after age 50. Hair grays as functioning melanocytes in hair decrease (Blair, 1990).

SENSORY CHANGES

Visual impairment, defined as vision loss that cannot be corrected by glasses or contact lenses, increases with age. Nearly 19 percent of older adults age 70 and older and 30 percent of those over 85 years of age have some degree of visual impairment (Desai, Pratt, Lentzner, Robinson, 2001). Visual impairment frequently leads to motor vehicle accidents, injurious falls, and functional decline.

Presbycusis, the bilateral hearing loss associated with advanced age gradually occurs after age 50 and is characterized by a decreased sensitivity to high frequency tones.

CARDIOVASCULAR CHANGES

Cardiovascular disease (CVD) is the leading cause of morbidity and mortality in postmenopausal women in the United States. One in two women will die of coronary heart disease (CHD) or stroke (American Heart Association, 1997). The efficiency and muscle contractility of the heart decreases with aging, and there is a reduced ability to increase heart rate with hemodynamic stresses or acute illness (Tully, 2002).

The changes in lipid components that accompany postmenopausal estrogen decline (see Table 15–1) favor the slow formation of atherosclerosis. These changes are compounded by elevated blood pressure, smoking, obesity, diabetes, and heredity. The lipid changes associated with increased CHD risk are as follows (National Cholesterol Education Program, 2001):

- Increased low density lipoproteins (LDL) > 160 mg/dL if client does not have CHD and has no risk than one other CHD risk factor.
- Increased LDL > 130 mg/dL if client does not have CHD but has two or more other CHD risk factors or other noncardiac vascular disease.

- Decreased high density lipoprotein (HDL) <40 mg/dL.

PULMONARY CHANGES

Lung expansion decreases gradually with aging, as the thorax becomes more rigid and tissues less elastic. Reductions occur in pulmonary reserve and in vital capacity, and there is a decline over time in arterial oxygen concentration (Blair, 1990). The elderly are able to compensate for age associated changes in the pulmonary system; however, they are vulnerable to acute respiratory infections.

GASTROINTESTINAL (GI) CHANGES

The GI system can handle food that is chewed properly, albeit more sluggishly with aging. For proper chewing, gums and teeth must be in good condition. Estrogen deficiency can cause atrophic changes in the gums and influence mastication, as can poor dental hygiene and gum disease. Generally, the amount of hydrochloric acid in the stomach decreases with age, as does pepsin. Peristaltic action and emptying times decrease, and absorption of certain substances, such as the B vitamins, iron, and calcium, is affected.

REPRODUCTIVE CHANGES

- *Vulva.* With the loss of estrogen, the vulva undergoes atrophy, and subcutaneous tissues diminish (Holfand & Powers, 1996). The labia majora become small and the labia minora almost nonexistent. The skin becomes thinner, and pubic hair loss is progressive. Dystrophies and pruritus are more frequent.
- *Vagina.* Epithelial maturation decreases. The failure to produce glycogen containing superficial cells causes an increase in the vaginal pH, which may predispose the woman to infection (Jacobs Institute of Women's Health, 2000). The vagina becomes shortened, thinned, and narrowed, with obliteration of the vaginal fornices and eventual loss of vaginal rugae. Sebaceous gland secretions decrease and the vagina loses most of its lubricating ability, especially in response to sexual stimulation. Changes may be prevented or slowed by the continuation of regular intercourse.

Over time, the uterus decreases in size and the endometrium atrophies. The cervix pales and shrinks with loss of the fornices so that the external os is

TABLE 15–1. Laboratory Values with Older Adults

Test	Unchanged/Same as Younger Reference	Decrease with Older Subjects	Increase with Older Subjects
CBC			
RBC	unchanged	or slight decrease	
Hgb	unchanged	or slight decrease	
Hct	unchanged	or slight decrease	
RBC indices	unchanged		
WBC count	unchanged		
Differential			
Basophils	unchanged		
Eosinophils	unchanged		
Myelocytes	unchanged		
Bands	unchanged		
Monocytes	unchanged		
Lymphocytes	unchanged	or slight decrease	
Platelets	unchanged		
ESR			slight increase
B_{12}		decrease	
Folate/folic acid		decrease	
TIBC/transferrin	unchanged		
Serum Fe	unchanged		
Blood chemistry electrolytes			
Na	unchanged	or slight decrease	
K	unchanged		or slight increase
Cl	unchanged		
Ca	unchanged	or slight decrease	
P	unchanged		
Mg		decrease	
Glucose			
FBS	unchanged		or slight increase
PPBS			increase
OGTT			increase
HgA_{1c}			increase
End products of metabolism			
BUN	unchanged		or slight increase
Creatinine	unchanged		or slight increase
Creatinine clearance		decrease	
Bilirubin	unchanged		
Uric acid			slight increase
Liver function tests			
ALAT (SGPT)	unchanged		
AST (SGOT)	unchanged		
LDH	unchanged		or slight increase
Alkaline phosphatase			gradual increase
Total protein	unchanged	or slight decrease	
Albumin		decrease	
Globulin	unchanged		
Lipoproteins			gradual increase
Total cholesterol			gradual increase
LDL			increase
HDL	unchanged	or slight decrease in women	or slight increase in men
Triglycerides			increase

(Continued)

TABLE 15–1. (*cont.*)

Test	Unchanged/Same as Younger Reference	Decrease with Older Subjects	Increase with Older Subjects
Thyroid function tests			
T_4	unchanged	or slight decrease	
T_3		decrease	
TSH			slight increase

Source: Reprinted by permission of the publisher from Interpretation of Laboratory Values in Older Adults, by K. D. Melillo, in Nurse Practitioner 18(7) 59–67. Copyright 1993 by Elsevier Science Publishing Co., Inc.

nearly flush with the vaginal wall. The endocervix becomes atrophic and the cervical canal stenotic. The ovaries and fallopian tubes atrophy and are usually not palpable on examination; in fact, any adnexal mass in a woman over 50 is considered malignant until proven otherwise.

◆ *Pelvic Floor.* The muscular tissue loses tone after menopause, causing increases in uterine prolapse, cystocele, and rectocele (Holfand & Powers, 1996). This loss of tone may be heightened by past pregnancy and vaginal delivery.

◆ *Breast.* Breast size tends to diminish as glandular breast tissue decreases and is replaced by fat; the breasts often hang lower on the chest (Bickley & Hoekelman, 1999).

URINARY CHANGES

Urinary tract changes are secondary to estrogen deficiency, aging, and past trauma from childbearing. The distal portion of the urethra shortens and thins and the opening shifts closer to the introitus. Bladder capacity decreases, and the bladder and urethral tissue lose tone. With age, there is an increase in uninhibited bladder contractions and postvoid residual volume (Bradway & Getman, 2002). Renal clearance diminishes, but the kidneys are able to maintain a proper fluid balance in the body, unless concurrent disease or severe stressors are imposed.

ENDOCRINE CHANGES

◆ *Thyroid.* Irregularity and nodularity of the thyroid increase with age (Feil & Cotter, 2002). Thyroid function appears to remain stable after menopause, although hyperthyroidism and hypothyroidism are more common in women, in general, and in the elderly (U.S. Preventive Services Task Force [USPSTF], 1996). See Table 15–1 for normal changes in thyroid values with aging.

◆ *Pituitary.* Adequate hormonal secretion continues despite decreased pituitary size.

MUSCULOSKELETAL CHANGES

Muscle tone is related to exercise. In the sedentary woman, normal tone and strength diminish. Atrophy occurs more rapidly with aging if muscles are not used (see Osteoporosis). The proportion of fat and water change with aging: Fat increases and water decreases.

NEUROLOGICAL CHANGES

Forgetfulness is not uncommon and may be related to neuron loss that begins when a woman is in her 20s. Some brain and spinal cord efficiency is lost, which is evident, for example, in slowed pupillary response. Sleep may be more easily disrupted. The incidence of Alzheimer's disease increases with age. The third leading cause of death in the United States is cerebrovascular accident (CVA). The principal risk factors are age, hypertension, smoking, coronary artery disease, and diabetes.

SEXUALITY AND AGING

Sexuality continues as an important component of a woman's life until her death. It represents a need to be accepted, a need for intimacy and companionship. Sexuality is influenced by many factors. Although most older adults continue to be sexually active, physical changes associated with aging, illness, and opportunity have major influence on the frequency and satisfaction of sexual behaviors. Physical changes in older women that may have a negative impact on sexuality include the following (Holfand & Powers, 1996):

◆ Thinning of vaginal walls
◆ Vaginal lubrication volume smaller

- Decreased labial sensation
- Change in libido from drugs, depression, medical, and relationship problems
- Dyspareunia from vaginal irritation, tissue friability, and anxiety
- Loss of elasticity, length, and width of vagina

Changes caused by hormonal deficiency may be lessened with estrogen or testosterone therapy. Other factors that affect sexuality, either positively or negatively, include longer life span; issues surrounding aging, such as physical and social losses and transitions; an increase in chronic illness; body image changes; effects of medications on libido; more time for intimacy; and freedom from worry about contraception/pregnancy. Sexuality is seldom considered in the counseling of midlife and aging women, yet women in this age group have a variety of concerns and information needs. Women need information about sexually transmitted diseases and "safer sex" (Letvak & Schoder, 1996). Whether single or married, women may desire information about common sexuality concerns, such as masturbation. They may also want information about male sexuality and aging and may need help adapting sexual practices to accommodate physical and emotional changes. Sensitivity to the needs and concerns of lesbian couples should be the same as for any other couple.

HYPOESTROGENIC CHANGES

The loss of estradiol with decreasing ovarian function results in a host of changes among postmenopausal women. The incidence and severity of complaints vary greatly, but most frequently, they involve vasomotor instability, vaginal and urinary tract changes, headaches, insomnia, and menstrual irregularity. Research suggests that the vasomotor instability and genitourinary changes are clearly related to the physiologic changes of menopause, but the impact of psychological, social, and cultural factors on other associated symptoms is less clear (Holfand & Powers, 1996; Shaw, 1997).

VASOMOTOR INSTABILITY

Vasomotor instability, better known as hot flashes or flushes, coincides with a surge of LH and decrease in estrogen level and is followed by a measurable increase in body surface heat and a fall in core temperature. The hot flash is an intense feeling of heat that begins in the upper chest or neck and proceeds up the face and head. It typi-

cally lasts for five to twelve minutes and concludes with profuse perspiration. Hot flashes and night sweats tend to increase at night. They can occur in the premenopause, but more frequently in postmenopause, lasting in most women for one to two years, but in some (10–15%) for longer than 10 to 15 years (Shaw, 1997).

Epidemiology

Hot flashes and flushes are the most consistently reported symptom of the menopause. As many as 60 percent of women experience hot flashes for less than five to seven years in the perimenopausal years; 10 to 15 percent of women experience them for more than ten to fifteen years (Shaw, 1997).

Subjective Data

Evaluate the client's menstrual history for changes suggestive of perimenopause, such as decreasing or increasing intervals between menses and dysfunctional/anovulatory bleeding patterns. The client will report episodes of feeling extreme warmth rising from the chest up to the face and head, followed by perspiration and sometimes chills. If these vasomotor symptoms occur at night, they disrupt sleep—causing insomnia, exhaustion, and irritability. Flushes can occur frequently during a 24-hour period, hence the client may report the need to change clothing and bed linens often.

Objective Data

Physical Examination. Findings are frequently absent, but may include vasodilation of peripheral blood vessels in the skin coupled with mild increase in pulse, but without alteration in blood pressure; increased digital temperature; and decreased intracore temperature with chills.

Diagnostic Tests and Methods

- *Serum FSH Level.* A level greater than 40 mIU/mL is diagnostic of menopause (AACE, 1999). FSH is less reliable during the perimenopause when there are irregular bursts of follicular function alternating with no ovarian response.
- *Client Diary of Episodes.* Confirms oral history.

Differential Medical Diagnoses

Hypothalamic/pituitary tumor, infection (viral illness, tuberculosis, systemic infection with fever, human immunodeficiency virus [HIV] infection), alcoholism, thyroid disease.

Plan

Psychosocial Interventions. Reassure the client that vasomotor instability is normal during the perimenopause. In addition, explain the physiology of menopause. Offer adaptive measures as follows.

- Adjust the room temperature; leave a window open; use a portable fan to accommodate an office environment.
- Wear clothing in layers for ease of removal; wear more cotton.
- Try stress management techniques such as relaxation exercises, meditation, and yoga.

Medication. Hormone Replacement Therapy (HRT) or Estrogen Replacement Therapy (ERT) are effective in greater than 90 percent of women. Adjust the dosage to accommodate client symptoms. Advise the client that HRT/ERT is more likely to be safe if used for less than five years. Alternative therapies may be tried first or introduced after HRT is stopped if symptoms continue. Herbal therapies, soy products, and vitamin E are the most common alternatives used by breast cancer survivors for menopause symptoms (Many US breast, 2002). A population-based survey of 886 women found that stress management, over-the-counter remedies, chiropractic therapy, massage therapy, dietary soy, acupuncture, naturopathic homeopathic remedies, and herbal remedies were reported as commonly used for menopause symptoms; and 89 to 100 percent found them somewhat or very helpful (Newton et al., 2002). (See Hormone Replacement Therapy, later in this chapter, for a complete description of administration, side effects, contraindications, evaluation outcomes, and teaching/counseling.)

Alternative Therapies. Alternative therapy is indicated if HRT or ERT is contraindicated. The following drugs may be offered to decrease vasomotor instability.

- *Clonidine.* Transdermal clonidine can be applied in a 0.1 mg dose or more at bedtime or the transdermal patch (AACE, 1999). Side effects include severe hypotensive episodes, dizziness, fatigue, nausea, and mood swings. There is limited evidence to support its use for vasomotor symptoms (Gass & Taylor, 2001). The side effects' discomfort often outweigh possible relief from this drug for women with hot flashes (Treating hot flashes, 2002).
- *Selective Serotonin-Reuptake Inhibitors (SSRIs).* Several small studies of low dose SSRIs have shown a 50 to 80 percent reduction in hot flashes (Gass & Taylor, 2001). In breast cancer survivors, venlafaxine (Effexor) 75 mg daily reduced hot flashes by 60 percent in four weeks; fluoxetine (Prozac) decreased the frequency and severity of hot flashes by 50 percent (Treating hot flashes, 2002). Side effects include nausea, dry mouth, drowsiness, dizziness for venlafaxine, and nausea, decreased libido, dry mouth, weight gain, and headaches for fluoxetine.
- *Gabapentin* (Neurontin): An anti-seizure drug, it reduced hot flash severity by 50 to 70 percent in nineteen women taking tamoxifen for breast cancer (Treating hot flashes, 2002). Side effects are nausea, tremor, drowsiness, blurred vision, and lack of muscular coordination.
- *Vitamin E.* Vitamin E can be prescribed at 100 IU daily, increasing over weeks or a few months to 600 IU, until relief of symptoms. In a randomized controlled study of breast cancer survivors taking tamoxifen, women taking Vitamin K 400 IU twice a day experienced one less hot flash per day than those taking placebo (Gass & Taylor, 2001).
- *Other Interventions.* Advise the client to limit her caffeine and alcohol intake and not to smoke. Drinking eight to ten glasses of water daily is also advised; drinking cold water at the beginning of a flush may help to alleviate the discomfort. Hot drinks and foods should be avoided. Separate bed sheets and blankets can be used, then taken off without disturbing the bed partner. Regular exercise every day may improve sleep; however, heavy exercise must be avoided immediately before bedtime.
- *Herbal Therapies.* Many herbal therapies are available that promise relief of symptoms. Advise caution in use as FDA approval is very limited for these substances and no standardization exists at present (Israel & Youngkin, 1997). Black cohosh has been shown to be effective in some studies in reducing hot flashes (Barclay, 2002; Jellin, 2002). Allow four weeks for symptoms to improve. The usual dose is 20 mg twice a day (Jellin, 2002). Side effects are GI upset, headache, dizziness, weight gain, and cramping due to estrogenic effect. Red clover and chaste berry are other herbs that also may offer some relief.
- *Soy and Isoflavones.* Most studies on hot flashes have used isoflavone amounts of 40 to 80 mg/day. There are inadequate data to recommend an amount to prevent osteoporosis or reduce cholesterol. Choosing whole soy foods rather than supplements or soy-enriched foods is preferred (ACOG, 2001; NAMS, 2000).

Follow-Up

Call the client to evaluate the effectiveness of therapy in relieving the signs and symptoms of perimenopause. (See Hormone Replacement Therapy for follow-up related to that therapy.) If therapy is ineffective, suggest referral to a gynecologist.

VAGINAL CHANGES

The vagina, composed of thick tissue with accordionlike folds (rugae) during the childbearing years, thins dramatically in the absence of estrogen. This process predisposes the woman to vaginal infection, trauma, and pain.

Epidemiology

Decreased estrogen, whether because of natural or surgical menopause, contributes to vaginal atrophy. Vaginal changes including vaginal wall friability, increase in pH, irritation, susceptibility to infection, dyspareunia, and related loss of sexual desire are common among postmenopausal women and often occur during perimenopause.

Subjective Data

A menstrual history will reveal symptoms of vaginal change, possibly including vaginal dryness, loss of lubrication with intercourse, pain or soreness with penile thrusting during intercourse, unusual vaginal discharge, infection, and postcoital bleeding.

Objective Data

Note: Postmenopausal bleeding is not normal and should be evaluated.

Physical Examination. Findings include thinning and paleness of vaginal epithelia, bloody vaginal discharge, brittle pubic hair, disappearance of rugae, and infection.

Diagnostic Tests and Methods

Serum FSH. FSH is less reliable during the perimenopause when there are irregular bursts of follicular function alternating with no ovarian response.

Papanicolaou (Pap) Smear. Maturation index for indication of estrogen deficiency (test is optional, not as diagnostic as FSH level is). Over 50 percent parabasal cells equates with a marked estrogen decline.

Gonorrhea Culture, Wet Mount, and Chlamydia Test. Performed if appropriate.

Differential Medical Diagnoses

Vaginitis and sexually transmitted diseases (bacterial, viral, fungal infection), leukoplakia, lichen sclerosis, malignancy, postmenopausal uterine bleeding, diabetes mellitus.

Plan

Psychosocial Interventions. Teach the client about the normal physiological changes of menopause, aging, and sexuality that may occur.

Medication. *Estrogen* cream (Premarin Vaginal Cream) is indicated to reverse vaginal atrophic changes (see Hormone Replacement Therapy for a general description of hormone use).

   Apply 1 g estrogen cream or the equivalent intravaginally daily for two to four weeks, then decrease to 1 g, two to three times weekly when symptom relief is achieved. Then decrease to one application per week or eliminate altogether based on symptoms. Vaginal absorption into the bloodstream is very efficient; therefore, a progestin to protect against endometrial hyperplasia is recommended. Oral hormone replacement therapy (HRT) is described later in this chapter.

   Another estrogen cream is Estrace estradiol cream 0.01%. The client uses 2 to 4 g per day for one to two weeks, then half that dose for another one to two weeks, then maintains with 1 g one to three times a week for three weeks, after which use can be tapered for maintenance or cessation if symptoms abate. Vagifem 25 mcg vaginal tablets may also be used with 1 tablet intravaginally daily for two weeks, then one tablet two times weekly. The vaginal ring, Estring, provides yet another source of local treatment for vaginal changes. The ring is inserted high in the vagina and replaced every ninety days. Any estrogen treatment is contraindicated for the same reasons as oral estrogen. Thus, the history is very important.

Other Interventions. Treat any vaginal infection as indicated, and educate the client about "safer sex" (see Chapters 9 and 11). Teach her Kegel's exercises, as these may help with arousal (see Chapter 21, Urinary Incontinence, Pelvic Muscle Exercises, for more detail). Offer the client suggestions or readings on sexual pleasuring to increase arousal (see Chapter 6). Advise her to use a water-soluble vaginal lubricant with intercourse to prevent trauma from penile thrusting and alleviate the discomfort of friction (lubricants will not reverse epithelial changes). Lubricant jellies, creams, and suppositories are available over the counter (without prescription). Vegetable oils or lotions without perfume may be suggested. Advise the client to wash her hands thoroughly before and after applying any vaginal lubricant.

Lubrin Vaginal Suppositories. Insert one suppository 5 to 20 minutes prior to intercourse as needed.

K-Y Jelly. Apply as needed.

Replens Vaginal Suppositories or Cream. Insert cream or suppository 5 to 20 minutes prior to intercourse. May be used as needed.

Astroglide. Apply intravaginally as needed.

Follow-Up

Advise the client to return to the health care provider if no relief occurs. Referral for sexual therapy may be indicated if the problem seems unrelated to physical changes in the vagina.

URINARY TRACT CHANGES

Urgency, nocturia, increased incidence of urinary tract infection, and incontinence are common among postmenopausal women and often occur during the perimenopause. The urethra and bladder have large numbers of estrogen receptors and subsequently atrophy during menopause. Detrusor instability (urge incontinence) and/or urethral sphincter incompetence (stress incontinence) are the most common causes of urinary incontinence in women over age 60. These conditions are influenced not only by hypoestrogenism but also by restricted mobility, medications, endocrine disorders, pelvic floor denervation, prolapse, excessive weight, and constipation (Bradway & Getman, 2002). (See Chapter 21, Urinary Incontinence.)

MENSTRUAL IRREGULARITY

As the number of ovarian follicles capable of producing estrogen decreases, a woman experiences irregularities of the menstrual cycle. Ideally her periods are shorter and less frequent, but often they are a mix of heavy, longer bleeding episodes that are closer together due to anovulation. With anovulation, the epithelium builds from unopposed estrogen stimulation with no progesterone to transpose it to a secretory state. Although irregular bleeding is common, endometrial cancer must be ruled out. Low-dose oral contraceptives help to regulate menses in perimenopausal women and control menstrual bleeding in postmenopausal women. Formulations as low as 20 mcg

of ethinyl estradiol are effective and better tolerated (AACE, 1999).

Subjective Data

The client's history indicates a change in the regularity of cycles and characteristics of menses (waxing and waning menses) or the absence of menses, and, often, other symptoms of hypoestrogenism.

Objective Data

Physical Examination. The physical and pelvic exam should be normal, and may or may not reveal changes suggestive of approaching meno-pause (see Chapter 8 for causes of abnormal menstrual bleeding and physical findings).

Diagnostic Tests and Methods. A pregnancy test must be used to rule out pregnancy as a cause of the bleeding. A serum FSH level of greater than 40 mIU/mL is diagnostic of menopause; FSH reaches a maximal level one to three years after menopause, then declines gradually. Endometrial abnormalities (hyperplasia and carcinoma) may be ruled out with an endometrial biopsy or ultrasound. If anemia is suspected, a hemoglobin and hematocrit may be done.

Differential Medical Diagnoses

Pregnancy, spontaneous abortion, anovulation, hyperplasia, carcinoma, infection, abnormalities of the uterus such as fibroids or polyps, endometriosis, adenomyosis, injury, ovarian abnormalities such as tumors or cysts.

Plan

Psychosocial Interventions. Reassure the client that bodily changes are normal, explain the physiology of menopause, and educate regarding methods of treatment, if indicated.

Medication. For the perimenopausal woman who is ovulating, recommended treatment is low dose oral contraceptives or continuous progestin, either oral or depot.

Endometrial Biopsy. Office-based endometrial biopsy or ultrasound has replaced dilation and curettage (D & C) as the method of choice for diagnosing endometrial abnormalities (AACE, 1999).

Follow-Up

Refer the client to a gynecologist for evaluation of suspected abnormalities, especially carcinoma. Any bleeding that does not respond to therapy also requires that the client be referred. Any postmenopausal woman who bleeds requires referral to rule out pelvic cancer, unless on HRT and the bleeding pattern is consistent for the therapy.

OVERVIEW OF CURRENT HORMONE REPLACEMENT THERAPY RESEARCH AND IMPLICATIONS FOR PRACTICE

In May 2002, the portion of the Women's Health Initiative (WHI) trial in which the health benefits of combined hormone replacement therapy with 0.625 mg conjugated equine estrogen (CEE) and 2.5 mg medroxyprogesterone (MPA) were being studied was ended before the planned 2005 completion. The "overall health risks exceeded benefits . . . for an average 5.2 year follow-up," according to the investigators (Writing Group, 2002, p. 321). Approximately half of the over 16,000 healthy postmenopausal women ages 50 to 79 years were randomly assigned to the oral HRT and the rest to oral placebo. Increased hazard ratios found an increased relative risk of 29 percent for coronary heart disease, 26 percent for breast cancer, 113 percent for pulmonary emboli (PE), and 41 percent for stroke in the women using combined therapy as compared to placebo. These findings equated to "absolute excess risks per 10,000 person-years attributable to estrogen plus progestin" of "7 more CHD events, 8 more strokes, 8 more PEs, and 8 more invasive breast cancers" (Writing Group, 2002, p. 321). Despite significant decreased risks of colorectal cancer, endometrial cancer, and hip fractures for the HRT users, the investigators felt the excesses in the aforementioned areas warranted discontinuation of the trial. Admitted limitations of the trial include the use of only one drug regimen so that results may not apply to lower doses of the same drugs, to other hormone formulations, or to other routes of administration. Also, though the findings related to coronary heart disease (CHD) and venous thromboembolism (VTE) supported those of the Heart and Estrogen/Progestin Replacement Study (HERS), no other clinical trials for breast cancer or colorectal cancer have been done, and there is limited trial data for fractures (Writing Group, 2002). Interestingly, the estrogen-only portion of the WHI trial was not ended, suggesting that this formulation may be safer than HRT. That will remain to be seen in this and future studies.

Reported simultaneously were the findings from the prospective Breast Cancer Detection Demonstration Project (BCDDP), saying that women "who used estrogen-only replacement therapy, particularly for ten or more years, were at significantly increased risk of ovarian cancer" (Lacey, Mink, Lubin, Sherman, et al., 2002, p. 334). Data were collected through four phases between 1979 and 1998 on 31,354 women who were menopausal or who became menopausal during this time. The relative risk of ovarian cancer in the estrogen/progestin-only group increased during the first two years, then decreased to below the risk for nonusers after two or more years (Lacey et al., 2002). However, the number of women using combined HRT was small, and a longer duration of time would be needed to determine if the original findings for HRT would hold true.

The Heart and Estrogen/Progestin Replacement Studies (HERS and HERS II) in which older, menopausal women with coronary disease were randomized to HRT or placebo found that the incidence of deep vein thrombosis (DVT) and pulmonary embolism (PE) increased two- to three-fold with HRT use in the HERS trial, but DVT incidence was no longer statistically significant in the HERS II segment (last 2.7 years of the total 6.8 years) (Hulley, Furberg, Barrett-Connor, Cauley, et al., 2002). Overall, the risk for DVT was significantly increased with HRT use. CVD rates were not more favorable in the hormone group either. In addition, the incidence of biliary risk for DVT was significantly increased with HRT use. Nor were CVD rates more favorable in the hormone group. In addition, the incidence of biliary tract surgery in HRT users was increased 48 percent. Cancer risk did not differ significantly between user and nonuser groups for breast, lung, or colon cancer, though cancers in general were 19 percent more frequent among hormone users. Hip fracture was more frequent in the user group, interestingly. Other trials to assess the effects of HRT on atherosclerosis progression support the HERS and HERS II trials findings (Petitti, 2002).

As expected, the resulting fallout from these studies has shaken current clinical practice related to menopause therapy significantly. What is clear is that long-term use of 0.625 mg CEE with 2.5 mg MPA must be reevaluated and prescribed very individually based on the client's history, needs, and risks (Kaunitz, 2002; Stevenson & Whitehead, 2002). Notelovitz (2002) suggests that each client's situation is different, and treatment for menopause-related conditions must be tailored to the individual, just as are therapies for other conditions, such as hypertension. He notes that hormone therapy, if customized to the woman and monitored, can be safe. Are there factors in the woman's history that indicate that an association with hormone therapy use could increase her risks? These must be assessed and considered in any therapy regimen. Notelovitz emphasizes that if risk factors are absent and the lowest effective dosage of the natural estrogen therapy 17-beta estradiol is used for a specific condition, such as to prevent osteoporosis and enhance the quality of life in early menopause, plus the client is effectively monitored, then use is safe. When women are older, have heart disease, an increased breast cancer risk, or other possible conditions that warrant careful consideration about use of hormones, the clinician must evaluate all factors in partnership with the woman, including if hormone therapy or some other therapy would be best, the length of such therapy, and the specific therapy regimen. Lower doses of hormones, particularly natural hormone regimens, are considered safer, preferred, and have been shown to provide effective clinical outcomes with fewer or no adverse effects (Notelovitz, 2002). Natural hormones suggested are 17-beta estradiol and prometrium, and the transdermal route is considered to be safest (Notelovitz, 2002).

Thus, the provider, in close partnership with the client, must consider all the factors in the client's history when determining a possible therapy. Kaunitz (2002) advises the following: (1) HRT is not indicated to treat/prevent CVD; (2) other measures must be considered, such as lipid-lowering therapies, as well as CV lifestyle changes for CVD prevention/treatment where risk or disease are present; (3) HRT may be preferred for certain women for vasomotor symptoms, but should be used less than five years; (4) use of a progestin/progesterone other than MPA is advised (norethindrone acetate, norgestimate, prometrium); (5) lower doses of both estrogen and progestin are prudent; (6) nonhormonal therapies should be considered and may be better for a client, such as bisphosphonates and SERMS; (7) other more traditional measures for prevention and treatment of osteoporosis must be used (e.g., aerobic and weight-bearing exercises, calcium, vitamin D, no smoking, moderate or no alcohol); (8) annual clinician breast exams and mammography are essential (and BSE should be added); and (9) local therapies for vaginal atrophy and dyspareunia, including estrogen creams, but not systemic hormone therapy, are advised.

The reader is asked to place hormone replacement therapy and these recent data in proper perspective when examining the subsequent sections on selected conditions and various therapies. Also, the rapidity with which information changes warrants close attention to new research findings as they unfold and their implications. Additional information on HRT and ERT are provided later in this chapter.

ALTERATIONS IN MOOD

A significant number of women report that changes in mood and concentration, irritability, nervousness, and depression occur during midlife. A number of psychosocial changes occur at this time of life, including relationship changes, loss of partner, bodily changes of aging, parents and/or children needing care, and role changes that may also impact mood. The relationships between hormonal changes and anxiety and depression in the perimenopausal woman remain to be clarified, however. Both the central and peripheral nervous systems contain 17-beta estradiol sensitive cells, and even the brain responds to withdrawal or absence of ovarian steroids. Estrogen influences the concentrations and availability of neurotransmitters, including serotonin, in the brain. Research has shown that estrogen increases the degradation of monoamine oxidase, the enzyme that catabolizes serotonin, regulates the amount of free tryptophan, the precursor for serotonin, and enhances the transport of serotonin (Sherwin, 1996). Very few clinical correlations are available.

EPIDEMIOLOGY

No single cause for mood alterations has been identified. Hormonal deficiency may play a role, but consideration must be given to other factors in the client's life, such as aging and how she feels about it. U.S. society reveres youth, and the reality of lost youth and changes in body image may upset some women. Other major life changes that are common for a woman of perimenopausal and menopausal age include one's children leaving home; death or disability of a spouse or partner; helping aging parents; realization that one may not have achieved all of one's life goals, loss of childbearing capacity; and concerns about retirement and finances. Psychological symptoms, including decreased concentration and memory, mood changes, mild and transient depression, and decreased sexual desire not related to vaginal changes, have been attributed to menopause (Jacobs Institute of Women's Health, 2000). Many of these symptoms may be interrelated to the physical symptoms of menopause, such as hot flashes causing insomnia, leading to loss of concentration from loss of sleep. The interrelationships among hormone levels, affective symptoms, and lifestyle factors, need further examination.

SUBJECTIVE DATA

The client's history may reveal periods of crying, anger, sadness, irritability, depression, anxiety attacks, family members' reports of mood swings, and expressions of suicide. If a psychological disorder is suspected, a referral to a mental health professional is indicated.

OBJECTIVE DATA

Physical Examination

Findings on physical examination may include decreased affect, lethargy, inappropriate responses, and crying. A complete examination is indicated to rule out systemic diseases, drug use, or other conditions that could affect physiological function and cause symptoms.

Diagnostic Tests and Methods

General diagnostic tests, such as complete blood cell (CBC) count, thyroid studies, FSH/LH, urinalysis, and blood chemistry analysis are indicated to determine normal baselines and deviations. Drug testing may also be indicated. Other tests that may be done are psychological scales and questionnaires, such as CAGE and MAST alcoholism questionnaires, and Zung, Beck, or Geriatric Depression scales (Beck & Beck, 1961; Mayfield, McLeod, & Hall, 1984; Selzer, 1980; Yesavage & Brink, 1983; Zung, 1965).

DIFFERENTIAL MEDICAL DIAGNOSES

Depression, anxiety disorders, neurological impairment, sexual dysfunction, psychiatric disorder.

PLAN

Psychosocial Interventions

Refer the client for psychological evaluation as appropriate; protect if the client is suicidal.

Life transitions, grief work, and affective and physical changes associated with perimenopausal transitions may require individual or group therapy and support. Educational programs focused on midlife and menopause that emphasize accurate information, positive attitudes, and connection with other women may reassure the client.

Medication

Hormone replacement therapy (discussed later in this chapter). Although women seek hormone therapy to help with their mood, concentration, or depressive symptoms, no hormone is FDA approved for these symptoms without other indications for use. (See Antianxiety and Antidepressant Therapy in Chapter 23 or other reference texts.)

Exercise

Advise the client to engage in regular aerobic exercise and resistance training to improve muscle strength, unless contraindicated. Exercise may improve the client's psychological outlook and reduce mood swings.

Balanced Diet

Advise the client to maintain a nutritionally balanced diet and to avoid simple carbohydrates, which can induce hypoglycemic reactions.

Stress Reduction Techniques

Relaxation exercises, yoga, meditation, and regular physical exercise may reduce stress.

FOLLOW-UP

If the client does not respond to lifestyle changes and/or medication therapy, she should be referred to an appropriate mental health professional for additional treatment.

COGNITIVE FUNCTION/ MEMORY LOSS/ ALZHEIMER'S DISEASE

Cognition encompasses the entire range of human intellectual functions, including learning and memory. Estrogen may enhance or preserve cognitive function by improving cholinergic function, neuronal survival, and cerebral blood flow. Some studies have suggested that estrogen may be associated with a decreased risk or delayed age of onset of AD, but several others have found that it has no protective effects and is ineffective in delaying the progression of AD (Mulnard et al., 2000;

Seshadri et al., 2001; Waring et al., 1999). Two ongoing randomized trials of estrogen for preventing AD are under way, but the results are unlikely to be available for a decade. Thus, estrogen as a treatment to prevent or slow the progression of AD is not recommended at this time.

SUBJECTIVE DATA

The client, or significant other, may report signs and symptoms of declining mental functioning, for example, forgetfulness, decreased concentration and attention, getting lost in familiar environments, and expressive or receptive language impairment.

OBJECTIVE DATA

A comprehensive history and physical examination, review of prescribed and over-the-counter medications are done to rule out reversible and potentially treatable causes of cognitive impairment. Screening for cognitive impairment can be done with instruments such as the Mini Mental Status Examination (MMSE), or Short Portable Mental Status Questionnaire (SPMSQ) (Folstein, Folstein, & McHugh, 1975; Pfeiffer, 1975).

DIAGNOSTIC TESTS

Recent guidelines from the American Academy of Neurology recommend the following diagnostic tests in the evaluation of dementia (Knopman, Dekosky, Cummings, et al., 2001): CBC, thyroid profile, B_{12} and folate levels, blood chemistry analysis, screening for depression, and CT or MRI of the brain.

DIFFERENTIAL MEDICAL DIAGNOSES

Mild cognitive impairment, vascular dementia, Alzheimer's disease, alcohol dementia, depression, delirium, toxic effects of medications, malignancy, infection, thyroid disorders.

PLAN

Psychosocial Interventions

Depending upon the duration and severity of cognitive impairment, refer the client for consultation with a neurologist, neuropsychologist, mental health professional, or other primary care provider for further evaluation. If symptoms are mild and complete evaluation, including cognitive screening, is normal, reevaluate in six to twelve months, and reassure the client about benign senescent forgetfulness. Individual and group therapy may be considered.

SLEEP DISORDERS

With aging, sleep stages 3 (early phase of deep sleep) and 4 (deep sleep and relaxation) decrease and brief arousals become more frequent (Blackman, 2000). Alterations in sleep patterns may be the result of hot flushes and night sweats. The need for overall sleep diminishes slightly with age; the average adult needs five to seven hours of sleep each day.

EPIDEMIOLOGY

Any number of factors may contribute to sleep disturbances in addition to estrogen decline: lack of exercise, excessive napping during the day, stress, depression, anxiety, illness, restless sleep partner, uncomfortable sleeping accommodations, excessive activity prior to bedtime, and stimulant drugs. Sleep disorders are common among the general population and increase in the perimenopausal and postmenopausal years. The exact incidence is unknown.

SUBJECTIVE DATA

The client reports signs and symptoms of menopause, as well as irritability, interrupted sleep, and feelings of tiredness.

OBJECTIVE DATA

Findings on physical examination include lethargy, dark circles under the eyes, and possible altered response time. Diagnostic tests are used to rule out other diseases that cause lethargy, fatigue, and insomnia, such as anemia, sleep apnea, or hypothyroidism. Be sure that obstructive sleep apnea, associated with significant daytime sleepiness and increased motor vehicle accidents, is not a factor. This condition is a risk factor for cardiovascular death (Harding, 2000).

DIFFERENTIAL MEDICAL DIAGNOSES

Neurological disorders, psychological disturbances.

PLAN

Reassure and educate the client about causes and remedies of sleep disorders. Referral to a sleep therapy specialist may be indicated. Consult current pharmacological therapy references for information on sedatives and sleeping medications, but only after giving nonpharmacological interventions a fair trial of several months.

Nonpharmacological Interventions

- *Evaluate naps.* Encourage ten- to thirty-minute naps during the daytime if the client is severely sleep deprived. If napping is interfering with night sleep, however, urge decreasing naps if possible.
- *Avoid caffeine.* Foods and beverages containing caffeine should be decreased or eliminated, especially after 5 P.M. Evaluate prescription and over-the-counter medications that might contain caffeine, for example, some cold remedies.
- *Limit alcohol intake.* Alcohol consumption should be less than 4 oz. per day or, preferably, eliminated altogether.
- *Avoid smoking.* Encourage the client to stop smoking. Offer literature and referral to a group for support.
- *Exercise before or in the early evening.* Exercising should occur no later than 7 P.M. (Aerobic exercise in late evening increases wakefulness.)
- *Arrange for a comfortable sleep environment.* Make suggestions concerning mattress comfort, soundproofing or earplugs, room darkening, sleeping clothes, room temperature, elimination of distractions.
- *Arrange quiet activity prior to bedtime.* Reading or listening to soothing music or environmental sounds may encourage sleep.
- *Avoid sleeping medications.* If the client is unable to sleep, advise her to get up and read or watch television, then try again in thirty to sixty minutes. Learning relaxation techniques, such as slow breathing from the diaphragm or playing mental games, and using them at bedtime may be beneficial. By setting aside a time to review concerns and activities of the day and coming up with solutions to problems before going to bed, the client may succeed in separating worries from the act of going to bed. (The bed should not be used as an office.) Taking warm baths, drinking milk (but not too much), and eating light (nonsugar) snacks before bedtime may also be helpful.
- *Limit food intake.* Heavy meals interfere with sleep; light snacks closer to bedtime are better.

- *Herbal remedies:* Valerian root has sedative-hypnotic qualities shown to improve sleep quality and the time it takes to fall asleep (Jellin, 2002). Short-term use is recommended. Effects may take several days to weeks before relief. Ingestion as a tea, tablet, or capsule about sixty minutes before bedtime is suggested. Warn clients of the unpleasant odor.

FOLLOW-UP

The client may require referral to a sleep disorder program.

HORMONE REPLACEMENT THERAPY (HRT): SPECIFIC INFORMATION

See the aforementioned section on hormone replacement therapy for a background on the most recent research findings. The discussions in the subsequent section on HRT provide information to help the clinician with decisions about use. Despite the concerns raised by the WHI study results, women have the option, unless medically contraindicated, of hormone replacement therapy (HRT) (estrogen and progestin therapy) during the perimenopause and after. The concerns related to an increased risk of endometrial cancer, which peaked during the 1970s, have been tempered by the realization that the addition of a progestin to estrogen replacement therapy (ERT) (unopposed estrogen) offers significant protection against progressive hyperplasia. This benefit of the progestin, however, must be weighed against its possible potential negative effects, such as symptoms similar to premenstrual syndrome (PMS), attenuation of HDL-cholesterol, or breast pathology. Thus, the decision to use HRT must be made by the informed client. As mentioned earlier, data from the WHI study indicated that HRT (one regimen only) increased the risk of cardiovascular events, stroke, and pulmonary embolus in healthy postmenopausal women. The HERS trial found that postmenopausal women taking 0.625 mg of estrogen and 2.5 mg of medroxyprogesterone acetate had an increased risk for coronary events in the first year by nearly 50 percent and, overall, no reduction in their rate of CHD events (Hulley et al., 1998). Herrington et al. (2000) found no cardiovascular benefit in the effect of estrogen alone or estrogen plus MPA on the progression of coronary atherosclerosis in women with coronary disease. On the other hand, Hodis et al. (2001) reported from the Estrogen in

Prevention of Atherosclerosis Trial (EPAT) that healthy women taking oral ERT (17-beta estradiol) had a slower rate of progression of subclinical atherosclerosis than women taking a placebo, and Grodstein, Manson, Colditz et al. (2000) found that the risk for coronary events was lower among HRT users without previous heart disease, though the risk of stroke was increased. An increased risk of VTE was associated with HRT use in the HERS trial (Grady et al., 2000). Viscoli et al. (2001) advised that estrogen therapy should not be prescribed to prevent cardiovascular disease after a stroke or ischemic attack because it increased the risk of fatal stroke in their randomized, controlled study of postmenopausal stroke patients. Rodriguez et al. (2001) found that all women in their study who used ERT had an overall reduction in CVD mortality by 30 percent, but thin women (BMI < 22 kg/m^2) had the most reduced risk, more than 50 percent.

CLIENT EDUCATION AND COUNSELING

The health care provider must provide the client with accurate, current information about the probable benefits and possible adverse effects of HRT. ACOG recommended (before the WHI results were announced) that HRT is one treatment to consider for vasomotor symptoms relief, atrophy of the genitourinary tract, reduction of osteoporosis risk, and potentially, cardiovascular disease (ACOG Committee on Gynecologic Practice, 2002). However, the new data indicate that HRT (CEE and MPA at dosages in the WHI study) should not be used for CVD prevention (Writing Group, 2002). The following factors have consistently demonstrated association with therapy adherence: client education, patient involvement in decision making and treatment monitoring, simplification of the treatment regimen, and reduction of side effects caused by medications (Jacobs Institute of Women's Health, 2000; Vastag, 2002). Generally, the following areas are included in discussion with the client.

Signs and Symptoms of Hypoestrogenism

Estrogen taken orally, transdermally, or vaginally is effective in relieving vasomotor and urogenital symptoms (dyspareunia, dysuria, and urinary tract infections). Brown et al. (2001), from the HERS research group, found no reduction in frequency of UTIs with HRT use, but the study population consisted of women with heart disease, which may have affected results. However, the Hormones and Urogenital Therapy Committee in Britain

concluded from a meta-analysis of studies that ERT was effective as a treatment for genitourinary atrophy (Cardozo et al., 1998) and that estrogen as beneficial in preventing recurrent UTIs in postmenopausal women (Cardozo et al., 2001). The dosage is individualized for relief of symptoms.

Osteoporosis. Bone loss begins in the third or fourth decade of a woman's life, and accelerates rapidly because of estrogen deficiency in the first postmenopausal decade. HRT helps prevent bone loss, but it must be taken continuously to preserve bone mass (Greendale, Espeland, Slone, Marcus, Barrett-Connor, for the PEPI Safety Follow-up Study [PSFS] Investigators, 2002). Because of HRT's serious side-effect profile, women are usually better off taking bisphosponates (alendronate and risedronate) or a selective estrogen receptor modulator (SERM) (tamoxifen and raloxifene) (Vastag, 2002). (Osteoporosis is discussed more fully later in this chapter.)

Endometrial Cancer. Both continuous and cyclic regimens of progestins prevent estrogen induced endometrial hyperplasia. The addition of a progestin, recommended for the client who still has a uterus, does not detract from the favorable estrogen effects on bone density, or most other hypo-estrogen complaints. Women should be told that any prolonged bleeding or any staining or bleeding after months or years of no bleeding warrants seeing the provider to rule out cancer.

Lipid Changes. Although estrogen alone positively impacts lipid fractions by lowering LDL and raising HDL, conflicting studies exist on the impact of estrogen-progestin combination on the lipid profile. Progestins, especially MPA, attentuate the HDL cholesterol-elevating properties of estrogens (The Writing Group, 1995). Because HRT is usually given in combination with progestin, the data concerning the cardioprotective effects are important. In several long-term studies, lowering of LDL and raising HDL cholesterol levels did not decrease cardio-vascular events (Herrington et al., 2000; Hulley et al., 1998).

Breast Cancer. Study results are mixed on the relationship of postmenopausal hormone therapy on breast cancer. Although approximately 55 observational studies have been done between 1994 and 1996, 90 percent did not demonstrate an increased risk of breast cancer (AACE, 1999). However, a small, but significant, increase in breast cancer is probably associated with long-term hormone therapy, whether estrogen alone or estrogen plus progestin (Chen, Weiss, Newcomb, Barlow, &

White, 2002). The health care provider and individual woman should weigh the benefits versus the potential side or adverse effects (ACOG, 2002).

Blood Pressure. In the PEPI trial, no significant effects on blood pressure were noted with either estrogen alone or in combination with a progestin.

Stroke. The WHI study supported the results of the study by Grodstein et al. (2000) that taking estrogen with progestin increases the risk of stroke. Grodstein's study also found that taking estrogen alone increased the stroke risk.

Cardiovascular Disease. The WHI HRT study results (Writing Group, 2002) significantly countered the many observational studies that implied that HRT reduced CHD risk (Grodstein et al., 1996; Stampfer et al., 1991). The PEPI trial in 1995 indicated some beneficial effects from HRT use on arterial wall smooth muscle, blood flow, platelet aggregation, and blood pressure (The Writing Group, 1995). However, results of the HERS and Estrogen Replacement and Atherosclerosis (ERA) randomized clinical trials failed to show a beneficial effect of ERT on survival for women with established CVD (Herrington et al., 2000; Hulley et al., 1998). These data, plus a meta-analysis of twenty-two trials, led the American Heart Association to not recommend ERT for secondary prevention of CVD or for primary prevention, even before the WHI study results were available (Mosca, Collins, Herrington, et al., 2001). The overall impact of ERT on cardiovascular health is complex. The ongoing randomized clinical trial with ERT alone from the WHI may resolve other important issues, but results will not be available until 2005. Cholesterol-lowering drugs such as statins, as well as low-dose aspirin (100 mg), have been shown to be effective in reducing overall morbidity and mortality in women with CVD (Brown, Brockenbrough, Zhao, et al., 1998; Collaborative Group of the Primary Prevention Project, 2001). ERT did not have an effect on the progression of atherosclerosis in women who were being treated with lipid-lowering drugs in the EPAT research (Hodis et al., 2001). Efforts to prevent or slow the progression of cardiovascular disease in women should focus on the woman's total cardiovascular risk profile and include exercise, weight control, healthy diet, BP control, diabetes prevention, and smoking cessation.

Gallbladder Disease. Both observational and randomized trials have now indicated that ERT and HRT increase the chances for gallstones and risk of biliary tract surgery in postmenopausal women (Hulley et al., 2002; Simon,

Hunninghake, Agarwal, et al., 2001; Uhler, Marks, & Judd, 2000). The primary cause of gallstones in women is obesity; cholesterol gallstones occur when cholesterol in the bile exceeds the normal range, and precipitates form stones. In women who are not obese, gallstones are caused by a reduced rate of production of bile salts and other substances. In evaluating each client, family history, current risk factors, and the need for preventive health measures are assessed.

Mood and Sleep. Many women report improved overall psychological well-being while taking estrogen, although studies are inconclusive (Jacobs Institute of Women's Health, 2000). However, Rexrode and Manson (2002) found that HRT offered improvement in mood and depression symptoms in postmenopausal women with hot flashes but offered no mental health benefits that were significant in women without hot flashes. In fact, the latter group reported a decline in physical activity and energy that was more rapid than in the placebo group. Bixler et al. (2001) found that HRT use in postmenopausal women was associated with a significantly lower risk of sleep apnea.

Venous Thromboembolism. The risk for DVT and PE is increased significantly in postmenopausal women taking oral estrogen or estrogen plus progestin without other risk factors for venous thromboembolism being present (Grady et al., 2000; Hulley et al., 2002; Writing Group, 2002).

Glucose Tolerance. Kaplan et al. (1998) found that the use of estrogen and MPA was associated with a decrease in the risk of developing diabetes, better glucose control, and a decreased risk of MI in women with diabetes. However, with the current findings from WHI related to CHD, stroke, and HRT use, consultation with a specialist and careful consideration of HRT use is advised for women with diabetes.

Bleeding Patterns. When a woman experiences irregular periods during the transition to menopause, the low-dose estrogen patch or birth control pill is recommended (Finkel, Cohen, & Mahoney, 2001). Therapy with cyclic progestin with an estrogen produces menstrual-like vaginal bleeding and spotting in many women. For some, this is an unacceptable side effect. Continuous combined regimens of estrogen and progestin reduce the incidence of unwanted bleeding.

Alzheimer's Disease. ERT or HRT use by postmenopausal women did not result in a reduced risk of developing Alzheimer's disease (Seshadri et al., 2001). One study did find that healthy postmenopausal women taking HRT had improved verbal and visual memory and ability to concentrate (Resnick & Maki, 2001). A large ancillary study to the WHI is underway to examine cognitive aging and HRT and SERMs. Whether the HRT arm of the study will be ended is not known at this writing.

Ovarian Cancer. Lacey et al. (2002) found a significant risk of ovarian cancer associated with estrogen-only use, especially if use was for ten or more years. Short-term HRT use was not associated with an increased risk, though the investigators urged further long-term studies of HRT use to assess effects on the ovary. See the aforementioned information.

Other. The risk of *obstructive sleep apnea* equals that of premenopausal women and is significantly lower in postmenopausal women who use HRT than in those who do not (Bixler et al., 2001). The risk of *dry eye syndrome* is significantly increased with the use of ERT or HRT (Schaumberg, Buring, Sullivan, & Dana, 2001).

REQUIRED ASSESSMENT BEFORE INITIATING HRT

Take a complete client history. Special emphasis is placed upon a personal history of heart disease, stroke, hypertension, diabetes, breast or reproductive system cancer, biliary disease, liver disease, tendency to have blood clots, other significant conditions, and symptoms of vasomotor dysfunction as well as any family history of osteoporosis, heart disease, hypertension, stroke, diabetes, clotting disorders, colon cancer, breast cancer, or other major disease. Personal characteristics that put the woman at risk for a condition that could be impacted by HRT or ERT would be important, such as a history of smoking or drinking alcohol. A complete physical examination is indicated. Note signs of hypoestrogenism in the presence or absence of menses. Note any abnormalities that would contraindicate hormone replacement use.

Diagnostic Tests and Methods

Complete evaluation per midlife and late life protocol includes determination of baseline values for common tests. The basic testing/evaluations done initially include cholesterol and lipid profile, urinalysis, complete blood count, thyrotropin stimulating hormone level, blood chemistry profile, a screen for colorectal cancer, cervical screening, and mammogram. Time intervals for testing are provided in the subsequent section on Women's Midlife and Late Life Health Care Program.

- Serum FSH level may be indicated, but a one-year period of amenorrhea is also diagnostic of ovarian failure.

- Bone density evaluation (DEKASCAN) is advised for all women with risk factors for osteoperosis. All women over 65 years of age, regardless of risk factors, should have a baseline DEXA. See Chapter 4 for further information. May be indicated if the reason for initiating therapy is to prevent osteoporosis.
- Endometrial biopsy or pelvic ultrasonography is indicated if dysfunctional bleeding is present.
- A menstrual diary and an accurate record of other bleeding episodes over several months may provide insights for diagnosis and treatment. The diary may also be helpful after HRT is begun.

Ovarian/pelvic ultrasound is indicated if there is a suspected enlarged ovary or pelvic mass, or if there is a family history of ovarian cancer.

TREATMENT CONSIDERATIONS

Hormone dosages, preparations, and schedules are individualized according to symptoms and client history and choice. In general, there are three protocols for administering hormone therapy: (1) estrogen only, (2) estrogen with addition of cyclic progestins, and (3) continuous estrogen with the addition of continuous progestins. Table 15–2 lists some of the more widely used preparations of estrogen, progestin, and testosterone and their dosages.

Absolute Contraindications to Estrogen Use

- Known or suspected cancer of the breast (undiagnosed breast mass)
- Known or suspected estrogen dependent neoplasia
- History of uterine or ovarian cancer
- History of coronary heart disease or stroke
- History of biliary tract disorder
- Undiagnosed, abnormal genital bleeding
- History of or active thrombophlebitis or thromboembolic disorders (A family history of thrombotic disease is a contraindication according to some experts)
- Pregnancy
- Migraine headaches and hypertension may be worsened

Absolute Contraindications to Progestin Use

- Active thrombophlebitis or thromboembolic disorders
- Liver dysfunction or disease
- Known or suspected cancer of the breast
- Undiagnosed abnormal vaginal bleeding
- Pregnancy

TABLE 15–2. Hormone Replacement Regimens

Cyclic Treatment Regimens (dose in mg)	
Estrogens	
Conjugated estrogen (Premarin)	0.3, 0.625, 0.9, 1.25, 2.5
Estropipate (Ogen, Ortho-Est)	0.625, 1.25, 2.5, 5.0
Micronized estradiol (Estrace)	0.5, 1.0, 2.0
Esterified estrogens (Estratab, Menest)	0.3, 0.625, 1.25, 2.5
Progestins	
Medroxyprogesterone acetate (MPA) (Amen, Cycrin, Provera)	2.5, 5.0, 10.0
Norethindrone	2.5, 5.0
Norethindrone acetate (Aygestin)	5.0, 10.0

Continuous Treatment Regimens (estrogen and progestin daily; dose in mg)	
Estrogens	
Conjugated estrogens	0.625
Estropipate	0.625
Miconized estradiol	1.0
Progestins	
Medroxyprogesterone acetate	2.5, 5.0
Norethindrone	0.35
Norethindrone acetate	1.0
Micronized progesterone (Prometrium)	100, 200

Combination Therapy (dose in mg)

Premphase
  Conjugated estrogens 0.625 for 14 days; conjugated estrogens 0.625 and MPA 5 for 14 days.

Prempro
  Conjugated estrogens 0.625 and MPA 2.5
  Conjugated estrogens 0.625 and MPA 5.0

Ortho-Prefest
  Estradiol 1.0 and estradiol 1.0 mg and norgestimate 0.09 in an alternating sequence of 3 tablets each

FemHRT 1/5
  Ethinyl estradiol 5 mcg and norethindrone acetate 1.0

Activella
  Estradiol 1.0 and norethindrone acetate 0.5

Estrogen and Testosterone Daily Regimens (dose in mg)

Estratest
  Esterified estrogens 1.25 and methyltestosterone 2.5
Estratest HS
  Esterified estrogens 0.625 and methyltestosterone 1.25
  Conjugated estrogen (Premarin) 0.625 and methyltestosterone 5
  Conjugated estrogen (Premarin) 1.25 and methyltesterone 10

Transdermal Estradiol (dose in mg/day)	
Alora	0.05, 0.075, 0.1 twice weekly
Climara	0.025, 0.05, 0.075, 0.1 once weekly
Estraderm	0.05, 0.1 twice weekly
Vivelle	0.0375, 0.05, 0.075, 0.1 twice weekly
Esclim	0.025, 0.0375, 0.05, 0.075, 0.1 twice weekly
Combipatch	
Estradiol 0.05 and norethindrone acetate 0.14 twice weekly	
Estradiol 0.05 and norethindrone acetate 0.25 twice weekly	

Vaginal Estrogen Creams and Tablets (daily, cyclically, or as directed)	
Estradiol (Vagifem)	25 mcg tablets
Estradiol (Estrace)	0.01 mg/g
Estropipate (Ogen)	1.5 mg/g
Conjugated estrogen (Premarin)	0.625 mg/g

Hormone Vaginal Ring	
Estrogen ring (Estring)	7.5 mcg released per 24 hours

FOLLOW-UP EVALUATION

Follow-up assessment on an annual basis for all clients on HRT should include the following: interim history, complete medical examination, including breast and pelvic examinations, mammography, and Papanicolaou smear, if indicated. Endometrial evaluation is indicated for clients on ERT without progestin, and those with prolonged bleeding (> 10 days), or persistent, irregular bleeding. Office-based endometrial biopsy and pelvic ultrasound are the standard methods of evaluation.

POSTMENOPAUSAL HORMONE REPLACEMENT THERAPY

Hormone replacement therapy (estrogen, progestin, and/or testosterone) is given orally, transdermally, and vaginally. Oral estrogens include natural, conjugated, and synthetic estrogens. Natural estrogens, such as micronized estradiol (Estrace) and estropipate (Ogen), are converted in the liver to estrone, which becomes the primary circulating estrogen. Oral estrogens all have a reduction in bioavailability because of the first-pass effect through the liver and less potency than transdermal delivery because they have to pass through the gastrointestinal tract. For osteoporosis, oral estrogen is effective for prevention and inhibition of bone loss with doses 0.5 mg to 0.75 mg of 17-beta estradiol, 0.625 mg of conjugated estrogen daily, and epidermal doses of 0.025 to 0.1 mg (AACE, 2001; NAMS, 2002). Oral esterified estrogen 0.3 mg/day without progestin for 2 years caused positive bone changes and no endometrial hyperplasia (NAMS, 2002). With any hormone therapy for osteoporosis prevention, 1200 mg of elemental calcium per day is needed and 400 to 600 IU of vitamin D. The most commonly used progestin has been MPA for many years, but the WHI data suggest other progestogens such as norethindrone, norethindrone acetate, or natural, micronized progestrone. The most commonly used progestin is medroxyprogesterone acetate (MPA) (Provera). Norethindrone is also frequently used. The most commonly used testosterone is methyltestosterone. Side effects of the hormonal components are estrogen or progestin or androgen related. Estrogen-related side effects include breast tenderness, nausea (usually subsides in three to six months), and headaches. Progestin-related side effects include nausea, acne, headaches, and PMS-like symptoms, such as irritability. Androgen-related side effects include acne and hirsutism. Lipid levels should be followed.

ORAL REGIMENS

Cyclic Estrogen/Progestin Therapy. Start with a low dose estrogen (see examples in Table 15–2). If hypoestrogenic symptoms persist after thirty days, increase the daily dosage incrementally. If the client has an intact uterus, add a progestin or progesterone on days 1 to 12 or days 13 to 25 of the month. A dosage equivalent to 5 to 10 mg of MPA is advised. A progestin or progesterone may also be given at two-, three-, or six-month intervals to aid in preventing endometrial hyperplasia (AACE, 1999). Prolonged withdrawal bleeding more than ten days may indicate the need for endometrial biopsy or ultrasound. If bleeding begins before day 10 of the progestin administration and is cyclic, increase dosage or duration of progestin to see if this regulates the bleeding pattern.

Advantages. Cyclic therapy is effective for relief of hypoestrogenic symptoms and prevention of osteoporosis in recently menopausal women (AACE, 2001).

Disadvantages. Withdrawal bleeding after the progestin is stopped may lead to decreased client compliance; however, dosing every three months may be less problematic (10 mg per day for twelve to fourteen days).

Continuous Daily Estrogen/Progestin Therapy. Start with a low-dose estrogen once daily. If the uterus is intact, a continuous progestin should be added, the equivalent of MPA 2.5 daily. If hypoestrogenic symptoms persist after thirty days, increase the estrogen incrementally. If the estrogen is increased, the progestin may need to be increased, such as MPA 2.5 mg daily to 5 mg daily.

Advantages. No cyclic bleeding occurs with the continuous therapy, and therapy is effective in preventing osteoporosis.

Disadvantages. The client may have acyclic bleeding during the first few months; this usually resolves by six months. The client may find the unpredictable bleeding pattern unacceptable; if so, switch to the cyclic option, and convert to the continuous method some years later. Endometrial evaluation by biopsy or ultrasound is required for prolonged and persistent bleeding, or if bleeding occurs once amenorrhea is established. Even slight staining calls for evaluation.

The most exhaustive data on efficacy have been collected on Premarin, but Table 15–2 also lists substitutes.

Transdermal Estrogen

Transdermal estradiol (Estraderm, Climara) delivers human 17-beta estradiol directly to the bloodstream, bypassing the liver. Patches are available in a variety of dosages: 0.025 mcg/d; 0.05 mcg/d; 0.075 mcg/d; and 0.1 mcg/d. If hypoestrogenic symptoms persist after thirty days, increase the dosage. If uterus is intact, add a progestin equivalent to MPA 10 mg/d for 12 days per month or add MPA 2.5 mg continuously as presented previously in the continuous daily estrogen/progestin therapy discussion.

Advantages. Among the advantages of transdermal estrogen are prompt relief of hypoestrogenic symptoms and delivery of natural 17-beta estradiol directly to target cells. Continuous levels are delivered without fluctuation. Improved compliance is noted among women who do not desire oral medication. Short-term data suggest that the patch (Climara 0.025 mg weekly, Vivelle 0.025 mg twice weekly, Estraderm 0.05 mg weekly) is equal to oral estrogens in the prevention of osteoporosis (AACE, 2001). The patch does not significantly affect clotting factors or any other liver functions, as if taken orally (Finkel et al., 2001).

Disadvantages. Skin irritation from the patch may occur; however, preventive measures can be taken.

- Make sure that the application area is clean, dry, and free of oil, powder, perfume, and soap.
- Leave the system open to the air (with protective covering off) for ten to fifteen minutes prior to application to allow some of the alcohol to evaporate.
- Rotate the patch with each change. Apply to upper outer quadrants of buttocks (less sensitive). Do not use on breasts.

Transdermal absorption of estrogen induces increased synthesis of triglycerides (AACE, 1999).

Transvaginal Estrogen

Vaginal application of estrogen is absorbed and enters the systemic circulation, though at lower blood levels of estrogen. It exerts a potent local effect, however, enhancing revascularization of the vaginal epithelium. Vaginal administration of estrogen is indicated for the treatment of atrophic vaginitis. One applicator of estrogen cream inserted twice weekly usually is adequate to relieve symptoms. Most of the side effects seen with oral estrogen can be experienced with vaginal estrogen systems, such as the ring or tablets, but usually are mild or not reported.

Testosterone Therapy

Esterified estrogens with methyltestosterone (Estratest tablets) or conjugated estrogens (Premarin) with methyltestosterone may be used when a client's primary complaint is loss of libido, in the absence of other medical and psychosocial factors. (Progestins must be added if the client has an intact uterus.)

Advantages. Improvement in libido with some women; prevention of osteoporosis, relief of hypoestrogenic symptoms.

Disadvantages. Androgenic side effects: acne, hirsutism, alopecia, clitoromegaly. Androgens may lower HDL levels. Side effects are infrequent and dose-related and usually resolve after discontinuation of therapy.

PERIMENOPAUSAL HORMONE REPLACEMENT THERAPY

Clients who are still ovulating may need contraception as they approach menopause, yet have indications for supplemental estrogen therapy as their estrogen level declines. The points to consider in continuing or initiating low dose contraceptive therapy are many.

- Estrogen may be necessary as the aging ovary begins to secrete lower levels of estradiol several years prior to the last menstrual period. The fluctuations in the estrogen levels during perimenopause are great. The client may have some beginning signs or symptoms of deficiency but continue to have regular menses. *Reference point:* Postmenopausal estrogens are about 1 percent as potent as ethinyl estradiol. Thus, 10 mcg of ethinyl estradiol (EE) is about equivalent to 1 mg of conjugated estrogen. It is necessary to change from oral contraception to postmenopausal hormone therapy because even with the lowest estrogen dose oral contraceptive available, the estrogen dose is fourfold greater than the standard postmenopausal dose, and with increasing age, the dose-related risks with estrogen become significant.
- Control of irregular or breakthrough bleeding may be required. The bleeding may occur because of inadequate production of luteal phase hormone or because of an estradiol peak without subsequent ovulation.
- HRT does not provide contraception. Elective abortion is highest among teenagers and second highest among women aged 40 years of age and older. 1.5

percent of elective abortions are in women over age 40 (CDC, 2000). Postmenopausal estrogens will not provide contraception, although they will ameliorate symptoms.

- No data suggest an increased risk of heart disease. Studies indicate no increased risk in women over age 40 using low-dose ethinyl estradiol (less than 35 mcg) oral contraceptives, provided they do not smoke (Hatcher & Guillebaud, 1998).
- Oral contraceptive (OC) users are at decreased risk to develop endometrial and ovarian cancer (Ness et al., 2000).
- Data from formal studies regarding the effect of OCs on cervical neoplasia lack consistency (Hatcher & Guillebaud, 1998). OC users are likely to be sexually active, often not using a barrier method, a risk factor for cervical cancer.
- Studies on the use of oral contraceptives do not demonstrate an increased risk of breast cancer, nor any protection against it (Collaborative Group on Hormonal Factors in Breast Cancer, 1996).
- The incidence of fibroids is 30 percent lower among OC users (Hatcher & Guillebaud, 1998).
- Pelvic inflammatory disease (PID) and ectopic pregnancy are less common among OC users (Hatcher & Guillebaud, 1998).

Therapy options to regulate anovulatory cycles for perimenopausal women include oral contraceptives containing less than 35 mcg of estrogen or low-dose progestational treatment. These may be used if no contraindications exist. Low-dose oral conjugated estrogen (0.3–0.625 mg Premarin) or an estrogen patch are options if contraception is not an issue. Progestin is added when the uterus is intact. Management includes annual screening exams—Pap smear, colorectal cancer screen, and FSH level evaluation. One suggested regimen is to begin annual FSH evaluation when the FSH level exceeds 40 mIU/mL on days 5 to 7 of a pill-free week, switch the client to ERT/HRT. (See subsequent section on the Women's Midlife and Late Life Health Care Program for other tests/diagnostic methods that may be indicated based on age and assessment findings.) Allay the fears of older clients about the increased risks of heart disease and stroke. Communicate to the client the contraindications to OC use: smoking, hypertension, diabetes, thromboembolic disorders, impaired liver function, and known or suspected estrogen dependent neoplasm (see Chapter 9).

OPTIONS AFTER HYSTERECTOMY/OOPHORECTOMY

Posthysterectomy (without Oophorectomy)

Hysterectomy promotes earlier ovarian failure; the surgery itself may compromise blood supply to the ovaries, and the uterus contributes hormonally to ovarian function (Grodstein & Stampfer, 1996). Monitor the client for hypoestrogenic symptoms. Measure the FSH level every one to two years.

Postoophorectomy

An abrupt, drastic fall in estradiol occurs following oophorectomy (no gradual adaptation is possible, as with natural menopause). The symptoms are often severe, particularly hot flashes and intestinal symptoms. Surgical menopause is a predisposing factor to osteoporosis, and it is known that bone is maintained by ERT. ERT is generally begun immediately postoperatively; high doses, such as 1.25 mg to 2.5 mcg per day of Premarin, may be needed for up to a year postoperatively (AACE, 1999).

INITIATING HRT AND FOLLOW-UP

Provide the client with written and oral information about HRT. Explain the risks and benefits as they apply to the client's own situation. Request that the client keep a menstrual calendar; educate her concerning what constitutes abnormal bleeding. Advise the client to telephone the health care provider immediately if she experiences any of the following:

- Unexpected bleeding.
- Abdominal pains, bloating.
- An increase in headaches.
- Symptoms not relieved or that increase.
- Visual disturbances.
- Shortness of breath or chest pain.
- Calf pain.

Obtaining written consent for hormone therapy from the client is optional but advised because consumers continue to be confused about ERT and HRT and their risks and benefits.

Adequate follow-up is critical in maximizing compliance and to evaluate the response to medications and side effects. A reasonable approach is to call the client in a month, and schedule a two- to three-month visit after therapy is initiated. Clients should be encouraged to call with questions or concerns at any time. Stress to the client that even if she experiences no problems, annual exams, routine tests, and communication are important.

CHANGING DOSAGE OR DISCONTINUATION OF THERAPY

Adjustment of ERT dosage may be needed to provide symptom relief. The dosage is increased gradually to find the minimum level needed for symptom relief. After six months of adequate relief at a dosage higher than 0.625 mg Premarin or equivalent, gradually decrease doses to 0.625 mg (see Table 15–2). (*Example:* 1.25 mg for 3 weeks, 0.9 mg for 1 week; if tolerated, 1.25 mg for 2 weeks, 0.9 mg for 1 week; 1.25 mg for 1 week, 0.9 mg for 1 week; stabilize at 0.9 mg for 2 weeks, then 0.9 mg for 3 weeks, 6.25 mg for 1 week, and so on.) The client may need and benefit from testosterone therapy as well.

Hormone replacement therapy (HRT) should be discontinued gradually. (*Example:* 7 tablets per week for 1 month; 6 tablets per week for 1 month; 5 tablets per week for 1 month, and so on until zero.)

WOMEN'S MIDLIFE AND LATE LIFE HEALTH CARE PROGRAM

Comprehensive health care, which includes traditional medical care, as well as health promotion and disease prevention, should be individualized for each client. The plan of care focuses on the existing health problems and projected long-range health outcomes, and each client's preferences concerning the risks and benefits of preventive measures. Emphasis is on health education, appropriate screenings for early detection of disease, and discussion of positive health behaviors. A holistic health care program includes education and appropriate evaluation and testing.

EDUCATION

Many women lack knowledge of the emotional, sexual, social, and medical aspects of the perimenopausal and postmenopausal phases of life; hence, client education must be comprehensive. Approximately half of all deaths occuring in the United States in 1990 may be attributed to factors such as tobacco, alcohol, and illicit drug use, diet and activity patterns, motor vehicles, and sexual behavior, and are potentially preventable by changes in personal health practices (USPSTF, 1996).

TABLE 15–3. Therapeutic Lifestyle Changes: Nutrient Composition of TLC Diet

Nutrient	Recommended Intake
Saturated fat	Less than 7% of total calories
Polyunsaturated fat	Up to 10% of total calories
Monounsaturated fat	Up to 20% of total calories
Total fat	25–35% of total calories
Carbohydrate	50–60% of total calories
Fiber	20–30 grams per day
Protein	Approximately 15% of total calories
Cholesterol	Less than 200 mg/day
Total calories (energy)	Balance energy intake and expenditure to maintain desirable body weight/prevent weight gain

Source: National Cholesterol Education Program (http://hin.nhlbi.nih.gov/ncep_slds/atpiii/slide45.htm)

Anatomy and Physiology

Explain the changes expected with the perimenopausal transition and postmenopausal period, including the most common signs and symptoms and usual nonmedical and medical methods of management.

Nutrition and Dental Health

Dietary excess and imbalance is associated with diseases such as breast and colon cancer, stroke, coronary heart disease, hypertension, and osteoporosis. Explain the dietary need to decrease fat, especially saturated fats (Table 15–3); increase complex carbohydrates and fiber; have a moderate protein intake; and increase dietary calcium or add a calcium supplement. Counsel clients to visit a dental care provider on a regular basis, floss daily, and brush their teeth daily with a fluoride containing toothpaste.

Exercise/Obesity

33.4 percent of adults aged 20 through 74 year were overweight (mean body mass index 26.3) according to the National Health Nutrition Examination Survey III (Kuczmarski, Flegal, Campbell, & Johnson, 2002). In a fourteen-year prospective study, middle-aged women with a body mass index greater than 23 but less than 25 had a 50 percent increase in risk of nonfatal or fatal CHD (Manson, Willett, Stampfer, Colditz, et al., 1995). Physical inactivity is also related to an increased risk of CHD. Research has shown a 50 percent lower risk of CHD in physically active women (American Heart Association, 1997). Encourage weightbearing, aerobic, flexibility, and joint mobility activities. Adults should be encouraged to increase activity gradually, with the goal of at least 30 minutes daily of physical activity of moderate intensity, (e.g., brisk walking, stair climbing); more strenuous activities such as slow jogging, cycling, field and court games, and swimming (AHA, 1997).

Smoking, Alcohol, and Drug Use

Communicate the need to stop all untoward substance use. Refer the client to a smoking cessation program, Alcoholics Anonymous, or drug treatment program as appropriate. Stress the need for caution with prescription drug use also (see Chapter 23 and Nonreproductive Health Concerns of Aging Women, end of Chapter 15).

Relaxation and Stress Reduction

Emphasize the need for awareness of one's stress level and the contributing factors. Promote the use of relaxation techniques and behavior modification, rather than alcohol or drugs.

Contraception

Give information about effective, safe birth control methods if the client desires protection during the transition before menopause (see Chapter 9).

Hormone Replacement Therapy

Tell the client about the risks, benefits, and side effects of HRT. Provide written information.

Sexuality

Discuss how the transition to menopause will affect sexuality, particularly the frequent vaginal changes and ways to counter them satisfactorily (e.g., regular sexual activity, lubrication, and Kegel's exercises). Assessing sexual function and counseling clients to prevent sexually transmitted diseases and HIV should be a routine part of the evaluation, regardless of age.

Accident Prevention

Counsel all clients to use auto safety belts, wear bicycle helmets, and refrain from driving while under the influence of alcohol or other drugs (see Accident Prevention, in Nonreproductive Health Concerns of Aging Women).

PERIODIC EVALUATION AND TESTING

Preventive services for the early detection of disease have been associated with reductions in morbidity and mortality. Periodic health evaluation and selected screening tests are recommended based on effectiveness of the specific test, age, and other individual risk factors of the client. A comprehensive health history that specifically addresses midlife or late life issues is invaluable. Domestic violence and abuse screening should be included. Screening for risk in all areas is available. A complete physical examination, also necessary, includes height, weight, integumentary, oral cavity, thyroid, cardiovascular and thoracic systems, breasts (including instruction in breast self-examination [BSE]), abdomen, extremities, and pelvic and rectal components.

Diagnostic Tests, Methods, and Screening

See also Chapter 4.

Cholesterol and/or Lipid Profile. (See Chapter 4 for general screening guidelines.) If no prior testing has been done, obtain a fasting lipoprotein profile (total cholesterol, LDL cholesterol, HDL cholesterol, and triglyceride) when HRT is initiated. If normal, repeat every five years to age 64, and then every three to five years thereafter. If cholesterol is 200 mg/dL or above, or HDL is < 40 mg/dL, a follow-up lipoprotein profile is needed for appropriate management based on LDL. Recent guidelines identify three categories of major risk factors to modify the goals and treatment of LDL-lowering therapy (National Cholesterol Education Program, 2001). For details, see http://www.nhlbi.nih.gov/guidelines/cholesterol/index.htm.

Dipstick Urinalysis. For preventive care perform yearly, as appropriate in all women.

Hemoglobin Levels. Routine screening for anemia is not recommended (Institute for Clinical Systems Improvement, 2001). For women with a history of excessive menstrual flow, and for women 65 years of age or older, hemoglobin levels should be measured as part of routine preventive care.

Blood Chemistry Profile. All major U.S. authorities do not recommend multiple blood chemistry screens for asymptomatic normal risk individuals (Institute for Clinical Systems Improvement, 2001).

Colorectal Cancer Screening. For women at normal risk, begin annual screening with a digital rectal exam, at age

40, annual fecal occult blood testing beginning at age 50, and colonoscopy every ten years beginning at age 50. Sigmoidoscopy every five years is another screening option, though the colonoscopy is considered the gold standard (American Cancer Society [ACS], 2001). For women at an increased risk of colorectal cancer, more frequent screening is recommended. What constitutes increased risk and the frequency of screening differs among authorities.

Cervical Screening. Annual Pap smear and pelvic exam are recommended for all women age 18 and older. If a client has three or more consecutive normal Pap smears, then the test may be done less frequently, at the discretion of the client and health care professional (ACS, 2001). In women aged 70 and older with at least two negative Pap smears, regular pelvic exams and Pap smears are probably not indicated (AGS, 2000b). Annual pelvic exams are warranted however, to evaluate other areas, for example, the ovaries. If the client has had a hysterectomy for benign disease, then repeat the Pap smear one year after surgery; if negative, then every two years. If the cervix was not removed, or if the client has ever had an abnormal Pap, then continue Pap smears as indicated.

Ovarian Cancer Screening. Bimanual pelvic examination is of unknown sensitivity in detecting ovarian cancer; small, early stage ovarian tumors are often not detected by palpation (ACS, 2001). Routine screening by transvaginal ultrasound or serum tumor markers is not recommended in asymptomatic women (ACS, 2001). There is insufficient evidence to conclude that women with hereditary cancer syndrome should undergo annual pelvic examinations, CA-125 measurements, and transvaginal ultrasound to screen for ovarian cancer (National Cancer Institute, 2002). However, improved survival has been shown with serum CA-125 and transvaginal ultrasonography, so more study is needed to assess use in reducing mortality (Alexander-Sefre, Menon, & Jacobs, 2002; Menon & Jacobs, 2000).

Endometrial Cancer Screening. Routine screening is neither cost effective nor warranted (ACS, 2001). A biopsy is indicated if abnormal uterine bleeding occurs.

Lung Cancer Screening. No suitable techniques are available, although some clinicians support annual chest x-rays for women 50 years and older who smoke more than a pack of cigarettes daily. All major U.S. authorities do not routinely recommend chest x-rays or sputum cytology for asymptomatic normal risk individuals (ACS, 2001). Advise the client to stop smoking, because of the in-

creased risks of breast disease, hypertension, osteoporosis, cervical cancer, early menopause, and lung cancer.

Breast Cancer Screening. Teaching and reinforcing BSE and encouraging an annual exam by a health care provider are important. A yearly mammogram and clinical breast examination by a health care professional and a monthly breast self examination are currently recommended for women age 40 and older (ACS, 2001). The American Geriatrics Society recommends that women over 65 years receive mammograms annually or biennially until at least 75 years of age, and biennially or every three years, with no upper age limit (AGS, 2000a). Mammography is not recommended in women with health conditions negatively affecting life expectancy such as terminal diagoses or advanced heart failure (AGS, 2000). Recommendations vary for women at increased risk of breast cancer (see Chapter 14).

Skin Cancer Screening. Skin cancer is the most common type of cancer in the United States and is virtually 100 percent curable if diagnosed and excised early (ACS, 2001). An examination should be performed yearly in women over 40 (ACS, 2001).

Cardiovascular Screening. All major U.S. authorities do not recommend routine screening electrocardiograms (ECGs) for asymptomatic, normal risk individuals (Institute for Clinical Systems Improvement, 2001). The risk of cardiovascular disease does increase with age, however, and the health professional may want to consider more regular ECG use in the later decades of a client's life.

Hearing Examinations. Hearing screening is not necessary for asymptomatic women under age 65, except for those exposed regularly to excessive noise, but women 65 years and older should be evaluated for hearing loss (Institute for Clinical Systems Improvement, 2001). An otoscopic exam and audiometric testing are practical methods to evaluate hearing loss.

Vision Screening. A comprehensive eye examination, including visual acuity and glaucoma screening, is recommended every three to five years (Institute for Clinical Systems Improvement, 2001).

Immunizations. Updated diphtheria and tetanus immunizations are needed every ten years. Annual influenza immunization beginning at age 50 and Pneumococcal vaccine every five years are recommended (Institute for Clinical System Improvement, 2001). Hepatitis B Virus (HBV) immunization is recommended for women ages 40 to 64 if not done previously and for ages 65 and over only in high-risk groups (Institute for Clinical System Improvement, 2001).

Bone Density Screening. Bone mineral density (BMD) measurements are currently recommended for all women with medical reasons for bone loss, such as steroid use for more than three months, poor lifetime calcium intake, hyperthyroidism, alcohol abuse, metastatic cancer, primary hyperparathyroidism, renal disease, multiple myeloma, leukemia, hepatic disease (Gordon & Speroff, 2002); for all women 65 years or older regardless of risk factors; and for younger postmenopausal women who have risk factors, including a history of non-traumatic fractures (AACE, 2001; NAMS, 2002) (see Osteoporosis). Bone density measurement is more reliable than clinical assessment, and may help the client and primary care provider make more informed decisions about the potential benefits and risks of therapies such as estrogen.

- Dual-energy x-ray absorptiometry (DEXA), or dual x-ray absorptiometry (DXA), is widely used in the clinical setting and is safe, accurate, and precise and recommended for diagnosis and monitoring of osteoporosis (AACE, 2001; NAMS, 2002). This measure is being used more frequently because it is less expensive and can be done rapidly.
- QCT densitometry—modified quantitative computerized tomography of the lumbar spine—calculates bone mass. This method is more costly and uses a higher dosage of radiation.
- Single photon absorptiometry (SPA) measures the density of cortical bone of the distal radius or calcaneus. SPA is accurate, less expensive, and predictive for future risk of nonspine fracture.

Diabetic Screening. Fasting plasma glucose level should be used to screen for diabetes. All women over the age of 45 should be screened every three years (American Diabetes Association, 2002) (see Chapter 21).

Endometrial Biopsy

- *With Hormone Replacement Therapy.* Routine screening for endometrial hyperplasia or cancer is not recommended for clients on HRT; however, if taking unopposed estrogen (ERT), endometrial biopsy or is recommended when clinically indicated. (See also DUB, which follows.)
- *With Dysfunctional Uterine Bleeding (DUB).* DUB is defined as any bleeding that occurs a year or more after a previous episode of perimenopausal bleeding (single episodes of spotting or blood tinged discharge are sig-

nificant), heavy or frequent bleeding episodes, or bleeding at inappropriate times with hormone replacement therapy (HRT), such as after six months of continuing combined therapy. Initially, the health are provider must rule out endometrial carcinoma; refer the client to a gynecologist for evaluation (see Chapter 8).

Blood Pressure Screening. Elevated blood pressure puts clients at risk for coronary artery disease, peripheral vascular disease, stroke, renal disease, and retinopathy. Blood pressure should be measured as part of the periodic evaluation, which should occur every three to five years or as appropriate (Institute for Clinical System Improvement, 2001).

Thyroid Dysfunction. Hypothyroidism and hyperthyroidism are more common in women, older adults, and clients with a family history of thyroid disease. Thyroid malignancy occurs twice as frequently in women as in men. Thyroid palpation should be part of the periodic evaluation, but screening for thyroid disease with thyroid stimulating hormone (TSH) levels is not recommended (Institute for Clinical System Improvement, 2001).

OSTEOPOROSIS

Osteoporosis is a condition characterized by low bone mass, deterioration of bone tissue leading to bone fragility, and consequent susceptibility to fracture. Bone mass peaks at age 30, and postmenopausal bone loss is most prominent during the first postmenopausal decade (AACE, 2001). The greatest loss occurs in the femoral neck and lumbar vertebrae comprised of trabecular bone, which is subject to future fracture. A long, silent, asymptomatic period (10 to 20 years postmenopause) is typical. Osteoporosis-related fractures commonly involve the proximal femur (hip), vertebral body, and distal forearm, of these sites, the proximal femur has the greatest effect on morbidity and mortality.

Osteoporosis and related skeletal fractures result in enormorous economic costs, considerable disability, and premature death. The perimenopausal and postmenopausal woman requires knowledge of the epidemiology, risk factors, screening tests, and treatment regimens for osteoporosis.

EPIDEMIOLOGY

Osteoporotic fractures in aging women are a major public health problem. In the United States, approximately 150,000 to 250,000 hip fractures occur annually in women over age 65, with 15 to 25 percent needing long-term home nursing care. Twelve percent to 20 percent of hip fracture victims will die within one year of fracture, and more than 50 percent of survivors will be incapacitated, many of them permanently (AACE, 2001). Estimates for vertebral fracture approach 650,000 cases per year, with a prevalence of 40 percent by age 80. There is good evidence that raloxifene and estrogen and two bisphosphonates (alendronate, risedronate) can reduce the rate of bone loss and improve bone mineral density in postmenopausal women. Greater benefit is achieved with current use, continued for three years, and therapy begun close to menopause; longer-term HRT use beyond three years does not lead to additional bone mineral density (BMD) gains (Greendale et al., 2002). Since slow bone loss resumes after these pharmocologic measures are discontinued, they may need to be taken indefinitely to provide maximal protection to age 75. ERT may be less likely to slow down bone loss or prevent fractures in women over 75 years (AACE, 2001). Women should be aware of the value of these agents in preventing osteoporosis to enhance long-term compliance.

SUBJECTIVE DATA

The client may report some of the risk factors listed in Table 15–4; these risk factors can help identify clients who are susceptible to fracture and to develop an osteoporosis prevention program, but fail to identify a substantial proportion of clients with low bone mass (AACE, 2001). The medical evaluation includes a family and a medical history. Medications or coexisting diseases that cause or aggravate bone loss need to be eliminated or appropriately treated.

TABLE 15–4. Risk Factors for Osteoporosis-Related Fractures

Advancing age

Prior low-trauma fracture as an adult

Low BMD

History of hip fracture in a first-degree relative

Smoking

Low body weight and weight loss

Increased likelihood of falling

Tallness

High bone turnover

Source: AACE. (2001) AACE 2001 Medical Clinical Guidelines for Practice for the Prevention and Management of Postmenopausal Osteoporosis. Endocrine Practice, 7(4), 294–312.

OBJECTIVE DATA

Physical Examination

A complete physical and gynecologic examination is indicated. Findings may include spinal injuries or other adverse effects such as loss of height and "dowager's hump" (curvature of the cervical and upper thoracic spine). Maintain a careful record of the client's height in centimeters, in order to detect any decrease.

Diagnostic Tests and Methods

Bone Mineral Density Measurements. (See also Bone Density Screening.) Currently, DXA, the preferred method for baseline and follow-up measurements, should be done for the following: (1) for risk assessment in perimenopausal or postmenopausal women who are concerned about osteoporosis and willing to accept interventions, (2) in women with x-ray findings that suggest osteoporosis, (3) in women beginning or receiving long-term glucocorticoid therapy, (4) for perimenopausal or postmenopausal women with asymptomatic hyperparathyroidism or other diseases or nutritional conditions associated with bone loss in whom evidence of skeletal loss would result in parathyroidectomy, (5) in women undergoing treatment for osteoporosis, as a tool for monitoring the therapeutic response, (6) for all women 40 years or older who have sustained a fracture, and (7) for all women beyond 65 years of age (AACE, 2001; NAMS, 2002).

Laboratory Tests. CBC, serum chemistry, urinary calcium excretion. Additional tests may be indicated if secondary causes for bone loss are suspected.

DIFFERENTIAL MEDICAL DIAGNOSES

Multiple myeloma, Cushing's syndrome, hyperparathyroidism, glucocorticoid use, thyrotoxicosis.

PLAN

Psychosocial Interventions

Discuss with the client the importance of preventing or inhibiting further bone loss during the perimenopausal and postmenopausal years. Stress diet, exercise, health, and medication regimens. Advise the client to eliminate or decrease her alcohol intake and eliminate smoking.

MEDICATION

Therapies approved by the FDA for osteoporosis prevention and treatment include estrogen (with or without MPA), raloxifene, alendronate, risedronate, and calcitonin. Calcium and vitamin D supplementation do not require FDA approval and are recommended. Sodium fluoride stimulates bone formation but has not been approved by the FDA for these indications.

Estrogen Replacement Therapy (ERT). Therapy may begin at the time of menopause or oophorectomy, although can be initiated any time after menopause. Evidence suggests that most women taking estrogen therapy for seven to ten years or longer have a 50 percent or greater reduction in the incidence of osteoporotic fractures (WHO, 1994). For the prevention and treatment of osteoporosis, continuous daily estrogen (oral or transdermal) is recommended. Again, appropriate precautions in using hormone therapy based on the personal history and characteristics of the woman are essential.

Selective Estrogen Receptor Modulators (SERMs). Raloxifene (Evista) is recommended for prevention and treatment of postmenopausal osteoporosis. It provides estrogen-benefits to bone without endometrial or breast adverse effects (NAMS, 2002). Raloxifene significantly increases BMD in the spine and hip with two years' use and reduces vertebra fracture risk. Women complain of hot flashes with use of raloxifene, and the risk of deep vein thrombosis is the same as for ERT/HRT.

Calcium. By itself, calcium does not significantly influence bone resorption (NAMS, 2001); however, adequate intake is necessary for a positive calcium balance. A negative balance pulls calcium stores from the bone. Calcium and vitamin D supplementation can be administered to most women for a lifetime.

- *Dietary calcium.* Optimal dietary calcium comes from dairy products and tofu (bean curd), derived from soy bean milk. Factors that interfere with absorption include being older than 35, taking aluminum-containing antacids, consuming caffeine, and a high protein diet. Generally, about 500 mg of calcium can be gained through the diet (see Table 15–5).
- *Calcium and Vitamin D supplements.* The recommended daily calcium intake for women 19 to 50 years of age is 1,000 mg per day 1,500 mg per day for all women older than 65 years (AACE, 2001).

TABLE 15–5. Calcium Content of Various Calcium-Rich Foods

Food	Serving Size	Calcium per Serving (mg)*
Dairy products:		
Milk[†]	1 cup	290–300
Swiss cheese	1 oz (slice)	250–270
Yogurt	1 cup	240–400
American cheese	1 oz (slice)	165–200
Ice cream or frozen dessert	1/2 cup	90–100
Cottage cheese	1/2 cup	80–100
Parmesan cheese	1Tb	70
Powdered nonfat milk	1 tsp	50
Other:		
Sardines in oil (with bones)	3 oz	370
Canned salmon (with bones)	3 oz	170–210
Broccoli	1 cup	160–180
Soybean curd (tofu)	4 oz	145–155
Turnip greens	1/2 cup, cooked	100–125
Kale	1/2 cup, cooked	90–100
Corn bread	2 1/2-inch square	80–90
Egg	1 medium	55
Calcium fortified food (bread, cereal, fruit juices)[‡]	1 serving	varies

*A simple formula for calculating dietary calcium assigns 300 mg for the dairy free diet, 300 mg for each serving of a dairy product (cup or slice), and 160 mg for each serving of calcium fortified food.

[†]All milks (skim, 1%, 2%, and whole) have the same calcium content.

[‡]Breads and cereals, unless fortified with calcium, are relatively low sources of calcium but still contribute substantially to calcium intake because these foods constitute such a large part of the diet.

Source: AACE (2001). 2001 Medical Guidelines for the Prevention and Management of Postmenopausal Osteoporosis. Endocrine Practice 7(4), 294–312.

Women 50 to 65 not using ERT need 1,500 mg/d. (NAMS, 2002). When dietary intake is insufficient, a supplement is indicated. Products with calcium carbonate, for example Tums, provide the most calcium for the money. To minimize gastrointestinal side effects and enhance absorption, clients should take calcium with meals and with a bedtime snack. Calcium supplementation is contraindicated in women who have a history of renal stones. Hypercalciuria is unusual at dosages of < 1.5 gm/day.

Bisphosphonates. These drugs inhibit osteoclast activity and decrease bone resorption (NAMS, 2002). Alendronate, risedronate, and etidronate are three such drugs, but etidronate is not approved in the United States for osteoporosis therapy. Alendronate increased spine and hip BMD significantly from baseline in early postmenopausal women treated for two to four years; it increased BMD 5 to 10 percent in the spine and hip in women with low BMD or osteoporosis (NAMS, 2002). Risedronate studies have shown similar increases, and both drugs have shown reduced risk of fractures of the vertebra and hip, though after age 80, risedronate did not lower the risk in women without confirmed osteoporosis. Risedronate is particularly useful with elderly women with diagnosed osteoporosis (McClung et al., 2001). With both drugs, the client should be instructed to take it in the morning at least least 30 minutes before the first food, beverage, or medication of the day, swallow whole with 6 to 8 oz. of water, and avoid recumbancy for at least 30 minutes after taking the dose. The drug should be stopped if symptoms of esophageal disease (e.g., heartburn, difficulty swallowing) develop.

Calcitonin. May be used alone or with hormone replacement therapy to decrease bone resorption. Calcitonin may produce an analgesic effect and is useful in the immediate postfracture phase. It is an alternative to ERT, raloxifene, and bisphosphonate therapy for postmenopausal women who cannot or will not take ERT or a bisphosphonate. The recommended dosage is 100 IU/day subcutaneously or 200 IU intranasally daily (NAMS, 2002).

Sodium fluoride. A study by Rubin et al. (2001) found that a sustained-release sodium fluoride oral medication decreased vertebral fracture risk in postmenopausal women with osteoporosis but did not show significant BMD changes. The 80 subjects were 65 years and older. Further study with fluoride is needed to learn if this is a viable treatment.

Parathyroid hormone. A new treatment under investigation is parathyroid hormone. Daily injections have been effective in postmenopausal women with prior vertebral fractures in reducing further fracture incidence.

Rortero. Under study is a therapy that may reduce osteoporosis through daily injections that build bone. As few as one to two injections a year may prove to be helpful.

Weightbearing Exercise

Weightbearing, muscle strengthening exercise stimulates new bone formation and maintains the mineral content of the bone in children and adolescents and may slow bone loss in older adults (AACE, 2001). For clients with established osteoporosis, referral to physical therapy can help prevent falls and develop a program for decreasing kyphotic posture and improving overall muscle strength and mobility.

FOLLOW-UP

Consultation with or referral to a gynecologic and/or orthopedic specialist or osteoporosis center is indicated for progressing disease.

Preventive measures in childbearing clients include adequate dietary or supplemental calcium, weightbearing exercise several times per week, and evaluation for estrogen deficiency during periods of amenorrhea longer than six months, particularly during adolescence.

HIRSUTISM/VIRILISM

Though this problem is not seen frequently in postmenopause, it is being addressed to help the provider in case the condition arises. Hirsutism (increased hair in unusual amounts and places) that develops after menopause is one sign of benign hyperandrogynism (the appearance of testosterone-stimulated characteristics). The signs include excess facial and abdominal hair of a coarse nature and oily skin or acne. Hirsutism often causes extreme distress in women. The more severe states of virilization (clitoromegaly, deepening of the voice, balding, and changes in body habitus) are rare and usually secondary to adrenal hyperplasia or androgen producing tumors (Speroff, Glass, & Kase, 1999).

EPIDEMIOLOGY

Androgens enter the blood from the adrenal glands, ovaries, and peripheral sites, such as the liver, spleen, and adipose tissue. After menopause, the level of androgens in the blood usually falls below half of that in childbearing women (Hacker & Moore, 1998). Benign rises in androstenedione and testosterone levels are caused by ovarian stromal hyperplasia that sometimes develops under the influence of high luteinizing hormone (LH) levels. Testosterone levels, however, decrease in all women between the third and fifth postmenopausal year. Hirsutism is usually associated with persistent anovulation. Estrogen-androgen combination therapy for treatment of menopausal women may produce masculinizing side effects. Side effects are usually dose dependent but can develop even with low-dose methyltestosterone.

SUBJECTIVE DATA

The client may report an increase in facial, areolar, abdominal, and chest hair, oily skin, and acne. An increase in libido may occur (Hacker & Moore, 1998).

OBJECTIVE DATA

During the physical examination, note any increase in facial, upper abdomen, chest, and upper back and shoulder hair. Virilization is suggestive by temporal scalp hair loss, deep voice, acne, increase in muscle mass, and clitoromegaly. On pelvic examination, palpate for the presence of bilaterally enlarged ovaries (ovaries should not be palpable in postmenopausal women).

Diagnostic tests include serum total testosterone level to rule out ovarian and adrenal tumors, and dehydroepiandrosterone sulfate (DHEA-S) level and 17-hydroxyprogesterone (17-OHP) to rule out adrenal tumor. If either serum testosterone or DHEA-S is elevated, refer the client immediately to a gynecologist to rule out an androgen-producing tumor. TSH and prolactin are advised for initial evaluation also (Gordon & Speroff, 2002).

DIFFERENTIAL MEDICAL DIAGNOSES

Ovarian or adrenal androgen-producing tumors, Cushing's syndrome, drugs such as anabolic steroids and androgenic progestogens, and polycystic ovary syndrome.

PLAN

Approaches to the management of hirsutism are based on the underlying pathophysiology. For the postmenopausal woman without pathology, reassure that the increased hair growth is not abnormal and that it may abate as testosterone levels decrease in a few years, and provide suggestions for its removal (e.g., electrolysis). Medications to suppress ovarian and adrenal production of androgen may be useful. Spironolactone (aldosterone antagonist) 25 mg q.i.d. *or* 50 mg b.i.d. may help to decrease androgen production and block the effect of testosterone on hair follicles. Cimetidine, generally used to treat ulcers and excess gastric acid, may also provide an antiandrogenic effect. For pathologic causes in younger or older women, the underlying problem must be determined before curative treatment may occur. Causes of hirsutism and virilization are complex and require evaluation by a specialist. For instance, hyperinsulinemia and hyperandrogenism are frequently associated, and elderly women may become hirsute from hyperinsulinemia, in which case a fasting glucose to insulin ratio is needed (Gordon & Speroff, 2002). With Cushing's syndrome, dexamethasone (corticosteroid) 1.0 mg q.h.s. has been used to suppress adrenal hyperfunction, but this drug can cause osteoporosis and suppression of the hypothalamic-pituitary-adrenal axis, so it should be used with caution. Confer with a gynecologist who specializes in endocrinology and consult a current pharmacotherapeutics reference before prescribing drugs to treat hirsutism.

Follow-Up

Immediate referral to a gynecologic specialist is required whenever androgen-producing tumors are suspected.

NONREPRODUCTIVE HEALTH CONCERNS OF AGING WOMEN

More women are taking a proactive role in health maintenance and the prevention of disease. Preventive health care is a major area that the health care provider must focus on with women, especially as they age. Menopause provides a unique opportunity for the provider to assist the woman in maintaining ongoing cost-effective health care that includes appropriate referrals if necessary. Many risk factors can be modified by adapting positive health measures, such as not smoking, eating a low fat, low cholesterol diet (Table 15–3), and exercising. The aging process, however, is affected by biologic, social, economic, and psychological influences. Assessment of all these factors is critical to the development of an effective health care strategy for older women. Certain areas pos-ing more serious problems for the aging woman that may negatively affect her health include the following.

HEALTH CARE INSURANCE AND INCOME

Older Americans spent 11 percent of their expenditures on health, as compared to 5 percent spent by all consumers (AOA, 2001). Women who have lost spouses through death, divorce, or separation are more likely to have only public health care coverage or no insurance. Making co-payments, payment for services not covered by Medicare, or payment of insurance deductible is often a hardship for elderly women. Medicare and Medicaid managed care plans are increasing in numbers to help meet the economic challenge of caring for older adults and controlling costs. Elderly women who live alone or who are of ethnic minority tend to be poorer than elderly men. Social Security benefits are the largest single source of income for elderly people. The median yearly income for older women in 2000 was $10,899 and was $19,168 for older men (AOA, 2001). Income disparities persist among various elderly subgroups: 8.9 percent of elderly whites, 22.3 percent of elderly African Americans, and 18.8 percent of elderly Hispanics were poor (AOA, 2001). White women are more likely to have private insurance than nonwhite women. Women are more likely to have health insurance than men are, except in the 45- to 64-year-old group. Out-of-pocket costs of health care, including medications, often increase with acute and chronic illness as the woman ages; and if a choice among rent, food, and medicine confronts the elderly woman, she may forgo her medication. More serious illness is a likely consequence. It is essential that the health care provider be aware of resources in her or his locale to use for referral that can aid the woman in maintaining her finances in health or illness. The Area Agency on Aging (AAA) is a good resource and available in every county in the United States.

SOCIAL SUPPORT

With a life expectancy of over 75 years, most U.S. women will live half of their adult lives after their last child has left home. Nearly one-quarter of women over age 70 have no surviving children. Approximately 28.8 percent of women 75 years of age and over live with a spouse; almost 20 percent of women 85 years and over live in nursing homes (AOA, 2001). In 2000, 74 percent of men and 43 percent of women were married (AOA, 2001). Since the

proportion of women to men increases after age 65, the likelihood of finding male partners is decreased. Thus, while most elderly men have a spouse for assistance, most elderly women do not. The lack of social support can be a source of serious concern and increasing health risks in the elderly. The health care provider must be sensitive to the social living conditions of the woman and work with her to find ways to enhance her support systems.

ELDER MISTREATMENT

Elder mistreatment, including physical, sexual, and psychological abuse, financial exploitation, and neglect, has reached alarming proportions in the United States. In assessing the older woman, the health care provider should always evaluate for signs of actual abuse or neglect. Dependency and increasing longevity put the elderly woman at risk for abuse and neglect. Although about 4 percent of elderly Americans are victims of abuse yearly, it is likely to be underreported (Pillemer & Finkelhor, 1998). Detection of mistreatment is often difficult and, if suspected, requires more substantial assessment. Assisting the woman to seek appropriate avenues for support, as well as reporting suspected abuse, are inherent in providing holistic health care.

CHRONIC ILLNESS

Chronic illnesses increase in women over age 60; women are likely to have at least one chronic condition or multiple conditions (AOA, 2001). As a result of aging and chronic illness, the client may experience limitations in functional capacities for managing daily living. A small minority, approximately 1 percent of persons 65 to 74 years of age live in nursing homes, compared to almost 20 percent of persons 85 years and older (AOA, 2001).

Common Chronic Problems

- ◆ Visual and hearing impairments
- ◆ Arthritis
- ◆ Hypertension
- ◆ Heart disease
- ◆ Diabetes
- ◆ Orthopedic problems
- ◆ Chronic respiratory disease

Heart disease, cancer, and stroke continue to be the leading causes of death among older women (National Vital Statistics, 2000).

FUNCTIONAL STATUS

The primary goal of health promotion and disease prevention in the elderly is to promote independent functioning as long as possible. All elderly clients should be asked about the level of independence in carrying out basic activities of daily living (ADL) including bathing, grooming, dressing, toileting, transferring, eating, and walking and instrumental activities of daily living (IADL). Issues of sexuality, attitudes toward menopause, and cultural variations must be considered. The IADLs, including meal preparation, shopping, housework, telephoning, money management, and medication management, are critical to maintaining independence in the community. Functional changes can be a warning sign of a beginning pathological process such as drug toxicities, early dementia, or acute illness (Schretzman & Strumpf, 2002).

DEPRESSION AND SUICIDE RISK

As well as assessing for physical changes, the provider must be alert to depressive symptoms in the aging woman. Depression is one of the most common emotional problems affecting older adults. Community-based surveys of older adults estimate that prevalence rates of significant depressive symptoms are 13 percent (Kurlowicz, 2002). Depression is associated with physical illness and disability at all ages, and older persons are at greater risk of concurrent depression and disability than younger adults (Kurlowicz, 2002). Preliminary data for 1999 for the United States indicated that persons age 65 and older had the highest suicide rate of any age group: 15.8 per 100,000 population (Eberhardt, Ingram, Makuc, et al. 2001, Table 47). Elderly women in this age group had a significantly lower incidence of suicide than men: 4.3 to 32.1 per 100,000 population. Women 75 to 84 years had a slightly higher rate than the other older age groups. Conwell (1994) found that the ratio of completed to attempted suicides rose from about 1 in 200 among young adult women to 1 in 4 among elderly person of both genders. Of all the risk factors for completed suicide, the most common is a single episode of major affective illness occurring at the time of suicide (Conwell, 1994).

Risk Factors for Depression

- Unrecognized or untreated affective disorders
- Physical illness
- Losses and changes in older age (decreases in physical vigor, mental agility, income, relocation, social roles)
- Bereavement
- Isolation
- Prior depressive episode

Depressed older women may present with multiple somatic complaints (e.g., insomnia, fatigue, constipation, anorexia) or with a lack of interest in self-care or a functional decline. The elderly seldom complain of a depressed mood or seek care for emotional symptoms (Martin, Fleming, & Evans, 1995). A detailed history and mental status examination can help to distinguish the thinking and behavioral changes associated with depression from those of dementia. Early and aggressive detection and treatment of depression among the elderly is critical because prognosis is good and it may be a life-saving treatment. Referral for psychiatric consultation is recommended.

POLYPHARMACY

Older adults are prescribed an average of thirteen to fifteen prescriptions per year and take an average of 4.5 prescription medications per day (French, 1996). This does not take over-the-counter medications, supplements, and herbs into account.

The elderly are at significantly high risk of drug-drug interactions, drug toxicity, and adverse drug reactions. Drug therapy may also play a role in accidents and injuries. Review of current prescription and nonprescription drug use should be done at each periodic health visit. Additionally, interactions with foods must be considered.

Herbal drug use is a concern as more older women seek to self-medicate with alternative therapies.

INJURY PREVENTION

Falls

Falls are the leading cause of nonfatal injuries and unintentional injury deaths among Americans 65 years and older in the United States (Baum, Capezuti, & Driscoll, 2002). Approximately 25 percent of community-dwelling elderly fall one or more times each year; in residential institutions, the proportion is higher, about 50 percent (Baum et al., 2002). Frail elderly persons, with the following multiple intrinsic risk factors are at high risk: postural instability, osteoporosis, gait disturbances, decreased muscle strength and proprioception, poor vision, cognitive impairment, multiple medications, and use of psychoactive and antihypertensive drugs. Extrinsic or environmental risk factors include stairs, cluttered furniture, slippery surfaces, inadequate lighting, incorrect footwear, and absence of assistive devices in the bathroom. Periodic fall assessment and education are recommended with elderly clients to prevent injuries.

Fires/Burns

Fires and burns are also leading causes of death in older adults. Older persons may be at increased risk of dying in residential fires because of impaired vision, hearing, mobility, or mental status. Cigarette smoking is a leading cause for burn injuries and deaths among the elderly; scald burns primarily involve hot tap water, food, and drinks. Measures to promote safety in the home are important, such as installing and maintaining effective smoke detectors, removal of hazardous heaters, and setting household water heaters at or below 120° F.

LIMITED ACCESS TO CARE

Decreasing vision and other physical impairments may limit an older woman's driving ability and access to care. Alternative transportation may create a financial burden, particularly if multiple health services at multiple sites are needed.

There may be a shortage of health care providers who are trained and interested in holistic care of perimenopausal and postmenopausal women, or who will accept Medicare and Medicaid. When family members and other caregivers are lacking, elders become dependent on the health care system, particularly nursing homes. But for the women of midlife who are the caretakers for elderly parents, stress is increased during the perimenopausal transition. Women's health care providers must emphasize preventive measures and appropriate use of early detection in order to address the problems of morbidity and chronic illness in the elderly. Health and social services for older women are often interdependent, providing a comprehensive, holistic approach.

REFERENCES

Administration on Aging. (2001). *A profile of older Americans: 2001.* Retrieved June 3, 2002 from http://www.aoa.gov/aoa/STATS/profile/2001/3.html

Alexander-Sefre, F., Menon, U., & Jacobs, I. (2002). Ovarian cancer screening. *Hospital Medicine, 63*(4), 210–213.

American Association of Clinical Endocrinologists (AACE). (1999). AACE medical guidelines for clinical practice for management of menopause. *Endocrine Practice,* 5(6), 355–366.

American Association of Clinical Endocrinologists (AACE). (2001). 2001 medical guidelines for clinical practice for the prevention and management of postmenopausal osteoporosis. *Endocrine Practice,* 7(4), 294–312.

American Cancer Society (ACS). (2001). *Cancer prevention and early detection worksheet for women.* Retrieved June 3, 2002 from http://www.cancer.org

American College of Obstetricians and Gynecologists (ACOG), Committee on Gynecologic Practice. (2002). ACOG committee opinion. Risk of breast cancer with estrogen-progestin replacement therapy. *International Journal of Gynaecology and Obstetrics, 76*(3), 333–5.

American College of Obstetricians and Gynecologists (ACOG). (2001). Use of botanicals for management of menopausal symptoms. *ACOG Practice Bulletin, 28,* 1–11.

American Diabetes Association. (2002). Screening for diabetes. *Diabetes Care, 25,* S21–S24.

American Geriatrics Society (AGS), Clinical Practice Committee. (2000a). AGS position statement: Breast cancer screening in older women. *Journal of the American Geriatrics Society, 48,* 842–844.

American Geriatrics Society (AGS), Clinical Practice Committee. (2000b). *AGS position statement: Screening for cervical carcinoma in older women.* Accessed June 3, 2002. http//:www.americangeriatrics.org/products/positionpapers/cer_carc_2000.

American Heart Association. (1997). Cardiovascular disease in women. *Circulation, 96,* 2468–2482.

Barclay, L. (2002, June 24). Black cohosh controls menopausal symptoms. *Medscape Medical News.* Report from Endo 2002: Abstracts p3-333, p3-317. June 21, 2002.

Baum, T., Capezuti, E., & Driscoll, G. (2002). Falls. In V. T. Cotter & N. E. Strumpf (Eds.), *Advanced practice nursing with older adults* (pp. 245–269). New York: McGraw-Hill.

Beck, A. T., & Beck, R. W. (1961). Screening depressed patients in family practice: A rapid technique. *Postgraduate Medicine, 52,* 81–85.

Bickley, S., & Hoekelman, R. A. (1999). *Bates' guide to physical examination and history taking* (7th ed.). Philadelphia: Lippincott.

Bixler, E. O., Vgontzas, A., Lin, H., Ten Have T, Rein, J., Vela-Bueno, A., & Kales, A. (2001). Prevalence of sleep-disordered breathing in women: Effects of gender. *American Journal of Respiratory Critical Care Medicine, 163,* 608–613.

Blackman, M. R. (2000). Age-related alterations in sleep quality and neuroendocrine function: Interrelationships and implications. *Journal of the American Medical Association, 284*(7), 879–881.

Blair, K. A. (1990). Aging: Physiological aspects and clinical implications. *Nurse Practitioner, 15*(2), 14–28.

Bradway, C., & Getman, G. (2002). Genitourinary problems. In V. T. Cotter & N. E. Strumpf (Eds.), *Advanced practice nursing with older adults* (pp. 83–102). New York: McGraw-Hill.

Brown, B. G., Brockenbrough, A., Zhao, X. Q., et al. (1998). Very intensive lipid therapy with lovastatin, niacin, and colostipol for prevention of death and myocardial infarction: A 10-year Familial Atherosclerosis Treatment Study (FATS) follow-up. *Circulation,* 98 (Suppl 1), 1–635 Abstract.

Brown, J. S., Vittinghoff, E., Kanaya, A. et al., for the Heart and Estrogen/Progestin Replacement Study Research Group. (2001). Urinary tract infections in postmenopausal women: Effect of hormone replacement therapy and risk factors. *Obstetrics and Gynecology,* 98, 1045–1052.

Cardozo, L., Bachmann, G., McClish, D., Fonda, D., & Birgerson, L. (1998). Metaanalysis of estrogen therapy in the management of uerogenital atrophy in postmenopausal women: Second report of the Hormones and Urogenital Therapy Committee. *Obstetrics and Gynecology,* 92(4 Pt 2), 722–727.

Cardozo, L., Lose, G., McClish, D., Versi, E., & de Koning Gans H. (2001). A systematic review of estrogens for recurrent urinary tract infections: Third report of the hormones and urogenital therapy (HUT) committee. *International Urogynecological Journal of Pelvic Floor Dysfunction,* 12(1), 15–20.

Centers for Disease Control and Prevention (CDC). (2000, December 8). *CDC surveillance summaries. MMWR,* 49 (SS-11).

Chen, C. L., Weiss, N. S., Newcomb, P., Barlow, W., & White, E. (2002). Hormone replacement therapy in relation to breast cancer. *Journal of the American Medical Association,* 287(6), 734–741.

Collaborative Group on Hormonal Factors in Breast Cancer. (1996). Breast cancer and hormonal contraceptives: Collaborative reanalysis of individual data on 53,297 women with breast cancer and 100,239 women without breast cancer from 54 epidemiological studies. *Lancet,* 347, 1713–1727.

Collaborative Group of the Primary Prevention Project. (2001, January 13). Low-dose aspirin and vitamin E in people at cardiovascular risk: A randomized trial in general practice. *Lancet,* 34–41.

Conwell, Y. (1994). Suicide in the elderly. In L.S. Schneider, C. F. Reynolds III, B. D. Lebowitz, et al. (Eds.), *Diagnosis and treatment of depression in late-life: Results of the NIH Consensus Development Conference.* Washington, DC: American Psychiatric Press.

Desai, M., Pratt, L. A., Lentzner, H., & Robinson, K. N. (2001). *Trends in vision and hearing among older Americans. Aging Trends. No. 2.* Hyattsville, MD: National Center for Health Statistics.

Eberhardt, M. S., Ingram, D. D., Makuc, D. M., et al. (2001). *Urban and rural health chartbook: Health United States, 2001.* Hyattsville, MD: National Center for Health Statistics. Table 47. Death rates for suicide, according to sex, race, Hispanic origin, and age: United States, selected years 1950–99.

Feil, M., & Cotter, V. (2002). Thyroid disorders. In V. T. Cotter & N. E. Strumpf (Eds.), *Advanced practice nursing with older adults* (pp. 127–139). New York: McGraw-Hill.

Finkel, M. L., Cohen, M., & Mahoney, H. (2001). Treatment options for the menopausal woman. *The Nurse Practitioner,* 26(2), 5–15.

Folstein, M. F., Folstein, S. E., & McHugh, P. R. (1975). Minimental state: A practical method for grading the cognitive state of patients for the clinician. *Journal of Psychiatric Research,* 12, 189–198.

French, D. G. (1996). Avoiding adverse drug reactions in the elderly patient: Issues and strategies. *Nurse Practitioner,* 21(9), 90–105.

Gass, M. L. S., & Taylor, M. B. (2001). Alternatives for women through menopause. *American Journal of Obstetrics and Gynecology,* 185, S47–56.

Gordon, J. D., & Speroff, L. (2002). *Handbook for clinical gynecologic endocrinology and infertility.* Philadelphia: Lippincott Williams & Wilkins.

Grady, D., Wenger, N. K., Herrington, D., Khan, S., Furberg, C., Hunninghake, D., Vittinghoff, E., & Hulley, S. (2000). Postmenopausal hormone therapy increases risk for venous thromboembolic disease: The Heart and Estrogen/progestin Replacement Study. *Annals of Internal Medicine,* 132(9), 689–696.

Greendale, G. A., Espeland, M., Slone, S., Marcus, R., & Barrett-Connor, E. for the PEPI Safety Follow-up Study (PSFS) Investigators. (2002). Bone mass response to discontinuation of long-term hormone replacement therapy: Results from the Postmenopausal Estrogen/Progestin Interventions (PEPI) safety follow-up study. *Archives of Internal Medicine,* 162(6), 665–672.

Grodstein, F., Manson, J. E., Colditz, G. A., Willett, W. C., Speizter, F. E., & Stampfer, M. J. (2000). A prospective, observational study of postmenopausal hormone therapy and primary prevention of cardiovascular disease. *Annals of Internal Medicine,* 133 (12), 933–941.

Grodstein, F., & Stampfer, M. J. (1996). Cardiovascular disease and impact of sex steroid replacement. In E. Y. Adashi, J. A. Rock, & Z. Rosenwalls (Eds.), *Reproductive endocrinology, surgery, and technology* (Vol. 2). Philadelphia: Lippincott-Raven.

Grodstein, F., Stampfer, M. J., Manson, J. E., Colditz, G. A., Willett, W. C., Rosner, B., Speizer, F. E., & Hennekens, C. H. (1996). Postmenopausal estrogen and progestin use and the risk of cardiovascular disease. *New England Journal of Medicine,* 335, 453–461.

Hacker, N. F., & Moore, J. G. (1998). *Essentials of obstetrics and gynecology* (3rd ed.). Philadelphia: W. B. Saunders Co.

Harding, S. M. (2000). Complications and consequences of obstructive sleep apnea. *Current Opinion in Pulmonary Medicine,* 6(6), 485–489.

Hatcher, R. A., & Guillebaud, J. (1998). The pill: Combined oral contraceptives. In R. A. Hatcher et al. (Eds.), *Contraceptive technology* (17th ed., pp. 405–466). New York: Ardent Media.

Herrington, D. M., Reboussin, D. M., Brosnihan, K. B., Sharp, P., et al. (2000). Effects of estrogen replacement on the progression of coronary-artery atherosclerosis. *New England Journal of Medicine, 343,* 522–529.

Hodis, H., Madk, W., Lobo, R., et al. for the Estrogen in Prevention of Atherosclerosis Trial (EPAT) Research Group. (2001). Estrogen in the prevention of atherosclerosis: A randomized, double-blind, placebo-controlled trial. *Annals of Internal Medicine, 135,* 939–953.

Holfand, S. L., & Powers, J. (1996). Sexual dysfunction in the menopausal woman: Hormonal causes and management issues. *Geriatric Nursing, 17,* 161–165.

Hulley, S., Furberg, C., Barrett-Connor, E., Cauley, J., Grady, D., Haskell, W., Knopp, R., Lowery, M., Satterfield, S., Schrott, H., Vittinghoff, E., Hunninghake, D., HERS Research Group. (2002). Noncardiovascular disease outcomes during 6.8 years of hormone therapy: Heart and Estrogen/progestin Replacement Study follow-up (HERS II). *Journal of the American Medical Association, 288*(1), 58–66.

Hulley, S., Grady, D., Bush, T., Furberg, C., Herrington, D., Riggs, B., & Vittinghoff, E. (1998). Randomized trial of estrogen plus progestin for secondary prevention of coronary heart disease in postmenopausal women. *Journal of the American Medical Association, 280*(7), 605–613.

Institute for Clinical Systems Improvement (Bloomington, MN). (2001). *Preventive services for adults.* Retrieved June 18, 2002, from http://www.guideline.gov/VIEWS/summary.a...mmary&view=brief_summary&sSearch_string=

Israel, D., & Youngkin, E. Q. (1997). Herbal therapies for perimenopausal and menopausal complaints. *Pharmacotherapy, 17*(5), 970–984.

Jacobs Institute of Women's Health Expert Panel on Menopause Counseling. (2000). *Guidelines for counseling women on the management of menopause.* Retrieved May 21, 2002, from http://www.jiwh.org/Menodownload.htm.

Jellin, J. M., Gregory, P., Batz, R., Hitchens, K., et al. (2002). *Pharmacist's Letter/Prescriber's Letter Natural Medicines Comprehensive Database* (4th ed.). Stockton, CA: Therapeutic Research Faculty.

Kaplan, R. C., Heckbert, S. R., Weiss, N. S., Wahl, P. W., Smith, N. L., Newton, K. M., & Psaty, B. M. (1998). Postmenopausal estrogens and risk of myocardial infarction in diabetic women. *Diabetes Care, 21,* 1117–1121.

Kaunitz, A. (2002). Use of combination hormone replacement therapy in light of recent data from the Women's Health Initiative. *Medscape Women's Health eJournal,* retrieved July 17, 2002 from http://www.medscape.com/viewarticle/438357?srcmp+wh-071202&WebLogicSession=pT4.

Knopman, D. S., DeKosky, S. T., Cummings, J. L., Chui, H., Corey-Bloom, J., Relkin, N., Small, G. W., Miller, B., & Stevens, J. C. (2001). Practice parameters: Diagnosis of dementia (an evidence-based review). Report of the Quality Standards Subcommittee of the American Academy of Neurology. *Neurology, 56,* 1143–1153.

Kuczmarski, R. J., Flegal, K. M., Campbell, S. M., & Johnson, C. L. (1994). Increasing prevalence of overweight among U.S. adults: The National Health and Nutrition Examination Surveys, 1960 to 1991. *Journal of the American Medical Association, 272,* 205–211.

Kurlowicz, L. (2002). Delirium and depression. In V. T. Cotter & N. E. Strumpf (Eds.) *Advanced practice nursing with older adults.* (pp. 141–162). NY: McGraw-Hill.

Lacey, J. V. Jr., Mink, P. J., Lubin, J. H., Sherman, M. E., Troisi, R., Hartge, P., Schatzkin, A., & Schairer, C. (2002). Menopausal hormone replacement therapy and risk of ovarian cancer. The Journal of the American Medical Association, 288(3), 334–341.

Letvak, S., & Schoder, D. (1996). Sexually transmitted diseases in the elderly: What you need to know. *Geriatric Nursing, 17*(4), 156–160.

Liberman, U., Weiss, S., Broll, J. et al. for the Alendronate Phase III Osteoporosis Treatment Study Group. (1995). Effect of oral alendronate on bone mineral density and the incidence of fractures in postmenopausal osteoporosis. *New England Journal of Medicine, 333,* 1437–1443.

Manson, J. E., Willett, W. C., Stampfer, M. J., Colditz, G. A., Hunter, D. J., Hankinson, S. E., Hennekens, C. H., & Speizer, F. E. (1995). Body weight and mortality among women. *New England Journal of Medicine, 333,* 677–685.

Many U.S. breast cancer survivors use alternatives to HRT. (2002). *Reuters medical news.* Retrieved July 17, 2002 from http://www.medscape.com/viewarticle/438322

Martin, L. M., Fleming, K. C., & Evans, J. M. (1995). Recognition and management of anxiety and depression in elderly patients. *Mayo Clinic Proceedings, 70,* 999–1006.

Mayfield, D., McLeod, G., & Hall, P. (1984). The CAGE questionnaire. *American Journal of Psychiatry, 131,* 1121.

McClung, M. R., Geusens, P., Miller, P., Zippel, H., et al. (2001). Effect of risedronate on the risk of hip fracture in elderly women. Hip Intervention Program Study Group. *New England Journal of Medicine, 344*(5), 333–340.

Menon, U., & Jacobs, I. (2000). Recent developments in ovarian cancer screening. *Current Opinions in Obstetrics & Gynecology, 12*(1), 39–42.

Mosca, L, Collins, P., Herrington, D. M., et al. (2001). Hormone replacement therapy and cardiovascular disease. *Circulation, 101,* 499–503.

Mulnard, R. A., Cotman, C. W., Kawas, C., et al (2000). Estrogen replacement therapy for treatment of mild to moderate Alzheimer's disease: A one-year randomized clinical trial. *Journal of the American Medical Association, 283,* 1007–1015.

National Cancer Institute (NCI). (2002). *Ovarian cancer: Screening.* Retrieved June 5, 2002, from http://www.nci.nih.gov/templates/page pr.

National Cholesterol Education Program. (2001). *Third report of the National Cholesterol Education Program (NCEP) Expert Panel on detection, evaluation, and treatment of high blood cholesterol in adults (Adult Treatment Panel III).* NIH Publication No. 01-3670. Retrieved May 21, 2002, from http://www.hin.nhlbi.nih.gov/ncep slds/atpiii

National Vital Statistics Report. (2002). Vol. 50, No. 6. March 21, 2000. Retrieved May 21, 2002, from http://www.cdc.gov/nchs/products/pubs/pudd/nvsr/50/50-pre.htm.

Ness, R., Grisso, J. A., Klapper, J., et al. and the SHARE Study Group. (2000). Risk of ovarian cancer in relation to estrogen and progestin dose and use characteristics of oral contraceptives. *American Journal of Epidemiology,* 152, 233–241.

Newton, K., Buist, D., Keenan, N., Anderson, L., & LaCroix, A. (2002). Use of alternative therapies for menopause symptoms: Results of a population-based survey. *Obstetrics & Gynecology,* 100(1), 18–25.

North American Menopause Society (NAMS). (2000). The role of isoflavones in menopausal health: Consensus opinion of The North American Menopause Society. *Menopause,* 7(4), 215–229.

North American Menopause Society (NAMS). (2001). The role of calcium in peri- and postmenopausal women: Consensus opinion of The North American Menopause Society. *Menopause,* 8(2), 84–95.

North American Menopause Society (NAMS). (2002). Management of postmenopausal osteoporosis: Position statement of The North American Menopause Society. *Menopause,* 9(2), 84–101.

Notelovitz, M. (2002). Why individualizing hormone therapy is crucial: Putting the results of the WHI trial in perspective. *Medscape Women's Health eJournal,* 7(4). Retrieved July 17, 2002 from http://www.medscape.com/viewarticle/438356 print.

Petitti, D. B. (2002). Hormone replacement therapy for prevention: More evidence, more pessimism. *Journal of the American Medical Association,* 288(1), 99–101.

Pfeiffer, E. (1975). A short portable mental status questionnaire for the assessment of organic brain deficit in elderly patients. *Journal of the American Geriatrics Society,* 23, 433–441.

Pillemer, K., & Finkelhor, D. (1998). The prevalence of elder abuse: A random sample survey. *The Gerontologist,* 28, 51–57.

Resnick, S. M., & Maki, P. M. (2001). Effects of hormone replacement therapy on cognitive and brain aging. *Annals of the New York Academy of Science,* 949, 203–214.

Rexrode, K. M., & Manson, J. E. (2002). Postmenopausal hormone therapy and quality of life: No cause for celebration. *Journal of the American Medical Association,* 287(5), 641–642.

Rodriguez, C., Calle, E., Patel, A., Tatham, L., Jacobs, E., & Thun, M. (2001). Effect of body mass on the association between estrogen replacement therapy and mortality among elderly U.S. women. *American Journal of Epidemiology,* 153(2), 145–152.

Rubin, C. D., Pak, C. Y., Adams-Huet, B., Genant, H. K., Li, J., & Rao, D. S. (2001). Sustained-release sodium fluoride in the treatment of the elderly with established osteoporosis. *Archives of Internal Medicine,* 161(19), 2325–2333.

Schaumberg, D., Buring, J., Sullivan, D., & Dana, M. (2001). Hormone replacement therapy and dry eye syndrome. *Journal of the American Medical Association,* 286, 2114–2119.

Schretzman, D., & Strumpf, N. E. (2002). Principles guiding care of older adults. In V. T. Cotter & N. E. Strumpf (Eds.), *Advanced practice nursing with older adults* (pp. 5–25). New York: McGraw-Hill.

Selzer, M. L. (1980). The Michigan Alcoholism Screening Test (MAST). *American Journal of Psychology* (revised), 25(3), 176–181, 197.

Seshadri, S., Zornberg, G., Derby, L. E., Myers, M. W., Jick, H., & Drachman, D. A. (2001). Postmenopausal estrogen replacement therapy and the risk of Alzheimer disease. *Archives of Neurology,* 58(3), 435–440.

Shaw, C. R. (1997). The perimenopausal hotflash: Epidemiology, physiology, and treatment. *The Nurse Practitioner,* 22(3), 55–66.

Sherwin, B. B. (1996). Hormones, mood, and cognitive functioning in postmenopausal women. *Obstetrics and Gynecology,* 87, 20S–26S.

Simon, J., Hunninghake, D., Agarwal, S., Lin, F., et al. (2001). Effects of estrogen plus progestin on risk for biliary tract surgery in postmenopausal women with coronary artery disease. The Heart and Estrogen/progestin Replacement Study. *Annals of Internal Medicine,* 135(7), 493–501.

Speroff, L., Glass, R. H., & Kase, N. G. (1999). *Clinical gynecological endocrinology and infertility.* Baltimore, MD: Williams and Wilkins.

Stampfer, M., Colditz, G. A., Willett, W. C., Manson, J. E., Rosner, B., Speizer, F. E., & Hennekens, C. H. (1991). Postmenopausal estrogen therapy and cardiovascular disease. Ten-year follow-up from the nurses' health study. *New England Journal of Medicine,* 325, 756–762.

Stevenson, J .S. (1977). *Issues and crises during middlescence.* New York: Appleton-Century-Crofts.

Stevenson, J. C. & Whitehead, M. I. (2002). Hormone replacement therapy. *British Medical Journal,* 325(7356), 113–114.

Treating hot flashes with drugs: An update. (2002). *Harvard Women's Health Watch,* 9(12), 6.

Tully, K. (2002). Cardiovascular disease in older adults. In V. T. Cotter & N. E. Strumpf (Eds.), *Advanced practice nursing with older adults* (pp. 29–65). New York: McGraw-Hill.

Uhler, M., Marks, J., & Judd, H. (2000). Estrogen replacement therapy and gallbladder disease in postmenopausal women. *Menopause, 7*(3), 162–167.

U.S. Census Bureau. (2000). *Current population survey.* Racial Statistics Branch, Population Division. Retrieved May 21, 2002, from http://www.census.gov/population/www/socdemo/race/ppl-142.html.

U.S. Department of Health and Human Services. (1999). *Health, United States, 1999 with health and aging chartbook.* Retrieved May 21, 2002, from http://www.cdc.gov/nchs/products/pubs/pubd/hus/2010/2010.htm.

U.S. Preventive Services Task Force. (1996). *Guide to clinical preventive services* (2nd ed.). Baltimore, MD: Williams & Wilkins.

Vastag, B. (2002). Hormone replacement therapy falls out of favor with expert committee. *Journal of the American Medical Association, 287*(15), 1923–1924.

Viscoli, C., Brass, L., Kernan, W., Sarrel, P., Suissa, L., & Horwitz, R. (2001). A clinical trial of estrogen-replacement therapy after ischemic stroke. *New England Journal of Medicine, 345*(17), 1243–1249.

Waring, S. C., Rocca, W. A., Petersen, R. A., O'Brien, P. C., Tangalos, E. G., & Kokmen, E. (1999). Postmenopausal estrogen replacement therapy and risk of AD: A population-based study. *Neurology, 52*(5), 965–970.

World Health Organization (WHO). (1994). *Assessment of fracture risk and its application to screening postmenopausal osteoporosis: Report of a WHO study group.* Technical Report Series 843. Geneva: Author.

The Writing Group for the PEPI trial. (1995). Effects of estrogen or estrogen/progestin regimens on heart disease risk factors in postmenopausal women: The postmenopausal estrogen/progestin interventions (PEPI) trial. *Journal of the American Medical Association, 273*(3), 199–208.

Writing Group for the Women's Health Initiative Investigators. (2002). Risks and benefits of estrogen plus progestin in healthy postmenopausal women: Principal results from the Women's Health Initiative randomized controlled trial. *Journal of the American Medical Association, 288*(3), 321–333.

Yesavage, J. A., & Brink, T. L. (1983). Development and validation of Geriatric Depression Scale: A preliminary report. *Journal of Psychiatric Research, 17,* 41.

Zung, W. W. K. (1965). A self-rating depression scale. *Archives of General Psychiatry, 12,* 63–70.

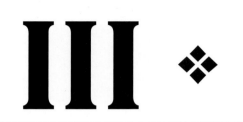

III ❖ Promotion of Women's Health Care During Pregnancy

CHAPTER 16

ASSESSING HEALTH DURING PREGNANCY

Kelly L. Cokely Yeong

A *National Insti- tutes of Health and Human Services expert panel . . . recommended that prenatal care begin prior to conception, pre- ferably within one year of a planned pregnancy.*

Highlights

- Barriers to Prenatal Care
- Preconception Counseling, Assessment
- Presumptive, Probable, and Positive Signs and Symptoms
- Sexuality during Pregnancy
- Initial Prenatal Visit, Subsequent Visits
- Progressing Physical Changes
- Commonly Recommended Tests
- Risk Assessment
    Genetic and Preterm Assessments
    Attachment
    Environmental, Occupational Hazards
- Psychosocial Assessment
    Domestic Violence
- Nutrition
- Major Theories of Maternal Role Development
- Preparation for Childbirth: Counseling and Classes
- Adolescent Pregnancy
- Delayed Pregnancy
- Nontraditional Families
- Substance Abuse Screening

❖   INTRODUCTION

Prior to the early 1900s few women received prenatal care or evaluation. The advent of consistent and comprehensive prenatal care, begun in early pregnancy, has markedly decreased both maternal and infant morbidity and mortality in the United States. Today prenatal care encompasses risk assessment, social services, client education, and medical care. Ideally this care should begin prior to conception (Scott, Hammond, Danforth, & DiSaio, 1999).

Despite advances in prenatal care, several barriers to initiating care exist (Scott et al., 1999).

Barriers to Prenatal Care

- *Unrecognized Pregnancy.* Pregnancy may go unrecognized because of lack of knowledge about the signs and symptoms of pregnancy, limited body awareness, a history of irregular menses, or obesity.
- *Denied Pregnancy.* Pregnancy may bedenied, particularly if unplanned, because of the woman's ambivalence regarding motherhood.
- *Limited Finances.* Financial constraints or limited health insurance may discourage a woman from securing prenatal care.
- *Inaccessibility of the Health Care System.* An inconvenient location of the health care facility, lack of transportation, lack of provider availability, or fear of the health care system may make it difficult for a woman to obtain prenatal care.
- *Lack of or Poor Support System.* The pregnant individual may be experiencing safety issues, particularly if she is in a situation involving domestic violence (ACOG, 1999a).
- *Language Barrier.* A woman with little or no ability to speak English (ACOG, 1999a).

Today many women have jobs outside the home both for financial reasons and for professional accomplishment. In two-income families, partners share childrearing responsibilities, and the male partner is expected to be active in the care and nurturing of offspring. Our concept of *family* has expanded to include nontraditional households, such as same sex relationships, single-parent families, and cohabitation.

The advent of consumerism in health care also has influenced our concept of pregnancy (Maloni, 1996). Current biostatistics indicate that the typical U.S. couple will have one or two children. Many women/couples make a conscientious effort to have a healthy pregnancy, and therefore couples with the availability of modern medical technology have greater expectations for a healthy pregnancy and infant.

Clients as consumers have come to expect an optimal outcome in pregnancy, and preconception counseling has become common. Throughout pregnancy, women may question the safety of various activities and the effects of substances on the developing fetus. Women and their partners are also increasingly included in the decision-making process, and frequently they participate in community prenatal classes. All of these changes make for a different experience of pregnancy and parenthood for today's women.

PLANNING FOR A HEALTHY PREGNANCY

PRECONCEPTION COUNSELING

Interest in preconception education and counseling began in the 1980s in the United States. In evaluating new information and reconsidering older data, many health care providers became convinced that pregnancy may be too late for expectant parents to correct unhealthy habits. A National Institutes of Health and Human Services expert panel reviewed the factors that contribute to good pregnancy outcomes for women and infants, and subsequently recommended that prenatal care begin prior to conception, preferably within one year of a planned pregnancy (ACOG, 2000a). The status of a woman's health can influence not only her ability to conceive, but also her ability to maintain the pregnancy (Cunningham, Gant, Leveno, Hauth, & Wenstrom, 2001).

At the time of conception, a woman should be in an optimal state of emotional and physical health. Health educators and health care providers have concluded that this directly improves pregnancy outcomes (Scott et al., 1999). The goal of preconception care and counseling is to maximize the health of the woman and the health of her potential infant. Ideally, preconception counseling is accompanied by a complete physical and psychosocial evaluation. Prior to conception, prospective parents have an opportunity to make informed decisions and ultimately to make lifestyle adjustments to maximize their chances of a successful outcome in pregnancy (ACOG, 2000a).

Teaching/Learning Methods

A healthy lifestyle can be promoted through individual teaching during routine examinations, community adult health education programs, or traditional classes with content directed toward prospective parents. Although current studies do not demonstrate that preconception education directly influences perinatal outcomes, new information can be acquired that enhances a positive perinatal outcome. Demonstrated statistical changes in the ultimate outcome for pregnancy may not be available for several generations of infants, thus long-term goals such as parental behavior changes and improved health status in someday parents needs to be the guiding philosophy for marketing these classes (ACOG, 2000a).

Reva Rubin investigated the relationship between social support and pregnancy outcomes and found that the mother's ability to identify with the developing fetus fostered attachment to the child. Hence, the quality of the social support given to a woman during pregnancy correlates positively with maternal-fetal attachment (ACOG, 1999a). In addition, enhancing a parent's knowledge about fetal growth and development promotes intrauterine bonding and subsequent parenting skills. These concepts reinforce the importance of programs directed toward preconception health promotion (Morrison, 2000).

Nonpregnant persons may not feel compelled to attend preparation classes; therefore, tools must convey the importance of preconception education and the potential for improved perinatal outcomes. Information should focus strongly on maternal and fetal health, timing of pregnancy, and how these factors influence the overall life plan (Cunningham et al., 2001). The normal physiological changes associated with pregnancy and their affect on the woman's body and self-image and legal/ethical issues, such as genetic and diagnostic testing, are other subjects that need to be covered in these classes. Moreover, pertinent information about community agencies and family services should be provided for those in need of follow-up support (Morrison, 2000).

PRECONCEPTION ASSESSMENT DATA

Preconception care and counseling are valuable in identifying risks in the client's medical history and current health status, and their potential impact on a pregnancy.

Assessment includes history taking and a physical examination, often augmented by laboratory/diagnostic testing (Morrison, 2000).

Subjective Data

During the evaluation, obtain a detailed medical, social, reproductive, and family history. By identifying problems early, it is sometimes possible to resolve them prior to conception and ultimately improve perinatal outcome (ACOG, 2000a).

A comprehensive screening tool such as the Preconceptional Health Assessment (see Figure 16–1) can facilitate risk assessment with prospective parents (Cefalo & Moos, 1995). This appraisal includes a checklist that assesses the health status of the prospective mother. Through it, information specific to the client's family, medical, reproductive, and drug histories can be obtained. Nutrition and lifestyle choices also can be evaluated.

In addition, it is important to assess human immunodeficiency virus (HIV) risk factors. These factors include history of homosexual activity, intravenous drug use, multiple sexual contacts, blood or blood product transfusion, or close contact with bodily fluids.

Objective Data

Physical Examination. A complete physical examination is needed, with special emphasis on the systems identified during the risk appraisal. A thorough pelvic examination should also be performed, including a Papanicolaou (Pap) smear, cultures for gonorrhea and chlamydia, and a wet smear evaluation (ACOG, 2000a).

Diagnostic Tests and Methods. These include rubella titer and antibody screen, serology for syphilis, complete blood cell (CBC) count with indices, blood type/Rh, random blood sugar, and urinalysis. Hemoglobin electrophoresis may be performed if sickle cell or thalassemia status is of concern. If positive, test the father for these traits also. Refer for genetic testing if both display traits. Screening for viral disease, such as HIV, hepatitis, cytomegalovirus (CMV), or toxoplasmosis, can be offered (Reynolds, 1998). The National Institutes of Health have suggested that health care providers offer a screening test for cystic fibrosis (CF) carrier status. Groups at high risk for CF include Caucasians, particularly Ashkenazi Jews, central or north Europeans, those with a partner with CF, and individuals with a family history of CF (Shulman & Elias, 2001). Encourage testing father for syphilis, HIV, hepatitis and blood type/Rh.

PRECONCEPTIONAL HEALTH ASSESSMENT

What is your main interest in seeking preconceptional counseling?

_____

_____

_____

So that we can address your specific interests and concerns, we ask that you complete the following questionnaire. You may use the back of the form to provide additional information when necessary.

Place an X next to any item that applies to you.

SOCIAL HISTORY

Do you

_____ drink beer, wine, or hard liquor

_____ smoke cigarettes or use any other tobacco products

_____ use marijuana, cocaine, or any recreational drugs

_____ use lead or chemicals at home or at work
If yes, list the specific chemicals if you know what they are:

_____

_____

_____ work with radiation

_____ participate in an exercise program

Are you

_____ 34 years of age or older

NUTRITION HISTORY

On the back of this sheet, list by meal everything you ate and drank yesterday, including the approximate amount; indicate snacks separately.

Do you

_____ practice vegetarianism

_____ eat unusual substances, such as laundry starch or clay

_____ have a history of bulimia or anorexia

_____ follow a special diet
If yes, describe:

_____

_____

_____ supplement your diet with vitamins
If yes, list vitamins and dosages:

_____

_____

FIGURE 16–1.   Preconceptional health assessment. *(Source: Reprinted with permission from the authors. Cefalo R.C., & Moos M.K. (1995) Preconceptual health care: A practical guide (2nd ed.). St. Louis, Missouri: Mosby-Year Book.)*

_____ take medications, including oral contraceptives

_____ have an intolerance for milk

MEDICAL HISTORY

Do you now have or have you ever had

_____ diabetes

_____ thyroid disease

_____ phenylketonuria (PKU)

_____ asthma

_____ heart disease

_____ high blood pressure

_____ deep venous thrombosis (blood clots)

_____ kidney disease

_____ systemic lupus erythematosus (SLE)

_____ epilepsy

_____ sickle cell disease

_____ cancer

_____ other health problems that require medical or surgical care
If yes, describe:

_____

_____

INFECTIOUS DISEASE HISTORY

Do you or your partner have a history of

_____ recurrent genital infections

_____ herpes simplex

_____ *Chlamydia* infection

_____ human papillomavirus (genital warts)

_____ gonorrhea

_____ syphilis

_____ viral hepatitis or high-risk behavior, including use of intravenous street drugs, intimate bisexual/homosexual contact, or multiple sexual partners

_____ acquired immunodeficiency syndrome (AIDS) or high-risk behavior, including use of intravenous street drugs, intimate bisexual/homosexual contact, or multiple sexual partners

_____ occupational exposure to the blood or bodily secretions of others

_____ blood transfusions

FIGURE 16–1 (*cont.*)

Do you

_____ own or work with cats

_____ have documented immunity to rubella

MEDICATION HISTORY

Do you

_____ routinely or occasionally take prescribed medications
If yes, list names and dosages:

_____

_____

_____ routinely or occasionally take over-the-counter medications
If yes, list names and dosages:

_____

_____

REPRODUCTIVE HISTORY

Do you have a history of

_____ uterine or cervical abnormalities

_____ two or more pregnancies that ended between 14 and 28 weeks of gestation

_____ one or more fetal deaths

_____ one or more infants who weighed less than 5½ lbs. at birth

_____ one or more infants who were admitted to a neonatal intensive care unit

_____ one or more infants with a birth defect

FAMILY HISTORY

Do you, your partner, or members of either of your families, including children, have

_____ hemophilia

_____ thalassemia

_____ Tay-Sachs disease

_____ sickle cell disease or trait

_____ phenylketonuria (PKU)

_____ cystic fibrosis

_____ a birth defect

_____ mental retardation

_____ Are you and your partner related outside of marriage (such as cousins)?

_____ Do you and your partner have the same ethnic or racial background, such as Ashkenazic Jewish, Mediterranean, or black?

FIGURE 16–1 (cont.)

Provide instruction in basal body temperature (BBT) assessment, charting, and timing of intercourse to interested couples (see Chapter 10). Also review menstruation and fertility awareness methods to enhance possibility of conception (see Chapter 8).

CLIENT EDUCATION AND COUNSELING

Preconception counseling and intervention for the client and her partner should focus on the following areas (ACOG, 2000a).

*   *Menstrual Cycles.* Advise the client to keep an accurate record of her menstrual cycles in order to help establish gestational dating.
*   *Adequate Exercise and Nutrition.* A vitamin/mineral supplement is often recommended to increase maternal nutrition stores. In September 1992, the U.S. Public Health Service Centers for Disease Control announced new recommendations regarding folic acid supplementation in the periconceptional period. These advise all women of childbearing age to consume 0.4 mg of folic acid per day for the purpose of reducing the risk of a neural-tube-defect affected pregnancy. Women with a history of an affected pregnancy are at particular risk in each subsequent pregnancy, and it is recommended that they should take 4 mg of folic acid daily. Folic acid supplementation is recommended at least one month prior to attempting conception and through the first three months of pregnancy (ACOG, 2000a). Folic acid supplementation is contraindicated in those women with pernicious anemia. Food sources of folic acid include broccoli, leafy green vegetables, eggs, and orange juice. Encourage overweight or underweight clients to attain an ideal weight prior to conception. Obesity increases the risk of perinatal mortality and morbidity. It may contribute to the development of hypertension and diabetes in pregnancy (Brown, 2001). Recent studies suggest that obesity increases the risk of neural tube defect regardless of folic acid intake (Werler, Louik, & Mitchell, 1999). Low pregravid weight increases the risk of premature birth and intrauterine growth retardation (Ramachandran, 2002). Beginning an exercise program prior to pregnancy will hopefully improve cardiovascular status and impart a feeling of overall well-being into the pregnancy as well. Exercise may also help the overweight woman attain close to ideal and ideal weight.

*   *Avoidance of Teratogens.* Warn the client that potential teratogens can be related to occupation and lifestyle, for example, cleaning solutions, hair colors/perms, photography solutions, radiation, aromatic hydrocarbons, and chemicals used in processing food and textiles.
*   *Affirmation of Pregnancy Decision.* Stress that the couple needs time to affirm the decision to attempt pregnancy.
*   *Readiness for Parenthood.* Assess the couple's social, financial, and psychological readiness for pregnancy and commitment to parenthood.
*   *Identification of Unhealthy Behaviors.* Assist the couple to identify and alter unhealthy behaviors, such as smoking, alcohol consumption, and drug use (i.e., prescription, over-the-counter, and illegal drugs).
*   *Treatment of Jeopardizing Conditions.* Ensure that medical conditions, i.e., hypertension, diabetes, hepatitis, sexually transmitted diseases, that may jeopardize the pregnancy outcome are evaluated. Refer the couple to a specialist as needed.
*   *Identify Genetic Risk.* When risks are identified, refer the couple for genetic counseling and laboratory testing to determine carrier status (see Figure 16–2).
*   *Effective Professional Relationship.* To encourage the client's early entry into prenatal care, initiate and nurture a positive professional relationship.
*   *Preconception Classes.* Where appropriate, refer the couple to community adult educational resources for preconception classes (e.g., March of Dimes).
*   *Laboratory Tests.* Order all appropriate laboratory tests, evaluate the results, and discuss the findings and their implications with the client.
*   *Appropriate Vaccinations.* If the client is not immune to rubella, administer the vaccine and advise the client to wait three months before attempting conception. Also vaccinate for tetanus, hepatitis, and varicella when indicated.
*   *Special Dietary Needs.* If the client has special dietary needs (e.g., vegetarian, cultural, overweight, underweight), refer her to a dietician. Use of megavitamin/mineral supplements are to be avoided. Assess for eating disorders, pica. Economic constraints may negatively affect dietary intake.
*   *Insurance Coverage.* With the advent of managed health care, and ever-changing insurance coverage, it is important for couples to evaluate their benefits. Many insurance policies have contracts designating preferred sites for care and delivery (ACOG, 2000a).

Name _____   Patient # _____   Date _____

1. Will you be 35 years or older when the baby is due?   Yes ___   No ___

2. Have you, the baby's father, or anyone in either of your families ever had any of the following disorders?
   • Down syndrome (mongolism)   Yes ___   No ___
   • Other chromosomal abnormality   Yes ___   No ___
   • Neural tube defect, spina bifida (meningomyelocele or open spine), anencephaly   Yes ___   No ___
   • Hemophilia   Yes ___   No ___
   • Muscular dystrophy   Yes ___   No ___
   • Cystic fibrosis   Yes ___   No ___
   If yes, indicate the relationship of the affected person to you or to the baby's father: _____

3. Do you or the baby's father have a birth defect?   Yes ___   No ___
   If yes, who has the defect and what is it? _____

4. In any previous marriages, have you or the baby's father had a child, born dead or alive
   with a birth defect not listed in question 2 above?   Yes ___   No ___
   If yes, what was the defect and who had it? _____

5. Do you or the baby's father have any close relatives with mental retardation?   Yes ___   No ___
   If yes, indicate the relationship of the affected person to you or to the baby's father: _____
   Indicate the cause, if known: _____

6. Do you, the baby's father, or a close relative in either of your families have a birth defect,
   any familial disorder, or a chromosomal abnormality not listed above?   Yes ___   No ___
   If yes, indicate the condition and the relationship of the affected person to you or to the
   baby's father: _____
   _____

7. In any previous marriages, have you or the baby's father had a stillborn child or three or more first
   trimester spontaneous pregnancy losses?   Yes ___   No ___
   Have either of you had a chromosomal study?   Yes ___   No ___
   If yes, indicate who and the results: _____
   _____

8. If you or the baby's father is of Jewish ancestry, have either of you been screened for
   Tay-sachs disease?   Yes ___   No ___
   If yes, indicate who and the results: _____
   _____

9. If you or the baby's father is black, have either of you been screened for sickle cell trait?   Yes ___   No ___
   If yes, indicate who and the results: _____
   _____

10. If you or the baby's father is of Italian, Greek, or Mediterranean background, have either of
    you been tested for ß-thalassemia?   Yes ___   No ___
    If yes, indicate who and the results: _____
    _____

11. If you or the baby's father is of Philipine or Southeast Asian ancestry, have either of you been
    tested for α-thalassemia?   Yes ___   No ___
    If yes, indicate who and the results: _____
    _____

12. Excluding iron and vitamins, have you taken any medications or recreational drugs since
    being pregnant or since your last menstrual period? (Include nonprescription drugs.)   Yes ___   No ___
    If yes, give name of medication and time taken during pregnancy: _____
    _____

Note: Any patient replying "YES" to questions should be offered appropriate counseling. If the patient declines further counseling or testing, this should be noted in the chart. Given that genetics is a field in a state of flux, alterations or updates to this form will be required periodically.

FIGURE 16–2. Sample prenatal genetic screen. *(Source: ACOG, 2001a).*

ASSESSMENT DURING PREGNANCY

Well woman's health care during pregnancy begins with a complete history and thorough physical examination during the initial visit. The initial visit is the ideal time to screen for particular risk factors suggesting preterm delivery or other poor outcomes (see Risk Assessment, later in this chapter). Since many women continue to experience unintended pregnancy, however, routine exams are also ideal for screening and education. Encourage the client to seek prenatal care early in pregnancy.

The health care provider and the client establish the foundation of a trusting relationship by jointly developing a plan of care for the pregnancy. This plan is tailored to the client's lifestyle preferences as much as possible and focuses primarily on education for overall wellness during pregnancy. The ultimate goal is early detection and prevention of potential problems in the pregnancy.

Return office visits include physical evaluation of the client and her fetus, client education, and the continuation of a holistic approach to pregnancy care.

SIGNS AND SYMPTOMS OF PREGNANCY

Signs and symptoms that may be reported by the pregnant client are traditionally categorized into three groups, defined as follows and summarized in Table 16–1.

- *Presumptive.* Signs or symptoms frequently reported with pregnancy, although not conclusive for pregnancy.
- *Probable.* Signs or symptoms that are more reliable indicators of pregnancy, often noted on the physical examination or with laboratory testing.

- *Positive.* Signs or symptoms noted when absolute confirmation of pregnancy is made.

Although these signs and symptoms assist in confirming pregnancy, they *cannot* enable the health care provider to differentiate an intrauterine pregnancy from an ectopic pregnancy.

OVERVIEW OF INITIAL PRENATAL VISIT

During the initial visit, the health care provider performs a complete assessment and counsels the client about risk factors and prenatal care. Several components are included (ACOG, 1997).

- *Confirmation of Pregnancy.* Perform a beta-human chorionic gonadotropin (β-hCG) urine test if seen prior to FHTs, ultrasound; if negative, retest using a radioimmunoassay (RIA) β-hCG serum test (see Table 16–5).
- *History.* Obtain a complete medical, psychosocial, family, and reproductive history (see Chapter 4). Several areas require more in-depth evaluation during pregnancy. Information obtained may help date the pregnancy (ACOG, 1997).
  - Menstrual history—last normal menses.
  - Contraceptive history—last time used, dates of unprotected intercourse.
  - Gynecologic history.
  - Sexual history—high-risk behavior.
  - Surgical history.
- *Physical Examination.* (See Chapter 5.) Assess the client's vital signs and perform a complete head-to-toe examination with particular attention to the pelvic evaluation. Establish the client's baseline

TABLE 16–1. Signs and Symptoms of Pregnancy

Presumptive	Probable	Positive
Amenorrhea	Abdominal enlargement	Auscultation of fetal heart sounds
Breast tenderness and enlargement	Ballottement	Palpation of fetal movements
Chadwick's sign	Braxton-Hicks contractions	Radiological and/or ultrasonic verification of gestation
Fatigue	Goodell's sign	
Hyperpigmentation	Hegar's sign	
Chloasma	Palpation of fetal contours	
Linea nigra	Positive pregnancy test	
Fetal movements (quickening)	Uterine enlargement	
Urinary frequency		
Nausea/vomiting		

Source: Adapted from Pillitteri (1999).

cervical status and perform clinical pelvimetry if it is part of the protocol in a particular setting. The normal pregnant cervix is usually 3 to 4 cm long, closed, firm in texture and usually mid to posterior in position. Testing the adequacy of the pelvis, if unproven by previous vaginal delivery, includes measurement of the diagonal conjugate from the posterior inferior edge of the symphysis pubis to the sacral promontory (normally 12.5 cm or greater), which estimates the inlet; the transverse diameter of the midpelvis includes evaluation of the ischial spines (sharp or blunt and degree of prominence) and of the anteroposterior diameter by the shape of the sacrum (curved or flat). The ischial tuberosities should be 8 cm or more apart.

◆ *Laboratory Tests.* Perform routine laboratory tests (Table 16–2) and additional testing as needed (Table 16–3).

◆ *Risk Assessment.* Refer the client for thorough risk assessment as indicated (see Table 16–3).

◆ *Prenatal Educational Materials.* Provide and review information about prenatal classes, nutrition, exercise, teratogens, sexuality, and choices in infant feeding.

◆ *Exercise during Pregnancy.* Exercise helps many women maintain a feeling of well-being. It is also helpful in keeping weight gain in control. ACOG supports the need for exercise and recommends 30 minutes of exercise most days of the week. It is important to carefully select the type of exercise, as well as individual medical and obstetric risk (ACOG, 2002).

◆ *Sexuality during Pregnancy.* See discussion that follows.

◆ *Schedule Follow-Up Visits.* Discuss the importance of continued prenatal care and work out a schedule for follow-up visits.

SEXUALITY DURING PREGNANCY

Physiological Changes

Table 16–4 gives a summary of physiological changes that may enhance pleasure or diminish a woman's sexual response during pregnancy. Second trimester changes, such as increased pelvic congestion and vaginal lubrication, may enhance sexual enjoyment. Opportunities arise to review the physiological changes that influence sexuality both during the initial prenatal visit and during subsequent visits.

TABLE 16–2. Routine Tests to be Performed on all Pregnancy Clients[a]

ABO blood group/Rh factor identification/Antibody screen
Complete blood cell count with indices (Hb, Hct, MCV, MCH, MCHC)
Rubella titer
Syphilis screening/VDRL, RPR
Hepatitis screening
Urinalysis
Chlamydia screening
Gonorrhea screening
Group Beta strep screening
Pap smear

[a]Values may vary according to the laboratory used.
Note: Hb = hemoglobin; Hct = hematocrit; MCV = mean corpuscular volume; MCH = mean corpuscular hemoglobin; MCHC = mean corpuscular hemoglobin concentration; VDRL = Venereal Disease Research Laboratories test; RPR = rapid plasma reagin; HIV = human immunodeficiency virus.
Sources: ACOG (1997); Gabbe, Niebyl, & Simpson (2002)

Psychosocial Changes

Pregnancy is often a time of profound emotional and developmental upheaval and can present a developmental crisis for both partners. Some couples experience increased intimacy and closeness from the bond pregnancy creates. Sexuality during pregnancy can be affected directly. The health care provider's role involves providing anticipatory guidance through sexuality education and assessment, both at the initial prenatal evaluation and during subsequent visits. Several concerns are often reported (Lim, 2002).

◆ Fear of causing miscarriage or harm to the developing fetus.

TABLE 16–3. Additional Tests Performed on the Basis of the Pregnant Client's History[a]

α-fetoprotein/triple screen
Antibody screening
Blood chemistry
Cystic Fibrosis screen
Cytomegalovirus titer
Fifth disease titer
Glucose tolerance tests
Hemoglobin A1C
Hemoglobin electrophoresis
Herpes culture
HIV screening
Serum iron studies
Toxoplasmosis titer
Thyroid studies
Urine culture
Tuberculin skin test

[a]Values may vary according to the laboratory used.
Sources: Cunningham et al. (2001); Gabbe et al. (2002).

TABLE 16–4. Physiological Changes in Pregnancy that Influence Sexuality

First Trimester	Second Trimester	Third Trimester
Fatigue and lethargy	Increased pelvic congestion	Physical discomfort, backache
Nausea and vomiting	Increased vaginal moisture	Increasing uterine irritability
Breast tenderness		Excessive pelvic congestion
Abdominal bloating		Vulvar/femoral varicosities
Increased urination		

Source: Adapted from Cunningham et al. (1999) and Pillitteri (1999).

- Need for modifications in positioning for coitus with advancing gestation.
- Fluctuating libido by both partners and the resulting effect on sexual desire and contact.
- The woman's perceived loss of attractiveness to her sexual partner, body image changes.
- Misinformation and misconception regarding sexuality, safety; the impact of religious taboos.
- A declining desire for intimacy as the woman withdraws or focuses on infant preparation.

Guidelines for Intervention

Take a sexual history early in the pregnancy to establish baseline information, e.g., frequency, monogamy, risk factors, about both partners. Knowledge of sexual activity since last normal menses may help with dating the pregnancy. To the extent that medical findings allow, give permission for the couple to be sexually active during and after pregnancy.

Contraindications to Sexual Intercourse

The following conditions may preclude sexual relations during a portion of the pregnancy (Cunningham et al., 1999).

- History of repeated miscarriage.
- History of cervical incompetence, without cerclage.
- Current possibility of threatened abortion.
- Placenta previa.
- Undiagnosed vaginal bleeding.
- Premature rupture of membranes, preterm labor.
- Severe vulvar varicosities.

SUBSEQUENT PRENATAL VISITS

At each subsequent prenatal visit, measure the client's weight and blood pressure; assess for quickening/fetal movement; evaluate the client's urine for blood, protein, ketones, nitrites, and glucose; determine fundal height; and assess fetal heart tones. Also at each visit, evaluate any client complaints and answer questions appropriately. Review appropriate nutrition and use of prenatal vitamin/mineral supplements. Leopold's maneuvers should be performed weekly after 35 weeks to determine fetal presentation and position. (Scott et al., 1999). Include the partner when possible in auscultation of fetal heart tones and palpation of fundal height changes. Share positive aspects of the exam, e.g., normal heart tones, good growth. Review with the couple the common discomforts of pregnancy and how they may influence sexuality. Encourage the partner's participation in the labor and delivery process to improve his ability to empathize during the postpartum period. As appropriate, offer the couple suggestions about sexual frequency, foreplay, and alternate forms of intimacy. As the pregnancy advances, offer advice on coital positioning.

Weeks 12 to 16

Review laboratory findings with the client and her partner. If appropriate order genetic testing, such as amniocentesis or alpha-fetoprotein tetra. Screen the father of the baby for sickle cell (hemoglobin electrophoresis) disease, blood type/Rh as indicated. If a woman chooses to have CF carrier testing performed, it can be done at any time during the pregnancy. Ideally, it should be performed in the preconception period. The results of this test take two weeks. If a woman is identified as a carrier, the father of the baby is then tested for carrier status, which would then take another two weeks for results.

Weeks 16 to 20

Assess for fetal movements (quickening). Ultrasound evaluation may be performed to confirm gestational age and assess fetal well-being. Encourage the couple to enroll in prenatal classes.

Weeks 24 to 28

If Rh negative, reevaluate the antibody screen titer. Perform glucose screening for gestational diabetes. Administer

RhoGAM immune globulin as indicated. Reactions to RhoGAM [Rh$_o$(D) immune globulin] are infrequent, mild, and primarily at the injection site. An occasional person may react more strongly. A few women may experience a slight temperature elevation. Retest hemoglobin and hematocrit. Evaluate the client for risk of preterm labor and perform a cervical assessment including cervical position, consistency, length, and dilation.

Weeks 28 to 32

Offer the client counseling regarding the choice of health care provider for the infant. Assess the client's breasts and discuss preparation for breast-feeding. Discuss the importance of daily fetal movement as an indicator of fetal well-being.

Weeks 32 to 34

Reassess the client for risk of preterm labor; assess the cervix as indicated.

Weeks 34 to 36

Review with the client the signs and symptoms of labor; provide a handout listing them. Obtain a vaginal/anorectal culture for GBS (group Beta strep) (Bloom & Ewing, 2001). According to setting protocol, begin weekly cervical cultures for active HSV (herpes simplex virus) in those with positive history. Retest for chlamydia and gonorrhea in those with infections earlier in pregnancy.

Weeks 36 to 40

Assess fetal position and presentation. Review and negotiate the client's birth expectations. Forward a copy of the client's prenatal records to the hospital labor area for future reference. Document the client's final choice of a pediatrician. Initiate fetal surveillance as indicated. A cervical examination may be performed per the protocol of the institution. For women at or beyond 36 weeks who are at risk for recurrent HSV infection, suppressive antiviral therapy may be considered. Suppressive therapy can include Acyclovir 400 mg twice a day, Valcyclovir 500 mg once daily, or Famcyclovir 250 mg twice a day (ACOG, 1999b). Review client desires for postpartal contraception. Reinforce preparation for breastfeeding. Arrange for infant car seat.

Week 40 and Beyond

Prepare the client for postdate pregnancy protocol. Perform a cervical assessment. Institute fetal surveillance, such as ultrasound, nonstress testing, and biweekly office visits. Check via ultrasound for AFV (amniotic fluid volume).

PROGRESSING PHYSICAL CHANGE

Several changes commonly occur during pregnancy (Scott et al., 1999).

- *Skin.* Increased vascularity; increased pigmentation of face (chloasma), areola, abdomen (linea nigra), and genitalia; striae of breasts and abdomen.
- *Head.* Mild changes in scalp; excessive oiliness or dryness.
- *Eyes.* Vessel dilation in the sclera.
- *Mouth.* Edematous, friable gums.
- *Chest/Cardiovascular.* Increased respiratory effort and rate; progressive elevation of the diaphragm; hand/pedal edema by third trimester.
- *Breasts.* Increased fullness, tenderness, enlargement, and excretion of colostrum are common by the third trimester.
- *Heart.* Exaggerated heart sounds, particularly functional murmurs in systole.
- *Abdomen.* Distention secondary to flatus and increased uterine size; diminished bowel sounds as peristaltic movements are slowed; enlarging uterus, which displaces abdominal organs.
- *Genitalia/Reproductive*
  - *External.* Increased pigmentation; pubic hair may lengthen. Near term, pelvic congestion and overall swelling of labia majora are common; vulvar varicosities may be noted.
  - *Vagina.* Increased pelvic congestion and hypertrophy; rugation of vaginal mucosa is prominent.
  - *Cervix.* Positive Chadwick's sign (bluish/purple color) is noted; may soften, dilate, and efface close to term. Positive Goodell's sign (softening with growth of cervical glands) may be noted.
  - *Uterus.* Positive Hegar's sign (softening of the lower uterine segment) often present by 6 weeks' gestation. At 12 weeks' gestation the fundus is noted at the symphysis pubis; at 16 weeks' gestation the fundus is midway between the symphysis and the umbilicus. Uterine enlargement occurs in linear fashion (1 cm per week). The uterine fundus can be palpated at the umbilicus at approximately 20 weeks and measures 20 cm. By the 36th week the fundus is just below the ensiform cartilage and measures approximately 36 cm; the fundal height drops slightly near term (lightening). Measurement

may then no longer correspond with week of gestation. The uterus maintains a globular/ovoid shape throughout pregnancy.

- *Adnexa.* Discomfort may be noted with exam due to stretching of the round ligaments throughout pregnancy. The ovaries are not palpable once the uterus fills the pelvic cavity at 12 to 14 weeks' gestation.
- *Urinary.* The bladder may be palpable; frequency and incontinence are common, particularly with multiparity.
- *Rectal.* Increased vascular congestion with resulting hemorrhoids is often noted.
- *Musculoskeletal.* Increased relaxation of pelvic structures, lordosis, sciatica, and discomfort at the symphysis pubis are common. Pain from round ligament syndrome often noted at sulcus of thighs.
- *Endocrine.* May have mildly enlarged thyroid; however, diffusely enlarged thyroid nodularity or increased firmness is abnormal.

DIAGNOSTIC TESTS AND METHODS

To assess the development of the fetus and the well-being of the mother, the health care provider may use a variety of invasive and noninvasive tests.

Pregnancy Tests

It is important to diagnose pregnancy as early as possible to maximize the benefits from health care and minimize risks to the developing fetus (see Table 16–5 for a description of pregnancy tests) (Cunningham et al., 2001; Hatcher, 1998).

Human chorionic gonadotropin (hCG) is detected in pregnancy at about the time of implantation. Levels in normal pregnancy usually double every 48 to 72 hours; by the first missed period, serum values reach 50 to 250 mIU per mL. Levels peak at approximately 60 to 70 days postfertilization, then decrease to plateau at 100 to 130 days of pregnancy. Tests vary in sensitivity, specificity, and accuracy—influenced by the length of gestation, concentration of specimen, proteins or blood present, and some drugs. Human chorionic gonadotropin is composed of alpha and beta subunits. The alpha subunit of hCG reacts with the alpha subunits of luteinizing hormone (LH), follicle stimulating hormone (FSH), and thyrotropin (TSH) due to similar molecular structure. Tests that are specific for beta subunit are more accurate; serum tests are generally more sensitive and specific than urine tests.

Quantitative, serial measurements of serum *beta-human chorionic gonadotropin* (β-*hCG*) are valuable in documenting the viability of the gestation. Serum and urine tests specific for β-hCG have accuracy rates of 99 percent, with few false positives. With urine testing, early gestational age and decreased specimen concentration may yield false negatives (Table 16–5).

Technological advances in *ultrasonic imaging* (see Chapter 19) have enabled accurate evaluation or monitoring of several aspects of pregnancy (Scott et al., 1999).

- Early first trimester identification of intrauterine pregnancy, ectopic, and/or multiple pregnancy.
- Demonstration of growth and viability of the embryo.
- Identification and evaluation of uterine, fetal, and placental anomalies.
- Serial measurements to evaluate fetal growth.
- Evaluation of amniotic fluid levels.
- Biophysical profile to evaluate fetal well-being in later stages of pregnancy. Commonly recommended tests are described in Tables 16–6 and 16–7 (ACOG, 1997; Chernecky & Berger, 2001; Cunningham et al., 2001; James, 2001; Scott et al., 1999).

ASSESSMENT OF COMMON CONCERNS

The pregnant client may report common concerns in a multitude of areas. These concerns are mainly physical (see Chapter 17) and may include nausea and vomiting, fatigue, backache, constipation, and edema. Psychological/developmental concerns (see Chapter 17) may include changes in libido, emotional lability, and nightmares.

RISK ASSESSMENT

Assessment of a maternity client for risk factors encompasses physical, historical, and psychosocial aspects. The client at risk is identified, evaluated, and observed, with special consideration given to the course and outcome of pregnancy. Screening is done to detect genetic defects, to determine the risk of preterm labor and delivery, and to assess parental-fetal attachment and hazards in the environment and workplace. Screening should ideally be done at the initial visit, during each remaining trimester, and whenever necessary.

Genetic Screening

The purpose of genetic screening is to identify those at risk for an inherited or acquired defect and to identify

TABLE 16–5. Pregnancy Tests

Type	Specimen Source	Sensitivity (mIU/mL)	Example	Comments
Beta Subunit Radioimmunoassay (RIA).	Serum	5	Used mainly in hospitals and large outpatient laboratories.	Radioisotopes. *Uses:* Quantifies β-hCG. Serial measurements useful in determination of pregnancy viability, trophoblastic disease, ectopic pregnancy. *Specificity:* For β-hCG. No cross-reaction with LH, FSH, TSH. *Reliable:* 7 days postconception. *Time:* 1 to 2 hours, usually run in batches.
Enzyme-liked immunosorbent assay (ELISA); immunometric test.	Serum urine	25–100	Clearview hCG (Wampole), Icon II hCG (Wampole), Precise (Becton-Dickinson), Quick Vue (Quick 1), Testpack Plus hCG (Abbot).	Monoclonal antibodies; enzyme coupling. *Uses:* Serum tests quantify β-hCG and hCG. Same as RIA if -hCG specific; urine tests qualify β-hCG. *Specificity:* No cross-reaction with LH FSH, TSH if β-hCG specific. *Reliable:* 7 to 10 days postconception. *Time:* 1–7 minutes.
Agglutination inhibition tests.	Urine	150–2500	Pregnospia (Organon, UCG-Beta Slide (Wampole), β-hCG (Ortho), Pregnosticon (Organon).	Agglutination of coated latex particles and hCG antibodies. Positive if no agglutination occurs. *Uses:* Qualifies pregnancy. *Specificity:* Varies; if β-hCG specific, no cross-reaction to LH, FSH, TSH. Sensitivity set at higher levels to decrease cross-reaction in test to whole hCG molecule. *Reliable:* 14 to 21 days postconception. *Test:* 2 minutes.

Sources: Cunningham et al. (2001); Hatcher (1998).

unrecognized defects in healthy individuals. (Cunningham, et al., 2001). Genetic defects account for most of all first trimester spontaneous abortion. It is estimated that 3 to 5 percent of infants in the United States have recognizable defects present at birth. Up to 15 percent of all live births will reveal defects when assessed five to ten years after delivery (Cunningham et al., 2001; Gabbe et al., 2002). Approximately one-third of children in pediatric hospitals are treated for conditions that have a genetic component. Approximately 25 percent of birth defects are attributed to genetic factors, 15 percent to environmental factors, 30 percent to a combination of these—leaving 30 percent unaccountable. It is estimated that 50 percent of spontaneous abortions and 5 to 7 percent of intrauterine fetal deaths are caused by chromosomal abnormalities (Cunningham, et al., 2001; Mange & Mange, 1998).

Clients with potential risks (Figure 16–2) should receive further counseling, testing, education, and guidance in decision making (ACOG, 2001a; Mange & Mange, 1998).

Tools for the Detection and Diagnosis of Genetic Defects (Also See Chapter 19)

- *Family Pedigree.* A graphic record of family medical history may reveal an inheritance pattern and help to identify whether further laboratory testing and clinical evaluation are needed (Mange & Mange, 1998).
- *Alpha-fetoprotein.* Levels of a α-fetoprotein circulating in maternal serum or amniotic fluid are evaluated in relation to gestational age, maternal age, weight, race, presence of diabetes, or previous history of neural tube defects. Increased levels may indicate neural tube defect (NTD), Turner's syndrome,

TABLE 16–6. Laboratory and Diagnostic Tests Often Performed during Pregnancy

Test	Nonpregnant Values	Pregnant Values	Implications for Mother/Fetus
Cervix-Vagina			
Chlamydia	Negative	Negative	Culture remains gold standard for diagnosis; neonatal infection; implicated preterm labor.
Gonorrhea	Negative	Negative	Culture remains gold standard for diagnosis; neonatal infection; implicated in preterm labor, spontaneous abortion, ectopic pregnancy, chorioamnionitis, IUGR.
Group beta strep	Negative	Negative	May be considered normal vaginal flora in a client who is not pregnant, however, neonatal infection can be fatal; implicated in preterm labor, chorioamnionitis, UTI, endomyometritis.
Herpes simplex genitalis	Negative	Negative	Neonatal infection can be fatal. Implicated in preterm labor and spontaneous abortions. Primary infection third trimester carries higher fetal/neonatal risk.
Listeria	Negative	Negative	Strong association with intrauterine fetal demise (IUFD); preterm delivery and chorioamnionitis. Congenital defects not widely noted. Found in unpasteurized dairy products.
Mycoplasma	Negative	Negative	May be considered normal vaginal flora in a client who is not pregnant; however, implicated in spontaneous abortions; controversial rare cause of anencephaly, stillbirth.
Bacterial vaginosis	Negative	Negative	Condition marked by shift in normal vaginal flora from predominence of lactobacilli to anaerobes. Implicated in PROM, preterm birth, endometritis.
Trichomonas	Negative	Negative	Controversial cause of LBW, PROM.
Serology			
Antibody screen	Negative	Negative	Positive screen indicates sensitization; done at initial and 28th week visits, and after maternal fetal blood exchange in Rh-negative woman.
Cytomegalovirus	Negative	Stable titer	Majority demonstrate immunity; maternal immunity does not prevent congenital infection; primary infection is more severe for fetus; cytomegalic inclusion disease is evident in 5–10 percent of those affected; overall fetal morbidity, cost factors, predictability of occurrence/recurrence limit use of this testing.
Hepatitis	Negative	Negative	If positive screen in HB_sAg or HB_cAg, IgM titer to assess active, chronic, convalescent states; the presence of anti-HB_c IgG indicates previous infection; anti-HB_s is positive only in those with successful vaccination; transplacental transmission is rare; neonatal infection can occur. Screen for HCV is those at risk.
Rubella	Immunity greater than 1:10	Stable titer	If nonimmune, vaccinate postpartum, compatible with breastfeeding. No evidence amassed of adverse consequence noted in infants or pregnancies inadvertently vaccinated first trimester. Infection during first trimester associated with high rates of spontaneous abortion and congenital malformation.
Syphilis	Nonreactive	Nonreactive	If reactive, perform FTA-ABS test or MHA-TP to confirm presence of *Treponema pallidum* organism; if woman is untreated, approximately 25 percent of offspring die in utero, 25 percent perinatally/neonatally, 40 percent develop syphilis; long-term sequelae beginning in newborn.
Toxoplasmosis (IgG titer)	Negative	Stable titer	If positive, repeat titer in 2 weeks: An 8-fold increase in IgG, or positive IgM titer, indicates active infection; more virulent if new infection during first trimester, but less frequent; less than 10 percent of infants infected third trimester display disease; for woman with risk of exposure to seropositive cats or uncooked meat and eggs.
HIV (ELISA)	Nonreactive	Nonreactive	Immunofloresence, Western Blot confirm diagnosis; mandatory in many states to offer testing; recent studies indicate AZT given in pregnancy to infected woman reduces vertical transmission to fetus; virus can be transmitted via breast milk to neonate. False negative confirmed by polymerase chain reaction (PCR) testing.

TABLE 16–6. (*cont.*)

Test	Nonpregnant Values	Pregnant Values	Implications for Mother/Fetus
Type/Rh	A+ A− B+ B− 0+ 0− AB+ AB−		If Rh negative, screen for antibodies; ABO incompatibility usually result of O woman carrying an A or B fetus; degree of hemolysis is usually mild.
Fifth disease (erythema infectiosum) IgM titer	Immune	Stable titer	Human parvovirus B19; controversial rare cause of fetal aplastic anemia and nonimmune hydrops; 50 percent of women are immune. Follow exposed, at risk women who are IgM positive, IgG negative, for perinatal sequelae.

Hematology

Test	Nonpregnant Values	Pregnant Values	Implications for Mother/Fetus
Red blood cell count	3.5–5.5/mm^3	Increases 20 percent by term	Stable during pregnancy.
White blood cell count	4.5–11/mm^3	5–12/mm^3; may increase	Values of up to 25 mm^3 have been noted during labor.
Hematocrit	37–47/percent	28.6–38.4 percent	Decreased values reflect overall 50 percent increase in plasma volume—physiological anemia.
Hemoglobin	12–16 g/dL	11–16 g/dL	Increased oxygen carrying capacity of red blood cells compensates for volume expansion.
Platelets	250,000–500,000/mm^3		May decrease with severe preeclampsia. Rule out immune thrombocytopenic purpura (ITP).
Hemoglobin A1c	4.0–8.2 percent	6.5 percent	Measure of long-term glucose control in identified gestational diabetic; changes are seen in 3–5 weeks after optimal diet and insulin control; not accurate in diabetics with chronic renal failure or disease that impairs erythrocytes.

Hemoglobin electrophoresis	HgbA1
	  96–98.5 percent;
	HgbA2
	  1.5–4.0 percent;
	HgbF
	  0–2.0 percent
		Same	Detects amounts of hemoglobin normally found and presence of HgbS HgbC; diagnosis of trait and disease is dependent on percentage of types to HgbA; screen all African American, Mediterranean, Asian women; occasionally noted in white population.

Blood Chemistry

Test	Nonpregnant Values	Pregnant Values	Implications for Mother/Fetus
Alkaline phosphatase (Total)	12–63 IU/L	May double	Elevated in liver conditions; increases due to placental involvement; in diseases involving connective tissue.
Blood urea nitrogen (BUN)	10–15 mg/dL	8–10 mg/dL	Pregnant values are lower due to increased glomerular filtration rate. In pregnancy induced hypertension (PIH), values increase to nonpregnant levels due to pathological arterial spasm and vasoconstriction.
Cholesterol	130–200 mg/dL	243–305 mg/dL	Accurate levels not reflected in pregnancy.
Creatinine	0.8 mg/dL	0.5–0.7 mg/dL	Pregnant values are lower due to increased glomerular filtration rate. In PIH, values increase to nonpregnant levels due to pathological arterial spasm and vasoconstriction.
Iron—serum	60–160 mcg/dL	Decrease	Iron demands increase during pregnancy.
Lactate dehydrogenase (LDH)	30–200 IU/L		Elevated in various conditions, especially those with tissue destruction, hypoxia, or an inflammatory process; seen in heparin therapy.
Serum alanine aminotransferase (ALT, SGPT)	3–35 IU/L		Used primarily to monitor the liver; may increase in severe preeclampsia.
Serum aspartate aminotransferase (AST, SGOT)	5–40 IU/L	May decrease	Elevated in conditions where cardiac or hepatic damage occurs; also elevated post IM injections; may also be depressed in diabetic ketoacidosis (DKA) and beriberi.
Thyroid panel: triiodothyronine (T$_3$)	24–35 percent	Decrease	Due to increase of thyroid binding globulins by estrogen.
Thyroxine (T$_4$)	5.3–14.5 mcg/dL	Increase	Basal metabolic rate increases by 25 percent; increased thyroid binding globulins.
Thyrotropin (TSH)	0.5–10 mcU/mL		Most sensitive indicator for hypothyroid/hyperthyroid states in pregnancy.

TABLE 16–6. (*cont.*)

Test	Nonpregnant Values	Pregnant Values	Implications for Mother/Fetus
Total iron binding capacity (TIBC)	250–460 mcg/dL	Increase	Estrogen increases ability for iron to bind to transferrin, which regulates transport in the body.
Uric Acid	4.2–6.0 mg/dL	3.0–4.2 mg/dL	Pregnant values are lower due to increased glomerular filtration rate. In PIH, values increase to nonpregnant levels due to pathological arterial spasm and vasoconstriction.

Urinalysis

Test	Nonpregnant Values	Pregnant Values	Implications for Mother/Fetus
Albumin	Negative	Less than 100 mg/24 h	Elevations seen in preeclampsia and urinary tract infections.
Chloride	170–250 mEg/24 h	Slight increase	Due to increased glomerular filtration rate.
Creatinine	1.0–1.8 g/24 h	Elevated	Due to increased glomerular filtration rate.
Glucose	120 g/24 h	Elevated	Due to decrease renal threshold and increased glomerular filtration rate.
Ketones	Negative	Same	Presence may indicate dehydration; starvation states; ketoacidosis in insulin-dependent diabetic; strenuous exercise.
White blood cells	Less than 1–3 per high power field	Same	Often vaginal contamination, urinary tract infection if other indicators.
Red blood cells	Less than 2–3 per high power field	Same	Presence may be due to violent exercise, kidney trauma, systemic or renal disease.
Bacteria	Greater than 100,000 colonies/mL	Greater than 10,000 colonies/mL	Infection if same species.
Nitrites	Negative	Negative	Some bacteria convert urine nitrates into nitrites in the bladder. Positive indicates infection. Urine must be retained in the bladder several hours for conversion to occur. Gram positive cocci do not produce nitrites, *E. coli* may.

Note: HCV = hepatitis C virus; IUGR = intrauterine growth retardation; UTI = urinary tract infection; PROM = premature rupture of membranes; LBW = low birth weight; HB$_s$Ag = hepatitis B surface antigen; HB$_c$Ag = hepatitis B core antigen; IG = immunoglobulin; FTA−ABS = fluorescent treponemal antibody absorption; MHA−TP = microhemagglutination assay for antibody to *Treponema pallidium*; PCR = polymerase chain reaction.

Sources: ACOG (1997), Chernecky & Berger (2001), Cunningham et al. (2001), James (2001), Scott et al. (1999).

oomphalocele, tetralogy of fallot. Decreased levels may indicate Down syndrome, trisomy 18. In decreased levels, a tetra serum of MSAFP, BHCG, unconjugated estrodial and dimeric inhibin A (DIA) increases the sensitivity of testing (Haddow et al., 1998; Mishell & Brenner, 2001).

◆ *Amniocentesis.* Fluid aspirated from the amniotic sac has multiple test applications such as chromosome analysis, karyotype, α-fetoprotein, deoxyribonucleic acid (DNA) markers, viral studies, biochemical linkage assays, and inborn errors of metabolism (Mange & Mange, 1998).

◆ *Chorionic Villus Sampling.* Transcervical aspiration of chorionic villi permits results for the same test as does amniocentesis, with the exception of -fetoprotein results (Mange & Mange, 1998).

◆ *Fetal Blood Sampling.* Improvements in ultrasound technology allow for percutaneous umbilical blood sampling (PUBS) of the fetus. Used to diagnose hemophilia A, various immunologic diseases in which fetal blood not contaminated with amniotic fluid is needed (Creasy & Resnick, 1998).

◆ *Level 2 Ultrasound/Fetal Scan.* Indirect visualization of the fetus enables evaluation of overt, structural changes; it is usually performed in a tertiary setting (Mange & Mange, 1998).

◆ *Fetoscopy.* Direct visualization of the fetus and placenta allows for tissue sampling or limited interventions with the fetus in life threatening situations. Fetoscopy is rarely used since the advent of recombinant DNA techniques and amniocentesis. The risk of miscarriage with fetoscopy is 3 to 5 percent higher than with amniocentesis or chorionic villus sampling (Gabbe et al., 2002; Scott et al., 1999).

Preterm Labor Screening

The demographic, historical, and psychosocial factors associated with increased incidence of preterm labor and delivery are assessed with preterm screening. *Preterm labor* is the presence of regular uterine contractions causing cervical dilation and effacement prior to 37 completed weeks' gestation and after 20 completed weeks. The etiology of preterm labor is unknown. Current

TABLE 16–7. Additional Tests Often Carried Out During Pregnancy

Test	Values	Significance	Implications
Cystic fibrosis Carrier testing profile	Tests for 34 of the most common CF mutations	Risk for cystic fibrosis carrier status	An abnormal value is followed by screening of the father of the baby. If the father of the baby is tested positive, chorionic villus sampling or amniocentesis can be performed to determine if the fetus is affected.
Maternal serum α-fetoprotein (MSAFP Tetra)	Less than 0.4 MOM (multiples of the mean	At risk for aneuploidy Down syndrome, trisomy 18	Relative to maternal weight, age, race, gestational dating, diabetic status, singleton vs. multiple gestation. A tetra screen aids in the detection of chromosomal abnormalities in low MSAFP. BHCG unconjugated estriol and Dimeric inhibin A (DIA) measurements viewed in relation to MSAFP value increase sensitivity of test.
	0.4–2.5 MOM	Normal range is 85 to 95 percent	Margin of error is 5–15 percent.
	Greater than 2.5 MOM	At risk for neural tube defect, Turners syndrome, abdominal wall defect, esophageal atresia. May indicate risk for PTB, IUGR, pregnancy loss.	All abnormal values should be evaluated selectively by ultrasound, fetal scan, and amniocentesis; identified strong family/maternal history of neural tube defect.
Fasting blood sugar (FBS)	70–105 mg/dL	≥ 105 mg/dL elevated	Not valuable in healthy pregnancy.
1-hour glucose tolerance test (GTT)	135–140 mg/dL	≥ 140 mg/dL elevated	Suspicious for diagnosis of gestation diabetes. Screening done at 24–28 weeks' gestation; screen earlier if H/O[a] 4000-g infant, history of gestational diabetes, or previous fetal death. Repeat 24–28 weeks if initial screen normal.
3-hour GTT			Diagnostic of gestational diabetes.
FBS	70–105 mg/dL	≥ 105 mg/dL elevated	Requires fasting 8 hours prior to testing. Carbohydrate loading of 200–300 gram/day for 3 days prior to testing increases sensitivity of test.
1 h	120–190 mg/dL	≥ 190 mg/dL elevated	Elevated FBS is indicator of probable need for insulin therapy.
2 h	120–165 mg/dL	≥ 165 mg/dL elevated	Criterion: Requires treatment if 2 of the 4 values are elevated.
3 h	70–145 mg/dL	≥ 145 mg/dL elevated	

[a]H/O = history of; PTB = preterm birth; IUGR = intrauterine growth retardation; BHCG = beta human chorionic gonadotropin

Sources: Chernecky & Berger (2001); Cunningham et al. (2001); Haddow, Palomaki, Knight, Foster, Neveux (1998); Mishell & Brenner (2001); Scott et al. (1999).

estimates are that preterm labor occurs in 8 to 17 percent of women (Gabbe et al., 2002). Perinatal morbidity/mortality increase as length of gestation decreases. Even with the most advanced technology, outcomes are poor for gestations of fewer than 26 weeks. Long-term sequelae such as chronic respiratory and neurological handicaps, blindness, learning disabilities, and financial strain are often reported (Creasy & Resnick, 1998; Cunningham et al., 2001). Parental emotional and financial strain may be significant.

The incidence of preterm labor and delivery may be reduced by early identification of risk factors, continuous assessment of physical changes, education, and treatment that reduces controllable risk factors. A screening tool is illustrated in Table 16–8 (Creasy & Resnick, 1998). If one or more major factors, or two or more minor factors, are present, the client is identified as belonging to a high risk group. (For further information on diagnosis and treatment, see Chapter 18.)

Assessment of Parental-Fetal Attachment

Assessing parental-fetal attachment may help to identify a family at risk for maladaptive behaviors in relation to the developmental tasks of pregnancy. The major developmental task for the family is achieving a strong sense

TABLE 16–8. Major and Minor Risk Factors in the Prediction of Spontaneous Preterm Labor

Major	Minor
Multiple gestation	Febrile illness
Diethylstilbestrol (DES) exposure	Bleeding after 12 weeks' gestation
Hydramnios	History of pylonephritis
Uterine anomaly	Cigarette smoking—more than
Cervic dilated more than 1 cm	10 per day
at 32 weeks' gestation	Second trimester abortion
2 second-trimester abortions	More than 2 first-trimester abortions
Previous preterm delivery	
Previous preterm labor	
Abdominal surgery during pregnancy	
History of cone biopsy	
Cervical shortening of less than 1 cm	
at 32 weeks' gestation	
Uterine irritability	
Cocaine abuse	

Note: Presence of one or more major factors and/or two or more minor factors places client in high risk group.

Source: Creasy & Resnick (1998).

of self (differentiation), while maintaining psychological and physical closeness (attachment). Another task is establishing a safe environment for the family unit (Lindigren, 2001).

Major risk factors for maladaptive behaviors are unintended pregnancy, marital discord or family violence, sexually transmitted disease, limited finances, substance abuse, positive HIV status, and adolescence. Other risk factors include poor social support system and educational background, adverse pregnancy outcome, or conditions that interfere with the ability to reason effectively (ACOG, 2001b; Cunningham et al., 2001; Lindigren, 2001). *All* women have the potential for maladaptive behaviors during pregnancy; therefore, interventions are directed toward reducing the effect of situations that lead to maladjustment.

Family assessment tools may provide a means for identifying women at risk for less than optimal maternal-fetal and maternal-infant attachment (Lindigren, 2001). These tools can be found in listed reference.

- *The Family Environment Scale* uses self-reporting to assess the internal family milieu.
- *The Card Sort Procedure* measures how family members relate to one another through a group problem-solving task.
- *The Support System Questionnaire* assesses the support system within the family, assesses outside influences on the family, and identifies family members at perinatal risk.

Assessment of Environmental and Occupational Hazards

The environmental and occupational factors that place mother and fetus at risk for injury or death need to be identified. Women of childbearing age comprise a significant proportion of the U.S. work force. Women are exposed to chemicals and infectious agents, demanding labor, and often less than ideal working conditions. Assessment should be made of the possible exposure to teratogens, physical demands of employment, and the workplace environment (Cunningham et al., 2001; Worthington, 2001).

Teratogens are substances or disorders with the potential to alter the fetus permanently in form or function (Worthington, 2001). Strongly suspected teratogens include various drugs, chemicals, infectious agents, heavy metals such as lead, and selected maternal disorders. Often the effect is dose related; the effect is greatest during fetal organogenesis (see Chapter 17).

Physically intensive employment increases the likelihood of low birthweight and preterm labor and delivery. Standing for long periods; increased pulling, pushing, or lifting of more than 10 to 25 pounds; and decreased rest periods also increase these risks (Cunningham et al., 2001). The physical setting needs to be assessed for risks of falling or being crushed; exposure to temperature extremes; and exposure to teratogens such as radiation, chemicals, or infectious agents (Worthington, 2001).

Recommended favorable working conditions for pregnant women include:

- Work only eight-hour shifts: no more than 48 hours per week, ideally less than 40 hours per week.
- Limit hours of work to between 6 A.M. and midnight.
- Take at least two 10-minute rest periods and one nutrition break per shift, with adequate rest facilities available.
- Avoid occupations that involve heavy lifting, hard physical labor, continuous standing, or constant moving about.
- Do not work in places where a good sense of balance is required for job safety, or where there is exposure to toxic substances.
- Be aware that substances permissible by state codes for a nonpregnant individual may be *unsafe* for a pregnant woman and a developing fetus. The Occupational Safety and Health Administration (OSHA) can answer questions about specific substances and situations (see Chapter 17).

PSYCHOSOCIAL ASSESSMENT AND INTERVENTIONS

During the first trimester, assess the meaning of pregnancy to the client and the positive, negative, or ambivalent feelings she may have, particularly if her pregnancy is unplanned (Sherwen, Scolveno, Toussie-Wengartan, 1999). Explore her feelings about this pregnancy, her economic concerns, and her level of anxiety. Validate the pregnancy with and help her to identify her support systems. Suggest childbirth education classes; begin anticipatory guidance counseling (see Chapter 17).

During the second trimester, assess the client's adaptation to pregnancy and to the body changes she has experienced. Explain how fetal growth/development and the client's own body/emotional changes will facilitate adaptation.

During the third trimester, determine how well the client is prepared for birth, delivery, and the physical needs of a newborn including infant feeding and child care needs. Explore her expectations about labor, birth, and the newborn—and her fears concerning motherhood, pain of labor, loss of control, and harm to herself or the fetus. Begin planning for postpartal contraception.

Domestic Violence

Throughout pregnancy, assess for subtle and overt signs of physical, sexual and emotional abuse (Durant, Colley, Saltzman, & Johnson, 2000; Huth-Bucks, Levendosky, & Bogat, 2002; McFarlane, & Parker, 1994; Price & Baird, 2001). The five-question *Abuse Assessment Screen* (Figure 16–3) may help to identify abused clients. The incidence of abuse is high but often goes unreported. It is estimated that abuse occurs in one out of six pregnancies, often occurring/escalating initially during pregnancy. The risk/incidence of abuse increases in the presence of alcohol and substance abuse.

Abused women are less likely to seek prenatal care or follow medical advice. Abuse places the mother and fetus at risk for perinatal complications, injury, homicide, and suicide.

DIETARY ASSESSMENT

A well-balanced diet is essential to optimal nutrition for maternal well-being and fetal growth (see also Chapter 17). Requirements during pregnancy include daily servings of dairy products, meat products, fruits/vegetables, and grains/bread. Routine dietary supplements also are required during pregnancy. Mega vitamin/mineral supplements are to be avoided.

It is always desirable that maternal weight gain and fetal growth be adequate; that appropriate weight be achieved by the neonate, depending on gestation age; that labor and delivery do not occur preterm; and that the mother be normotensive with stable hemoglobin. However, inadequate nutrition may place the client at risk for having a low birthweight infant, preterm labor, pregnancy induced hypertension, and anemia with resulting sequelae (Ramachandran, 2002; Scott et al., 1999).

PREPARATION FOR SURGICAL INTERVENTION

Complications related to fetal distress and failure for labor to progress at delivery are the primary reasons for surgical intervention. Surgical options include cesarean section, episiotomy, and forceps birth. Maternal medical conditions unrelated to pregnancy, such as appendicitis, also may necessitate surgery. Counsel clients at risk about the reasons for an episiotomy at delivery and the care involved; discuss cesarean birth with clients whose medical conditions predispose them to this type of delivery. For those needing forceps delivery, instruction is given at the time of delivery. *Providing in-depth education concerning surgical intervention to clients not at risk may add to their anxiety level.*

Cesarean Birth

Any condition that prevents the safe passage of the fetus through the birth canal or that seriously compromises maternal-fetal well-being may be an indication for cesarean birth. Examples include breech and transverse presentations, maternal-fetal hemorrhage, fetal distress, active genital herpes infection, severely impaired maternal cardiac status, cephalopelvic disproportion, placenta previa, and placental abruption (Creasy & Resnick, 1998; Cunningham et al., 2001).

Implications. It is estimated that one out of five deliveries in the United States is by cesarean birth. Statistics vary regionally. Several factors may explain the increase that has occurred.

◆ Reduced parity with greater numbers of nulliparous women.
◆ Electronic fetal monitoring (EFM), which facilitates detection of fetal distress.
◆ Repeat cesarean deliveries, usually with prior classical incision.

ABUSE ASSESSMENT SCREEN

1. Have you **ever** been emotionally or physically abused by your partner or someone important to you?

YES ☐ NO ☐

2. **WITHIN THE LAST YEAR,**
   have you been hit, slapped, kicked, or otherwise physically hurt by someone?   YES ☐ NO ☐
   If YES, by whom?_____ Total number of times_____

3. Since you've been pregnant, were you hit, slapped, kicked, or otherwise
   physically hurt by someone?   YES ☐ NO ☐
   If YES, by whom?_____ Total number of times_____

MARK THE AREA OF INJURY ON THE BODY MAP. SCORE EACH INCIDENT ACCORDING TO THE FOLLOWING SCALE:

SCORE

1= Threats of abuse including use
   of a weapon

2= Slapping, pushing; no
   injuries and/or lasting pain

3= Punching, kicking, bruises,
   cuts and/or continuing pain

4= Beating up, severe
   contusions,
   burns, broken bones

5= Head injury, internal injury,
   permanent injury

6= Use of weapon; wound from
   weapon

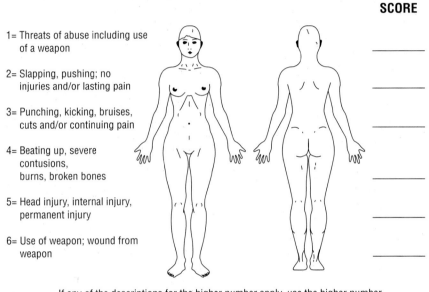

If any of the descriptions for the higher number apply, use the higher number.

4. **WITHIN THE LAST YEAR,**
   has anyone forced you to have sexual activities?   YES ☐ NO ☐
   If YES, who? _____ Total number of times _____

5. Are you afraid of your partner or anyone you listed above?   YES ☐ NO ☐

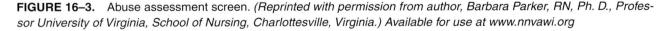

Developed by the Nursing Research Consortium on Violence and Abuse. Readers are encouraged to reproduce and use this assessment tool.

FIGURE 16–3. Abuse assessment screen. *(Reprinted with permission from author, Barbara Parker, RN, Ph. D., Professor University of Virginia, School of Nursing, Charlottesville, Virginia.) Available for use at www.nnvawi.org*

- ◆ Fewer forceps deliveries.
- ◆ More advanced-age pregnancies.
- ◆ Greater threat and incidence of legal malpractice suits.

Surgery is done under regional or general anesthesia with combination cold-knife, electrocautery techniques. Vaginal birth after cesarean birth (VBAC) is common today, as most surgeons employ a low transverse uterine incision to deliver the infant. The vertical, or classical, incision requires cesarean birth for subsequent births, as the uterus is more likely to rupture during active labor.

Side Effects and Adverse Reactions. The side effects of a cesarean birth are related to infection, hemorrhage, embolus, injury to proximal organs, and anesthesia. Studies in maternal mortality statistics vary, with approximately 5 to 40 per 100,000 cesarean births. Select studies show substantially lower rates of maternal mortality related to the cesarean section itself.

Contraindications. Vaginal delivery is preferred in cases of maternal coagulopathies, or when the fetus has died or is too premature to survive outside the uterus.

Counseling. Inform the client about the procedure and its rationale, anesthesia, recovery, and postoperative care. Explain how the surgery will affect the newborn, breastfeeding, and activities of daily living. Also explain that signs of infection/complication will be monitored.

THE DEVELOPMENTAL STAGES OF PREGNANCY

Maternal role attainment is not an inevitable, instinctive event initiated by the act of birth; instead it is an active process requiring personal motivation. It is believed that the "roots" of this role develop during childhood. During pregnancy a woman actively works on assuming the behaviors she believes encompass the "ideal" mother (Attrill, 2002; Gay, Edgil, & Douglas, 1988; Rubin, 1984; Sherwen et al., 1999).

MAJOR THEORIES OF MATERNAL ROLE DEVELOPMENT

Two leading theorists in maternal role development are Reva Rubin and Regina Lederman.

Reva Rubin's contributions to maternity nursing provide valuable insights into the biopsychosocial experience of childbearing. Rubin developed a framework for the process of maternal role assumption in 1967, although she published from 1961 to 1984. Her early publications *Basic Maternal Behaviors* and *Maternal Touch* are considered classics in maternity nursing (Gay et al., 1988).

Rubin's writings include concepts about body image, self-esteem, and thought process during pregnancy, as well as assumption of the maternal role prior to and after delivery (Gay et al., 1988). Without the desire for children, there is no active motivation to assume a maternal role. Rubin identified maternal tasks and behaviors normally seen during the antepartum and postpartum periods. Assessment of those behaviors can be used to evaluate the mother's progress toward assumption of a maternal role (see Table 16–9) (Gay et al., 1988; Rubin, 1984; Sherwen et al., 1999). Rubin concluded that if the mother perceived a threat to her pregnancy, such as HIV infection or miscarriage, then she was less likely to bond with her infant and therefore was at risk for poor attachment.

When Rubin made her initial observations of maternal behaviors, strong consumer participation in childbirth education and health care was in its infancy. Today, childbearing couples have the option of knowing the gender of their fetus, see their fetus through the technology of ultrasound, and are more knowledgeable and less passive than

TABLE 16–9. Reva Rubin Theory: the Antepartum Phase

Trimester	Maternal Task/Behavior	Nursing Significance
First	"Who me?" "Pregnant?" "Now?"	Question of identity—conception thought to be a surprise—resulting ambivalence related to the reality of pregnancy. Incorporation of concept of fetus into self. Acceptance of pregnancy/fetus by self and significant others.
Second	Seeking safe passage for self and child. Ensuring the acceptance of the child fetus. Protective behaviors by the mother for the child.	Acceptance of growing fetus by self, others. Willingness to "house" fetus even with body/role/ego changes. Passage of socially accepted values, behaviors, attitudes, skills from mother to child.
Third	Mother's binding-in to her unknown child. Learning to give of self.	"Binding-in" developed from initial maternal-fetal bonds to adult-child companionship. These bonds include fetal movements, maternal anatomic changes. Nurturant behaviors given from mother to child.

Sources: Gay et al. (1988), Rubin (1984), Sherwen (1999).

parents of previous generations. Ultimately, some of Rubin's observations may have less relevance for contemporary women, but they are a timeless framework for family-centered maternity care. Using Reva Rubin's three postpartum developmental phases, a mother's progress during the postpartum period may be assessed (Gay et al., 1988; Rubin, 1984; Sherwen et al., 1999). (The three phases and their characteristic behaviors are described in Table 16–10.)

Regina Lederman views maternal role assumption as identification with motherhood; namely, as part of the larger process of psychosocial development in pregnancy that includes taking the developmental step from being a woman without child to being a woman with child (Lederman, 1996). This process is a progressive change in thinking for the mother, away from concerns about self and more toward concern for the mother-infant unit. Two important factors come into play to achieve this goal: motivation and the degree of preparation for the mothering role.

According to Lederman, motivation for motherhood is reflected by the degree to which one expresses the interest and the ability to nurture and empathize with a child. This encompasses the perception of motherhood as a life fulfilling event (Lederman, 1996). The woman's motivation for pregnancy is questioned if her thoughts toward the child (fetus) are infrequent, aversive, avoided or denied, or if the woman desires the pregnancy but not the child.

Preparation for motherhood involves acquiring the ability to see oneself as a mother (Lederman, 1996). This is accomplished through *fantasizing/dreaming,* which is an arena for rehearsing motherhood skills. The woman relies on her life experiences of being nurtured and on her ability to identify with other women in their positive role as mothers. According to Lederman, all women bring conflicts to a pregnancy. But if the conflicts are not re-solved through preparation and bargaining during pregnancy, then the woman may find the motherhood role unrewarding, thereby increasing her feelings of inadequacy.

Lederman describes a woman's relationship with her own mother as the final aspect of maternal role development. The availability of the client's own mother, her acceptance of that pregnancy, her respect for the daughter's autonomy, and her willingness to share her previous childbearing/childrearing experiences all impact the outcome of preparation (Lederman, 1996).

Rubin's and Lederman's frameworks are generally considered compatible, although they use different names for similar concepts. Absence of these processes or inability to pass through them satisfactorily may impede the progress of maternal role development (Lederman, 1996; Rubin, 1984; Sherwen et al., 1999). This recognition is fundamental for nursing assessment during pregnancy and the postpartum period.

Implications of Rubin's and Lederman's Theories

- ◆ Identify whether the client is at higher risk for maladaptation at initial and ongoing prenatal visits.
- ◆ Monitor the client's progress by observing for expected role behaviors.
- ◆ When maladaptive behaviors are identified, refer the client for appropriate counseling.

PREPARATION FOR CHILDBIRTH: COUNSELING AND CLASSES

The prospect of having a problem-free pregnancy and healthy baby is aided by early and complete prenatal education. Maternal expectations of labor and delivery based on prenatal experience/knowledge are predictive of postpartum maternal-infant attachment. The primary goal of

TABLE 16–10. Reva Rubin Theory: The Postpartum Phase

Phase	Behaviors
Taking in	Passive, receptive, dependent infant mode; sleep, food are paramount. Often thought to be a process of regeneration. Mother spends time claiming her infant, bringing the infant into her social fabric. Mother begins with initial touching activities: first fingertips then to whole-hand touching within days 1 to 5 postdelivery.
Taking hold	Increased autonomy, independence usually begin on third day postpartum. Characterized by accomplishing what must be done over the next 2 to 3 weeks of the postpartum period. Mother demonstrates mastery of her own body's functioning, readiness to master some of her many tasks of motherhood.
Letting go	Starts during second and third weeks postdelivery. Mother begins to separate herself from the symbiotic relationship she and her infant enjoyed during pregnancy/delivery. Prior to this point, guilt was predominate feeling for the mother when separated from her infant.

Sources: Gay et al. (1988), Rubin (1984), Sherwen et al. (1999).

childbirth education classes is to reduce the fear-pain-tension cycle and make the childbirth experience a positive one—and thereby facilitate maternal-infant attachment (ACOG, 2001b).

Prior to the 19th century, childbirth was a social event, centered in the home with family members and friends. That changed, but by the 1960s women began to question the extensive procedures and strong medications often used for hospital managed labor and delivery. Women began to change the rigid structure of medical practice.

Society was finally ready for the 1944 classic by Grantley Dick-Read, *Childbirth without Fear,* which espoused that the pain of labor could be eliminated by reducing the fear, apprehension, and tension associated with childbirth. The underlying principle behind childbirth education is that the woman can use skills and intellect to control her body during childbirth (ACOG, 1997; Lederman, 1996).

STRATEGIES FOR PREPARATION

In *childbirth preparation classes,* accurate information is provided about the physiological and psychological adaptations that occur during parturition (ACOG, 1997; Pillitteri, 1999; Sherwen, 1999). Only information pertinent to managing labor and delivery process is included. In *prenatal parenting classes,* on the other hand, discussions may include a variety of topics surrounding parenting. In addition, comprehensive formats may be presented as re-

TABLE 16–11. Subjects Commonly Covered in Prenatal Classes

Anatomy and physiology of reproduction
Physiological and psychological changes during pregnancy
Sexuality during pregnancy
Nutritional needs
Teratogens and their impact on the fetus
Danger signs in pregnancy
Fetal growth and development
Role of the father and siblings
Prenatal exercise
Signs and stages of labor
Preparation for labor and delivery
Cesarean delivery
Postpartum support groups/parenting skills
Infant care
Infant safety/first aid/cardiopulmonary resuscitation (CPR)
Postpartum family planning

Sources: ACOG (1997), Lederman (1996), Sherwen et al. (1999).

fresher courses. How many clients pursue some form of prenatal education with their first baby is not known.

The education may be sought in a traditional classroom, from a resource book at the library, or from group sessions organized by local health departments. Programs are also offered by hospitals, community agencies and groups, or individuals qualified to teach childbirth education. The participation of health care providers and obstetric staff nurses as educators is desirable to ensure continuity of care and consistency of childbirth preparation instruction (see Table 16–11). To help ensure that a client is adequately prepared for childbirth, the health care provider may implement various strategies.

- During the initial prenatal evaluation, encourage enrollment in a prenatal class.
- Provide the client with resources according to her assessed knowledge level and financial ability.
- Provide prenatal counseling on an individual basis during ongoing prenatal visits.
- Supply pertinent pamphlets regarding pregnancy concerns throughout antepartum care.
- Act as role model and client advocate to encourage the client's educational responsibility.
- Periodically evaluate the client's knowledge deficits and intervene when appropriate.

CHILDBIRTH METHODS

Some couples will need help choosing birth preparation classes; they may be confronted with many alternatives. Childbirth education classes, such as Bradley (partner coached) and Lamaze (psychoprophylactic) techniques serve the dual purpose of explaining the birth process and dispelling fears concerning labor and delivery (ACOG, 1997; Caton, Corry, Frigoletto et al, 2002).

The Lamaze Method

Classes in the Lamaze method or "prepared childbirth classes" are the most popular. This method uses techniques that focus the mother's attention on breathing and relaxation exercises as well as massage (ACOG, 1997; Caton et al., 2002). Consequently, the perception of pain is lessened, as is the amount of medication needed for pain relief. The father's presence and active support during the birthing process can heighten the sense of family at the moment of birth, thereby increasing the perception of a positive birthing experience. Partner or coach involvement is a fundamental cornerstone of both methods.

The Bradley Method

The primary goal of the Bradley method is a completely unmedicated labor and delivery. The training techniques are directed toward the coach, not the mother. The coach is educated in massage/comfort techniques to use during labor and delivery.

Hypnobirthing

Hypnobirthing is not unlike other childbirth techniques. The program teaches women how to use their natural ability to give birth. Hypnobirthing involves relaxation techniques and natural childbirth education enhanced by hypnosis. The education program can involve classes, which use video demonstration as well as professional instruction, and also audiotapes on self-hypnosis (Mongan, 2002).

Other Options

The Read method, or "natural" childbirth, is also based on relaxation and breathing technique; the Wright method, based on psychoprophylaxis but with less active breathing than that in the Lamaze method, is also called "new childbirth." Sheila Kitzinger's psychosexual method includes chest breathing and simultaneous abdominal release. Yoga can also be used to aid in childbirth.

In counseling the client regarding the many approaches to childbirth education, it is paramount to consider her readiness to learn, knowledge base, attitudes and fears about pregnancy, and the support systems available to her. It is an ongoing process, begun at the initial prenatal evaluation.

ADOLESCENT PREGNANCY

Adolescent pregnancy is usually defined as pregnancy occurring between the age of menarche and 19 years of age, but it also can be viewed in relation to emotional maturity and financial independence. Most adolescent pregnancy is unintended. Often adolescent mothers and their babies form a nontraditional family (nontraditional families are discussed later in this chapter). Perinatal/maternal morbidity is significantly higher in pregnancies of adolescent mothers, which is in part due to incomplete maternal growth and the increased psychological needs of adolescent women. "Magical" thinking, feelings of invincibility, and limited abstract thought processes contribute significantly to the incidence of unintended pregnancy (ACOG, 2001b; Cunningham et al., 2001; Janke, 1996; Sherwen et al., 1999).

FACTS ABOUT ADOLESCENT PREGNANCY

- Adolescent pregnancy can be related to cultural norms, peer interaction, immature cognitive abilities, psychological needs, increasing societal acceptance, unprotected coitus, birth control failure or misuse.
- It is estimated that 23 percent of females are sexually active by age 15; 71.4 percent by age 19.
- Less than 40 percent of sexually active adolescents attempt some form of birth control; use is often sporadic.
- Adolescents are typically sexually active for six to twelve months prior to seeking birth control services or choosing a method of contraception.
- Among 15- to 19-year-old sexually active women, one of ten will become pregnant during a calendar year; among that group (estimated at 1 million), 39 percent will end their pregnancies in abortion. A significant number will conceive again shortly thereafter.
- Many young women deny signs and symptoms of pregnancy, feel embarrassed to admit their inability to use birth control, or feel embarrassed to use birth control.
- One in three pregnant adolescents will drop out of high school.
- Pregnant adolescents are less likely to seek early, regular prenatal care.
- As they age, women who give birth during adolescence have approximately half of the median family income noted in those who have their first child mid-20s and older.
- One out of five pregnant adolescents experiences emotional, sexual, or physical abuse (Abu-Heija, Ali, & Al-Dakheil, 2002; Stevenson, Maton, & Teti, 1999).

OBJECTIVE DATA

A physical exam will reveal changes similar to those seen during an adult physical exam, particularly during the breast, abdominal, and pelvic evaluations. Evaluate Tanner staging (see Chapter 4), as young adolescents may be physically immature, which would significantly impact growth and development in pregnancy. A final area of evaluation would be for evidence of eating disorders, substance abuse, or depression (ACOG, 2001b; Cunningham et al., 2001).

DIFFERENTIAL MEDICAL DIAGNOSIS

Ectopic pregnancy, endometrial regression, polycystic ovary disease, immature hypothalamic-pituitary-gonadal axis with primary amenorrhea, secondary amenorrhea, pseudocyesis, anorexia/eating disorders, ovarian tumors (ACOG, 2001b; Scott et al., 1999).

PLAN

Pregnant adolescents, especially those younger than 16 years, are at risk for having low birth-weight infants and preterm births. Moreover, they are at increased risk for cesarean births. Cephalopelvic disproportion may result from immature skeletal development of the pelvis. It remains the primary goal of the health care provider to promote the best possible pregnancy outcome through client evaluation and education. Therefore, focus education on general health maintenance and how pregnancy needs will change health status. The cognitive abilities of adolescents vary, however, as do their abilities to assimilate information. Foster behaviors that will promote independence in adolescent development (ACOG, 2001b; Janke, 1996).

Encourage the client to maintain peer interactions and continue to meet educational needs. Help her to clarify the father's role, make use of family support systems, and set realistic goals. Assess the client's cognitive abilities (e.g., concrete versus abstract). Encourage behaviors that foster parenting skills such as attending classes for this, and demonstration of what has been learned. Be aware of the increased rate of suicide among adolescents, the risk of substance abuse, and the need to promote a nonjudgmental atmosphere in which the client may express views about the pregnancy.

Health care providers need to assess their own value system, particularly to avoid stereotyping. The foundation for a trusting relationship is based on mutual acceptance, caring, and a nonjudgmental approach. Assisting the client to achieve the developmental tasks of adolescence, such as financial, emotional, and physical independence, is the underlying task for the health provider (ACOG, 2001b; Janke, 1996). Remember that despite increasing public awareness and concern, adolescents continue to

need support from the community in the areas of wellness, education, finance, and family planning.

MEDICATION

Stress the importance of *no* medication use without the consent of a health care provider.

DIET

The adolescent diet is notoriously inadequate. Because of the increased risk for inadequate nutrition, it is imperative to stress normal, adequate nutrition and the value of daily prenatal vitamins and iron supplementation. Educate the client on what constitutes appropriate nutritional choices. Changing body image and the increased demands of fetal growth and development place adolescent mothers at further risk for eating disorders. Careful periodic assessment during prenatal care will aid the health care provider in early detection of inadequate nutrition.

Adolescent dietary needs include 38 to 50 kcal/per kg of body weight, and 1.5 to 1.7 grams of protein per kilogram of body weight per day is recommended. A twenty-five- to thirty-pound weight gain depending on prepregnant weight is recommended (ACOG, 2001b; Sherwen et al., 1999). Encourage a balanced diet from the food pyramid and limiting nonnutritional foods or snacks. Instruction in good nutrition is related to maternal/fetal growth needs and should reinforce the need for adherence on the part of the adolescent mother (see Chapter 17).

SMOKING

Although the harmful effects of smoking cigarettes are well documented, adolescents continue to smoke at alarming rates; adolescent females smoke more than adolescent males. Cigarette smoking is highly correlated to early sexual activity; it is often seen as a display of "adult" behavior, rebellion, or peer pressure (Creasy & Resnick, 1998; Janke, 1996).

Smoking increases the risk of spontaneous abortion, preterm labor and birth, hypertension, placenta previa/abruptio, low birthweight infants, perinatal death, Sudden Infant Death Syndrome (SIDS), and long-term developmental delays in offspring (ACOG, 2001b; Gabbe et al., 2002). Direct counseling strategies toward decreasing or cessation of smoking and investigating support groups for that purpose. Education must be appropriate for the client's knowledge level and address both the immediate and long term impact of tobacco on the client and her offspring. Another strategy to help a client stop smoking is to encourage other outlets, such as chewing gum, sugarless candy, handiwork, and exercise.

SELF-CARE

Emphasize proper hygiene techniques. Advise the client to avoid contact sports but maintain physical activity by walking, swimming, and participating in prenatal exercise classes. Stress the importance of not consuming chemical substances during pregnancy without knowledge or direction of a health care provider.

EDUCATION

Encourage the client to remain in school during pregnancy or to obtain her general equivalency diploma. Home tutoring and schools for pregnant adolescents are also viable options, although peer interaction is decreased.

FINANCES

Financial concerns are heightened if education is interrupted as a result of pregnancy. Three areas of assessment may be helpful: insurance coverage; government assistance through such programs as Women/Infant/Children (WIC) or Aid to Dependent Children (ADC); job benefits (if employed).

FAMILY PLANNING

Frequent conception is common with adolescent mothers; as many as 40 to 50 percent conceive again within 24 months. Discuss motivation, maturity, and physical and financial practicality of contraceptive methods. Advise the client to choose a reliable method prior to completion of pregnancy. Explore the client's options for contraception, sexual responsibility, and risk behaviors for sexually transmitted disease.

FOLLOW-UP

Adolescent mothers are at higher risk for inflicting child abuse, being victims of domestic violence, conceiving frequently, contracting sexually transmitted disease (including HIV), having education disrupted, and having maladaptive peer interaction. Evaluate such situations when they become evident and initiate intervention in areas of greatest concern.

DELAYED PREGNANCY

Any woman who completes her pregnancy on or after her 35th birthday is referred to as a mother of advanced maternal age (Scott et al., 1999). Extensive literature in medicine and genetics has debated whether any significant risks are associated with childbearing after age 35. These risks generally stem from preexisting medical conditions, infertility, chromosomal abnormalities, or nutritional deficits. With proper control of underlying medical conditions, most women can have successful pregnancy outcomes. The highest absolute risk and sharpest rise in maternal mortality, however, occurs after the age of 40. Older gravidas are more likely to experience gestational diabetes, preeclampsia, placenta previa, pulmonary embolus, and exacerbation of underlying medical conditions. The woman over 40 is at increased risk for cesarean and operative vaginal delivery, as well as ectopic pregnancy, spontaneous abortion, multiple gestation, preterm labor, abnormal labor patterns, and neonatal intensive care unit admissions (De La Rochenbrachard & Thonneau, 2002).

Women may delay childbearing for medical or economic reasons or because of career or personal relationship choices. By postponing childbearing, women have increased their life experiences and psychological stability (Heinenen & Saarikoski, 2002). This may better equip them to rear children. A major influence on a woman's parenting behavior is the type and number of roles she has undertaken in life. Taking on multiple roles is thought to be either self-enhancing (promoting self-esteem and personal fulfillment) or personally divisive (increasing stress and anxiety) (Heinenen & Saarikoski, 2002). Older mothers may particularly cherish the ability to have children, and if these mothers have higher salaries, they may be better able to provide for their children financially (Heinenen & Saarikoski, 2002). Society encourages increased paternal involvement; consequently, the financial and emotional needs of parenting are shared more by both partners. Furthermore, postponing parenthood or choosing not to have children has gained acceptance, as well as delaying subsequent pregnancies.

Delayed parenting is probably influenced to the greatest degree by the increasing availability of effective contraception. Advances in contraceptive techniques have enabled greater freedom to time the birth of the first child. An additional reason for delayed childbearing may be the steady increase in late or second marriages. Moreover, for women who previously suffered from infertility, the prospect of bearing a child has improved with advances in reproductive technology.

HISTORY AND PHYSICAL EXAMINATION

For women whose pregnancy occurs later in life, the history and physical examination are the same as for other pregnant clients. Devote particular attention to nutritional and immunization status; reproductive, medical, occupational, and social histories; chemical substance use; and genetic concerns. Offer the client referral for genetic counseling and a review of available genetic testing. Identify any occupational hazards.

DIAGNOSTIC TESTS AND METHODS

The minimum standard tests are needed; medical conditions may require additional individual assessment. The American College of Obstetricians and Gynecologists (ACOG) recommends genetic testing for all women who are 35 years of age or older at the time of delivery. If the client elects genetic testing after counseling has been completed, scheduling for amniocentesis or chorionic villus sampling follows.

PLAN

Initiate discussions of pregnancy and encourage the client's questions. Several subjects may require review and counseling (Heinenen & Saarikoski, 2002).

- ◆ Normal physiology of pregnancy.
- ◆ Pertinent medical history findings.
- ◆ Genetic concerns and the testing available.
- ◆ Occupational hazards; exposure to teratogens.
- ◆ Nutrition and weight control.
- ◆ Warning signs in pregnancy; client dos and don'ts.
- ◆ Substance use/abuse.
- ◆ Exercise, travel, and leisure activities.
- ◆ Sexuality.

Make referrals where appropriate and encourage the client to explore educational resources within the community (e.g., prenatal classes). Tailor follow-up visits to pertinent medical findings and individual needs.

NONTRADITIONAL FAMILIES

The U.S. family has made several remarkable changes in the past twenty-five years. Today's U.S. families include the "typical" nuclear family and nontraditional families, including one-parent households, same-sex parents, single-by-choice parents, unmarried heterosexual couples living together, and those choosing to remain childfree. These patterns are the result of profound social and demographic changes in the United States and are becoming increasingly accepted. The contraceptive revolution of the 1960s greatly influenced family structure by changing the role of women. Selective fertility has played a fundamental role in economic shifts within households.

THE RISKS

Increased stress and maladaptive behaviors are reported among many nontraditional families. For health care providers, particular attention to the client's lifestyle choices may help in identifying her particular needs prior to pregnancy. Often women in nontraditional families have greater financial, education, and legal concerns. They may make many requests of their health care provider or they may feel reluctant to share their private lives. As always, the establishment of a trusting relationship is vital for both health care provider and client.

Though all behaviors cross boundaries, a higher incidence of the following maladaptive behaviors has been reported among some nontraditional mothers (Fasouliotis & Schenker, 1999; Gabbe et al., 2002; Price & Baird, 2001).

- ◆ Suicide (adolescents).
- ◆ Alcoholism/chemical abuse (lesbians, adolescents).
- ◆ Greater dependency on welfare monies (adolescents).
- ◆ Domestic violence (nontraditional families).
- ◆ Higher incidence of noncompliance with health care advice due to mistrust of "the system" (lesbians, adolescents).

HISTORY AND PHYSICAL EXAMINATION

History taking during the initial workup is important in identifying nontraditional family units. Several areas need to be explored.

- ◆ Sexual preference/practices.
- ◆ Legal status of relationship (i.e., paternity).

◆ Length of relationship and overall support systems for pregnancy.

◆ Employment setting, income, and how loss of income would impact pregnancy.

◆ Social ramifications of role modeling as a parent in a nontraditional household.

◆ Dietary practices (provide nutritional counseling and referral where appropriate) (Mishell & Brenner, 2001).

During the initial prenatal examination, carefully observe for signals of physical or chemical abuse (e.g., bruises, unusual marks, history of numerous bone fractures or excessive "accidents"). Women in nontraditional lifestyles may be at risk for maladaptive behaviors.

DIFFERENTIAL MEDICAL DIAGNOSES

Intrauterine pregnancy, substance abuse, dysfunctional adolescence, battering (Scott et al., 1999).

PLAN

Counseling, support, anticipatory guidance, and education are among the psychosocial interventions (ACOG, 2001a; Gabbe et al., 2002).

◆ Counsel the client about feelings of anger, hostility, fear, anxiety, aversion, and ambivalence throughout the pregnancy.

◆ Provide a calm, supportive, nonjudgmental environment for improved communication.

◆ Give anticipatory guidance regarding common stressors of pregnancy, both physical and emotional.

◆ Counsel about general wellness issues such as hygiene and breast self-exam (BSE), anatomy and physiology, and prevention of sexually transmitted diseases and HIV infection.

◆ Provide resource/referral information when domestic violence or substance abuse is a potential or identified risk, or when financial concerns are great.

FOLLOW-UP

Periodically throughout pregnancy and postpartum, reevaluate the client for continued risk. In addition, periodically evaluate the strength of the client's support systems.

SUBSTANCE ABUSE SCREENING IN PREGNANCY*

Screening is done to detect the use or misuse of any substance known or suspected to exert a deleterious effect on the client or her fetus (Koren, 2001). The effects of specific drugs are difficult to assign, because often multiple drugs are used and nutritional status is poor. The use of multiple drugs is associated with intrauterine growth retardation (IUGR) and increased anomalies. Factors that may impact a drug's effects are duration of use, dosage, timing in gestation, and use of other drugs (Gilstrap, Little, & Brent, 1998; Koren, 2001). Ideally, counseling a client concerning substance abuse begins prior to conception. Open discussions may make a client aware of the need to prevent pregnancy and to obtain counseling if necessary. Clients who use substances only occasionally need to be aware of the potential teratogenic effect of even one exposure.

Ascertain whether the mother and fetus have been exposed to harmful substances, assess the mother's need for counseling, and design intervention that targets and eliminates the abuse and decreases potential harm to mother and fetus. Being nonjudgmental is a key to success; a client is more apt to trust and reveal patterns of abuse if the health provider does not display dismay or disgust.

Initially, the goal of the health care provider is to prevent complications of pregnancy and in utero exposure, thereby minimizing permanent sequelae. Behavioral problems, learning disabilities, and physical anomalies may be present in the newborn. If multigenerational drug use is to be prevented, a link in the chain of addiction must be broken. Getting the client into treatment may help to identify her needs as an individual, teach her how to cope with the stresses that lead to drug use, and perhaps introduce skills for coping and potential parenting. In turn, these measures may enhance parent-child bonding and reduce the incidence of emotional, physical, or sexual abuse and neglect, which are often a common experience among children of substance abusers (Kissen, Srikis, Morgan, & Huang, 2001; Walton-Moss & Campbell, 2002).

It is important to stop drug abuse during pregnancy to prevent the potential for parents to give their infant or child drugs in food or a bottle as a means of consoling, or for a mother to breastfeed her infant while continuing to

*The author wishes to acknowledge the contributions of Marion Fuqua, RNC, MS, OGNP, to this section.

use illicit drugs. Accidental ingestion of drugs may occur if drugs are in the house. Current studies do not suggest that drug or alcohol use by the father of the baby influences the outcome of the pregnancy. Concern over chromosomal damage caused by hallucinogens and cannabinoids is also unwarranted. Drug use by the father, however, may be indicative of other factors that adversely affect outcomes (Koren, 2001).

SCREENING QUESTIONS

The questions below may aid the health care provider evaluate a client who is at risk for substance abuse during pregnancy. Using accepting terminology may encourage honest answers without fear of reproach. Some clients may be offended by assumption of use, however, in terms such as "How often do you use."

1. Have you ever used recreational drugs? If so, what, when, and how much?
2. Have you ever taken a prescription drug other than as intended? If so, what, when, and how much?
3. Have you used any legal or recreational drugs during this pregnancy? What, when, and how much?
4. How often do you drink alcohol? What, when, how much?
5. How often do you smoke cigarettes? How many per day?
6. What are your feelings about drug use during pregnancy?

ASSESSMENT

The following overview briefly describes only a few side effects of specific drug use. Further reading is encouraged concerning other substances and sequelae documented in research.

Smoking

Smoking increases the risk of spontaneous abortion, preterm labor and delivery, maternal hypertension, placenta previa, abruptio placenta, low birthweight infant, perinatal death, and possibly long term developmental delays in offspring (ACOG, 2000b; Cunningham et al., 2001; Faden & Graubard, 2000; Gabbe et al., 2002). The perinatal death rate among infants of smoking mothers is 20 to 35 percent higher (Gabbe et al., 2002). Central apnea, intrauterine growth retardation, and increased incidence of childhood respiratory infections have been noted (Faden & Graubard, 2000). Nicotine reduces fetal blood flow, and this may be related to the transient decrease in fetal movement associated with maternal smoking. There is an association between maternal smoking and increased risk of congenital urinary tract anomalies (Faden & Graubard, 2002). Alcohol and smoking combined increases the risk for adverse perinatal outcomes. They both are frequently associated with use of other chemicals in pregnancy. Prenatal exposure and passive exposure after birth may be a risk factor for sudden infant death syndrome (SIDS) (Gabbe et al., 2002).

In counseling a client, present measures to decrease smoking cues and behaviors; provide information about support groups for smoking cessation; stress the immediate and long-term impact of tobacco use on her and her fetus; encourage her to seek appropriate outlets to replace smoking, such as chewing gum, eating sugarless candy, doing handiwork or exercising. Use of nicotine gum is contraindicated in pregnancy. The adverse effects of smoking appear to be dose related. The pregnant client who smokes twenty or more cigarettes per day may benefit from a nicotine transdermal patch. Circulating levels of nicotine from smoking cigarettes would be reduced as would exposure to other toxins found in cigarettes such as carbon monoxide (Faden & Graubard, 2000).

Counsel the patient that smoking cessation may decrease the risk of infant and fetal mortality by 10 to 50 percent. The greatest impact is seen if cessation occurs in the first trimester (Faden & Graubard, 2000).

Cocaine

Decreased plasma cholinesterase activity in the pregnant woman, fetus, and newborn increases the risk of cocaine toxicity. Cocaine use produces vasoconstriction, tachycardia, and hypertension in both the mother and fetus (Gabbe et al., 2002; Kissin et al., 2001). Uteroplacental insufficiency may result secondary to reduced uterine blood flow and placental perfusion. Studies suggest that perinatal cocaine use increases the risk for spontaneous abortion, preterm labor with rupture of membranes and delivery, intrauterine growth retardation, intrauterine fetal distress and demise, seizures, withdrawal, cerebral infarcts, and complications of the neonatal course. Cocaine may increase the risk of placental abruption, uterine rupture, SIDS, and congenital anomalies (ACOG, 2000b; Creasy & Resnick, 1998; Gabbe et al., 2002; Kissin et al., 2001; Koren, 2001).

Alcohol

Excessive alcohol use remains a major public health issue in the United States. Underreporting of alcohol intake makes it difficult to estimate the rate of alcohol use in pregnancy. Maternal-fetal effects of alcohol usage appear to be dose related. Fetal alcohol syndrome (FAS) is generally thought to occur in infants born to women who consume six standard drinks per day and is estimated to occur in 1 to 2 per 1000 live births. Characteristics of FAS include craniofacial dysmorphia, intrauterine growth retardation, microcephaly, and congenital anomalies such as limb abnormalities and cardiac defects. Long-term sequelae include postnatal growth retardation, attention deficits, delayed reaction time, and poor scholastic performance. FAS is the most common cause of mental retardation in the United States.

Other adverse outcomes of alcohol usage in pregnancy include intrauterine fetal demise and an increased rate of spontaneous abortion (Gabbe et al., 2002; Kissin et al., 2001; Koren, 2001). Fetal alcohol effects (FAE) are less severe and are noted in those consuming two to six standard drinks per day. Though some studies failed to demonstrate adverse consequences with fewer than two standard drinks per day, no known safe threshold for alcohol consumption exists. Alcohol and smoking combined have an additive risk for adverse perinatal outcomes (Koren, 2001).

LSD

Usage of lysergic acid diethylamide in pregnancy is not known to increase perinatal morbidity or mortality. Long-term effects on development, however, are not known (Creasy & Resnick, 1998; Gabbe et al., 2002).

Opiates/Narcotics

Opiates such as heroin may induce intense addiction in both mother and neonate. Neonatal withdrawal occurs in up to 95 percent of neonates exposed in utero (Gabbe et al., 2002).

An increased incidence of sudden infant death syndrome (SIDS) has been found among these infants (Gabbe et al., 2002). Intrauterine growth retardation, increased fetal distress, and persistently small fetal head circumference have also been noted.

Though not teratogenic alone, opiates may become so when "cut" with other substances. Reported complications in addicts also include preeclampsia, premature rupture of membranes, placental abruption, and meconium staining. When compared with drug-free children, opiate-exposed children had deficits ranging from poor motor performance to hyperactivity and impulsiveness (Kissin et al., 2001).

A woman's withdrawal from opiates has been associated with fetal demise (Kissin et al., 2001). Methadone

substitution has been successful during pregnancy but must be used in a closely supervised treatment program (Kissin et al., 2001). Narcotic antagonists, such as Narcan® (Naloxone), Nubaine® (Nalbuphine), and Stadol® (Butorphanol) (frequently given in labor) can precipitate withdrawal symptoms. Narcan® may be used to reverse narcotic overdose (Gabbe et al., 2002).

Methamphetamines

Methamphetamines produce some of the same effects as cocaine, such as increased risk for abruption, hemorrhage, preterm labor, eclampsia, increased perinatal mortality, fetal distress, and intrauterine growth retardation. Evidence exists that exposure may also increase the incidence of cerebral hemorrhage, infarction, or cavitation. Use of methamphetamines does not increase risk of congenital defects (Gilstrap et al., 1998; Koren, 2001).

Marijuana

In the general population, marijuana is the most frequently used illicit drug. Fetal levels are several times lower than maternal. Use of marijuana is highly correlated with use of alcohol and cigarettes. Usage may lead to preterm delivery and intrauterine growth retardation; however, marijuana is not considered teratogenic (Gabbe et al., 2002).

Organic Solvents/Aromatic Hydrocarbons

Organic solvents/aromatic hydrocarbons (AHC) are present in paints, glue, enamel, varnish, lacquer, and resins. They are easily absorbed through the skin, lungs, gastrointestinal tract, and easily cross the placenta. Exposure may occur in the workplace or be recreational ("huffing" or "sniffing"). Toluene is the most popular AHC for this purpose. Usage during pregnancy may lead to intrauterine growth retardation, microcephaly, hydrocephaly, limb anomalies, and craniofacial dysmorphia similar to FAS. Toluene exposure places the mother and fetus at risk for hyperchloremic metabolic acidosis (Gabbe et al., 2002; Koren, 2001).

Physical Examination

The physical examination of a woman abusing a chemical substance may reveal fresh needle or track marks, a dazed appearance, inappropriate behavior or affect, extreme agitation or stupor, frequent conjunctivitis, tremors, flecks of paint around the mouth and nose, fetal/maternal tachycardia, or poor maternal weight gain (or weight loss) not attributed to underlying maternal disease. (See Chapters 18 and 23 for evaluation, diagnosis, and treatment.)

Plan

Client counseling must continue into the postpartum period. During that time, her problem may worsen if the infant is not feeding, sleeping only for short intervals, crying shrilly, difficult to console, and avoiding eye contact. For some women addicts, fear of legal action may deter them from getting any form of prenatal care, and they may choose to forgo hospital delivery. Recidivism is high (Gabbe et al., 2002; Kissin et al., 2001).

A drug screen should be done to identify all drugs that a client is using, since multiple drug usage is common. Assist the client to enroll in a drug rehabilitation program that offers her ease of accessibility and provides optimum social support. (Be aware that resources for treating pregnant substance abusers are often limited and have long waiting lists.) Management includes dietary counseling, ideally by a nutritionist. The client should be seen perhaps every one to two weeks and begin nonstress tests by 30 weeks' gestation. Serial ultrasounds are indicated to assess fetal growth patterns and placental health.

Constant encouragement and motivation are required to reinforce the need for compliance. Be honest about drug effects, but do not humiliate the client. Be open and direct with questions while being supportive of her efforts. Some women do not see their infant as part of themselves, nor do they care to. Most, however, genuinely do not want to harm their child. Consequently, those who can only focus on the present may benefit from counseling on the immediate effects of substance use on both mother and baby. Discussion of long-term effects may heighten compliance and promote a sense of maternal responsibility for the fetus and infant. The mother may consider her own needs first when she is making a decision about continuing to use drugs (Kissin et al., 2001). Most importantly, clients need to understand and value consistent prenatal care.

REFERENCES

Abu-Heija., Ali, A., & Al-Dakheil, S. (2002). Obstetrics and perinatal outcome of adolescent nulliparous pregnant women. *Gynecologic and Obstetric Investigation, 53*(2), 90–2.

American College of Obstetricians and Gynecologists (ACOG). (1997). *Guidelines for perinatal care.* Washington: Author.

American College of Obstetricians and Gynecologists (ACOG). (1999a). Psychosocial risk factors: Perinatal screening and intervention. *Compendium of Selected Publications,* 211–217.

American College of Obstetricians and Gynecologists (ACOG). (1999b). Management of herpes Herpes in pregnancy. *Compendium of Selected Publications,* 363–370.

American College of Obstetricians and Gynecologists (ACOG). (2000a). *Planning your pregnancy.* Washington: Author.

American College of Obstetricians and Gynecologists (ACOG). (2000b). *Drugs and pregnancy.* Washington: Author.

American College of Obstetricians and Gynecologists (ACOG). (2001a). Prenatal diagnosis of fetal chromosomal abnormalities. *Compendium of Selected Publications,* 457–467.

American College of Obstetricians and Gynecologists (ACOG). (2001b). *Having a baby.* Washington: Author.

American College of Obstetricians and Gynecologists (ACOG), Committee of Obstetric Practice. (2002). ACOG committee opinion: (267), Exercise during pregnancy and the postpartum period. *Obstetrics and Gynecology, 99*(1), 171–173.

Attrill, B. (2002). The assumption of the maternal role: A developmental process. *Australian Journal of Midwifery, 15*(1), 21–5.

Bloom, K., & Ewing, C. (2001). Group B streptococcal (GBS) disease screening and treatment during pregnancy: Nurse-midwives' consistency with 1996 CDC recommendations. *Journal Midwifery Women's Health, 15*(1), 17–23.

Brown, G. (2001). Maternal mortality: Clinical implications of international perspectives. *Journal of American Medicine Women's Health 46*(1), 191–2.

Caton, D., Corry, M., Frigoletto, F., Hopkins, D., Lieberman, E., Mayberry, L., Rooks, J. Rosenfield, A., Sakala, C., Simkin, P., & Young, D. (2002). The nature and management of labor pain: Executive summary. *American Journal of Obstetrics and Gynecology, 186*(5), S1–15.

Cefalo, R., & Moos, M. (1995). *Preconceptional healthcare: A practical guide* (2nd ed). St. Louis: Mosby.

Chernecky, C., & Berger, B. (2001). *Management of common problems in obstetrics and gynecology* (4th ed.). Boston: Blackwell.

Creasy, R., & Resnick, R. (1998). *Maternal-fetal medicine: Principles and practice* (4th ed.). Chicago: Harcourt Brace and Company.

Cunningham, F., Gant, N., Leveno, K., Hauth, J., & Wenstrom, K. (2001). *Williams obstetrics* (21st ed.). Norwalk, CT: Appleton & Lange.

De La Rochenbrochard, E., & Thonneau, P. (2002). Paternal are and maternal age are risk factors for miscarriage: Results of a multicentre European study. *Human Reproduction, 17*(6), 1649–1656.

Durant, T., Colley, G., Saltzman, L., & Johnson, C. (2000). Opportunities for intervention: Discussing physical abuse during prenatal care visits. *American Journal of Preventive Medicine, 19*(4), 238–244.

Faden, V., & Graubard, B. (2000). Maternal substance use during pregnancy and developmental outcome at age three. *Journal of Substance Abuse, 12*(4), 329–340.

Fasouliotis, S., & Schenker, J. (1999). Social aspects of assisted reproduction. *Human Reproduction Update, 5*(1), 26–39.

Gabbe, S., Niebyl, J., & Simpson, J. (2002). *Obstetrics: Normal and problem pregnancies.* Philadelphia: Churchill Livingston.

Gay, J., Edgil, A., & Douglas, A. (1988). Reva Rubin revisited. *Journal of Obstetric Gynecologic and Neonatal Nursing, 17,* 394–399.

Gilstrap, L., Little, B., & Brent, R. (1998). *Drugs and pregnancy* (2nd ed.). New York: Elsevier.

Haddow, J., Palomaki, G., Knight, G., Foster, D., & Neveux, L. (1998). Second trimester screening for Down's syndrome using maternal serum Dimeric inhibin A. *Journal of Medical Screening, 5*(3), 115–19.

Hatcher, R. (1998). *Contraceptive technology* (17th ed.). New York: Irvington.

Heinenen, S., & Saarikoski, S. (2002). Reproductive risk factors, pregnancy characteristics and obstetric outcome in female doctors. *British Journal of Obstetrics and Gynecology, 109*(3), 261–264.

Huth-Bucks, A., Levendosky, A., & Bogat, G. (2002). The effects of domestic violence during pregnancy on maternal and infant health. *Violence Victim, 2,* 169–185.

James, D. (2001). Maternal screening and treatment for group B streptococcus. *Journal of Obstetric, Gynecologic and Neonatal Nursing, 30*(6), 659–666.

Janke, S. (1996). Teen pregnancy. *Childbirth educator* (2nd quarter), 14–16, 37.

Kissin, W., Srikis, D., Morgan, G., & Huang, N. (2001). Characterizing pregnant drug-dependent women in treatment and their children. *Journal of Substance Abuse and Treatment, 21*(1), 27–34.

Koren, G. (2001). *Maternal-fetal toxicology* (3rd ed.). New York: Marcel Dekker.

Lederman, R. (1996). *Psychosocial adaptation in pregnancy* (2nd ed.). Englewood Cliffs, NJ: Prentice Hall.

Lim, P. (2002). Pregnancy and sexuality. *Midwifery Today: International Midwifery, 62,* 36–38.

Lindigren, K. (2001). Relationship among maternal fetal attachment, prenatal depression and health practices in pregnancy. *Research and Nursing Health, 24*(3), 203–217.

Maloni, J. (1996). Transforming prenatal care: Reflections on the past and present with implications for the future. *Journal of Obstetric, Gynecologic and Neonatal Nursing, 25,* 17–23.

Mange, E., & Mange, A. (1998). *Basic human genetics* (2nd ed.). Sunderland, Massachusetts: Sinauer Associates, Inc.

McFarlane, J., & Parker, B. (1994). Preventing abuse during pregnancy: An assessment and intervention protocol. *Maternal Child Nursing, 19,* 321–324.

Mishell, D., & Brenner, P. (2001). *Management of common problems in obstetrics and gynecology* (4th ed.). Boston: Blackwell Scientific Publications.

Mongan, M. (2002). *Hypnobirthing: A celebration of life.* Retrieved May 9, 2002 from www.hypnobirthing.com.

Morrison, E. (2000). Preconception care. *Primary Care, 27,* 1–12.

Pillitteri, A. (1999). *Care of the childbirthing and childrearing family* (3rd ed.). Philidelphia: J. B. Lippincott.

Price, S., & Baird, K. (2001). Domestic violence in pregnancy. *Practice of Midwifery, 4*(7), 12–14.

Ramachandran, R. (2002). Maternal nutrition: Effect on fetal growth and outcome of pregnancy. *Nutrition Review, 60*(2), 526–534.

Reynolds, H. (1998). Preconception care: An integral part of primary care for women. *Journal of Nurse Midwifery, 43*(6), 445–458.

Rubin, R. (1994). *Maternal identity and the maternal experience.* New York: Springer.

Scott, J., Hammond, B., Danforth, D., & DiSaio, P. (1999). *Danforth's obstetrics and gynecology* (8th ed.). Philadelphia: Lippincott.

Sherwen, L., Scolvino, M., & Toussie-Wengartan, C. (1999). *Maternity nursing care of the childbearing family.* Englewood Cliffs, NJ: Prentice Hall.

Shulman, L., & Elias, S. (2001). Cystic fibrosis. *Clinical Perinatology, 28*(2), 383–393.

Stevenson, W., Maton, K., & Teti, D. (1999). Social support, relationship quality among pregnant adolescents. *Journal of Adolescence, 22*(1), 109–201.

Walton-Moss, B., & Campbell, J. (2002). Intimate partner violence, implications for nursing. *Online Journal Issues Nursing, 7,* 1–6.

Werler, M., Louik, C., & Mitchell, A. (1999). Achieving a public health recommendation for preventing neural tube defects with folic acid. *American Journal of Public Health, 89*(11), 1637–1640.

Worthington, K. (2001). Reproductive hazards on the job. *American Journal of Nursing, 101*(10), 104.

CHAPTER 17

PROMOTING A HEALTHY PREGNANCY

Maryellen C. Remich

*T*he issues of concern to pregnant women involve safety, comfort, and uncertainty about what to expect during pregnancy, labor, and delivery.

Highlights

- Nutrition and Weight Gain
- Immunization
- Common Complaints
- Anticipatory Guidance
    Chemical Use, Radiation
    The Workplace
    Sexual Activity
    Exercise
    Dental Care
    Travel
    Accidents, Blows to the Abdomen
    Infant Care
    Sibling Rivalry
    Family Planning
- Danger Signs: First, Second, and Third Trimesters
- Initial Assessment in Labor

❖ INTRODUCTION

The ultimate goal of pregnancy is the birth of a healthy infant into a healthy and nurturing family who can provide for his or her physical, psychological, emotional, and spiritual needs. During pregnancy, many normal physiological changes lead to discomfort or concern for the mother. Health care providers must differentiate between normal and pathological changes, educate clients about changes, and help them to recognize and respond appropriately to signs of pathology and labor. In addition, health care providers need to individualize client education about prenatal nutrition and weight gain.

NUTRITION AND WEIGHT GAIN

Good nutrition before and during pregnancy decreases the risks of significant health problems for the client and her infant. Studies have shown that the influence of maternal nutrition lasts into the infant's adulthood (Reifsnider & Gill, 2000). Pregnant women with poor dietary habits are at increased risk for anemia, preeclampsia, obesity, and osteoporosis with associated morbidity and mortality. Women who are underweight or who gain little weight during pregnancy are more likely to have small-for-gestational-age infants. Women who are obese or whose weight gain is excessive are at risk for pregnancy-induced hypertension and gestational diabetes (Reifsnider & Gill, 2000; Thadhani, Stampfer, Hunter, et al., 1999). Ideally, issues of nutrition and weight gain should be addressed during preconception counseling (see Chapter 16). Because most women are highly motivated to eat properly during pregnancy (Clark & Ogden, 1999), the nutrition instruction that they receive during pregnancy could result in positive and sustained dietary changes for the entire family.

SUBJECTIVE DATA

Several points are assessed during the first prenatal interview and reassessed as necessary at subsequent visits.

- ◆ Nutrition knowledge.
- ◆ A recall of the client's diet, ideally seven-day, though 24-hour is often more attainable (See Figure 17–1).
- ◆ Food storage and preparation capabilities.
- ◆ Portion of income spent for food.
- ◆ Food-buying practices.
- ◆ Cultural and religious preferences.
- ◆ Food aversions or allergies (e.g., lactose intolerance).
- ◆ Meanings attached to eating (e.g., celebration).
- ◆ Prepregnancy weight; and body mass index (see Figure 17–2).

- ◆ Activity level and any change since pregnancy.
- ◆ Lactation during or just prior to pregnancy.
- ◆ Reproductive age (number of years menstruating).
- ◆ High gravity and parity (two or more pregnancies within two years or five or more total deliveries).
- ◆ Megavitamin herbal, or vitamin supplement use.
- ◆ Nicotine, alcohol, medication, or drug abuse.
- ◆ Psychosocial disorders (e.g., depression, bulimia).
- ◆ Discomforts from pregnancy (e.g., dyspepsia).
- ◆ Complications during past pregnancies (e.g., small-for-gestational-age neonate, preterm delivery, perinatal loss, gestational diabetes) (Kline, 2000).
- ◆ Nutritional risk factors, for less than optimal pregnancy outcomes (see Table 17–1).

OBJECTIVE DATA

Physical Examination

Clients with nutritional risk in pregnancy are reviewed in Table 17–1. Table 17–2 provides an overview of vitamin and mineral deficiencies and toxicity symptoms that may require additional work up.

Later in pregnancy, abnormal weight gain patterns, abnormal uterine size to dates, increased blood pressure, and nondependent edema are signs that indicate nutritional risk.

Diagnostic Tests and Methods

- ◆ Height, weight with body mass index (Figure 17–2).
- ◆ Complete blood cell count (CBC) to screen for anemia.
- ◆ One-hour 50 g Glucola to rule out gestational diabetes.
- ◆ Urine dipstick to detect proteinuria (suggestive of pregnancy induced hypertension), glycosuria (suggestive of gestational diabetes), and ketonuria (suggestive of hyperemesis gravidarum).

Food Frequency Form

Please check the column that shows how often you eat the following foods.
Check only one column for each food.

Name _____ Date _____	2–4 Times A Day	Once Daily	2–4 Times A Week	Once Weekly	Hardly Ever or Never
Beef, pork, ham, hamburger					
Luncheon meats, hot dogs					
Chicken, turkey, poultry					
Fish, seafood					
Eggs					
Dried peas or beans (legumes)					
Peanut butter					
Nuts					
Cereals (dry or cooked)					
Grains					
Breads, rolls, biscuits					
Tortillas					
Crackers					
Rice					
Pasts, noodles, spaghetti, macaroni					
Milk					
Cheese					
Yogurt, pudding, custard					
Fruits					
Fruit juices					
Vegetables					
Water					
Added fat					
Coffee, tea, cocoa					
Sodas, fruit-flavored drinks					
Alcohol: beer, wine, whiskey					
Candy, sweets					
Cakes, pies, cookies, donuts, sweet rolls					
Potato chip, pretzels, corn/tortilla chips					
Ice cream					

WEEKLY TOTALS:

Meat _____   Fruits & Juices* _____   Cakes, pies _____
Poultry_____   Vegetables*_____   Chips_____
Fish_____   Dairy products_____   Ice Cream _____
Legumes_____   Water_____   Candy_____
Eggs_____   Sodas_____   Fats_____
Breads & Cereal_____   Alcohol_____   Other _____
Rice & Pasta _____   *Ask types to determine if they are high in vitamin A or C

FIGURE 17–1.   Food Frequency Form. *(Used with permission from Kline, D.A. (2000).* Nutrition for women: Part 1 Sexual and Reproductive Health *(5th ed.). Eureka, CA: Nutrition Dimension.)*

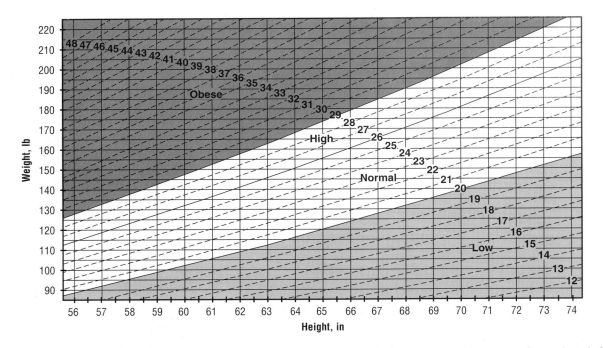

FIGURE 17–2.   Chart for Estimating Body Mass Index (BMI) Category and BMI. To find BMI category (e.g., obese), find the point where the woman's height and weight intersect. To estimate BMI, read the bold number on the dashed line that is closest to this point. *(Courtesy of the Food and Nutrition Board, Institute of Medicine. Copyright 1992 by the National Academy of Sciences, Washington, DC.)*

◆ Other less commonly used laboratory assays available to diagnose other nutritional deficiencies (normal values in pregnancy differ from nonpregnant values) (see Chapter 16).

◆ History, physical, and laboratory tests may reveal symptoms of vitamin or mineral deficit or toxicity (see Table 17–2).

DIFFERENTIAL MEDICAL DIAGNOSES

Normal nutrition in pregnancy, ruling out overweight or underweight; anemia; gestational diabetes; drug, alcohol, or nicotine abuse; eating disorders; problems affecting nutrition (e.g., cultural, economic, psychosocial); and complications of pregnancy and medical conditions requiring dietary intervention.

PLAN

Psychosocial Interventions

Encourage the client to verbalize any physical and psychosocial problems and explore interventions with her. Interventions for the normal physiological changes that may interfere with a woman's ability to eat an adequate diet are described later in the chapter (see Common Complaints).

Dietary Interventions

Assuming the client's dietary intake was adequate before conception and her weight is within a normal range, protein intake should increase by 10 g per day and caloric intake (kcal) should increase by 300 in the last two trimesters. Normal weight gain is 25 to 35 pounds (Figure 17–3). (Kline, 2000). Educate the client about the dietary adjustments needed to supply nutrients, taking into account the client's cultural, religious, and personal preferences, as well as lifestyle, food preferences, intolerances, and aversions.

High or low activity levels require adjustment of calorie and protein intake. The goal is appropriate weight gain patterns. Variable energy needs of pregnant clients make advising total calorie needs difficult. Exercise calorie needs are added to the 300 kcal/day. The client with very low prepregnant weight may need more than 300 kcal/day added to her diet. The best advice is to eat to appetite with quality food choices (Kline, 2000).

TABLE 17-1. Nutritional Risk Factors for Less than Optimal Pregnancy Outcomes

I. Preconception Risk Factors
   A. Body Mass before Pregnancy
      Underweight (BMI less than 19.8)
      Overweight (BMI of 26–29)
      Obese (BMI greater than 29)
II. Past Medical History

Age of less than 18 or 4 reproductive years	Cancer/AIDS
Diabetes	Gastrointestinal disease or surgery (i.e., stomach stapling, liver disease)
Hypertension	Endocrine diseases (thyroid dysfunction)
Chronic renal disease	Contraceptive methods
Heart disease	

III. Past Obstetrical History
   Multiparity (5 or more pregnancies)
   Closely spaced pregnancies (less than 12 months)
   Gestational diabetes
   Preeclampsia
   Preterm labor or delivery
   Recurrent miscarriage
   Small or large for gestational age infant
   Congenital anomaly
IV. Current Pregnancy
   A. Psychosocial Factors
      Low income
      Cultural factors
      Food preferences/intolerances (e.g., lactose intolerance)
      Food access/storage/preparation restrictions
      Substance abuse (e.g., nicotine, alcohol, drugs)
      Medication use (over-the-counter or prescription)
      Megavitamin/mineral use
      Herbal supplements
      Eating disorders
      Pica, ptyliasm, changes in taste and smell
      Psychological disorders (depression, mental retardation)
   B. Obstetrical Factors
      Hyperemesis gravidarium
      Anemia
      Inadequate or excessive weight gain
      Gestational diabetes
      Pregnancy-induced hypertension
      Breastfeeding during pregnancy
      Bed rest secondary to obstetrical complications
V. Dietary Factors
   A. Inadequate or excessive intake of

Protein	Calcium/Phosphorus
Calories	Magnesium
Fat	Fiber
Sodium	Folic acid
Zinc	Vitamins B_6, B_{12}, C, A
Iron	Water

Adapted from Kline, D.A. (2000). Nutrition for women Part 1: Sexual and reproductive health (5th ed.). Eureka, CA: Nutrition Dimensions. Laedwig, P.W., London, M.L., Moberly, S., & Olds, S.B. (2002). Contemporary Maternal-Newborn Nursing Care (5th ed.). Upper Saddle River, NJ: Prentice-Hall.

TABLE 17–2. Vitamins and Minerals: Symptoms of Deficit and Toxicity

	RDA in Pregnancy	Symptoms of Deficit	Symptoms of Toxicity
Fat-Soluble Vitamins			
A	800 RE (retinol equivalents)	night blindness, skin lesions	nausea, vomiting, abdominal pain, headache papilledema, lethargy, hypomenorrhea, hypercalcemia
D	10 mcg	bone pain, muscle pain, weakness	constipation, diarrhea, fatigue, anorexia, nausea, vomiting, headache, metallic taste in mouth
E	12 mcg	hyporeflexia, ataxia, anemia, myopathy	blurred vision, diarrhea, dizziness, nausea, headache
K	65 mcg	increased bleeding	excessive bruising, abnormal bleeding
Water-Soluble Vitamins			
C	95 mg	irritability, pain with touch, scurvy	unlikely with water-soluble vitamins
B_1 (Thiamin)	1.6 mg	peripheral neuritis, muscle weakness, depression, memory loss, anorexia, dyspnea	
B_2 (Riboflavin)	1.8 mg	sore throat, stomatitis, sore tongue, anemia, facial dermatitis	
B_3 (Niacin)	20 mg	skin eruption, stomatitis, headache, dizziness, insomnia, memory problems, dementia	
B_6 (Pyridoxine)	2.2 mg	stomatitis, skin lesions, seizures, peripheral neuritis	
B_9 (Folic acid)	400 mcg	megoblastic anemia	
B_{12}	2.6 mcg	irreversible nervous system damage, ataxia, paresthesia, memory loss, confusion, dememtia, abnormal hematopoiesis	
Biotin	*	scaly skin, muscle pain, pallor, anorexia, nausea, fatigue, high cholesterol	
Pantothenic Acid	*	anorexia, abdominal pain, arm and leg pain, depression, muscle spasms, neuromuscular degeneration	
Minerals			
Calcium	1200 mg	convulsions, osteomalacia	decreased neural function, calcium deposits in soft tissue, kidney stones
Potassium	*	muscle weakness, paralysis, nausea, vomiting, heart failure, tachycardia	parenthesis, muscle weakness, cardiac abnormalities
Sodium	*	nausea, abdominal pain, muscle cramps, convulsions	hypertension, edema
Chloride	*	alkalosis, muscle cramps, cramps, apathy	vomiting
Iron	30 mg	anemia, fatigue, apathy, irritability, tachycardia, palpitations	metabolic acidosis, gastrointestinal mucosal erosion, liver and kidney dysfunction, lethargy
Zinc	15 mg	poor wound healing, decreased taste & smell, anorexia, dermatitis, alopecia, depressed immune function, altered reproductive function	rare
Magnesium	320 mg	anorexia, muscle spasms, weakness, depression, hypertension, confusion, convulsions, nausea, poor coordination	rare

*No RDAs for these nutrients

Adapted from National Academy of Sciences. (1989). Recommended daily allowance. Washington, DC: National Academy Press.

National Academy Press and Institute of Medicine (Food and Nutrition Board). 1998. Recommended levels for individual intake, 1998, B vitamins and choline. Washington, DC: National Academy Press.

Institute of Medicine (Food and Nutrition Board) (1997). Dietary references for calcium, phosphorus, magnesium, vitamin D and flouride. Washington, D.C.: National Academy Press.

Somer, E. (1995). Essential Guide to Vitamins and minerals. New York: Harper-Collins.

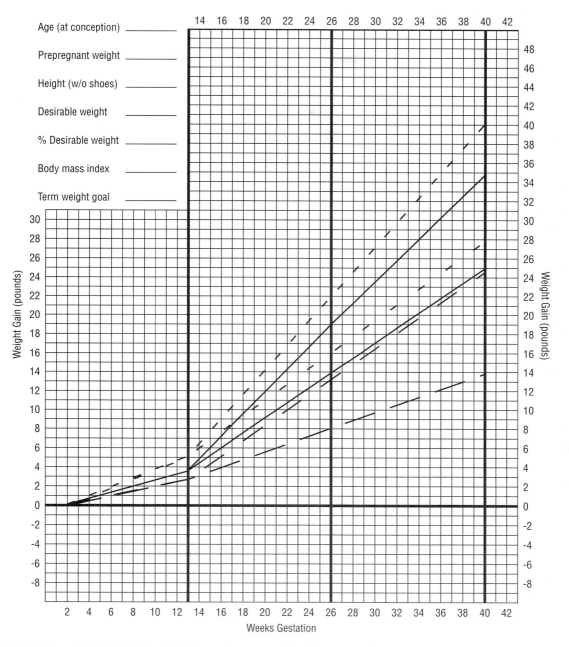

Age (at conception) _____

Prepregnant weight _____

Height (w/o shoes) _____

Desirable weight _____

% Desirable weight _____

Body mass index _____

Term weight goal _____

Weight Gain (pounds)

Weeks Gestation

FIGURE 17–3. Prenatal Weight-Gain Grid. Normal to overweight clients should maintain weight between the solid lines, underweight clients between the short dashed lines, and overweight clients between the long dashed lines. Young adolescents, African American women, and smokers should strive for gains at the upper end of the recommended ranges. Short women (< 62 inches) should strive for gains at the lower end of the range (*Source: Adapted with permission from Nutrition during Pregnancy, copyright 1990 by the National Academy of Sciences. Courtesy of the National Academy Press, Washington, DC.*)

Inadequate calcium intake has been implicated in pregnancy induced hypertension along with magnesium, iron and omega-3-fatty acids (Kline, 2000). Advise clients with lower than optimal intake of calcium to increase their dietary calcium with dairy products, green leafy vegetables, tofu, canned salmon, egg yolks, whole grains, legumes, and nuts. Juices and foods with calcium supplementation have recently become available. A calcium carbonate or citrate supplement may be necessary. Clients with lactose intolerance may benefit from taking lactase supplements (e.g., Lactaid), eating lactose-reduced dairy products (yogurt, cheese, milk, or cottage cheese), or eating dairy products in small quantities (Kline, 2000). Omega-3 fatty acids are in fish and fish oils. Magnesium sources are meat, nuts, dark green leafy vegetables, and dairy products. Iron is supplemented with the prenatal vitamin and found in meat and dark green leafy vegetables (Kline, 2000).

Vegetarians choose this lifestyle for cultural, religious, personal, or philosophic reasons. Types of vegetarians' diets vary: excluding all animal food sources; including milk, eggs, fish, and/or poultry; fruit as a main dietary staple; or macrobiotics who eat mainly cereals. In most cases, with the help of a registered dietician, these clients can plan a diet that meets their pregnancy needs (see Table 17–3). These clients are particularly advised to use a prenatal vitamin and mineral supplement (Cunningham et al., 2001; Kline, 2000).

If the client's body weight at conception is above or below her normal range, counsel her to adjust her caloric intake appropriately. Figure 17–3 shows the desirable weight range (normal), weights that are low, weights that are high, and weights that are obese. Recommended weight gain is 28 to 40 pounds if low, 25 to 35 pounds if normal weight, 15 to 25 pounds if high weight, and 15 pounds if obese (ACOG, 2000).

Adolescents have nutritional needs not only of the pregnancy but also of their own growth. Pregnant teens, those within four years of menarche, need 40 to 47 kcal/day per kg of body weight plus 1 gm of protein per day per kg of body weight. Additional adjustments are needed for activity levels. Weight gain should start early, closely monitored for appropriate patterns and adjusted as needed. Supplementation with vitamins is recommended (Kline, 2000).

For clients with a twin pregnancy, data indicate that a weight gain of 35 to 45 pounds is ideal (ACOG, 2000). Although recommendations for calorie, protein, or calcium intake are lacking, prudence suggests that increases in these nutrients are needed.

For the client with five or more pregnancies or with pregnancies that are closely spaced, emphasize optimal nutrition in all areas but particularly protein, calcium, iron, and folic acid. Vitamin supplementation is advised (Kline, 2000).

Risk factors for iron-deficiency anemia include menorrhagia, vegetarian diet (particularly with the exclusion of eggs), diets lacking red meat or low in vitamin C, multiple gestation, more than three blood donations per year, and chronic aspirin use. In pregnancy, anemia is present with a hemoglobin of less than 11.0 g/dL in the first and third trimester and 10.5 g/dL in the second trimester

TABLE 17–3. Daily Food Guide During Pregnancy

Food Group	Examples	Nutrients	Recommended Servings
Meat and meat alternatives	beef, poultry, fish, eggs, nuts, dry beans	protein, iron, magnesium, folate, B vitamins, zinc, phosphorus	3–4/day (2 oz = serving) 2 eggs, 4 tbsp nut butters, $1/2$–$2/3$ c. nuts, 1 c. dry beans
Milk	milk, yogurt, cheese	calcium, riboflavin, Vitamin B_{12}, magnesium, Vitamins A, E, D	4/day (serving = 8 oz. Milk, 1.5 oz. cheese, 2 c. cottage cheese, $1 1/2$ c. ice cream, 1 c. pudding/yogurt)
Fruits	variety is important	Vitamins A, C, folate, fiber, potassium	2–4/day, 1 serving a high vitamin C fruit (serving = 1 small piece, $1/2$ c. juice, $1/2$ c. berries)
Vegetables	variety is important	Vitamins A, C, folate, fiber, magnesium	3–5/day, 1 serving a high vitamin C vegetable, 1 serving high in folate (dark green, leafy), (1 serving = 1 c. raw, $3/4$ c. cooked)
Breads, cereals	whole grain breads, cereals, rice, pasta	thiamine, niacin, iron, zinc, fiber, folate, if fortified	7–11/day (1 serving = 1 slice, 1 muffin, $1/2$–$3/4$ c. cereals, etc.)
Fats, oils, sweets	soda, cookies, desserts	calories	as needed for calories for protein sparing

Source: Adapted from Kline, D.A. (2000). Nutrition in women Part 1. Sexual and reproductive health *(5ᵗʰ ed.). Eureka, CA: Nutrition Dimension.*

(Cunningham et al., 2001). Encourage a diet that includes foods high in iron (e.g., liver, lean red meats, oysters, dark green vegetables, peas, iron-fortified cereals, dried beans, and blackstrap molasses). Iron supplementation is recommended in the second and third trimester. Calcium and magnesium, if given with iron, decrease absorption. Vitamin C and administration between meals enhances absorption (Kline, 2000).

If the client has been diagnosed with hyperemesis gravidarum, optimal nutrition is essential for the remainder of pregnancy. Weight gains in the second and third trimesters have the greatest impact on fetal growth (see Chapter 18) (Kline, 2000).

Omega-3 (essential) fatty acids are a vital component of cell membranes and cannot be synthesized. The maternal liver converts essential fatty acids into long chain polyunsaturated fatty acids that are used for fetal brain, nervous system, and cell membrane development. Inadequate levels of essential fatty acids have been associated with pregnancy-induced hypertension, preterm birth, low birthweight, low head circumference and body length in the neonate. Omega-6 fatty acids are plentiful in most diets. Omega-3 fatty acids are found in fish and fish oils (Kline, 2000). One prenatal vitamin (Prima-Care) supplies essential fatty acids.

Neural tube defects incidences can be reduced by an estimated 50 percent if women consume adequate folic acid prior to conception. Smoking and alcohol use decrease serum folate levels. Other factors influencing neural tube defect development include maternal obesity, diabetes mellitus, hyperthermia, and exposure to trihalomethanes in water, paternal exposure to solvents, or use of medication for seizure control (valporic acid and carbamazipine) (Tinkle & Sterling, 1997). High intake of vitamin A (over 10,000) of retinol, not beta-carotene, should be avoided to reduce risk of head, brain and spinal cord defects (Kline, 2000). Combination hormonal contraceptives decrease the B_6 levels. If combination hormonal contraceptives were used 2–3 months before conception supplementation with 2 mg of Vitamin B_6 daily is advised (Kline, 2000). Zinc deficiency is common. Alcohol use, cigarette smoking, and a vegetarian diet can produce lower zinc levels. Zinc is essential for normal organogenesis in the first trimester. Iron interferes with zinc absorption. Zinc should be supplemented in the first trimester, iron in the last two trimesters (Kline, 2000).

Medication

Prenatal Vitamin/Mineral Supplements. Although needed only by those whose diet is inadequate or otherwise at nutritional risk, supplements are usually prescribed for all pregnant women.

- *Administration.* One tablet by mouth daily. Each supplement should contain 15 mg zinc, 2 mg copper, 250 mg calcium carbonate or citrate, 2 mg B_6, 400 mcg folate, 50 mg vitamin C, 200 IU vitamin D, 15 IU vitamin E and 100 to 320 mg magnesium. 30 mg of elemental iron is added in the last trimester. Prescription prenatal vitamins contain 1 mg of folate (Kline, 2000).
- *Side Effects and Adverse Reactions.* Gastric upset, constipation, diarrhea.
- *Contraindications.* None are known.
- *Anticipated Outcomes on Evaluation.* The client's hemoglobin level is within normal range, and neither the client nor the infant develops pathology related to vitamin or mineral deficiencies.
- *Client Teaching and Counseling.* Inform the client of the need for a healthy, balanced diet even when taking a prenatal supplement. To maximize the absorption of iron in the supplement, the tablet should be taken when the stomach is empty, with a drink high in vitamin C content, not with coffee, tea, or milk. The client should discontinue other vitamin supplementation (Kline, 2000).

Iron Supplementation. If the client is not anemic, a supplement of 30 mg elemental iron is recommended during the second and third trimesters, usually supplied in the prenatal vitamin. If the client is iron deficient, supplementation of 60 to 120 elemental mg iron is recommended (Kline, 2000).

- *Administration.* 30 to 60 mg of elemental iron twice a day, as 150 mg ferrous sulfate, 300 ferrous gluconate, or 100 mg ferrous fulmate (Kline, 2000).
- *Side Effects and Adverse Reactions.* Gastric upset, constipation, diarrhea.
- *Contraindications.* Some hemoglobinopathies (e.g., β-thalassemia without a dietary deficiency in iron; see Chapter 18).
- *Anticipated Outcomes on Evaluation.* Hemoglobin levels above 11.0 g/dL in the first and third trimester and 10.5 g/dL in the second trimester. Elevated reticulocyte count indicates response to treatment (Cunningham et al., 2001).
- *Client Teaching and Counseling.* Advise the client to take the iron supplement on an empty stomach, separate from the prenatal vitamin, and with liquids containing vitamin C (e.g., orange, cranberry, or tomato

juice), not with milk, tea, or coffee. The addition of 15 mg of zinc and 2 mg copper is recommended because high levels of iron interfere with absorption of those minerals (Kline, 2000).

Calcium Supplement. A calcium supplement may be recommended. Women younger than 25 years whose calcium intake is less than 600 mg receive 600 mg of supplemental calcium per day (Kline, 2000). Ten mcg (400 IU) of vitamin D is recommended if the client does not use dairy products.

- *Administration.* Calcium carbonate or citrate is recommended. Advise avoiding oyster shell calcium, dolomite, or bone meal because these may contain heavy metals.
- *Side Effects and Adverse Reactions.* Increased intestinal gas.
- *Contraindications.* History of kidney stones.
- *Anticipated Outcome on Evaluation.* Neither the client nor the infant develops pathology related to inadequate calcium intake.
- *Client Teaching and Counseling.* Advise the client to split the calcium supplement into 250 to 300 mg doses and take with a light meal or snack to enhance absorption. Calcium should not be taken at same time as an iron supplement (Kline, 2000).

Follow-Up

Weight gain should be assessed at each visit. The gain should be steady and in the parameters described (see Figure 17–3). Maternal weight is gained primarily in the first half of the pregnancy. Fetal weight gain is primarily in the third trimester. Each client's weight gain should be evaluated with that knowledge. Abnormal weight gains should be evaluated by ruling out pregnancy induced hypertension and by assessing diet quality, activity levels, food preferences and intolerance, and socioeconomic and psychologic factors. Refer to a dietitian any client at nutritional risk (see Tables 17–1 and 17–2) with a drug or alcohol abuse problem, a chronic medical problem that requires a therapeutic diet, gestational diabetes, or a vegetarian diet. If psychosocial problems are affecting the client's diet or appetite, refer her to a mental health care provider. If the client has inadequate financial resources, refer her to a social workers for advice about government and private programs (e.g., Women, Infants, and Children [WIC]).

IMMUNIZATION

BEFORE PREGNANCY

Clients should have all childhood immunizations before conception to protect the fetus from an illness that could produce congenital anomalies and from the theoretical risk of exposure to immunizations. The health care provider should be aware of the measles, mumps, and rubella (MMR) immunization schedule, which may require the client to receive an additional MMR immunization. Hepatitis B vacines are available. Diphtheria/tetanus boosters are required every 10 years (Leccese, 1999). Varicella vaccination is recommended for seronegative, nonpregnant clients (McCarter-Spaulding, 2001). These issues should be addressed at the preconception checkup (see Table 17–4).

DURING PREGNANCY

Rubella

Despite large-scale immunization of preschool-age children, a resurgence of rubella and congenital rubella syndrome occurred between 1988 and 1991. The risk of congenital rubella syndrome is related to the gestational age of the fetus at the time of maternal infection. One study showed a fetal infection rate of 80 percent between 7 and 17 weeks, 45 to 50 percent at 13 to 16 weeks, 6 percent at 14 to 20 weeks, and 0 percent after 20 weeks (Signore, 2001).

Administering serum immunoglobulin to a pregnant client with rubella reduces her symptoms but does not alter the risk or severity of congenital rubella syndrome in the fetus. A theoretical risk of congenital rubella syndrome from immunization just prior to pregnancy or during the first trimester exists, but the observed risk is 0 percent (Signore, 2001).

If the client has a positive serological test, then there is no risk to the fetus if she is exposed to rubella. *All prenatal clients should be tested.* If seronegative, they should be cautioned to avoid anyone with a rash or viral illness.

All nonimmune clients should be immunized postpartum. Breastfeeding is not a contraindication. If Rho(D) immune globulin (human) (RhoGAM) is given seroconversion should be checked at the postpartum visit. Theoretically, RhoGAM could block antibody development (Signore, 2001).

All preschool children should be immunized even if a pregnant woman is in the household. Furthermore, all

TABLE 17–4. Recommendations for Immunizations During Pregnancy

Live Virus Vaccines	Inactivated Bacterial Vaccines
Measles—contraindicated Mumps—contraindicated Varicella-zoster—contraindicated	Pneumococcal—same as nonpregnant Meningococcal—same as nonpregnant Hempophilus—same as nonpregnant Cholera—risks verses benefits
Inactivated Viral Vaccines	**Live Bacterial Vaccines**
Rabies—same as nonpregnant Influenza—after the first trimester Hepatitis A & B—same as nonpregnant Enhanced poliomyelitis (IPV-e)—risk of exposure Japanese encephalitis—risks verses benefits	Poliomyelitis—no longer recommended Typhoid (Ty21a)—risks verses benefits Yellow fever—high risk areas only
Toxoids	**Hyperimmune Globulins**
Tetanus-diphtheria—same as nonpregnant	Hepatitis B—postexposure prophylaxis; Give along with vaccine initially then vaccine alone at one and six months. Rabies—postexposure prophylaxis Tetanus—postexposure prophylaxis Varicella-zoster—consider for postexposure prophylaxis within 96 hours
Pooled Immune Serum Globulins	
Hepatitis A—postexposure prophylaxis Measles—postexposure prophylaxis	

Source: Reproduced with permission from Cunningham, F.G., Gant, N., Leveno, K.J., Gilstrap (II) L.C., Hauth, J.C., & Wenstrom, K.D. (2001). Williams' obstetrics (21st ed.). New York: McGraw-Hill.

nonpregnant persons of unknown immunity status should be immunized, particularly health care providers, Hispanic women, women entering higher education facilites, and international travelers. Because of theoretical risk, women of childbearing age should not become pregnant for three months following immunization (Signore, 2001).

Hepatitis B Virus

Infection with hepatitis B virus (HBV) carries significant sequelae if the client becomes a chronic carrier. Infection can lead to chronic hepatitis, cirrhosis, or primary hepatocellular carcinoma. Infants whose mothers test positive for hepatitis B surface antigen (HBsAg) may become infected and are at 90 percent risk for disease. Certain populations are at high risk for HBV infection, but limiting screening to persons in those groups results in failure to identify 50 percent of women who are HBV carriers (Stevenson, 1999).

All clients should be screened for HBsAg prenatally or, if not then, when they are admitted to the hospital. If HBsAg is positive, further testing of the client, her children, and her sexual partner is advised. The pediatrician should be advised of the mother's positive status and is responsible for appropriate care of the infant.

If a client is HBsAg and HBsAb (antibody to HBsAg) negative and at risk for infection, immunization is encouraged as pregnancy is not a contraindication (ACOG, 1998) (Ingardia, Kelley, Steinfeld, & Wax, 1999). Groups at risk include women of Asian, Pacific Island, or Eskimo descent, no matter where they were born; women born in Haiti or sub-Saharan Africa; women with work histories in public safety or health care (especially those exposed to blood); women who live with HBV carriers or hemodialysis clients; or women who have a history of intravenous drug use or sexual partners who have used intravenous drugs. Others at risk are women with a history of acute or chronic liver disease, women who work or live in institutions for the mentally disabled, women who have been rejected as blood donors, women with a history of blood transfusion, or women with multiple sexually transmitted disease (STD) episodes, multiple sexual partners, or whose partner has multiple sexual partners.

Influenza Vaccine

Pregnancy increases the morbidity of influenza infection, particularly clients with chronic medical illness, immunosuppressed clients, foreign travelers, and health care and chronic care providers. Some studies have suggested fetal infection may increase congenital anomalies and schizophrenia. More study is needed. Influenza vaccine is inactivated and generally considered safe. The Centers for Disease Control and Prevention recommend that the flu vaccine be offered to all pregnant clients in the second and third trimester. High-risk clients may receive the vaccine the first trimester (Kashyap & Gruslin, 2000).

Immunizations

Routine immunizations are usually not indicated during pregnancy. The decision to immunize should be made only after the risk of disease has been weighed against the risk of vaccination for mother and fetus.

Determination of susceptibility should include a history of prior illness, previous vaccinations, and, most important, serological tests. Other information is helpful, but *only serological tests can prove immunity.* The Centers for Disease Control (CDC) have developed definitions of susceptibility, which may be obtained through the Advisory Committee on Immunization Practices.

Risk of exposure is reduced by avoiding travel to endemic areas, practicing appropriate hygiene, and avoiding infected persons. This strategy is preferred to immunization.

Pregnancy may alter the rate of maternal complications in some diseases and cause special health problems.

In general, live vaccines are to be avoided; killed vaccines are safer (see Table 17–4) (Stevenson, 1999).

Varicella Vaccine

Varicella vaccine is recommended for all non-immune clients. Avoiding pregnancy for one month after immunization is recommended (McCarter-Spaulding, 2001). One study demonstrated no increase in congenital varicella syndrome or congenital anomalies in inadvertently exposed fetuses (Shields, Galil, Seward, et al., 2001) Varicella-zoster immunoglobulin (VZIG) is recommended for susceptible exposed pregnant women within 96 hours of exposure. VZIG will reduce the maternal complications of varicella but not the rates of fetal or newborn infection (McCarter-Spaulding, 2001).

COMMON COMPLAINTS

Many symptoms that are frequently reported to health care providers are most often attributable to pregnancy but must be evaluated to rule out other pathology.

FIRST TRIMESTER

Nausea and Vomiting

Etiology. Physiological changes that cause nausea and vomiting during pregnancy are unknown; however, unusually high levels of estrogen and progesterone and the introduction of human chorionic gonadotropin (hCG) have been studied (Cunningham et al., 2001). Vitamin B_6 deficiency has also been explored with little support in the studies (Steele, French, Gatherier-Boyles, et al., 2001). Multiple gestation and molar pregnancies are associated with higher incidences of nausea and vomiting. 60 to 70 percent of women experience nausea and vomiting. Symptoms generally last until the second trimester of pregnancy and are usually associated with a positive pregnancy outcome (Cunningham et al., 2001; Steele et al., 2001). Huxley (2000) theorized that nausea and vomiting in early pregnancy stimulated placental growth resulting in normal weight neonates with heavier placentas.

Subjective Data. Nausea and/or vomiting are reported by the client between the fourth and sixteenth weeks of pregnancy. It may or may not be limited to certain times of the day (Cunningham, et al., 2001). The history should *not* include fever, lethargy, muscle aches, abdominal pain, cramping, diarrhea, jaundice, back pain, dark urine, changes in the shape or color of bowel movements, vaginal bleeding, head injury, headache, projectile vomiting, vomiting blood, excessive thirst, neurological signs, ataxia, chest pain, ear pain or ringing, or psychosocial distress, as these symptoms/signs indicate other conditions that may require medical or other appropriate follow-up (Seller, 2000).

Objective Data. Physical examination and vital signs are within normal limits. Significant negatives include the absence of signs of dehydration and vaginal bleeding. A hydatidiform gestation may present with hyperemesis and possible prolonged vaginal spotting. Multiple pregnancies often cause severe nausea and/or vomiting.

Uterine size should be appropriate for dates. Fetal heart tones should be audible at 12 weeks' gestation.

Weight loss, dehydration, urine acidosis, blood alkalosis, and hypokalemia suggest hyperemesis gravidarum (Cunningham et al., 2001).

Urine ketone and specific gravity tests are used to rule out dehydration. Tests specific to disease suggested by physical and history should be obtained.

Differential Medical Diagnoses. Nausea and vomiting related to pregnancy ruling out hyperemesis gravidarium, multiple gestation, hydatidiform gestation, gastrointestinal disease (e.g. appendicitis, gastroenteritis), endocrine disease (e.g., hyperthyroidism), neurological disease (e.g. migraines), cardiorespiratory disease, nutritional disease (e.g., pica, vitamin deficiencies, food poisoning) medication overdose, emotional disease (e.g., eating disorders, depression) (Cunningham et al., 2001; Seller, 2000).

Plan

Psychosocial Interventions. Explain to the client that nausea and vomiting usually are limited to the first trimester and are usually related to positive pregnancy outcomes. Advise her to notify the health care provider if any symptoms ruled out during history-taking occur in the future.

Medication

- Phosphorated Carbohydrate Solution (Emetrol)
  - *Indications.* To reduce smooth muscle contractions of hyperactive gastric muscles.
  - *Administration.* Emetrol 1 to 2 tablespoons. Repeat every 15 minutes up to five times until nausea and vomiting are relieved.
  - *Side Effects and Adverse Reactions.* None are known.
  - *Contraindications.* Diabetes or hereditary fructose intolerance.
  - *Anticipated Outcome on Evaluation.* Decreased nausea and vomiting.
  - *Client Teaching and Counseling.* Instruct the client never to dilute this medication or drink fluids of any kind immediately before or after taking a dose (Physician's Desk Reference, 2001).

Lifestyle Changes

- Ask the client to keep a diary listing when and for how long nausea and vomiting occur and what activities, associated factors, or foods trigger or improve symptoms. Interventions suggested by this diary are most likely to succeed.
- Advise the client to rest when the nausea occurs, avoid stress, avoid sights and smells that trigger nausea, refrain from wearing clothing that is tight and constricting about the abdomen, and reduce work loads. Support and assistance from the client's partner may also improve symptoms.
- Suggest hypnosis, acupressure (e.g., Seabands) (Stule et al., 2001), or cold compresses to the throat.

- Describe relaxation techniques that may help: progressive relaxation (systematic tensing and relaxing of muscle groups), autogenic training (using suggestions such as "My right arm is heavy"), meditation (repeating a sound or gazing at an object while clearing the mind of all distractions), visual imagery (visualizing self in a relaxing place), and touching/massage.

Dietary Interventions

- Symptoms may be relieved by eating small, frequent meals that do not allow the stomach to become too empty or full, including high-carbohydrate or high-protein, easily digested meals and snacks; sipping carbonated drinks, including foods that tend to neutralize stomach acid (e.g., apples, milk, bread, potatoes, calcium carbonate tablets); eating crackers on arising; drinking fluids between meals instead of with meals; and avoiding foods that may irritate the stomach (e.g., spicy or fatty foods). Lemonade and potato chips have more nutrients and may be more effective than soda and crackers.
- Sit upright after eating.
- If a vitamin/mineral supplement is causing nausea, it may be discontinued until the client is less nauseated, often after about 14 to 16 weeks of pregnancy. Folic acid supplementation is advised (ACOG, 2000). A balanced diet would provide all necessary vitamins and minerals, except iron needed in the second and third trimester (see Nutrition and Weight Gain).
- Remind the client of the need for adequate hydration (6 to 8 glasses per day). Sipping lukewarm fluids every five minutes is tolerated better than drinking an entire glass of fluid at one time.
- Ginger, 250 mg four times/day, was shown in one study to decrease nausea and vomiting early in pregnancy with no adverse affects on pregnancy noted (Vutyavanich, Kraisarin, & Ruangsri, 2000).

Follow-Up. Refer to a physician any client who is unable to hold down liquids for more than twelve hours, who loses five pounds or more, who has ketonuria or any symptoms of dehydration or pathology.

Constipation

Etiology. Large amounts of circulating progesterone cause decreased contractility of the GI tract, resulting in slow movement of chyme and increased water reabsorption from the bowel. The large bowel is also mechanically compressed by the enlarging uterus, most noticeably in the first and third trimesters. The client may have changed her food and fluid intake or exercise level in response to nausea and vomiting, fatigue, culturally prescribed expectations of pregnant women, or medically prescribed treatment (ACOG, 2000). Prenatal vitamins with iron or calcium can also be constipating (Kline, 2000).

Subjective Data. The client may report abdominal cramping, flatulence, or increasing difficulty with bowel movements or intervals between them. Stools may be small, hard, round, and dark. Often the client has a history of constipation before pregnancy. Her diet may be high in refined carbohydrates and low in bulk and fluids, and she may rarely exercise. The client may have taken antacids, calcium, iron supplements, anticholinergics, tricyclic antidepressants, or codeine medications. These can constipate. The history should *not* include change in stool (i.e., color, shape, or pattern), diarrhea, abdominal pain, fever, weight loss, anorexia, periumbilical pain, rectal bleeding, pus or mucus in bowels, emotional distress, or excessive laxative use, because these symptoms/signs may indicate other conditions requiring medical or other appropriate follow-up (Seller, 2000).

Objective Data. Physical examination and vital signs are within normal limits, although hyperactive bowel sounds, constipated stool in the rectum, a sausage-shaped mass in the lower left quadrant that disappears after bowel movements, hemorrhoids, or hemorrhoidal tags may be revealed.

The *stool for occult blood* test is used to detect the presence of blood in the stool. A stool sample is collected during a digital rectal examination. The stool is applied to the card provided, and a drop of developer is placed on the card. If the card turns bright blue, blood is present.

Client teaching in preparation for the test includes diet information. For the most accurate results, the client should eliminate meats, fish, poultry, and green leafy vegetables for three days prior to the test. Aspirin or NSAIDs should not be consumed during that same three-day period. Hemorrhoids, anal fissures, and vaginal bleeding may also result in positive readings.

Differential Medical Diagnosis. Constipation related to pregnancy ruling out preterm labor, pica, gastrointestinal disease (e.g., irritable bowel syndrome, appendicitis) chronic laxative use, use of medications known to cause constipation (e.g., codeine), or anal pain (Seller, 2000).

Plan

Psychosocial Interventions. Explain to the client how pregnancy exacerbates the symptoms of constipation and that

symptoms should improve after delivery. Advise her to notify the health care provider if any symptoms ruled out during history-taking occur in the future.

Medication. Advise the client to avoid mineral oil, as it will decrease the absorption of fat-soluble vitamins. Cathartics are contraindicated in pregnancy.

Review with client what other medication (e.g., calcium supplements, iron) she is taking to determine whether constipation is a side effect—then help her to reduce their use if possible.

- Bulk-forming, nonnutritive laxatives (e.g., Metamucil, Fibercon)
  - *Indications.* Constipation caused by low dietary bulk.
  - *Administration.* Available in tablets or granules. Take per package instructions.
  - *Side Effects and Adverse Reactions.* If taken without adequate fluids, may swell in throat or esophagus, causing choking.
  - *Contraindications.* Fecal impaction or intestinal obstruction.
  - *Anticipated Outcome on Evaluation.* Softer stools with decreased constipation.
  - *Client Teaching and Counseling.* Instruct the client to drink 8 oz of water or more with each dose. Do not use if having difficulty breathing or swallowing, chest pain, or vomiting. If these occur, advise to seek immediate medical attention. She may need to continue treatment for two to three days before maximum effect is noted (PDR, 2001).

Lifestyle Changes. Encourage the client to exercise regularly (according to ACOG guidelines), establish a time of day to defecate, avoid prolonged attempts to defecate, and elevate her feet on a stool while defecating to avoid straining.

Dietary Interventions. Advise the client to eat foods high in bulk (e.g., fresh fruits and vegetables, whole-grain breads and cereals), drink fluids (6 to 8 glasses of water per day above that drunk with meals), decrease refined carbohydrates, and drink warm fluids on arising to stimulate bowel motility. Explain that if she takes her vitamin/mineral supplement every second or third day or changes to a supplement without iron and calcium temporarily, then constipation may be less of a problem. If any foods or juices (e.g., bran, prune juice) have helped the client in the past, encourage their use (ACOG, 2000; Seller, 2000).

Follow-Up. If prenatal vitamins or iron are discontinued, monitor the client for anemia. Folic acid should be supplemented in the first trimester. If purging or psychosocial stress is causing constipation, refer the client to a mental health care provider. If symptoms of a pathological condition develop, refer the client to a physician.

Hemorrhoids

Etiology. Hemorrhoids occur when the vascular submucosa in the rectoanal canal bulges and becomes congested with varicosities. They become significant only when they become symptomatic. Hemorrhoids are exacerbated during pregnancy by increased intravascular pressure in veins below the uterus, constipation, and straining at stool (ACOG, 2000; Curtis & Schuler, 2000).

Subjective Data. The client may report a history of constipation, hemorrhoids before pregnancy, multiparity, increased age, or a family history of hemorrhoids. She may notice swelling, fullness, or a lump at her anus; bright red, painless bleeding on the stool surface during defecation; or increased mucus with defecation. If an anal fissure develops, defecation is often painful.

Objective Data. Physical examination and vital signs may be within normal limits, or hemorrhoids may be visible externally or palpated internally. Anal fissures or hemorrhoidal tags may be noted. Thrombosed hemorrhoids are a painful, shiny, bluish or purple clot-containing mass near the anus.

Diagnostic tests and methods include evaluation of the *hemoglobin level* in the blood. The hemoglobin level may be decreased if bleeding is extensive or prolonged. Stool for occult blood is the other diagnostic tool (see Constipation).

Differential Medical Diagnosis. Hemorrhoids exacerbated by pregnancy; rule out abscessed or thrombosed hemorrhoids (Cunningham et al., 2001), rectal lesions (e.g., condyloma acuminato, cancerous lesions), all of which may require more extensive medical referral and intervention.

Plan

Psychosocial Interventions. Explain to the client the underlying changes that created or exacerbated the hemorrhoids and assure her that the condition will improve or resolve after pregnancy. Encourage her to contact a health care provider if any symptoms occur in the future.

Medication

♦ Topical anesthetics (e.g., Preparation H, Anusol)
  • *Indications.* To shrink the swelling of hemorrhoids and reduce itching.
  • *Administration.* Apply cream, freely as needed, to hemorrhoids up to four times per day: in the morning, at night, and after each bowel movement. If a suppository is used, insert it into the rectum after cleaning and drying the anal area, six times per day as needed after bowel movements.
  • *Side Effects and Adverse Reactions.* Occasional burning of irritated tissues.
  • *Contraindications.* Client sensitivity to components of the medication. Heart disease, hypertension, thyroid disease, and diabetes are contraindications to suppository use.
  • *Anticipated Outcomes on Evaluation.* Decreased swelling, pain, or itching of hemorrhoids.
  • *Client Teaching and Counseling.* Instruct the client in cream or suppository use. Clean and pat the anus dry. With the suppository, remove the foil wrapper before insertion. If soft, hold under cold water (in foil) for two to three minutes. With the cream, use a dispensing cap: Attach the cap to the tube and fill it by squeezing the tube. Lubricate the tip, gently insert it into the anus, and squeeze the tube to deliver cream into the rectum. Clean the cap with soap and water after use (PDR, 2000).

Lifestyle Changes. Advise the client to try to avoid constipation by following the measures described in the preceding section (see Constipation). Encourage her to use warm or cool sitz baths (Epsom salts may be added), witch hazel pads (e.g., Tucks), and ice packs or cold compresses to reduce the size of the hemorrhoids (ACOG, 2000). Furthermore, advise her to avoid straining by elevating her feet on a stool while attempting to defecate. Applying petroleum jelly around the anus before defecating will help reduce pain and bleeding. Resting with feet and hips elevated for at least an hour daily plus avoiding prolonged sitting or standing can be helpful (ACOG, 2000; Curtis & Schuler, 2000).

Kegel's exercises will improve circulation. To learn the feel of tightening the pubococcygeal (Kegel) muscles, first have the client sit on the commode and start and stop her urine flow. To do the exercise, squeeze and tighten 10 seconds each, ten to twenty times. Repeat the entire series three times a day (ACOG, 2000). Gentle self-digital replacement of hemorrhoids if possible and careful perineal cleansing habits are also helpful.

Refer the client to a physician if she has symptoms of thrombosed hemorrhoids, does not respond to interventions, or has symptoms of other pathology.

Flatulence

Etiology. The physiological changes that result in constipation also may result in increased flatulence.

Subjective Data. A client may report increased passage of rectal gas, abdominal bloating, constipation, or belching, but not abdominal pain, epigastric pain, use of food or medications that cause gas, change in bowels, greasy bowel movements, anxiety or depression (Seller, 2000).

Objective Data. Often, hyperactive bowel sounds or abdominal distention is detected on physical exam.

Differential Medical Diagnoses. Flatulence; rule out irritable bowel syndrome, lactose or food intolerance, medication side effects, hyperventilation or other gastrointestinal disease (e.g., malabsorption syndromes).

Plan

Psychosocial Interventions. Reassure the client that increased flatulence is related to pregnancy and should resolve afterward.

Lifestyle Changes. Teach the client measures to avoid constipation. Help her to recognize the symptoms of hyperventilation or air swallowing in order to alleviate flatulence. The client may find that she is breathing fast, sighing, or feeling the need for frequent deep breaths. She may feel tingling in her fingers, toes, or lips, dizziness, or confusion. Rebreathing air that is exhaled into a paper bag or cupped hands may help decrease symptoms. Because stress often causes hyperventilation, becoming aware of areas in her life that cause stress may be helpful for the client. Avoiding gum chewing, large meals, and smoking also will reduce flatulence.

Dietary Interventions. Advise the client to limit gas-forming foods (e.g., carbonated beverages, cruciferous vegetables, baking soda, cheese, beans, bananas, peanuts, calcium carbonate supplements). Pasta, corn, and whole grains when cooked, refrigerated, or frozen then reheated form gas-producing substances. Each cooling and reheating makes them more potent. Mint can increase abdominal gas.

Follow-Up. Refer her to a mental health care provider if symptoms of psychosocial stress are evident.

Fatigue

Etiology. Fatigue during pregnancy occurs primarily during the first and third trimesters (the highest energy levels often occur during the second trimester). First-trimester fatigue may be caused by physical changes (e.g., increased oxygen consumption, progesterone and relaxin levels, and fetal demands) and psychosocial changes (e.g., reexamination of roles). Mood swings, multiple role fulfillment, and depression may also cause insomnia. Third-trimester fatigue is usually caused by sleep disturbances that result from increased weight, physical discomforts, and decreased exercise. Fatigue, in particular, can be a symptom in most pathological problems—emotional, physical, or dietary (ACOG, 2000).

Subjective Data. The client may report fatigue despite normal amounts of sleep or insomnia due to difficulty in getting comfortable, fetal movements, urinary frequency, vivid dreams, increased stress, or emotional problems. Her family or work situation may not allow her to rest during the day. The history should *not* include depression, anxiety, difficulty with concentration, anorexia, anemia, use of medications known to cause drowsiness, exercise intolerance, chest pain or discomfort, change in bowel habits, flulike symptoms, sore throat, coughing, or dyspnea, or other symptoms/signs indicating other conditions requiring medical or other appropriate follow-up (Seller, 2000).

Objective Data. The physical examination and vital signs are within normal limits.

A *complete blood count* (CBC) is used to evaluate the client for signs of anemia, infection, or blood dyscrasias. The procedure involves venipuncture and withdrawal of blood, which is sent to laboratory for evaluation. The client may apply pressure to the venipuncture site until bleeding stops. Hematoma formation at the site is common and will resolve.

Differential Medical Diagnosis. Fatigue due to pregnancy ruling out other pathological states.

Plan

Psychosocial Interventions. Explain to the client that increased fatigue is expected in the first trimester and insomnia is common in the third. Encourage her to contact the health care provider if she develops other symptoms.

Encourage verbalization of psychosocial problems and explore appropriate interventions. Encourage the client to accept offers of help. Advise the client to avoid, if possible, major life stresses (e.g., moving) during pregnancy.

Medication. Supplemental iron may be appropriate if anemic. No sleeping medications are prescribed.

Lifestyle Changes. Encourage adequate sleep and rest periods; help the client to arrange work, child care, and other activities to permit additional rest.

Encourage good posture, wearing of low-heeled shoes, and pelvic rock exercises to ease backaches. Pelvic rock exercises are taught to the client by having her stand against a wall, bend knees slightly, and insert her hand behind the small of her back. Move the pelvis to roll her uterus up toward her chest and push her buttocks toward the floor. This should push her hand against the wall. Encourage her to do this while standing, walking, and sitting.

Suggest ways to increase comfort and reduce insomnia (e.g., placing pillows behind her back, raising the head of the bed up on blocks).

Establishing a regular sleep time and routine may induce sleep.

Demonstrate exercises that consume less energy (isometric instead of aerobic exercises). Have the client avoid exercise during the two hours prior to sleep.

Recommend exercise for sedentary clients (see Exercise, later in chapter).

Relaxation techniques may help.

Measures to reduce leg cramps may decrease their occurrence (see Leg/Muscle Cramps).

Dietary Interventions. Correct nutritional inadequacies, paying attention to total nutrient intake and distribution of those nutrients throughout the day (see Nutrition). Advise client to avoid caffeine after midday and heavy meals at the end of the day. Suggest that warm milk may induce sleep. Encourage higher fluid intake earlier in the day, decreasing in the evening. Avoiding high-sugar diets may be helpful (Curtis & Schuler, 2000).

Follow-Up. Refer the client to a physician if symptoms of pathology are evident. When severe psychosocial stress, anxiety, or depression are noted, referral to a mental health care provider is appropriate.

Urinary Frequency or Incontinence

Etiology. A physiologic change during the first trimester that causes urinary difficulty is the enlargement of the uterus, which compresses the bladder. In the second trimester, however, as the uterus becomes an abdominal organ, these symptoms improve. In the third trimester, fetal presenting parts often compress the bladder. This, in addition to hyperplasia and hyperemia of the pelvic organs and increased kidney output, leads to urinary frequency and incontinence (ACOG, 2000; Curtis & Schuler, 2000).

Subjective Data. The client may report increased urination, nocturia, or involuntary loss of urine. The history should *not* include back pain, fever, flulike symptoms, hematuria, dysuria, urgency, dark, cloudy or blood urine, dribbling, suprapubic pain, polyuria, polydipsia, polyphagia, history of perineal or abdominal trauma, as these symptoms/signs indicate other conditions requiring more thorough follow-up and possible medical referral. She may report use of alcohol or caffeine (ACOG, 2000; Curtis & Schuler, 2000).

To differentiate urine loss from rupture of membranes (ROM), know that ROM may be described as fluid from her vagina that cannot be controlled with Kegel exercises or as fluid that does not smell of urine and that may increase while she is lying down, gush at first when she stands, then decrease after standing.

Objective Data. Physical examination and vital signs are within normal limits. The costal vertebral angle and suprapubic area are not tender. Vaginal exam does not reveal pooling of amniotic fluid but may reveal a cystocele. Abdominal exam does not reveal contractions or uterine irritability.

Urinalysis and culture and sensitivity tests are used to detect urinary tract infection, renal and metabolic diseases. The test procedure first involves obtaining the best specimen. Instruct the client to wash her hands, then separate her labia. Provide three cleansing wipes and have her wipe from front to back once with each wipe, on the right side, then the left side, and then the middle. She should start to urinate in the commode, then catch a small amount of urine midstream in a sterile cup, and finish urinating in the commode. She should replace the lid on the cup tightly without touching the inside or top edge. Client teaching should stress that failing to follow this procedure jeopardizes the accuracy of the test.

The urine can be poured over a urine dipstick. Presence of nitrites, or 3–4 plus protein, suggests a urinary tract infection, plus glucose suggests ruling out diabetes (see Chapter 21).

The *nitrazine test* is one test that may help discriminate between vaginal discharge and amniotic fluid. Use of a sterile technique reduces the possibility of introducing infection if the membranes have ruptured. A sterile cotton-tipped applicator is used to remove discharge from the vaginal pool. It is placed on nitrazine paper and the color change is compared with the chart. If the pH is 3.5 to 5, the fluid is normal vaginal discharge. If the pH is 7, the discharge may be amniotic fluid, Note that blood and vaginal discharge associated with certain vaginal infections (e.g., bacterial vaginosis and trichomonas vaginitis) may give a higher than normal pH reading.

The *fern test* also discriminates between vaginal discharge and amniotic fluid. Again, a sterile speculum is used. The sample of vaginal discharge is placed on a clean slide and allowed to dry. Amniotic fluid forms a fernlike pattern under microscopic examination. Inform the client that the nitrazine and fern tests are the best way to discriminate between vaginal discharge and amniotic fluid. Differentiation is important because premature rupture of membranes can cause amniotitis or preterm labor. The practitioner may also look for fluid leaking from the cervix, which may not necessarily be amniotic fluid, but would certainly raise suspicion.

A screening 50 g glucola test that is negative (see Chapter 16) reduces the likelihood of diabetes.

Differential Medical Diagnosis. Urinary frequency/incontinence due to pregnancy, ruling out urinary tract infection, pyelonephritis, kidney stone, stress urinary incontinence, gestational diabetes, preexisting diabetes mellitus, hypokalemia, and spontaneous rupture of membranes (Curtis & Schuler, 2000).

Plan

Psychosocial Interventions. Show the client diagrams of female anatomy. Often when a client can view the anatomical changes that occur during pregnancy, she understands the reason for urinary frequency and incontinence. Reassure her that these symptoms should improve after delivery. Advise the client to notify the health care provider if any symptoms ruled out during history-taking occur in the future.

Lifestyle Changes. Resting and sleeping in the lateral recumbent position enhance kidney function. Kegel exercises increase perineal muscle tone.

Dietary Interventions. Advise the client to maintain an adequate fluid intake (6 to 8 glasses of water) to decrease the incidence of urinary tract infections. Water intake should decrease two to three hours before bedtime. In addition, advise the client to discontinue drinking beverages that contain alcohol or caffeine (ACOG, 2000).

Follow-Up. A client with urinary tract infection (UTI) must be treated appropriately. Refer clients with symptoms of pathology, such as frequently repeated UTIs, to a urologist.

Varicosities of Vulva and Legs

Etiology. Physiologic changes during pregnancy that exacerbate varicosities are the increased venous stasis caused by the pressure of the gravid uterus and the vasodilation resulting from hormonal changes. Women who develop varicosities often have a genetic predisposition, are inactive, obese, and have poor muscle tone. Prolonged standing or sitting aggravates the condition (Cunningham, et al., 2001; Curtis & Schuler, 2000).

Subjective Data. The client may report aching, throbbing, swelling, or heaviness in the legs or vulvar area, often worse at night. The client may also report multiparity, prolonged standing or sitting, or decreased activity. She may note increased symptoms as she becomes older. A family history of varicosities may be reported. The history should *not* include calf pain, clotting, swelling, redness, or tenderness, or a white, cold, numb leg, as these symptoms/signs indicate other conditions requiring immediate medical follow-up.

Objective Data. Diagnostic tests are not necessary. Physical examination and vital signs are within normal limits. Knotted, twisted, and swollen veins, however, are visible in the legs or vulva with possible edema below the varicosities. Peripheral pulses are normal. Significant negatives include no inflammation over the varicosities, equal pedal and femoral pulses; no firm, cordlike feel; no dependent cyanosis; no positive Homan's sign; no deep pain on palpation; no distention of veins on the dorsal side of the foot after it is elevated 45 degrees; and no restlessness, fever, or tachycardia (Seller, 2000).

Differential Medical Diagnosis. Varicosities of legs and/or vulva exacerbated by pregnancy ruling out vascular disease (e.g., deep vein thrombosis), edema from pregnancy-induced hypertension, physiologic edema of pregnancy, or other musculoskeletal disease.

Plan

Psychological Interventions. Explain to the client the reasons for the varicosities and inform her that the varicosities will not resolve until after delivery. Advise the client to notify the health care provider if any symptoms ruled out during the history-taking occur in the future.

Any surgical intervention would be delayed until after delivery or, optimally, until after childbearing is complete.

Lifestyle Changes. Some lifestyle changes may help to relieve discomfort. Teach the client proper application of support hose and compression stockings: Have her lie flat and raise her legs to drain the veins. While her legs are elevated, have her roll the stockings on. Advise the client to do this before she rises in the morning and to leave the stockings on until she goes to bed at night.

Instruct the client to avoid crossing her legs and not to wear knee-high stockings or a constrictive band around the legs.

Because orthostatic hypotension is common, tell the client to change position gradually when rising to avoid dizziness.

Explain the importance of elevating the legs above the level of the heart at least twice a day. Advise the client to wear comfortable shoes and to avoid prolonged standing or sitting, altering position frequently (ACOG, 2000; Curtis & Schuler, 2000).

Instruct the client in the use of perineal pads with a sanitary belt or maternity girdle to compress vulvar varicosities.

Explain to the client the need to avoid leg or vulvar injury, as hemorrhage may result.

Dietary Interventions. Warn the client to avoid excess weight gain during pregnancy and encourage weight loss during the postpartum period.

Follow-Up. Refer a client with symptoms of pathology to a physician.

Headache

Etiology. Physiologic changes during pregnancy that cause headaches include increased circulatory volume, vasodilation caused by high levels of circulating progesterone, tissue edema resulting from vascular congestion, stress, fatigue, sinus congestion, caffeine withdrawal, and low blood sugar. Other causes include muscle spasm, allergens, hyperventilation, or noxious fumes. Headaches not caused by pathology are very common in pregnancy. Women who had headaches prior to pregnancy frequently improve; 15 to 20 percent will have migraines (Curtis & Schuler, 2000). Headache can be a symptom of serious illness, which must be ruled out.

Subjective Data. Focus on the nature, frequency, intensity, location, description of the pain; factors that trigger, worsen, or alleviate it; and changes that have occurred during pregnancy in the quality of the headaches. The client may report a past or family history of headaches or increased stress. The history should *not* include injury to the head, neck, or back; nausea, vomiting, diarrhea, fever; migraine aura; occupational exposure to chemicals; consumption of alcohol, chocolate, or aged cheese; unbalanced intake of calories; fatigue, as these symptoms/signs may indicate other conditions requiring medical or other appropriate follow-up. Pathology may also be present if there is a history of increasing intensity and frequency of headaches, increase with coughing or straining, worse in morning, disrupts sleep; facial edema; changes in the level of consciousness; memory changes; depression, anxiety, motor, visual, or sensory changes; nausea, vomiting; stiff neck; fever; ear or eye pain; rhinitis; flulike symptoms; injury; or prodomata (i.e., visual, auditory, or sensory changes preceding a headache) (Seller, 2000).

Objective Data. Physical examination and vital signs, particularly blood pressure, weight gain pattern, ophthalmoscopic examination, and ear, nose, throat, neurological, musculoskeletal, and upper respiratory exams are within normal limits.

A *urine dipstick test* that is negative for protein and ketones reduces the possibility of pregnancy-induced hypertension and dehydration from vomiting.

The *serum glucose test* (to rule out hypoglycemia) procedure begins with venipuncture; blood is withdrawn into a tube containing chemicals that stabilize the glucose. The tube is sent to a laboratory. Another method involves performing a fingerstick to withdraw a drop of blood that is then placed on a reagent strip. The strip is then analyzed in a machine or read against a scale (least accurate method).

Teach the client that a hematoma is common at the venipuncture site and will resolve. Tenderness at the fingerstick is common. Accurate interpretation of the results depends on obtaining an accurate history of food intake during the time preceding the test. This test is often performed after the client fasts or ingests a measured amount of glucose.

A complete blood count is another diagnostic test used (see Fatigue).

Differential Medical Diagnosis. Benign vascular headache of pregnancy ruling out pregnancy-induced hypertension, HELLP syndrome, infectious process (e.g., sinus infections), cardiovascular diseases, muscloskeletal disease (e.g., muscle tension headache), neurological disease (e.g., cluster or vascular headache) hypoglycemia, caffeine withdrawal (Seller, 2000). Chapter 22 has additional discussion about headaches. Caution is advised with the use of the medications described because several are not recommended in pregnancy.

Plan

Psychosocial Interventions. Explain to the client the physiologic changes that are causing the headache and that it may improve in the second trimester. Advise the client to notify the health care provider if any symptoms ruled out during the history-taking occur in the future.

Ask the client to keep a diary of activities, foods, and environmental stimuli that occur around the time of the headache. This may reveal triggering factors.

Teach the client symptoms of pregnancy-induced hypertension (headache that is different in nature, visual changes, photophobia, confusion, swelling in the face or hands, severe swelling in the feet, epigastric pain) and encourage immediate contact with a physician.

Medication. Acetaminophen is indicated for headache and other pain.

- *Administration.* 325 to 650 mg every four hours as needed for pain.
- *Side Effects and Adverse Reactions.* None are known.
- *Contraindication.* Sensitivity to acetaminophen, consuming three or more alcoholic drinks a day, history of liver damage.
- *Anticipated Outcome on Evaluation.* Reduced headache pain.
- *Client Counseling.* Instruct the client to notify the health care provider if headache pain continues. Overdose of acetaminophen requires prompt attention. It has been associated with liver damage. Advise against chronic use (PDR, 2000).

Lifestyle Changes. Advise the client to avoid activities and situations that may trigger headaches (stress, smoking, smoke-filled rooms, blinking lights, sleeping late). Advise her to reduce stress as much as possible, get adequate sleep, have her neck and shoulders massaged with heat or cold applied.

Encourage the client to practice relaxation techniques (see Nausea and Vomiting).

Dietary Interventions. Advise the client to eat a regular, balanced diet and to avoid intake of food that triggers headaches (e.g., caffeine, chocolate, nitrites, hard aged cheese, alcohol—especially red wine). Drink 6 to 8 glasses of water daily (Curtis & Schuler, 2000).

Refer the client to a physician if the headache is severe, does not respond to interventions, requires strong pain killers, or demonstrates other signs of pregnancy-induced hypertension, pathology, or eye strain. If caffeine withdrawal is causing headache, advise weaning off caffeine gradually. If signs of severe psychosocial stress are present, refer the client to a mental health care provider. Referral to a pain center may help severe headache that is not due to pathology.

Breast Pain, Enlargement, and Changes in Pigmentation

Etiology. Physiologic changes that underlie these complaints are the increased levels of estrogen and progesterone, which cause the fat layer of breasts to thicken and the numbers and development of milk ducts and glands to increase. As a result, the breasts, especially the area round the areola, increase in size, weight, and tenderness, and bluish veins appear on the chest. The nipples become erect, melatonin causes the areolae to darken, the Montgomery tubercles enlarge, and there is a slight colostrum discharge (ACOG, 2000; Curtis & Schuler, 2000).

Subjective Data. The client may report increasing tenderness, weight, and size of the breasts, darkening of the areolae, leakage of colostrum from the nipples. The history should not include pain and redness localized in one area of the breast, fever, flulike symptoms, injury, masses, dimples, bloody discharge, changes in skin texture, or changes in breast or nipple size, shape, symmetry, as these symptoms/signs may indicate other conditions requiring medical follow-up. Some medications are known to cause galactorrhea (Seller, 2000).

Objective Data. No diagnostic tests are necessary. Physical examination and vital signs are within normal limits. Areas of induration, inflammation, or heat; masses; skin dimpling; skin changes; enlarged nodes; or unilateral or bloody nipple discharge should not be present.

Differential Medical Diagnosis. Breast tenderness, enlargement, and pigment changes due to pregnancy ruling out mastitis, fibrocystic breast tissue, breast injury, and breast cancer (Seller, 2000).

Plan

Psychosocial Interventions. Explain to the client the reasons for the breast changes. Inform her that pain often improves in the second trimester but the other changes will remain until after lactation ends. Advise the client to notify the health care provider if any symptoms ruled out during the history-taking occur in the future.

Lifestyle Changes. Advise the client to examine her breasts in the same way as before pregnancy, except that no special time of month is indicated. If instruction is necessary, provide it (see Chapter 14).

In addition, the client may need to constantly wear a supportive bra. Correct fit is important as breast size changes in pregnancy. She may find wearing a bra while sleeping more comfortable.

Dietary Interventions. Advise the client to avoid the use of caffeine.

Follow-Up. Clients with symptoms of mastitis must be treated appropriately (see Chapter 14). Refer the client with symptoms of pathology to a physician.

Menstrual-like Cramping

Etiology. The physiologic changes underlying the sensation of cramping may be the increased vascular congestion in the pelvis, the pressure exerted by the presenting fetal part, or stretching of the round ligaments. Many women report such cramping during the first one or two months of pregnancy and again at the end of pregnancy.

Subjective Data. The client reports sensations similar to those she experienced just prior to her menses, before she was pregnant. The history should *not,* however, include severe cramping, unilateral right lower quadrant or suprapubic abdominal pain, contractions, vaginal bleeding, vaginal discharge, rupture of membranes, bowel or urinary tract symptoms (see Urinary Frequency or Incontinence and Constipation), as these symptoms/signs may indicate other conditions which may require medical follow-up (ACOG, 2000; Curtis & Schuler, 2000).

Objective Data. Physical examination and vital signs are within normal limits. There is no vaginal bleeding, cervical dilatation, adnexal masses, tenderness, or vaginal pooling of amniotic fluid. Uterine size equals dates. There is no suprapubic tenderness.

Serum β Human chorionic gonadotropin-quantitative (hCG) is evaluated to identify and monitor pregnancy and to diagnose certain pregnancy-related complications (e.g., abortion, ectopic pregnancy, hydatidiform gestation). A blood sample is withdrawn by venipuncture and sent to a laboratory. In normal pregnancies, the hCG level is expected to double every other day. A deviation could indicate a complication of pregnancy and requires further testing (Curtis & Schuler, 2000).

Nitrazine and *fern tests* and *urinalysis and culture and sensitivity* may also be indicated (see Urinary Frequency and Incontinence).

Differential Medical Diagnosis. Normal menstrual-like cramping in pelvis ruling out ectopic pregnancy, abortion, premature labor, gastrointestinal disease (e.g., constipation), and urinary tract infection.

Plan

Psychosocial Interventions. Explain to the client the physiologic changes that underlie the sensations. In addition, inform the client that no signs of imminent abortion or labor exist and that the sensations should decrease in the second trimester but may return again in the third. Advise the client to notify the health care provider if any symptoms ruled out during the history-taking occur in the future.

Follow-Up. Refer the client with symptoms of pathology to a physician.

SECOND TRIMESTER

Backache

Etiology. Physiologic change underlying a backache is the shift in the center of gravity caused by the enlarging uterus. Muscle strain results. In addition, a high level of circulating progesterone softens cartilage and loosens once-stable joints, thereby increasing discomfort. Upper back pain can also be caused by increased breast size (ACOG, 2000; Curtis & Schuler, 2000). Night backache may result from pressure on the lower back from venous stasis and the gravid uterus.

Subjective Data. The client reports dull, aching pain in the upper or lower back that increases as the day goes on. Ask the client to describe the location, nature, and duration of the pain, exacerbating and relieving factors, the changes in pain that occur with movement. She may be wearing improperly fitting or high-heeled shoes. The client may have gained excessive weight, report being obese before pregnancy, must stand or sit for long time periods or be fatigued. She may be large busted and/or wear an improperly fitting or poorly supporting bra. Many clients lift heavy objects by bending from the waist rather than bending the knees; low back muscles are strained as a result of this movement (ACOG, 2000; Curtis & Schuler, 2000). There should be *no* history of back injury, surgery, or symptoms of urinary tract infection, gastrointestinal symptoms, vaginal infection, ruptured membranes, uterine contractions, pain or numbness in buttocks, legs, or hips, or neurologic deficit (Seller, 2000).

Objective Data. No diagnostic tests are done. Physical examination and vital signs are within normal limits; however, lordosis, abnormal gait, or tenderness along paraspinous muscles may be revealed. Significant negatives include no costal vertebral angle tenderness; no pain with straight-leg raises; normal patellar, deep tendon, and plantar reflexes; and a normal neurologic exam. No urinary tract or gastrointestinal symptoms (see Urinary Frequency and Incontinence), no abnormal vaginal discharge (see Leukorrhea), and no uterine contractions are detected.

Differential Medical Diagnoses. Backache ruling out uterine contractions, genital infections, urinary tract infections, gastrointestinal disease, kidney stone, pancreatitis, ulcer, musculoskeletal back disorders, including muscle sprain or strain (Seller, 2000).

Plan

Psychosocial Interventions. Explain to the client the changes underlying the backache, and inform her that it should decrease or resolve after pregnancy. Advise the client to notify the health care provider if any symptoms ruled out during the history taking occur in the future.

Medication. Acetaminophen (see Headache).

Lifestyle Changes. Instruct client in the pelvic tilt exercise (see Fatigue). Proper body mechanics, particularly when lifting require her to keep her back straight when lifting and to bend her knees, keeping the object close to her body; if she must hold her breath to lift an object, it is too heavy. Advise her to avoid excessive twisting, bending, and stretching. Back rubs may help. (ACOG, 2000)

Inform the client that an exercise program encourages general fitness.

Pelvic tilt (see Fatigue) helps to relieve back pain by relieving muscles often tired from the excessive lordosis of pregnancy.

Advise the client, when standing for long periods, to rest one foot on a low stool, and when sitting for long periods, to rest her feet on a low stool, to raise her knees above the hips and to sit with her back firmly against the back of the chair. While driving, she should sit straight and position the seat so that her knees are slightly bent when using the pedals.

Advise the client to avoid excessive walking or standing. Uterine support with a maternity girdle or belt may offer some relief (ACOG, 2000).

Inform the client that a firm, supportive mattress may be helpful. Advise her to assume a lateral recumbent position while sleeping, with pillows supporting the back and legs. Sleeping in this position promotes comfort. Some clients sleep better on the couch.

Advise the client with upper back pain to wear a good, supportive bra.

Warm tub baths may be soothing. Advise the client to be careful when rising from the tub, as she may experience dizziness. She should have someone's help or hold on to some other support. Do not recommend tub baths for clients in whom rupture of membranes is suspected.

Inform the client that massage and relaxation techniques, as well as use of a heating pad (do not sleep with) or cold applications for short periods, may promote comfort.

Dietary Interventions. Advise the client to avoid gaining excessive weight.

Follow-Up. If severe pain does not respond to intervention, refer the client to a physical therapist. Refer any client who requires strong pain medication or who has symptoms of pathology to a physician.

Syncope

Etiology. The physiologic changes underlying syncope (feeling dizzy or faint) are related to pooling of blood in the lower extremities, expansion of blood volume, and compression of the vena cava and lungs by the gravid uterus (Curtis & Schuler, 2000). True vertigo is often described as the room spinning or disorientation in relation to space. Syncope is also caused by hypovolemia, low blood sugar, anemia, substance abuse, hyperventilation, postural hypotension, vena cava compression, and illness.

Subjective Data. The client reports lightheadedness or dizziness that lasts a minute or less when she is standing, lying on her back, or changing position. She may report low or sporadic intake of calories. There should be *no* history of loss of consciousness; use of medications; exposure to toxic agents; substance abuse; sinus, hearing, or ear problems, numbness or tingling in the digits or around the mouth; nausea or vomiting; melena; heart palpitations; shortness of breath; neurological symptoms or anxiety or depression as these symptoms/signs may indicate other conditions that may require medical or other appropriate follow-up (Seller, 2000).

Objective Data. Physical examination and vital signs are within normal limits. *Hemoglobin* tests may reveal anemia. Blood sugar level is in normal limits.

Differential Medical Diagnosis. Syncope related to the hemodynamic changes in pregnancy, ruling out orthostatic hypotension, compression of vena cava, hyperventilation, anemia, hypoglycemia, dehydration, substance abuse, exposure to a toxic agent, psychosocial stress, or central nervous system, cardiac, respiratory, endocrine, eye, ear, or sinus pathology.

Plan

Psychosocial Interventions. Explain to the client the physiologic changes causing syncope. Advise the client to notify the health care provider if any symptoms ruled out during the history-taking occur in the future.

Advise the client to avoid stressful situations. Teach her to recognize hyperventilation. Encourage her to verbalize problems and explore appropriate responses.

Lifestyle Changes. Advise the client to rest in the lateral recumbent position; to change position gradually, holding on to something when rising; or to lower her head below the level of the heart if feeling faint.

To reduce blood pooling in the extremities, instruct the client to apply compression stockings before getting out of bed and to perform leg pumping exercises (flexing and extending the ankle several times).

If being in a crowd induces symptoms, advise the client to move to an open window or go outside and loosen or remove layers of clothing.

Dietary Interventions. Advise the client to eat regularly throughout the day. Assess her diet for adequate calorie and fluid intake and distribution.

Follow-Up. Refer a client with symptoms of pathology to a physician.

Leukorrhea

Etiology. The physiologic changes underlying leukorrhea arise from the high levels of estrogen that cause increased vascularity and hypertrophy of cervical glands as well as vaginal cells (Cunningham et al., 2001). As a consequence, leukorrhea production increases; the discharge is white or yellow, thin, and more acidic than normal vaginal discharge (ACOG, 2000).

Subjective Data. The client reports increased vaginal discharge. History should *not,* however, include green, watery, bloody, itchy, or irritating discharge that smells foul or fishy; fever; flulike symptoms; abdominal pain: bleeding after intercourse; dysuria or dyspareunia. Ask the client if she has multiple or new sexual partners, recently resumed sexual activity, performed douching, had abnormal Pap smears in the past, or recently used antibiotics.

Objective Data. Physical examination and vital signs are within normal limits: however, the pelvic exam may show increased but normal-appearing vaginal discharge.

A *normal saline and potassium hydroxide test* (wet mount) is used to determine whether candida, trichomonads, clue cells, white or red blood cells, or bacteria are present in the vaginal discharge. A Q-tip is used to obtain some vaginal, not cervical, discharge which is placed on two clean, dry microscope slides. A drop of normal saline is placed on one and a drop of potassium hydroxide on the other. Coverslips are used and the specimens are examined under the microscope. Candida, trichomonads, clue cells, and abnormal numbers of coccal bacteria, red cells, and white blood cells may indicate a vaginal infection.

A *Papanicolaou smear* is done to detect changes in the cervical or endocervical cells that could indicate dysplasia, carcinoma, or human papillomavirus. Signs of vaginal infection or herpes simplex may also be noted.

Both tests are speculum exams; that is, cervical and endocervical cells are collected using a wooden or preferably plastic spatula and cytobrush (though during pregnancy, a Q-tip is preferred to reduce cervical bleeding from the collection procedure), placed on a microscope slide, sprayed with a fixative, and sent to a pathology laboratory for examination.

Inform the client that the Pap smear is a screening test used to determine which clients require additional testing. Advise the client that she should not douche, use vaginal medications, or have intercourse for 24 hours before the test. The procedure may cause slight spotting up to 24 hours afterward.

The *nitrazine* and *fern tests* are also used (see Urinary Frequency and Incontinence).

Differential Medical Diagnoses. Physiologic leukorrhea of pregnancy, ruling out ruptured membranes, vaginitis, cervicitis, urinary tract infection, condyloma acuminatum, genital herpes, sexually transmitted diseases, and cervical dysplasia or neoplasia.

Plan

Psychosocial Interventions. Reassure the client that increased leukorrhea is normal and will decrease postpartum. Advise the client to notify the health care provider if any symptoms ruled out during the history-taking occur in the future.

Lifestyle Changes. Advise the client to keep the vulva clean and dry; to avoid pantyhose and other tight or layered clothing; to wear cotton underwear and a nightgown without underwear at night; and if using panty liners to use unscented/nondeodorant ones, changing them frequently. Also, advise her to avoid douching and tampon use unless otherwise instructed by the health care provider. Feminine sprays, powders, etc. should not be used.

Dietary Interventions Some clients have recurrent monilia during pregnancy. Instruct these clients to avoid large amounts of carbohydrates in their diets. If an antibiotic has been prescribed, advise the client to take acidophyllus (may be obtained over the counter) or consume a sugar-free yogurt containing active cultures.

Follow-Up. Refer all clients with abnormal Pap smears or symptoms of pathology for appropriate follow-up. Clients with symptoms of vaginitis require appropriate treatment (see Chapter 11).

Epistaxis and Epulis

Etiology. The physiologic change underlying epistaxis and epulis is the high level of circulating estrogen. The nasal mucosa and gums become hypertrophic and hyperemic and, as a result, bleed more easily (ACOG, 2000; Curtis & Schuler, 2000).

Subjective Data. The client reports that her nose or gums bleed easily, but she is able to control a nosebleed within 15 minutes. Nosebleeds are usually preceded by blowing the nose, picking at the nose, or overexertion. Gums bleed after teeth brushing or flossing, but the bleeding stops quickly. The client reports continuing her dental care during pregnancy. She has no history of hypertension, bleeding problems, menorrhagia, sinus symptoms, upper respiratory infection, swollen glands, fever, trauma, cocaine or chronic nasal spray use. She may report a history of nasal stuffiness, postnasal drip, or hay fever.

Objective Data. Physical examination and vital signs, particularly blood pressure, are within normal limits. The nasal mucosa may be swollen and dull red or pink, and clotted blood may be observed. Increased vascularization may be evident as may postnasal drip. The gums may show evidence of trauma caused by a toothbrush or floss and may look swollen and inflamed. Nasal polyps, growths, and evidence of cocaine use should not be observed. A *complete blood count* is the diagnostic test performed (see Fatigue).

Differential Medical Diagnoses. Epistaxis and/or epulis of pregnancy ruling out upper respiratory infection (e.g., sinusitis, nasal polyps), hypertension, anemia, bleeding disorders, cocaine or chronic nasal spray use, gingivitis, or other dental disease.

Plan

Psychosocial Interventions. Explain to the client the underlying physiologic changes that cause the problem and inform her that the condition should resolve after pregnancy. Advise the client to notify the health care provider if any symptoms ruled out during the history-taking occur in the future.

Lifestyle Changes Advise the client, when nosebleeds occur, to loosen clothing around the neck, sit with her head tilted forward, pinch her nostrils for ten to fifteen minutes, and apply ice packs to her nose. Light packing of the nose with sterile gauze may help. Inform her that applying petroleum jelly to the nostrils will lubricate and protect the mucosa. Advise the client to avoid overheated air, excessive exertion, and nasal sprays. A cool mist vaporizer may help humidify the air. Do not use if allergic to molds or mildew (ACOG, 2000; Curtis & Schuler, 2000).

Inform the client that the reduced air pressure at high altitudes may precipitate nosebleeds. Instruct the client to blow her nose gently, one nostril at a time and not to pick at her nose.

Advise clients with epulis to practice good oral hygiene, using a soft toothbrush and flossing regularly and gently. Instruct clients that warm saline mouthwashes relieve discomfort. Regular dental care is advised. Dental x-rays while shielding the abdomen and use of local anesthesia are safe (ACOG, 2000; Curtis & Schuler, 2000).

Dietary Interventions. Advise the client to maintain a healthy diet; to avoid sugary, sticky, or starchy food; and to cut food that is difficult to chew into small pieces to reduce gum trauma.

Follow-Up. Refer clients with gum and tooth disease to a dentist. Clients whose nose bleeds cannot be controlled within fifteen minutes or who have high blood pressure or symptoms of pathology should be referred to a physician.

Muscle Cramps in the Calf, Thigh, or Buttocks

Etiology. The physiologic change underlying muscle cramps in pregnancy is uncertain. An imbalance in the phosphorus/calcium ratio has been postulated, but a correlation with calcium intake has not been established (ACOG, 2000). Cramps occur primarily in the second and third trimesters and could be related to the pressure of the gravid uterus on pelvic nerves and blood vessels (Curtis & Schuler, 2000).

Subjective Data. The client reports calf, thigh, or buttocks cramps that occur mostly at night or in the early morning. She may report a similar history with previous pregnancies, excessive exercise or walking, or wearing of high-heeled or poorly supporting shoes. There should be *no* history of deep-vein thromboembolytic disease, recent trauma or surgery, swelling, lower back pain, muscle strain, arthritis, increased pain or limping with walking.

Objective Data. Physical examination and vital signs, particularly Homan's sign, and pulses are within normal limits. No redness, tenderness, heat, swelling, coldness, numbness, or whiteness appears in a calf or leg (Seller, 2000).

Diagnostic tests are not done unless pathology is suspected.

Differential Medical Diagnoses. Calf, thigh, or buttocks cramps, ruling out thromboembolytic disease, (e.g., varicosities) dehydration, musculoskeletal disease (e.g., sciatica, arthritis).

Plan

Psychosocial Interventions. Explain to the client the physiologic changes that could possibly cause muscle cramping and inform her that the condition should improve after delivery. Advise the client to notify the health care provider if any symptoms ruled out during the history-taking occur in the future.

Lifestyle Changes. Advise the client to avoid stretching her legs, pointing toes, walking excessively, and lying on her back and to wear low-heeled shoes.

Instruct the client in calf stretching: Have the client stand three feet from a wall and lean toward it to rest the lower arms against the wall, keeping her heels on the floor. Advise her that performing this exercise ten to twelve times before going to bed may reduce cramping.

Dietary Interventions. Assure adequate hydration.

Follow-Up. Refer a client with symptoms of pathology to the physician.

Ligament Pain

Etiology. The physiologic change underlying ligament pain is the growth of the uterus, which causes ligaments in the pelvis to stretch (ACOG, 2000; Curtis & Schuler, 2000). The round ligaments attach to the uterus at the top of the fundus, extend anteriorly and inferiorly to the oviducts, through the inguinal canal, and attach at the labia majora. Other ligaments attach at the upper fundus, extend bilaterally to the upper labia majora and from the posterior cervix to the sacrum. (Cunningham, et al., 2001).

Subjective Data. Usually in the second trimester, the client reports sharp or dull pain on either or both sides of the uterus. The pain often starts or worsens with twisting, stretching, or quick movements (ACOG, 2000). The history however, does *not* include contractions, constipation, diarrhea, vomiting, vomiting blood, changes in stools, low-grade fever, anorexia, periumbilical pain, right lower abdominal or flank pain, urinary tract infection symptoms, a tender lump in the groin that tends to worsen the longer she stands, or one-sided constant pain that increases (if the pregnancy is less than 14 to 16 weeks). These symptoms may indicate problems other than ligament pain, and require further evaluation (Seller, 2000).

Objective Data. Physical examination and vital signs are within normal limits. Tenderness at the supravaginal insertion site or laterally to the uterus may occur on pelvic exam. Significant negatives include no contractions, cervical dilatation, effacement or softening, rupture of membranes, adnexal or abdominal masses, hernias, hyperactive or underactive bowel sounds, rebound tenderness, jaundice, or tenderness on abdominal palpation other than along the affected ligament.

Differential Medical Diagnoses. Stretching of ligaments, ruling out preterm labor, ectopic pregnancy, rupture of an ovarian cyst, gastrointestinal disease (e.g., appendicitis) urinary tract disease (e.g., kidney stone, infection) and inguinal hernia (Seller, 2000).

Plan

Psychosocial Interventions. Explain to the client the underlying physiologic change causing the pain and inform her that the pain will resolve after pregnancy. Advise the client to notify the health care provider if any symptoms ruled out during history-taking occur in the future.

Lifestyle Changes. Advise the client to avoid sudden twisting or stretching movements. Inform her that getting out of bed by turning onto her side and pushing up with her arm will reduce abdominal muscle and back strain.

Fingertip massage, warm bath, or heat to the affected area may provide relief. Heating pads should not be used over fifteen minutes. Advise her to avoid excessive exercise, standing, or walking. Frequent, short rest periods during the day may help (ACOG, 2000; Curtis & Schuler, 2000).

Follow-Up. Refer clients with symptoms of pathology to a physician.

Excessive Salivation and Bad Taste in Mouth

Etiology. The etiology of oral changes is not known. It is theorized that eating starchy foods may stimulate the salivary glands (Cunningham et al., 2001).

Subjective Data. The client reports increased salivation or a bitter taste in her mouth. History should *not* include a sore throat, fever, flulike symptoms, heat, pain or lesions in the mouth, bad breath, upper abdominal pain, bloating, lethargy, dental problems, or pica. In addition, the client practices good dental hygiene and does not have symptoms of a psychiatric disorder.

Objective Data. No diagnostic tests are necessary. Physical examination and vital signs, particularly the condition of the mouth and teeth, are within normal limits. Occasionally, perioral irritation, red-coated tongue, swollen glands, drooling, or salivation interfering with speech may occur.

Differential Medical Diagnoses. Excessive salivation related to pregnancy ruling out dental problems, upper gastrointestinal problems (e.g., stomatitis), upper respiratory disease (e.g., pharyngitis) and pica.

Plan

Psychosocial Interventions. Reassure the client that the complaint is related to pregnancy and that the condition should resolve after the pregnancy. Also, inform the client that her breath does not smell unpleasant. Advise the client to notify the health care provider if any symptoms ruled out during the history-taking occur in the future.

Lifestyle Changes. Advise the client to maintain good oral hygiene.

Dietary Interventions. Advise the client to avoid excessive starch intake and to maintain a good diet and adequate hydration. Inform her that sucking hard candy or breath mints or chewing gum may improve the taste in her mouth but increase gas.

Follow-Up. Refer a client with symptoms of pathology to a physician. Refer a client with symptoms of dental disease to a dentist.

Discomfort in the Upper Extremities

Etiology. Postural changes caused by the enlarging breasts may cause a flexion of the neck and slumping shoulders. This plus the retention of fluids can cause aching, numbness, and weakness of the upper extremities. Carpal tunnel syndrome results from swelling in the wrists, causing numbness, tingling, weakness, and pain in the first through third digits (Cunningham et al., 2001).

Subjective Data. The client may report pain, numbness, weakness, or tingling in the upper arms or hands. History does not include cardiac symptoms; symptoms of hyperventilation (numbness around mouth with nausea or sweating), loss of sensation in the extremities, loss of ability to grip, history of trauma to neck, shoulder, arm or wrist, recent chest trauma or surgery, or arthritis. She may report a past history of carpal tunnel syndrome (ACOG, 2000; Seller, 2000).

Objective Data. The fingers may exhibit decreased sensation during neurological testing. The hands may be edematous. Pain produced by forced flexion at wrist or tapping on the carpal tunnel indicates carpal tunnel syndrome. Otherwise the physical examination and vital signs are within normal limits (Seller, 2000).

Differential Medical Diagnoses. Pain, numbness, tingling, or weakness in the upper extremities, ruling out carpal tunnel syndrome, musculoskeletal disease (e.g., arthritis), cardiac problems, or psychosocial problems causing hyperventilation.

Plan

Psychosocial Interventions. Assure the client that the discomfort is related to pregnancy and will resolve after the pregnancy is over.

Lifestyle Changes. Wearing a wrist splint especially to bed at night to prevent sleeping on flexed wrists. During the day, if the hands are affected, raise hands above the head and pump the fists. At night, put the hands over the side of the bed and shake. Avoid aggravating movements, especially fine motor movements (e.g., typing, writing).

Advise wearing a well-supporting bra. Avoid slumping.

Dietary Interventions. See Edema for interventions to reduce swelling.

Follow-Up. Refer any client with symptoms of pathology to a physician. Any client with recurrent hyperventilation should be referred for counseling.

Pica and Changes in Taste and Smell

Etiology. The physiologic change underlying pica (i.e., eating nonnutritive substances) is unknown. Pica has been ameliorated with correction of anemia in some clients (Cunningham, et al., 2001). Many clients notice a change in their senses of taste and smell probably due to high estrogen levels (Kline, 2000).

Subjective Data. The client reports changes in her senses of taste and smell. Common changes include those in the taste of coffee, tobacco, alcohol, milk, eggs, and red meats. The client may report cravings for nonfood items (pica) or state that eating specific items is important for a healthy pregnancy, delivery, and baby and not eating them may cause harm or birthmarks.

Pica may lead to constipation, bowel obstruction or perforation, parotid gland obstruction, anemia, lead intoxication, or parasitic infection (Kline 2000).

Clients may also report financial problems affecting the food budget.

Objective Data. Physical examination, particularly of the abdomen and mouth, and vital signs are within normal limits.

Diagnostic tests include the *urine dipstick,* which if negative for ketones rules out ketonuria, and a *complete blood count* to rule out anemia.

Differential Medical Diagnoses. Changes in taste and smell related to pregnancy, ruling out pica. If pica is diagnosed, rule out anemia, ketonuria, obstruction, parasitic intestinal problems, poor nutrition, and lead poisoning (Kline, 2000).

Plan

Psychosocial Interventions. Reassure the client that the changes in taste and smell should resolve after the pregnancy and may improve as pregnancy advances. While respecting cultural variations, explain that eating nonfood items (e.g., starch) may hurt rather than protect the mother or fetus. Advise the client to notify the health care provider if any symptoms ruled out during the history-taking occur in the future.

Dietary Interventions. Evaluate the client's diet to determine its adequacy. A high iron diet with iron supplements may be needed with anemia. If pica is diagnosed, explain the need to maintain a healthy diet and that problems could occur if the craved substance either is substituting for nutritious food, blocking nutrient absorption, or is harmful to the mother or fetus (Kline, 2000).

Follow-Up. Refer a client with symptoms of pathology to a physician or a client eating an inadequate diet to a dietitian. A client without adequate financial resources may be referred to a social worker.

THIRD TRIMESTER

Braxton-Hicks Contractions

Etiology. In early gestation, the uterus begins painless, irregular contractions known as Braxton-Hicks contractions. No cervical dilatation occurs. The contractions are thought to increase the tone of uterine muscles in preparation for labor. (ACOG, 2000; Cunningham et al., 2001; Curtis & Schuler, 2000).

Subjective Data. The client may report a sudden tightening or pressure in the uterus, without the sensation of building, that lasts from 30 seconds to 2 minutes. The contractions may decrease with position change or emptying of the bladder. History does *not* include regular contractions, vaginal bleeding, bloody show, leaking or rupture of membranes, symptoms of urinary tract infection, constipation, diarrhea, fever, flulike symptoms, or cramping, as these symptoms/signs may indicate other conditions requiring medical follow-up. Increased vaginal discharge may signal cervical dilatation (ACOG, 2000; Cunningham et al., 2000).

Objective Data. Physical examination and vital signs are within normal limits. The pelvic exam, particularly cervical dilatation, effacement, and station, is within normal limits. No bleeding from the cervical os or pooling of amniotic fluid is evident. Vaginal discharge is negative for ferning and nitrazine demonstrates a pH of 3 to 3.5. The abdominal exam does not reveal regular contractions, rigid, tender uterus, or suprapubic tenderness. Bowel sounds are normal. The fetus should be normally active.

Differential Medical Diagnoses. Braxton-Hicks contractions, ruling out preterm labor, premature rupture of membranes, urinary tract infection, pyelonephritis, gastroenteritis, constipation, and normal fetal activity.

Plan

Psychosocial Interventions. Reassure the client that Braxton-Hicks contractions are normal. Teach the client to differentiate between Braxton-Hicks and labor contractions. Labor contractions grow longer, stronger, and closer together and occur at regular intervals. Often, activity strengthens labor contractions, but decreases Braxton-Hicks contractions. Labor is differentiated from Braxton-Hicks contractions by the presence of cervical changes.

Advise the client to notify the health care provider if any symptoms ruled out during the history-taking occur in the future.

Lifestyle Changes. Advise the client to empty her bladder frequently, though she must stay well hydrated. Inform her that resting in a lateral recumbent position, walking, or exercising lightly may relieve contractions.

Lamaze breathing may ease the discomfort of contractions. Teach the client to breathe slowly and deeply at about half her normal rate. Make sure that she is inhaling and exhaling approximately equal amounts of air. Advise the client to contact the health care provider if contractions become strong or different in character from previous contractions.

Follow-Up. Refer a client with possible preterm labor, premature rupture of membranes, or symptoms of pathology to a physician.

Dyspnea

Etiology. The physiologic change underlying dyspnea is the enlarging uterus, which presses up against the abdominal organs and diaphragm, preventing full expansion of the lungs. The woman has an increased awareness of the need to breathe. Dyspnea can occur when the client lies supine and the pressure of the gravid uterus against the vena cava reduces venous return to the heart (ACOG, 2000).

Subjective Data. The client reports shortness of breath dizziness, or lightheadedness. There should be *no* history of headache, sore throat, coughing, flulike symptoms, perioral numbness, fever, night sweats, wheezing, chest pain, palpitations, indigestion, exercise intolerance, vomiting, sweating, hyperventilation, or anxiety. Neither does the client smoke or have a history of respiratory or cardiac problems (Seller, 2000).

Objective Data. Physical examination, particularly of the upper respiratory tract, heart, lungs, and vital signs are within normal limits. Hemocrit may reveal anemia.

Differential Medical Diagnosis. Dyspnea related to pregnancy, ruling out upper respiratory infection pulmonary or cardiac problems, and anemia.

Plan

Psychosocial Interventions. Reassure the client that her dyspnea is related to normal physiologic changes of pregnancy and that it will improve when the fetus drops into the pelvis. Inform her that it is not an indication that she or the fetus is receiving insufficient air. Advise the client to notify the health care provider if any symptoms ruled out during history-taking occur in the future.

Lifestyle Changes. Advise the client to avoid exercise that precipitates dyspnea, to rest after exercise, and to avoid overheating and very warm environments and to move slowly. Instruct her not to wear restrictive clothing. Inform the client that sitting up very straight or elevating her head with pillows may help relieve dyspnea (ACOG, 2000). Lying in the lateral recumbent position displaces the uterus off the vena cava and improves breathing efforts.

Follow-Up. Refer a client with symptoms of pathology to a physician.

Edema

Etiology. The physiologic change underlying edema is increased capillary permeability caused by elevated hormone levels. Sodium and water are retained. Thirst increases. Plasma osmolarity is lowered and the osmoreceptors for vasopressin are suppressed. Edema occurs most often in dependent areas. Moreover, the pressure of the gravid uterus slows down venous return to the heart. Consequently, more fluid passes into intracellular spaces (Cunningham, et al., 2001).

Subjective Data. The client reports mild edema in her hands and feet that worsens as the day progresses. Warm weather or prolonged sitting and standing may increase edema. It should improve by morning. Advise the client not to wear constrictive bands on her legs. Question her about her diet; a diet deficient in protein, calories, or fluids or high in sodium, fat, or sugar may increase edema.

The history does *not* include numbness, loss of sensation or muscle strength in the fingers of either or both hands. Edema is dependent and improves after a night's sleep. There is *no* report or evidence of facial edema, edema in one extremity, especially one leg, confusion, headache, visual changes, fatigue, nausea, vomiting, dyspnea, hives, upper abdominal pain, decreased fetal movement, decreased urine output, or rapid weight gain (i.e., more than 2 pounds per week) (Curtis & Schuler, 2000).

Objective Data. Physical examination, particularly of the heart, lungs, extremities, and abdomen, and vital signs are within normal limits. No protein is seen in urinanalysis. Although edema is no longer a diagnostic criteria for hypertensive disorders complicating pregnancy, gestational hypertension leads to a fluid shift from intravascular to intracellular spaces, causing generalized edema. Physiologic edema in pregnancy is not associated with significant proteinuria, nor with blood pressure elevation or quick or significant weight gain. Physiologic edema of the extremities is 0 (no swelling) to +1 (after pressing skin for 5 seconds, the indentation is slight and the contour normal). Deep tendon reflexes are also normal. Jaundice, upper abdominal pain, or headache are not noted.

The *urine dipstick for protein* should be no greater than a trace (Cunningham et al., 2001).

Differential Medical Diagnoses. Physiologic edema of pregnancy ruling out gestational hypertension; renal, liver, cardiac, or vascular disease; local trauma or infection to extremities; allergic reaction; carpal tunnel syndrome.

Plan

Psychosocial Interventions. Reassure the client that edema in pregnancy is normal and will resolve after pregnancy. Advise the client to notify the health care provider if any symptoms ruled out during the history-taking occur in the future.

Lifestyle Changes. Advise the client to lie in a lateral recumbent position for one to two hours twice a day and to sleep in that position at night. Also advise her to avoid long periods of sitting or standing. If a client must sit for extended periods, she should also stand—preferably walk—10 minutes every one to two hours. Regular aerobic exercise may improve blood flow to legs.

Instruct the client not to wear constrictive bands on the legs and arms; however, she should wear maternity support pantyhose.

Inform the client that raising arms and legs above the level of the heart for short periods and pumping hands and feet may decrease edema. Advise her not to curl her hands under her head or pillow at night if they are swollen or numb. Use of wrists supports would decrease swelling and numbness.

Dietary Interventions. Advise the client to eat adequate protein and calories, drink 6 to 8 glasses of water a day (reducing fluids does not reduce edema), and avoid high intake of sugar and fats (they can cause water retention). Sodium intake should be moderate; a low intake may be detrimental to the pregnancy and a high intake may increase water retention.

Follow-Up. Refer a client with symptoms of pregnancy-induced hypertension or with symptoms of pathology to the physician. A dietitian may assist with special dietary needs.

Dyspepsia

Etiology. The physiologic changes underlying dyspepsia are the increase in levels of circulating progesterone that causes decreased gastrointestinal peristalsis and the relaxation of the hiatal sphincter. In addition, the pressure of the gravid uterus against the intestines and stomach increases the reflux of gastric contents into the esophagus (ACOG, 2000; Curtis & Schuler, 2000).

Subjective Data. The client reports heartburn and bloating. The client may be under stress, depressed, swallowing air, or overweight. History does *not* include chest pain; shortness of breath; exercise intolerance; palpitations; sweating; anxiety; upper abdominal pain, especially after heavy, fatty, or spicy meals; fatty, foul-smelling stools; anoxia; nausea, diarrhea, constipation, or vomiting; pain in right shoulder, fever, or flulike symptoms, as these symptoms/signs may indicate other conditions requiring medical follow-up (Seller, 2000).

Objective Data. No diagnostic tests are necessary. Physical examination, particularly of the heart and abdomen, and vital signs are within normal limits.

Differential Medical Diagnoses. Dyspepsia related to pregnancy ruling out cardiac and gastrointestinal disease (e.g., cholelithiasis, irritable bowel syndrome).

Plan

Psychosocial Interventions. Reassure the client that dyspepsia is related to pregnancy and should improve or disappear after pregnancy. Advise the client to notify the health care provider if any symptoms ruled out during history-taking occur in the future.

Medication. *Calcium carbonate* is indicated for hyperacidity. One to two tablets are recommended every hour, as needed (see Nutrition section). Abdominal bloating may occur in some clients. Inform the client that calcium carbonate is an additional source of calcium (Kline, 2000).

◆ Cimetidine (Tagamet), Ranitidine (Zantac)

• *Administration.* Take one tablet orally daily (200 mg of cimetidine or 75 mg of rantidine). For prevention of symptoms, take with water 30 to 60 minutes before a meal. The same dose will alleviate symptoms.

- *Side Effects and Adverse Reactions.* May affect serum levels of theophylline, warfarin, phenytoin, or triazolam.
- *Contraindications.* Allergy to cimetidine, ranitidine, or other acid relievers.
- *Anticipated Outcomes on Evaluation.* Relief of dypspepsia.
- *Client Teaching and Counseling.* Contact the health care provider with persistent abdominal pain, hemoptysis, or difficulty swallowing. If taking consistently for two weeks, contact health care provider (PDR, 2001).

Lifestyle Changes. Advise the client not to lie down, bend, or stoop for two hours after eating. Inform her that for sleeping, the head of the bed can be elevated six inches. Instruct the client not to wear restrictive clothing around the abdomen or waist.

Teach the client to recognize her hyperventilation and swallowing of air, which may aggravate dyspepsia.

Advise the client to stop smoking.

Dietary Interventions. Advise the client to avoid hot, spicy, fatty, gas-forming foods; coffee; alcohol; and gum chewing. Instruct her to eat small, frequent meals and to chew slowly and thoroughly. Inform her that sipping water, milk, hot tea, or a tablespoonful of heavy cream, yogurt, or half-and-half may help dyspepsia. Drink fluids between meals (ACOG, 2000).

Advise the client to avoid excessive weight gain.

Follow-Up. Refer any client with symptoms of pathology to a physician.

Joint Pain/Ache

Etiology. The physiologic changes underlying joint discomfort are hormonal. Hormone changes increase the mobility of all joints, particularly the sacroiliac, sacrococcygeal, and pubic joints. This slightly increases the size of the pelvis in preparation for delivery. The increased mobility of the joint is often painful and more prone to injury (ACOG, 2000).

Subjective Data. The client reports pain in the pelvis or hip joints. Sciatic nerve pain is felt in the buttocks and down the back or side of the affected leg. It can be excruciating (Curtis & Schuler, 2000). Pain often increases after fetal engagement. The history does *not* include contractions, symptoms of urinary tract infection, or

swelling, stiffness, or redness in the joints, pain radiating down legs, intermittent claudication, or fever, abnormally cold and/or white digits and other flulike symptoms, as these symptoms/signs indicate other conditions requiring medical follow-up. There is no history of tick bites or being in a wooded area where ticks could bite (Curtis & Schuler, 2000; Seller, 2000).

Objective Data. Physical examination, pulses, and vital signs, particularly the joints and musculoskeletal system, are within normal limits; however, tenderness may be noted when palpating the symphysis pubis. There are no signs of labor.

Differential Medical Diagnoses. Joint pain, ruling out urinary tract infection, contractions, Lyme's disease, or other rheumatic, vascular, or joint diseases.

Plan

Psychosocial Interventions. Reassure the client that the discomfort is limited to pregnancy. Advise her to notify the health care provider if any symptoms ruled out during the history-taking occur in the future.

Medication. Acetaminophen may be taken.

Lifestyle Changes. Advise the client to avoid excessive walking, high-heeled shoes, jarring movements, high-impact activities, or other movements that can cause pain. Inform her that she may apply a heating pad or warm moist heat to the painful area for 15 to 20 minutes and that good posture is helpful. Cold to the affected buttock with sciatic nerve pain may be more effective. Lie on the opposite side (Curtis & Schuler, 2000). Instruct the client that she may place pillows between the thighs and underneath her abdomen to support and align the back while sleeping.

Follow-Up. Refer any client with symptoms of pathology to a physician.

Emotional Lability/Anxiety/Depression

Etiology. The physiologic change underlying lability is the constant rising and falling of hormonal levels during pregnancy. Progesterone has a depressant effect on the central nervous system. Fears about personal and fetal vulnerability, labor and delivery, increased responsibility, new and changing roles often produce anxiety (ACOG, 2000).

Subjective Data. The client may report emotional instability, mood swings, feeling blue, depressed, fatigue, or frequent crying. She may have sleep disturbances. She has adequate support systems and denies fatigue and physical or psychosocial problems.

Objective Data. Physical examination and vital signs are within normal limits with a normal affect and weight gain pattern.

Differential Medical Diagnoses. Emotional lability or anxiety from pregnancy, ruling out fatigue and physical or emotional disorders (e.g., depression abuse).

Plan

Psychosocial Interventions. Psychosocial interventions should be considered.

- Reassure the client that mood swings are common and should improve after the postpartum period (see Chapter 20).
- Explain the normal introversion that occurs in pregnancy and its role in mood swings.
- Assess the adequacy of the client's support systems, including support and communication between partners. Encourage her to discuss her feelings with a trusted person.
- Teach the client communication techniques: use of "I" statements, describing the feelings of the speaker without transferring blame to or labeling the feelings of the listener (e.g., "I am embarrassed by your behavior" rather than "You embarrassed me with that behavior"). Encourage both the client and her significant other to observe the accompanying body language ("I'm OK" while crying indicates that the speaker may not be OK). Encourage clarification and guard against not fully listening to the speaker but instead formulating a response while listening. Instruct the client to use reflective responses for clarification (i.e., reword and reflect what the listener has said). Advise her to use silence to encourage the speaker to continue or clarify his or her thoughts.
- Encourage the client to participate in pleasurable activities and to take time for rest, sleep, exercise, and grooming.
- Encourage the client to express her concerns, listening in a nonjudgmental environment. Explore ideas and solutions for problems.
- Childbirth classes and a birth plan may help the client to express her fears surrounding labor and delivery and to construct a method of coping with them.
- All explanations to the client should be clear, concise, simple, and honest because she may have difficulty concentrating.

- Address all the physical discomforts experienced by the client to enhance her ability to rest (Davis, 1996).
- Encourage socialization.

Dietary Interventions. Assess the adequacy of the client's diet and that caloric intake is spread throughout the day.

Follow-Up. Refer a client with symptoms of mental illness to a mental health care provider. Couples may also need specialized interventions.

Altered Body Image

Etiology. The physiologic changes underlying body image alterations result from hormonal fluctuations and the growing uterus. Chloasma, uneven brown patches across the nose or cheeks and around the eyes, can appear lighter on black or brown skin. The areolae, vulva, and upper and inner thighs darken. The normally vertical, pale line that stretches from the umbilicus to the mons darkens (linea nigra). Some women experience acne as a result of increased levels of circulating progesterone, whereas others note improvement. Striae are stretch marks on the skin. Mild pruritus from dryness, as well as stretching, is frequent. Some clients develop spider nevi and palmar erythema. Skin tags and moles may appear or change. Breasts enlarge in preparation for lactation. The abdomen enlarges with the growing fetus (Curtis & Schuler, 2000).

Subjective Data. The client may report any of the previously described changes. Severe, generalized itching; jaundice; upper abdominal pain; bloating; malaise; constipation; diarrhea; change in stool color or shape; change in a mole and severe psychosocial stress are *not* reported.

Objective Data

- Physical examination and vital signs are within normal limits.
- A *bile acid* (*cholyglycine*) *test* is done with severe abdominal pruritus to determine the level of bile acids in the serum. A venipuncture is performed and blood withdrawn for laboratory evaluation. The client must be instructed to fast for 8 hours before the test. The bile acid level is significantly elevated in pruritus gravidarum.

Differential Medical Diagnoses. Changes in skin, breasts, and/or abdomen, ruling out liver disease, pruritis gravidarum, and dermatologic or emotional problems.

Plan

Psychosocial Interventions. Psychosocial interventions are predominantly to encourage verbalization of concerns.

♦ Reassure the client that changes are due to pregnancy and will either fade (e.g., striae) or gradually disappear (e.g., nipple darkening, linea nigra) after delivery.

♦ Encourage the client to verbalize her concerns, including her perception of her partner's reaction to the pregnancy and body changes. Encourage her to communicate with her partner. (See Emotional lability.)

Lifestyle Changes. Lifestyle changes may improve body image.

♦ If acne is a problem, advise the client to wash her face carefully, use a topical astringent, avoid wearing makeup that clogs pores, and apply a strong sunblock when in the sun. A strong sunblock may minimize chloasma.

♦ Moisturizing lotions may reduce itching, but will not help striae.

♦ Advise the client to avoid irritating soaps (e.g., those with fragrance, antibacterial properties, or deodorants), long, hot showers, and other drying agents.

♦ Encourage regular exercise to control weight gain if no contraindications to exercise exist.

♦ Encourage the client to consider breastfeeding, emphasizing that it will induce faster involution of the uterus and easier postpartum weight loss.

Dietary Interventions. Advise the client to maintain a well-balanced diet (see Nutrition) with adequate fluids, which may help reduce acne breakouts and minimize unnecessary weight gain.

Follow-Up. Refer a client with symptoms of pathology to the physician. All changes in moles should be evaluated by a physician. A client with severe relationship or psychosocial stress may be referred to a mental health care provider.

ANTICIPATORY GUIDANCE DURING PREGNANCY

The issues of concern to pregnant women involve safety, comfort, and uncertainty about what to expect during pregnancy, labor, and delivery.

CHEMICAL USE AND SAFETY

Tobacco

Smoking is related to bleeding, preterm rupture of membranes, abruptio placenta, placenta previa, spontaneous abortion, premature birth, low birthweight, Sudden Infant

Death Syndrome (SIDS), lags in developmental milestones, and low IQ in the child. The adverse effects of smoking increase with the number of cigarettes smoked each day and with the years that the client has smoked. Recent research demonstrates increased rates of SIDS with prenatal and postnatal exposure that is dose related. A slight decrease in fetal birthweight with secondhand smoke exposure has been demonstrated. Encourage the client and all household members to stop smoking (ACOG, 2000; ACOG Educational Bulletin, 2000; Curtis & Schuler, 2000; Nusbaum, Gordon, Nusbaum, et al., 2000). Refer to a smoking cessation clinic. Use of nicotine replacement products or other medications should only be used only if other methods have failed and the risks of smoking outweigh the risk of nicotine replacement interventions. *Smoking and Pregnancy* (ACOG Educational Bulletin, 2000) presents a smoking cessation program for pregnant women.

Alcohol

Alcohol use can cause low birthweight, fetal alcohol syndrome (intrauterine growth retardation, malformations, characteristic facial features, behavior and learning problems), and fetal alcohol exposure (learning and behavior disabilities only). (See Table 17–5.) As little as 1 oz of alcohol per day (e.g., one beer, glass of wine or shot of liquor) has been implicated. (ACOG, 2000; Curtis & Schuler, 2000). Currently, the best advice for a pregnant woman is complete abstinence from alcohol. Data supports the idea that the earlier use of alcohol is stopped, the less likely are the affects on the fetus (Cunningham et al., 2001). Dose of alcohol per day was less important in studies than alcohol consumed per event. Binge drinking, even infrequent, could lead to fetal damage (Cunningham et al., 2001).

Over-the-counter cough and cold medications can have up to 25 percent alcohol (ACOG, 2000; Curtis & Schuler, 2000).

Artificial Sweeteners

Aspartame (Nutrasweet) is a Category B substance. This sweetener is composed of two naturally occurring amino acids, phenylalanine and aspartic acid. Clients with phenylketonuria, though, are not able to use it. Saccharin is a Category C substance (Hale, 2000).

Caffeine

Though caffeine has not been shown to be teratogenic, it may increase risk of spontaneous abortion (Cnattingius, Signorello, Annerén, et al., 2000). It is a diuretic, often

TABLE 17–5. Known or Suspected Teratogens

- Alcohol
- ACE inhibitors
- Phenytoin
- Carbamazephine
- Tremethadione
- Paramethodione
- Valproic acid
- Warfarin compounds
- Retinol
- Isotretinoin (Accutane)
- Etretinate
- Tretinoin
- Testosterone
- Anabolic steroids
- DES
- Androgenic steroids
- Danocrine
- Cyclophosphamide
- Methotrexate
- Aminopterin
- Tetracycline
- Aminoglycosides
- Sulfonamides
- Trimethoprim
- Griseofulvin
- Ribavirin
- Tobacco
- Thalidomide lead
- Mercury
- Benzene
- Toluene
- Xylene

Infections

- Varicella-zoster
- Coxsackie and other enterovirus strains
- Parvovirus
- Rubella
- Cytomegalovirus
- HIV
- Listeriosis
- Lyme disease
- Toxoplasmosis
- Malaria
- Group A and B streptococcus
- Salmonella and shigella
- Hansen disease

Source: Adapted from Cunningham et al. (2001); Frattarelli & Moore (1998).

displaces more nutritious food choices, can exacerbate mood swings, disturb rest, and cause fetal or newborn heartbeat irregularities. (Curtis & Schuler, 2000).

Inform the client of caffeine sources: coffee, tea, chocolate, some sodas, and some over-the-counter pain and cold medications. Explain the physical effects of caf-feine withdrawal (e.g., lethargy, irritability, headache) and their usual duration (3 to 4 days). Mixing decaffeinated and caffeinated products in increasing ratios to wean from caffeine use may reduce these effects.

Illegal Drugs

The risks of using illegal drugs include fetal addiction, prematurity, low birthweight, placental abruption, still-birth, and hepatitis B and HIV infection. Advise clients to stop using drugs. Refer clients using illegal drugs to a drug detoxification center specializing in the needs of pregnant women or to a mental health care provider whose expertise is drug abuse (see Chapter 18) (Curtis & Schular, 2000).

Over-the-Counter Medications/Vitamins/Herbs

Health care providers do recommend specific over-the-counter medications for minor complaints, such as headaches. Some medications are not advised during pregnancy. Herbs have not been well studied. Advise the client not to take any medication/vitamin/herb without first consulting a health care provider. Also advise her that megadoses of vitamins (e.g., vitamins A and D) could harm both her and the fetus; she should take only a vitamin/mineral supplement advised by a health care provider.

Prescription Drugs

Some prescription drugs are harmful to the fetus. Advise the client to report all medications she is taking to her health care provider for evaluation prior to use (see Table 17–5).

Environmental Exposure

In order to be teratogenic, a substance must cross the placenta in high enough doses to expose the fetus at a critical stage of development. Genetic predisposition may also be a factor. Some substances are potentially teratogenic. The best advice is to avoid chemical exposure before and during pregnancy, particularly when organogenesis is occurring in the first trimester (Cunningham et al., 2001).

The client can be exposed to various chemicals in her work setting, home, or other environments. To reduce exposure when using chemicals (e.g., household cleaning items), the client should ensure that work areas are well ventilated and wear protective gloves. Advise the client to avoid inhaling chemical fumes, particularly from paint or turpentine, and to wash off any chemicals on the skin immediately. Also advise her if she is in doubt about the toxicity of a chemical to which she has been exposed, she should notify a health care provider, call a poison control center, or go to an emergency room.

Knowledge about teratogens is growing. To obtain the most current information, several hotlines are available.

- Reproductive Toxicology Center is a subscription service available to professionals (www.reprotox.org)
- National Pesticide Information Center (1-800-858-7278)
- Occupational Safety and Health Administration (www.osha.gov/SLTC/reproductivehazards)
- Material Safety Data Sheets (MSDSs) are required to be available whenever chemicals are used in the workplace. Pregnancy issues are addressed.

Lead Poisoning

Homes built before 1980 potentially could be a source of lead contamination from water pipes, construction materials, and paints. Other sources of lead include solder, batteries, wood preservatives, and cigarette smoke (Cunningham et al., 2001; Curtis & Schuler, 2000). Advise the client to avoid lead exposure and discuss with her health care provider her concerns.

THE WORKPLACE

In general, women may continue to work until delivery if their pregnancy is uncomplicated and the jobs present no special hazards (ACOG, 2000). These hazardous jobs include health care workers, day care providers, some industrial jobs,—laboratory technician, artists, printing jobs, chemists, painters, car cleaning services, veterinary work, orthotics manufacturing, funeral home workers, and carpenters. Jobs requiring strenuous work, heavy lifting, climbing, carrying, prolonged standing—can create problems. Shift or night work plus significant fatigue from work can increase risk of preterm birth, small for gestational age infants, or pregnancy-induced hypertension (ACOG, 2000; Cunningham et al., 2001; Khattak, K-Moghtader, McMartin, et al., 1999; Mozurkewich, Luke, Avni, & Wolf, 2000).

Modifications

Some modifications may be needed in employment.

- The client should not work longer than 8 hours per day, 48 hours per week, avoiding shift and night hours.
- The client should take two 10-minute breaks and one meal break each 8-hour shift.
- The client should have a place to rest on her side and should be able to elevate her legs and use the restroom.
- Jobs should be modified if safety may be compromised by dizziness, loss of balance, nausea, and vomiting.
- Jobs with strenuous workloads—heavy lifting, prolonged standing, shift or night work—should be modified to reduce or eliminate these stressors (Frattarelli & Moore, 1998; Mozurkewich et al., 2000).
- Jobs where workers are exposed to extreme temperatures, high humidity, smoke, irritating gases and chemicals should be modified to avoid these stressors (Frattarelli & Moore, 1998).
- Health care workers exposed to ionizing radiation, chemotherapy, anesthetic agents, and infective diseases should be protected (Frattarelli & Moore, 1998).
- Day care providers, animal care providers, and meat handlers should be protected from diseases known to cause fetal defects (see Contact with Diseases).
- Hobbies of stained glass, ceramics, and pottery making should be avoided (Frattarelli & Moore, 1998).
- Advise avoiding painting and refinishing.
- Each pregnancy should be evaluated to assess the risk of continued working. Factors to assess include past pregnancy complications and outcomes, medical complications of the current pregnancy, obstetrical complications, and the characteristics of the work environment.
- Clients have certain rights that are protected by law. The Pregnancy Discrimination Act requires the employer to treat pregnancy as any other disability would be treated. The Occupational Safety and Health Administration ensures that employers either provide a workplace free of hazards likely to cause death or serious harm or provide information about dangerous chemicals or substances. The Family and Medical Leave Act requires employers of more than 50 persons to give 12 weeks of unpaid leave with

birth, adoption or foster care of a child, care of a spouse, child, parent with a serious health condition, or if unable to perform the job because of any disability including pregnancy. Vacation and sick pay must be given if earned, and health benefits cannot be changed. The same or equal job must be available upon return to work (ACOG, 2000).

CONTACT WITH DISEASE

Ideally, clients should avoid persons with disease. In addition, immunizations should be up-to-date prior to pregnancy. The client should also be assessed for susceptibility to hepatitis B, rubella, toxoplasmosis, cytomegalovirus, and varicella-zoster before pregnancy or early in the prenatal period (see Chapter 16).

Toxoplasmosis

Advise clients to avoid *Toxoplasmosis* infection by not handling raw meat or gardening without gloves and avoiding outdoor sandboxes and litter boxes. If the client must change a cat's litter, she should wear gloves. Afterward, hands are washed well (Curtis & Schuler, 2000).

Cytomegalovirus

Fifty to 85 percent of U.S. and Western European women have been exposed to cytomegalovirus (CMV). Antibodies do not protect from reinfection but primary infection during the first half of pregnancy carries the greatest risk of fetal infection. It affects 0.5 to 3 percent of newborns. Day care providers should avoid contact with saliva, respiratory secretions, urine, and feces with hand washing and cleaning of toys and cooking, eating, and drinking utensils (Damato & Winnen, 2002).

Fifth's Disease (Parvovirus B19)

Clients are advised to avoid exposure to children with undiagnosed rashes. Fifth's disease can, though rarely, cause fetal hydrops in a client who contracts the disease while pregnant (McCarter-Spaulding, 2000).

Varicella-Zoster

Chickenpox can rarely affect the fetus if the client becomes infected during the first half of the pregnancy. Adults, particularly if pregnant, are at much greater risk of developing severe complications. If infected close to term, the greatest danger lies in the newborn's developing the disease before the mother has developed antibodies and transferred them to the fetus transplacentally. Any client without a history of chickenpox exposure is advised to avoid exposure. Immunization prior to pregnancy is advised. Avoid pregnancy for one month (McCarter Spaulding, 2002). If exposure occurs, immunity can be tested and immune globulin is advised within 96 hours of exposure. She should contact her health care provider immediately (ACOG, 2000).

Mumps

If contracted during pregnancy, mumps can cause uterine contractions leading to miscarriage or preterm labor. If not immune or vaccinated, the client should avoid exposure and receive vaccination postpartum (ACOG, 2000).

Measles

Rubeola is not linked to fetal defects but may cause miscarriage or preterm labor. Infection close to term could result in the fetus's developing the disease without sufficient antibodies to protect it. Avoidance of exposure is advised and contacting the health care provider immediately upon exposure is recommended because an immune gamma globulin is available. Vaccination postpartum recommended (Cunningham et al., 2001).

Lyme Disease

Lyme disease can be transmitted to the fetus through the placenta. Antibiotics will cure the client with early stage Lyme disease. Its effect on the fetus is unknown. Advise avoiding tick bites by wearing long pants tucked into boots and long sleeves in grassy or wooded areas. Insect repellant can be applied to the clothes but not directly to the skin. A skin check for ticks is recommended after potential exposure. Contact a health care provider with suspected exposure (ACOG, 2000; Cunningham et al., 2001; Curtis & Schuller, 2000).

Rubella

German measles can cause significant harm to the fetus if the client contracts it in the first half of her pregnancy. All clients should be tested prenatally and, ideally, preconceptionally. If nonimmune, advise the client to avoid exposure to anyone with an undiagnosed rash. Advise vaccination preconceptually then wait three months to conceive. If exposed contact the health care provider immediately. Nonimmune clients should be vaccinated immediately postpartum (see Immunizations) (ACOG, 2000).

Listeriosis

Listeriosis is caused by bacteria infecting unpasteurized milk, soft cheese, raw unwashed vegetables, and shellfish. If contracted early in the pregnancy, miscarriage is more likely. Babies infected at birth can have fever and feeding, and breathing problems, which may not develop until they are several weeks old. The symptoms are flulike. To avoid listeriosis do not eat unpasteurized dairy products; undercooked meat, poultry, fish, or eggs; raw or cold meat, eggs, or seafood (ACOG, 2000). Advise clients to contact their health care provider if flulike symptoms occur.

Tuberculosis

The incidence of tuberculosis is rising. If client is exposed, a skin test or chest x-ray is advised. Refer to a physician if she tests positive. She can be treated during pregnancy. The newborn can be exposed at birth. Advise contact with the health care provider if exposure is suspected (ACOG, 2000).

Sexually Transmitted Diseases

Sexually transmitted diseases (STDs) pose a health threat to the fetus. Assess the client for a history of STDs; ask about the number of sexual partners she has and her use of condoms. Advise her to use condoms if she has multiple partners or a new partner, if she is unsure of her partner's sexual or drug use history, or if her partner has multiple sexual partners.

Educate clients to recognize symptoms of infection and if exposed to high-risk sexual partners to contact a health care provider as soon as possible (see Chapter 11).

SEXUAL ACTIVITY

Many fluctuating factors—physical, hormonal, and psychosocial—influence sexual desire and sexual response throughout pregnancy.

Normal Sexual Activity

Normal sexual activity is permissible, unless history of miscarriage exists, bleeding occurs, preterm labor is a risk, infection develops, intercourse is painful, placenta previa exists, or membranes rupture or are suspected of rupturing.

Assure the couple that the fetus will not be injured by intercourse nor is the fetus able to understand what is happening.

Encourage the couple to experiment with positions that may be more comfortable (e.g., woman on top, side lying) (ACOG, 2000).

Communication

A couple may require help adjusting to changes brought about by pregnancy. Some women have increased sexual desire, some less. The woman, though, often has an increased need for closeness during pregnancy. She should communicate all of these concerns to her partner. Emphasize to the couple that closeness and cuddling need not always culminate in intercourse. A mental health care provider may be consulted if necessary.

Alternative Forms of Sexual Expression

Cunnilingus is safe if the partner does not blow air into the vagina. Air embolisms may be fatal (Cunningham et al., 2001). Condoms are advised with anal sex. Advise changing the condom if vaginal intercourse is then desired. If intercourse is prohibited, specify what is meant: orgasm, vaginal penetration, or unprotected penetration. Other forms of sexual expression (e.g., cuddling, kissing, masturbation) may be advised.

EXERCISE

Regular exercise during pregnancy increases a client's sense of well-being, improves sleep, helps to control weight gain, tone muscles, and, after delivery, hastens recovery.

General Guidelines

A client who was physically active before conception should be able to engage in the same activities throughout pregnancy. You may need to advise clients not to take up new activities or sports if this activity requires balance because their sense of balance is decreased and their joints are looser, which increases the risk of injury.

Many exercise programs for pregnant women exist but because exercise specialists are not regulated, advise clients to consult their health care provider and to check the credentials of the instructor.

- ◆ The client should exercise three to four times per week, not sporadically.
- ◆ The client should drink water before, during, and after exercise to replace what is lost during exercise.

Eat a light snack before exercising rather than exercising on an empty stomach. Be sure calorie intake includes exercise expenditure.

- The client should not exercise in hot, humid conditions or when feeling ill.
- The client should make a five- to ten-minute warmup of stretching exercises routine. Exertion should be moderate, stopping if fatigued, breathless, profusely sweating, or unable to converse. After a five- to ten-minute cooldown period of stretching, the heart rate should be under 100 beats per minute. The length and intensity of the program are built gradually, though often must decrease in the third trimester.
- The client should exercise on a floor that absorbs impact (e.g., rug-covered or wooden floor). The client should wear clothes that are loose or stretch and a well-fitting support bra. Sneakers are supportive and absorb impact. Deep knee bends should be avoided as should pointing toes, full situps, double leg raises, and straight toe touches; these exercises may injure joints or cause cramps.
- To avoid dizziness, the client should rise slowly following exercise.
- The client should avoid high-impact exercises (jumping, jerking, rapid direction changes), exercises that may force air into the vagina (upside-down bicycles), exercises that stretch the adductor muscles of the legs (putting soles of feet together and pushing down or bouncing legs), exercises that require uncomfortable positions, and exercises that exaggerate the normal curvature of the spine.
- After the first trimester, the client should not lie on her back for more than a few minutes at a time.
- Weight lifting exercise may be continued if started preconceptually, without increasing the weight. Use of circuit machines or spotter is advised.
- The client should modify the exercise program as the physical load of pregnancy increases.
- The client should stop exercising and contact a health care provider if any of the following occur: pain, bleeding, suspected membrane rupture, dizziness that does not resolve quickly after rising, shortness of breath (unable to talk comfortably), palpitations, faintness, tachycardia, back pain, pelvic pain or pressure, or difficulty walking (ACOG, 2000).

Prohibited Sports

Advise the client not to participate in snow or water skiing, surfing, diving, scuba diving, horseback riding, or any sport performed at high altitude, where oxygen depri-vation (e.g., mountain sickness) or abdominal trauma are possible because they pose a risk of serious injury to mother and fetus (Curtis & Schuler, 2000). Other sports are safe if the client is skilled and very careful. These include in-line skating, tennis, and jogging. Good exercise suggestions for previously sedentary clients include walking, cycling (if they know how), swimming, prenatal yoga, and low-impact or water aerobics (ACOG, 2000).

Pregnancy Complications

Several complications of pregnancy may prohibit exercise. These include premature labor (current or past pregnancies) pregnancy-induced hypertension, threatened abortion, a history of three or more spontaneous abortions, incompetent cervix, intrauterine growth retardation, multiple fetuses, small for gestational age, client is underweight or has inadequate weight gain, and medical and cardiac diseases. Clients at risk should speak with a physician. Toning and stretching exercises, however, reduce the complications of bedrest. (ACOG, 2000; Cunningham et al., 2001; Curtis & Schuler, 2000).

SAUNAS, HOT TUBS, WHIRLPOOLS, TANNING BEDS

Advise clients not to use such equipment. The high water temperature could raise body temperature above 39°C (102.2°F), which is not considered safe (ACOG, 2000). In addition, because blood is shunted to the skin in the sauna or whirlpool, the heart has difficulty maintaining circulation. Syncope could result. Tanning is not advised due to risk of serious sunburn, dehydration, and skin cancer.

RADIATION EXPOSURE

Ionizing Radiation (X-Ray, Radiation Therapy)

Dosage of ionizing radiation less than 5 rad does not harm the fetus. The greatest risk of fetal harm is between 8 and 15 weeks of gestation. Total exposure during an intravenous pylogram series is 0.6 to 1.4 rad. Several guidelines are suggested that pertain to exposure to diagnostic x-rays.

- Avoid unnecessary x-rays or wait until after 15 weeks, or use ultrasound. Magnetic resonance imaging is not recommended in the 1st trimester due to lack of information. With all testing, weigh risk vs. benefits, waiting if possible.

- Advise the client to inform anyone ordering or taking an x-ray that she is pregnant, and to insist on lead shielding of the abdomen (Cunningham et al., 2001).
- Advise the client to follow exactly the directions of the technician to avoid having to retake x-rays.
- Advise a regularly inspected facility staffed with certified technicians and supervised by a radiologist.

Microwaves

Emissions from microwave ovens are very low. For safety, advise following manufacturer's directions and don't stand close to the oven while in use (Curtis & Schuler, 2000).

Ultrasound

The use of ultrasound, high-frequency sound waves, has not demonstrated fetal or maternal harm in over thirty years of use (ACOG, 2000).

Nuclear Medicine

Fetal exposure to radiation during nuclear medicine studies can be calculated. Consultation with a specialist is advised (Cunningham et al., 2001).

DENTAL CARE

Regular dental care is important during pregnancy. The dentist must be told of the pregnancy and x-rays performed with an abdominal shield. Local anesthesia is usually safe (ACOG, 2000).

TRAVEL

Generally, a client without medical or obstetrical complications can travel until 36 weeks. Travel is best undertaken during the second trimester when risk of complications is low and the client is feeling her best (Jothivijayarani, 2002).

General Guidelines

- The client should check with her health care provider prior to traveling. Travel may be contraindicated with certain complications: risk for preterm labor, repeated spontaneous abortions, gestational hypertension, placental abnormalities, bleeding, intrauterine growth retardation, or a medical condition, e.g., cardiac disease, sickle cell anemia/trait, (ACOG Committee Opinion No. 264, 2002).

- If planning to fly, the client should check with the airline about restrictions, usually starting at 36 weeks. Pregnant women should not fly in unpressurized planes above 8,000 feet. (ACOG Committee Opinion No. 264, 2002)
- The client should walk for 10 minutes every two hours while traveling. If driving, she should plan to make stops; if flying or traveling by train or bus, she should arrange for an aisle seat.
- To exercise while seated, take a deep breath, extend lower legs, flex feet, wiggle toes, and contract abdominal and buttocks muscles. With swollen hands, stretch above head and open and close fists.
- The client should drink adequate fluids and urinate every two hours to increase comfort. Light snacks may help reduce nausea.
- The client should not take medication for motion sickness or constipation without first consulting a health care provider.
- Seat belt should be worn over the pelvis at all times while flying.
- Most sea cruise liners will allow travel up to seven months of pregnancy.
- The client should be provided with names of obstetricians in the area to which she will be traveling and given a copy of her prenatal record in case of unexpected complications.
- Travelers to high altitudes or where additional immunization is required should consult their health care provider for individual risk assessment (ACOG Committee Opinion No. 264, 2002; Jothivijayarani, 2002).

Foreign Travel Guidelines

- Immunizations required for travel should be received at least 3 months before conception (see Immunizations).
- Use of chloroquine during pregnancy (to prevent malaria) is safe. Advise the client to start the medication one to two weeks before traveling to the risk area. Covering exposed skin, mosquito netting, and spraying bug repellents on clothing reduce chance of being bitten. In some areas (East Africa, Thailand), the strains of malaria are resistant to chloroquine. Mefloquine is used in latter pregnancy. Because malaria during pregnancy carries increased risk to the mother and fetus, travel to these destinations should be postponed until after delivery.

- In areas where water has been known to be contaminated, clients should avoid drinking it, as well as eating raw fruits and vegetables and using ice made from contaminated water or glasses washed in it. Water purification tablets containing iodine are not safe for pregnant women. The pregnant woman should drink only boiled or bottled water, soft drinks, or bottled fruit juices. Advise the client which medications and antibiotics to use if she should develop nausea, vomiting, or diarrhea and prescribe them for her if necessary.
- All meat should be thoroughly cooked.
- The American College of Obstetricians and Gynecologists publishes a directory of board-certified obstetricians practicing in foreign countries.
- The International Association for Medical Assistance to Travelers (1-716-754-4883) (*www.iamat.org*) can assist finding English-speaking doctors worldwide. The International SOS Assistance (1-800-523-8662) (*www.internationalsos.com*) will provide medical information and assistance 24 hours/day. Both organizations require membership (ACOG Committee Opinion No. 264, 2002; Jothivijayarani, 2002).

Seat Belts

Advise the client to use shoulder and lap belts when traveling in a car. Correct positioning of a seat belt requires that the lap portion be placed below the abdomen, across the upper thighs. The shoulder belt should rest between the breasts. Both belts should be worn snugly (ACOG, 2000; Jothivijayarani, 2002).

CHILDBIRTH PREPARATION

Although all pregnant women do not have the same goals for their labor and delivery experience, most clients in their first pregnancy benefit from prepared childbirth classes. A birthing partner assists the client during her labor and delivery. The partner may be her husband, the baby's father, a friend, her parent, a sibling, or a paid birthing attendant.

Three Philosophies

- Grantly Dick-Read uses education and relaxation techniques to reduce the fear-tension-pain cycle.
- Bradley teaches exercise to prepare muscles, relaxation techniques, and inward focusing with deep abdominal breathing to achieve labor and delivery without medication.
- Lamaze uses relaxation techniques and breathing techniques, outward focusing, and conditioned response to relax during labor (Curtis & Schuler, 2000).

Many classes adapt parts of the three philosophies. Classes usually comprise five to six couples, employ varied media to present materials, permit discussion, and ultimately prepare the client and her partner for many different experiences during labor and delivery, including use of pain medication (Curtis & Schuler, 2000).

VIVID DREAMS AND FANTASIES

Vivid dreams and fantasies are common, healthy, and normal during pregnancy. Recurrent themes may indicate an area of concern for the client. Assess the need for intervention. Reassurance of the normalcy of vivid dreams is often all the client requires.

CONCERN FOR BABY

Reassure the client that her concern about whether the baby will be normal is not unusual. The many tests that are available to diagnose problems prenatally may be discussed, if appropriate. If her concern seems excessive, refer the client for counseling.

ACCIDENTS OR BLOWS TO THE ABDOMEN

Reassure the client that the amniotic fluid and abdominal structure protect the fetus, although a very serious blow to the abdomen could cause injury (e.g., hitting the steering wheel during an auto accident). Recommend that she contact a health care provider if an abdominal blow should occur. Danger signs include vaginal bleeding or fluid, abdominal pain, uterine contractions, or fewer or no fetal movements (Curtis & Schuler, 2000). Abusive relationships may intensify during pregnancy. If a woman is in a potentially abusive relationship, abuse may begin once she is pregnant. Refer her to a mental health care provider if abuse is suspected (see Chapter 23).

FETAL HICCUPS

Hiccups are common and do not harm the fetus.

BATHING

Advise the client that she may take tub baths if ruptured membranes are not suspected and if she takes safety precautions in case she experiences syncope. Late in pregnancy, a woman may need help rising out of a low tub.

INFANT SAFETY SEATS

By state law in many cases, most hospitals do not discharge infants unless the parents' car is equipped with an infant safety seat. These seats can be rented or purchased and sometimes are available from charitable organizations and government social service offices. Hospitals, car dealers, baby stores, and consumer safety councils have the information.

FEEDING METHOD

Whether to breastfeed or bottle feed is a woman's personal choice, although breast milk is the ideal infant food.

Breastfeeding

Advantages. Breast milk is ideally suited for the newborn and changes as the infant grows, adjusting to fulfill his or her nutritional needs, particularly a premature baby. The milk is digestible, economical, and always ready. Breastfeeding encourages bonding between mother and child, speeds up uterine involution, suppresses ovulation (although not a reliable method of birth control), and helps weight loss. The sucking motion of nursing helps to develop the infant's jaws, teeth, and palate. Antibodies, hormones, enzymes, and growth factors in breast milk provide protection against disease, reduce the development of allergies and aid growth and development. Any adverse reaction to breast milk is usually related to the mother's diet, and removing the offending food often solves the problem. Special techniques and equipment help mother and baby to have a successful nursing experience in unusual or difficult situations (e.g., mouth deformities, Down syndrome, or breast abnormality (ACOG, 2000). Many mothers successfully continue nursing after returning to work by pumping and storing milk.

Disadvantages. Breast discomfort, sore or leaking nipples, increased incidence of mastitis, engorgement, less personal time than if bottle feeding, vaginal dryness, and decreased libido are often cited as disadvantages.

Contraindications. Breastfeeding is prohibited in the face of serious illness, very low maternal weight, certain in-

fections (e.g., active, untreated tuberculosis: HIV disease or AIDS; hepatitis B; herpes lesion on the areola). Breastfeeding is also contraindicated if the mother is taking certain medications or abusing drugs, or if the infant has certain metabolic disorders (e.g., phenylketonuria) (ACOG, 2000).

Preparation for Breastfeeding. Educating a mother about breastfeeding will increase the likelihood of a successful breastfeeding experience. Encourage the client to attend a class (e.g., those offered by La Leche League), to read a good reference book about lactation, and to find a support person (a woman who had a successful nursing experience) (ACOG, 2000).

Nipple preparation is unnecessary unless nipples are inverted and do not become erect when stimulated. Assess for this by placing the forefinger and thumb above and below the areola, compressing behind the nipple. It should become erect and protrude. If it flattens or inverts, advise the client to wear breast shells during the last two months of pregnancy (Curtis & Schuler, 2000). These are worn inside the bra with the nipples centered in the hole and a plastic dome fitted over it. The client should begin wearing the breast shells one hour a day for one week and increase wearing time one hour each day until she is wearing the shells eight hours a day. The client should maintain this schedule until after delivery, and then wear the shells 24 hours a day until the baby latches on easily when they are not used.

The nipples should not be rubbed roughly with a towel or rolled. No drying agents (e.g., alcohol, witch hazel, or soap) should be applied.

Bottle Feeding

Advantages. The client can return to work more easily, go on a strict reducing diet, and have others share in the baby's feeding.

Preparation for Bottle Feeding. If the client has chosen bottle feeding, emphasize that infant formula is recommended for the entire first year. Many formulas are available, for example, modified cow's milk and soy-based formulas with varied levels of iron and calories. Formulas are also designed for infants with special dietary needs. The pediatrician will advise the mother about the best formula for her baby. Formulas can be purchased in various forms: concentrated (need to be diluted with equal amounts of water), powdered (to be mixed with water), ready to use (poured directly into bottles), and prepackaged (ready to use in disposable bottles). Advise the client to follow directions carefully and never over- or under-dilute the formula.

If a clean water source is available, bottles and nipples need only be cleaned carefully with soap and water and stored away from sources of contamination.

Infants should always be held during feedings. The bonding that occurs while an infant is held is essential to her or his emotional growth. The bottle should not be propped up against the infant. Propping can cause a newborn to aspirate formula (ACOG, 2000).

CIRCUMCISION

Circumcision is not recommended or discouraged. Studies have shown decreased incidence of phimosis, paraphimosis, balanoposthitis, and penile cancer. The risk of local injury and infection is low. Parents are encouraged to consider religious, cultural, and ethnic traditions in their decision. Informed consent is important (Cunningham et al., 2001).

SIBLING RIVALRY

Many parents need reassurance that sibling rivalry is normal.

Techniques to Minimize Rivalry

Parents can use the following techniques to minimize rivalry.

- Enroll the older child(ren) in sibling classes.
- Encourage the older child(ren) to verbalize emotions and acknowledge those emotions.
- Role play with a doll safe handling of a newborn.
- Expect and tolerate some regression.
- If the older child(ren) is to be moved from a crib to a bed or into another room to accommodate the baby, do so before the baby is born, preferably two to three months before.
- If the older child(ren) desires, buy a gift that she or he can give to the new infant. Be sure that the gift is safe for an infant and request that it be placed in the bassinette (purchase an item that can be cleaned or sterilized). The older child(ren) can then identify the infant in the nursery.
- The first time the child(ren) comes to visit, have the infant in the bassinette. Give the older child(ren) individual attention until he or she expresses an interest in the infant.
- It may also help to have a gift from the infant to the older child(ren).

- Encourage grandparents and visitors to pay attention first to the older child(ren) and to have her or him introduce the baby.
- Find time every day to be alone with the older child(ren).

GRANDPARENTING

The grandparents of the newborn must go through developmental changes, which can either result in a closer, supportive relationship with their children or widen the communication gap. Much new information about pregnancy, feeding—particularly breastfeeding—and child rearing has emerged. The grandparents may or may not desire to be active participants in the newborn's life. Role changes must occur, adult children now being considered equals. New parents lack confidence in their parenting skills, wanting their parents' support without criticism. Grandparents have life experiences, traditions, knowledge, time, and often money the new parents don't have. They can provide stability and unconditional love to the older siblings. Grandparents not infrequently have taken the parenting role when the parent is unable or unwilling to do so.

Assess the communication skills, role expectations, and support skills of the parents and grandparents. Encourage the grandparents to learn about new parenting, feeding, and child rearing skills their children may use. Teach good communication skills. Encourage attendance at grandparenting classes if available.

FAMILY PLANNING WITH BREASTFEEDING

Encourage the client to begin thinking about family planning methods before delivery.

Spacing Births

Ideally, women should space births at least eighteen months apart to allow their bodies to recover and replace nutritional reserves.

Lactational Amenorrhea Method

The lactational amenorrhea method of birth control is probably effective for ten weeks if fully or nearly fully breastfeeding (at least fifteen feedings a day lasting at least 10 minutes each) and amenorrheic. If any of these criteria are not met, a complementary form of birth control should be used (Cunningham et al., 2001).

Oral Contraceptives

Progestin-only oral contraceptives are very effective when used during breastfeeding, and some progestins may increase milk supply. These may be used immediately postpartum. Combination contraceptives—oral, patch, and ring—are not contraindicated while nursing but often reduce milk supply. For this reason, they are not prescribed until at least three months postpartum and often after weaning (ACOG, 2000).

Depo-Provera

Depo-Provera has shown no effect on lactation in many studies (Cunningham et al., 2001).

Subdermal Implants

At writing this method of birth control is not available.

Barrier Methods

Foam, suppositories, and lubricated condoms are recommended if a client has intercourse. They also counteract the normal vaginal dryness that occurs postpartum and with breastfeeding.

Condoms are always recommended to reduce STD exposure risk, as well as to provide for contraception.

Diaphragm and Cervical Cap

If the client used a diaphragm or cervical cap prior to conception and wants to use it again, it must be refitted (ACOG, 2000).

Intrauterine Devices

Intrauterine devices (IUDs) are usually inserted eight weeks postpartum or after a menstrual period (Cunningham et al., 2000).

Nonhormonal IUDs have long been used by lactating women without adverse effect on their milk supply. Although Mirena, a new progesterone IUD, in the package insert does not recommend use with breastfeeding, other progesterone-only methods have been used successfully (see Chapter 9).

Ovulation and Sympto-Thermal Methods

If these methods are desired, refer the client and her sexual partner to classes. Advise them that the first ovulation following pregnancy can occur at any time; they should wait until menses normalize before using this method (ACOG, 2000).

Sterilization

If a client desires sterilization, the procedure may be done on the first postpartum day, during a cesarean birth, or after her postpartum visit (ACOG, 2000). General anesthetic agents may sedate the infant temporarily if nursing.

Vasectomy

If the woman's partner decides to have a vasectomy, the procedure can be done at any time. Both partners, however, must be aware that a man is not sterile until his sperm count is zero. A second sperm count to confirm is recommended (Hatcher, Trussell, Stewart, et al., 1998).

DANGER SIGNS AND SYMPTOMS

Potential problems in pregnancy may be indicated by the development of particular signs or symptoms. Should she recognize such a sign, the client should contact the health care provider as soon as possible.

FIRST TRIMESTER

Signs and symptoms in the first trimester including spotting or bleeding, cramping, painful urination, severe vomiting, and/or diarrhea, fever higher than 100°F, low abdominal pain located on either side or in the middle, lightheadedness, and dizziness, particularly if accompanied by shoulder pain. Any accident with abdominal trauma should be evaluated (Curtis & Schuler, 2000).

SECOND TRIMESTER

Signs and symptoms in the second trimester include all those noted for the first trimester plus regular uterine contractions; pain in one leg or calf, often increased with foot flexion and redness, heat, and tenderness, or coldness, numbness, and whiteness; symptoms of vaginal infection or sexually transmitted disease; sudden gush of fluid that cannot be controlled by Kegel exercises; absence of fetal movement for more than 24 hours after quickening; a sudden weight gain; periorbital or facial swelling; or severe upper abdominal pain or headache with visual changes and/or photophobia.

THIRD TRIMESTER

Signs and symptoms in the third trimester (after 26 weeks) include all those noted for the first and second trimesters plus a decrease in the daily fetal movement indexes (see Chapter 19). If movement is insufficient, she should contact the health care provider immediately (Curtis & Schuler, 2000).

INITIAL ASSESSMENT IN LABOR

PRELABOR

The prelabor stage can begin one month to one hour before labor begins. It is a period of cervical softening, effacement, and descent of the presenting part into the pelvis. Dilatation of the cervix can also occur during this time.

Subjective Data

Lightening, dropping, or engagement occurs when the presenting part descends into the pelvis. The client notes easier breathing but increased pelvic pressure, cramping, low back pain, and more frequent urination. Among primiparas, lightening can occur two to four weeks before labor and, among multiparas it may be as late as during labor. Either increasing (nesting) or decreasing energy levels are noted. Vaginal discharge increases and thickens. The client may notice loss of the mucous plug (a thick red or brown plug) and/or bloody show (a pink-tinged mucous discharge). Braxton-Hicks contractions may increase and become more intense. They are irregular, feel high and in front, occur suddenly without buildup, and decrease after urinating or changing position.

Labor contractions are felt in the back, legs, or lower abdomen, and frequently are accompanied by menstrual-like or gastrointestinal cramping sensations. With walking or over time, they grow longer, stronger, regular, and close together (ACOG, 2000).

Objective Data

Physical examination reveals a weight loss of 1 to 2 pounds since the last visit. Softening of the cervix, effacement, and possibly some dilatation occur; dilatation is occasionally as much as 4 cm. The cervix moves more anterior. With descent of the presenting part into the pelvis, the fundal measurement may decrease and presenting part may palpate vaginally.

DECISION TO GO TO HOSPITAL OR BIRTHING CENTER

Subjective Data

Usually, when contractions are 3 to 5 minutes if a primipara, or 5 to 8 minutes apart if a multipara, lasting 45 to 60 seconds with the characteristics of true labor, the client should go to the hospital/birthing center. Each client, though, should be individually assessed based on her pregnancy risk and the distance the client lives from the hospital. Also, if the client was scheduled for a cesarean birth, has a history of precipitous labor, or has a high-risk pregnancy, she may need to go to the hospital/birthing center earlier.

Signs indicating a client should be in the hospital as soon as possible include a significant decrease in fetal movement; menstrual-like bleeding; constant, severe contractions without relief; and fever or rupture or suspected rupture of membranes. If the umbilical cord is in the vagina (see Chapter 18) the client should call an ambulance and assume a knee-chest position.

Objective Data

If the cervix is dilated 4 cm or greater, if amniotic fluid is present in the vagina, if the presenting part is not vertex and the client is having contractions (see Chapter 18), and if the uterus is hard and tender without relaxation, the client should be in the hospital.

Palpation of the umbilical cord during a pelvic exam signals a life-threatening emergency. The health care provider should attempt to push the presenting part back into the uterus while the physician is contacted immediately (see Chapter 18).

REFERENCES

American College of Obstetricians and Gynecologists (ACOG). (2000, September). *Smoking and pregnancy.* Educational Bulletin No. 260. Washington, DC: Author.

American College of Obstetricians and Gynecologists (ACOG). (2000). *Planning for your pregnancy and birth* (3rd ed.). Washington, DC: Author.

American College of Obstetricians and Gynecologists (ACOG). (2002, December) *Air travel during pregnancy.* Committee Opinion No. 264. Washington, DC: Author.

American College of Obstetricians and Gynecologists (ACOG). (1998). *Viral hepatitis in pregnancy* (Educational Bulletin No. 248). Washington, D.C.: Author.

Clark, M., & Ogden, J. (1999). The impact of pregnancy on eating behaviors and aspects of weight concern. *International*

Journal of Obesity and Related Metabolic Disorders, 23(1), 18–24.

Cnattingius, S., Signorello, L.B., Annerén, G., Clausson, B., Ekbon, A., Ljuner, E., Blot, W.J., McLaughlin, J.K., Petersson, G., Rane, A., & Granath, F. (2000). Caffeine intake and the risk of first trimester spontaneous abortion. *The New England Journal of Medicine, 343*(25), 1839–1845.

Cunningham, F.G., Gant, N., Leveno, K.J., Gilstrap II, L.C., Hauth, J.C., & Wenstrom, K.D. (2001). *Williams' obstetrics* (21st ed.). New York: McGraw-Hill.

Curtis, G.B., & Schuler, J. (2000). *Your pregnancy week by week* (4th ed.). Tucson, AZ: Fisher Books.

Damato, E.G., & Winnen, C. (2002) Cytomegalovirus infections: Perinatal implications. *Journal of Obstetric, Gynecological and Neonatal Nursing, 31*(1), 86–92.

Davis, D. (1996). The discomforts of pregnancy. *Journal of Obstetrics and Gynecology, 25*(1), 73–81.

Frattarelli, J.L., & Moore, G.R. (1998). Workplace hazards during pregnancy. *Primary Care for OB/GYN, 5*(1), 54–59.

Hale, T. (2000). *Medications and mother's milk* (9th ed.). Amarillo, TX: Pharmasoft Publishing.

Hatcher, R.A., Trussell. J., Stewart, F., Cates, W., Stewart, G.K., Guest, F., & Kowal, D. (1998). *Contraceptive technology* (17th ed.). New York: Ardent Media.

Huxley, R. (2000). Nausea and vomiting in early pregnancy: Its role in placental development. *Obstetrics and Gynecology, 95*(5), 779–782.

Ingardia, C.J., Kelley, L., Steinfeld, J., & Wax, J. (1999). Hepatitis B vaccination in pregnancy: Factors influencing efficacy. *Obstetrics and Gynecology, 98*(6), 983–986.

Jothivijayarani, A. (2002). Travel considerations during pregnancy. *Primary Update for OB/GYN, 9*(1), 36–40.

Kashyap, S., & Gruslin, A. (2000). Influenza vaccination during pregnancy. *Primary Care Update for OB/GYN, 7*(1), 7–11.

Khattak, S., K-Moghtader, G., McMartin, K., Barrera, M., Kennedy, D., Koren, G. (1999). Pregnancy outcome following gestational exposure to organic solvents: A prospective controlled study. *Journal of the American Medical Association, 281*(12), 1106–1109.

Kline, D.A., (2000). *Nutrition for women: Part 1 Sexual and reproductive health* (5th ed.). Eureka, CA: Nutrition Dimension.

Laedwig, P.W., London, M.L., Moberly, S., & Olds, S.B. (2002). *Contemporary material-newborn nursing care* (5th ed.). Upper Saddle River, NJ: Prentice Hall.

Leccese, C. (1999). Calling the shots without calling them shots. *Advance for Nurse Practitioners, 2,* 51–54.

LeMone, P. (1999). Vitamins and minerals. *Journal of Obstetrical, Gynecologic and Neonatal Nursing, 28*(5), 520–532.

McCarter-Spaulding, D.E. (2001). Varicella infection in pregnancy. *Journal of Obstetric, Gynecologic and Neonatal Nursing, 30*(6), 667–673.

Mozurkewich, E.L., Luke, B., Avni, M., & Wolf, F.M. (2000). Working conditions and adverse pregnancy outcome: A meta-analysis. *Obstetrics and Gynecology, 95*(4), 623–634.

Nusbaum, M.L., Gordon, M., Nusbaum, D., Mc Carthy, M.A., & Vasilakis, D. (2000). Smoking alarm: A review of the clinical impact of smoking on women. *Primary Care Update for OB/GYN, 7*(5), 207–214.

Physicians' Desk Reference (PDR) for Nonprescription Drugs and Dietary Supplements (22nd ed.). (2001). Montvale, NJ: Medical Economics Company.

Reifsnider, E., & Gill, S.L. (2000). Nutrition for the childbearing years. *Journal of Obstetrical, Gynecological and Neonatal Nursing, 29*(1), 43–55.

Seller, R.H. (2000). *Differential diagnosis of common complaints.* Philadelphia: W.B. Saunders.

Shields, K.E., Galil, K., Seward, J., Sharrer, R.G., Cordero, J.F., & Slater, E. (2001). Varicella vaccine exposure during pregnancy: Data from the first 5 years of the pregnancy registry. *Obstetrics and Gynecology, 98*(1), 14–19.

Signore, C. (2001). Rubella. *Primary Care Update for OB/GYN, 8*(4), 133–139.

Somer, E. (1995). *Essential guide to vitamins and minerals.* New York: Harper-Collins.

Steele, N.M., French, J., Gatherier-Boyles, J., Neuman, S., & LeClaire, S. (2001). Effects of acupressure by sea-bands on nausea and vomiting of pregnancy. *Journal of Obstetric, Gynecologic and Neonatal Nursing, 30*(1), 61–70.

Stevenson, A.M. (1999). Immunizations for women and infants. *Journal of Obstetric, Gynecologic and Neonatal Nursing, 28*(5), 534–544.

Thadhani, R., Stampfer, M.J., Hunter, D.J., Manson, J.E., Solomon, C.G., & Curhan, G.C. (1999). High body mass index and hypercholesterolemia: Risk of hypertensive disorders of pregnancy. *Obstetrics and Gynecology, 94*(4), 543–550.

Tinkle, M.B. & Sterling, B.S. (1997). Neural tube defects: A primary prevention role for nurses. *Journal of Obstetric, Gynecologic and Neonatal Nursing, 26*(5), 503–512.

Vutyavanich, T., Kraisarin, T., & Ruangsri, R. (2001). Ginger for nausea and vomiting in pregnancy: Randomized, double-masked, placebo-controlled trial. *Obstetrics and Gynecology, 97*(4), 577–582.

CHAPTER 18

COMPLICATIONS OF PREGNANCY

Joan Corder-Mabe

*T*he advanced prac-
tice role in high
risk care includes several
functions: assessment,
anticipating concerns,
education, advocating
for the client, and coun-
seling.

Highlights

- Infections
    - Hepatitis
    - Rubella
    - Varicella-Zoster
    - Cytomegalovirus
    - Parvovirus B19
    - Toxoplasmosis
    - HIV/AIDS
    - Sexually Transmitted Diseases Affecting
      Pregnancy
    - Pyelonephritis
    - Intra-amniotic Infection
- Bleeding
    - Spontaneous Abortion
    - Ectopic Pregnancy
    - Gestational Trophoblastic Disease
    - Placenta Previa
    - Abruptio Placentae
- Anemias
    - Iron Deficiency Anemia
    - Folic Acid Deficiency
    - Thalassemia
    - Sickle Cell Anemia
- Hyperemesis Gravidarum
- Gestational Hypertension
- Diabetes
- Preterm Labor and Birth
- Substance Abuse
- Multiple Gestation

❖ INTRODUCTION

A high-risk pregnancy is one in which a condition exists that jeopardizes the health of the mother, her fetus, or both. The condition may be pre-existing or may have occurred solely because of the pregnancy. Between 1900 and 1980, the maternal mortality rate was drastically reduced. Since the 1980s, the rate of decline has slowed. In 1999, of the almost 4 million live births in the United States, there were over 300 maternal deaths; approximately 3.3 per 100,000 women died annually (ACOG Today, 1999; Ventura, et al., 2001). Yet one statistic raises much concern and many questions: The maternal mortality rate among African American women and women of color is more than four times that of white women (ACOG Today, 1999; Koonin, MacKay, Berg, et al., 1997) Women of high parity and older women are also at increased risk (Abel, Kruger, & Burd, 2002; Bai, Wong, Bauman, & Mohsin, 2002; Seoud, Nassar, Usta, et al., 2002).

Prenatal care has long been known to influence perinatal outcome because it allows timely and appropriate intervention to prevent or lessen the impact of untoward occurrences. Even though more women are receiving prenatal care in the first trimester, in 1998, 17.2 percent of pregnant women had little or no prenatal care (Guyer et al., 1999). The early receipt of prenatal care varies substantially among racial and ethnic groups. Lack of or late prenatal care is associated with low birthweight infants who are at increased risk of neonatal mortality. The reasons that women frequently give for not seeking prenatal care are lack of money, no transportation, and not being aware of their pregnancy. Moreover, increased stress levels and inadequate support systems have been associated with complications of pregnancy. Is it the lack of prenatal care or the social and behavioral factors associated with inadequate care that contribute to the increased maternal and fetal morbidity and mortality?

Infant mortality is frequently used as a benchmark of the health status of nations and/or communities. In the United States, the infant mortality has gradually declined in the past twenty years, mostly due to increased technology of caring for the sick neonate. The black infant mortality rate was 2.4 times the white infant mortality rate in 1998, a ratio that has persisted for several years (Guyer et al., 1999). In 1992 and 1993, the United States ranked twenty-second among industrialized nations. Even with all of our advances and increased resources spent for maternal and child health care, the United States has steadily fallen behind other nations. Birthweight is the single most important predictor of infant survival. In the United States, most infant deaths are associated with low birthweight. As with infant mortality rates, racial disparities persist in low birthweight categories, with black infants being much more likely than white infants to be of low birth weight. (Guyer et al., 1999; Vintzileos, Ananth, Smulian, et al., 2002).

Optimal perinatal health care involves effective systems to assess all obstetrical clients for risk factors and to identify those women who are at risk. Appropriate interventions and procedures must then be implemented to minimize perinatal mortality or morbidity. Many perinatal centers have established antenatal care units to provide this specialized medical and nursing care. Home care programs have also been developed that provide cost-effective personal care to high-risk pregnant women in surroundings that are familiar to them. Social marketing is increasingly being used by public health to build community awareness of health issues and prompt women to seek women's health services, particularly prenatal care (Josten, Wedeking, Block, et al., 1997). Much needs to be learned about the effectiveness and efficiency of these strategies (Koniak-Griffin, Anderson, Verzemnieks, & Brecht, 2000; Lowry, Hays, Lopez, & Hernandex, 1998).

The advanced practice role in high-risk care includes several functions: assessment including the woman's perception of her risk status (Gupton, Heaman, & Cheung, 2001), anticipating concerns, education, advocating for the client, and counseling. The practitioner assesses the physical and emotional health of the woman; assists the family to activate its own strengths and develop strategies to deal with stressors of high-risk pregnancy; anticipates the needs and concerns the family may have and assists family members to make appropriate plans to meet their needs; educates the woman and her family about all aspects of the treatment and care so that they can actively participate in the management; advocates for the woman and assists her to communicate and interact with the health care system; and counsels the client throughout her pregnancy.

Even with comprehensive, high quality prenatal care, many of the conditions discussed in this chapter will continue to occur with less than optimal outcome. Many of these complications arise from underlying conditions that impact the etiology and severity of the current pregnancy (Misra, Grason, & Weisman, 2000). The goal of care at all times is the best possible outcome for the woman and her family; the ultimate goal is a healthy mother with a healthy infant.

INFECTIONS

HEPATITIS

Hepatitis is an acute, systemic, viral infection and the most frequent cause of jaundice during pregnancy. It occurs as hepatitis A (HAV); hepatitis B (HBV); non-A, non-B, which includes hepatitis C (HCV), hepatitis G (HGV or GBV-C), and hepatitis E (HEV); and hepatitis D (delta hepatitis). Hepatitis A is an RNA virus formerly known as infectious hepatitis, because it causes an acute, mild, self-limiting hepatitis without major risk to health. Liver enzymes are temporarily affected and the woman does not become a carrier. Hepatitis B, formerly known as serum hepatitis, is a DNA virus that causes an acute, more severe infection. Thirty-five percent of all cases of hepatitis are caused by the hepatitis B virus (Duff, 1998). Among its sequelae are chronic hepatitis, cirrhosis, and hepatocellular cancer. Pregnancy does not affect the severity or outcome of the disease. Non-A, non-B hepatitis is a viral syndrome that behaves much like hepatitis A and is transmitted either by parenteral (hepatitis C) or enteric (hepatitis E) routes (Duff, 1998). It does not, however, have markers for hepatitis A or hepatitis B. Hepatitis G can occur through perinatal transmission and is commonly found with hepatitis B, hepatitis C, or Human Immunologic Virus (HIV). It can be identified in serum by polymerase chain reaction (PCR) (Duff, 1998). Hepatitis D is a hybrid particle with a delta core and a hepatitis B surface antigen coat. It can only occur with hepatitis B. Transmission is similar to hepatitis B. Generally, a coexisting infection is not more virulent except in homosexuals and parenteral drug abusers when fatality can approach 5 to 10 percent. Hepatitis B vaccination seems reasonable to prevent hepatitis D in the mother and therefore neonatal infection.

Epidemiology

Hepatitis A: HAV infection is acquired primarily by the fecal-oral route by either person-to-person contact or ingestion of contaminated food, particularly milk and shellfish, or polluted water. High risk populations are American Indians, Alaskan Natives, and those women living in western states. The rates are highest in children and employees in day care centers (Duff, 1998).

Hepatitis B: Traditionally, risk populations for hepatitis B were defined by ethnic origin and historical data. Asians, Pacific Island residents, Eskimos, and certain African peoples are at increased risk. Hepatitis B virus (HBV) is transmitted through contaminated blood and blood products and through sexual intercourse. Skin punctures with contaminated needles, syringes, or medical instruments can also transmit the virus. Perinatal transmission does occur. The fetus is not at risk for the disease until it comes in contact with contaminated blood at delivery.

Incidence reports reveal that the hepatitis B carrier state affects 5 percent of the world population, with a higher percentage in tropical areas and Southeast Asia.

Hepatitis C: Risk factors for obstetric population include women with sexually transmitted diseases such as HIV and hepatitis B, multiple sexual partners, history of blood transfusions, and history of intravenous drug use. The prevalence in prenatal to women is 1 to 2 percent (Duff, 1998).

Hepatitis D: Occurring as co-infection with hepatitis B, it has the same transmission and risks (Duff, 1998). Perinatal transmission has been reported, but immunoprophylaxis for hepatitis B has been effective in preventing neonatal infection (Duff, 1998).

Hepatitis E: Although rare in the United States, hepatitis E is endemic in developing countries and is transmitted by fecal/oral route (ACOG Educational Buttetin, 1998). Risk to obstetric population involves women who travel to developing countries. Once the pregnant woman recovers from the acute phase of infection, perinatal transmission does not occur.

Subjective Data

Hepatitis A produces flulike symptoms with malaise, fatigue, anorexia, nausea, pruritus, fever, and upper right quadrant pain. Symptoms of hepatitis B are similar to those of hepatitis A but with less fever and skin involvement. The older the woman is, the more severe her symptoms. Infection may be inapparent to the woman or the provider. Most clients with hepatitis C, D, or E are asymptomatic or have general flulike symptoms similar to hepatitis A.

Objective Data

Physical examination may reveal a normal general appearance. Jaundice of the skin, sclera, or nail beds may be present.

Hepatitis A: Serological testing to detect IgM antibody is done to confirm acute infection, which becomes detectable five to ten days after exposure and can remain positive for up to six months.

Hepatitis B: The immunoglobulin M antibody response occurs three to four weeks after exposure to the virus and before elevation of liver enzymes. When the IgM level is elevated in the absence of IgG elevation, then acute infection is suspected. The level of IgM usually returns to normal in eight weeks. Explain to the client that the test will differentiate acute infection from chronic disease.

The immunoglobulin G antibody response occurs about two weeks after the IgM response begins. The level of IgG increases rapidly and slowly returns to normal. The IgG level may remain elevated for years. When the IgG is elevated in the absence of IgM elevation, chronic disease is suspected.

Hepatitis B virus antigens and antibodies are identified in a laboratory screening. The testing for HBsAg should be included in the initial prenatal assessment for all clients and repeated later in pregnancy for women in high risk groups (Wong, Chan, Yu, & Ho, 1999). HBV, also called the Dane particle, consists of an inner core and an outer surface capsule. Laboratory screening is used to identify the presence of hepatitis B surface antigen in the blood, as well as antibodies to the virus surface or core. The hepatitis B surface antigen (HBsAg) screening test is most commonly performed, as a rise in HBsAg appears at the onset of clinical symptoms and generally indicates active infection. If HBsAg persists in the blood, the client is identified as a carrier. The hepatitis B surface antibody (HBsAb) appears four weeks after the surface antigen and indicates immunity. Elevation of hepatitis B core antibody (HBcAb) occurs in the period between disappearance of HbsAg and appearance of HBsAb. HBcAb is the only marker in this period that indicates a recent hepatitis infection.

Prepare the client for repeat testing, as HBV screening tests may also be used to monitor the progression of infection.

Serum levels of glutamic-pyruvic transaminase (SGPT) and serum glutamic-oxaloacetic transaminase (SGOT), cellular enzymes found in the liver, are evaluated to determine liver damage. When liver damage occurs, increased amounts of these enzymes are released into the bloodstream.

As these enzymes are evaluated as part of a complete panel of blood work, usually following a positive screening for HBV or clinical signs of illness, inform the client that enzyme levels will be retested to monitor the severity and progression of disease.

Hepatitis C: Confirmed by the identification of anti-C antibody performed with an enzyme immunoassay (EIA). Testing for hepatitis C is not widely recommended at present except in known exposure (Dillman, 1999).

Hepatitis D: For acute infection, serologic test will have positive antigen and positive IgM antibody (Duff, 1998).

Hepatitis E: Confirmation done through electron microscopy of stool sample; fluorescent antibody blocking assay and Western blot assay are also available (Duff, 1998).

Hepatitis G: It can be identified in serum by polymerase chain reaction (PCR) (Duff, 1998).

Differential Medical Diagnoses

Fatty liver disease, pregnancy-induced hypertension with HELLP (hemolysis, elevated liver enzymes, and low platelets) syndrome, secondary syphilis, drug-induced hepatitis.

Plan

Psychosocial Interventions. Reassure the client that the fetus is at minimal risk if other risk factors are absent. Family members should be encouraged to assist with household and child care duties to allow the client to rest.

Medication. *Hepatitis A:* Immune globulin (gamma globulin) or immune-specific globulin (ISG) is indicated for any pregnant woman exposed to HAV to provide passive immunity through injected antibodies. All household contacts should also receive gamma globulin. Gamma globulin is given intramuscularly. Immune globulin intravenous (IGIV) is available to provide passive immunity.

Hepatitis B: Immune globulin (HBIG) contains a high titer of hepatitis B surface antigen (HBsAg), which provides passive immunity to hepatitis B. Pregnant women with definite exposure to HBV should receive HBIG as soon as possible after contact and again thirty days later. Any household or sexual contact should be tested and, if negative, receive immunoprophylaxis with HBIG. Those individuals should also receive the vaccination series. The newborn of a woman positive for HBV should be given HBIG within twelve hours of delivery. If a woman is suspected of having an acute infection during pregnancy, serial HBsAg tests are done. Disappearance of HBsAg indicates that the fetus is no longer at risk. Close contacts of women with HBV should also receive HBIG, if not already immunized.

Hepatitis B vaccine is indicated for the newborn of a woman who has tested positive for HBsAg to stimulate the newborn's active immunity. It should be given as soon as possible after birth up to seven days of life, and again at thirty and sixty days. The Centers for Disease Control and Prevention (CDC) recommend routine vaccination of all newborns. Dosage recommendations depend upon the status of the mother. The vaccination is not contraindicated during pregnancy. Recombivax HB and Energix-B are the two approved products for hepatitis B vaccination (Duff, 1998).

Hepatitis C, D, and E: No current licensed vaccine for use with hepatitis C or D infection is available. Passive immunization with immunoglobulin may be provided to the pregnant woman positive for hepatitis C, but the benefit to the neonate has not been demonstrated. This has not become standard practice (Cunningham, Gant, Leveno, et al., 2001). Testing and follow-up for the newborn is recommended.

Hygienic Measures. All caregivers, whether health care providers or family members, should use universal precautions at all times. Stress to the client and her family that hepatitis A, C, D, and E are highly contagious. Explain the mode of transmission in the instruction and advise family and friends concerning good hand washing and hygiene.

Diet. Recommend a bland diet with additional fluids, depending on the extent of a client's nausea and vomiting. Intravenous fluid hydration may become necessary.

Breastfeeding. Infants who have received prophylaxis at birth and are currently on the immunization schedule should continue breastfeeding.

Follow-Up

Frankly discuss and assess possible drug use, as hepatitis is frequently associated with substance abuse. In addition, as hepatitis is sexually transmitted, recommend the use of condoms throughout the remainder of the pregnancy, and arrange to repeat screening tests for sexually transmitted diseases, especially human immunodeficiency virus (HIV) infection.

RUBELLA

Commonly called German measles or three-day measles, rubella is an acute, mild, contagious disease caused by the rubella virus.

Epidemiology

The etiology and risk factors of rubella are important in relation to pregnancy because of the potential teratogenic effects of the virus on the fetus, particularly in the first trimester. When infection occurs in the first four weeks of conception, 50 percent of fetuses have signs of rubella infection; in the second four-week interval following conception, 25 percent of fetuses will be affected; in the third month, 10 percent of fetuses will be affected; and beyond the first trimester only 1 percent of fetuses will be infected. In recent years, the epidemiology of rubella has shifted from children to women more than 15 years of age and foreign-born women. Most cases occurred in persons from Mexico and Central America (CDC, 2001b). Other countries report the same trend with the increased prevalence of congenital rubella occurring in the immigrant population from less developed nations (Sheridan, Aitken, Jeffries, et al., 2002). The disease occurs worldwide, more frequently in springtime, and is more likely among adolescents and young adults.

Transmission occurs by direct contact with urine, stool, or nasopharyngeal secretions with an incubation period of two to three weeks. Infected individuals can transmit the infection for several days without experiencing the characteristic symptoms or rash. The disease is transmitted to the fetus through transplacental infestation.

The low incidence of rubella and related congenital anomalies is attributed to the availability of rubella vaccine since 1969. It is estimated that 5 to 15 percent of women of childbearing age are susceptible to rubella.

Subjective Data

The client reports a nonpruritic rash, fever, and a feeling of general malaise. She has no history of the disease or vaccination.

Objective Data

Postauricular and occipital lymphadenopathy is present early in process. Fever may range from 99.5 to 101.7°F, and conjunctival erythema (mild conjunctivitis) may be noted. The characteristic maculopapular rash starts on the face, spreads to the trunk, and disappears by the third day.

The diagnostic test used is hemagglutination inhibition (HI). A serum sample is obtained and sent for laboratory evaluation. Antibodies are usually not present in the serum until after the rash has developed. When confirmation of rubella infection is important, as it is in pregnancy, an HI antibody titer is drawn immediately after exposure to the virus and repeated in two to three weeks. An initial titer of 1:8 indicates absence of previous rubella infection. A fourfold rise in antibody titer in two to three weeks indicates infection. Prepare the client for repeat testing.

When rubella affects the fetus, it is termed *rubella syndrome;* defects of the eyes (cataracts, retinopathy, glaucoma), ears (degenerative changes in inner ear, hearing loss), and heart (patent ductus arteriosus, pulmonary artery stenosis) may result. Also associated with the syndrome are decreased head circumference, mental retardation, and poor childhood growth and language and motor development. Seizures related to encephalitis from central nervous system damage also may occur (CDC, 2001b).

Differential Medical Diagnoses

Rubeola, scarlet fever, drug reaction.

Plan

Ideally, all women have been vaccinated and have adequate immunity; however, it is recommended that all women be screened during the initial prenatal visit. Assessment of rubella status should be included in a preconception visit. If negative, vaccination should be done a minimum of three months prior to conception. Counsel clients who do not have adequate immunity to avoid situations where they may come in contact with infected persons. Vaccination is recommended during the immediate postpartum period. Breastfeeding is not a contraindication to vaccination (CDC, 2001b).

If active disease occurs during the first trimester, counsel the client concerning the risks to her fetus. Support her decision to continue or terminate the pregnancy.

VARICELLA-ZOSTER (CHICKENPOX)

Varicella-zoster is a highly contagious infection caused by a virus of the same name (varicella-zoster virus or VZV) (Chapman, 1998). Varicella is a member of the herpes virus family and, like herpes, varicella can lay dormant in the dorsal root ganglia and reactivate later. Less than 10 percent of occurrences are in individuals over 10

years of age. It is a common benign childhood disease that can be more serious in adulthood. In pregnant women, the severity of the disease may be further increased, particularly if there is pulmonary involvement. Once an individual is infected, immunity is usually lifelong. Therefore, varicella is rare in pregnancy; 95 percent of pregnant women have antibodies to VZV. Immunization is available and may be used prior to conception if indicated.

Epidemiology

Pregnant women are at risk for developing varicella when they come in close physical contact with children who have active infection. (Most adults have had chickenpox.) The virus is transmitted through direct contact with respiratory tract secretions with an incubation period of ten to fourteen days. Individuals are infectious the 24 hours prior to the rash until all cutaneous lesions have crusted. Complications of varicella infection in children are rare, but encephalitis and pneumonia are life-threatening complications that occur in adult infection (Chapman, 1998; Hackley, 1999)

The major consequence of varicella in pregnancy is infection in the neonate. Ten to 20 percent of infants of mothers who had acute varicella infection during pregnancy develop varicella through dissemination of the virus across the placenta. Neonatal signs appear within five to ten days postdelivery. The symptoms are variable including nothing but scattered skin lesions to more generalized rash with visceral infection and possible pneumonia. Prior to treatment with acyclovir, neonatal mortality was 20 to 30 percent (Chapman, 1998). Infection during the first half of pregnancy is associated with low birth weight, limb hypoplasia, microcephaly, chorioretinitis, and cataracts (Cottrell & Carter, 1998).

Subjective Data

The client reports fever, malaise, and a generalized pruritic rash predominantly on the trunk. Usually, her history reveals exposure during the previous two weeks.

Objective Data

Physical examination of the client reveals a characteristic rash. Fluid from the vesicles may be examined for diagnosis and several antibody tests performed.

Diagnosis of varicella is usually made by clinical exam alone (Chapman, 1998). Physical examination shows a maculopapular rash on the trunk. The rash quickly progresses to vesicles that erupt and then crust over. New vesicles form daily for two to three days. Consequently, a mixture of red papules, vesicles, and scabs appears at one time. Fever of 101 to 103°F may be present. Prenatal infection can lead to varicella embryopathy or varicella in the newborn. Congenital anomalies associated with varicella are limb atrophy, microencephaly, cortical atrophy, motor and sensory manifestations, and eye problems such as cataracts, chorioretinitis, microphthalmia, and Horner's syndrome.

Diagnostic methods include clinical evaluation of the virus isolated from vesicular fluid. Several antibody tests are also used to detect infection: complement fixation (CF), radioimmunoassay (RIA), latex agglutination (LA), enzyme-linked immunosorbent assay (ELISA), fluorescent antibody against membrane antigen (FAMA), and immune adherence hemagglutination (IAHA). None of these tests is in widespread use for screening at this time, but the two most useful are the FAMA and ELISA.

Medical Differential Diagnoses

Rubella, rubeola.

Plan

Psychosocial Interventions. Focus on identifying women who are at risk prior to or shortly after exposure to the virus. Counsel any woman who has been exposed and has not previously had the infection to be tested for VZV antibody.

The primary care provider must educate all pregnant women to avoid situations where they may come in contact with varicella (Chapman, 1998; Hackley, 1999). When infection does occur, women require instructions on how to avoid spread of infection and how to relieve the discomforts of skin eruptions.

Medication. Medication is given for symptomatic relief of pruritic; acetaminophen is given to control fever. For severe varicella infection in pregnancy involving pneumonia and high fever, intravenous acyclovir may be recommended. Acyclovir has demonstrated safety and can be used in all trimesters of pregnancy.

Varicella zoster immune globulin (VZIG) is administered as soon as possible after a woman who has not had varicella infection or who has not been previously immunized is exposed to the virus. A newborn whose mother had an onset of varicella five days before or two days after delivery should receive VZIG (Chapman, 1998; Cottrell & Carter 1998).

Immunization. Women of reproductive age should be assessed for varicella immunity prior to pregnancy and offered the vaccine, Varivax. The vaccine is administered in two subcutaneous doses, four to eight weeks apart (Hackley, 1999). Pregnancy should be avoided for a minimum of three months following the last vaccination. Effects of the varicella virus on the fetus are unknown; therefore, pregnant women should not be vaccinated (Chapman, 1998). If a pregnant woman is vaccinated, she should be advised of the potential effects on the fetus. Because the risks are small, the decision to terminate a pregnancy should not be based on whether vaccine was administered during pregnancy.

Breastfeeding. Most live viruses are not secreted in breast milk. Whether attenuated varicella vaccine is excreted in breast milk or causes infection is not known. Attenuated rubella vaccine has been detected in breast milk but only produces asymptomatic infection in the nursing infant. Therefore, varicella virus vaccine may also be considered for a nursing mother (Hackley, 1999).

Other Interventions. Institute measures to prevent the spread of infection. Isolate the client until the rash has disappeared, which is usually about seven days. Take respiratory and skin precautions if the client is in labor and in the hospital. Following delivery, she should be isolated with her neonate in a private room.

CYTOMEGALOVIRUS

Cytomegalovirus (CMV) is a DNA virus that is widely spread throughout the human population (Brown & Abernathy, 1998). Congenital infection is different from perinatal infection. Congenital CMV infections, especially those that occur in the first twenty weeks of gestation, are associated with symptomatic disease at birth and possible long-term problems of mental retardation, microencephaly, intracranial calcification, chorioretinitis, hearing loss, or cerebral palsy. The most common cause of hearing loss in children is perinatal CMV (Brown & Abernathy, 1998; Damato & Winnen, 2002). Acute congential effects of the neonate include hepatosplenomegaly, thrombocytopenia, hepatitis with jaundice, and/or anemia.

Epidemiology

The etiology of congenital disease involves in utero infection. Congenital CMV infection results from hepatogenous dissemination of virus across the placenta secondary to primary maternal CMV infection. In women, the likelihood of seropositivity has been correlated with low socioeconomic status, older age, multigravidity, large number of sexual partners, and a first pregnancy before age 15. Women who fit these criteria are at most risk for primary CMV infection. Perinatal CMV is acquired through intrapartum exposure to secretions or postpartum exposure to CMV in breast milk or blood transfusions.

Pregnant women acquire active disease mostly from sexual contact, blood transfusions, and contact with children in daycare centers. Reactivation of previous infection can also occur and cause congenital CMV. Incidence reports reveal that congenital CMV occurs among 0.5 to 2.9 percent of all infants. In women who acquire primary disease during pregnancy, 50 percent of those infants will be affected (Brown & Abernathy, 1998).

Subjective Data

Most women with primary infections are asymptomatic. Women may, however, report flulike symptoms, including myalgia, chills, and malaise (Damato & Winnen, 2002).

Objective Data

Lymphadenopathy and hepatosplenomegaly may be present. Blood work demonstrates leukocytosis and lymphocytosis; liver function tests are elevated. Diagnosis is most often made by means of antibody tests, including hemagglutination inhibition, ELISA, and fluorescent antibody. A positive CMV-specific IgM test confirms that infection occurred during the previous sixty days. A fourfold rise in IgG antibody titer indicates recent infection (Brown & Abernathy, 1998). Other laboratory findings will include atypical lymphocytes on differential WBC, low platelet count, and elevated serum transaminase concentrations (Brown & Abernathy, 1998).

Differential Medical Diagnoses

Mononucleosis, HIV disease.

Plan

No therapy prevents or treats CMV infection. Screening for CMV using cervical cultures or blood tests is not recommended. Women with documented active infection during pregnancy may elect termination of their pregnancy, depending on the gestational age. Discuss the risks and be sensitive to the client's concerns and anxiety. A live attenuated vaccine has been developed, but concerns exist about the ability of the virus to reactivate when shed through the cervix or during breastfeeding. The vaccine is yet to be recommended (ACOG Practice Bulletin, 2000b).

Teaching all pregnant women about good hygiene and handwashing helps decrease the spread of disease. Advise pregnant women to avoid exposure to individuals with CMV infection (e.g., persons with AIDS). Explain that CMV is sexually transmitted and advise the use of condoms and limiting sexual partners as strategies that reduce the transmission of the infection.

PARVOVIRUS B19 OR ERYTHEMA INFECTIOSUM (FIFTH DISEASE)

This type of virus (parvovirus B19) usually does not cause infection in humans. When, however, acute infection does occur during pregnancy, particularly before eighteen weeks of gestation, fetal infection and stillbirth are possible.

Epidemiology

The prevalence of infection among pregnant women and fetuses is not known. Among adults, 30 percent are carriers of antibodies for parvovirus. Infection is spread transplacentally, by oropharyngeal route in casual contact, and through infected blood components. Estimating risk is impossible because studies are limited. Erythema infectiosum is a self-limiting disease and complete recovery usually occurs (Bukowski & Saade, 2000).

The most significant effect of human parvovirus on the fetus is the occurrence of fetal hydrops. The hydrops develops as a result of the aplastic anemia secondary to the viral infection and subsequent congestive heart failure. (Markenson & Yancey, 1998). The incidence of hydrops is varied from 0 to 38 percent, with most researchers reporting 15 to 27 percent. (Markenson & Yancey, 1998; ACOG Practice Bulletin, 2000b).

Schoolteachers, day care workers, and women living with school-age children are at highest risk for being seropositive for parvovirus B19, especially if a recent outbreak has occurred in those settings. These women may benefit from a baseline serologic test to determine their susceptibility to infection. Prevention is the best strategy and includes routine hand washing when handling children, cleaning of toys and hard surfaces in contact with infected children, and avoiding the sharing of food or drinks (McCarter-Spaulding, 2002).

Subjective Data

A client may report a facial rash and sometimes arthritic pain of the hands, wrists, and knees.

Objective Data

The most characteristic sign of parvovirus B19 infection is the "slapped-face" rash, a macular rash that may also be found on the trunk. The rash may subside only to return in response to stress, exercise, sunlight, or bathing.

Viral infection of the bone marrow causes destruction of red blood cell precursors so blood work reveals a transient aplastic crisis. The crisis usually happens only in women who have an underlying hemoglobinopathy. IgG shows a 30 percent rise with acute infection. The serum maternal α-fetoprotein is also elevated. Parvovirus B19 has not been implicated in preterm birth (Koga et al., 2001). When there is a history of parvovirus B19 in the first trimester, a level II sonogram is ordered between 20 and 22 weeks to evaluate fetal structures and to detect the presence of hydrops. If there are no signs of hydrops, no further testing is necessary (Bukowski & Saade, 2000). With hydrops, fetal edema and ascites are observed. There have been reports of subsequent sonograms that revealed resolution of previously detected hydrops (Bukowski & Saade, 2000; Markenson & Yancey, 1998).

Medical Differential Diagnoses

Rubella, rubeola, roseola, scarlet fever.

Plan

Sonography. A Level II sonogram should be done in any woman with suspicion of parvovirus infection. Serial sonograms should be ordered after acute infection to monitor for the occurrence of hydrops. Prognosis for hydrops may not be as grave as earlier believed; normal sonographic findings have been reported in some pregnancies. The health care provider should share what information is available and be sensitive to the client's concerns.

TOXOPLASMOSIS

Toxoplasmosis is a common infectious disease caused by the intracellular protozoan parasite *Toxoplasma gondii*. Primary infection during pregnancy is associated with stillbirth or congenital infection. Symptoms usually appear at birth. About 10 percent of infected infants manifest severe disease characterized by chorioretinitis, cyanosis, pneumonia, hepatosplenomegaly, jaundice, and thrombocytopenia purpura. Infants who survive sustain some permanent neurological damage.

Epidemiology

Risk factors for maternal infection include eating raw or undercooked meats and living in rural areas.

Usual transmission is through ingestion of tissue cysts in contaminated meat or through contact with oocytes in feces of infected cats or farm animals, or eating unwashed fruit, berries, or vegetables with contagious oocytes on their surface. Chances of transplacental transmission to the fetus increases depending upon when the acute maternal infection occurs. During the first trimester, about 10 percent of the fetuses will be affected, but the chance increases to 60 percent if infection occurs in the third trimester (ACOG Practice Bulletin, 2000b; Beazley & Egerman, 1998). Any history of maternal infection affords permanent immunity. Spontaneous abortion, stillbirth, or severe congenital infection occurs in 10 to 15 percent of pregnancies complicated with toxoplasmosis. Serious congenital infection is more likely to occur when maternal infection occurs in the third trimester.

Women who are positive for HIV or who are on immunosuppressive therapy following transplantation will be more susceptible to toxoplasmosis.

The overall incidence is 0.25 to 1.0 per 1000 live births. About 30 percent of the U.S. population has been infected with toxoplasma organism, which is a lower prevalence compared to other areas such as England, France, Africa, and countries in Central America (Beazley & Egerman, 1998).

Subjective Data

Although most women are asymptomatic, the client may report fatigue, fever, rash, depression, malaise, headache, and sore throat. Infection occurs one to two weeks after exposure, and the client may remain symptomatic for as long as several months.

Objective Data

Physical examination reveals lymph node enlargement, particularly in the posterior cervical chain.

Diagnosis is made by means of serial toxoplasma antibody tests (two or more) done three weeks apart. The second sample shows significantly higher levels of antibodies if active infection is present. An indirect fluorescent antibody test of 1:512 or greater correlates with active infection. Recently, testing for toxoplasma DNA in amniotic fluid has been used to determine presence of fetal infection. Ultrasound is also used to detect findings such as intracranial calcifications, intrauterine growth retardation, microcephaly, neonatal ascites, hepatosplenomegaly, and cardiomegaly, which can all be associated with toxoplasmosis infection (ACOG Practice Bulletin, 2000b).

Some countries screen all pregnant women for toxoplasmosis during the initial prenatal visit. That is not currently an acceptable approach in this country.

Differential Medical Diagnosis

Infectious mononucleosis.

Plan

Psychosocial Interventions. Educate prenatal clients about the risk of toxoplasmosis and discuss prevention. Advise pregnant women to avoid handling cat litter, to wear gloves when gardening, to always wash their hands well after handling cats, and to avoid eating undercooked or raw meats. Prevention of disease is the key to management.

If primary infection occurs in the first trimester, discuss the option of terminating the pregnancy with the client and her family.

Medications. Pregnant women with toxoplasmosis should be treated with spiramycin. Once in utero infection is detected, sulfadiazine, pyrimethamine, and folinic acid are given together to treat the fetus (ACOG Practice Bulletin, 2000b; Beazley & Egerman, 1998). Pyrimethamine is not recommended in the first trimester because of possible teratogenicity (Beazley & Egerman, 1998). Clindamycin or azithromycin are acceptable alternatives if the woman is allergic to sulfonamides (Beazley & Egerman, 1998). Treatment has shown to decrease the fetal findings and pregnancy outcomes have been good (ACOG Practice Bulletin, 2000b).

A newborn whose mother was treated antenatally for toxoplasmosis should be treated prophylactically with a combination of pyrimethamine and sulfadiazine (antimalarial drug). An infant with symptoms or an asymptomatic infant with positive cerebrospinal fluid should also be treated.

HUMAN IMMUNODEFICIENCY VIRUS (HIV)*

Human Immunodeficiency Virus (HIV) attacks the T4 cells, decreases the CD-4 cell count, and disables the immune system. As the CD-4 cell count decreases, immune system dysfunction occurs. Organs such as the kidney and liver can suffer tissue damage before major system dysfunction is apparent. The condition progresses to a severe immunosuppressed state termed Acquired Immunodeficiency Syndrome (AIDS). Recent reports indicate that pregnancy does not accelerate the progression of HIV to AIDS and/or death. (Public Health Service Task Force, 2002). The CDC definition of AIDS is an HIV-infected person with a specific opportunistic infection or a CD-4 count less than 200 mm.

Epidemiology

The disease was not recognized until the early 1980s and there is no reliable data collection system for the number of HIV-positive individuals. Historically, HIV/AIDS was a disease of homosexual males. Now, the incidence of HIV/AIDS has increased in women. Fifty percent of all the HIV/AIDS cases worldwide now occur in women, compared to 19 percent in 1995 (CDC, 2002b). HIV infection is the third leading cause of death among all U.S. women aged 25 to 44 years and the leading cause of death among black women in this age group. Most of the women affected by HIV have male partners who use injectable drugs or who are bisexual men. Women who use drugs themselves or are prostitutes are more likely to be HIV affected. After 1995, the mortality associated with HIV infection decreased by 71 percentage due to the introduction of new and combined drug therapy (Guyer et al., 1999).

An estimated 7,000 infants are born to HIV-infected women in the United States each year. Most cases of infant HIV infection are due to perinatal transmission. The chances of a woman's having an infant who has HIV infection varies from 5 to 60 percent with an average of 20 to 30 percent. The large variance reported in transmission statistics relates to advances in treatment being developed over the short time that women are beginning to be represented in the HIV positive population. Using prenatal drug treatment has been able to decrease verti-

---

*Refer to Chapter 12 for a more complete discussion of HIV/AIDS.

cal transmission from 30 percent to 8 percent (PHSTF, 2002). Vertical transmission is affected by the viral load of the mother, status of the maternal immune system, route of delivery, general health of the fetus, presence of maternal infection, and exposure to genital secretions. Usually, the greater the viral load of the mother, the more likely that vertical transmission of the virus will occur (PHSTF, 2002). Women with AIDS and the suppressed immune system are more likely to transmit the virus to the fetus. A first twin during vaginal delivery also has increased risk to contract the virus because of its longer exposure to cervical/vaginal secretions. Any delivery complication such as forceps delivery, lacerations, or episiotomy add to fetal risk for the same reason. Placental vasculitis (chorioamnionitis) facilitates the spread of the virus.

Most HIV infections in the United States are HIV-1, but HIV-2 is endemic in other countries such as Africa.

HIV infection is acquired by sexual contact, exposure to blood or bodily fluids, vertical transmission to the fetus, perinatal exposure at delivery, and breastfeeding. Historically, HIV/AIDS was associated with the male homosexual community and intravenous drug abusers. The prevalence of HIV infection and AIDS is now increasing more rapidly among women than among men (Lyon & Younger, 2001). Most women with AIDS have acquired the disease through heterosexual contact, and a majority of those women are mothers. Pregnancy rates among women infected with HIV remain high. The implications to discuss this disease in women's and infants' health are obvious.

The relationship between pregnancy and HIV infection is difficult to separate because so many of the women with HIV/AIDs have other risks associated with complications of pregnancy. Many of these women affected by HIV also have problems with drug addiction, lack of access to prenatal care, inadequate nutrition, poverty, and increased incidence of sexually transmitted diseases. Considering these factors, women affected by HIV also have increased risk for preterm delivery, premature rupture of membranes, intrauterine growth retardation, postpartum endometritis, and increased perinatal mortality (PHSTF, 2002).

The risk of acquiring HIV through heterosexual contact is greater for women because semen has high concentration of the virus, and coitus causes more breaks in the vaginal lining as compared to the penile skin. The presence of other genital infections increases those chances.

Subjective Data

Most people remain asymptomatic after exposure to the virus. Within the first few months of being infected, many persons experience an acute viral infection similar to mononucleosis with complaints such as weight loss, fever, night sweats, pharyngitis, rash, and lymphadenopathy. These symptoms resolve within a few weeks and are frequently not perceived by the client as significant.

The woman may experience several episodes of discrete illnesses such as weight loss or an infection with a definitive beginning and end. Once the symptoms subside, the woman returns to a prediagnosis level of function. At some point, these illnesses become chronic and, even though controlled, are not cured. Usually, at this time the woman is on prophylaxis drug therapy. The symptoms experienced at this point are varied and reflect which organ systems are most affected by the virus. Common symptoms include dyspnea and fatigue, decreased muscle strength, cramping pain in the extremities, nausea and vomiting, and recurrent vaginal yeast infections (Holzemer, 2002). Because these are also common complaints associated with pregnancy, identifying onset of illness may be difficult.

Objective Data

The enzyme linked immunosorbent assay (ELISA) detects antibodies to the virus that develop within twelve weeks of exposure. It is the screening test for exposure to HIV and, if reactive on two separate tests, is followed by the Western blot assay. The Western blot is the confirmatory diagnostic test.

With advancing technology, ways of assessing the status of the immune system and level of invasion of the virus are being developed. Monitoring of CD-4 cell count assesses a person's status as to the invasion of the virus, and RNA levels or viral load assessments are used as a staging indicator of the disease. Symptoms experienced by the woman are not correlated with the determined viral loads or CD-4 counts. A decrease in viral load does not coincide with resolution of symptoms of the disease (Holzemer, 2002; PHSTF, 2002). (Refer to Chapter 12 for more detailed information on screening and monitoring status of HIV.)

Differential Medical Diagnosis

Refer to Chapter 12.

Plan

Prevention. Major media campaigns have educated citizens on the need to protect themselves from the spread of HIV. "Safer sex" has become the focus of many national and local campaigns including advice to reduce the number of sexual partners, avoid partners with high-risk histories (multiple partners, homosexual relations, intravenous drug users), and use latex condoms during all sexual encounters. Abstinence-based educational campaigns have also emerged.

In February 1994, the National Institutes of Health announced findings of a study sponsored by the Pediatric Clinical Trials Group (PACTG), which found that administering Zidovudine (ZDV) during pregnancy, labor, and delivery and during the neonatal period reduced perinatal transmission of HIV by two-thirds. Epidemiological studies have since confirmed this finding (PHSTF, 2002). Women with advanced HIV disease or previous antiretroviral therapy were not included in this study. The PACTG recommended the development of national policies and protocols for the counseling and screening of all pregnant women (PHSTF, 2002). Since then, much effort by governmental agencies, professional groups, and concerned citizens has occurred to educate women about this potential preventive strategy.

Numerous reports indicate that women know about HIV and its transmission. There are only a few studies that specifically report the knowledge, attitudes, and practices of pregnant women. The problem now is that many pregnant women, particularly minority and women of other cultures, may have inadequate knowledge about the treatment and perinatal transmission of HIV/AIDS. Reports vary as to the percentage of pregnant women who are offered and tested for HIV prenatally (Lansky, Jones, Frey & Lindegren, 2001; Royce, Walter, Fernandez, et al., 2001, Stringer, Stringer, Cliver, et al., 2001). In the past, education programs targeted homosexual males and intravenous drug users. Because women constitute the fastest growing population affected by HIV/AIDS, educational programs designed for minority and women of other cultures are necessary to be effective in reducing the incidence of HIV (Flake, 2000).

Prenatal Screening. Initially, selected testing based upon assessment of risk behaviors in pregnant women was standard, but it was later discovered that significant numbers of women who tested HIV positive had not given any history of risk behaviors. Some groups, including the American Medical Association, have proposed national

policies to mandate testing for all pregnant women. The 1998 Institute of Medicine report recommended universal testing of pregnant women with notification (IOM, 1998). In 2000, ACOG adopted the IOM recommendation (ACOG Practice Bulletin, 2000b). Some groups feel that mandatory testing would deter many of the affected women from seeking prenatal care and have proposed mandatory counseling and informed consent for testing. Many states have passed legislation directing prenatal HIV testing, but there is variation as to mandatory testing versus mandatory counseling with offering of testing (Flake, 2000; Frank, Esch, & Margeson, 1998; Royce et al., 2001; Sinclair, 1999; Stringer et al., 2001). The prenatal counseling recommendation is to discuss with the pregnant woman how HIV is acquired, strategies to reduce transmission, perinatal transmission, and strategies to prevent transmission to the fetus. Pharmaceutical treatment should be offered. At present, federal funds to states for HIV programs include stipulations encouraging statewide systems to promote interview screening of all pregnant women for HIV. As knowledge is gained in the prevention of perinatal transmission and treatment of HIV/AIDS, recommendations about prenatal screening may become clearer.

Women who are seropositive for HIV should be counseled about the risk of perinatal transmission and potential for obstetric complications. A discussion of the options on continuing the pregnancy, medication, risks, perinatal outcomes, and treatments is warranted.

Prenatal Care. Women affected by HIV warrant comprehensive prenatal care that can be provided by the local obstetrical care delivery system. Community-based care with appropriate consultation and guidance from the appropriate referral center is preferred. The usual screening tests done in normal pregnancy should also be done with emphasis on sexually transmitted diseases. Screening for gonorrhea, chlamydia, herpes, hepatitis B, C, and D, and syphilis are particularly important. Testing for antibody to CMV and toxoplasmosis is also recommended. If not routinely done for the normal pregnant women in the prenatal setting, a tuberculin skin test with follow-up chest x-ray as indicated for the woman who is HIV positive. Vaccinations for hepatitis B, pneumococcal infection, hemophilus B influenza and viral influenza should be done to offer protection for opportunistic infections. Close scrutiny and follow-up of suspicious Pap smear results are prudent because of the increased risk of cervical changes associated with HPV and HIV (Dole, 2001).

Newborn Screening. Many states anonymously test all newborns for HIV in order to assess the prevalence of the virus. Some states have taken efforts to make these records available to women or to pediatricians as deemed necessary. Prior to the ACTG 076 protocol, some professionals were calling for mandatory newborn screening. At present, mandatory screening of newborns is occurring in two states.

Medication. Nucleoside analog reverse transcriptase inhibitors, non-nucleoside reverse transcriptase inhibitors, and protease inhibitors are available and are being used in the treatment of persons positive for HIV (see Table 18–1). Much research continues as to when treatment is initiated, which drugs to choose, and in what combination. Over time, resistance to the drugs occurs and, therefore, it is not clearly known when changes to other drugs are most advantageous (Esch & Frank, 2001; PHSTF, 2002). The nucleoside analog reverse transcriptase inhibitors inhibit the binding site of the reverse transcriptase enzyme, the key enzyme in transforming viral RNA to DNA. They do not kill the virus but inhibit viral replication. Azidothymidine (AZT), the most popular, remains the initial therapy is most cases. The non-nucleoside reverse transcriptase inhibitors (NNRTI) alter the shape of the active site on the binding site of the reverse transcriptase enzyme (PHSTF, 2002). The protease inhibitors work by inhibiting the HIV protease enzyme, a necessary enzyme for formation of the protein capsule surrounding the viral RNA in mature viruses (Esch & Frank, 2001 PHSTF, 2002). Treatment with protease has reduced HIV replication and increased CD-4 cell counts better than the other categories of drugs. The use of these drugs during pregnancy is being investigated and usage varies by geographical areas. At present several protocols are recommended (PHSTF, 2002).

Zidovudine (ZDV) chemoprophylaxis has shown to be effective in reducing perinatal transmission, and now combination drug therapy is the current standard of care for pregnant women (Newshan & Holt, 1998; PHSTF, 2002). Specific protocols regarding the individual drugs, dosage, and side effects are changing quickly and thus continuous monitoring of the latest recommendations is warranted. The pregnant woman positive for HIV needs to be monitored by both the perinatal and infectious disease specialists. The most recent information is available on HIV/AIDS Treatment Information Service (ATIS) website *http://www.hivatis.org.* The decision to use any antiretroviral drug during pregnancy should be discussed with the woman, including the known and unknown benefits and risks to her and her fetus (PHSTF, 2002).

Since the release of the protocol, there are reports of the relationship of the maternal viral load to success of treatment with ZDV. ZDV has a protective effect prenatally but may not be as effective late in the third trimester or intrapartally if the viral load is increasing or is high at that time of administration (Newshan, Holt, 1998; PHSTF, 2002). The major sign of toxicity is bone marrow suppression, so hematocrit, white cell count, and platelet count should be done periodically. Those women on Zidovudine during pregnancy should also be monitored by a monthly complete blood cell count and liver function tests (PHSTF, 2002). Trimethoprim-sulfamethoxazole is the drug of choice for prophylaxis for pneumonia carinii infection, a common opportunistic infection associated with AIDS. This regimen also provides protection against toxoplasmic encephalitis (Newshan, Holt 1998). The CD-4 and T-lymphocyte count should be monitored each trimester to determine need for initiation of prophylaxis for opportunistic infections.

Physical Concerns. Fatigue or decreased physical endurance has been identified by HIV-positive clients and their caregivers as a major health care problem. Exercise has been proposed as a strategy to increase endurance and improve mental outlook. Direct positive effect on the immune system has been theorized but as yet has not been demonstrated. Effects of exercise, including prenatal

TABLE 18–1. Available Antiretroviral Drugs

Nucleoside Analog Reverse Transcriptase Inhibitors

Azidothymidine (AZT)—Retrovir, Zidovudine
Didanosine (ddI)—Videx
Zalcitabine (ddC)—Hivid
Stavudine (d4T)—Zerit
Lamivudine (3TC)—Epivir
Abacavir—Ziagon

Non-Nucleoside Reverse Transcriptase Inhibitors (NNRTIS)

Delavirdine—Rescriptor
Nevirapine—Viramune
Efavirenz—Sustiva

Protease Inhibitors

Saquinavir—Invirase
Indinavir—Crixivan
Ritonavir—Norvir
Nelfinavir—Viracept
Ammeravir—Agenerase
Lopinavir/Ritonavir—Kaletra

exercises and prepared childbirth, have not been studied for their effects on the HIV-positive pregnant woman.

Psychosocial Issues. The issues of women who are positive for HIV are complex and difficult. Women are more likely to be involved in full-time caregiving roles, living in poverty, and less able to access health care. Even when the diagnosis of HIV positive is made, the woman is usually not symptomatic and, therefore, is likely to react with denial. Because of this denial, discussions about planning for the future, accepting preventive treatment for perinatal transmission, and reducing the transmission of HIV to present partners is difficult. Previous experience and general mental health will attribute to the women's ability to cope with the disease and/or the pregnancy. With the emphasis on prenatal screening, many of these women are having to deal with an initial diagnosis of a fatal disease as well with stressors of a pregnancy. Those women who abuse drugs are even more difficult to help because of the nature of their lifestyle, which is usually disorganized and without adequate family or community support. A discussion about the option of termination of the pregnancy may be appropriate.

Women who have progressed to AIDS face a daily risk of developing an opportunistic infection, are challenged dealing with normal activities of daily living with compromised energy level and decreased physical endurance, overwhelmed by financial burdens of medical and drug therapies and emotional responses to a life-threatening condition as well as concern regarding who will care for their infants if they become ill. A home care model with the appropriate supportive care including nutritional services, counseling, nursing, homemaker, and spiritual care is the most effective, client-oriented, and cost-effective approach (Josten et al., 1997). Case management involves being able to identify the strengths of the woman and develop a plan of care that provides comprehensive care while maintaining the woman's independence as long as possible (Bovo, 2001).

As the disease progresses, the woman affected by HIV who is trying to cope with the stresses of the illness and treatment is at increased risk for clinical depression and suicide (Lyon & Younger, 2001). The applicability of this observation to pregnant and postpartum women is unknown.

Many community-based multicultural organizations have developed programs throughout the country to address the various issues regarding HIV/AIDS. Many communities have AIDS service directories, volunteer organizations, and academically based and/or federally funded projects to assist HIV-affected women access resources. The national AIDS hotline 1-800-342-AIDS is an excellent source of information for clients and providers.

Education/Counseling. The HIV-positive pregnant woman will need education concerning infection control issues at home, safer sex precautions, stages of the HIV disease, and treatment modalities at these various stages. She will need information about the preventive drug therapies for her unborn child. Much national attention supported with federal funds has been spent to disseminate the prevention of HIV message.

Health care provider attitudes and fears may compromise care given to HIV-affected women. It has been reported that professionals with negative attitudes about the HIV-affected person reflect that anxiety and concern about contracting the disease through exposure to that person (Katz, 2001). Rejection and avoidance have been documented. Education about HIV has been shown to reduce the fear and resentment toward HIV-affected persons and has been associated with less rejection and avoidance behavior. Nationally supported educational programs have been established across the country through Ryan White funds to address specific issues regarding HIV, including pregnant women (Newshan & Holt, 1998). Childbirth educators and prenatal care providers should educate all pregnant women about the risks and treatment for HIV (Ruiz & Molitor, 1998).

Delivery. Some reports suggest that cesarean birth may decrease the risk of HIV transmission (PHSTF, 2002). It has been shown that the risk of HIV transmission increases when the fetal membranes have been ruptured more than four hours before delivery, which may attribute to lower transmission rates in cesarean births. For that reason, fetal membranes should remain intact until delivery. Efforts to reduce instrumentation such as avoiding use of episiotomy, fetal scalp electrodes, and scalp pH are necessary to decrease the newborn's exposure to maternal vaginal secretions and blood.

Newborn. With the increased use of combination therapy, more fetuses are being exposed without clear understanding of the impact. Comprehensive follow-up and monitoring of these newborns is recommended (PHSTF, 2002).

Breastfeeding. Even though there have been only a few cases of transmission of HIV to an infant through breastfeeding, the Public Health Service recommends women who are HIV positive avoid breastfeeding (PHSTF, 2002). In addition, the Committee on Pediatric AIDS recommends women with known risks for HIV be counseled specifically regarding the appropriateness of breastfeeding.

Postpartum Contraception. In some groups, rates of pregnancy in HIV-affected women are high. Reasons women continue to be at risk for pregnancy are complex and multifactorial. Reasons include denial of illness and its meaning, positive secondary gains related to the pregnancy, perception of the low risk of transmission to the child, ethical and cultural beliefs about contraception and conception, lack of access to health care including family planning services, or the inability to negotiate with partner for safer sex practices including pregnancy prevention practices. For the woman who is also abusing drugs, pregnancy may be a low priority issue for her. Intrauterine devices (IUDs) are usually not advised in these women because of the risk of pelvic infection. All other methods are viable options with emphasis that latex condoms should be used in addition to reduce transmission to the partner. Surgical sterilization may be desired and should be discussed. Contraceptive services including sterilization should be available and affordable. Important to any discussion of contraception regarding HIV-affected women is sensitivity to the woman's choice. The provider's responsibility is to ensure the client makes an informed decision based upon current knowledge. Even though effective contraception seems to be logical for the provider, directive counseling on contraception, especially sterilization, is inappropriate.

Legal Issues. Because of the previous documented discrimination that has occurred in HIV-positive persons, maintaining confidentiality is critical to the woman and her family. Legal issues regarding a positive HIV include insurance coverage, job security, documentation policies, state testing and reporting protocols, and guardianship of surviving children. The provider must maintain current knowledge of local laws and policies that affect the health care of the HIV-affected woman and her newborn. Referral to community legal services is appropriate.

SEXUALLY TRANSMITTED DISEASES AFFECTING PREGNANCY

Many sexually transmitted infections, including HIV, are known to have fatal or severely debilitating effects on the fetus. Table 18–2 summarizes the infections most commonly faced by providers in prenatal care. For early treatment and prevention of vertical transmission, screening for many sexually transmitted diseases is done at the initial prenatal visit. Refer to Chapter 11 for a more detailed discussion of these diseases and their impact on women's health.

PYELONEPHRITIS

Acute pyelonephritis in pregnancy is a common renal disorder defined as the presence of actively multiplying bacteria in the upper urinary tract. It usually, although not always, follows a previous asymptomatic bacteriuria (ASB). *Escherichia coli* (*E. coli*) is the most common organism for ASB.

Epidemiology

In normal pregnancy, the ureters become dilated and compressed secondary to the influence of progesterone and compression of the gravid uterus. In addition, the renal plasma flow increases about 35 percent during pregnancy. The glomerular filtration rate (GFR) rises 50 percent after the first trimester and remains elevated through delivery. This increased ratio of the glomerular filtration ratio leads to an increase in electrolytes, glucose, and other filtered substances reaching the renal tubules. Reabsorption of sodium usually is maintained, but glucose reabsorption does not increase proportionately. Glucosuria during pregnancy is not unusual and contributes to an environment conducive to bacterial growth. Increase in the GFR accelerates the excretion of creatinine, urea, and uric acid, which manifest in a fall in the blood urea nitrogen (BUN) and serum creatinine values. Secondary to pressure from the gravid uterus, the bladder loses muscle tone, becomes more easily distended, and predisposes to lower urinary tract infection. All of these factors contribute to the incidence of urinary tract infections in pregnancy.

Acute pyelonephritis occurs in up to 2 percent of all pregnancies and is the most common nonobstetrical reason for antepartum admissions (Gilstrap & Ramin, 2001). Ascension of bacteria to the kidney will lead to pyelonephritis. Effects on the mother include bacterial endotoxemia leading to endotoxin shock and acute renal dysfunction leading to acute renal failure. Pyelonephritis in pregnancy has been reported to be associated with small-for-gestational age babies and preterm delivery, but recent studies have not corroborated that finding. Transient renal failure, Adult Respiratory Distress Syndrome, sepsis, and shock are all associated with pyelonephritis in pregnancy (Gilstrap & Ramin, 2001). There have also been conflicting reports of a link between pyelonephritis and hypertension and anemia. It occurs more frequently

TABLE 18–2. Sexually Transmitted Diseases Affecting Pregnancy

Organism	Incidence in Pregnancy	Affect on Pregnancy	Medications	Other Concerns
Herpes simplex virus (HSV)	About 20 % of the adult population have been diagnosed with HSV and about 2 % of women acquire HSV during pregnancy. Infants born to women infected with HSV have a 30–50 % chance of acquiring infection. Infants with skin, eye, and mouth infection showed no mortality, but more seriously affected infants with systemic infection have a 60 % mortality.	The same painful vesicular lesions appear as In the nonpregnant client. Initial viremia in the first trimester of pregnancy is frequently associated with spontaneous abortion. Not all infants born through an infected birth canal become infected, in fact, most infected infants are not born to women with a history of herpes genitalis. Perinatal transmission is more likely if the initial infection is near the time of delivery. Infants manifest HSV in localized form by lesions on the skin, eyes, or oral cavity. In more severe systemic forms shown by lethargy, poor feeding, fever, irritability, convulsions, jaundice, apnea, shock, and possible death.	Oral and topical Acyclovir have been used. Usual regimen is 200 mg orally 5 times day for 7–10 days until lesions resolve. Hospitalization for intravenous administration of Acyclovir or valacyclovir have been used to decrease chances of infant becoming infected or treat life-threatening maternal infections including encephalitis, pneumonitis, or hepatitis. Some HSV experts recommend prophylactic therapy using Acyclovir, valacyclovir, or famciclovir starting at 36 weeks, but definitive evidence as to the risks to the fetus are still inconclusive.	Instructions for the client include symptomatic relief measures as nonpregnant women. Cool perineal compressors, sitz baths, loose-fitting clothes help to alleviate pain. Cesarean delivery is not necessary for every client with a history of herpes: only recommended when active lesions are present. Infants born through an HSV-infected birth canal should be monitored carefully for neonatal complications. Women need to be instructed to avoid intercourse in the third trimester with partners known or suspected of having HSV. Viral cultures collected during pregnancy are not able to predict viral shedding at delivery. Thus, routine cultures on women with a history of HSV are not recommended. Breastfeeding is allowed if contact with the active lesions is avoided.
Syphilis (Treponema pallidum)	40–50% of infants of infected mothers contract congenital syphilis 20.6 congenital syphilis cases per 100,000 live births in 1998.	Syphilis unaltered by course of pregnancy. Chance often unnoticed and/or internal and not diagnosed during pregnancy. Treponemas cross placenta as early as 9 weeks of gestation, but fetal involvement rare prior to 18 weeks of gestation. Maternal infection increases risk of endarteritis, stromal hyperplasia, and immature villi. Increased risk of premature labor and birth. Congenital syphilis signs and symptoms: hepatosplenomegaly, osteochondritis, jaundice, rhinitis, anemia, lymphadenopathy, nervous system involvement, periostitis, ocular abnormalities, nonimmune hydrops, IUGR, pseudoparalysis of an extremity.	Benzathine penicillin G 2.4 million units IM. No known alternative to penicillin treatment in pregnancy. Treat pregnant women with penicillin after desensitization. Some experts recommend a second dose 1 week after initial treatment when woman in third trimester. Erythromycin should not be used because it cannot be relied upon to cure an infected fetus. Erythromycin estolate should NOT be given in pregnancy because of possible hepatotoxicity.	All pregnant woman should be screened in early pregnancy. Serologic test should be reported in third trimester in populations with high incidence or women at high-risk. Infant diagnosed with congenital syphilis should be placed in isolation until treatment administered. All women infected with syphilis should be tested for HIV. Any woman who delivers a stillborn infant after 20 weeks gestation should be tested for syphilis. No infant should leave the hospital without documentation of results of maternal syphilis test.

Disease	Incidence	Signs/Symptoms	Treatment	Comments
Gonorrhea (Neissaeria gonorrhea)	Estimated 600,000 cases a year in the U.S.	85% of infected women have no symptoms. Ophthalmium neonatorum: results from delivery through infected birth canal. Pelvic inflammatory disease is complication of gonorrhea infection.	Ceftriaxone, 125 mg IM in a single dose or cefixime, 400 mg p.o. in a single dose followed by presumptive treatment for chlamydia. Erythromycin base or stearate 500 mg p.o. qid × 7 days or Erythromycin ethylsuccinate 800 mg p.o. qid × 7 days. Pregnant women who cannot tolerate a cephalosporin should receive Spectinomycin 2 gm IM (single-dose)	Gonorrhea screening should be done at initial prenatal visit and repeated in the third trimester. Test of cure not recommended when using drug of choice and woman asymptomatic. Test for syphilis with positive gonorrhea. All states have mandated prophylaxis in the first hour of life. Newborn prophylaxis: Tetracycline or erythromycin ointments, silver nitrate ophthalmic drops, and penicillin GM have all been used as prophylaxis. Partners must be treated. Avoid coitus until both partners are cured.
C Trachomatic (Chlamydial cervicitis)	Most common STD. Occurs in 5% of pregnant women with a range of 3–37%. More prevalent in adolescents and young women.	Frequently the woman is asymptomatic. It is a common cause of mucopurulent cervicitis. Chlamydial infection during pregnancy is associated with prematurity and stillbirth. Urinary tract infection caused by Chlamydia untreated may progress to pyelonephritis. Infants born vaginally to infected women have a 10–20 % chance of acquiring conjunctivitis. The newborn may also develop a pneumonia type of infection with congestion, wheezing, and cough up to 12 weeks of age. It may also cause a middle ear infection in the infant.	Tetracycline, Doxycycline, ofloxann are contraindicated in pregnancy. Erythromycin 500 mg qid for 7 days. (See Gonorrhea) Azithromycin 1g orally Amoxicillin 500 mg tid for 7 days	Fluoroquinolone resistance to N. gonorrhea is spreading in parts of Asia, the Pacific, and the U.S. west coast. If women, who have previously been diagnosed and treated with a recommended regimen, have recurrent symptoms, culture and sensitivity are necessary prior to further treatment. Treatment is essential for the sexual partner. Encouragement of abstinence during treatment is important to prevent reinfection. Treatment prior to delivery will eradicate maternal cervical chlamydial infection and prevent vertical transmission to the newborn. Many states mandate the use of erythromycin topical eye ointment within the first one hour of birth to prevent both gonorrhea and chlamydial infection. All women positive for chlamydia need to be screened for other STDs.
Trichomonas	Occurs in 20–30% of all pregnant women.	Women may experience diffuse, malodorous, yellow-green discharge or may be asymptomatic. Associated with premature rupture of membranes, preterm delivery, and low birthweight. Recent reports suggest association between any prenatal vaginal infections and preterm delivery.	Metronidazole 2 g initial treatment. Metronidazole 500 mg bid × 7 days. The treatment of asymptomatic Trichomonas has not lessened poor outcomes. Avoidance of using Metronidazole in the first trimester has been a common practice because of concern of teratogenicity. Recent multiple studies have not demonstrated that association.	Partners need treatment. Instruct client to avoid sexual intercourse until she and her partner have completed therapy. Screening for Trichomonas during pregnancy is not recommended but treatment of symptomatic women recommended.

Sources: ACOG Practice Bulletin, (1999); Burst, (1998); CDC (2002b); Donahue (2002); Hollier & Cox (1998); Klebanoff et al., (2001); Tiller (2002); Whiteside, Katz, Anthes, et al., (2001); Wyckoff (2000).

in women affected by sickle cell disease and diabetes (Gilstrap & Ramin, 2001).

Subjective Data

Maternal symptoms include fever, shaking chills, malaise, flank pain, nausea and vomiting, headache, increased urinary frequency, and dysuria. Symptoms of mild cough to severe respiratory distress syndrome are present when severe cases lead to pulmonary dysfunction.

Objective Data

Traditionally, all pregnant women are screened by urine culture on the initial prenatal visit and monitored throughout pregnancy with a dipstick method for presence of nitrites.

For the symptomatic woman, a urine culture is necessary. Bacteriuria, with pyuria and white blood cell casts will be present in urine examination. A count of 1 to 2 bacteria per high power field in spun urine or more than 20 bacteria in the sediment of a centrifuged specimen of urine collected by bladder catheterization is diagnostic. Hematuria may be present. Urine culture is necessary for diagnosis and determination of causative agent. Determining the causative agent is important in monitoring recurring episodes. Also, if the causative organism is Group Beta Streptococcus, intrapartum chemoprophylaxis is recommended to reduce neonatal Group Beta Streptococcal Disease.

Differential Medical Diagnoses

Acute cystitis, urinary calculi, glomerulonephritis, labor, choreoamnionitis, appendicitis, abruptio placentae.

Plan

Prevention. The incidence of pyelonephritis can be significantly reduced by screening and treating asymptomatic bacteriuria during prenatal visits. Acute pyelonephritis will occur in 25 percent of those women untreated for bacteriuria. Clean catch urine cultures are recommended at the initial prenatal visit for all pregnant women. If on the client's initial prenatal visit, urine culture reveals > 100,000 organisms per millimeter, the client should be treated regardless of the presence of symptoms. It is important to do a repeat urine culture following treatment because 25 percent of women treated for bacteriuria will experience recurrence and 34 percent will develop acute pyelonephritits (Gilstrap & Ramin, 2001). For those women treated for bacteriuria during

pregnancy, prophylaxis antibiotic maintenance may be ordered by some providers throughout the remainder of the pregnancy. Close monitoring and urine screening for all pregnant women at each routine prenatal visit are recommended.

Medication. For the initial episode of pyelonephritis, a first-generation cephalosporin is the drug of choice 1 to 2 g every six hours. Ampicillin plus gentamicin is used for recurrences. Antibiotic suppression is continued throughout the remainder of the pregnancy after an episode of pyelonephritis. Nitrofurantoin 100 mg once or twice daily is a common suppression regimen (Gilstrap & Ramin, 2001). Sulfa drugs need to be avoided in late pregnancy because of the increase risk of neonatal hyperbilirubinemia. Antipyretic agents are used as necessary for fever.

Hospitalization. Historically, all pregnant women with a diagnosis of pyelonephritis were admitted to the hospital for antibiotics and hydration. Intravenous antibiotic therapy continues for 24 to 48 hours after the woman becomes afebrile, and costovertebral angle tenderness subsides. The complications, even though uncommon, are severe and can be life threatening. Recently, outpatient protocols have been developed in an attempt to provide safe and effective outpatient care of these women. The outpatient model includes intravenous (IV) hydration, 2 g of IV ceftriaxone, observation for 24 hours and discharge once the woman is afebrile. Women with high-risk factors such as signs of sepsis, allergies, respiratory compromise, preterm labor, gestation greater than 37 weeks, history of substance abuse, or known fetal malformations are not recommended to be managed outside of the hospital (Wing, Hendershott, Debuque, & Millar, 1999). Most providers are continuing to manage pregnant women with initial hospitalization.

Postpartum. About 2 to 4 percent of women develop a lower urinary tract infection postdelivery secondary to factors such as birth trauma, expected bladder hypotonia, residual urine, catheterization, anesthesia, and vaginal examinations. Pyelonephritis can be a likely sequelae to these infections if not treated adequately. Antibiotic therapy for these infections continues for up to ten days. Education of the new mother should include the importance of completing all medication to decrease incidence of recurrence. Since *E. coli* is the causative organism in most cases, sulfonamides, nitrofurantoin, ampicillin, or ephalosporins are used. Breastfeeding while taking sulfonamides is controversial, but the risk is low in healthy full-term infants.

Women who experienced recurrent urinary tract infections or pyelonephritis during pregnancy need radiographic evaluation of the upper urinary tract three months postpartum to assess for structural abnormality. Urine for culture and sensitivity should be obtained at the routine postpartum visit.

INTRA-AMNIOTIC INFECTION

Intra-amniotic infection (IAI) is any infection within the intrauterine structures. Although in the past, the terms *chorioamnionitis* and *amnionitis* were used interchangeably, each is a specific diagnosis dependent on the structures affected. The conditions are frequently not detected until after delivery.

The organisms most often isolated from the amniotic fluid of infected women are Group B streptococci, *Bacteroides* species, *Bacteroides bivius, Escherichia coli, Clostridium,* peptostreptococci, and *Fusobacterium. Mycoplasma hominis* and *Listeria monocytogenes* have also been isolated, but not necessarily from infected women. How these organisms may affect preterm labor and neonatal sepsis is not clear. Group B streptococci are currently the most common cause of sepsis and meningitis in neonates and young infants. Group A streptococci are not usually associated with neonatal sepsis.

Perinatal Group B Streptococcal Disease

Group B streptococcus (GBS) is a leading cause of neonatal infection in the United States and a significant cause of maternal illness. GBS is a gram positive bacterium that colonizes in the vagina and when present during pregnancy attributes to maternal and/or neonatal infection (McKenna & Iams, 1998).

Epidemiology

In most populations studied, from 10 to 30 percent of pregnant women were colonized with GBS in the vaginal or rectal areas (McKenna & Iams, 1998). Colonization rates can differ among ethnic groups, geographic areas, and by age; however, rates are similar between pregnant and nonpregnant women. The incidence of GBS is higher in African American women and women under 20 years of age (McKenna & Iams, 1998). The amniotic cavity usually protects the fetus from ascending pathogens; however, with rupture of the membranes and onset of labor, ascending infection from the lower genital tract can occur. Infants born to women who have positive GBS cultures prenatally have a significant increase in early onset disease compared to infants born to women whose prenatal cultures were negative (McKenna & Iams, 1998).

The incidence of neonatal sepsis is only 1 to 2 percent; however, infection can be fatal or lead to permanent neurodevelopmental defect (Chandran et al., 2001; McKenna & Iams, 1998; Mitchell, Steffenson, Hogan, & Brooks, 1997). The origin of group B streptococci in the genital tract is unclear, but the gastrointestinal tract seems the likely source. Reinfection is common through either autoinfection or sexual intercourse.

Subjective Data

Women with colonies of group B streptococci in the genital tract are asymptomatic. With intra-amniotic infection, however, the client may report vague symptoms of fever and malaise, usually in the third trimester after membranes have ruptured.

Objective Data

Early diagnosis is difficult because symptoms do not occur until infection has progressed substantially and caused amniotis.

The earliest sign of infection is most likely fever. Uterine tenderness, foul-smelling amniotic fluid, maternal leukocytosis, and tachycardia are detected late in the infectious process.

Cultures can be done to isolate group B streptococci, but a minimum of 24 hours is needed for test results. Gram stains can provide immediate results but are not specific or reliable for group B streptococci (McKenna & Iams, 1998). Routine antenatal screening has not been effective in detecting women at risk for delivering an infected neonate. Maternal colonization is frequently transient and intermittent; therefore, a positive antenatal culture does not indicate that a culture will be positive at the time of labor (McKenna & Iams, 1998).

Differential Medical Diagnoses

Pyelonephritis, bacterial vaginosis, gonorrhea.

Plan

Prevention. Research has focused on either inducing protective immunity in the neonate or eradicating colonization from the mother and/or neonate (chemoprophylaxis). Several vaccines to induce antibodies against GBS are being developed but may have limited effectiveness due to reduced transplacental transport of protective antibody before 32 to 34 weeks' gestation. Controversy has surrounded the screening, timing, and treatment of GBS to reduce neonatal GBS infection.

Psychosocial Interventions. All pregnant women need education, especially in the third trimester, on the potential for GBS infection. They also need to be aware of risk factors and screening recommendations. It is unclear whether a woman who has had a child with neonatal sepsis is truly at risk during a subsequent pregnancy, but emotionally she is clearly at risk. Any history of neonatal sepsis can cause apprehension. The provider must recognize this and be sensitive to the client's concerns and questions.

Screening. In May 1996, Centers for Disease Control and Prevention (CDC) in collaboration with the American College of Obstetricians and Gynecologists (ACOG) and the American Academy of Pediatrics (AAP) released recommendations on the prevention of perinatal Group B Streptococcal Disease. Both a screening-based and a risk-factor-based approach have been appropriate. Studies over the past years have demonstrated a reduction in the incidence of neonatal Group B Streptococcal infection due to the more widespread usage of routine testing and prophylactic treatment (CDC, 2000a, 2000b; Schrag et al., 2000). A revision of the guidelines, which is predicted to recommend that routine testing be done at 37 weeks of gestation, is expected late in 2002. A provider can access the most current information on screening at the CDC web site *www.cdc.gov/ncidod/dbmd/gbs*. The screening-based approach recommends all pregnant women be screened at 35 to 37 weeks' gestation for anogenital GBS colonization. Obtain one or two swabs from the vaginal introitus and anorectum without using a speculum. Cervical cultures are not acceptable. Appropriate nonnutritive moist swab transport systems (e.g., Amies') are commercially available. Those women positive for GBS should be offered intrapartum penicillin. The other approach is to provide intrapartum chemoprophylaxis for women with risk factors without screening. Much effort has been given into developing a rapid test for identification of GBS colonization at the time of admission in labor (Bergeron et al., 2000). Thus far, no test has been proven sensitive enough to warrant routine use in place of bacterial culture.

Medication. Antibiotic treatment of women who are colonized during prenatal screening is not effective in eliminating the organism or preventing neonatal disease. Antibiotic treatment prenatally is not recommended. Intravenous penicillin G is the drug of choice for intrapartum chemoprophylaxis in women with a documented

positive culture for GBS. Ampicillin is an acceptable alternative as well as other agents such as Clindamycin when used if clinical amnionitis is present. Women who are treated based upon risk factors include those who (1) had a previous infant with invasive GBS disease, (2) had GBS bacteriuria during current pregnancy, (3) are less than 37 weeks' gestation, (4) have ruptured membranes 18 hours or more, or (5) have temperature equal to or greater than 38°C (100.4°F) (Chandran et al., 2001; McKenna & Iams, 1998). The presence of multiple gestation alone is not a criteria for intrapartum chemoprophylaxis but because of its frequent association with preterm birth may necessitate consideration for treatment. If the prenatal screening results are unknown at the onset of labor, chemoprophylaxis should be given based upon intrapartum risk factors (Chandran et al., 2001).

Delivery. Critical to the implementation of the CDC guidelines is the notification of staff caring for the woman during the intrapartum period. A positive prenatal screening for group B streptococcus needs to be clearly documented on the chart. The woman needs to be counseled to the importance of knowing her GBS status and, if positive, needs to know to communicate that to staff in the intrapartum unit. Neonatal colonization usually occurs at the time of delivery, but cesarean birth does not reduce the vertical transmission or infection rates. Presence or suspicion of GBS is not an indicator for surgical delivery.

Neonatal Follow-Up. Routine use of prophylactic antibiotic agents for infants born to mothers who received intrapartum prophylaxis is not recommended. For infants symptomatic of sepsis, several management approaches are being used. Close observation and assessment for sepsis is critical. Routine workups may not be necessary (Mitchell et al., 1997; Mullaney, 2001).

Implications for Providers. Even with release of guidelines by national groups, controversy continues among professionals. Providers need to maintain current on the recommendations and accepted approaches within their practice sites. Clear documentation of any screening results and management plans are critical. Table 18–3 summarizes risks associated with GBS disease. Systems for communicating prenatal culture results to intrapartum physician and nursing staff must be established. Brochures have been developed by numerous public and private organizations to assist the provider counsel and educate women and their families. Providers need to be assured that any patient educational materials being used in the practice reflect the current recommended guide-

TABLE 18–3. Risks Associated with Delivering an Infant with Perinatal Group B Streptococcal Disease

Prenatal
< 20 years of age
African American ethnicity
Positive 35–37 week GBS culture
Previous delivery of GBS infected neonate (early onset)
Treatment of GBS bacteriuria in current pregnancy

Intrapartal
Membrane rupture > or = 18 hours
Fever > or = 38°C (100.4°F)
< 37 weeks' gestation

Source: Adapted from McKenna & Iams (1998). Chandran et al. (2001);

lines. Compliance with the existing guidelines has not been demonstrated so providers need to communicate and use the guidelines consistently for all pregnant women (Chandran et al., 2001; Mitchell, 1997).

Implications for Parents. Women and their families need to be aware of the strategies for the early detection, treatment, and prevention of Group B Streptococcus transmission to the neonate. One volunteer organization, Group B Strep Association, has been formed to educate expectant parents about the implications of Group B Streptococcus on neonatal outcome.

BLEEDING

Bleeding any time during pregnancy is serious and potentially life threatening. It occurs in 10 to 20 percent of all pregnancies (Krause & Graves, 1999). The amount of bleeding and the time it occurs determine the urgency and management plan.

SPONTANEOUS ABORTION

Spontaneous abortion is the termination of pregnancy before the point of fetal viability. Gestation should not be more than 20 weeks and conceptus should not weigh more than 500 g or be longer than 16.5 cm, crown to rump. *Miscarriage* is the lay term for spontaneous abortion.

Types of abortion are categorized according to signs and symptoms.

- A *threatened abortion* is possible pregnancy loss; however, pregnancy may continue without further problems. Slight bleeding usually occurs, and some uterine contractions are felt as abdominal cramping.

Uterine size is compatible with dates, the cervical os is closed, and no products of conception are passed. Prognosis is unpredictable.

- An *inevitable abortion* is a pregnancy that cannot be salvaged. Moderate bleeding and moderate to severe uterine cramping occur, and the cervical os is dilated. Uterine size is compatible with dates. The products of conception are not passed. Prognosis is poor.
- In an *incomplete abortion,* some products of conception are passed. Moderate to severe uterine cramping and heavy bleeding occur. Uterine size is compatible with dates; the cervical os is dilated. Prognosis is poor.
- In a *complete abortion,* all products of conception are expelled. Bleeding may be minimal and uterine contractions have subsided. The uterus is normal prepregnancy size; the cervical os may be opened or closed.
- A *missed abortion* occurs when the embryo is not viable but is retained in utero for at least six weeks. Uterine contractions are absent. Bleeding may initially be absent, but spotting begins and later becomes heavier.
- *Habitual abortion* is the experience of three or more consecutive spontaneous abortions.

Epidemiology

A precise etiology of spontaneous abortion does not exist, but varied maternal and fetal factors are attributed to its incidence. Maternal age greatly increases the risk, i.e., a 40-year-old woman carries twice the risk of a 20-year-old. Genetic abnormalities are the most common. Endocrinologic disorders—specifically, elevated levels of luteinizing hormone—have also been associated with pregnancy loss. Low levels of fibrinogen and Factor VII antigen have been associated with increased chance of spontaneous abortion (Nelson, Ness, Grisso, & Cushman, 2001). Prior pregnancy loss is associated with increased risk for pregnancy loss, but consideration of the genetic and endocrinological factors makes this relationship unclear. Frequently, the embryonic sac is empty or a degenerated fetus is found; both conditions are referred to as *blighted ovum.* Another cause of spontaneous abortion is maternal infections. Both viral and bacterial infections can cause local infection of the conceptus, endometritis, or more generalized pelvic disease, all of which can lead to fetal death and abortion.

In addition, anatomic abnormalities of the reproductive tract are associated with abortion, usually in the second trimester. Some chronic diseases, such as diabetes, nutritional deficiencies, renal diseases, and lupus erythematosus, also affect a woman's ability to maintain her pregnancy. Moreover, lifestyle practices, such as smoking, substance abuse, and exposure to environmental hazards, are related to early pregnancy loss. Incidence reports reveal that about 20 percent of all pregnant women experience some cramping and bleeding in early pregnancy. About one-half of those women continue through an uneventful pregnancy; the other half suffer pregnancy loss.

Subjective Data

Varying degrees of vaginal bleeding, low back pain, abdominal cramping, and passage of products of conception are reported. Usually the severity of cramping progresses, and a change is seen in the type of blood lost.

Many women in early pregnancy report "spotting," a brown-red vaginal discharge that stains underwear or toilet tissue. Vaginal bleeding that becomes bright red is usually significant. The amount of bleeding is ascertained by the saturation of sanitary napkins and the frequency with which the napkins must be changed. Saturation of one sanitary napkin every hour is significant.

Objective Data

Data are established using categorizations based on the client's signs and symptoms and diagnostic test results.

Uterine size is less than the expected gestational size.

Fetal heart tones are reassuring and dictate a conservative management plan; their absence beyond the tenth week of gestation may indicate a missed abortion.

Cervix may be dilated, soft or products of conception noted at the os; bleeding may be seen.

Real-time sonography will determine the presence of an embryonic sac and detect fetal cardiac motion, which is reassuring and dictates a "wait-and-see" management approach. If the β-hCG is greater than 1000 mIU/ml and if the pregnancy is intrauterine, the gestational sac should be visualized by transvaginal ultrasound (Krause & Graves, 1999). Transabdominal ultrasound of the gestational sac may not be visualized until the B-hCG reaches 6000 mIU/ml. Absence of the embryonic sac in the uterus may indicate ectopic pregnancy and must be investigated further.

Serial β-*subunit human chorionic gonadotropin* (β-*hCG*) measurements scheduled at least two days apart correlate with appropriate rise in β-hCG. Blood is collected for each measurement and sent to the laboratory.

β-hCG levels should double every two days in early pregnancy, peak at about 10 weeks, then gradually decrease during the remainder of pregnancy. Doubling of levels every two days indicates viability and favorable prognosis (Cunningham et al., 2001). Failure of the β-hCG level to double is suspicious of ectopic pregnancy or abortion. Although the client requires no specific instructions for this test, waiting the two days between specimens may be distressing to her.

Some providers use *progesterone* in addition to β-hCG levels to determine presence of a viable pregnancy. Progesterone levels equal to or greater than 25 ng/ml are suggestive of a viable intrauterine pregnancy (Krause & Graves, 1999).

Differential Medical Diagnoses

Malignancy, cervicitis, ectopic pregnancy, gestational trophoblastic disease (hydatidiform mole).

Plan

Psychosocial Interventions. Provide information for the client and her partner throughout all phases of threatened or eventual abortion. Reasons for blood tests and sonograms should be openly discussed. Explain to the client that precautions of bed rest and/or pelvic rest will continue until an asymptomatic period of at least 48 hours has elapsed.

The health care provider should be understanding of the many different responses to pregnancy loss. A response may be influenced by the value of the pregnancy to the client or couple, the desire for pregnancy, the length of gestation, history of other pregnancy losses, the couple's relationship, their social network and support, and religious beliefs. Expressions of anger directed toward the care provider are common. Sensitive listening, counseling, and anticipatory guidance is important to assist the woman and her family adjust to the pregnancy loss (Fox, Pillai, Porter, & Gill, 1997; Krause & Graves, 1999; Swanson, 1999) (refer to Chapter 10, Infertility).

Medication. In some cases, progesterone supplementation via vaginal suppositories has been used successfully for women with known luteal phase defect associated with spontaneous abortion defect.

Specific Interventions. Threatened abortion requires conservative "wait and see' management, unless symptoms threaten the life of the mother. Bedrest is not shown to affect outcome in threatened abortion but is commonly prescribed. The client at home on bedrest and/or pelvic rest should be instructed to maintain adequate hydration and report ominous signs or symptoms. The client should be evaluated weekly in the health office to determine complete blood count, serial β-hCG levels, any signs of infection, or a missed abortion.

- Bedrest requires that the woman be away from her job, have limited or no child care responsibilities at home, and rest in a horizontal position, except when bathing or using the toilet.
- Pelvic rest means no sexual intercourse; no douching or inserting anything into the vagina.
- Instructions for hydration are to drink a minimum of 32 ounces of noncaffeinated fluid every 24 hours.
- Clients are taught the signs and symptoms of infection and how uterine contractions and vaginal bleeding may progress.

Inevitable, incomplete, or missed abortion should be treated more aggressively as soon as a definitive diagnosis is made. To prevent infection and uterine hemorrhage, the uterus should be emptied of all products of conception. Whether instrumental evacuation is necessary in cases of complete abortion is controversial. Conservative management using misoprotol is now being proposed as a reasonable alternative to surgical intervention (Chung, Lee, Cheung, et al., 1999). If some products of conception remain in the uterus as evidenced by cramping and bleeding, enlarged and/or soft uterus, or fever, suction curettage is recommended. Removal of necrotic decidua decreases the incidence of postabortion bleeding and shortens the recovery period.

Missed abortion usually progresses to inevitable abortion, but a "wait-and-see" approach can be emotionally intolerable for some women. In such cases, suction curettage is recommended during the first trimester. In the second trimester, dilatation and evacuation may be performed or labor may be induced with an intravaginal prostaglandin E_2 (PGE$_2$) suppository. Some primary care providers use a laminaria to dilate the cervix overnight prior to the procedure, thereby facilitating a less stressful dilatation procedure. For some women, delaying the definitive diagnosis and treatment plan is necessary to help them accept the situation emotionally.

Follow-Up

Instruct the client about the danger signs of infection or incomplete evacuation of the uterus: fever, foul-smelling lochia, excessive bleeding, back or abdominal pain. The Rh factor should be assessed and immunoglobulin administered to Rh-negative, unsensitized women.

Inform the client that she will need to use contraception for at least four to six months to allow for complete maternal healing and regeneration of endometrial lining. Advise her to have a gynecological exam within two to three weeks of the abortion.

If a woman has had repeated pregnancy losses, complete evaluation is recommended to determine possible causes; appropriate treatment may be instituted prior to future pregnancies (refer to Chapter 10, Infertility).

ECTOPIC PREGNANCY

Ectopic pregnancy is the implantation of a fertilized ovum outside the uterine cavity (Cunningham et al., 2001). Most ectopic pregnancies occur in a fallopian tube, but may also occur in the cervix, on an ovary, or in the abdominal cavity. Following implantation, the embryo grows, but no decidua is present. The structure of the implantation can sustain some growth; however, rupture is usually inevitable. Early signs of pregnancy, including uterine changes and amenorrhea, are present, secondary to hormonal influence. Ectopic pregnancy is a potentially life-threatening condition and involves pregnancy loss.

Epidemiology

The etiology of extrauterine implanatation originates with an interference in normal ovum transport. Women at risk are those who have used an intrauterine device or who have a history of infertility, pelvic inflammatory disease, tubal surgery (e.g., ligation or reconstruction), or ectopic pregnancy, the most common being history of tubal infection (Mashburn, 1999).

Some risk, although low, is associated with abdominal or pelvic surgery, postacute appendicitis, intrauterine exposure to diethylstilbestrol (DES), or use of drugs that slow ovum transport (e.g., minipill). Cesarean birth is not an associated risk factor (Cunningham, et al., 2001).

Incidence worldwide has increased but varies significantly among populations. In the United States, ectopic pregnancy occurs in approximately 1 in 50 pregnancies and is a leading cause of maternal mortality (Cunningham et al., 2001; Mashburn, 1999). It is more prevalent in poor, less advantaged countries. Although maternal mortality has decreased in the United States, the actual number of ectopic pregnancies has increased. The increased incidence appears to be related to factors associated with infertility, such as chronic salpingitis, earlier detection by ultrasound, and sensitive β-hCG assays.

Subjective Data

Classical and atypical presentations are used in diagnosis. The classical clinical presentation includes many of the early signs of pregnancy: one to two months of amenorrhea, nausea, breast tenderness. The most common presenting symptoms are abdominal pain and irregular vaginal bleeding. Abdominal pain can be unilateral, and mild vaginal bleeding is possible. The client is motivated to seek emergency care when her pain becomes sharper and she experiences more generalized discomfort. She may report gastrointestinal disturbances and feelings of malaise and syncope. She may faint. Classically, pain is referred to the shoulder as the hemorrhage becomes extensive and irritates the diaphragm.

Atypical clinical presentations are not so clearly evident. Many clients report vague or sub-acute symptoms. They may report menstrual irregularity. Amenorrhea may not be obvious, as intermittent spotting or mild vaginal bleeding may mimic normal menses. Ectopic pregnancy should be considered in diagnosis when any woman of childbearing age reports mild or severe abdominal symptoms. Symptoms do not necessarily correlate with the severity of the condition; mild signs and symptoms may occur with massive hemorrhage (Hick, Rodgerson, Heegaard, Sterner, 2001; Mashburn 1999).

Objective Data

Any sexually active woman with a missed menses is at risk for ectopic pregnancy. Use of current diagnostic methods has provided the early detection of ectopic pregnancy before symptoms occur or become severe. When symptoms do occur, they mimic other problems with similar complaints.

Physical examination may reveal symptoms of shock especially after hemorrhage. The woman in early gestation may appear in little discomfort. General signs of shock include cool, clammy skin and poor skin color and turgor. Late signs are hypotension and tachycardia. Abdominal examination may reveal some unilateral adnexal tenderness. A pelvic exam reveals a normal-appearing cervix, but marked tenderness is noted. The vaginal vault may be bloody, usually brick red to brown in color. There may be vaginal tenderness. A tender adnexal mass may be palpated, and the uterus may be slightly enlarged and soft.

Levels of serial β-hCG are used to diagnose ectopic pregnancy. A small amount of functioning trophoblastic tissue, as is found in ectopic pregnancy, will produce a small amount of β-hCG without the amount of expected doubling increases associated with normal pregnancy. In a normal intrauterine pregnancy, hormone levels should double every two to four days with a predictable slope of increase. Low β-hCG levels are therefore suggestive of an ectopic pregnancy and should be followed by a repeated quantitative radio-immunoassay.

A sonogram is used to determine if the pregnancy is intrauterine, to assess the size of the uterus, and to detect presence of fetal viability. (Mashburn, 1999). If the β-hCG is greater than 1000 to 2000 mIU/ml at 35 days of gestation, and the pregnancy is intrauterine, a gestational sac should be visualized by transvaginal ultrasound (Mashburn, 1999). Absence of an intrauterine gestational sac is diagnostic of ectopic pregnancy.

Culdocentesis may be done to detect intraperitoneal blood, which will be present following tubal pregnancy rupture. This procedure is carried out during a pelvic exam. The health care provider inserts a needle through the vaginal wall into the cul-de-sac and withdraws whatever fluid is present. Nonclotted blood indicates hemorrhage. The source of bleeding is then identified by means of laparoscopy or laparotomy, and measures are taken to control bleeding.

Differential Medical Diagnoses

Pelvic inflammatory disease, ovarian cyst, ovarian tumor, intrauterine pregnancy, recent spontaneous abortion, early hydatidiform degeneration, acute appendicitis, and other bowel-related disorders.

Plan

Psychosocial Interventions. Inform the client about procedures and support her as early diagnosis and appropriate medical referral are pursued. Because laparoscopy is frequently necessary for a definitive diagnosis, prepare the woman for safe and timely transfer to a hospital. Information about the procedure and management plan should be clearly stated for the client and her partner, a family member, or friend.

Medication. Methotrexate, prostaglandins, RU 486 (misoprotol), and actinomycin have been used in the non-surgical management of ectopic pregnancy. These therapies are new for this condition and have been administered successfully muscularly, via local infiltration, or orally. It clears remaining trophoblastic tissue and may avoid the need for laparotomy. (Cunningham et al., 2001; Luciano, Roy, & Solima, 2001; Mashburn, 1999). The client eligible for medical therapy must be hemodynamically stable and the mass must be unruptured, measuring fewer than 4 cm determined by ultrasound. The severe side effects of bone marrow suppression, hepatotoxicity, stomatitis, pulmonary fibrosis, alopecia, and photosensitivity from methotrexate are uncommon in short-term therapy for ectopic pregnancy, but need to be administered with appropriate caution. Single dose methotrexate is 50 mg/m² of body surface area intramuscularly. Another regimen is methotrexate, 1 mg/k of body weight intramuscularly every other day, alternating with Leucovorin, 0.1 mg/kg intramuscularly every other day, for a total of 8 days (Cunningham, et al., 2001). Treatment continues until the β-hCG drops equal to or greater than 15 percent in 48 hours or 4 doses of methotrexate has been given. Serum β-hCG should be monitored weekly until undetected; blood count, platelet count, and liver enzyme levels should also be monitored weekly (Mashburn, 1999). Colicky pain secondary to the stomatitis can mimic ectopic rupture and must be differentiated by assessment for hypotension, tachycardia, or falling hematocrit indicating hemorrhage. Clients should avoid gas-producing foods such as beans or cabbage, which may also mimic ectopic rupture. Clients should also avoid sun exposure while taking the methotrexate because of the photosensitivity of the drug.

Surgical-Evacuation of Conceptus. Immediately after ectopic pregnancy is diagnosed, the conceptus is surgically evacuated. The success of conservative surgery is influenced by the condition of the client and the affected organ (e.g., fallopian tube, ovary), location of the conceptus, and the client's desire for future fertility. Two problems associated with surgery are uncontrolled bleeding and residual trophoblastic tissue. Because of the bleeding, a salpingectomy is necessary for many tubal ectopic pregnancies. A laparotomy should only be indicated in the case of uncontrolled hemorrhage or hemodynamic instability. Historically, treatment focused on prevention of death, but with the ability to perform linear salpingostomy, emphasis is now on facilitating rapid recovery, preserving fertility, and reducing costs (Cunningham et al. 2001).

Follow-Up

Postoperatively, all Rh-negative unsensitized clients should be given Rh immunoglobulin. Discuss the normal body changes the client will experience. Instruct her concerning contraception, danger signals (e.g., signs of postsurgical infection or hemorrhage), and any further follow-up testing. The emotional needs of clients will vary. Pregnancy may not have been realized prior to diagnosis, and learning about the pregnancy and pregnancy loss in

such a short period can be overwhelming (Minnick-Smith & Cook, 1997). Pregnancy should be acknowledged and its meaning discussed. Explain to a client that having one ectopic pregnancy increases her chances for future ectopic pregnancies; however, the risk is less with the use of methotrexate. Review the signs and symptoms of repeated ectopic pregnancy with her. Advise her to practice contraception for at least two months to allow for adequate healing and tissue repair. In 20 percent of cases treated with methotrexate, residual tissue remains and causes hemorrhage and other complications. Weekly blood tests for β-hCG levels should be monitored until β-hCG becomes undetectable. The initial follow-up visit should include discussion of the need for follow-up blood testing, emotional responses to the ectopic pregnancy, risk factors, and need for contraception.

Prevention of ectopic pregnancies through screening and client education is essential. Preventing tubal damage from, for example, sexually transmitted disease, can decrease the incidence of the disorder. Encouraging the use of condoms can decrease the incidence of many infections responsible for tubal scarring. Early detection and prompt treatment of gonorrhea and chlamydia, when they do occur, can decrease morbidity.

Selection of an appropriate contraceptive method is important. Because IUD use may be associated with infections and tubal pregnancy, women need to be informed of the risk and effect of an IUD on future pregnancies.

GESTATIONAL TROPHOBLASTIC DISEASE

Gestational trophoblastic disease is a group of neoplastic disorders that originate in the human placenta. Gestational tissue is present but pregnancy is nonviable.

- *Hydatidiform mole.* The most common type of gestational trophoblastic disease, hydatidiform mole is a benign neoplasm of the chorion in which chorionic villi degenerate and become transparent vesicles containing clear, viscid fluid. Recently, two types of molar gestations have been distinguished: partial and complete. No fetus or amnion is found in the complete mole, but in the partial mole, a fetus or evidence of an amniotic sac is present.
- *Invasive mole* (chorioadenoma destruens). Invasive mole is a complete molar gestation that has invaded the myometrium, metastasized to other tissues, or both. Karyotyping reveals abnormal genetic material resulting from an empty egg or diploid sperm.

♦ *Choriocarcinoma*. This rare chorionic malignancy may follow any type of pregnancy, even years later. Half of choriocarcinomas occur following hydatidiform molar pregnancy.

Epidemiology

Etiology may be influenced by nutritional factors, such as protein deficiency. Such deficiencies would explain some of the race and geographical differences associated with gestational trophoblastic disease.

The incidence of molar pregnancy varies markedly around the world. Incidence in the Far East and Southeast Asia is five to fifteen times greater than that in Western industrialized nations. The true incidence of partial mole is unknown, because many are diagnosed as spontaneous abortions and tissue karyotyping is not done. Moles do recur in subsequent pregnancies. Age is also a factor; older women have a greater incidence of molar pregnancy.

Subjective Data

Presenting symptoms are similar to those of spontaneous abortion. The client usually reports signs of early pregnancy (amenorrhea, breast tenderness, morning sickness) and presents with vaginal bleeding around the twelfth week of gestation. Bleeding may begin as spotting, usually brownish rather than bright red. Some women experience severe nausea and vomiting and are treated for hyperemesis gravidarum. Fluid retention and swelling, similar to what is associated with gestational hypertension later in a pregnancy, may occur with molar pregnancy in the second trimester (Cunningham et al., 2001). Uterine cramping may or may not be present.

Objective Data

Physical examination may reveal what is sometimes a first sign of molar pregnancy: expulsion of grapelike vesicles with or without a history of vaginal bleeding. Vital signs are usually stable; no medical emergency exists. The abdomen is soft and nontender; in the vagina, bloody or clear vesicles may be present. The uterus is usually enlarged beyond the point of expected gestation and has a "doughy" consistency (Cunningham, et al., 2001). Ovaries may be enlarged and tender secondary to theca lutein cysts, which develop from ovarian hyperstimulation of high human chorionic gonadotropin levels. No fetal heart tones or fetal activity is detected.

The sonogram shows the absence of the gestational sac and characteristic multiple echogenic regions within the uterus (Cunningham et al., 2001).

Human chorionic gonadotropin levels are extremely high in molar pregnancies and continue to rise 100 days after the last menstrual period. No single value is diagnostic; therefore, serial values must be evaluated and compared with the normal pregnancy curve for β-hCG.

Differential Medical Diagnoses

Normal pregnancy, threatened abortion: error in dates, uterine myomas, polyhydramnios, multiple gestation.

Plan

Prompt identification of gestational trophoblastic disease and appropriate referral are essential to management.

Psychosocial Interventions. Explain the diagnostic procedures and follow-up blood work to the client. Explore the meaning of the client's pregnancy with her and her partner, a family member, or friend. Support them in their grieving. Accounting for religious beliefs and cultural practices is crucial in counseling women during treatment concerning the necessity of contraception. Reassurance about future pregnancies is appropriate, because prognosis is good even for women with invasive molar pregnancies (Berkowitz, Tuncer, Bernstein, & Goldstein, 2000).

Medication. If β-hCG levels either rise or plateau after evacuation, *chemotherapy* is indicated for potential metastatic disease. For women who wish to protect their fertility, single-agent therapy is used, usually methotrexate administered orally (Wong, Ngan, Cheng, & Ng, 2000).

Other Interventions. Evacuation of the uterus is necessary as soon as the diagnosis is made. *Dilatation and curettage* (suction curettage) is the safest, most effective method of emptying the uterus. Labor induction with prostaglandins or oxytocin is not recommended because these agents are inefficient in emptying the uterus of all trophoblastic tissue (Cunningham et al., 2001). Hospital admission is necessary for adequate anesthesia and nursing surveillance.

A *chest x-ray* is ordered to establish a base-line if there is any question later of invasive disease.

Serial monitoring of β-hCG levels is done weekly until normal for three weeks and then monthly for six months after the evacuation procedure. Levels of β-hCG are used to detect residual trophoblastic tissue. If any tissue remains, β-hCG levels will not regress. A rising β-hCG level could indicate the presence of a new gestation and must be investigated prior to any extensive diagnostic imagining or therapeutic intervention.

No further intervention is necessary if β-hCG levels decrease to normal, that is, become nondetectable. Pregnancy may be allowed after β-hCG levels remain normal for a minimum of one year (Cunningham et al., 2001; Lan, Hongzhao, Xiuyu, Yang, 2001). *Reliable contraception* must be used during this time because a positive pregnancy test cannot differentiate normal early pregnancy from beginning invasive disease. Reliable and safe contraceptives such as oral contraceptives, medroxyprogesterone acetate (Depo-provera), or barrier methods are desirable.

PLACENTA PREVIA

In placenta previa, the placenta becomes implanted in the lower segment of the uterus and obstructs the presenting part prior to or during labor. When the cervix begins to dilate, the placenta is pulled away from the endometrial wall and bleeding can occur. Any significant bleeding that leads to hemorrhage can endanger the mother and, if allowed to persist, can interfere with uteroplacental sufficiency.

The three types of previa (total, incomplete, and marginal) are classified by the amount of cervix involved.

◆ In *total or complete previa,* the entire internal os is covered with placenta.

◆ In *incomplete (or partial) previa,* the internal os is only partially covered by the placenta.

◆ In *marginal or low lying previa,* the edge of the placenta is at the cervical os but does not obstruct any part of it.

The amount of cervical dilation can affect the classification system. Other systems are based on the amount of placental encroachment over the os at the point of full dilation.

Epidemiology

The etiology of placenta previa is unknown, but certain women are at greater risk than others. Parity is the most common risk factor; old fundal implantation sites are scarred and not suitable for implantation. Other uterine surgical scars, such as those from cesarean birth or myomectomy, increase the chance of placental malimplantation (McMahon, Li, Schenck, et al., 1997). Advanced maternal age, maternal smoking, and a history of induced or spontaneous abortion have also been reported

to be risk factors for placenta previa (McMahon, Li, Schenk, Olsham, & Royce, 1997). Maternal complications such as hysterectomy, intrapartum and postpartum hemorrhage, septicemia, and thrombophlebitis have been noted in the women diagnosed with placenta previa (Crane, Van den Hof, Dodds, et al., 2000)

Incidence seems to vary with gestation, although the condition is reported in 1 of every 200 pregnancies. Better diagnostic techniques have revealed gestational differences. For example, in the second trimester, placenta previa is a prevalent finding on sonogram, but as pregnancy progresses the incidence falls. In the third trimester, the lower uterine segment stretches and develops, making the placenta seem to migrate away from the internal os, and the previa resolves.

Subjective Data

The characteristic symptom of placenta previa is painless bleeding during the third trimester of pregnancy. Bleeding may occur as early as 20 weeks of gestation and without any precipitating event. Previa should be suspected in any bleeding that occurs after 24 weeks of gestation. Blood is usually bright red. A woman may experience symptoms of shock, such as syncope. The first bleed, however, is usually not a significant amount.

Objective Data

Vital signs are stable; fetal heart tones are normal, and fetal activity is present. The uterus is non-tender with a normal resting tone. Bright red blood is evident on sanitary napkins.

Diagnosis is best made by sonogram. No pelvic exam is done to avoid dislodging any clot that may have formed at the cervix. Historically, a sterile vaginal exam was done in a surgical suite to determine the diagnosis; if catastrophic bleeding occurred during the procedure, an emergency cesarean was performed. Now, however, with noninvasive accurate sonograms, such examination is rarely necessary or recommended (Cunningham et al., 2001).

Differential Medical Diagnoses

Abruptio placentae, genital lacerations, excessive show, cervical lesions and/or severe cervicitis, nonvaginal bleeding (urinary or rectal), ectopic pregnancy (Rees & Paradinas, 2001).

Plan

The role of the primary care provider lies primarily in the early detection of placenta previa. Referral for appropriate intervention is necessary.

Medication. Not indicated.

Management. The medical plan depends on the extent of hemorrhage and length of gestation. If gestation is less than 36 weeks, an attempt is made to stabilize the mother, administer transfusions as needed, and maintain the pregnancy. Strict hospital bed rest is employed, and the mother and fetus are closely monitored. If bleeding stops and the hematocrit is greater than 30 percent, then gradual ambulation may be allowed. Some women may be allowed to return home with limited activity until further problems arise or labor begins.

Provide the client with clear instructions about pelvic rest and what to do if signs of impending labor or bleeding begins.

During the "wait-and-see" period, amniocentesis may be done weekly after 36 weeks to document fetal maturity. In addition, serial sonograms are done to determine placement of the placenta and to note any migration. Later in the pregnancy, placental problems can lead to uteroplacental insufficiency and intrauterine growth retardation.

Sonography. Serial sonograms are also used to monitor fetal growth. If bleeding continues or recurs, then operative delivery may be forced.

Delivery. The amount of bleeding, general fetal condition, fetal presentation and gestation will affect delivery decisions. Once fetal maturity is accomplished, delivery is planned. When gestation is less than 36 weeks and previa is coexisting with preterm labor, some clinicians are successfully using an expectant approach using tocolysis. This practice needs further study before it becomes a standard recommendation for management (Towers, Pircon, & Heppard, 1999). The extent to which the os is covered by the placenta determines if vaginal delivery is considered. Cesarean delivery is usually recommended (Cunningham et al., 2001).

Postpartum Follow-Up. It is the same as for other postpartum women. The amount of blood loss is associated with perinatal outcome, even though the number of bleeding episodes does not increase perinatal mortality or morbidity. A mother usually recovers readily from anemia and fluid loss. During the first month of life, the infant is at increased risk for death, compared with infants of the same gestational age and birth weight. The increased risk is probably related to transient episodes of fetal hypoxia.

ABRUPTIO PLACENTAE

Abruptio placentae is the partial or complete detachment of a normally implanted placenta at any time prior to delivery. Detachment occurs more frequently during the third trimester, but may occur anytime after 20 weeks of gestation. The proposed mechanism is that maternal arterioles become thrombosed and lead to degeneration of decidua and, subsequently, to rupture of one vessel. The resultant bleeding forms a retroplacental clot, which increases pressure behind the placenta and adds to the separation process.

The classification of abruptio placentae is based on the signs and symptoms of abruption in combination with selected laboratory findings.

Epidemiology

The etiology of abruptio placentae is unknown. Maternal smoking, poor maternal nutrition, chorioamnionitis, and use of cocaine are risk factors for premature separation. Until recently, maternal age and multiparity have also been associated with increased incidence of abruption, but recent reports fail to show that relationship. There are reports that multiple gestation is also associated with abruption (Ananth, Smulian, Demissie, et al., 2001). Conditions with underlying vascular involvement, particularly hypertension, can predispose a woman to abruption. (Witlin, Saade, Mattar, & Sibai, 1999). Severe trauma, such as an automobile accident or injury secondary to domestic violence, has also been associated with abruption. (Pearlman, Klinich, Schneider, et al., 2000). The incidence of battering of women has grown and the incidence of battering during pregnancy is reported to be higher than other times, even though there is no evidence to support this observation (Ballard, Saltzman, Gazmararian, et al., 1998; Moore, 1999).

The true incidence is unknown because abruption occurs in varying degrees. Incidence is reported to be 1:120 births per year (Witlin, Saade, Mattar, & Sibai, 1999).

Subjective Data

Symptoms of abruptio placentae can vary significantly depending on the extent and location of separation. The client may report labor pains with some continual cramping. With more severe abruption, severe, sudden, knife-like pain may be described. The client may experience no bleeding, a small amount of dark old blood, or profuse bleeding. Depending on the amount of blood lost from the systemic circulation, she may experience symptoms of shock, such as syncope.

Objective Data

Physical Examination. May reveal vaginal bleeding (dark old blood or bright red blood), uterine tenderness (local or generalized), increased uterine tone, occasional board-like quality with little or no relaxation between contractions, lack of fetal heart tones, or signs of fetal distress (such as tachycardia, loss of beat-to-beat variability, or late decelerations). No vaginal or rectal exam is done until placenta previa is eliminated as a diagnosis. (Witlin, Saade, Mattar & Sibai, 1999).

Sonogram. Frequently used to locate a retroplacental clot. A clot may not be seen on the sonogram in an early abruption, but if symptoms are severe, time is critical and diagnosis must be made on presumptive signs.

Differential Medical Diagnoses

Placenta previa, placenta accreta, hematoma of rectus muscle, ovarian cysts, appendicitis, degeneration of fibroids.

Plan

Immediate identification of possibility or suspicion of abruptio placentae dictates prompt referral for appropriate stabilization and treatment.

Psychosocial Interventions. Allay the anxiety of the woman and her family. They need to be informed about impending diagnostic tests, possible hospitalization, and surgery.

Management. Maintain respiratory and cardiovascular support (intravenous fluid, oxygen), as needed, until the client is transported to the hospital. Because of the potential for hemorrhage, development of a coagulopathy disorder is a risk. Hemorrhage, which if not corrected by delivery of the fetus and the placenta, will lead to depletion of the clotting factors and can be life-threatening (Cunningham et al., 2001). Hemorrhage may occur into the postpartum period.

Delivery. Delivery is necessary if severe symptoms are present and condition is life-threatening for the mother or fetus. Whether the fetus is to be delivered by cesarean or vaginal birth will depend on the assessment of the mother and the fetus. If the mother's condition is stable, but the fetus is not viable, cesarean birth is not indicated. Cesarean delivery is indicated when there are signs of fetal distress, maternal hemorrhage, maternal coagulopathy, or poor progress of labor. Fetal well-being is assessed by electronic fetal monitoring. If both mother and fetus are stable, assessment for fetal maturity is done to assist in decisions of the timing of delivery.

Follow-Up

After delivery, care for women with abruptio placentae is the same as that for other postpartum women. It may be necessary to deal with pregnancy loss or in some cases, when the infant survives, maternal grieving may occur over loss of a "normal" pregnancy or delivery. Infants may need care in a newborn intensive care unit, which adds to family stress.

ANEMIAS

Anemia is the reduction of hemoglobin to below normal quantity (Dixon, 1997). In a normal pregnancy, concentrations of erythrocytes and hemoglobin fall because of a disproportional increase in the ratio of plasma volume to erythrocyte volume (physiological anemia of pregnancy). During pregnancy, plasma volume increases as much as 45 to 50 percent, but erythrocyte volume increases only 25 percent. Many women have borderline hemoglobin levels before pregnancy; therefore, they do not have the reserve necessary to support physiological changes. Hemoglobin concentration decreases after eight weeks, drops to its lowest level at midpregnancy, and rises slightly or stabilizes near term. Hemoglobin and hematocrit values are expected to return to prepregnancy level by six weeks postdelivery unless there was severe blood loss during the intrapartal or postpartal period. Anemia is not a disease, but a symptom of an underlying condition.

IRON DEFICIENCY ANEMIA

In iron deficiency anemia, the hematocrit is less than 32 percent. The hemoglobin concentration is less than 11 g/dL in the first and second trimester or less than 10.5 g/dL in the third trimester (Cunningham et al., 2001). Many providers initiate treatment with a hematocrit of 34 percent.

Epidemiology

The cause of iron deficiency anemia is an inadequate iron supply, usually secondary to poor dietary intake. Teenagers and women of low socioeconomic status are at greatest risk because of the likelihood of inadequate or improperly balanced diets (Cunningham et al., 2001). Women with short intervals between pregnancies or who have histories of prolonged heavy menses are also at risk.

The incidence of iron deficiency anemia is highest among pregnant women. Approximately 30 to 50 percent of all women are anemic in pregnancy.

Subjective Data

A woman may experience some fatigue or lassitude that may affect her ability to perform activities of daily living. In the second and third trimesters of pregnancy, she may notice shortness of breath on exertion.

Objective Data

All prenatal clients should be screened in the first trimester for anemia. Physical examination of a pregnant woman may suggest iron deficiency anemia; blood tests confirm it.

Physical examination may reveal pale conjunctiva and mucous membranes. Grade II systolic heart murmur may also be detected. Fetal iron stores are protected at the expense of maternal stores (Cunningham et al., 2001). Consequently, fetal effects are not noted unless the maternal hemoglobin level is below 7 g/dL.

Diagnostic tests show decreased serum iron levels; the number of reticulocytes is low. A complete blood count (CBC) with indices is done showing mature red cells as microcytic and hypochromic. The mean corpuscular volume (MCV = 80–95 u^3) will be decreased; the mean corpuscular hemoglobin (MCH = 27–31 pg) will be decreased; the mean corpuscular hemoglobin concentration (MCHC = 32–36 percent) will be decreased; and the reticulocyte count (0.5–3.1 percent) will be either normal or low. Two very sensitive and reliable laboratory tests for diagnosis of iron deficiency are serum ferritin (concentration of less than 12 mcg/L) and free erythrocyte protoporphyrin (FEP).

Differential Medical Diagnoses

Folate deficiency, thalassemia, sickle cell disease, aplastic anemia, HELLP syndrome.

Plan

Psychosocial Interventions. Inform the client of her need to eat a well balanced diet, emphasizing foods that are high in iron. Explain how iron-rich foods are important for her health during and after pregnancy.

Medication. Supplemental iron is administered. Whether it should be given to all pregnant women is controversial. The recommended daily dose of elemental iron for U.S. nonpregnant women is 60 mg. Most prenatal vitamins contain that amount of iron. Women with a hematocrit level of less than 32 percent should be treated for iron deficiency anemia.

The recommended dosage when deficiency is diagnosed is 180 to 200 mg of elemental iron per day in separated doses; this amount is equivalent to the iron contained in two or three 300 mg tablets of ferrous sulfate. Total iron supplementation per day should include iron contained in prenatal vitamin and not exceed the 200 mg of elemental iron daily. For women who cannot tolerate oral iron therapy, parenteral administration may be necessary (Bayonumeu, Subiran-Buisset, Baka, et al., 2002).

A side effect of iron supplementation is gastrointestinal disturbance. To enhance its absorption, iron should be taken thirty minutes prior to a meal, preferably with a source of vitamin C. Taking iron with milk, tea, or antacids should be avoided. This timing, however, may lead to gastrointestinal effects, disturbances that can be decreased by taking the iron after meals. For pregnant women, taking iron following meals is less problematic because dietary iron absorption is much more efficient during pregnancy. Instruct the client to drink extra fluids (not tea) to offset problems with constipation. Some clients may not be able to tolerate the maximum daily dose. To maximize the woman's compliance, individualize administration and dosage. Spacing the doses throughout the day may also help absorption because only so much can be absorbed at one time.

Follow-Up

Schedule a repeat reticulocyte count in about two weeks. The count should rise significantly. All anemic women should be closely monitored for infection and signs of intrauterine growth retardation. Following delivery, these women should remain on iron therapy and be monitored for recovery at least 3 months. Routine postpartum hemoglobin testing to assess for anemia is not recommended unless indicated because of excessive blood loss during delivery (Swaim, Perriatt, Andres, et al., 1999). More than two years may be needed to replenish iron stores from dietary sources. It has been reported that intervals between pregnancy of less than six months are associated with increased risk of poor maternal outcomes. One of the factors contributing to these outcomes is the lack of time for the body to recover from blood loss and physiologic anemia associated with pregnancy and delivery (Conde-Agudelo & Belizan, 2000). Counseling women about this period is important if other pregnancies are planned.

FOLIC ACID DEFICIENCY

Folic acid is a B-complex vitamin essential for cell growth and division. It promotes the maturation of red blood cells. Folic acid is stored in the liver for four to six weeks. Consequently, overt deficiency does not manifest until late in pregnancy or during the postpartum. Maternal folic acid deficiency in the first eight weeks of gestation is associated with neural tube defects (Botto, Moore, Khoury, & Erickson, 1999).

Epidemiology

Folic acid deficiency is due to an inadequate iron supply usually secondary to poor dietary intake of folic acid. It is the most common cause of megaloblastic anemia (Cunningham et al., 2001).

Teenagers and women of low socioeconomic status are at greatest risk for folic acid deficiency because of the likelihood of inadequate or improperly balanced dietary intake. Green vegetables, peanuts, and animal proteins, especially liver and red meats, are good sources of folic acid. Also at risk are women with hemoglobinopathies or those with a multiple pregnancy or pregnancies with a short interval between. Women taking hydantoin or ingesting ethanol are also at risk.

Folic acid deficiency in the United States is usually diet related. It is not unusual for folic acid deficiency to coexist with iron deficiency anemia.

Subjective Data

A client with folic acid deficiency may experience symptoms, including nausea, vomiting, and anorexia during pregnancy, and possibly experience symptoms of iron deficiency if it coexists.

Objective Data

Physical examination may reveal pale conjunctiva and mucous membranes, as well as a grade II systolic heart murmur. Signs of folic acid deficiency cannot be distinguished from those of iron deficiency anemia, as the two conditions are usually concurrent.

Diagnostic tests include determination of serum folate and RBC folate levels. Levels normally fall during pregnancy; however, a fasting folate level of less than 3 ng/mL in an anemic woman is a presumptive sign for diagnosis. Hypersegmented neutrophilic leukocytes and macrocytic red cells on peripheral smear are diagnostic, but definitive diagnosis is made by bone marrow examination. This should seldom be necessary. The reticulocyte count will be depressed in the folic acid deficient client, but reticulocytosis usually occurs within three days after administration of a folic acid supplementation.

Differential Medical Diagnoses

Iron deficiency anemia, thalassemia, sickle cell anemia.

Plan

Prevention. For those women who have no history of neural tube defects (NTD), consumption of folate 0.4 mg/day is recommended (Swain & St. Clair, 1997; Tinkle, 1997; Tinkle & Sterling, 1997). As of 1996, food sources such as breads and cereals are now being fortified with folic acid (Honein, Paulozzi, Mathews, et al., 2001; Mills & England, 2001; Tinkle, 1997). With the aggressive public education by public health officials and the March of Dimes and food fortification, there has been a 19 percent reduction in neural tube defects reported in the United States (CDC, 1998; Honein, Paulozzi, Mathews, Erickson, & Wong, 2001; Mills & England, 2001).

Psychosocial Interventions. Provide the client with information about foods that are high in folic acid. Explain to the client the importance of eating healthful foods every day to benefit herself and her fetus.

Treatment in Pregnancy. Prophylactic medication, a prenatal vitamin that contains 0.5 to 1.0 mg of folate, is given to most pregnant women. Prenatal vitamins that require a prescription usually contain 1 mg of folic acid. A full 1.0 mg per day is needed, if there is a deficiency. Women with significant hemoglobinopathies, on anticonvulsants such as Phenytoin, or have multiple gestation are advised to supplement with 1.0 mg daily of folic acid. Women who have had a previous infant affected by neural tube defect should be advised to supplement their diet with daily folate 4 mg/day two to three months prior to pregnancy. These women should continue folate 4 mg/day during pregnancy (Swain & St. Clair, 1997).

Follow-Up

The measures used for clients with folic acid deficiency are the same as those for women with iron deficiency anemia. The appropriate screening for iron deficiency should be performed and iron supplementation initiated when indicated.

THALASSEMIA

Thalassemia is an autosomal recessive genetic disorder that causes a reduction in or the absence of the alpha or beta globin chain in hemoglobin. Symptoms will depend upon the number and location of the missing proteins on the gene (ACOG Technical Bulletin, 1996). Either α- or β-thalassemia can occur.

Homozygous α-thalassemia or α-thalassemia major diagnosed women have short life expectancies and need expert obstetrical management. Women with α-thalassemia have signs and symptoms of hemolytic anemia, namely, hemosiderosis, a condition characterized by deposition in organs of the iron containing pigment hemosiderin, which is derived from hemoglobin degeneration. Symptoms may include chills, fever, hypotension, tachycardia, anxiety, nausea, vomiting, renal failure, and shock. Hydrops fetalis and stillbirth are associated with this condition (ACOG Technical Bulletin, 1996).

Heterozygous α-thalassemia carrier. Normal outcome is expected for mother and infant. Iron supplementation is given for documented iron deficiency anemia. If Asian, the partner should be screened for hemoglobinopathies due to the possibility of fetus being homozygous for α-thalassemia.

Heterozygous β-thalassemia minor (β-thalassemia carrier). Normal outcome is expected for mother and infant; is sometimes first identified in pregnancy. Women with the disorder are at risk for iron deficiency anemia and pregnancy-induced hypertension. Folic acid and iron supplementation are necessary, only if indicated. Parenteral iron is contraindicated because of the possibility of exogenous hemosiderosis. This disorder is more common in the African American, Italian, and Asian populations. Some forms can produce a child with major disease; therefore, partner should be screened for any hemoglobinopathies.

β-*Thalassemia major (Cooley's anemia)*, which is homozygous β, is rare and can be a life-threatening condition. Previously, these affected young women were not expected to survive into the childbearing years. Other countries are now reporting programs that have been following these young men and women into adulthood and report normal vocational, social, sexual, and reproductive goals. The impact of the disorder on pregnancies occurring in these groups is unknown (Psihogios, Rodda, Reid, et al., 2002).

Management

Asymptomatic thalassemia carriers do not require any special testing but should receive serial ultrasounds to monitor fetal growth. Nonstress testing is also suggested to evaluate fetal well-being. A good outcome is expected for both mother and infant. Administration of oral iron supplementation is controversial because hemosiderosis is possible (Cunningham et al., 2001). Parenteral administration is contraindicated. Further discussion is beyond the scope of this chapter; however, medical referral and genetic counseling is necessary.

SICKLE CELL ANEMIA

Sickle cell anemia is an autosomal recessive inherited disease that results from abnormal hemoglobin (hemoglobin SS) synthesis. Persons with sickle cell trait, on the other hand, are heterozygous (AS) for hemoglobin and may go undiagnosed because of the lack of symptoms. *Sickle cell trait (AS)*, however, may be identified with routine prenatal screening. *Hemoglobin C (Hemoglobin SC disease)* is another variant in hemoglobin formation and in women who are heterozygous for both the S and C genes have hemoglobin SC disease. All women in high risk groups should be screened during the initial prenatal visit.

In sickle cell trait, anemia and crisis states do not usually occur except in extreme cases. There is no increased risk for the fetus.

Hemoglobin C is a common disorder and occurs in women of African descent. Unless it occurs in combination with other hemoglobin variants, there are no adverse effects including anemia during pregnancy (ACOG Technical Bulletin, 1996).

Epidemiology

Sickle cell disease (sickle cell anemia) involves periods of hypoxia that lead to destruction of red blood cells, hemolytic anemia, and occlusion of blood vessels by abnormally shaped cells. Pregnancy can predispose to periods of hypoxia and trigger a crisis state. Infections, such as pyelonephritis, pneumonia, and osteomyelitis, occur more frequently among pregnant women with sickle cell disease. Other adverse effects that the disease has on pregnancy include an increased incidence of abortion, preterm labor, intrauterine growth retardation, and stillbirth (Koshy, 1999). Sickle cell disease is found almost exclusively in African Americans, but also among Greeks, Italians, Middle Easterners, and Asian Indians. Infants with sickle cell anemia will not show any signs of disease until the fetal hemoglobin has fallen to adult levels. In fact, some affected children do not demonstrate signs until adolescence.

Women with hemoglobin SC disease have less perinatal mortality than women with sickle cell anemia; there is an increased incidence of early spontaneous abortion and pregnancy induced hypertension (Koshy, 1999).

Sickle cell anemia is inherited as an autosomal recessive disorder. The disease occurs in 1 in 700 adult African Americans. The sickle cell trait is carried by 1 in 12 African Americans. Clinically significant hemoglobin SC disease occurs in 1 in 833 adult blacks in the United States (Koshy, 1999). The trait for hemoglobin SC occurs in 1 in 40 adult blacks (Koshy, 1999). One in every 625 black children born in the United States is homozygous for hemoglobin S.

Subjective Data

Women with sickle cell trait are usually asymptomatic.

The client with sickle cell anemia reports multifocal pain, dyspnea, malaise, neurological symptoms, and gastrointestinal upset.

The crisis state is characterized by pain, dyspnea, and malaise. Pain can be multifocal, occurring in the extremities, chest, abdomen, or back. It frequently occurs in bones and joints. Neurological symptoms include headache, visual changes, and seizures. Liver and spleen involvement results in gastrointestinal symptoms, including nausea and vomiting or severe abdominal cramping.

Women with hemoglobin SC disease have only mild symptoms and frequently are undiagnosed until they experience more pronounced symptoms in pregnancy.

Objective Data

Physical examination of the mother in sickle cell crisis reveals symptoms in several systems.

- Skin is pale and possibly jaundiced.
- Visual acuity and peripheral vision may decrease.
- Signs of distress are apparent. The client experiences shortness of breath and possibly signs of pulmonary embolus or pneumonia.
- Abdomen may be distended with hepatomegaly and palpable spleen. Fundal height may be equal to or less than expected, depending on the client's general health prior to the episode.
- Kidneys are unable to concentrate urine and signs of kidney failure may be evident.
- Fetal heart tones, if present, may be elevated or lack variability.

With hemoglobin SC disease, a dramatic fall in hematocrit occurs in a crisis secondary to a marked sequestration of a large volume of RBCs in the spleen. During pregnancy these women may have a mild thrombocytopenia associated with increased splenic activity (Telen, 2001).

A blood hemoglobin electrophoresis is done to determine the hemoglobin type. Electrophoresis confirms hemoglobin SS, AS or SC. During their initial prenatal visit, all African American women, women of Greek, Italian, Middle Eastern, or Asian Indian ancestry should be screened or have documentation of S and C hemoglobin. (ACOG Technical Bulletin, 1996; Chasen, Loeb-Zeitlin, & Landsberger, 1999; Yost, 2001)

Differential Medical Diagnoses

Malabsorption syndromes, alcoholic cirrhosis, hookworm infestation.

Plan

Psychosocial Interventions. Involve the client's family in every aspect of care. Provide information and clarification about the disease and its implication for pregnancy, delivery, and the fetus. The provider must be sensitive to the woman's possible fear of dying or fear of losing her infant. A crisis is painful and may be life-threatening.

Education. Make the client with sickle cell anemia aware of the need to recognize symptoms of crisis or complication as soon as possible. Immediate attention can defer the effect on the fetus and frequently decrease the intensity of symptoms. Instruct the client to seek care at the first sign of a crisis. Teach the client the danger signs of pregnancy-induced hypertension and signs and symptoms of infection. Early treatment of common infections, particularly vaginitis and cystitis, may decrease the incidence of more advanced infections, such as pyelonephritis and osteomyelitis. Information to women is provided by several organizations such as the Sickle Cell Disease Association, *http://sicklecelldisease.org,* the Sickle Cell Information Center *www.emory.edu/PEDS/SICKLE,* and many local coalitions (Day & Wynn, 2000; Mitchell, 1999).

Genetic Referral. The partner of the woman with sickle cell anemia, sickle cell trait, or hemoglobin SC should be tested and, if both are affected and/or carriers, prenatal diagnosis of the fetus should be offered. Hemoglobin S can be identified through hemoglobin electrophoresis and DNA analysis of fetal blood.

Preconception Counseling. Ideally, those women affected by hemoglobinopathies are screened and are aware—prior to conception—of the risks of sickle cell anemia and hemoglobin SC disease to themselves and to a pregnancy. Determining both her own and the partner's status can assist the couple in making appropriate reproductive decisions for them.

Medication. There is no specific medication for sickle cell disease or the crisis state. Antibiotics are used for infection. Analgesics are used for pain during a crisis. Iron therapy should be initiated only if anemia is present. Some authorities are concerned about iron overload; therefore, iron supplementation is not given unless indicated by serum iron and ferritin levels. Folate supplementation with good dietary habits and folic acid 1 mg/daily is recommended throughout the pregnancy.

Other Interventions. *Prophylactic transfusions* have been used throughout pregnancy with some success, but the practice is controversial (Koshy, 1999).

Blood samples are taken throughout pregnancy to closely monitor cardiac, renal, and liver function. This procedure is especially critical during and after crises.

A urine culture and sensitivity should be performed at least once each trimester for women with sickle cell trait. Sickling can occur in the renal medulla, leading to reduced oxygen, necrosis of kidney tissue, and renal tubular dysfunction (Koshy, 1999). These factors predispose to an increased risk for bacteriuria, which, if undiagnosed, can progress to pyelonephritis.

An early sonogram is recommended to confirm dates; serial sonograms to assess fetal growth. Starting at 30 weeks, sonograms should be done weekly or biweekly to assess fetal well-being and amniotic fluid volume.

Sickle cell crisis requires hospitalization, enabling administration of transfusions, oxygen, intravenous therapy for hydration, and sedation and analgesia.

Delivery. Depends on the condition of both mother and fetus in relation to gestation and the risks and benefits that are presented. After 36 weeks, delivery should be initiated as soon as fetal lung maturity is documented. Vaginal delivery is preferred, if possible, and general anesthesia should be avoided because of the risk of hypoxia. During labor, fluid overload must be avoided and the woman should remain in the left lateral recumbent position as much that can be tolerated. Oxygen therapy may be necessary.

Follow-Up

After delivery, recommend genetic counseling to assist the client and her family to plan future pregnancies (Koshy, 1999). The newborn is screened within the first few days of life. The woman is observed closely for postpartum hemorrhage.

Women with hemoglobin SC disease need the same program of prenatal care as outlined above for the woman with sickle cell anemia. Several contraceptive methods—including oral contraceptives, barrier methods, and tubal ligation—are safe and acceptable options for women of childbearing age with sickle cell disease (Koshy, 1999). Depo-Provera (medroxyprogesterone) has been shown to be another acceptable alternative, and has been associated with reduced anemia and incidence of painful crisis (ACOG Practice Bulletin, 2000).

HYPEREMESIS GRAVIDARUM

Hyperemesis gravidarum is the persistant vomiting of pregnancy differentiated from the common nausea and vomiting of pregnancy by weight loss of more than 5 percent of the prepregnant weight, dehydration, and electrolyte imbalance (Miller, 2002). There is debate if this condition represents a disease or just an accelerated function of a normal process. The occurrence of hyperemesis usually peaks around the fourth or fifth week of pregnancy, continues until the twelfth week, and then dissipates.

Epidemiology

It is reported that between 50 and 80 percent of all pregnant women experience the nausea of pregnancy and of that group 1 to 2 percent develop hyperemesis. The occurrence of hyperemesis interferes with the woman's normal lifestyle and is reported to be uncomfortable and annoying. Women report loss of efficiency at work, requirements for time off, negative effect on the relationship with their partner, and some reported feelings of depression (Attard, Kohli, Coleman, et al., 2002; Miller, 2002). Because of these negative consequences of the symptoms, the financial burden on society is estimated at $130,000 million per year in the United States.

The cause of nausea and vomiting in pregnancy is unknown, but more than likely, it is associated with the rise in human gonadotropin and/or estrogens associated with early pregnancy. The significant rise in human gonadotropin being produced by the placenta correlates with the occurrence of hyperemesis (Furneaux, Langley-Evans, & Langley-Evans, 2001). The occurrence of hyperemesis is theorized to be related to the pregnant woman's response to these triggers based upon her underlying vestibular, gastrointestinal, olfactory, and emotional status (Black, 2002; Buckwalter & Simpson, 2002; Goodwin, 2002; Heinrichs, 2002; Koch, 2002). Historically, much discussion described the deep-rooted distress of pregnancy, which was being transformed into physical symptoms. There is no scientific evidence to support these discussions, but a woman's stress level and personal situation may contribute to her ability to cope and deal with this condition (Buckwalter & Simpson, 2002).

Subjective Data

The woman reports severe nausea and episodes of uncontrolled vomiting and retching.

Objective Data

There is no diagnostic test available to determine hyperemesis. There have been some efforts to develop a reliable assessment tool to determine the severity of the symptoms in order to assist in clinical management. The Motherisk—PUQE (pregnancy-unique quantification of emesis and nausea) has been investigated in Canada but no acceptable tools are used in the United States (Koren, Boskovic, Hard, et al., 2002).

The enigma of this disorder is that these women have normal upper endoscopy exams and normal computed tomographic exams of the abdomen (Koch, 2002). The uterine, breast, and skin changes are all within normal limits of pregnancy. Electrolytes will indicate dehydration if the vomiting persists beyond 24 hours.

Differential Medical Diagnosis

Gastroenteritis, gastroesophageal reflux disease, cholecystitis, pancreatitis, gastric and duodenal peptic disease, irritable bowel disease, hepatitis, pyelonephritis, and appendicitis.

Plan

There is some positive evidence that women who take a multivitamin that includes vitamin B_6 and B-complex prior to pregnancy is afforded protection from experiencing hyperemesis (Black, 2002). There are no prospective, double-blind comparative studies done on the treatment of hyperemesis. Treatment approaches are based upon empirical knowledge and practices.

The provider must be sure to eliminate the other serious possibly life-threatening gastrointestinal disorders before proceeding with what is a conservative approach to managing this disorder.

In 1983, Bendectin (doxylamine-vitamin B_6 combination) was the only drug approved for the treatment of nausea and vomiting in pregnancy. In response to litigation that Bendectin causes birth defects, it was removed from the market by the manufacturer. A comparable drug is available in Canada and has been used without increase risks of teratogens (Niebyl & Goodwin, 2002). Some providers instruct women experiencing nausea and vomiting to use a combination of an over-the-counter sleep aid (doxylamine) and vitamin B_6 (Niebyl & Goodwin, 2002) Other antiemetics such as Promethazine are used to control vomiting (Koren & Levichek, 2002).

Dietary counseling is usually added to any medication therapy. The diet can consist of liquids that contain salt, glucose, and potassium such as sports drinks and bouillon. The woman must be able to consume a minimum of 1.0 to 1.5 liters of fluid in order to prevent dehydration. If liquids are not tolerated, intravenous therapy is warranted. In some areas, the woman may be able to obtain intravenous therapy in an office setting, ambulatory care, or emergency room. Hospitalization is avoided if possible. Once the woman is tolerating liquids, the diet is advanced to brothy soups with noodles or rice. If tolerated, solid starches such as potatoes or pasta are added. Chicken or fish are preferred protein sources. Fatty foods such as creamed soups are avoided because they will delay gastric emptying (Koch, 2002).

Other alternative therapies such as acupuncture, acupressure wrists bands, biofeedback, and hypnosis have been used by women with some success (Buckwalter & Simpson, 2002; Smith, Crowther, & Beilby, 2002; Steele, French, Gatherer-Boyles, et al., 2001).

GESTATIONAL HYPERTENSION

Gestational hypertension is characterized by hypertension with proteinuria after 20 weeks of gestation and a return of the blood pressure to normal postpartum. Previously, gestational hypertension was known as pregnancy-induced hypertension or toxemia of pregnancy. Gestational hypertension is characterized by a blood pressure of 140/90 or greater, either systolic, diastolic or both, on two occasions at least six hours apart.

Eclampsia refers to a convulsive state. Previously, if the blood pressure rose 30 mmHg systolic or more than

15 mmHg diastolic above the woman's baseline, she was considered preeclamptic. This definition has not shown to be a reliable predictor of outcome. The National High Blood Pressure Education Program Working Group, which has recommended standard language and management of high blood pressure, no longer use this variation as a criterion but warns that women experiencing these changes warrant close observation (ACOG Practice Bulletin, 2002). To be diagnosed with severe preeclampsia, a woman must demonstrate the elevated blood pressure and proteinuria as defined as urinary excretion of 0.3 g protein or higher in a 24-hour urine specimen.

In severe preeclampsia, the blood pressure is higher than 160/110 on two occasions at least six hours apart. Proteinuria is greater than 500 mg in 24-hour urine collection, and oliguria (less than 500 mL in 24 hours) is detected. Severe preeclampsia is diagnosed if pulmonary edema or thrombocytopenia with or without liver damage is present. Cerebral or visual disturbances, epigastric or right upper-quadrant pain, or fetal growth retardation may also be noted.

Chronic hypertension in pregnancy is defined as elevation in blood pressure prior to the twentieth week of gestation or hypertension before the current pregnancy. Mild hypertension is described as 140 mmHg systolic or above or 90 mmHg diastolic or above. Severe chronic hypertension would be described as a blood pressure above 180/110 mmHg (ACOG Practice Bulletin, 2001)

Endothelial Damage. The true cause of gestational hypertension continues to allude researchers. Much has been learned regarding the physiological changes. The latest theory focuses on the activation of the coagulation system and subsequent endothelial injury. Subsequent to an immunological disturbance triggered by abnormal placental implantation, substances are released that activate or injure endothelial cells. The effect of endothelial injury explains the multiorgan system involvement. Endothelial damage leads to subsequent platelet adherence, fibrin deposition, and the presence of schistocytes. The fluid shift from intravascular to intracellular spaces causes generalized edema. Hemoconcentration occurs because of the decreased blood volume in the intravascular space. Decreased blood flow to the liver leads to microembolization, ischemia, possible infarct, and tissue damage. Subcapsular hemorrhage may occur.

Thromboxane/Prostacyclin Imbalance. One explanation describes hypertension developing secondary to an imbalance in placental prostacyclin and thromboxane production. Prostacyclin is a potent vasodilator and inhibitor of platelet aggregation. A deficiency during pregnancy contributes to the occurrence of preeclampsia. Thromboxane, on the other hand, is a potent vasoconstrictor and stimulates platelet aggregation.

In normal pregnancy, thromboxane is increased: Maternal plasma levels are higher late in pregnancy than in midpregnancy. In normal pregnancy, prostacyclin and thromboxane levels are equal, but in a preeclamptic woman, the placenta produces seven times more thromboxane than prostacyclin. Vasoconstriction, platelet aggregation, and reduced uteroplacental blood flow result. This observation may explain some of the hematologic changes associated with gestational hypertension but does not identify the primary etiology of the disease.

Vasospasm. The disease is characterized by generalized vasospasm and a constant degree of tension in the vascular system. As a result, blood pressure rises and blood flow to target organs is reduced, giving rise to the various signs and symptoms of gestational hypertension. (Riskin-Mashiah, Belfort, Saade, & Herd, 2001). In addition to the vascular system, the organs most affected are the brain, liver, kidneys, placenta, and lungs. Decreased blood flow to the brain leads to fluid shift, cerebral edema, and changes in sensorium. Cerebral edema also leads to central nervous system irritability, which can predispose to convulsions. These effects are of particular interest in the placenta. The severity of the hypertension may be associated with the degree of involvement of the trophoblasts. Women with clinically observed severe gestational hypertension have an increased rate of vascular lesions of the placenta (Many, Schreiber, Rosner, et al., 2001). Other genetic variances in normal placental function may also contribute to the severity of the condition (Gratacos, Casals, Gomez, et al., 2000; Knerr, Beinder, & Rascher, 2002).

Kidneys. Decreased blood flow to the kidneys normally initiates production of renin and angiotensin I, which is converted to angiotensin II, the pressor agent that causes vasoconstriction, and stimulates production of increased aldosterone. Aldosterone stimulates the reabsorption of sodium. In normal pregnancy, plasma renin and angiotensin II are elevated, but vasoconstriction does not occur because of the increased aldosterone. The higher levels of aldosterone indirectly increase blood volume and offset vasoconstriction. In gestational hypertension, the kidney becomes compromised.

Fetus. Prolonged vasoconstriction can contribute to intrauterine growth retardation and premature separation of the placenta (abruptio placentae) (ACOG Practice Bulletin, 2002; Buchbinder, Sibai, Caritis, et al., 2002; Vatten, Odegard, Nilsen, et al., 2002). The relationship between the reduced uteroplacental blood flow and the incidence of low birthweight has recently been challenged (Campbell & MacGillivray, 1999; Xiong, Demianczuk, Saunders, et al., 2002). Antepartum surveillance recommendations are based upon the assumption that the changes secondary to hypertension in the placenta negatively impact fetal outcome.

Lungs. Fluid shift in the lungs leads to pulmonary edema. Again, these changes help describe the events associated with gestational hypertension, but are not unique occurrences to this disease and do not explain a primary etiology.

Calcium. Recently, studies have reported an inverse relationship of maternal blood pressure and calcium intake. Women with preeclampsia have been hypocalcuric due to increased kidney reabsorption of calcium. Calcium supplementation has been shown to reduce both systolic and diastolic blood pressure. So far, there is no direct evidence that calcium supplementation affects long-term fetal outcome. Studies are presently in progress to determine the role of calcium supplementation in the prevention of gestational hypertension. Recently, other researchers have reported the use of antioxidant therapy with 1,000 mg per day of Vitamin C and 400 mg per day of vitamin E. No large randomized studies have supported this recommendation (ACOG Practice Bulletin, 2002).

Epidemiology

Although it is not known why gestational hypertension occurs, acceptable explanations are affected by several important observations.

- Gestational hypertension occurs more frequently in primigravidas.
- Gestational hypertension occurs more frequently with excessive placental tissue, as is seen in women with diabetes, gestational trophoblastic disease, and multiple gestation.
- Gestational hypertension seems to have a genetic component. Some evidence has been found that the genetic composition of fetal tissue may predispose a woman to the development of eclampsia. An increased incidence of eclampsia among female relatives has been noted, but no conclusions have been drawn so far.

- Symptoms usually do not become evident until the third trimester, but there is evidence the process begins as early as the first trimester.
- Symptoms progress; early identification of symptoms and subsequent intervention can decrease the severity of disease and improve perinatal outcome.

Five to 7 percent of all pregnant women experience gestational hypertension but wide variation is reported across the United States. (ACOG Practice Bulletin, 2002). It is responsible for more than 25,000 deaths annually. Women at risk for developing gestational hypertension include those at extreme ends of the childbearing age range (teenagers and women older than 40), women with preexisting vascular or renal disease, obese women, and women with lupus erythematosus.

Subjective Data

The two most significant signs of gestational hypertension (proteinuria and hypertension) occur without the woman's awareness. By the time symptoms occur, gestational hypertension can be severe. A woman may report headache, visual disturbances, facial, ankle, and finger edema, or severe heartburn with abdominal pain. Generalized edema may be observed but is not considered a sign of gestational hypertension. Therefore, frequent prenatal visits for all pregnant women are recommended for blood pressure and proteinuria screening. All women should be informed of the danger signals and directed to seek evaluation immediately.

Objective Data

Neurological. Woman may exhibit a decreased attention span, disorientation, sleepiness, or decreased alertness. Brisk reflexes or clonus may herald an imminent convulsive state; however, many normal women have hyperactive reflexes. Assessment may thus be helpful in monitoring drug therapy, but it cannot be diagnostic for determining status of gestational hypertension.

Retinal Changes. May include edema and arteriolar spasm.

Lungs. Rales and rhonchi can be heard in affected lobes when pulmonary edema is present.

Liver. Hepatomegaly or upper right quadrant tenderness, or both, may be present.

Kidneys. Oliguria (less than 500 mL of urine in 24 hours) is associated with severe hypertension.

Fundal Height. Usually as expected by dates. A nonreactive nonstress test may indicate fetal compromise.

Blood Pressure. Must be carefully and consistently measured to be meaningful. Consistent measurements are those obtained in the same arm with the client in the same position, using appropriate size cuff, and taken at least six hours apart (ACOG Practice Bulletin, 2002).

Measurements are done to detect changes in blood pressure and urine. The mean arterial pressure (MAP), or the average pressure in the arteries, is calculated from a blood pressure reading using the formula MAP = ⅓ S + ⅔ D, where D is diastolic pressure, and S is systolic pressure.

In normal pregnancy, cardiac output increases, but peripheral resistance decreases. Arterioles relax to compensate for increased blood volume. MAP should decrease, particularly in the second trimester. An elevated MAP is important to note but is not a valid predictor of impending gestational hypertension or eclampsia.

- MAP should be 82 mmHg or lower in the first and second trimesters and 89 mmHg or lower in the third trimester.
- Weight is determined every visit; the client should gain no more than 4 pounds per month, or fewer than 2 pounds per week.
- A urine dipstick is done at every prenatal visit to screen for proteinuria; normal is negative or trace.
- The hematocrit is monitored to detect hemoconcentration; should not be greater than 42 percent.

Convulsive State. An emergency situation and can occur at any time, although the client has usually exhibited signs of severe gestational hypertension. Convulsive facial twitching and tonic-clonic contractions of the body occur. Gradually, movements subside, but the client may remain in a coma for an indefinite period. Following seizure, the client is hypoxic and acidotic and requires stabilization before delivery.

Differential Medical Diagnoses

Diseases that mimic severe gestational hypertension or HELLP syndrome (see subsequent discussion), including cholecystitis, viral hepatitis, idiopathic thrombocytopenia, hemolytic uremic syndrome, microangiopathic syndrome, fatty liver disease pregnancy, and peptic ulcer. Other hypertensive disorders may occur and become evident during pregnancy. Other conditions with similar presenting symptoms such as appendicitis, kidney stones, pyelonephritis, and gastroenteritis are other possibilities.

Chronic Hypertension. In this disorder, a blood pressure of 140/90 or higher develops before pregnancy, is recognized before 20 weeks of gestation, or continues indefinitely postpartum. Chronic hypertension is seen more frequently in multiparous older women who had hypertension in previous pregnancies. African American women are overrepresented in the incidence of maternal hypertension. Fetal survival is related to clinical course, maternal renal function, and gestation at delivery. Clinical signs are different from those of gestational hypertension.

- Edema is usually absent.
- Proteinuria is absent.
- Hyperflexia does not occur.
- Weight gain is within normal limits.
- Physical signs associated with hypertension, such as retinal changes (arteriosclerosis and hemorrhages), occur.
- Fundal height may lag behind normal expectations, indicating possible intrauterine growth retardation.

Chronic Hypertension with Superimposed Gestational Hypertension. Signs of gestational hypertension can occur in a woman who already has underlying hypertension. Proteinuria may or may not occur. Perinatal mortality increases significantly.

Late, Transient, Gestational Hypertension. Some women experience elevated blood pressure late in the third trimester, intrapartally, or within the first 24 hours postpartally. Other signs of preeclampsia or chronic hypertension are absent, and blood pressure usually returns to normal limits by ten days postpartum. Whether the occurrence is a sign of underlying chronic hypertension is unclear but is unlikely (Terrone, Rinehart, May, et al., 2001).

HELLP Syndrome. HELLP is an acronym for hemolysis, elevated liver enzymes, and low platelets. Controversy surrounds the terminology, incidence, cause, diagnosis, and management of this syndrome. It is, however, considered a variant of severe preeclampsia and can develop prenatally, intrapartally, or postpartum (ACOG Practice Bulletin, 2002).

Symptoms and signs of HELLP syndrome include nausea (with or without vomiting), epigastric pain, upper quadrant tenderness, demonstrable edema, and hyperbilirubinemia. Blood tests reveal elevated serum glutamate-oxaloacetate transaminase (SGOT = 5–40 IU/L); elevated serum glutamate-pyruvate transaminase (SGPT = 5–35 IU/L); normal serum electrolytes; elevated blood urea nitrogen (BUN = 10–20 mg/dl), and creatinine (0.5–1.1 mg/dl); normal prothrombin time (PT = 11–12.5 seconds), partial prothrombin time (PPT = 60–70 seconds), and fibrinogen; a peripheral blood smear indicating burr cells, schistocytes, or both; and thrombocytopenia (platelet count below 100,000/mm^3). Proteinuria is 2+ or greater (ACOG Practice Bulletin, 2002).

Disseminated Intravascular Coagulopathy. Disseminated intravascular coagulopathy is associated with severe gestational hypertension and HELLP syndrome. Most authors, however, do not consider HELLP syndrome a variant of disseminated intravascular coagulopathy because coagulation parameters in HELLP (PT, PTT, and serum fibrinogen) are usually within normal limits. Opinions vary, but the true relationship between these two processes is unclear.

Plan

Prevention. Since the etiology of gestational hypertension/preeclampsia is unknown, efforts to prevent or reduce the incidence have been unsuccessful. The goal in management of gestational hypertension/preeclampsia is in the early detection and stabilization of the symptoms. There have been attempts to prevent the disease through dietary manipulation. In the past, high protein or low salt diets were used to correct abnormalities. Other dietary adjustments are being examined.

- *Calcium.* Calcium supplementation of 1500 to 2000 mg/d used in clinical trials in the hopes to reduce overall incidence; initiated prior to 20 weeks' gestation and continued throughout pregnancy. Results of clinical trials have not shown effectiveness.
- *Magnesium.* Because of long successful history of using magnesium sulfate in treatment of gestational hypertension and eclampsia, magnesium deficiency proposed as possible cause; studies have been conflicting; magnesium supplements are not recommended to prevent eclampsia.
- *Zinc.* Historically, zinc deficiency has been associated with gestational hypertension and eclampsia, preterm delivery, and intrauterine growth retardation. At present, no adequate data support strong relationship between zinc deficiency and the prevention of gestational hypertension or eclampsia.

Psychosocial Interventions. The major role of the primary care provider in working with a client with a hypertensive disorder in pregnancy is providing education and support. Teaching about a healthy, balanced diet is impor-

tant. The client may need to be taught to take her blood pressure or perform a dipstick urine test. All clients need to know the danger signals of gestational hypertension.

The provider must also be sensitive to the client's anxieties and concerns about the expected outcome and health of her unborn child. Women with gestational hypertension should be assisted and encouraged, within safety limits, to continue normal preparation for birth and the newborn.

Medication. Drugs are given to decrease seizure activity and reduce blood pressure.

Aspirin. Low dose aspirin therapy has been instituted if mild gestational hypertension is diagnosed because it is believed to decrease thromboxane production and platelet aggregation and may decrease the incidence of preeclampsia and fetal growth retardation. No increased maternal or fetal risks have been demonstrated after administration of 60 to 80 mg of aspirin daily late in the third trimester in the woman at high risk for developing gestational hypertension. Women at high risk are those with chronic hypertension, a history of placental abruption, gestational hypertension in a previous pregnancy, or lupus erythematosus. More research is needed to define the effectiveness, length of therapy, and the appropriate high-risk client for this therapy (Coomarasamy, Papaioannou, Gee, & Khan, 2001). Aspirin therapy in normotensive women has not shown to be of benefit and is not recommended by the American College of Obstetricians and Gynecologists (ACOG) (ACOG Practice Bulletin, 2002). The primary care provider should be in consultation with the obstetrician/obstetrical specialist if aspirin therapy is being considered.

Magnesium Sulfate. The drug of choice to control or prevent seizure activity is magnesium sulfate (see Table 18–4). It is usually given as a bolus and subsequently in continuous intravenous infusion. Because magnesium sulfate readily crosses the placenta, the newborn will be affected by the sedative properties of the drug. The

TABLE 18–4. Monitoring Needed to Administer Magnesium Sulfate

Activity to Monitor	Sign of Toxicity
Deep tendon reflexes	Hypoactivity
Respirations	< 12 rpm
Urinary output	< 25 mL/h
Blood pressure	Significant drop (> 15 mm Hg)
Pulse	Tachycardia—sign of shock

Source: ACOG Practice Bulletin (2002).

newborn may exhibit hypotonia, suppressed respiratory effort at delivery, and poor sucking. These effects subside as the newborn excretes drug over the following three to four days. Other anticonvulsive medications such as diazepam or phenytoin have been used for control of eclampsia, but magnesium sulfate remains the drug of choice.

Antihypertensive Therapy. Initiated to decrease blood pressure enough to protect maternal organs without causing hypotension and threatening fetal oxygen supply. Cardiotoxicity is possible and, therefore, electrocardiographic monitoring during administration is recommended. Because of the known teratogenic effects during pregnancy, confining its use to the intrapartum period is necessary.

Hydralazine. The drug used most often, hydralazine relaxes smooth muscle and causes vasodilation. Blood pressure drops quickly; therefore, the client must be closely watched every two to five minutes until stabilization occurs, which is within one hour. If not controlled or corrected, blood pressure can drop rapidly, leading to fetal hypoxia and subsequent distress. Labetalol is also being used as an alternative to hydralazine without any differences in perinatal outcome.

Whether pregnant women with chronic hypertension should be treated with antihypertensive agents is controversial. Most specialists agree that therapy should be continued for women who are already on a treatment regimen, including the possible use of diuretics. Therapy for women on reserpine or propranolol should, however, be changed because of their fetal side effects. For women not taking a drug, hydralazine (Apresoline) or methyldopa

(Aldomet) is recommended. Treatment is generally initiated when the blood pressure is 150/110. Management is planned after accurate dates of pregnancy are determined (ACOG Practice Bulletin, 2001b).

Conservative Treatment. Intermittent bed rest, an adequate diet, and close monitoring are recommended for women with mild gestational hypertension. Bed rest assists the cardiovascular return of fluid from the extremities and increases blood flow to the heart and subsequently to the uterus, causing uterine relaxation. Bed rest, preferably in the left lateral position at least intermittently throughout the day, and limited physical activity induce diuresis and, usually, a drop in blood pressure. Sustained bed rest produces major side effects and should be avoided. Home care is successful when family support is adequate to afford the client appropriate rest. A client who is not hospitalized should visit the health office two to three times a week for evaluation. Antepartal self-monitoring needs to be taught to the client (see Table 18–5).

Antepartal monitoring of pregnant women with known chronic hypertension involves obtaining baseline serum creatinine, uric acid, and creatinine clearance. In addition, a baseline sonogram is done to confirm dates; sonograms are repeated in the second and third trimesters, and fundal height is carefully determined at regular prenatal visits. Moreover, the client must be taught how to take her blood pressure twice a day.

Delivery. The only cure for gestational hypertension is delivery of the fetus. Primary goal of management is to allow pregnancy to progress as far as possible without jeopardizing maternal or fetal well-being. Timing and

TABLE 18–5. Antepartal Monitoring of Pregnant Woman with Mild Gestational Hypertension

Home	Office Visit
Check blood pressure once or twice a day	Check blood pressure
Check weight every day	Check weight
Perform urine dipstick twice daily	Perform urine dipstick (protein)
Observe symptoms: occipital headaches, blurred vision, irritability or emotional tension, scotoma, epigastric pain, or any signs and symptoms of labor	Assess symptoms: occipital headaches, blurred vision, irritability or emotional tension, scotoma, epigastric pain, or any signs and symptoms of labor
Record fetal movements daily	Obtain baseline serum creatinine, uric acid, creatinine clearance, total urinary protein. Repeat twice every week
	Obtain baseline liver enzymes, hematocrit, platelet count—twice a week
	Auscultate fetal heart tones, baseline fundal height, and weekly measurements
	Perform baseline nonstress test (NST) twice weekly
	Perform contraction stress test if NST is nonreactive
	Obtain baseline and serial sonograms
	Arrange for amniocentesis near term, starting at 33 weeks

Sources: ACOG Practice Bulletins (2001b, 2002); Barton, Barton, O'Brien, et al. (2002).

mode of delivery depend on stability of the maternal-fetal unit, gestation, and the cervix. For the woman with eclampsia, delivery should occur as soon as possible after the woman and fetus are stabilized. If the cervix is favorable and other factors are controlled, labor is induced with intravenous oxytocin. Concurrently, magnesium sulfate therapy is administered to control or prevent seizures. Cesarean delivery is initiated if immediate delivery is indicated.

Some controversy exists as to use of epidural anesthesia. With proper blood pressure control, it can provide satisfactory anesthesia and permit the mother to be awake for delivery (Head, Owen, Vincent, et al., 2002).

Hospitalization. Hospitalization is usually essential in the treatment of chronic hypertension with superimposed gestational hypertension. The intrauterine environment becomes increasingly hostile to the fetus, and each day is a delicate balance between the risks and benefits of intrauterine and extrauterine existence.

Severe gestational hypertension is treated aggressively, as hypertension poses an immediate threat to mother and fetus. Aggressive therapy includes maternal and fetal assessments, medications to prevent seizure activity and stabilize blood pressure, and preparation for delivery. Because of the need for intensive and sometimes invasive monitoring techniques such as invasive hemodynamic monitoring, hospitalization is required with critical obstetrical care provided by appropriate medical and nursing staff (ACOG Practice Bulletin, 2002).

System Support. For the client with eclampsia, airway maintenance and oxygen are necessary. Hemodynamic monitoring is useful for appropriate fluid management.

Follow-Up

The prognosis for pregnancy depends on the severity of symptoms. Some reports suggest gestational hypertension is a predictor of hypertension later in life (Lindeberg & Hanson, 2000; Marin, Gorostidi, Portal, et al., 2000). With aggressive screening, identification, and treatment, maternal and fetal morbidity and mortality have decreased. Following delivery, most women recover quickly without any sequelae. The presence of contributing factors dictates the type of follow-up necessary. If underlying chronic hypertension or lupus erythematosus is suspected, then postpartal referral to an internist for assessment is needed.

Many women do not have problems with elevated blood pressure in subsequent pregnancies; however, all women should be informed of the possibility and the need for early prenatal care and evaluation.

DIABETES

Diabetes is a chronic disease characterized by a relative lack of insulin or absence of the hormone, which is necessary for glucose metabolism. In normal pregnancy profound metabolic alterations occur to support the growth and development of a fetus. Maternal basal metabolism increases as a response to fetal growth. The increase contributes to increased glucose utilization and the risk of maternal acidosis. Glucose rapidly moves from maternal circulation to the fetus by simple diffusion; insulin does not cross the placental membrane.

Insulin, however, is present as early as 12 weeks in the fetal pancreas; it is stimulated by glucose from the maternal circulation. The increase in glucose to the fetus results in accelerated growth of the fetus. Human placental lactogen (HPL) and growth hormone (somatotropin) increase in direct correlation with the growth of placental tissue; it rises throughout the last twenty weeks of pregnancy and causes an increase in insulin resistance. HPL stimulates the mobilization of free fatty acids for maternal use, which can lead to maternal ketoacidosis. The hormonal changes of pregnancy have conflicting but carefully balanced effects on carbohydrate metabolism. The increased estrogen acts as an insulin antagonist. Progesterone, on the other hand, augments insulin secretion while diminishing its peripheral effectiveness. In most cases, the maternal pancreas is able to increase insulin production to maintain normal glucose levels (Illsley, 2000; Yamashita, Shao & Friedman, 2000).

The woman with undiagnosed diabetes is not able to cope with changes in metabolism resulting from insufficient insulin. The woman with suboptimal function who is not diabetic may not experience difficulty early in the pregnancy, but when pregnancy related hormones are produced by the enlarging placenta and reach certain levels, her pancreas will not be able to accommodate the increased insulin demand. The increased need for insulin and the tendency toward hyperglycemia emerge most often between 20 and 30 weeks of gestation.

In an attempt to predict client outcome and to establish treatment guidelines for diabetic clients, several classification systems are used. White's classification was based on age at onset of disease and degree of vascular involvement, but because of improved technology to monitor and treat mother and fetus, the classification is

TABLE 18–6. Classification of Diabetes

A. Insulin-dependent type (type I)
B. Non-insulin-dependent type (type II)
  1. Nonobese
  2. Obese
C. Other types (secondary diabetes)
  1. Pancreatic disease
  2. Hormonally induced
  3. Chemically induced
  4. Insulin receptor abnormalities
  5. Certain genetic syndromes
  6. Others
D. Impaired glucose tolerance (subclinical diabetes)
E. Gestational diabetes (pregnancy-induced glucose intolerance)

Source: ACOG Practice Bulletin, (2001c).

infrequently used. A simpler classification developed from the National Diabetes Data Group Classification of Diabetes Group is now used (see Table 18–6).

Diabetic Woman's Response During Pregnancy

A woman with diabetes may have several problems during pregnancy as a result of her diabetes, such as hypoglycemia, urinary tract infection, hypertension, hydramnios, and retinopathy.

Hypoglycemia. Hypoglycemia occurs primarily in the first trimester in insulin-dependent, controlled diabetics. Because of its accelerated growth, the fetus uses glucose available in the maternal circulation, thereby decreasing the diabetic woman's need for insulin. Women accustomed to a consistent diet and insulin intake are not able to adjust to their reduced need for insulin. Consequently, they commonly develop hypoglycemia in the first trimester (Rosenn & Miodovnik, 2000).

Urinary Tract Infection. Urinary tract infection is common in diabetics because more glucose is filtered due to their increased glomerular filtration rate. Glycosuria predisposes to bacterial infection (Rosenn & Miodovnik, 2000).

Hypertension. Hypertension is related to the same factors that cause gestational hypertension. Diabetics have a predisposition to hypertension in pregnancy (Roach, Hin, Tam, et al., 2000).

Hydramnios. Ten to 20 percent of diabetics have hydramnios. The reason is poorly understood, but it is explained as caused by fetal glycosuria. The urine in amniotic fluid attracts water to balance the high osmolarity of the fluid (Uvena-Celebrezze & Catalano, 2000).

Retinopathy. Diabetes is associated with retinal changes that may exacerbate during pregnancy and become more symptomatic (Rosenn & Miodovnik, 2000).

Effects on Fetus and Neonate

The fetus who remains in an environment of maternal hyperglycemia may demonstrate macrosomia, teratogenesis, or death.

Macrosomia. The accelerated fetal growth that occurs when the mother has poorly controlled diabetes leads to a macrosomic or large-for-gestational-age infant (Langer, 2000; Uvena-Celebreeze, Catalano, 2000).

Teratogenesis. If significant maternal hyperglycemia continues, it can lead to maternal ketoacidosis and to movement of ketones across the placental membrane. These ketones have been associated with teratogenesis. Although rare, agenesis has been linked with ketosis between 5 and 6 weeks gestation. Cardiac anomalies also occur. Ideally, preconception and early pregnancy glycemic control will prevent excess rates of congenital anomalies (Reece & Homko, 2000). There is need for increased planning for pregnancy in diabetic women.

Death. Among mothers who develop ketoacidosis, 50 percent of infants die. Early first trimester ketosis may cause early pregnancy loss. Hyperinsulinemia in the fetus may lead to delayed surfactant production in the lung and contribute to the incidence of respiratory distress syndrome.

Other Effects. Neonates of diabetic women have more problems with hypoglycemia, hypocalcemia, polycythemia, and hyperbilirubinemia in the first days of life (Uvena-Celebreeze & Catalano, 2000).

Epidemiology

Diabetes is thought to have more than one cause. Insulin deficiency may be associated with damage to the pancreatic cells that make insulin, inactivation of insulin by antibodies, or increased insulin needs, as in pregnancy and obesity.

A genetic component, possibly an autosomal recessive trait, may exist but is not clearly understood. Diabetes is more prevalent in some families than others. Ethnicity may also be a factor.

It is estimated that 2 to 3 percent of all pregnant women have diabetes mellitus; 90 percent of them have gestational diabetes. The prevalence of gestational diabetes is reported between 1 and 14 percent and does vary by ethnic groups (ACOG Practice Bulletin, 2001c). Today, maternal mortality is negligible, but fetal mortality is 10 to 20 percent. Excluding death due to major congenital malformations, the perinatal mortality rate among newborns of diabetic women who receive optimal care approaches that observed during normal gestation (Landon, 2000). In the early 1970s, 30 percent of all diabetic women died from complications related to diabetes in pregnancy; 65 percent of their infants died (Feudtner & Gabbe, 2000).

Subjective Data

Insulin-Dependent Diabetes. A woman who is insulin dependent may experience more problems with nausea during early pregnancy. Insulin management is more difficult if she is nauseous and vomiting because eating patterns and insulin dosage are disrupted. If care is not taken, she may experience shock, coma, or both.

Gestational Diabetes. The client with gestational diabetes may be asymptomatic throughout the pregnancy.

Objective Data

Certain signs are common in women with diabetes in pregnancy.

- Insulin-dependent women may have retinal changes that occurred during a previous pregnancy. Retinal changes are also seen in older women or women who have been diabetic since early childhood. Gestational diabetes does not generally cause retinal changes.
- Fundal height may be greater than, equal to, or less than expected by dates, depending on the uteroplacental unit. Beginning in the second trimester, fundal height will exceed expected height by dates. Evidence of excessive uterine fluid is a tympanic, tight abdomen.
- Excessive weight gain is common.
- Glycosuria is present.

Women with gestational diabetes may be asymptomatic throughout pregnancy or have only subtle signs. Therefore, earlier testing (prior to the 26 to 28 weeks' gestation) of symptomatic women will facilitate prompt intervention. Identification is a three-step process.

The first step is to identify the population at risk. The client's history may suggest gestational diabetes and warrant screening in the second trimester at 18 to 20 weeks' gestation. Some clinicians have suggested screening women at high risk of GDM at the initial prenatal visit,

but this is controversial and has not been a reliable detection of GDM. High-risk historical factors include the following:

- Family history of diabetes.
- Poor obstetrical history, such as unexplained stillbirths or spontaneous abortions.
- Previous unexplained birth of preterm or low birthweight infant.
- Previous newborn weighing 4000 g or more.
- Previous infant with major congenital anomaly.
- Previous history of gestational diabetes.

Risk factors in the current pregnancy: If any of these risk factors are present at any point in the pregnancy, the glucola screening should be considered.

- Maternal age more than 25 years.
- Obesity (weight more than 200 pounds) or body mass index greater than 25.
- Recurrent monilial vaginitis.
- Glycosuria determined with urine dipstick on two consecutive occasions.
- Hydramnios.
- Excessive weight gain or fundal height greater than expected, or both.

Finally, screen all prenatal clients either through assessment of high-risk factors, patient history, or laboratory screening for glucose tolerance (ACOG Practice Bulletin, 2001c). Universal screening of all pregnant women has not shown to be justified because screening of high-risk women will identify most of the affected women (Coustan, 2000). The American Diabetes Association, ACOG, and the Fourth International Workshop Conference on Gestational Diabetes recommend screening of risk groups. In actual practice, most private physicians and academic centers practice universal screening (ACOG Practice Bulletin, 2001c). A reliable, specific, and cost effective screening for gestational diabetes is the 1-hour post-50-g glucola plasma screen. Optimal time is between 26 and 28 weeks of gestation (ACOG Practice Bulletin, 2001c).

If the 1-hour plasma glucola is between 130 and 140 mg/dL, the client should undergo a 3-hour glucose tolerance test (GTT) to establish the diagnosis. Experts in some countries are challenging all screening programs, but in the United States, universal screening has become standard practice with exception for some low-risk populations such as teens. In clients with a 1-hour glucola screen above 185–190 mg/dl, the glucose tolerance test is unnecessary. Some experts suggest that treatment should be initiated immediately without performing the GTT. Other experts suggest performing a fasting blood glucose, and if that level is 105 mg/dl or greater, treat the woman for GDM. Two elevated values on the 3-hour GTT are diagnostic of gestational diabetes. There is recent consideration for lowering the criteria values for diagnosis but consensus does not exist at present (ACOG Practice Bulletin, 2001c; Coustan, 2000). If one value is elevated, repeat the screening at 32 to 34 weeks.

Differential Medical Diagnoses

Pancreatitis, malabsorption syndrome, hyperemesis gravidarum, hyperthyroidism.

Plan

Preconceptional Counseling. Because of the teratogenic effects of uncontrolled glucose in the first trimester of pregnancy, women with already existing diabetes need to be advised to obtain glucose control prior to pregnancy. Women on oral hypoglycemic agents should discontinue those agents and use insulin for glucose control prior to conception. Those on insulin may need to adjust doses in order to obtain closer glucose regulation than allowed in the nonpregnant condition.

Psychosocial Interventions. The primary care provider can play a major role in educating a client with diabetes and helping achieve healthy outcome. Encourage the client to continue preparing for birth of the child. Do not discourage her from attending childbirth classes. Because of the frequent prenatal visits and additional testing, the client may require help in rearranging and adjusting work responsibilities. Much depends on the maturity and motivation of the client. Normal daily activity should be continued.

Educating the client about treatment is critical to the successful management of diabetes. With appropriate counseling and information, the client and her family will be able to deal with all changes in her body as well as in her lifestyle.

Medication. The main goal of treatment is control of blood glucose levels. Ideally blood glucose should remain between 60 and 90 mg/dL fasting and 120 mg/dl two hours after meals; levels above 150 mg/dL have been associated with increased perinatal morbidity (Jovanovic, 2000). Glucose levels can be lowered through diet control and insulin administration if indicated.

Insulin requirements for the previously diagnosed diabetic woman frequently decline in the first trimester and then gradually increase during the remaining months of pregnancy.

For a woman who has gestational diabetes, insulin therapy is initiated if, on more than two episodes within a two-week interval, glucose levels are above 120 mg/dL. Women who receive insulin should monitor their glucose levels at home daily; this includes a fasting level and at least one two-hour postprandial level. Currently, insulin therapy is not recommended for all gestational diabetics, but it may be in some centers.

A mixture of intermediate and regular insulin is given in one to two subcutaneous doses daily. Beef and pork insulin have been replaced by semisynthetic human insulin preparations (Jovanovic, 2000). Because of less immunogenic properties of human insulin products compared to animal insulin, they are preferred during pregnancy. Amounts are adjusted on the basis of daily glucose levels. Insulin dosages frequently are split between the morning and evening to provide around-the-clock coverage. Pregnant diabetics require a larger dose of insulin, and their needs increase throughout pregnancy. A decrease in insulin needs during the third trimester may signal placental dysfunction, not stabilization of the diabetic process. The use of the open-loop continuous subcutaneous insulin infusion pump therapy is gaining acceptance for pregnant women. Bolus amounts are necessary to cover meals and are determined by self-monitoring but, at all other times, the pump provides generally close to 1 unit of insulin per hour continuously. Insulin lispro, an analog of regular human insulin, has recently been used to assist in lowering postprandial glucose concentration. Studies are still in progress (Jovanovic, 2000; Langer, 2000).

Most oral hypoglycemic agents have historically been associated with teratogenesis, and their use has not been recommended. Some researchers are evaluating the usefulness of some of the newer oral hypoglycemic agents (Langer, 2000). Ideally, women with diabetes on oral hypoglycemic agents should be counseled about their specific drug and evaluated as whether to continue. There are some promising results using these agents, such as metformin for treatment of polycystic ovarian syndrome (insulin resistance) with resulting increased ovulation fertilization and birth without teratogenesis. Use of some of these agents may become common (Glueck, Wang, Gold-enberg, & Sieve-Smith, 2002).

Diet. To accommodate pregnancy, 300 calories should be added to the diet of any woman each day. Diet counseling is initiated immediately after diagnosis of gestational diabetes. Ideally, a nutritionist should be available for instruction initially and consultation throughout pregnancy. The diet should contain 30 calories per kilogram of maternal weight (plus 300 calories for pregnancy) for the normal weight woman, 24 calories per kilogram for the overweight woman, and 12 calories per kilogram for the morbidly obese woman. Have 35–40 percent of the calories derived from complex carbohydrates (Jovanovic, 2000). Additional fiber may help control glucose.

Some clients maintain adequate control of their diabetes with dietary changes alone. Differences occur in how to monitor glucose accurately in these clients. Some systems use weekly office visits and fasting blood sugar and two-hour post-prandial levels to monitor glucose. Other centers teach clients home glucose monitoring, which may be ordered two to four times a day, daily, or intermittently throughout the week. The provider must be sensitive to the women's ability to cope with frequent self-monitoring techniques required for glucose management. For some women, acceptance of the diagnosis and perception of the impact of GDM on herself and fetus will affect adherence to treatment regimes.

Exercise. Exercise can be a healthy adjunct in controlling glucose levels if it is not prolonged, over strenuous, or contraindicated for other reasons. It must be tailored to the individual's glucose-insulin balance with proper timing, intensity, and duration. The client should not exercise during states of fasting or hyperinsulinemia (Carpenter 2000).

Monitoring Techniques. Several tests may be done throughout pregnancy to provide information about maternal and fetal health.

The *glycosylated hemoglobin* A_{1c} *(HbA$_{1c}$) test* measures glucose saturation of red blood cells, that is, the amount of glucose that will last the cell's lifetime. The test reflects serum glucose levels over the previous four to six weeks. Prolonged periods of hyperglycemia are evident in an elevated HbA_{1c}. The test is useful in evaluating past glucose control and client compliance. Any value less than 6.1 percent indicates good diabetic control; 6.1 to 8 percent, fair control; and 8 percent or higher, poor control. HbA_{1c} does not correlate well with fetal well-being.

Routine urine screening is necessary because diabetic clients are predisposed to urinary tract infections.

An eye examination is recommended for established diabetics because of the proliferative retinopathy that occurs. Exacerbation occurs in about 15 percent of diabetics during pregnancy; laser coagulation may be required to control the process and prevent the possibility of blindness. Because GDM usually does not affect the retina, history of GDM alone does not warrant retinal examination.

An early *sonogram* is recommended to confirm dates so that care may be planned and carried out at appropriate intervals. For established diabetics, *serial sonograms* are done based upon the risk, but usually starting at 26 to 28 weeks in four to six week intervals, in order to help in monitoring fetal growth (ACOG Practice Bulletin, 2001c; Landon, 2000). All women with diabetes have several sonograms to assess fetal size, amniotic fluid volume, and status of the placenta. Exams can detect fetal macrosomia, the most common reason for shoulder dystocia at delivery. Sonographic measurements of fetal abdominal circumference assist in detecting fetal macrosomia.

Maternal assessment of *fetal activity* is also used to assess fetal well-being. The interval of maternal detection of cessation of fetal activity and fetal death is shorter than in other complications of pregnancy. The woman should monitor fetal activity daily starting at 25 weeks gestation. (See section on fetal movement counts Chapter 19.)

α-*Fetoprotein (AFP) (tetra screen)* should be determined at 16 to 18 weeks of gestation to screen for spinal cord defects and Down syndrome. There is an increased incidence of neural tube defects in pregnant diabetics. Normal values of AFP for diabetic women are lower than for the nondiabetic population (ACOG Practice Bulletin, 2001c).

Fetal echocardography is done at 20 to 22 weeks' gestation in women with IDDM to detect presence of cardiac lesions, especially those of the great vessels and cardiac septum.

Serial nonstress testing (NST) should start at 32 weeks and continue until delivery. If the client has other vascular risks or is in poor glucose control, the NSTs should be started prior to 32 weeks' gestation and be done more frequently during the week. If the NST is nonreactive, the contraction stress test (CST) or biophysical profile (BPP) is done (Landon, 2000). Although the contraction or oxytocin challenge test (CST) is a more sensitive means of detecting fetal problems, most centers rely on biweekly NSTs because the CST carries the risk of preterm labor. The BPP is not superior to the NST alone, but does provide further information and assurance in order to allow continuation of the pregnancy. Doppler umbilical artery velocimetry studies are being used in some centers for antepartum fetal surveillance; more investigation is required for these studies to be used for reliable decision making regarding the pregnant woman with IDDM or GDM (Landon, 2000).

Delivery. Decisions concerning delivery can be difficult. Historically, the incidence of fetal death in the third trimester was decreased by arbitrary delivery at 36 to 37 weeks of gestation. Although infants survived, the incidence of respiratory distress syndrome and the complications of premature birth increased.

Newer technologies are used to document fetal maturity prior to delivery. The lecithin/sphingomyelin (LS) ratio of the amniotic fluid of diabetic women is not a reliable determinant of fetal lung maturation; however, determining the presence of phosphatidylglycerol (PG) strongly correlates with maturity and enhances the reliability of the test. Because PG is associated with false immature rate, other more dependable tests are being evaluated (Landon, 2000). Samples are obtained by amniocentesis.

Increased chance of shoulder dystocia and cephalopelvic disproportion secondary to fetal macrosomia is associated with traumatic birth and asphyxia in diabetic women. Vaginal delivery is attempted unless the fetus is estimated by sonogram to weigh more than 5000 g. In that case, a cesarean delivery may be initiated (Landon, 2000).

Today, with more adequate assessment of fetal weight and well-being, clients may progress to term and deliver as normally as possible.

The key to intrapartum management of diabetic women is control of blood sugar within strict parameters. Clients are monitored with fingerstick blood samples every one to two hours and intravenous insulin is administered if necessary. An epidural is acceptable analgesia and anesthesia.

Follow-Up

After delivery, insulin needs drastically decrease. The established diabetic may not need to return to insulin therapy for a few days. She should, however, resume her usual prepregnant glucose monitoring routine. The gestational diabetic who has been taking insulin will not need to continue. Screen the gestational diabetic with a 100-g five-hour glucose tolerance test at the six-week postpartum exam to assess for underlying diabetes (MacNeill, Dodds,

Hamilton, et al., 2001). Encourage the diabetic women to breastfeed, as it helps use glucose (Kjos, 2000).

The primary health care provider must discuss future childbearing plans and contraception with clients. The risks should be discussed candidly. The gestational diabetic can return to whatever contraceptive method she prefers. The hormones contained in oral contraceptive do not impair glucose metabolism or increase risk for cardiovascular disease as earlier theorized; therefore, the diabetic woman can safely use low dose oral contraceptives as long as she is otherwise healthy. Oral contraceptives are contraindicated in women who are over 35 years old, smoke, have hypertension, or show signs of retinopathy, neuropathy, or other vascular changes (ACOG Practice Bulletin, 2000a). The low dose combination pill or mini-pill may be used by well controlled diabetics. There is some evidence of deterioration in carbohydrate tolerance in depomedroxyprogesterone acetate (Depo-Provera) users. These are acceptable alternatives but are not suggested as first line choices (Kjos, 2000). Historically, intrauterine devices have been contraindicated for insulin dependent diabetics because of their association with infection, but this has recently been challenged. There are no contraindications for the use in the woman with a history of gestational diabetes (ACOG Practice Bulletin, 2000a).

Suggest sterilization if the woman has completed her family or the risks of future pregnancies warrant the procedure.

PRETERM LABOR AND BIRTH

A preterm birth is one that occurs prior to 37 completed weeks of gestation (Cunningham, et al., 2001). Premature/preterm labor has its onset prior to 37 completed weeks of gestation (Cunningham, et al., 2001). The onset of labor, which is poorly understood no matter when it occurs, involves complex interaction among fetal, hormonal/endocrine, structural, and maternal changes. Low birthweight (LBW) infants weigh fewer than 2500 gm at birth, regardless of gestational age. Very low birthweight (VLBW) infants weigh fewer than 1500 gm at birth. In many discussions of preterm birth, low birthweight is used interchangeably. Infant weight has traditionally been used as the indicator for gestational age. Evaluation of programs, drug therapy, research, and policies have been developed using birth-weight as the defining variable for prematurity. With the advent of sensitive pregnancy tests in correlation with accurate menstrual history and improved technology with sonography, gestational age can be accurately determined and differentiated from the premature infant. Low birth-weight infants can be the result of prematurity, in some instances a result of a poor intrauterine environment, or a combination of those factors. There is no one explanation for the incidence of low birthweight or prematurity. Until preterm labor is better understood, prevention and treatment will be inadequate. Many of the factors are known, but how these factors interact and in what order is yet unclear. A premature, or preterm birth, can occur spontaneously or by medical intervention. The spontaneous delivery includes delivery that spontaneously occurs after preterm labor, premature rupture of membranes, or premature dilation of the cervix. When a medical or obstetrical disorder is present such as diabetes, gestational hypertension, placenta previa, abruptio placentae, or intrauterine growth retardation, medical intervention may be necessary for the sake of improving the outcome for both mother or fetus and preterm birth may occur by choice. This form of indicated preterm birth is not the focus of this section.

Theories of Labor

Human labor is a complex multifaceted interaction between the mother and fetus. Term labor is initiated by the activation of phospholipase, which releases arachidonic acid from the fetal membranes and is a precursor to the prostaglandin synthesis. Many organisms produce phospholipase A2 and thus may initiate labor. Several theories to explain the onset and maintenance of labor have been proposed; but no one theory by itself has adequately explained the process.

Uterine Stretch. The uterine stretch theory suggests that once the uterus reaches a certain size, it begins to contract to empty itself. The fact that premature labor occurs in most multiple gestations supports this theory; however, the theory does not explain why some women have excessively large newborns without premature labor or why women with small-for-gestational-age newborns have preterm birth.

Progesterone Withdrawal. It was believed that progesterone decreased immediately prior to birth and triggered labor. Clinically, however, the decrease has not been demonstrated; administration of progesterone does not slow or stop labor.

Oxytocin Sensitivity. Oxytocin causes increased uterine activity but not necessarily cervical changes. It plays a

major role in the second stage of labor and postpartum but not in the initiation of labor.

Prostaglandins. The release of prostaglandins from the endometrium stimulates uterine activity, and has a significant role in the initiation of labor. Use of prostaglandins any time during gestation induces labor.

Preterm Labor Syndrome. This approach suggests that in response to an inflammatory insult, whether it be an infection or ischemia, the fetal membranes and decidua produce cytokines. These cytokines, endogenous cell mediators produced in response to inflammation, then stimulate the production of the precursors to prostaglandins, which stimulate the myometrial contractions and release the proteases that injure the membranes and underlying decidua. The result is cervical ripening, dilatation, and/or membrane rupture. An important concept is that the more advanced gestational age correlates with the responsiveness of the uterus to this insult, i.e., the women after 30 to 32 weeks' gestation will be more susceptible to this syndrome than the women at 22 weeks' gestation (Lu & Goldenberg, 2000; Norwitz & Robinson, 2001). In addition, it has been felt that a closed cervix with the mucous plug intact has protected the amniotic sac from invasion from bacteria. It has been observed that *Escherichia coli* can permeate living chorioamnionic membranes and lead to inflammation (Lu & Goldenberg, 2000).

Fetal Influence. The fetus, which has been observed to produce platelet-activating factor into the amniotic fluid, may play a synergistic role in the initiation of labor. This factor is responsible for activating the cytokine network.

The risk to the fetus for preterm birth is associated with the immaturity of the organ systems. Conditions common in the premature infant are respiratory distress syndrome, intraventricular hemorrhage, bronchopulmonary dysplasia, patent ductus arteriosus, necrotizing enterocolitis, sepsis, apnea, and retinopathy of prematurity. Some of the long-term effects are increased risk for neuro-developmental handicaps such as mental retardation, cerebral palsy, seizure disorder, blindness, and deafness. These births account for 70 percent of the mortality and nearly 50 percent of the long-term morbidity associated with childbirth (Lu & Goldenberg 2000; Mauldin & Newman, 2001).

Epidemiology

The incidence of LBW and VLBW deliveries has changed little in the past 30 years, even though infant mortality has drastically decreased. Black infants have twice the risk as caucasian infants to be born at LBW. The reason for this remains unclear (CDC, 2000c).

The causes of preterm labor are unknown, although several complications and conditions of pregnancy are associated with preterm birth (see Table 18–7).

Demographic risks for preterm labor include age under 17 years or greater than 34 years, African American ethnicity, and poor socioeconomic status. These risk factors are probably not causative but do contribute to preterm labor because of their association with inadequate prenatal care, poor nutrition, or lifestyle.

TABLE 18–7. Principal Risk Factors for Preterm Labor and Birth

Demographic Risks
Age: < 17 years or > 34 years
Low socioeconomic status
Unmarried
Race: African American
Low educational level

Medical Risks Predating Pregnancy
Parify: 0 or > 4
Nonimmune status for selected infections (e.g., rubella)
Genitourinary anomalies/surgery
Low birthweight, preterm birth
Multiple spontaneous abortions
Low weight for height
Selected diseases (e.g., hypertension)
Poor obstetric history
Maternal genetic factors
Short interpregnancy interval

Medical Risks in Current Pregnancy
Multiple gestation
Hypotension
Hypertension/preeclampsia
First or second trimester bleeding
Spontaneous premature rupture of membranes
Anemia or hemoglobinopathy
Fetal anomalies
Hyperemesis gravidarum
Poor weight gain
Short interpregnancy interval: < 1 year
Selected infections
Placental problems
Oligohydramnios or polyhydramnios
Isoimmunization
Incompetent cervix
Assisted Reproductive Technology (Schieve)

Behavioral and Environmental Risks
Smoking
Alcohol and other substance abuse
High altitude
Poor nutritional status
Exposure to diethylstilbestrol and other toxic compounds

Sources: ACOG (2001a), CDC (2000), Lu & Goldenberg (2000), Norwitz & Robinson (2001), Robinson, Regan & Norwitz (2001), Schieve et al. (2002).

Medical risks, such as hypertension and genetic disorders, which were present before a pregnancy occurred, are associated with indicated preterm birth. The most predictive risk factor for preterm delivery is history of previous preterm delivery.

Medical risks initiated by the current pregnancy constitute a considerable list. Renovascular disorders, such as abruptio placentae, are linked with preterm labor. Conditions that enlarge the uterus excessively, such as multiple gestation and macrosomia, are also associated with preterm labor. Any infection is a risk factor. Pyelonephritis during pregnancy has long been recognized as a risk factor (see Table 18–7).

Bacterial infection of the lower genital tract and amnion may lead to rupture of membranes and preterm labor. The most common causative organisms are ureaplasma, urealyticum, mycoplasma hominis, Bacteroides, and *Gardnerella vaginalis*. It is unclear whether premature cervical dilatation and uterine activity lead to rupture of membranes or whether rupture of membranes from other factors leads to preterm labor. *It has been proposed that infection promotes the release of prostaglandins, which stimulate uterine activity and cervical change.* Data are not conclusive as to whether treating maternal infection will subsequently prevent preterm labor, but recent studies suggest that aggressive identification and treatment of bacterial vaginosis can reduce rates of premature delivery (ACOG Practice Bulletin, 2001a; Paige, Augustyn, Adih, et al., 1998).

Behavioral and environmental risks include smoking, alcohol consumption, and substance abuse. Such activities inject possible toxins into the maternal-fetal unit and possibly induce prostaglandin production. Many studies have linked occupational factors, especially prolonged periods of standing or walking, to the occurrence of preterm delivery and low birth-weight infants (Heaman, Sprague, & Stewart, 2001; Magann, Evans, Weitz, & Newman, 2002).

Subjective Data

Some women fail to recognize the signs and symptoms of preterm labor perhaps because the symptoms of pelvic pressure, increase in vaginal discharge, backache, and menstrual-like cramps mimic symptoms that occur in normal pregnancy (Weiss, Sakes, & Harris, 2002). Uterine contractions persistently occur with or without pain or discomfort. Clients may complain of low backache, a sense of lower abdominal pressure, or lower abdominal or thigh pain. Some women experience a change in vaginal discharge from creamy white to more mucoid, blood-tinged, or watery.

Objective Data

Cervical changes that indicate ripening (effacement, dilatation, or anterior position) and that occur prior to 35 weeks of gestation are signs of preterm labor. Cervical assessment has both objective and subjective qualities. Cervical dilatation of 3 cm or more is fairly straightforward but cervical consistency described as soft or firm is highly subjective and not reproducible among examiners. Any uterine activity assessed by electronic monitor or by palpation should be timed and considered preterm labor until shown otherwise. Early engagement and zero station of presenting part may also be observed.

The diagnostic tests depend on the physical findings. A *transabdominal sonogram* may be ordered to confirm gestational dates and assist in decisions about timing delivery. Sonogram assessment will include placental location, estimation of fetal weight, and amniotic fluid volume to assess fetal well-being. Serial sonograms can help identify a growth-retarded infant who may not necessarily be preterm but, instead, small-for-gestational-age.

Transvaginal sonogram assessment of the length of the cervix has also been used to predict early labor since shortened cervical canal length is associated with preterm delivery (Naim, Haberman, Burgess, et al., 2002). A cervical length of 30 mm or more using transvaginal sonography is evidence that effacement has not occurred (Lu & Goldenberg, 2000, Norwitz & Robinson, 2001). When the internal os has begun to open, the external os is closed, and the cervical canal is fewer than 18 mm, there is a funneling effect apparent on a transvaginal sonogram. These observations are superior to digital examination in predicting which women will deliver prematurely.

Recently, testing for *fetal fibronectin* has shown to be helpful in predicting women with preterm contractions at high risk for preterm delivery (Lu & Goldenberg, 2000, Norwitz, & Robinson 2001). The presence of fetal fibronectin, in the cervix or vagina is associated with chorioamionitis. The presence of the fetal fibronectin which normally is not detected in normal vaginal secretions after 22 weeks of gestation, indicates evidence of bacterial related membrane breakdown and associated preterm delivery (Cunningham, et al. 2001; Lu & Goldenberg, 2000; Norwitz & Robinson, 2001). A positive fetal fibronectin is associated with premature delivery within seven to fourteen days. Therefore, a positive fetal fibronectin may need a more immediate aggressive treatment and monitoring while a negative fibronectin warrants a wait and see approach (ACOG Practice Bulletin, 2001a).

Other assessments such as the presence of *meconium-stained amniotic fluid or elevated amniotic fluid white blood count* have been linked to intrauterine infection and, thus, preterm delivery. Implications of these two tests for the diagnosis or prognosis of preterm labor is unknown.

Sometimes, true preterm labor is diagnosed in *retrospect.* With the use of new tests, the goal is to improve the reliability and specificity of diagnosing preterm labor. Significant numbers of women experience painful regular contractions during pregnancy without having a preterm birth.

Criteria have been developed for defining preterm labor.

- Gestational age of 20 to 37 weeks.
- Documented regular contractions on fetal monitor: at least four in 20 minutes or eight in 60 minutes.
- Cervix at least 3 cm dilated or 80 percent effaced compared to initial cervical length (fewer than 30 mms).

Differential Medical Diagnoses

False labor/Braxton-Hicks contractions, urinary tract infection.

Plan

The primary care provider works with several team members in managing the care of a client in preterm labor. Because preterm labor is a multi-faceted problem, it requires a multidisciplinary approach. All members of the team provide information and support to encourage the client to participate in her care. All work toward the term delivery of a normal infant.

Psychosocial Interventions. The best treatment for preterm labor may be its prevention (Maloni, 2000; Moore & Freda, 1998). To meet that end, providing general health education about pregnancy, birth, and prenatal care is essential. Generally, to address the risk of having a low birth-weight infant, it is necessary to improve family planning services and provide accessible prenatal care for any woman regardless of her financial status. A client often needs assistance with lifestyle changes. Many of these risk factors, such as smoking, substance abuse, poor nutrition, and job-related activities, are amenable to change. Educating and counseling women about these issues prior to and during pregnancy could have beneficial effects on the incidence of preterm labor (Heaman, Sprauge, & Stewart, 2001; Weiss, Saks, & Harris, 2002). In addition, helping the client to deal with stress, whether it is related to physical exertion from specific physical activities, occupational requirements, or emotional and financial factors, may lower the incidence of preterm labor (Janke, 1999). Currently, however, the correlation between stress and preterm labor is unclear. All of these areas are difficult to research and only minimal attention has been given to them.

Identifying Infection. The incidence of preterm labor is linked with genital tract infection. Any client showing possible preterm labor should have cervical, vaginal, and urinary cultures done and be treated with appropriate antibiotics. The screening and antimicrobial treatment of *bacterial vaginosis* and bacteriuria have been reported to reduce the occurrence of preterm labor and birth (Goldenberg, 1998; Paige, et al., 1998). Any client with suspicion of preterm labor should have a sterile speculum examination for pH, ferning, and pooled vaginal fluid to rule out premature rupture of membranes. Cultures should be collected from the outer one-third of vagina and perineum for group *Beta streptococcus,* from the cervix for chlamydia and *N. gonorrhoea,* and from the external cervical os and posterior vaginal fornix for fibronectin. Metronidazole is recommended for bacterial vaginosis because it is effective, does not eradicate the normal lactobacillus, and avoids issues related to penicillin allergies (Goldenberg, 1998; Paige, Augustin, Adin, Witter, & Chang, 1998). Prophylactic administration of antibiotic therapy is not recommended.

Premature rupture of membranes (PROM) is the leaking of amniotic fluid prior to the onset of labor contractions, and this discussion refers to PROM prior to 37 weeks of gestation. PROM associated with preterm labor is differentiated from PROM at term in that infection of the choriodecidual membranes has preceded the PROM as compared to chorioamniotitis, which occurs with rupture of the membranes at term. The most common presenting symptom is history of a sudden gushing fluid from the vagina followed by persistent, uncontrolled leakage. A sterile vaginal exam is done to collect fluid for testing. When applied to a dry slide, amniotic fluid will dry into a microscopic crystallization in a "fern" pattern. It can accurately confirm premature rupture of membranes in 85–98 percent of cases. The pH of amniotic fluid if present will be blue-green and range from 6.5 to 7.75. A sonogram to determine amniotic fluid volume, fetal presentation, estimated fetal weight, and gestational age is done to prepare for delivery.

Diagnosing Preterm Labor. The diagnosis is frequently uncertain and, because the treatment incurs added risks, accurate diagnosis is critical but challenging because of lack of definitive tests. When cervical dilatation is 3 cm or more, the diagnosis of preterm labor is confirmed and the woman is a candidate for tocolysis. If the cervix is less than 3 cms, then the diagnosis is not confirmed; repeat the cervical exam in 30 to 60 minutes. There must be a cervical change of at least 1 cm, a dilation of 2 cm long, or a positive fibronectin assay before preterm labor is confirmed in the woman with persistent contractions. When the cervix is fewer than 2 cm long, monitor contraction frequency with external monitor, assay fibronectin, and repeat cervical examine in one to two hours. Research thus far has not demonstrated usefulness of uterine home monitoring in detecting or preventing preterm labor and currently ACOG does not recommend.

Some are using transvaginal ultrasound assessment as early as 15 weeks of gestation to detect risk of preterm labor. This procedure requires special expertise and therefore routine usage is not feasible. Thus far, transvaginal ultrasound assessment has not led to early effective treatment modalities or have preterm labor and pregnancy outcomes improved. Ultrasound assessment in combination with fetal fibronectin may be useful in detecting preterm labor but are not recommended for usage in routine screening (ACOG Practice Bulletin, 2001a).

Tocolytic Medication. Several types of drugs have been tried to interrupt preterm labor and prevent premature birth. At present, the role of any tocolysis is questionable. Studies are inconclusive and debatable; placebos have a high rate of effectiveness. Overtreatment is probably occurring in women in whom preterm labor has been misdiagnosed. There is evidence that tocolysis can delay delivery up to 48 hours and allow for the mother to be transferred to a setting where more risk-appropriate care can be provided, if necessary. This delay also provides an opportunity to administer steroids to the mother.

Many drug therapies involve some type of home monitoring system once the client stabilizes. The question that arises is whether self-palpation (which she must be taught) is as effective in detecting uterine contractions as use of a uterine monitoring device. Most programs employing devices also include home visits or phone calls from nurses. It is difficult to determine which is more effective: the uterine monitor or nursing contact. More research is needed. (Heaman, Sprague, & Stewart, 2001)

Magnesium sulfate competes with calcium in smooth muscle and reduces the force and frequency of uterine contraction. The client with premature contractions must be hospitalized and the magnesium sulfate administered parenterally, usually intravenously. The loading dose is usually 6 g magnesium sulfate in 10 to 20 percent solution over 15 minutes. Maintenance dose is 2 g/hr magnesium sulfate added to 1 liter dextrose with saline. The client must be closely monitored by specially trained personnel while receiving magnesium sulfate and be carefully weaned when therapy is discontinued. Side effects of magnesium sulfate are hypotension, nausea, headache, weakness, pulmonary edema, cardiorespiratory arrest, and hypocalcemia. If labor is arrested, the woman is weaned from the magnesium and placed on another tocolytic drug orally.

Beta sympathomimetics, including ritodrine and terbutaline, are the most promising drugs currently available. They suppress the contractile response of the uterus.

* Ritodrine (Yutopar), the only drug approved by the Food and Drug Administration for use in preterm labor, relaxes the uterus. Side effects are related to stimulation of the sympathetic nervous system: bronchial relaxation leads to pulmonary edema, hypotension can lead to fetal stress, glycogenolysis can lead to hyperglycemia, and cardiac stimulation leads to tachycardia. Ritodrine administration is initiated by intravenous therapy and requires hospitalization
* Terbutaline (Brethine) like ritodrine, is administered for uterine relaxation. Initially, it is given by subcutaneous injection 0.25 mg every three hours. Oral maintenance doses are continued unless uterine contractions return. Some evidence suggests that clients can learn to use a subcutaneous infusion pump and continue parenteral therapy at home; however, the advantage of the pump over oral dosing has not been substantiated

Antiprostaglandins, or prostaglandin synthetase inhibitors (e.g., indomethacin [Indocin]), have been tried for some clients resistant to beta-adrenergic drugs. The usual dose is a 50 mg loading dose orally or 50 to 100 mg dose rectally. Subsequently, 25 to 50 mg is administered orally every four to six hours, depending upon client response. Because prostaglandin is a strong stimulant of the uterine myometrium and indomethacin reduces the synthesis of prostaglandins, it has promise in the cessation of labor. They have limited use in short-term intervals because of their association with closure of the ductus arteriosus, neonatal pulmonary hypertension, and oligohydramnios (Norwitz, & Robinson, 2001).

Calcium channel blockers have been used to a limited extent to inhibit myometrial contractions. Oral nifedipine (Procardia) is being used with success for some women who do not respond to other therapies. It has become the drug of choice for some centers because of the low incidence of maternal side effects and ease of administration. Fetal side effects are not a concern. It cannot be given in combination with magnesium sulfate.

Oxytocin antagonists are being sought as an effective tocolytic. Atosiban (Antocin) is being studied in a number of trials across the United States. Atosiban displaces oxytocin and vasopressin from their receptor sites and thus reduces uterine contractility. There are minimal side effects, but effectiveness beyond 48 hours is doubtful. The oxytocin antagonists may be helpful in decreasing uterine irritability, maternal anxiety, and telephone calls and useless trips to the hospital, but they have not shown usefulness in treating preterm labor (Norwitz & Robinson, 2001).

In general, tocolytic medications are not indicated when maternal conditions warrant early delivery for the benefit of the woman or the fetus. Tocolytics would be contraindicated in women with cardiac disease, significant hypertension related to chronic or pregnancy induced hypertension, or the occurrence of antenatal hemorrhage. From the fetal perspective, tocolysis is not indicated in gestation 37 weeks or greater, cervical dilatation greater than 3 cm, birth weight of 2500 gms or more, fetal distress, intrauterine growth retardation, or maternal infection. Tocolysis is also contradicted in the case of fetal demise or lethal anomaly.

Risk Screening. Although not proven reliable or sensitive in predicting preterm labor, risk screening is used by most primary health care providers to try to identify at risk women and intervene to prevent preterm birth. Risk screening should be done at every prenatal visit. In fact, women who seek early and continuous prenatal care have longer gestation pregnancies and larger babies (McCormick & Siegel 1999). A uniform tool for risk screening is not currently available. (See section on epidemiology for list of risk factors.) Cervical fetal fibronectin has limited value as a predictor of preterm delivery in a low-risk population. A negative fibronectin is highly correlated with those women at low risk for delivering within fourteen days. A positive test may be a predictor of delivery, but the full clinical implication is controversial and thus the provider should not rely on this test for the management of preterm labor (ACOG Practice Bulletin, 2001a).

Education. The major component of a program to prevent preterm labor is education of the client and staff. Comprehensive assessments and timely interventions throughout pregnancy by appropriate professionals are critical to improve the perinatal outcome in the general population (Weis et al., 2002).

Client education includes instruction about a variety of preventive measures. Information is provided about the *signs and symptoms of labor.* All pregnant women should be instructed to notify the health care provider if leaking of fluid begins, vaginal spotting or bleeding develops, or uterine contractions occur every 10 minutes or more frequently. The client may need instruction to *time contractions* from the beginning of one contraction to the beginning of the next contraction.

A client may need to learn self-care strategies to differentiate true uterine contraction from the common cramps or abdominal discomfort associated with pregnancy. When uterine activity occurs, she should first lie down, preferably on her left side, drink fluids (at least 8 oz), palpate the uterus, and time contractions. The client must be instructed that if contractions do not subside in 30 to 60 minutes, she must be evaluated by a health care provider. The reliance on bed rest and hydration to manage preterm labor is misguided and may be dangerous because there is no statistical evidence that it is effective (Urbanski, 1997).

The client must also be informed about the specific *drug therapy* being administered, when and how to take it properly, and the side effects.

The staff must be educated to be sensitive to a client's complaints and not to dismiss low backache, cramps, or descriptions of "the baby balling up" as normal discomforts of pregnancy. Emergency room caregivers and answering services should be apprised of the special needs of a preterm labor client (Weiss et al., 2002).

Home Uterine Monitoring. Home uterine activity monitoring has been used in an effort to identify preterm labor for the purpose of diagnosing, monitoring, or adjusting tocolytic therapy. Review of studies fails to demonstrate the effectiveness of uterine monitoring in the reduction of preterm birth (Iams, Newman, Thom, et al., 2002).

Traditional Approach. The traditional plan of care comprises bed rest, hydration, and sedation.

- Bed rest assists the cardiovascular return of fluid from the extremities and increases blood flow to the

heart and subsequently to the uterus, causing uterine relaxation. Bed rest remains one of the most widely prescribed medical interventions for preterm labor, even though it is costly, disruptive to families, and may either have no effect or negative effects on fetal outcomes (Maloni, Brezinshi-Tomasi, & Johnson, 2001; Maloni & Kutil, 2000; McCormick & Siegel, 1999). Bed rest produces major side effects in every major organ system including cardiovascular deconditioning, diuresis with accompanying fluid, electrolyte, and weight loss, muscle atrophy, and psychological stress. Because of these physiological and psychological side effects of bed rest, the provider needs to anticipate and intervene to allay these effects. Assisting the woman and her family to arrange family activities and responsibilities to accommodate at least three to four periods of 20-minute rest in the recumbent position can relieve fatigue and pressure on the cervix. Home care including medical and nursing assessment, child care, homemaker services, supportive counseling, and instruction in stress relaxation are all interventions being utilized to assist preterm mothers in labor to maintain bed rest (Cunningham, E., 2001) Hospitalization to ensure bed rest is sometimes utilized but is not always effective (Cunningham, E., 2001).

- Sedation reduces the client's anxiety and helps her to rest. If, however, delivery is imminent, sedation poses the risk of neonatal respiratory suppression.

- Hydration also increases blood flow to the uterus. Even though commonly prescribed, the effectiveness of hydration has not been well established and needs further investigation (McCormick, & Siegel, 1999; Urbanski, 1997).

Ultrasound. Transabdominal ultrasounds are used to assist in the diagnosis and monitoring of the woman with preterm labor. Sonography is done to assess placental location, determine amniotic fluid volume, estimate fetal weight and presentation, and assess fetal well-being. Information from sonography assists in making delivery decisions. Transvaginal assessment of cervical length has also been used to identify women at risk for preterm birth. A cervical length of fewer than 30 mm at 24 to 28 weeks has been postulated to predict the occurrence of preterm birth. At present, this observation has not been tested in relation with any program of intervention.

Cerclage. Cerclage late in pregnancy for excessive dilation (CLIPED) historically has not been used but may be appropriate in some cases to delay delivery. Clients must be free of infection and greater than 21 weeks of gestation.

Delivery. If labor is not halted, delivery management is based on fetal size and presentation. Delivery mode should be as atraumatic as possible; cesarean section is frequently performed with breech presentations. Cesarean sections should only be performed for the usual fetal and maternal indications.

Corticosteroid Administration. It is recommended to administer corticosteroids to the mother prior to delivery to stimulate surfactant production in the fetus and decrease the incidence of respiratory distress syndrome, intraventricular hemorrhage, and overall neonatal mortality. To be effective, corticosteriods must be given between 24 and 34 weeks of gestation, maternal infection must not be present, and membranes should be intact (Goldenburg, 1998). Administrating steroids in the case of rupture of membranes is controversial. Women at risk for premature delivery are usually given dexamethasone 5 mg intramuscularly every 12 hours for 4 doses. Giving additional or rescue doses remains controversial (Cunningham, F. C. et al., 2001). The major maternal side effect is potential pulmonary edema when given concurrently with tocolytics. Follow-up of children whose mothers have prenatal corticosteroids has not shown any untoward effects (Goldenberg, 1998). In addition to corticosteroids, most centers are using surfactant replacement in the newborn to prevent or decrease the problems of respiratory distress syndrome (McCormick & Siegel, 1999). Exogenous replacement surfactant is even more effective when given to infants of mothers treated prenatally with corticosteroids. Neither of these treatments replaces the natural lung maturity that occurs in utero.

Preterm labor is not stopped if severe uterine bleeding or maternal disease or infection is present. Premature rupture of membranes is associated with preterm labor and genital tract infection; therefore, once rupture is suspected, cervical cultures, including those for group beta streptococci, mycoplasma, gonorrhea, and chlamydia, should be obtained. Decision making with respect to delivery must balance the risk of prematurity with that of maternal/neonatal sepsis. Currently, the conservative approach of delaying delivery is more common, unless infection cannot be controlled with antibiotic therapy.

The client is hospitalized. Her temperature is monitored throughout the day, and the leukocyte count is evaluated every two to three days. An amniocentesis is con-

sidered to rule out subclinical infection. Tocolysis is contraindicated when chorioamnionitis is present.

SUBSTANCE ABUSE

Research has documented a causal relationship between a woman's health behaviors and the health of her unborn child. Ingestion of certain chemicals, legal and illegal, can be teratogenic. Indeed, the use of illegal chemicals (those that have no medically sanctioned use) is rising at an alarming rate in the United States. Cocaine, an amphetamine, is one example. Unfortunately, improper use of tobacco, alcohol, and caffeine is common and tolerated in our society. In addition, certain controlled substances, such as sedatives, amphetamines, and narcotics, are misused.

Pregnancy affects a woman's response to certain drugs. Consequently, an amount of drug taken during pregnancy may have different, more unpleasant effects than it would in the nonpregnant state. Drugs cross the placenta but may not be able to cross back. The fetus, which usually requires more time to detoxify and excrete drugs, becomes a reservoir.

The timing of drug ingestion may also determine the type and severity of damage. Because many women are polyusers, the problem is compounded. Mixed drug abuse may increase the incidence of adverse effects. It certainly complicates the primary care provider's ability to predict outcome and the counseling needs of clients. Research on drug abuse has been extensive, but inconsistent and, in many cases, inconclusive. To assess clients effectively and intervene appropriately so as to promote and maintain health, however, the provider must be knowledgeable about current, accurate information.

Epidemiology

Trying to explain or predict human behavior is a complex, usually unsuccessful endeavor. Because so many variables interact, research becomes difficult; however, research suggests that combination of biological, sociological, and psychological factors interact to determine the onset and severity of substance abuse. Addiction may have a genetic basis.

The *psychic pain theory* states that drug use is an attempt to relieve "psychic pain." Feelings of depression, loneliness, or anger may lead persons to self-medicate. Some describe the use of drugs as a way to control their lives, which otherwise seem out of control or to combat feelings of powerlessness and helplessness. (Lindenberg, Solorzano, Krantz, et al., 1998; Washington, 2000). Other researchers have proposed that women's *inability to develop adequate relationships as children* is linked to later substance abuse (Cosden & Cortez-Ison, 1999). Substance abuse may be a harmful health behavior triggered in response to a major life stress or trauma. It has been reported that 70 percent of women report being raped or sexually abused prior to their substance abuse (Haller, Knisely, Elswick, et al., 1997).

In several recent studies of obstetrical populations, 10 to 15 percent of clients reported their drug use during pregnancy. According to national estimates from the National Institute on Drug Abuse, 5 percent of all pregnant women use an illicit drug in pregnancy (Howell, Heiser, & Harrington, 1999). Black women are more likely to use drugs than are white or Hispanic women (Ehrmin, 2001; Grason, Hutchins, & Silver, 1999). In reality, however, the incidence of drug use is higher, as many women deny use. Routine prenatal toxicology has been proposed to increase the identification of women abusing drugs during pregnancy. The intent has been to anticipate the medical treatment for complications of pregnancy, such as preterm labor, and provide the appropriate education and referral (Corrarino, Williams, Campbell, et al., 2000). There is much variance to the accuracy and usefulness of present urine and blood toxicology tests. Some states have enacted laws mandating prenatal drug screening and treatment, but there are legal/ethical pitfalls to this approach. Coerced treatment has not shown to be effective in reducing perinatal substance abuse and has been challenged as to its legal justification.

Subjective Data

A client with substance abuse problems does not usually seek health care expressing her abuse as a chief complaint. Her complaints are usually vague, frequently cloaked by other problems for which she desires some relief. Often, she seeks prenatal care late or not at all. The client may arrive at the emergency room in labor or experiencing a complication of pregnancy that involves pain or bleeding.

Symptoms of withdrawal that may motivate a woman to seek care include nausea and vomiting, nervousness, tremors, and abdominal cramps. A woman abusing drugs often has a history of sexually transmitted disease. Because many of the same lifestyle factors for drug use are also the same risk factors for HIV, a history of positive HIV status is associated with substance use in women. Other clues that place a woman at risk for substance

abuse include a history of a low birthweight infant, prostitution, poor self-care, parent or sexual partner who abuses drugs, or family violence (Lindenberg et al., 1998; Savitz, Henderson, Dole, et al., 2002).

Objective Data

Effects of selected drugs in pregnancy and signs of recent drug use are listed in Tables 18–8 and 18–9, respectively. (See Chapter 23 for more details on drug use.)

Drug use is an important part of a client's history. The primary care provider must remember that the client may be involved in illegal activities, such as drug selling and prostitution, and may fear repercussions of seeking care. She often denies substance abuse. A caring, concerned manner is therefore critical to help the client feel "safe" and respond honestly. Indeed, many clients feel relieved because they want to discuss their problem. Pregnancy is the motivator for some who want to try treatment. In settings where routine testing is done, the provider needs to inform the woman in a positive manner that routine testing will be done to assist in providing quality care and assuring for healthy outcome.

It is essential in discussions with clients about substance abuse to clarify the type of drug taken, the time during gestation when the fetus was exposed, and the amount of drug taken, it is necessary also to assess the client's concerns, level of knowledge, and fears. Such assessment depends on the adeptness of the provider. Questionnaires are available through drug and alcohol abuse centers to help the provider assess the type(s) and severity of an abuse problem (Allard-Henderson, 2000). Assessment tools to assess alcohol usage include the MAST (*Michigan Alcoholism Screening Tool*), the CAGE (*Cut Down Annoyed Guilt Eyeopener*), and the T-ACE (*Tolerance Annoyed Cut Down Eyeopener*) (Henderson-Martin, 2000). The *Substance Abuse Subtle Screening Inventory* (SASSI) is another effective clinical tool, which has been positively compared to using urine toxicology. The *Addiction Severity Index* (ASI) is a 180-item scale used for diverse groups including pregnant women to assess the frequency and intensity of drug use (Corrarino et al., 2000).

Ideally, the initial prenatal visit should provide an opportunity for all women to complete a confidential questionnaire that will provide a baseline for discussion. The provider should review the findings with the client in a private setting.

The provider must not be judgmental toward clients who are abusing drugs. Many women use drugs to fill a

TABLE 18–8. Incidence and Effects of Use of Certain Drugs in Pregnancy

Substance	Incidence	Possible Effect on Pregnancy
Nicotine	20–30% of women of childbearing age	Vasoconstriction: decreased uteroplacental blood flow, decreased birth weight, prematurity, abortion, abruptio placentae.
Alcohol	96% of population at some time	Decreased folic acid and thiamine, inadequate weight gain, second-trimester abortion, fetal alcohol syndrome, which is the leading cause of mental retardation, and alcohol-related birth defects.
Sedatives (barbiturates)	Widespread, not known	Teratogenic effects not known, newborn withdrawal, maternal seizures in labor.
Amphetamines (cocaine)	5–28% newborns reported exposed to cocaine	Vasoconstriction: pregnancy-induced hypertension, abruptio placentae, abortion; maternal starvation: ketosis and dehydration, "snow-baby syndrome," neonatal cerebral hemorrhage, preterm birth, increased incidence of sudden infant death syndrome, neural tube defects, failure to thrive.
Narcotics heroin morphine codeine meperidine opium	< 1% of pregnant women	Maternal and fetal withdrawal, abruptio placentae, abnormal presentation, preterm labor, premature rupture of membranes, intraamniotic infections, postpartum endometritis, urinary tract infection, septic thrombophlebitis, increased incidence of pregnancy-induced hypertension, intrauterine growth retardation, small-for-gestational-age infant, neonatal jaundice, congenital anomalies, including cardiac and genitourinary newborn infection.
Marijuana (cannabis)	10% of all 18- to 25-year-olds	"Amotivational syndrome," altered neonatal behavioral patterns, increased neonatal tremors, hyperactive startle reflex, inability to focus on an object, and decreased hand-to-mouth coordination.

Sources: Bauer (1999), Bishai & Koren, (1999), CDC (2002a), Eyler & Behnke (1999).

need in their lives; they already suffer from low self-esteem and guilt feelings. Showing disapproval may increase their guilt, and the only way they may be able to deal with guilt is by using more drugs. Prosecution has not been effective in reducing addiction (Ehrmin, 2001; Folley, 2002; Lindenberg et al., 1998; Ondersma, Simpson, Brestan, & Ward, 2000). The goal of therapy is to help the client deal with pregnancy by developing a trusting relationship with a person instead of the drug(s). Providing a full spectrum of medical, social, and emotional care is mandatory (Egelko, Galanteer, Dermatis, & DeMaio, 1998; Haller, Knisely, Ellswick, Dawson, & Schnoll, 1997; Howell, Heiser, & Herrington, 1999).

TABLE 18–9. Signs of Recent Drug Use

Sedatives	Unsteady gait, odor of fresh or stale alcohol, nystagmus, slurred speech
Amphetamines	Anxiety, paranoia, tracks or needle marks, tattoos or self-scarring over arms (to disguise needle marks), nasal irritation, frequent purposeless movements, excessive fetal activity
Narcotics	Depressed mood, nodding, pinpoint pupils, tracks or needle marks, tattoos, skin abscesses/cellulitis, fingertip burns (diminished pain sensation)
Hallucinogens	Paranoia, anxiety, thought disorders, impaired judgment, fingertip burns

Sources: Bishai & Koren (1999), Savitz et al., (2002).

The interview should be done in a matter-of-fact manner. Questions should be phrased in a fashion that assumes drug use to decrease the client's defensiveness, for example, How many times do you drink beer in one week? In addition, the provider should ask about drinking and drug use prior to pregnancy (Henderson-Martin, 2000). Evasive answers may indicate a problem. It is not necessary or wise for the primary care provider to seek a detailed account of drug usage at this initial interview. Referral and follow-up with substance abuse clinicians are ideal.

Differential Medical Diagnoses

Medical problems associated with substance abuse in pregnancy may include the following: sexually transmitted diseases including HIV infection and AIDS; uncertain date of last menstrual period; hepatitis; skin abscesses and cellulitis; anemia and malnutrition; tuberculosis; and urinary tract infections.

Plan

Substance abusers are not going to stop because of any one intervention or because someone tells them to stop. The success rates of treatment programs are dismal. Nevertheless, many women can be helped, as can their children, and that is the focus of the primary care provider.

Multifaceted programs are needed to more adequately promote the health of these women and their unborn children (Haller et al., 1997; Howell & Chasnoff, 1999).

Psychosocial Interventions. The dangers of drug use in pregnancy need to be conveyed. Preconceptional counseling should include information about alcohol, smoking, caffeine, medications, and all other drugs, legal and illegal. The primary care provider should be supportive, yet provide clear directions to pregnant and prepregnant clients about avoiding smoking, drinking, and drugs (Egelko, Galanteer, Dermatis, & DeMaio, 1998; Howell et al., 1999). Substance abuse crosses all socioeconomic and cultural groups; screening is not limited to low socioeconomic groups. Lack of insurance, lack of child care, lack of transportation, or homelessness are identified as barriers to substance abusing women seeking or staying in care. Removal of these barriers is important to any treatment intervention (Howell & Chasnoff, 1999).

Medication. See Chapter 23.

Legal Issues. Providers need to be aware of the laws and practices within their state and settings. Issues such as charting, confidentiality, and responsibilities for reporting vary by state.

Psychological Therapy. Once abuse has been identified, therapy should begin with the primary caregiver. Although the client may resist referral to a specialist and her personal freedom must be protected, adequate treatment is important. In addition to appropriate individual and/or group psychological therapy, a comprehensive program includes routine prenatal medical care, prenatal education, substance abuse education, parenting education, vocational training, housing if needed, and integration into self-help programs. Specialized programs for pregnant women are designed to deal with substance abuse as well as the high risk nature of pregnancy and birth. Case management and home visiting by caring, knowledgeable professionals have enhanced the effectiveness to perinatal substance abuse treatment (Corrarino et al., 2000).

Preparation for both delivery and infant care is a positive activity and should be encouraged. Special classes will help the client to prepare. Historically, these women do not receive gratification from infant care, but the programs preparing them for childbirth include strategies to boost self-esteem by helping the woman successfully parent her child.

A client should not be separated from her children, but instead should be involved in child care in a supportive, healthy environment. Children also need referral for close pediatric care.

Prenatal Care Issues. The types of drugs being used in pregnancy have variable effects on the women and her fetus.

Nicotine. Smoking cessation during pregnancy can reduce the risk of complications of pregnancy and incidence of low birthweight. One of the most effective strategies to assist people to quit smoking is having the medical professional advise cessation. Communities should have smoking cessation programs targeting pregnant women available at low or no charge from organizations such as the American Lung Association, the American Cancer Society, or the March of Dimes (refer to Chapter 23).

Alcohol. Heavy drinking is a risk to the fetus throughout the pregnancy, so reduction or elimination of alcohol at any time during gestation is beneficial to the fetus. Alcohol is associated with fetal alcohol syndrome and related birth defects. Fetal alcohol exposure is the leading cause of mental retardation. Referral to appropriate counseling including self-help groups such as Alcoholics Anonymous can be helpful (refer to Chapter 23).

Sedatives (Barbiturates and Benzodiazepines). When these drugs have been ingested in high doses prenatally and stopped abruptly, the withdrawal can be life-threatening to mother and fetus. Cessation of these drugs should be done gradually under the supervision of the physician. The withdrawal symptoms are similar to opiate withdrawal.

Amphetamines (Cocaine). Advise immediate cessation of subsequent drug; cocaine causes its effect quickly on the maternal system and fetus. Abruptio placentae is commonly associated with cocaine usage in pregnancy. Cocaine has been associated with stillbirths, prematurity, premature rupture of membranes, abruptio placentae, impaired infant growth, and central nervous system problems such as microcephaly. Many of these reports are inconclusive (Bishai & Koren, 1999). Reports of long-term effects on children as toddlers and young children are now more promising. Studies of these older children who were exposed prenatally to cocaine exhibit few cocaine effects when compared to similar control groups. These children continue to exhibit difficulty with developmental tasks and learning, mostly related to inadequate parenting from drug-addicted parents (Tronick & Beeghly, 1999).

Narcotics (Heroin, Morphine, Meperidine, Opium). Usually these women who are addicted to narcotics ingest periodic doses inconsistently. These peaks and nadirs of drug level create periods of fetal withdrawal and possible hypoxia. Methadone maintenance is given to stabilize the maternal addictive behavior and prevent periods of fetal binge and withdrawal. Methadone maintenance requires the women to be in a drug treatment program under the supervision of appropriate personnel. Hospitalization for initial stabilization and orientation to the methadone is ideal but may not be available in many communities. Most women require 80 to 120 mg/day of methadone to achieve the therapeutic effect to reduce the need for heroin (Joseph, Stancliff, & Langrod, 2000). Some programs are available in outpatient settings. The initial dose is usually 10 to 20 mg with additional doses of 5 mg every four to six hours, depending on evidence of withdrawal symptoms. Enrolling pregnant women in a methadone maintenance program can reduce obstetrical complications, increase chance for participation in prenatal care, and enhance the opportunity to engage them into drug treatment program. Neonates of women using narcotics including methadone will demonstrate signs and symptoms of neonatal abstinence syndrome (NAS). NAS includes generalized disorders of the gastrointestinal tract, respiratory, and central nervous systems. Paregoric, phenobarbital, and diazepam are used to alleviate the withdrawal symptoms in the neonate. Outcomes of the neonates exposed prenatally to methodone exhibited developmental delays, decrease attention, and irritability similar to the heroin exposed infants (Eyler & Behnke, 1999).

Marijuana. Effects on pregnancy and fetus are not clear; advise to discontinue usage.

Delivery. Ideally, women who are abusing drugs in pregnancy are identified, and plans for continuation of care carry into the intrapartum period. Either urine or blood toxicology screening may be done upon admission. Use of hair assays and testing of meconium is being explored in several institutions to screen for possible drug usage (Savitz et al., 2002). Frequency and type of maternal and fetal monitoring will be determined by the type and amount of prenatal drug(s) used.

Child Follow-Up. In general, infants born to mothers abusing drugs during pregnancy are at greater risk to experience lack of adequate parenting, possibly child neglect and abuse, as a result of attachment difficulties and mothers' disorganization and unpredictability (Shieh & Kravitz, 2002). The incidence of long-term effects of developmental delays and learning disabilities of in utero exposure to drugs is controversial. Because of the many confounding factors associated with these women and their unstable, often impoverished lifestyle, establishing a causative link to the in utero exposure to drugs and subsequent behavior is impossible.

MULTIPLE GESTATION

Several complications of pregnancy are associated with multiple gestation. Spontaneous abortion, for example, is more than twice as common in multiple gestation. Visualization of twins on an early sonogram of a woman who later delivered a single newborn has occurred and is known as the vanishing twin syndrome. It is believed that one or more embryos can be reabsorbed without jeopardizing the remaining embryo (Dickey, Taylor, Lu, et al., 2002). Low weight infants especially in the primigravida are more likely in multiple gestation (Blickstein, Goldman, & Mazkereth, 2000). Women with multiple gestation experience increased risk of other complications such as diabetes and gestational hypertension (Campbell & MacGillivray, 1999). There are reports of maternal deaths that arise from the complications associated with multiple gestation. Fatty liver disease and pulmonary edema are also more frequent in multiple gestation (Blickstein, 1997).

Overdistention can interfere with sustained functional labor contractions and affect dilatation and effacement; ineffective uterine activity results. It may also lead to uteroplacental insufficiency and fetal stress. Consequently, cesarean delivery is more common (Persad, Baskett, O'Connell, & Scott, 2001). Varied factors related to gestational age, general maternal health, labor pattern, and the maternal-placental unit determine fetal compensation in labor. Multiple gestation occurs in 3 percent of all births in the United States (Keith & Oleszczuk, 1999; Warner, Kiely, & Donovan, 2000). The incidence of postpartum hemorrhage from uterine atony is significantly increased secondary to overdistention of the uterus during pregnancy.

Development

Monozygotic (MZ) twins, also called identical twins, arise from a single fertilized ovum that divides during the early development phase into two embryos with identical genetic material The time of division determines fetal and placental morphology. Division occurring late, between eight and twelve days' postfertilization, will result in incomplete separation and, thus, conjoined twins.

Dizygotic (DZ) twins, also called fraternal twins, arise from multiple ova that are fertilized by multiple sperm. Multiple ovulation results from excessive gonadotropin stimulation. Fraternal twins are not true twins but siblings who share the same intrauterine environment. High-order multiple gestations (more than three fetuses) can result from monozygotic, dizygotic, or mono- and dizygotic division.

With a multiple gestation, blood volume increases 500 mL more than a single gestation; the volume of amniotic fluid in twin gestation may reach 10 L.

Epidemiology

Twin and higher-order births have been on the rise for the past decade to an incidence of 28.9 per 1,000 births in 1999, which represents a 50 percent increase from 1980. It is reported that the increased availability of assisted reproductive technology and the overall aging of the maternal cohort are the contributing factors (CDC, 2001a; Keith & Oleszczuk, 1999). The frequency of monozygotic twins is constant across the world at one set per 250 births. There is variation in the frequency of dizygotic twins among races, ethnic groups, maternal age, parity, and the use of fertility drugs and other assisted reproductive technologies (Warner et al., 2000). Incidence of multiple gestation varies among countries and races. Africa has the highest reported incidence and Japan has the lowest incidence. The risk of congenital anomalies in multiple gestation is three times greater than in a single gestation.

With identification of the vanishing twin syndrome, the incidence may be higher than previously thought. Early diagnosis by sonography has documented multiple gestations that resulted in single births (Keith & Oleszczuk, 1999).

Subjective Data

During early pregnancy, a woman with multiple gestation may experience more severe nausea and vomiting, which may last well into the second trimester. Hyperemesis gravidarum, probably related to increased human chorionic gonadotropin levels, may be the only diagnostic clue in the first trimester. The client may later experience excessive fetal movements. Neither sign, however, is reliable or helpful in early diagnosis.

Objective Data

The data used to diagnose the presence of a multiple gestation are collected by physical examination, maternal serum α-fetoprotein testing, and sonography.

In the second trimester, examination may reveal signs suggestive of multiple gestation. The most common early sign is a fundal height greater than expected for dates. More than one heartbeat may be heard. Palpation of more than one fetus is not usually possible until the third trimester.

Maternal serum α-fetoprotein is measured between 15 and 18 weeks of gestation. If the α-fetoprotein level is elevated, multifetal gestation is suspected. Sonography is used for definitive diagnosis and to identify the number of fetuses.

Differential Medical Diagnoses

Anemia, hyperemesis gravidarum, hyperthyroidism, gestational trophoblastic disease, gestational diabetes.

Plan

Clinical goals are to prevent premature birth and to detect fetal growth retardation early. The incidence of preterm delivery in multiple gestation is 20 to 50 percent (Warner et al., 2000). Fetal growth is usually satisfactory until 30 to 32 weeks of pregnancy but discordant growth has been observed as early as 22 weeks (Warner, Kiely, & Donovan, 2000). From 32 weeks onward, the total weight gain of fetuses is similar to the total weight gain of a single fetus. (Blickstein, 1997; Warner et al., 2000). Head circumference is similar, but fetuses have a low weight.

Psychosocial Interventions. Support the client during diagnostic testing. Clarify the critical nature of such testing. Explain to her that a late diagnosis of multiple gestation is associated with a greater risk of poor perinatal outcome.

Maternal Assessment. Carefully evaluate the usual pregnancy changes with particular attention to signs and symptoms of pregnancy induced hypertension and preterm labor. In late pregnancy the incidence of gestational hypertension increases three-fold; it also occurs earlier in pregnancy and is more severe (Lynch, McDuffie, Murphy, et al., 2002).

The larger increase in maternal blood volume associated with multiple gestation increases the incidence of iron deficiency anemia.

Fetal Surveillance. Sonography and a nonstress test are among the tests that may be carried out.

Sonography is done early in the second trimester to assess fetal structures for anomalies, to determine placental placement, and to identify chorionicity and amnionicity. Fetal anomalies occur more frequently in monozygotic twins.

After 28 weeks, sonograms are done every two to three weeks to assess fetal growth by measuring the biparietal diameter, but biparietal diameter alone is an inadequate predictor of growth. Recent studies consider birthweight and gestational age as better predictors of birth outcomes (Baker, Beach, Craigo, et al., 1997; Hanley, Ananth, Shen-Schwarz, et al., 2002; Warner et al., 2000). Intrauterine growth retardation must be differentiated from discordant growth. Growth discordant twins have lower Apgar scores, longer hospitalization, and higher perinatal death rates.

Malpresentation, which is common, is detected by sonogram. The most likely presentation is vertex/vertex; however, interlocking fetal parts can affect delivery. Crowding provokes less desirable presentations, such as vertex/breech, breech/breech, vertex/transverse, or several other combinations. Cord prolapse and cord entanglement are usually associated with malpresentation. Also diagnosed by sonogram is twin transfusion syndrome. Twin transfusion syndrome is uncompensated, unidirectional blood flow from one fetus to another. The donor twin becomes hypovolemic with suboptimal growth; the recipient becomes hypervolemic and hydropic.

Nonstress tests start at 28 weeks and are done weekly. Each fetus should be monitored separately if possible.

Other tests that may be done are chorionic villus sampling and amniocentesis. These tests are carried out for the same reasons as for a single gestation pregnancy. Preterm labor, if present, is treated as usual. The lecithin/sphingomyelin ratio is used to make a decision about the timing of delivery, for example, in the case of a woman with twins and gestational hypertension. As no significant difference is found in the lecithin/sphingomyelin ratio among sacs of laboring women, only one sac needs to be tapped.

Selective Termination. Selective termination, the voluntary reduction of the number of embryos in a high-order multiple gestation, is performed as early as possible in the first trimester, if desired. The intent is to increase the chance for survival for the remaining embryos. Among the various methods used is injection of potassium chloride into the embryonic sac to allow natural reabsorption. The number of embryos to be terminated is controversial but reduction to twins is preferred because of the improved outcomes (Yaron, Bryant-Greenwood, Dave, et al., 1999). Because the perinatal outcome is significantly less favorable for more than two fetuses, most recommend reduction to two embryos. Many ethicolegal questions

arise. The client and her family must have a thorough knowledge and understanding of the procedure and its implications.

Comfort Measures. To address the intense discomfort associated with the exaggerated physiological changes of multiple gestation, various measures may be implemented. Nausea and vomiting may require intravenous hydration. Constipation, heartburn, sleeping disturbances, and low back pain interventions can be reviewed as usual. The overdistended uterus mechanically blocks the lower extremities, causing dependent edema and varicosities in the legs and labia. Maternity support hose may be recommended early in pregnancy. A maternity "sling" girdle has been helpful for some women to help support the gravid uterus and alleviate lower backstrain associated with multiple gestation. Exercises, particularly those to stretch and strengthen the lower back muscles, may be suggested.

Although excessive fetal movement is reported, it does not warrant intervention.

The health care provider can assist women in controlling and coping with changes with anticipatory guidance and education (Maloni & Kutil, 2000; Ruiz, Brown, Peters, & Johnston, 2001; Schroeder, 1998; Watson-Blasioli, 2001).

Diet. In addition to foods that are rich in iron, recommend a supplement of 60 to 80 mg elemental iron per day. Encourage daily intake of prenatal vitamins with 1.0 mg folic acid. Monitor the woman's weight gain at each office visit.

Bed Rest. Bed rest for women with a multiple gestation has been studied extensively with inconclusive results (Schroeder, 1998; Watson-Blasioli, 2001). Although bed rest has not prevented preterm birth, some evidence suggests that bed rest initiated at 26 to 32 weeks may increase birthweight and thereby improve perinatal outcome. Most providers limit a woman's activity based on her lifestyle and general health. When a woman with multiple gestation is placed on bed rest, referral to a support group may assist her in dealing with the many physical and emotional changes she may experience (Maloni & Kutil, 2000; Ruiz, Brown, Peters, & Johnston, 2001, Schroeder, 1998; Watson-Blasioli, 2001).

Preparation for Childbirth. Classes should be begun earlier than usual, as immobility can be a problem in the later weeks of gestation.

Preterm Labor. Preterm labor is treated if signs occur. The use of tocolytic drugs to prevent preterm labor has not proven successful. Prophylactic cervical cerclage has also not been beneficial, unless the client is experiencing premature cervical dilatation.

Delivery. Decisions concerning delivery are based on gestational age, estimated fetal weights, presentations in relation to each other, and availability of adequate intra-partum monitoring. Cesarean birth is performed frequently because of malpresentations and because of concern for the ability of preterm and low birthweight fetuses to tolerate a difficult vaginal birth. An intrapartal sonogram is necessary to identify fetal presentations and establish a management plan for delivery.

Follow-Up

Because of the increased chance of uterine atony and early hemorrhage following a multiple birth, caution is exercised to identify and treat it as soon as possible.

Although breastfeeding decisions are based on the same reasoning as that used following the birth of a single infant, a woman with more than one newborn will probably need additional education and support. More patience and time are needed to establish adequate lactation and feasible routines. Lactation consultants, lay groups such as the La Leche League, and informed nurses within the health care system are available for referral.

Attachment may take longer when more than one infant is involved. Neonatal illness and separation can also interfere in parent-child bonding. Other factors affecting attachment include the meaning of the pregnancy to the couple, maternal health, and the general living conditions. If one or more of the siblings is hospitalized, ill, or dies, parents experience ambivalence in trying to grieve and at the same time celebrating the survival of one or more infants.

Most communities have lay groups of parents who have had multiple births, such as Mothers of Twins and Mothers of Multiples. These groups provide sympathetic counseling, practical suggestions on how to cope with more than one infant at a time, directions for obtaining equipment and supplies, and referral for financial assistance, which is frequently needed (Watson-Blasioli, 2001).

REFERENCES

Abel, E.L., Kruger, M., & Burd, L. (2002). Effects of maternal and paternal age on caucasian and Native American preterm births and birth weights. *American Journal of Perinatology, 19*, (1), 49–54.

ACOG Educational Bulletin. (1998, July). Viral hepatitis in pregnancy. No. 248. Washington, DC: American College of Obstetricians and Gynecologists.

ACOG Practice Bulletin. (1999, October). Management of herpes in pregnancy. No. 8. October. Washington, DC: American College of Obstetricians and Gynecologists.

ACOG Practice Bulletin. (2000a, July). The use of hormonal contraception in women with coexisting medical conditions. No. 18. Washington, DC: American College of Obstetricians and Gynecologists.

ACOG Practice Bulletin. (2000b, September). Perinatal Viral and Parasitic Infections. No. 20. Washington, DC: American College of Obstetricians and Gynecologists.

ACOG Practice Bulletin. (2001a, October). Assessment of risk factors for preterm birth. No. 31. Washington, DC: American College of Obstetricians and Gynecologists.

ACOG Practice Bulletin. (2001b, July). Chronic hypertension in pregnancy. No. 29. Washington, DC: American College of Obstetricians and Gynecologists.

ACOG Practice Bulletin. (2001c, September). Diabetes and pregnancy. No. 30. Washington, DC: American College of Obstetricians and Gynecologists.

ACOG Practice Bulletin. (2002, January). Diagnosis and management of preeclampsia and eclampsia. No. 33. Washington, DC: American College of Obstetricians and Gynecologists.

ACOG Technical Bulletin. (1996, February) Hemoglobinopathies in pregnancy. No. 220. Washington, DC: American College of Obstetricians and Gynecologists.

ACOG Today. (1999). Maternal mortality: No improvement since 1982. American College of Obstetricians and Gynecologists. 43 (7) 1, 6–7.

Allard-Henderson, R. (2000). Alcohol use and adolescent pregnancy. *American Journal of Maternal/Child Nursing, 25* (3), 159–162.

Ananth, C.V., Smulian, J.C., Demissie, K., Vintzileos, A.M., & Knuppel, R.A. (2001). Placental abruption among singleton and twin births in the United States: Risk factor profile. *American Journal of Epidemiology, 153* (8), 771–778.

Attard, C.L., Kohli, M.A., Coleman, S., Bradley, C., Hux, M., Atanackovic, G., & Torrance, G.W. (2002). The burden of illness of severe nausea and vomiting of pregnancy in the United States. *American Journal of Obstetrics and Gynecology, 185* (Supple), 220–227.

Baker, E.R., Beach M.L., Craigo, S.D., Harvey-Wilkes, K.B., & D'Alton, M.E. (1997). A comparison of neonatal outcomes of age-matched, growth-restricted twins and growth-restricted singletons. *American Journal of Perinatology, 14* (8), 499–502.

Bai, J., Wong, F.W.S., Bauman, A., & Mohsin, M. (2002). Parity and pregnancy outcomes. *American Journal of Obstetrics & Gynecology, 186,* 274–278.

Ballard, T.J., Saltzman, L.E., Gazmararian, J.A., Spitz, A.M., Lazorick, S., & Marks, J.S., (1998). Violence during pregnancy: Measurement issues. *American Journal of Public Health, 88* (2), 274–276.

Bauer, C.R. (1999). Perinatal effects on prenatal drug exposure. *Clinics in Perinatology, 26* (1), 87–104.

Bayoumeu, F., Subiran-Buisset, C., Baka, N.E., Legagneur, H., Monnier-Barbarino, M., & Laxenaire, M.C. (2002). Iron therapy in iron deficiency anemia in pregnancy: Intravenous route versus oral route. *American Journal of Obstetrics and Gynecology, 186* (3), 518–522.

Barton, C.B., Barton, J.R., O'Brien, J.M., Bergauer, N.K., & Sibai, B.M. (2002). Mild gestational hypertension: Differences in ethnicity are associated with altered outcomes in women who undergo outpatient treatment. *American Journal of Obstetrics* and Gynecology, *186,* 896–898.

Beazley, D.M., & Egerman, R.S. (1998). Toxoplasmosis. *Seminars in Perinatology, 22* (4), 332–338.

Bergeron, M.G., Ke, D., Menard, C., Picard, F.J., Gagnon, M., Bernier, M., Quellette, M., Roy, P.H., Marcoux, S., & Fraser, W.D. (2000). Rapid detection of group B streptococci in pregnant women at delivery. *The New England Journal of Medicine, 343* (3), 175–179.

Berkowitz, R.S., Tuncer, Z.S., Bernstein, M.R., & Goldstein, D.P. (2000). Management of gestational trophoblastic diseases: Subsequent pregnancy experience. *Seminars in Oncology, 6,* 678–685.

Bishai, R., & Koren, G. (1999). Maternal and obstetric effects of prenatal drug exposure. *Clinics in Perinatology, 26,* 75–86.

Black, F.O. (2002). Maternal susceptibility to nausea and vomiting of pregnancy: Is the vestibular system involved? *American Journal of Obstetricics and Gynecology, 185* (Supple), 204–209.

Blickstein, I. (1997). Maternal mortality in twin gestations. *The Journal of Reproductive Medicine, 42* (11), 680–684.

Blickstein, I., Goldman, R.D., & Mazkereth, R. (2000). Risk for one or two very low birth weight twins: A population study. *Obstetrics and Gynecology, 96* (3), 400–402.

Botto, L.D., Moore, C.A., Khoury, M.J., & Erickson, J.D. (1999). Neural-tube defects. *The New England Journal of Medicine, 341,* 1509–1519.

Bovo, C. (2001). Adjustment to chronic illness among HIV-infected women. *Journal of Nursing Scholarship, 33* (3), 21223.

Brown, H.L., & Abernathy, M.P. (1998). Cytomegalovirus infection. *Seminars in Perinatology, 22* (4), 260–266.

Buchbinder, A., Sibai, B.M., Caritis, S., MacPherson, C., Hauth, J., Lindheimer, M.D., et al. (2002). Adverse perinatal outcomes are significantly higher in severe gestational hypertension than in mild preeclampsia. *American Journal of Obstetrics and Gynecology, 186,* 66–71.

Buckwalter, J.G., & Simpson, S.W. (2002). Psychological factors in the etiology and treatment of severe nausea and vomiting in pregnancy. *American Journal of Obstetrics and Gynecology, 186* (Supple), 210–214.

Bukowski, R., & Saade, G.R. (2000). Hydrops fetalis. *Clinics in Perinatology, 27* (4), 1010–1031.

Burst, H.V. (1998). Sexually transmitted diseases and reproductive health in women. *Journal of Nurse-Midwifery, 43* (6), 431–444.

Campbell, D.M., & MacGillivray, I. (1999). Preeclampsia in twin pregnancies: Incidence and outcome. *Hypertension in Pregnancy, 183,* 197–201.

Carpenter, M.W. (2000). The role of exercise in pregnant women with diabetes mellitus. *Clinical Obstetrics and Gynecology, 43* (1), 56–64.

CDC. (1998). Use of folic acid-containing supplements among women of childbearing age—United States, 1997. *MMWR, 47* (47), 131–134.

CDC. (2000a). Early-onset group B streptococcal disease—United States, 1998–1999. *MMWR, 49* (35), 793–797.

CDC. (2000b). Hospital-based policies for prevention of perinatal group B streptococcal disease—United States, 1999. *MMWR, 49* (41), 936–940.

CDC. (2000c). State-specific changes in singleton preterm births among black and white women—United States, 1990 and 1997. *MMWR, 49* (37), 837–840.

CDC. (2001a). Births: Final data for 1999. *National Vital Statistics Reports, 49* (1), 1–3.

CDC. (2001b). Control and prevention of rubella: Evaluation and management of suspected outbreaks, rubella in pregnant women, and surveillance for congenital rubella syndrome. *MMWR, 50,* (N. RR-12), 1–23.

CDC. (2002a). Alcohol use among women of childbearing age—United States, 1991–1999. *MMWR, 51* (13), 273–276.

CDC. (2002b). Semiannual HIV/AIDS surveillance report, 13 (2). (Dec. 31, 2001). Retrieved Dec. 31, 2002 from www.cdc.gov/hiv/stats/htm.

CDC. (2002c). Sexually transmitted diseases treatment guidelines. *MMWR, 51,* 1–78.

Chandran, L., Navaie-Waliser, M., Zulqarni, N.J., Batra, S., Bayir, H., Shah, M., & Lincoln, P. (2001). Compliance with group B streptococcal disease prevention guidelines. *American Journal of Maternal/Child Nursing, 26* (6), 313–319.

Chapman, S.J. (1998). Varicella in pregnancy. *Seminars in Perinatology, 22* (4), 339–346.

Chasen, S.T., Loeb-Zeitlin, S., & Landsberger, E.J. (1999). Hemoglobinopathy screening in pregnancy: Comparison of two protocols. *American Journal of Perinatology, 16* (4), 175–180.

Chung, T.K., Lee, D.T.S., Cheung, L.P., Haines, C.J., & Chang, A.M.Z. (1999). Spontaneous abortion: A randomized, controlled trial comparing surgical evacuation with conservative management using misoprostol. *Fertility and Sterility, 71* (6), 1054–1059.

Conde-Agudelo, A., & Belizan, J. (2000). Maternal morbidity and mortality associated with interpregnancy interval: Cross sectional study. *British Medical Journal, 321,* 1255–1259.

Coomarasamy, A., Papaioannou, S., Gee, H., & Khan, K.S. (2001). Aspirin for the prevention of preeclampsia in women with abnormal uterine artery doppler: A meta-analysis. *Obstetrics and Gynecology, 98,* 861–866.

Corrarino, J.E., Williams, C., Campbell, W.S., Amrhein, E., LoPiano, L., & Kalachik, D. (2000). Linking substance-abusing pregnant women to drug treatment services: A pilot program. *Journal of Obstetric, Gynecologic, and Neonatal Nursing, 29,* 369–376.

Cosden, M., & Cortez-Ison, E. (1999). Sexual abuse, parental bonding, social support, and program retention for women in substance abuse treatment. *Journal of Substance Abuse Treatment, 16* (2), 149–155.

Cottrell, B.H., & Carter, C. (1998). Health care professionals: Have you had the chicken pox? *AWHONN Lifelines, 2* (4), 33–38.

Coustan, D.R. (2000). Making the diagnosis of gestational diabetes mellitus. *Clinical Obstetrics and Gynecology, 43* (1), 99–105.

Crane, J.M.G., Van den Hof, M.C., Dodds, L., Armson, B.A., & Liston, R. (2000). Maternal complications with placenta previa. *American Journal of Perinatology, 17* (2), 101–105.

Cunningham, E. (2001). Coping with bed rest. *AWHONN Lifelines, 5* (5), 51–55.

Cunningham, F.G., Gant, N.F., Leveno, K.J., Gilstrap, L.C., Hauth, J.C., & Wenstrom, K.D. (2001). *Williams obstetrics* (21st ed.). New York: McGraw-Hill.

Damato, E.G., & Winnen, C.W. (2002). Cytomegalovirus infections: Perinatal implications. *Journal of Obstetric, Gynecologic, and Neonatal Nursing, 31* (10), 86–92.

Day, S.W., & Wynn, L.W. (2000). Sickle cell pain and hydrooxyurea. *American Journal of Nursing, 100* (11), 34–39.

Dickey, R.P., Taylor, S.N., Lu, P.Y., Sartor, B.M., Storment, J.M., Rye, P.H., et al. (2002). Spontaneous reduction of multiple pregnancy: Incidence and effect on outcome. *American Journal of Obstetrics and Gynecology, 186* (1), 77–82.

Dillman, C.M. (1999). Hepatitis C: A danger to healthcare workers. *Nursing Forum, 34,* 23–28.

Dixon, L. (1997). The complete blood count: Physiologic basis and clinical usage. *Journal of Perinatology and Neonatology Nursing, 11* (3), 1–18.

Dole, P.J. (2001). Primary care of HPV management in HIV-infected women. *Nurse Practitioner Forum, 12* (4), 214–222.

Donahue, D.B. (2002). Diagnosis and treatment of herpes simplex infection during pregnancy. *Journal of Obstetric, Gynecologic, and Neonatal Nursing, 31* (1), 99–106.

Duff, P. (1998). Hepatitis in pregnancy. *Seminars in Perinatology, 22* (4), 277–283.

Egelko, S., Galanteer, M., Dermatis, H., & DeMaio, C. (1998) Evaluation of a multisystems model for treating perinatal cocaine addiction. *Journal of Substance Abuse Treatment, 15* (3), 251–259.

Ehrmin, J.T. (2001). Unresolved feelings of guilt and shame in the maternal role with substance-dependent African American women. *Journal of Nursing Scholarship, 33* (1), 47–52.

Esch, J.F., & Frank, S.V. (2001). HIV drug resistance and nursing practice. *American Journal of Nursing, 101* (6), 30–35.

Eyler, F.D., & Behnke, M. (1999). Early development of infants exposed to drugs prenatally. *Clinics in Perinatology, 26* (1), 107–143.

Feudtner, C., & Gabbe, S.G. (2000). Diabetes and pregnancy: Four motifs of modern medical history. *Clinical Obstetrics and Gynecology, 43* (1), 4–16.

Flake, K.J. (2000). HIV testing during pregnancy. *AWHONN Lifelines, 4* (1), 13–16.

Folley, E.M. (2002). Drug screening and criminal prosecution of pregnant women. *Journal of Obstetric, Gynecologic, and Neonatal Nursing, 31* (2), 133–137.

Fox, R., Pillai, M., Porter, H., & Gill, G. (1997, November/December). The management of late fetal death: A guide to comprehensive care. *Neonatal Intensive Care,* 56–66.

Frank, S., Esch, J.F., & Margeson, N.E. (1998). HIV mandatory testing of newborns: The impact on women. *American Journal of Nursing, 98* (10), 49–51.

Furneaux, E.C., Langley-Evans, A.J., & Langley-Evans, S.C. (2001). Nausea and vomiting of pregnancy: Endocrine basis and contribution to pregnancy outcome. *Obstetrics and Gynecology Survey, 56* (12), 775–782.

Gilstrap III, L.C., & Ramin, S.M. (2001). Urinary tract infections during pregnancy. *Obstetrics and Gynecology Clinics of North America, 28* (3), 581–591.

Glueck, C.J., Wang, P., Goldenberg, N., Sieve-Smith, L. (2002). Pregnancy outcomes among women with polycystic ovarian syndrome treated with metformin. *Human Reproduction, 17* (11), 2858–2864.

Goldenberg, R.L. (1998). *Low birthweight in minority and high-risk women.* Patient Outcomes Research Team (PORT) Final Report. AHCPR Pub. No. 98-N005.

Goodwin, T.M. (2002). Nausea and vomiting of pregnancy: An obstetric syndrome. *American Journal of Obstetrics and Gynecology, 185* (Supple), 184–189.

Grason, H., Hutchins, J., & Silver, G. (Eds.). (1999). *Charting a course for the future of women's and perinatal health.* Timonium, MD: Printing Corporation of America.

Gratacos, E., Casals, E. Gomez, O., Aibar, C., Cararach, V. Alonso, P.L., & Fortuny, A. (2000). Inhibin A serum levels in proteinuric and nonproteinuric pregnancy-induced hypertension: Evidence for placental involvement in gestational hypertension? *Hypertension in Pregnancy, 19* (3), 315–321.

Gupton, A., Heaman, M., & Cheung, L.W.K. (2001). Complicated and uncomplicated pregnancies: Women's perception of risk. *Journal of Obstetric, Gynecologic, and Neonatal Nursing, 30* (2), 192–201.

Guyer, B., Hoyert, D.L., Martin, J.A., Ventrua, S.J., MacDorman, M.F., & Strobino, D.M. (1999). Annual summary of vital statistics—1998. *Pediatrics, 104* (6), 1229–1246.

Hackley, B.K. (1999). Immunizations in pregnancy. *Journal of Nurse-Midwifery, 44* (2), 106–117.

Haller, D.L., Knisely, J.S. Elswick, R.K., Dawson, K.S., & Schnoll, S.H. (1997). Perinatal substance abusers: Factors influencing treatment retention. *Journal of Substance Abuse Treatment, 14* (6), 513–519.

Hanley, M., Ananth, C.V., Shen-Schwarz, S., Smulian, J.C., Lai, Y.L., & Vintzileos, A.M. (2002). Placental cord insertion and birth weight discordancy in twin gestations. *Obstetrics and Gynecology, 99,* 477–482.

Head, B.B., Owen, J., Vincent, R.D., Shih, G., Chestnut, D.H., & Hauth, J.C. (2002). A randomized trial of intrapartum analgesia in women with severe preeclampsia. *Obstetrics and Gynecology, 99,* 452–457.

Heaman, M.I., Sprague, A.E., & Stewart, P.J. (2001). Reducing the preterm rate: A population health strategy. *Journal of Obstetric, Gynecologic, and Neonatal Nursing, 30,* 20–29.

Heinrichs, L. (2002). Linking olfaction with nausea and vomiting of pregnancy, recurrent abortion, hyperemsis gravidarum, and migraine. *American Journal of Obstetrics and Gynecology, 185* (Supple), 215–219.

Henderson-Martin, B. (2000). No more surprises: Screening patients for alcohol abuse. *American Journal of Nursing, 100* (9), 27–32.

Hick, J.L., Rodgerson, J.D., Heegaard, W.G., & Sterner, S. (2001). Vital signs fail to correlate with hemoperitoneum from ruptured ectopic pregnancy. *American Journal of Emergency Medicine, 19* (6), 488–491.

Hollier, L.M., & Cox, S.M. (1998). Syphilis. *Seminars in Perinatology, 22* (4), 323–331.

Holzemer, W.L. (2002). HIV and AIDS: The symptom experience. *American Journal of Nursing, 102* (4), 48–52.

Honein, M.A., Paulozzi, L.J., Mathews, J.J., Erickson, J.D., & Wong, L.Y.C. (2001). Impact of folic acid fortification of the U.S. food supply on the occurrence of neural tube defects. *Journal of the American Medical Association, 285* (23), 2981–2986.

Howell, E.M., & Chasnoff, I.J. (1999). Perinatal substance abuse treatment findings from focus groups with clients and providers. *Journal of Substance Abuse Treatment, 17* (1–2), 139–148.

Howell, E.M., Heiser, N., & Harrington, M. (1999). A review of recent findings on substance abuse treatment for pregnant women. *Journal of Substance Abuse Treatment, 16* (3), 195–219.

Iams, J.D., Newman, R.B., Thom, E.A., Goldenberg, R.L., Mueller-Heubach, E., Moawad, A., et al. (2002). Frequency of uterine contractions and the risk of spontaneous preterm delivery. *The New England Journal of Medicine, 346* (4), 250–255.

Illsley, N.P. (2000). Placental glucose transport in diabetes pregnancy. *Clinical Obstetrics and Gynecology, 43* (1), 116–126.

Institute of Medicine (IOM). (1998). *Reducing the odds: Preventing perinatal transmission of HIV in the United States.* Washington, DC: National Academy Press.

Janke, J. (1999). The effect of relaxation therapy on preterm labor outcomes. *Journal of Obstetric, Gynecologic, & Neonatal Nursing, 28,* 255–263.

Joseph, H., Stancliff, S., & Langrod, J. (2000). Methadone maintenance treatment (MMT): A review of historical and clinical issues. *Mt. Sinai Journal of Medicine, 67,* 347–364.

Josten, L., Wedeking, L., Block, D.E., Savisk, K., & Vincent, P. (1997). Linking high-risk, low-income, pregnant women to public health services. *Journal of Public Health Management Practice, 3* (2), 27–36.

Jovanovic, L. (2000). Role of diet and insulin treatment of diabetes in pregnancy. *Clinical Obstetrics and Gynecology, 43* (1), 46–55.

Katz, A. (2001). HIV screening in pregnancy: What women think. *Journal of Obstetric, Gynecologic, and Neonatal Nursing, 30* (2), 184–191.

Keith, L., & Oleszczuk, J.J. (1999). Iatrogenic multiple birth, multiple pregnancy and assisted reproductive technologies. *International Journal of Gynecology and Obstetrics, 64,* 11–25.

Kjos, S.L. (2000). Postpartum care of the woman with diabetes. *Clinical Obstetrics and Gynecology, 43* (1), 75–86.

Klebanoff, M.A., Carey, J.C., Hauth, J.C., Hillier, S., Nugent, R.P., Thom, E.A., Ernest, J.M., Heine, R.P., Warner, R.J., Trout, W., Moawad, A., & Leveno, K.J. (2001). Failure of metronidazole to prevent preterm delivery among pregnant women with asymptomatic *Trichomonas vaginalis* infection. *New England Journal of Medicine, 345* (7), 487–493.

Knerr, I., Beinder, E., & Rascher, W. (2002). Syncytin, a novel human endogenous retroviral gene in human placenta: Evidence for its dysregulation in preeclampsia and HELLP syndrome. *American Journal of Obstetrics and Gynecology, 196,* 210–213.

Koch, K.L. (2002). Gastrointestinal factors in nausea and vomiting of pregnancy. *American Journal of Obstetrics and Gynecology, 185* (Supple), 198–203.

Koga, M., Matsuoka, T., Katayama, K., Takeda, K., Nakata, M., Sase, M., et al. (2001). Human parvovirus B19 in cord blood of premature infants. *American Journal of Perinatology, 18* (5), 237–240.

Koniak-Griffin, D., Anderson, N.L.R., Verzemnieks, I., & Brecht, M.L., (2000). A public health nursing early intervention program for adolescent mothers: Outcomes from pregnancy through 6 weeks postpartum. *Nursing Research, 29* (3), 130–138.

Koonin, L.M., MacKay, A.P., Berg, C.J., Atrash, H.K., & Smith, J.C. (1997). Pregnancy-related mortality surveillance—United States, 1987–1990. *MMWR, 46,* 17–36.

Koren, G., Boskovic, R., Hard, M., Maltepe, C. Navioz, Y., & Einarson, A. (2002). Motherisk-PUQE (pregnancy-unique quantification of emesis and nausea) scoring system for nausea and vomiting of pregnancy. *American Journal of Obstetrics and Gynecology, 185* (Supple), 228–231.

Koren, G., & Levichek, Z. (2002). The teratogenicity of drugs for nausea and vomiting of pregnancy: Perceived versus true risk. *American Journal of Obstetrics and Gynecology, 185* (Supple), 248–252.

Koshy, M. (1999). Sickle cell disease and pregnancy. *Hematology, American Society of Hematology,* 33–38.

Krause, S.A., & Graves, B.W. (1999). Midwifery triage of first trimester bleeding. *Journal of Nurse-Midwifery, 44* (6), 537–548.

Lan, Z., Hongzhao S., Xiuyu, Y., & Yang, X. (2001). Pregnancy outcomes of patients who conceived within 1 year after chemotherapy for gestational trophoblastic tumor: A clinical report of 22 patients. *Gynecology Oncology, 83*(1), 46–48.

Landon, M.B. (2000). Obstetric management of pregnancies complicated by diabetes mellitus. *Clinical Obstetrics and Gynecology, 43* (1), 65–74.

Langer, O. (2000). Management of gestational diabetes. *Clinical Obstetrics and Gynecology, 43* (1), 106–115.

Lansky, A., Jones, J.L., Frey, R.L., & Lindegren, M.L. (2001). Trends in HIV testing among women: United States, 1994–1999. *American Journal of Public Health, 91* (8), 1291–1293.

Lindeberg, S.N., & Hanson, U. (2000). Hypertension and factors associated with metabolic syndrome at follow-up at 15 years in women with hypertensive disease during first pregnancy. *Hypertension in Pregnancy, 19* (2), 191–198.

Lindenberg, C.S., Solorzano, R.M., Krantz, M.S., Galvis, C., Baroni, G., & Strickland, O. (1998). Risk and resilience: Building protective factors. *American Maternal/Child Health Nursing, 23* (2), 99–104.

Lowry, L.M., Hays, B.J., Lopez, P., & Hernandez, G. (1998). Care paths: A new approach to high-risk maternal-child home visitation. *MCN 23* (6), 322–328.

Lu, G.C., & Goldenberg, R.L. (2000). Current concepts on the pathogenesis and markers of preterm births. *Clinics in Perinatology, 27* (2), 263–283.

Luciano, A.A., Roy, G., & Solima, E. (2001). Ectopic pregnancy from surgical emergency to medical management. *Annals of New York Academy of Science, 943,* 235–254.

Lynch, A., McDuffie, R., Murphy, J., Faber, K., & Orleans, M. (2002). Preeclampsia in multiple gestation: The role of assisted reproductive technologies. *Obstetrics and Gynecology, 99* (3), 445–451.

Lyon, D.E., & Younger, J.B. (2001). Purpose in Life and Depressive Symptoms in Persons Living with HIV Disease. Journal of Nursing Scholarship. 33(2), 129–133.

MacNeill, S., Dodds, L., Hamilton, D.C., Armson, B.A., & VandenHof, M. (2001). Rates and risk factors for recurrence of gestational diabetes. *Diabetes Care, 24,* 659–662.

Magann, E., Evans, S.F., Weitz, B., & Newman, J. (2002). Antepartum, intrapartum, and neonatal significance of exercise on healthy low-risk pregnant working women. *Obstetrics and Gynecology, 99,* 466–472.

Maloni, J.A. (2000). Preventing preterm birth. *AWHONN Lifelines, 4* (4), 26–33.

Maloni, J.A., Brezinski-Tomasi, J.E., & Johnson, L.A. (2001) Antepartum bed rest: Effect upon the family. *Journal of Obstetric, Gynecologic, and Neonatal Nursing, 30* (2), 165–173.

Maloni, J.A., & Kutil, R.M. (2000). Antepartum support group for women hospitalized on bed rest. *American Journal of Maternal/Child Nursing, 25* (4), 204–210.

Many, A., Schreiber, L., Rosner, S., Lessing, J.B., Eldor, A., & Kupferminc, M.J. (2001). Pathologic features of the placenta in women with severe pregnancy complications and thrombophilia. *Obstetrics & Gynecology, 98,* 1041–1044.

Marin, R., Gorostidi, M., Portal, C.G., Sanchez, M., Sanchez, E., & Alvarez, J. (2000). Long-term prognosis of hypertension in pregnancy. *Hypertension in Pregnancy, 19* (2), 199–209.

Markenson, G.R., & Yancey, M.K. (1998). Parvovirus B19 in pregnancy. *Seminars in Perinatology, 22* (4), 309–317.

Mashburn, J. (1999). Ectopic pregnancy: Triage do's and don'ts. *Journal of Nurse-Midwifery, 44* (6), 549–557.

Mauldin, J.G., & Newman, R.B. (2001). Preterm birth risk assessment. *Seminars in Perinatology, 25* (4), 215–222.

McCarter-Spaulding, D. (2002). Parvovirus B19 in pregnancy. *Journal of Obstetric, Gynecology, and Neonatal Nursing, 31* (1), 107–112.

McCormick, M.C., & Siegel, J.E. (Eds.). (1999). *Prenatal care effectiveness and implementation.* Cambridge, UK: Cambridge University Press

McKenna, D.S., & Iams, J.D. (1998). Group B streptococcal infections. *Seminars in Perinatology, 22* (4), 267–276.

McMahon, M.J., Li, R., Schenck, A.P., Olshan, A.F., & Royce, R.A. (1997). Previous cesarean birth. A risk factor for placenta previa? *The Journal of Reproductive Medicine, 42,* 409–412.

Miller, F. (2002). Nausea and vomiting in pregnancy: The problem of perception—is it really a disease? *American Journal of Obstetrics and Gynecology, 185* (Supple), 182–183.

Mills, J.L., & England, L. (2001). Food fortification to prevent neural tube defects. *Journal of the American Medical Association, 285*(23), 3022–3023.

Minnick-Smith, K., & Cook, F. (1997). Current treatment options for ectopic pregnancy. *American Journal of Maternal/ Child Nursing, 22,* 21–25.

Misra, D.P., Grason, H., & Weisman, C. (2000). An intersection of women's and perinatal health: The role of chronic conditions. *Women's Health Issues, 10* (5), 256–266.

Mitchell, A., Steffenson, N., Hogan, H., & Brooks, S. (1997). Neonatal group B streptococcal disease. *American Journal of Maternal/Child Nursing, 22,* 249–253.

Mitchell, R. (1999). Sickle cell anemia. *American Journal of Nursing, 99,* 36.

Moore, M. (1999). Reproductive health and intimate partner violence. *Family Planning Perspectives, 31* (6), 302–312.

Moore, M.L., & Freda, M.C. (1998). Reducing preterm and low birthweight births: Still a nursing challenge. *American Journal of Maternal/Child Nursing, 23* (4), 200–208.

Mullaney, D.M. (2001). Group B streptococcal infections in newborns. *Journal of Obstetric, Gynecologic, and Neonatal Nursing, 30* (6), 649–658.

Naim, A., Haberman, S., Burgess, T., Navizedeh, N., & Minkoff, H. (2002). Changes in cervical length and the risk of preterm labor. *American Journal of Obstetrics and Gynecology, 186,* 887–889.

Nelson, D.B., Ness, R.B., Grisso, J.A., & Cushman, M. (2001). Influence of hemostatic factors on spontaneous abortion. *American Journal of Perinatology, 18* (4), 195–201.

Newshan, G., & Holt, M.J. (1998). Use of combination antiretroviral therapy in pregnant women with HIV disease. *American Journal of Maternal/Child Health, 23* (6), 307–312.

Niebyl, J.R., & Goodwin, T.M. (2002). Overview of nausea and vomiting of pregnancy with an emphasis on vitamins and ginger. *American Journal of Obstetrics and Gynecology, 185* (Suppl), 253–255.

Norwitz, E.R., & Robinson, J.N. (2001) A systematic approach to the management of preterm labor. *Seminars in Perinatology, 25* (4), 223–235.

Ondersma, S.J., Simpson, S.M., Brestan, E.V., & Ward, M. (2000). Prenatal drug exposure and social policy: The search for an appropriate response. *Child Maltreatment, 5* (2), 93–108.

Paige, D.M., Augustyn, M., Adih, W.K., Witter, F., & Chang, J. (1998). Bacterial vaginosis and preterm birth: A comprehensive review of the literature. *Journal of Nurse-Midwifery, 43* (2), 83–89.

Pearlman, M.D., Klinich, K.D., Schneider, L.W., Rupp, J., Moss, S., & Ashton-Miller, J. (2000). A comprehensive program to improve safety for pregnant women and fetuses in motor vehicle crashes: A preliminary report. *American Journal of Obstetrics and Gynecology, 182,* 1554–1564.

Persad, V.L., Baskett, T.F., O'Connell, C.M., & Scott, H.M. (2001). Combined vaginal-cesarean delivery of twin pregnancies. *Obstetrics and Gynecology, 98,* 1032–1037.

Psihogios, V., Rodda, C., Reid, E., Clark, M., Clarke, C., & Bowden, D. (2002). Reproductive health in individuals with homozygous B-thalassemia: Knowledge, attitudes, and behavior. *Fertility and Sterility, 77* (1), 119–127.

Public Health Service Task Force (PHSTF). (2002, February 4). *Recommendations for use of antiretroviral drugs in pregnant HIV—1-infected women for maternal health and interventions to reduce perinatal HIV-1 transmission in the United States.* Washington, DC: Author.

Reece, E.A., & Homko, C.J. (2000). Why do diabetic women deliver malformed infants? *Clinical Obstetrics and Gynecology, 43* (1), 32–45.

Rees, H.C., & Paradinas, F.J. (2001). The diagnosis of hydatiform mole in early tubal ectopic pregnancy. *Histopathology, 38* (5), 409–417.

Riskin-Mashiah, S., Belfort, M.A., Saade, G.R., & Herd, J.A. (2001). Cerebrovascular reactivity in normal pregnancy and preeclampsia. *Obstetrics and Gynecology, 98,* 827–832.

Roach, V.J., Hin, L.Y., Tam, W.H., Ng, K.B., & Rogers, M.S. (2000). The incidence of pregnancy-induced hypertension among patients with carbohydrate intolerance. *Hypertension in Pregnancy, 19* (2), 183–189.

Robinson, J.N., Regan, J.A., & Norwitz, E.R. (2001) The epidemiology of preterm labor. *Seminars in Perinatology, 25* (4), 204–214.

Rosa, C. (1998). Rubella and rubeola. *Seminars in Perinatology, 22* (4), 318–322.

Rosenn, B.M., & Miodovnik, M. (2000). Medical complications of diabetes mellitus in pregnancy. *Clinical Obstetrics and Gynecology, 43* (1), 17–31.

Royce, R.A., Walter, E.B., Fernandez, M.I., Wilson, T.E., Ickovics, J.R., & Simonds, R.J. (2001). Barriers to universal prenatal HIV testing in 4 U.S. locations in 1997. *American Journal of Public Health, 91* (5), 727–733.

Ruiz, J.D., & Molitor, F. (1998). Knowledge of treatment to reduce perinatal human Immunodeficiency Virus (HIV) transmission and likelihood of testing for HIV: Results from two surveys of women of childbearing age. *Maternal and Child Health Journal, 2* (2), 117–122.

Ruiz, R.J., Brown, C.E., Peters, M.T., & Johnston, A.B. (2001). Specialized care for twin gestations: Improving newborn outcomes and reducing costs. *Journal of Obstetric, Gynecologic, and Neonatal Nursing, 30* (1), 52–60.

Savitz, D.A., Henderson, L., Dole, N., Herring, A., Wilkins, D.G., Rollins, D., & Thorp, J.M. (2002). Indicators of cocaine exposure and preterm birth. *Obstetrics and Gynecology, 99* (3), 458–465.

Schieve, L.A., Meikle, S.F., Ferre, C., Peterson, H.B., Jeng, G., & Wilcox, L.S. (2002). Low and very low birth weight in infants conceived with use of assisted reproductive technology. *The New England Journal of Medicine, 346* (10), 731–737.

Schrag, S.J., Zywicki, S., Farley, M.M., Reingold, A.L., Harrison, L.H., Lefkowitz, L.B., Hadler, J.L., Danila, R., Cieslak, P.R., & Schuchat, A. (2000). Group B streptococcal disease in the era of intrapartum antibiotic prophylaxis. *The New England Journal of Medicine, 342* (1), 15–20.

Schroeder, C.A. (1998). Bed rest in complicated pregnancy. *The American Journal of Maternal/Child Nursing, 23,* 45–49.

Seoud, M.A.F., Nassar, A.H., Usta, I.M., Melhem, Z., Kazma, A., & Khalil, A.M. (2002). Impact of advanced maternal age on pregnancy outcome. *American Journal of Perinatology, 19* (1), 1–7.

Sheridan, E., Aitken, C., Jeffries, D., Hird, M., & Thayalesekaran, P. (2002). Congenital rubella syndrome: A risk in immigrant populations. *The Lancet, 359,* 674–675.

Shieh, C., & Kravitz, M. (2002). Maternal-fetal attachment in pregnant women who use illicit drugs. *Journal of Obstetric, Gynecologic, and Neonatal Nursing, 31,* 156–164.

Sinclair, B.P. (1999). The dilemma of HIV in women. *AWHONN Lifelines, 3* (2), 9–10.

Smith, C., Crowther, C., & Beilby, J. (2002). Acupuncture to treat nausea and vomiting in early pregnancy: A randomized controlled trial. *Birth, 29,* 1–9.

Steele, N.M., French, J., Gatherer-Boyles, J., Newman, S., & Leclaire, S. (2001). Effect of acupressure by sea-bands on nausea and vomiting of pregnancy. *Journal of Obstetric, Gynecologic, and Neonatal Nursing, 30* (1), 61–70.

Stringer, E.M., Stringer, J.S.A., Cliver, S.P., Goldenberg, R.L., & Goepfert, A.R. (2001). Evaluation of a new testing policy for Human Immunodeficiency Virus to improve screening rates. *Obstetrics and Gynecology, 98,* 1104–1108.

Swaim, L.S., Perriatt, S., Andres, R.L., Paradissis, J., & Watson, M.N. (1999). Clinical utility of routine postpartum hemoglobin determinations. *American Journal of Perinatology, 16* (7), 333–337.

Swain, R.A., & St. Clair, L. (1997). The role of folic acid in deficiency states and prevention of disease. *The Journal of Family Practice, 44* (2), 138–144.

Swanson, K. (1999). Effects of caring, measurement, and time on miscarriage impact and women's well-being. *Nursing Research, 48* (6), 288–298.

Telen, M.J. (2001). Principles and problems of transfusion in sickle cell disease. *Seminars in Hematology, 38* (4), 315–323.

Terrone, D.A., Rinehart, B.K., May, W.L., Martin, R.W., & Martin, J.N. (2001). The myth of transient hypertension: Descriptor or disease process? *American Journal of Perinatology, 18* (2), 73–77.

Tiller, C.M. (2002). Chlamydia during pregnancy: Implications and impact on perinatal and neonatal outcomes. *Journal of Obstetric, Gynecologic, and Neonatal Nursing, 31* (1), 93–98.

Tinkle, M. (1997). Folic acid and food fortification: Implications for the primary care practitioner. *The Nurse Practitioner, 22* (3), 105–114.

Tinkle, M.B., & Sterling, B.S. (1997). Neural tube defects: A primary prevention role for nurses. *Journal of Ostetric, Gynecologic, and Neonatal Nursing, 26* (5), 503–512.

Towers, G.V., Pircon, R.A., & Heppard, M. (1999). Is tocolysis safe in the management of third-trimester bleeding? *American Journal Obstetrics and Gynecology, 180,* 1572–1578.

Tronick, E., & Beeghly, M. (1999). Prenatal cocaine exposure child development, and the compromising effects of cumulative risk. *Clinics in Perinatology, 26* (1), 151–167.

Urbanski, P. (1997). How does hydration affect preterm labor? *AWHONN Lifelines, 1* (3), 25.

U.S. Department of Health and Human Services. (1998). *Low birthweight in minority and high-risk women. Patient Outcomes Research Team (PORT) final report.* AHCPR Pub. No. 98-N005. Rockville, MD: Author.

Uvena-Celebrezze, J., & Catalano, P.M. (2000) The infant of the woman with gestational diabetes mellitus. *Clinical Obstetrics and Gynecology, 43* (1), 127–139.

Vatten, L.J., Odegard, R.A., Nilsen, S.T., Salvesen, K.A., & Austgulen, R. (2002). Relationship of insulin-like growth factor-1 and insulin-like growth factor binding proteins in umbilical cord plasma to preeclampsia and infant birth weight. *Obstetrics and Gynecology, 99,* 85–90.

Ventura, S.J., Martin, J.A., Curtin, S.C., Menacker, F., & Hamilton, B.E. (2001). Births: Final data for 1999. *National Vital Statistics Reports, 49* (1), 1–4.

Vintzileos, A.M., Ananth, C.V., Smulian, J.C., Scorza, W.E., & Knuppel, R.A. (2002). Prenatal care and black-white fetal death disparity in the United States: Heterogeneity by high-risk conditions. *Obstetrics and Gynecology, 99,* 483–489.

Warner, B.B., Kiely, J.L., & Donovan, E.F. (2000). Multiple births and outcome. *Clinics in Perinatology, 27* (2), 347–361.

Washington, O.G.M. (2000). Effects of group therapy on chemically dependent women's self-efficacy. *Journal of Nursing Scholarship, 32* (4), 347–352

Watson-Blasioli, J. (2001). Double-take. *AWHONN Lifelines, 5* (2), 34–42,

Weiss, M.E., Saks, N.P., & Harris, S. (2002). Resolving the uncertainty of preterm symptoms: Women's experiences with the onset of preterm labor. *Journal of Obstetric, Gynecologic, and Neonatal Nursing, 31,* 66–76.

Whiteside, J.L., Katz, T., Anthes, T., Boardman, L., & Peipert, J.F. (2001). Risks and adverse outcomes of sexually transmitted diseases. *Journal of Reproductive Medicine, 46* (1), 34–38.

Wing, D.A., Hendershott, C.M., Debuque, L., & Millar, L.K. (1999). Outpatient treatment of acute pyelonephritis in pregnancy after 24 weeks. *Obstetrics and Gynecology, 94* (5), 683–688.

Witlin, A.G., Saade, G.R., Mattar, F., & Sibai, B.M. (1999). Risk factors for abruptio placentae and eclampsia: Analysis of 445 consecutively managed women with severe preeclampsia and eclampsia. *American Journal of Obstetrics and Gynecology, 180,* 1322–1329.

Wong, L. Ngan, H.Y., Cheng, D.K., & Ng, T.Y. (2000). Methotrexate infusion in low-risk gestational trophoblastic disease. *American Journal of Obstetrics and Gynecology, 183* (6), 1579–1582.

Wong, S., Chan, L.Y., Yu, V., & Ho, L. (1999). Hepatitis B carrier and perinatal outcome in singleton pregnancy. *American Journal of Perinatology, 16* (9), 485–488.

Wyckoff, M.M. (2000). Neonatal herpes simplex virus type II. *American Journal of Maternal/Child Health, 25* (2), 100–103.

Xiong, X, Demianczuk, N., Saunders, L.D., Want, F.L., & Fraser, W.D. (2002). Impact of preeclampsia and gestational hypertension on birth weight by gestational age. *American Journal of Epidemiology, 155,* 203–209.

Yamashita, H., Shao, J., & Friedman, J.E. (2000). Physiologic and molecular alterations in carbohydrate metabolism during pregnancy and gestational diabetes mellitus. *Clinical Obstetrics and Gynecology, 43* (1), 87–98.

Yaron, Y., Bryant-Greenwood, P.K., Dave, N., Moldenhauer, J.S., Kramer, R.L., Johnson, M.P., & Evans, M.I. (1999). Multifetal pregnancy reductions of triplets to twins: Comparison with nonreduced triplets and twins. *American Journal of Obstetrics and Gynecology, 180* (5), 268–271.

Yost, N.P., (2001, March). Diagnosing and managing sickle cell disease in pregnancy. *Contemporary OB/GYN,* 45–61.

CHAPTER 19

ASSESSING FETAL WELL-BEING

Marion Herndon Fuqua

*I*t is often a dilemma *for the client to make the choices presented by screening and assessment tests.*

Highlights

- Psychological Needs of Clients
- Indications for Fetal Assessment
- Sequencing Advanced Fetal Testing
- Fetal Movement Counts
- Fetal Heart Rate Assessment
- Nonstress Test and Contraction Stress Test
- Screening for Size/Dates Discrepancies
- Screening and Prevention of RhD Alloimmunization
- Maternal Serum Screening
- Ultrasonography
- Biophysical Profile
- Doppler Flow Studies
- Amniocentesis and Chorionic Villus Sampling
- Percutaneous Umbilical Blood Sampling
- Development of Screening Technology

❖ INTRODUCTION

The assessment of fetal well-being is both a subjective and an objective task, the success of which depends on open communication between the health care provider and the client. Very simple noninvasive assessments, such as perception of fetal movement and fundal height measurement, have been used for years. Technological advances in assessing the fetus and improving the chances of fertility not only for older women but also for women with disease have required that the health care provider gain increasing knowledge and skill. Allowing advanced practice nurses to perform antepartum testing not only provides continuity of care by providing education and medical care to the mother and fetus but also provides access to care in outlying areas where care would not be available.

Technological advances in assessing the fetus may initiate a number of questions, often leaving the health care provider with further questions and a client with new fears and anxieties about her pregnancy. Asking one question always leads to another, as Pandora's box is opened. As one author stated, "There is as yet an untested possibility that the reduction in mortality could be overshadowed by a higher incidence of long-term handicap because of a possible increase in the number of planned preterm deliveries of sick babies" (Alfirevic & Neilson, 1995). It will continue to be a struggle to decrease perinatal mortality without increasing the rate of inappropriate obstetric intervention.

PSYCHOLOGICAL NEEDS OF CLIENTS

Diagnosis, interpretation, and management or referral often are foremost in providing quality fetal assessment. Counseling, support, and education for mother and family are critical care elements that reduce anxiety about the unknown developing fetus and enable the health care provider to achieve continuity of care.

Interestingly, Kowalcek, Muhlhoff, Bachmann, and Gembruch (2002) found that stress experienced by the client or her partner while undergoing prenatal diagnosis was not related to the invasiveness of the procedure. They assessed that the ability of the test to provide an accurate assessment of normalcy in a timely fashion was fundamental to providing emotional relief to the client, whether chorionic villus sampling (CVS), amniocentesis, or ultrasound was used. Ultrasonographic scanning, even with its limitations as compared to diagnostic chromosomal analysis, provided greater psychological relief to clients and their spouses since immediate visualization of the fetus and positive verbal confirmation of fetal normalcy (within the realm of fetal scanning) were possible. This reveals that the anxiety experienced by clients and their families is often related to waiting for confirmation of normal test results and not to fear of an invasive procedure, as was previously thought. Clinicians need to be aware that even the simplest of tests raises concerns and possible anxiety for the client and her family.

Of utmost importance is to take into account racial-ethnic differences when counseling clients: One study revealed African American and Latina women to be less likely to use prenatal diagnosis as compared to white and Asian women, suggesting beliefs about testing, termination, and raising a disabled child may be unique to each racial-ethnic group; attitudes may be specific for the racial-ethnic group as opposed to socioeconomic status (Kupperman, Gates, & Washington, 1996). Cultural differences concerning pregnancy and disability do exist and need to be appreciated in order to provide information that enables the client to make an informed decision about fetal assessment. Variations in knowledge and access to prenatal diagnostic services influence a client's decisions as well and need to be assessed with each individual.

The following list of guidelines for emotional support, though by no means complete, does give insight into the time and attention needed for "supportive" care. Because the guidelines listed here apply to most of the tests described in this chapter, they are not repeated with the descriptions of the tests. Although only one or a few specific applications may be given in this list, there are many other situations that are applicable.

EMOTIONAL SUPPORT

- *Counsel the client before and after each test.* Prior to any test, ensure that the nature of the test, the information that it will provide, and the possibility of further intervention or testing are explained to the client. Counseling occurs before optional screening or testing to investigate a perceived risk to the client or fetus. Any risks to the client or fetus also are reviewed. To reinforce discussions and reduce anxiety, provide written information and answer questions thoroughly. Tell the client when test results are expected.

If maternal or fetal risk is the indication for assessment—for example, in cases of diabetes mellitus—the client needs to understand the particular risk, how it affects her pregnancy, and why various tests are important to assess fetal well-being. Depending on the clinical situation, several testing modalities are used. Often a client may become frustrated when one test cannot provide the necessary information, and it may be difficult for her to appreciate why different tests are required. If the health care provider explains the need for assessment, the benefits for both fetus and client, and encourages her to voice her opinions in the decision making process, the client will see herself as part of the solution, not the problem. Hence, the client is able to positively participate in the plan of care.

It is often a dilemma for the client to make choices presented by screening and assessment tests. Known as "optimistic bias," clients tend to perceive their own risks as being less than the risks of others, and abnormal results are often unanticipated by the client (Kowalcek et al., 2002). If the client is upset over the need for tests or the results of tests, she may not "hear" what is being said. Therefore, include the support person or significant other in the counseling and, if possible, wait until the client is ready to hear available options. A support person can later help the client to recall the plan of care when her anxiety eases.

◆ *Acknowledge the normalcy of feelings of guilt.* A client may feel guilty if she feels inconvenienced by testing but realizes its importance. Having to put the fetus first for nine months can be stressful during a healthy pregnancy, much less a complicated one requiring invasive or time-consuming procedures. With isoimmunization, for example, a client may feel guilty about her body "rejecting" or "harming" the fetus. Allow her to express those feelings. Reinforce the fact that she cannot control the actual isoimmunization process but can work with the health care team to provide the best care possible for her fetus and by doing so is helping her fetus.

◆ *Provide support when an infant has a chromosomal or structural anomaly.* The parents of a fetus with an abnormality may resent the invasive, lengthy procedures and wonder why they are necessary. The health care provider must be prepared to respond in such situations. The client must be informed of diagnoses and, where appropriate, referred to support groups for additional information. Support groups can be extremely helpful in assisting the client with the transition from being pregnant to caring for an infant with an abnormality. In addition, the client needs to grieve the loss of a "perfect child."

Hoeldtke and Calhoun (2001) have written an excellent article concerning perinatal hospice and the subsequent psychological care families need once a fetus is diagnosed with a lethal anomaly. The reader is referred to the source for an in-depth discussion of caring for the client and family.

◆ *Provide support if the client chooses termination.* A client who chooses to terminate her pregnancy for any reason also needs support. This may be particularly true if termination is performed during the first or second trimester when the client has started "showing," heard the fetal heartbeat, felt movement, seen the fetus with ultrasound, and perhaps confided to friends and family that she is pregnant. The decision to terminate a pregnancy is likely to be a very difficult one (Rillstone & Hutchinson, 2001; Schechtman, Gray, Baty, & Rothman, 2002).

◆ *Be aware of spiritual distress.* Spiritual distress may be encountered when the client or fetus requires blood (as with isoimmunization) or blood products (Rhogam). Although it is difficult, the client and health care provider may need to consult with legal sources concerning client and fetus rights. Spiritual distress may also be encountered with termination of a pregnancy, spontaneous abortion, fetal demise, or neonatal death. Clients who have a fetus with a structural or chromosomal anomaly may feel this is due to punishment for something they have done "wrong" or as a reflection upon their value as an individual. This can have significant repercussions within the family unit. There may be situations in which the health care provider may not be able to attend to the needs of the client. Further psychological, spiritual, or financial intervention may be necessary. The health care provider can be a valuable mediator in such instances, especially by ensuring that appropriate follow-up for abnormal test results is made available to the client *before* she undergoes various tests (Lewis, 2002).

INDICATIONS FOR FETAL ASSESSMENT

ROUTINE ASSESSMENT

Routine fetal assessment begins at the first prenatal visit. Fundal height is measured or a bimanual examination is performed to assess uterine size. If applicable, the fetal heartbeat is auscultated and the client's perception of fetal movement is determined.

This routine standard of care continues for all pregnancies until delivery. Some women begin pregnancy with risk factors (e.g., diabetes) that warrant further fetal surveillance. Complications of fetal or maternal origin may arise during pregnancy and require fetal testing. Surveillance or testing is done to monitor a fetus that may be at risk for poor outcome. Some tests, such as a α-fetoprotein, should be offered to all women as a screening method; a risk factor need not be present.

ADVANCED ASSESSMENT

In general, advanced assessment is indicated when there is the risk of uteroplacental insufficiency, but it also can be indicated because of fetal factors, such as decreased movement. Each clinical situation is individualized for client and fetus. While some risk factors can be identified at the initial prenatal visit, a significant percentage of problems arise in pregnancies without any risk factors. Not all health care providers believe that each of the following conditions warrants testing. Moreover, protocols concerning the onset and frequency of indications that warrant particular tests vary among institutions. As technology progresses and the etiology of fetal compromise is further understood, the list may grow (AAP and ACOG, 1997; ACOG, 2001a; Druzin, Gabbe, & Reed, 2002; Walsh, 2001).

Fetal Conditions

- Premature rupture of membranes
- Isoimmunization
- Decreased fetal movement
- Any irregularity of fetal heart rate
- History or presence of congenital anomalies
- Intrauterine growth retardation, presence or history of
- Abnormal amniotic fluid volume
- Premature rupture of membranes
- Combination of one major or two minor ultrasound markers of Down syndrome, or presence of choroid plexus cyst

Maternal Conditions

- Advanced maternal age (for genetic screening)
- Unexplained vaginal bleeding
- Postdate pregnancy
- Multiple gestation with significant growth discrepancy
- Abnormal triple screen
- Poor obstetric history, history of fetal loss
- Maternal substance abuse
- Nutritional and eating disorders
- Uterine structural anomalies
- Antiphospholipid syndrome

Maternal and Paternal Conditions

- Biological mother or father of the fetus with a chromosome translocation, carrier of a chromosome inversion or parental aneuploidy

Significant Maternal Disease

- Chronic hypertension
- Diabetes mellitus, insulin dependent or gestational
- Pregnancy induced hypertension
- Hemoglobinopathies
- Cardiac, renal, pulmonary, or connective tissue disease
- Hyperthyroidism
- Systemic lupus erythematosus

ADVANCED ASSESSMENT FOR PREGNANCIES AT RISK

The American Academy of Pediatrics and The American College of Obstetricians and Gynecologists (1997) states that "the goals of antepartum fetal surveillance include reducing the risk of fetal demise after 24 weeks gestation, delaying the need for intervention and prolonging gestation in pregnancies at risk for preterm delivery." Therefore, the clinician must take into consideration the severity of maternal disease, the risk of fetal death, and the risk of complications of an unnecessary premature birth due to intervention based upon possible false positive results.

Disagreement exists about when advanced fetal assessment should begin, but the following guidelines generally can be used.

- *Have an accurate estimation of gestational age for the high-risk pregnancy.* For example, a client with a previous ectopic pregnancy should have an ultrasound done early in the first trimester to confirm an intrauterine pregnancy. Accurate dating is also important for clients with chronic diseases such as diabetes and hypertension, or a history of an intrauterine-growth-restricted (IUGR) infant.

♦ *Begin as complications arise*. For example, once intrauterine growth retardation or pre-eclampsia is diagnosed, fetal surveillance should begin.

♦ *Anticipate events*. Begin assessment prior to the time the problem arose during the previous pregnancy. Weeks and colleagues (1995) suggest, however, that surveillance begin at 32 weeks with a history of demise, unless the fetal loss was before this in the previous pregnancy; then begin assessment two weeks prior to the diagnosis of the previous demise. In the case of RhD alloimmunization, if the previous pregnancy was affected, then amniocentesis or cordocentesis is suggested four to eight weeks prior to the point in gestation at which problems began to arise, perhaps earlier than 20 weeks gestation (ACOG, 1996).

♦ *Begin at 32 to 34 weeks of gestation for at-risk clients*. However, clients with high-risk conditions such as chronic hypertension with IUGR, should begin surveillance at 26 to 28 weeks. Initiation of testing is based on maternal and fetal status and options available (AAP and ACOG, 1997; ACOG, 1999). Manning (1999) has researched the use of the biophysical profile on fetuses younger than 24 weeks to predict asphyxia. Vintzileos (2000) published a recent article highlighting the use of specific algorithms for specific indications. The gestational age in which to initiate testing varied, as well as the assessment method. For example, in the presence of maternal vascular disease, ultrasound for growth and anatomy was performed at 18 to 20 weeks, followed by ultrasound, amniotic fluid volume and Doppler flow studies at 24 to 26 weeks. The reader is referred to the source for review. Assessment methods will increase as the age of viability decreases with technological advancements.

♦ *Assess the postdate fetus (gestational age greater than 40 weeks)*. If the only indication for assessment is postdates, then weekly surveillance is usually acceptable. The frequency of assessment ranges from daily to weekly depending on diagnosis severity (if applicable) and fetal and maternal status. Many centers begin testing at 41 weeks (Divon, 2002).

♦ *Frequency of testing*. This is based on the clinical condition of the mother and fetus. Some diseases dictate frequent testing as fetal compromise could be sudden, as in insulin dependent diabetes, where testing is usually twice weekly. If the potential for compromise is rapid, such as with isoimmunization, testing may be daily or twice daily (ACOG, 1999; Devoe, 1999).

♦ *Assess in the first trimester if fetal therapy possible*. First trimester screening allows for medical therapy to address conditions of the infant. Currently, there are several fetal conditions that can be successfully treated in utero through medical management of the mother. These include metabolic and endocrinologic disorders as well as toxoplasmosis. Treatment consists of medicating the mother for the specific condition; assessment to evaluate therapeutic fetal drug levels can be evaluated through percutaneous blood sampling (Evans, Harrison, Flake, & Johnson, 2002). Surgical fetal therapy is being researched to correct potentially lethal anomalies and neural tube defects, but is still investigational (ACOG, 2001a; Evans et al., 2002; Lyerly, Gates, Cefalo, & Sugarman, 2001). Computer software has been developed to perform case-specific "virtual surgery" prior to actual procedures enhancing favorable outcome in fetal surgery (Wilson, 2002). With advances in technology, intervention on the behalf of the fetus does not necessarily indicate delivery.

Stem cell transplantation therapy for the fetus is also under investigation. While research has centered on the treatment of childhood malignancy and adult disease, there is a focus on fetal therapy (ACOG, 1997a; Evans & Wapner, 2001; Touraine, 2001). Stem cells are a unique group of bone marrow cells capable of self-renewal, multilineage proliferation, and differentiation (Evans & Wapner, 2001). These cells have been found in bone marrow, peripheral blood, fetal cord blood, and the fetal liver. They could be infused into the fetus early in gestation intraperitoneally or via cordocentesis prior to target organ damage (Evans & Wapner, 2001). Stem cell therapy has been successful in treating severe combined immunodeficiency disorder. Treatment of other disorders is being researched, and stem cell therapy may be potentially able to treat other immunodeficiencies, and inborn errors of metabolism and hematology (Evans & Wapner, 2001).

SEQUENCING ADVANCED FETAL TESTING

Testing can begin for a variety of reasons at any gestational age. Some tests are more appropriate than others. Figure 19–1 provides an algorithm of fetal testing that might be used once problems arise. It is one of many available frameworks to be adjusted within institutional

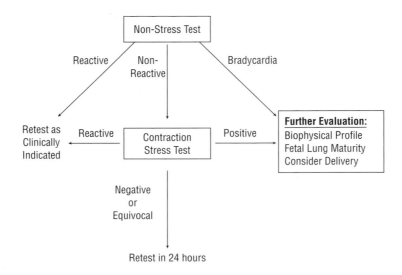

FIGURE 19–1. An Algorithm for Fetal Testing. *Adapted with permission from Druzin, M., Gabbe, S., & Reed, K. (2002). Antepartum fetal evaluation. In S. Gabbe, J. Niebyl, & J. L. Simpson (Eds.),* Obstetrics: Normal and problem pregnancies *(pp. 313–352). New York: Churchill Livingstone.*

protocols. As previously mentioned, Vintzeleos (2000) has developed twelve different algorithms using an indication-specific testing methodology. The reader is referred to the source for a review. No single test can be regarded as the exclusive choice for assessing fetal well-being as each test reveals different parameters of fetal pathophysiology, often in a complementary manner.

FETAL ASSESSMENT

FETAL MOVEMENT

Maternal perception of fetal movement correlates with fetal well-being. Fetal movement is usually perceived by the client at 16 to 20 weeks' gestation. By the use of ultrasound, fetal movement has been noted as early as 7 to 8 weeks (Cunningham, Gant, Leveno, et al., 2001). A normal fetus has coordinated movements by 16 to 20 weeks of gestation. Perceived fetal movement is most often related to trunk and limb motion and rollovers, or flips (Walsh, 2001). Generally, during the second half of pregnancy, fetal movement becomes more organized, and weaker movements are replaced by stronger movements (Christensen & Rayburn, 1999). Near term, the fetus spends 85 to 95 percent of its time in an quiet or active sleep state, where movement still occurs. Up to 80 percent of gross fetal movement can be perceived by the mother (Druzin et al., 2002). Maternal perception of

movement may also diminish, as a result of decreasing amniotic fluid volume, improved fetal coordination, fetal sleep cycles, and increased fetal size, thereby decreasing uterine volume (Cunningham et al., 2001).

Significance of Fetal Movement

Decreased fetal movement may be indicative of asphyxia and intrauterine growth retardation (Christensen & Rayburn, 1999). The compromised fetus decreases oxygen requirements by decreasing activity; documented cessation of activity is a possible indication of impending demise, and a decrease in activity is usually due to chronic, as opposed to acute, fetal distress (Christensen & Rayburn, 1999). It has been reported that decreased fetal movement may occur prior to fetal death by several days (ACOG, 1999).

Even with a reassuring fetal heart rate, decreased fetal movement is a sensitive indicator of fetal distress. It should be a red flag to the clinician when the client reports decreased fetal movement, even in the presence of normal electronic fetal monitoring. Clients with underlying "silent" problems but no obvious risk factors may be identified only through decreased fetal movement. Approximately 50 percent of fetuses with decreased fetal movement are stillborn, tolerate labor poorly, or require resuscitation at birth (Christensen & Rayburn, 1999; Lyndsey, 1999).

Factors That Decrease Fetal Movement

Maternal use of barbiturates, alcohol, methadone, narcotics, or cigarettes may decrease fetal movement (Cunningham et al., 2001; Walsh, 2001). The drug's effect depends on the amount used, concurrent use of other drugs, and the route by which the drug is taken (i.e., intravenous injection, inhalation, or oral).

Decreased movement, however, may be due to fetal sleep cycles or to inactivity during a particular time of day. Most fetal activity occurs between 9 P.M. and 1 A.M. with periods of inactivity of 20 to 75 minutes in normal pregnancies (Cunningham et al., 2001; Walsh, 2001). Research has shown that fetal activity does not increase after meals; in fact, movement increases with falling maternal glucose levels from 9 P.M. to 1 A.M. (Druzin et al., 2002).

Fetal factors associated with decreased fetal movement or abnormal patterns of fetal movement include hydrocephalus, bilateral renal agenesis, and bilateral hip dislocation. Most fetuses with congenital anomalies may have patterns of movement similar to those of normal fetuses (Christensen & Rayburn, 1999). A fetus with severe intrauterine growth retardation (characterized by fetal weight below the fifth for the given gestational age) may have diminished activity. Mild growth retardation, on the other hand, does not appear to reduce the number of fetal movements (Christensen & Rayburn, 1999).

FETAL MOVEMENT COUNTS (FMCs)

Procedure

Instruct all clients to perform fetal movement counts (FMCs) after 28 weeks' gestation. To heighten client awareness of fetal movement, instruct her to do FMCs daily using a protocol such as the following; several other counting methods have been devised (Christensen & Rayburn, 1999).

- Record the start time, then lie in the left lateral position when the fetus is most active. A quiet location is best. You may also sit or stand if you are able to detect movement.
- Place a hand over the abdomen to palpate movement.
- Remain in this position until you have counted ten fetal movements.
- Record the end time.

To ensure continuity, FMCs should be done at approximately the same time each day. If 10 movements are not obtained within 1 hour, then further testing is indicated. Fetal surveillance should be initiated within 12 hours of a client's perception of decreased activity; consider a nonstress test (NST) (Christensen & Rayburn, 1999). Participation in FMCs is heightened when less than 1 hour is spent each day counting fetal movements.

Advantages and Disadvantages

Performing FMCs is simple, inexpensive, and does not require machinery. The client may proceed at her own convenience and in privacy. FMCs can promote maternal-fetal bonding. Fetal compromise is often first realized when FMCs are initiated. Presence of adequate fetal movement offers some assurance of lack of fetal compromise.

There are also disadvantages to FMCs. A pregnant woman who is busy throughout the day and unable to lie quietly and focus on her fetus may feel less movement. An obese woman may feel less movement, although this has not been well documented. A client may become anxious if movement is difficult to palpate or perceive, particularly if the pregnancy is problematic or if there is a history of fetal demise.

Client Teaching and Counseling

Provide the client with detailed information concerning FMCs, including the significance of decreased fetal movement and the need to inform the health care provider promptly of any irregularity. Inquire about the client's FMCs at each visit to enhance the provider/client relationship and to stress the importance of FMCs.

FETAL HEART RATE ASSESSMENT

Fetal heart rate should be auscultated by 10 to 12 weeks of gestation with a doptone device or at 17 to 19 weeks with DeLee fetoscope (Walsh, 2001). Auscultate the fetal heart rate (FHR) at each prenatal care visit for one full minute to note rate and rhythm. Take care not to mistake placental flow or maternal heart rate for FHR. Placental flow or souffle is a swishing sound different from the actual fetal heartbeat, which is a very distinct, clear beat. To ensure that the maternal heart rate is not confused with the FHR, palpate the client's pulse at the wrist while simultaneously auscultating the fetal heart through the abdomen with a doptone device or fetoscope.

Procedure

Place a small amount of gel (with a water-soluble base) on the abdomen or directly on a doptone device. A fetoscope, which also can be used, does not require gel. Early in gestation (12 to 14 weeks), FHR is best auscultated just above the symphysis with the Doppler. As pregnancy progresses, the fetal heart is usually heard in the lower abdominal quadrants; however, toward the end of pregnancy if the fetus is not in the vertex position, the FHR is often auscultated near or above the umbilicus. It is easiest to locate FHR with the client on her back, if she is able to tolerate that position. Most women can tolerate being supine for a few minutes. If the FHR is not found quickly, it may help to locate the fetal back by performing Leopold's maneuvers.

Leopold's maneuvers are as follows (Cunningham et al., 2001):

- Facing the client, gently outline the uterus with warm hands. Ascertain what part of the fetus is at the fundus: Fetal breech feels nodular and large, and the fetal head feels hard, rounded, and generally more movable.
- Facing the client, gently but firmly palpate the sides of her abdomen using the palms of your hands. The fetal back will be a hard, resistant structure; the opposite palm should feel nodularity of the extremities, such as knees or elbows. If the fetus is not completely on its side, an additional moment of palpation may be needed to determine fetal orientation.
- Facing the client, grasp the lower portion of the maternal abdomen just above the symphysis pubis. If the presenting part is not engaged, it will be mobile. With careful palpation, noting cephalic prominence, it may be possible to determine whether the fetal head is extended or flexed.
- Facing the client's feet and using the tips of the first three fingers of each hand, gently but firmly palpate toward the axis of the pelvic inlet. If the fetal head presents, then the cephalic prominence will be noted first with one hand while the other hand will be able to descend more deeply into the pelvis.

In vertex presentation, the cephalic prominence will be on the same side as the arms and legs, thereby confirming flexion of the fetal head. Cephalic prominence on the same side as the back suggests extension of the fetal head, or face presentation. The ease with which the cephalic prominence is noted provides information regarding descent: If the cephalic prominence is palpable, then the vertex has not reached the level of the ischial spines.

These movements may be difficult to interpret if the placenta is anterior or if the client is obese (Cunningham et al., 2001).

Interpretation of FHR

The FHR should be 110 to 160 beats per minute (bpm), with allowance for variations in normal accelerations (Walsh, 2001). A normal fetal heart rate at twenty weeks' gestation is 150 to 170 bpm (Tucker, 2000). As the fetus matures, so does the parasympathetic and sympathetic nervous systems, thereby decreasing the fetal heart rate. A normal heart rate for a term fetus is 110 to 160 bpm. However, a fetus of more than 40 weeks will have a heart rate of 110 to 120 bpm due to the greater influence of the parasympathetic system (Tucker, 2000). Bradycardia is a baseline heart rate of less than 110 bpm for more than 10 minutes; tachycardia is a baseline heart rate of 160 to 180 bpm for more than 10 minutes (Tucker, 2000). Decelerations or variables may be heard, but they are identified and validated only with external FHR monitoring.

If fetal heart rate or rhythm abnormalities are heard, then a nonstress test is warranted to ascertain the FHR baseline and any periodic patterns. Ultrasound is used to assess cardiac function and note any anomalies. If FHR is absent, a second doptone device or fetoscope (if applicable) may be helpful. Ultrasound is indicated to document fetal viability if the FHR is not heard by 12 weeks' gestation with a doptone device, 19 weeks with a DeLee fetoscope, or if it is absent after previously being documented (Walsh, 2001).

Factors That Influence Fetal Heart Rate Detection

FHR may be heard earlier than 12 weeks with Doppler if the uterus is anteflexed, as opposed to being retroflexed, and if the client has little adipose tissue. Adipose tissue may make it more difficult to hear the fetal heart early in gestation or later using a fetoscope. The type and age of the doptone device used may also affect ability to hear the fetal heart early in gestation.

Advantages and Disadvantages

The procedure is noninvasive, and most clients enjoy hearing the fetal heart. Listening promotes bonding for mother, father, and siblings and may enable the mother to conceptualize her pregnancy early in gestation, prior to fetal movement. Often fetal movement can be heard with the doptone device and aids the client in recognizing fetal movement.

On the other hand, the client may be anxious if the fetal heart is not detected immediately or is not heard at all or if the fetus moves and the FHR is temporarily lost.

Client Teaching and Counseling

Inform the client of the normal range of heart rate to decrease her anxiety; many women are unaware that FHR should be 110 to 160 bpm and worry that the fetal heart is beating too fast. Reassurance usually suffices.

NONSTRESS TEST AND CONTRACTION STRESS TEST

The nonstress and contraction stress tests both reflect the status of fetal cardiac physiology, as well as the fetal status of the central, peripheral, and autonomic nervous systems through heart rate monitoring (Devoe, 1999). The tests were developed to assess any indication of uteroplacental insufficiency, thereby predicting the fetus' ability to endure the stress of labor or the need for premature delivery if the fetus is distressed and could be better cared for outside the uterus.

NONSTRESS TEST

Reactivity is present in over 85 percent of fetuses tested using electronic fetal heart rate monitoring at 28 to 32 weeks (ACOG, 1999). The nonstress test (NST) can be performed reliably after 28 weeks of gestation when the aforementioned fetal systems, particularly the autonomic nervous system, usually reach acceptable maturity and can be assessed; the 24 to 28 week fetus is unlikely to have a reactive pattern (ACOG, 1999). As technology expands, and the age of viability becomes earlier, ultrasound may become the primary method of assessment. Because it is a noninvasive and simple procedure, the NST is appropriate for many clinical indications. In cases of serious fetal or maternal disease, additional tests may be performed.

Procedure

Ideally, the client has not been fasting and has not smoked recently as this may affect test results (ACOG, 1999). The procedure involves the use of a fetal heart monitor. Two belts are secured around the abdomen; one holds the tocodynameter over the fundus, which measures any uterine activity. The other belt holds a transducer over the fetal heart, which measures the fetal heart rate. Preferably, the client lies on her left side to avoid supine hypotension. Fetal heart rate, fetal movement, and uterine contractions (if they occur) are assessed over 20 minutes and recorded on a monitor strip. The client notes fetal movement by using a handheld "event marker" or by pushing a button on the monitor that marks the strip. Perceived fetal movement is thereby correlated with FHR. Fetal movement without an acceleration is atypical, and further workup is warranted.

Interpretation

The NST may be interpreted as reactive or nonreactive. A *reactive NST* is characterized by two fetal heart rate accelerations that last 15 seconds and reach 15 beats above baseline FHR in 20 minutes (15-by-15 criterion). If a reactive NST cannot be obtained after 20 minutes, then monitoring is continued another 20 minutes in order to take the fetal sleep-wake cycle into account (ACOG, 1999; Lyndsey, 1999).

Prior to 32 weeks, an acceptable acceleration is 10 beats above baseline lasting 10 seconds or more. Many fetuses prior to 32 weeks will meet the 15-by-15 criterion, and once this is documented, the fetus should be "held" to this standard in subsequent evaluations (Baird & Ruth, 2002).

Factors that influence reactivity include maternal sedatives, smoking, fetal sleep cycles, maternal or fetal disease, and the recent administration of corticosteroids, namely betamethasone (Baird & Ruth, 2002, Devoe, 1999; Oncken, Kranzler, O'Malley, et al., 2002). Lengthening the NST another 30 minutes, or choosing another assessment method may be reasonable to rule out *some* of these variables (Baird & Ruth, 2002; Devoe, 1999; Oncken et al., 2002).

When the NST is reactive, or "negative," it can be repeated at weekly intervals; in most cases, fetal well-being can be relatively assured for one week. Some clinical situations involving the client or the fetus may dictate more frequent testing, such as type I diabetes, IUGR, PIH, or postdates (ACOG, 1999). The ideal interval for surveillance has not been established; weekly, biweekly, and daily testing are utilized, depending on the clinical situation; however, even with daily testing, fetal demise is encountered on rare occasions (Devoe, 1999). Frequency of testing is left to the discretion of the clinician, taking into account the clinical aspects of disease that affect maternal and fetal well-being.

A *nonreactive NST* is characterized by the absence of two fetal heart rate accelerations using the 15-by-15 criterion in a 20-minute time frame. Other questionable patterns, such as lack of variability and presence of decelerations may be noted, however. Additional testing, such as a contraction stress test (CST) or biophysical profile, should be considered (Devoe, 1999).

Periodic patterns that may be viewed during NSTs and CSTs and require evaluation include fetal bradycardia, tachycardia, decelerations, and lack of variability. The following definitions (variability, acceleration, deceleration, sinusoidal pattern), although helpful in understanding the fundamentals of interpreting FHR tracings, will neither replace diagnostic manuals nor diminish the expertise gained through experience in reading FHR tracings.

Variability

Short-term variability (STV), considered the most important indicator of fetal well-being, is the fluctuation of FHR from beat to beat, giving rise to a saw-toothed tracing. Variability reflects the pathway between the autonomic nervous system and the heart, and is a sensitive indicator of fetal oxygenation (Tucker, 2000). Short-term variability, however, can only be truly documented by using internal, not external, monitoring.

Long-term variability (LTV) is the fluctuation of FHR over 1 minute. It is assessed by noting the difference between maximum and minimum FHR, excluding accelerations, decelerations, and patterns exhibited during contractions.

The National Institute of Child and Human Development (NICHD, 1997) does not distinguish between LTV and STV as in practice they are usually evaluated as a unit and excludes the sinusoidal pattern.

Classification of Variability (NICHD, 1997)

- *Absent.* FHR changes are undetectable.
- *Minimal.* FHR changes are < 5 bpm.
- *Average/Moderate.* FHR changes are 6 to 25 bpm.
- *Marked.* FHR changes of > 25 bpm.

Essentially, FHR changes of 6 to 25 bpm are reassuring; however, minimal or marked variability does not always imply fetal distress. *Questionable tracings always require a second opinion concerning intervention or further diagnostic testing, such as CST or biophysical profile.*

Acceleration

Accelerations are increases in FHR over baseline, specifically a 15 bpm increase for 15 seconds; an acceleration lasting longer than 10 minutes is a baseline change (Tucker, 2000).

Deceleration

Decelerations are decreases of FHR below baseline; they can be early, late, or variable. *Early decelerations* usually occur as a vagal response to increased intracranial pressure with fetal head compression. An early deceleration is uniform in shape with a contraction, beginning and ending with the contraction. It is shallow and symmetrical and usually seen in the active phase of labor, between 4 and 7 cm (Tucker, 2000).

Late decelerations are symmetrical decreases in the FHR beginning at or after the peak of the contraction; FHR does not recover until contraction ends. Uteroplacental insufficiency should be questioned. Markedly compromised fetuses frequently display subtle, shallow decelerations (Tucker, 2000).

Variable decelerations are usually due to cord compression. Variable decelerations have variable shape, depth, and duration and may occur at any time. Severe decelerations last more than 60 seconds with FHR fewer than 70 bpm. Isolated or recurrent variable decelerations not associated with fetal movement may suggest oligohydramnios or cord compromise and require follow-up with an ultrasound to assess amniotic fluid volume (Devoe, 1999).

Sinusoidal Pattern

A sinusoidal pattern is characterized by a smooth, undulating FHR pattern, usually with an absence of variability. Oscillations are 2 to 6 cycles per minute, with an amplitude of up to 30 bpm. Reactivity is absent, and the pattern lasts beyond 10 minutes. The pattern may be seen with severe chronic, as opposed to acute, fetal anemia, and severe hypoxia and acidosis. Sinusoidal patterns have also been noted with the use of analgesics and in this circumstance do not indicate fetal compromise. The situation may be corrected with Narcan (Tucker, 2000).

Use of Vibroacoustic Stimulation

An artificial larynx, or acoustic stimulator, can be used to achieve a reactive tracing and reduce the length of the NST. No deleterious effects have been assessed, although research continues (Lyndsey, 1999). If accelerations or fetal movement are not noted within 10 minutes during the NST, vibroacoustic stimulation is applied to the woman's abdomen over the fetal head for 1 to 3 seconds. Acceptable accelerations usually result. One or two additional stimuli may be applied at one- to two-minute intervals if necessary. Induced accelerations appear to be valid in assuring fetal well-being (Devoe, 1999).

Advantages and Disadvantages

The advantages of the NST are that it is easily performed and noninvasive. Furthermore, hearing and seeing the FHR recorded on the tracing may promote maternal-fetal bonding.

A disadvantage of the NST is that it requires someone with expertise to read the results, particularly suspicious patterns. There is current investigation into the use of computerized analysis of fetal heart rate (Devoe, 1999). This provides an objective reading of the "tracing" or "strip," as well as providing accurate measurements of the various numerical parameters of the fetal heart rate. Computerized systems would refine interpretation of fetal heart rate patterns (variability, accelerations, decelerations, and baseline rate) (Bracero, Morgan, & Byrne, 1999; Devoe, 1999).

The NST can be a lengthy procedure, particularly if a protocol is not in place for the use of acoustic stimulation. However, the auditory brainstem response in the fetus is not functional until 26 to 28 weeks; only 20 percent or less of fetuses will respond to acoustic stimulation prior to 26 weeks (Baird & Ruth, 2002; Lyndsey, 1999). Continuous FHR tracing may be difficult to obtain if the client is obese or if the fetus is less than 28 weeks. The NST is only reactive 50 percent of the time prior to 28 weeks (ACOG, 1999).

Client Teaching and Counseling

Initially, to avoid client confusion and undue concern, explain the tracings of uterine activity and FHR. The client should also be told what the average FHR is and that variability is normal. Many women are alarmed when the FHR fluctuates (particularly with accelerations), or frightened if the FHR is temporarily "lost" as a result of a fetal or maternal position change. Explaining the different aspects of FHR monitoring can alleviate many fears. If vibroacoustic stimulation is used, have the client feel and hear the stimulus before applying it to the abdomen.

CONTRACTION STRESS TEST

This test is performed to note fetal response to uterine contractions, using the principle of induced stress to assess placental insufficiency. It is theorized that if the fetus is hypoxic or has uteroplacental insufficiency, late decel-erations will occur with uterine contractions (ACOG, 1999; Lyndsey, 1999).

Contraindications

Absolute contraindications are history of classical cesarean section, placenta previa or abruptio placentae, premature rupture of membranes, premature labor, multiple gestation, incompetent cervix. Relative contraindications are polyhydramnios or a condition that prohibits adequate uterine monitoring, such as obesity (Devoe, 1999; Lyndsey, 1999).

Procedure

The test procedure is much the same as that for the NST. The client is placed in a semi-Fowler's position to prevent supine hypotension. Attain an initial reading of blood pressure, pulse, and respirations. Blood pressure readings are taken every 10 to 15 minutes; maternal hypotension can decrease uteroplacental perfusion, and therefore lead to false-positive results (Lyndsey, 1999). The tocodynameter is applied to the fundus, and the transducer placed over the fetal heart. In obese clients, the transducer may have to be hand held to maintain a constant reading of the fetal heart rate. A baseline tracing of the fetus is obtained for 15 to 20 minutes. Contractions are achieved by means of nipple stimulation, which causes the release of endogenous oxytocin, or through the use of intravenous oxytocin. Nipple stimulation usually achieves adequate contractions, eliminating the need for intravenous oxytocin and shortening testing time (ACOG, 1999). Spontaneous contractions are acceptable, provided criteria are met. Protocols vary among institutions.

To perform nipple stimulation, the client brushes one nipple with the palmar surface of the fingers, or rolls the nipple between the thumb and index finger through her clothing. Stimulation is stopped after two minutes and restarted after five minutes if adequate contractions are not obtained. Stimulation is repeated in this cyclic manner for up to four cycles. If this is unsuccessful, one nipple can be stimulated for ten minutes, stopping when contractions begin and restarting when contractions stop. If needed, both nipples can be stimulated simultaneously for ten minutes (Tucker, 2000).

If no contractions are obtained, or are not sufficient to interpret a CST, an oxytocin infusion is begun. An intravenous line is started with a 21-gauge butterfly needle using half normal saline. The oxytocin infusion is begun at 0.5 to 1.0 mU/min. The rate is doubled every twenty minutes until uterine response is noted. Once adequate contractions are achieved, the infusion is discontinued. Regardless of the method used, the client is monitored until uterine activity returns to baseline; if late decelerations are noted, monitoring continues until the tracing is reactive (Lyndsey, 1999; Walsh, 2001).

Interpretation

Interpreting a CST requires three contractions, lasting at least 40 seconds each, within a ten-minute period. Since contractions are recorded through external monitoring, the only criteria they must meet in regards to strength is that they are clearly recorded in order to interpret the tracing. It is also important to note other aspects of the fetal heart rate strip, including reactivity (Lyndsey, 1999).

◆ *Positive CST*. Late decelerations in more than 50 percent of contractions, regardless of contraction frequency. Delivery should be considered or further tests pursued, as the CST has a 30 percent false-positive rate. If delivery is chosen, and reactivity is absent as well, abdominal delivery is considered as the fetus may not be able to tolerate the stress of labor (ACOG, 1999; Devoe, 1999; Lyndsey, 1999).

◆ *Equivocal CST with Hyperstimulation*. FHR decelerations in the presence of hyperstimulation (more than five contractions in ten minutes or contractions lasting longer than 90 seconds). Retesting should be done in 24 hours, or other tests pursued, such as a BPP (ACOG, 1999; Lyndsey, 1999).

◆ *Equivocal Suspicious*. Intermittent late decelerations noted or significant variable decelerations (ACOG, 1999). A suspicious test can be extended by obtaining 10 additional contractions. Extension may decrease a false-positive rate in the presence of a reassuring tracing. Repeat in 24 hours or select another fetal assessment method if extended testing remains questionable (Devoe, 1999; Lyndsey, 1999).

◆ *Negative or Normal CST*. No late or variable decelerations. Subsequent testing is based on fetal and maternal conditions and the protocol of the institution (ACOG, 1999).

◆ *Unsatisfactory CST*. Failure of adequate contractions to occur with either nipple stimulation or oxytocin infusion or an uninterpretable tracing (ACOG 1999). Consider a biophysical profile or repeat CST in 24 hours (Lyndsey, 1999).

Advantages and Disadvantages of the Contraction Stress Test

The CST determines fetal ability to endure labor. If the fetus cannot tolerate the stress of contractions in a controlled testing environment, then it is unlikely the fetus could tolerate labor. Therefore, this screening helps to avoid fetal distress.

Nipple stimulation is less costly than oxytocin infusion and does not carry the possible complications associated with venipuncture, such as phlebitis and bruising. Hence, the client may prefer nipple stimulation if she is comfortable touching her breasts in a clinical situation. Providing the client with privacy may reduce feelings of self-consciousness.

Theoretically, the CST carries the potential to induce labor; therefore, it is contraindicated if contractions are to be avoided. In the event that contractions induce fetal distress, immediate intervention should be initiated. Another disadvantage is that the CST may take longer than the NST. Clients may become upset with the invasive procedure of oxytocin infusion, if needed.

Client Teaching and Counseling

Review those points included in the discussion of the NST. In addition, inform the client about the possible use of intravenous oxytocin. Clients should be aware that in most cases "manufactured" contractions do not prompt actual labor, but they may cause slight discomfort. Often contractions are painless.

SCREENING FOR SIZE/DATE DISCREPANCIES

The developing fetus has a genetically predetermined potential for growth but can be influenced by the mother's health, placental function, maternal substance use and abuse, nutrition, and perinatal infection (Walsh, 2001).

When gestational age does not correlate with the apparent size of the uterus or fetus, further evaluation is indicated. The discrepancy may be noted during a bimanual exam or fundal height measurement at a regular prenatal visit, or at delivery when the Dubowitz examination is performed to estimate gestational age of the newborn. If the infant appears smaller or larger than would be expected for the dates, it is very important to determine the actual gestational age of the infant to the best of one's ability. This can impact decisions for interventions if needed. Regardless of when the discrepancy is detected, its cause should be investigated.

PROCEDURES

It is helpful to have good estimates of gestational age by means of pelvic examination or ultrasound in the first or second trimester. The last normal menstrual period is recorded and used as the basis for actual gestational age if the client is certain she remembers the first day of her last normal period and if her cycles are about 28 days long.

At each prenatal visit, fundal height is measured or uterine size is assessed to correlate size with gestational age. A measuring tape calibrated in centimeters is used; the distance between the top of the symphysis pubis and the top of the uterine fundus is measured. The general rule is to consider ultrasound if uterine size is three weeks above or below the calculated gestational age, or fundal height is 3 cm above or below the calculated gestational age (Walsh, 2001). Fundal height is most accurate when the bladder is empty.

Gestational age can be determined and the fetus assessed for abnormalities using ultrasound. A discrepancy in size may simply be the result of incorrect menstrual dates. It is, however, important to rule out other etiologies.

All clients who are at risk for IUGR should have an early ultrasound at 18 to 20 weeks and serial ultrasounds done thereafter, since fundal height measurement alone will miss one-third of IUGRs (Vintzileos, 2000). A single ultrasound in late pregnancy cannot detect IUGR (ACOG, 2000a).

DIFFERENTIAL MEDICAL DIAGNOSES

Small-for-Gestational-Age (SGA). SGA is a clinically generic term that describes an infant whose weight is less than 10th percentile without reference to etiology (ACOG, 2000a). Eighty percent of SGA babies are small but normal fetuses. Such fetuses are not at an increased perinatal risk and therefore do not require intervention (Manning, 2001).

Intrauterine Growth Restriction. Intrauterine growth restriction (IUGR) manifests as a fetal weight below the 10th percentile for age, but has clinical evidence of abnormal or dysfunctional growth. IUGR fetuses are at risk for perinatal compromise and death, depending on the gestational age, etiology of the IUGR, and severity and

progression of maternal disease (ACOG, 2000a). Twenty-six percent of stillbirths can be related in some way to IUGR (ACOG, 2000a). IUGR infants often have thermoregulatory difficulties and hypoglycemia, not to mention that many IUGR babies are born prematurely, therefore having to cope with the sequellae of preterm birth as well. The perinatal mortality and morbidity are significant.

The etiology of IUGR can also be divided into three categories (ACOG 2000a):

Maternal—inadequate substrate is available as seen with smoking, malnutrition, and severe chronic disease.

Placental—inadequate transfer of substrate due to placental insufficiency such as seen with essential hypertension or circumvallate placenta.

Fetal—adequate substrate is present from the mother, and the placenta is functioning normally, but the fetus is unable to use the substrate, as seen with intrauterine infection or congenital anomalies.

Growth restriction can be asymmetric or symmetric:

Asymmetrical growth restriction is related to inadequate substrates for fetal metabolism and occurs primarily in the latter part of pregnancy when growth is related to increase in cell size instead of cell number. Muscoloskeletal and head dimensions are spared but the abdominal circumference is decreased due to decreasing liver size and subcutaneous fat. Asymmetric IUGR is often due to decreased placental perfusion and maternal vascular disease (Manning, 2001; Resnik, 2002).

Symmetrical growth restriction occurs with fetal insult during the first trimester, when fetal growth is related to increase in cell number. There is inadequate growth of both the head and the body, all organs are proportionately reduced in size, and the absolute growth rate is decreased. The etiology of the insult may be infection such as cytomegalovirus, maternal drug use or abuse, and chromosomal or congenital anomalies (Resnik, 2002). However, with a normal interval rate of growth, this fetus may be representative of a small but normal fetus with small but normal parents (ACOG, 2000a; Resnik, 2002).

Large-for-Gestational-Age. An infant may be large for gestational age (LGA), or macrosomic, because of a pathological process, such as diabetes, or because of genetic reasons (e.g., parents of large stature). An LGA infant weighs more than 4,500 g at birth or above the 90th percentile for age (Walsh, 2001).

Risk factors include previous history of macrosomia, maternal prepregnancy weight, weight gain during pregnancy, gestational or insulin dependent diabetes, multiparity, male fetus, postdates, ethnicity, maternal birth weight, maternal height, maternal age less than 17 years, and an abnormal 50 g glucose screen with a resulting normal three-hour OGTT (ACOG, 2000c; Cunningham et al., 2001).

The complications of an LGA fetus for the mother include increased risk of cesarean birth, postpartum hemorrhage and puerperal infection despite the route of delivery, and long-term sequellae of pelvic floor injury attained during a difficult second stage of labor (Pryde & Kay, 2002). The macrosomic infant is at risk for birth trauma, most notably brachial plexus injuries and fractures of the clavicle and humerus associated with shoulder dystocia, as well as asphyxia. Severe asphyxia, while rare, can result in death during a difficult delivery secondary to shoulder dystocia (Pryde & Kay, 2002).

Differential Diagnoses. Increased uterine size may indicate twins, inaccurate dating, polyhydramnios, or uterine fibroids. Decreased size may indicate fetal demise or oligohydramnios. Both polyhydramnios and oligohydramnios may signify serious fetal anomalies (Walsh, 2001).

DIAGNOSIS AND INTERVENTION

Intrauterine Growth Restriction (IUGR). Diagnosis of IUGR requires ultrasound assessment. The standard indices used are abdominal circumference (AC), head circumference (HC), biparietal diameter (BPD), and femur length (FL). Amniotic fluid volume is assessed as well. These parameters are converted to estimate fetal weight (EFW) using standardized formulas and tables. The diagnosis of IUGR should be based on two ultrasound assessments, two to four weeks apart (ACOG, 2000a; Resnik, 2002). An AC that is within normal limits reliably excludes IUGR; a repeat ultrasound is performed in two to four weeks for confirmation (ACOG, 2000a).

Depending on the ultrasound assessment and maternal status, further evaluation of the client and fetus may include fetal karyotyping, maternal serum studies for evidence of viral infection, observation of the client for preeclampsia, and evaluation of the congenital and acquired thrombophylic disorders, particularly if a previous pregnancy was complicated by preeclampsia (Resnik, 2002).

Three variables are involved with treatment of IUGR: fetal environment, fetal assessment, and timing of delivery. This is important because IUGR infants have a greater risk of perinatal mortality and morbidity (Resnik, 2002).

Improving the fetal environment involves consideration of bed rest and stopping work (to increase uterine blood flow), cessation of drug use (alcohol, street drugs, smoking), and aggressive treatment of maternal disease (cardiac and renal conditions, hypertension, malabsorption syndrome) (ACOG, 2000a; Bernstein, Gabbe, & Reed, 2002). Smoking is the most important risk factor for IUGR and cessation of smoking, even in late pregnancy, provides benefit. Women who quit smoking as late as the seventh month still had infants that weighed more at birth than those women who smoked the entire pregnancy (ACOG, 2000a). Nutritional supplementation, low-dose aspirin therapy, and maternal oxygen therapy have not been shown to be of value (ACOG, 2000a; Resnik, 2002). Short-term oxygen therapy during labor may improve fetal acid base balance at the time of delivery (Resnik, 2002).

Tests assessing fetal well-being are fetal movement counts, biophysical profile, Doppler flow studies, amniotic fluid volume assessment, NST, or any combination of these tests (Resnik, 2002). Weekly fetal surveillance is indicated in IUGR, although biweekly assessment is considered with moderate IUGR. Daily surveillance may be indicated, depending on the condition of the mother or fetus (ACOG, 2000a, Devoe, 1999).

Doppler flow studies have become important in assessing the IUGR fetus and decreasing perinatal death and unnecessary induction of the preterm IUGR fetus. While ACOG (2000a) does not recommend the use of Doppler flow to diagnose IUGR, its use in managing an IUGR fetus has been documented. Abnormal results in assessment, particularly absent or reverse diastolic flow, should prompt the consideration for delivery, regardless of gestational age (ACOG, 2000a; Resnik, 2002).

Currently delivery is an optimal treatment for the mature IUGR fetus; the risks and benefits must be weighed for the immature fetus. The use of corticosteroids to decrease neonatal pulmonary and central nervous system morbidity is advised if delivery is likely to occur before 34 weeks of gestation (ACOG, 2000a; Resnik, 2002).

Large-for-Gestational-Age Fetus. Diagnosis of *fetal* (as opposed to infant) macrosomia is an estimated weight of greater than 4,500 g. Methods to predict birthweight include assessment of maternal risk factors, clinical exam using Leopold's maneuvers, and ultrasound estimation (ACOG, 2000c). However, ultrasound estimation is limited with an error rate of 10 to 15 percent and higher (ACOG, 2000c; Pryde & Kay, 2002). Future research may focus on measuring soft tissue mass to diagnose fetal macrosomia, such as humeral soft tissue thickness or quantifying fetal shoulder width and maternal pelvic dimensions to predict shoulder dystocia (Pryde & Kay, 2002).

If the diagnosis of fetal macrosomia is made, the client is screened for gestational diabetes if this has not already been done. Repeating an OGTT may be prudent even if the client had a normal OGTT.

Management is based on the glycemic status of the client. For nondiabetic clients, dietary counseling has been advocated but not thoroughly studied (ACOG, 2000c). In a nondiabetic client, awaiting spontaneous labor is the rule, and induction is not advised. Cesarean delivery is considered if EFW is 5,000 g or greater (ACOG, 2000c).

Establishing euglycemia through dietary counseling or insulin use in diabetic clients can reduce the prevalence of macrosomia (ACOG, 2000c; Pryde & Kay, 2002). In pregnancies complicated by diabetes with an EFW of < 4,250 g, induction may be considered after establishing fetal lung maturity, although induction is debated (ACOG, 2000c; Pryde & Kay, 2002). In pregnancies complicated by diabetes with an EFW of 4,250–5,000 g, elective cesarean delivery is considered (ACOG, 2000c; Pryde & Kay, 2002).

Client Teaching and Counseling

Describe to the client the interventions that are to be carried out. Emphasize that these interventions will increase the chances of a healthy, term infant (if possible) and may heighten her participation with the proposed plan of care. For a client whose fetal growth restriction is due to drug use, further discussion about drug use is necessary (see Chapter 18, Substance Abuse).

Many clients believe that a large infant is a sign of good health and that the mother has adequately cared for herself and her infant. The opposite, however, can be true for the mother of a small infant. When counseling clients, it may be difficult to overcome the negative connotations associated with a small infant. Educating the client concerning the underlying processes of abnormal growth patterns may encourage her participation in care.

After delivery, if the cause of the SGA or LGA infant is diagnosed, appropriate intervention or counseling should be initiated. For instance, a mother of an LGA baby should be screened for undiagnosed diabetes, even if previous screens were negative. Both the mother of an LGA or IUGR baby should be encouraged to seek early prenatal care with subsequent pregnancies to establish accurate dating and to follow the growth of the fetus serially to assess any abnormal growth patterns. If maternal conditions exist that can be modified or controlled, such as eating disorders or maternal substance abuse, then the postpartum period is an excellent time for preconceptional counseling. Open discussions concerning substance use may make the client aware of the need to prevent pregnancy and to seek counseling if she is dependent on a substance. Clients who use substances occasionally need to be aware of the potential teratogenic effect of one exposure.

SCREENING AND PREVENTION OF RhD ALLOIMMUNIZATION

Maternal sensitization, or alloimmunization, may occur with exposure to blood or blood products that contain an antigen not found in maternal blood cells. Exposure potentially prompts production of antibodies to that antigen. Sensitization can occur following transfusion or exposure to fetal blood containing factors inherited from the father. The incidence of Rh alloimmunization has decreased because of the administration of anti-D immune globulin (Rhogam) to unsensitized women. However, 1 percent of Rh-D negative women are alloimmunized (Neal, 2001). It may increase due to sharing of needles among drug users, or an Rh-negative woman may unknowingly abort an Rh-positive fetus (Tabsh & Theroux, 1998). Fetal sensitization can also occur according to the "grandmother" theory: an Rh-negative fetus is exposed to enough maternal Rh-positive red blood cells during delivery to cause fetal sensitization (Tabsh & Theroux, 1998).

Rh STATUS

Rh status refers to presence (Rh-positive) or absence (Rh-negative) of Rh antigen on the red blood cell. More than 400 antigens of the Rh factor have been identified. They can all cause hemolytic disease; however, the D antigen causes the majority of Rh alloimmunization. *Other antigens have various effects on fetuses as a result of diversified antibody responses and should be managed individually* (Cunningham et al., 2001). Because the vast majority of cases of alloimmunization are due to the D antigen, in the remainder of this section the D antigen is used as an example.

Initial Screening

For all clients, determine blood type, Rh status, and atypical antibody titer (indirect Coombs test) at the first prenatal care visit.

Interpretation of Results and Management. If the client is D-negative or has a positive antibody screen, determine the father's blood type and Rh and antigen status. If the father is D-negative and has no antigens to the corresponding antibodies that the mother has, then no further consideration is needed (ACOG, 1999). If, however, the father is Rh-positive and has a negative antigen screen, or if testing the father's blood is not possible, draw a maternal antibody titer at 28 weeks. If D antibody is absent, then give Rhogam.

Rhogam is given specifically to prevent alloimmunization to D antigen. Rhogam is comprised of anti-D IgG antibodies and, while not clearly understood, acts by binding with Rh-positive fetal cells if they are present in the maternal circulation. Through various means, it blocks maternal antigen processing (Jackson & Branch, 2002). Rhogam is of no value when alloimmunization has occurred. Rhogam is again given within 72 hours of delivery if the fetus is Rh-positive. There is debate as to whether one should give Rhogam to Rh-negative clients who undergo bilateral tubal ligation after delivery, because in the future they may decide to have the ligation reversed (ACOG, 1999; Neal, 2001). Breastfeeding is not a contraindication to administration of Rhogam.

If the client has a positive antibody screen and the father is positive for antigen, maternal antibody should be characterized and the titer determined. Titers must be followed through gestation if it is determined that antibodies are IgG; IgG can cross the placenta and cause hemolytic disease in the fetus. A rising or elevated titer (greater than or equal to 1:8 or 1:16, depending on the laboratory) indicates the need for further clinical assessment (see Management of an Isoimmunized Pregnancy later in this section) (ACOG, 1996; Jackson & Branch, 2002).

Of clinical importance is the need to notify the blood bank of the client's irregular antibody in the event a transfusion is needed at delivery.

It is possible to determine fetal blood type through polymerase chain reaction (PCR) using amniocytes or chorionic villi obtained during procedures for standard obstetric indications (Neal, 2001; Stockman, 2001). For example, a 40-year-old Rh-negative client requests CVS

for genetic screening. Villi obtained can be used for chromosomal analysis and to determine fetal blood type. Fetal cells have also been isolated from maternal blood; determining fetal blood type early in pregnancy would decrease the need of obtaining repeated maternal antibody titers as well as invasive and noninvasive fetal testing. If the fetus is Rh-negative, no further intervention is necessary. More research is needed to give consistent accuracy to avoid mistyping an Rh-positive fetus as an Rh-negative fetus (Wachtel, Shulman, & Sammons, 2001).

Other Indications for Administration of Rhogam During Pregnancy. Rhogam should be given anytime there exists a potential for mixing Rh-positive fetal and Rh-negative maternal blood. *If there is ever any doubt as to whether to give Rhogam, then it should be given* (ACOG, 1999).

- Chorionic villus sampling
- Therapeutic or spontaneous abortion
- Ectopic pregnancy
- Molar pregnancy
- Amniocentesis
- Antepartum hemorrhage
- Cordocentesis or other percutaneous fetal procedures
- External cephalic version
- Fetal death
- Fetal surgery
- Transfusion of D-positive blood to D-negative mother

Hemorrhage. If at any time during the pregnancy a large fetal-to-maternal hemorrhage is suspected, or copious bleeding occurs at delivery, as with manual removal of the placenta, the Kleihauer-Betke test is performed on a sample of maternal blood to measure fetal blood in the maternal system. If fetal blood is present in maternal blood, then 10 mcg of Rhogam is given per milliliter of fetal blood in the maternal system. The standard dose is 300 mcg, which is effective for 30 mL of fetal blood. If more than 30 mL of blood is present in the maternal system, then the volume of fetal red cells can be estimated by analysis of maternal blood; the dose of Rhogam is adjusted accordingly (ACOG, 1999).

Many physicians do not give anti-D immune globulin to a client with a live fetus in the presence of a *threatened* abortion up to 12 weeks of gestation (ACOG, 1999).

PROCESS OF ALLOIMMUNIZATION

If the client does not receive Rhogam and is exposed to D antigen on fetal cells, she will produce anti-D IgM antibodies. This initial response usually is not problematic (unless the exposure is massive), as IgM antibodies do not usually cross the placenta. A second exposure to fetal cells with the D antigen will cause the development of IgG antibodies. No amount of prophylaxis at this point will prevent a hemolytic response (Cunningham et al., 2001).

Anti-D IgG antibodies cross the placenta readily, coat fetal cells if they have D antigen, and cause hemolysis. The fetus compensates by increasing its production of red blood cells, but if hemolysis is severe, the fetus maximizes red blood cell production in the liver and spleen. The increased demands on the fetal liver result in enlargement, altered function, and decreased albumin production, which lead to leakage of fluid from the fetal vasculature. Ascites and effusions thereby develop. As hemolysis continues, anemia worsens. Ultimately, cardiovascular collapse and fetal death occur. These events describe the process of fetal hemolytic disease, or hydrops fetalis (Cunningham et al., 2001; Redman & Berry, 2002).

Management of an Alloimmunized Pregnancy

Management begins with assessment of maternal blood type, presence or absence of Rh factor, and any atypical antibody titers at the first prenatal visit. Information from the client about a prior pregnancy, if applicable, or actual prenatal records from a previous pregnancy are helpful. If the client has had a previously affected pregnancy, the severity of hemolytic disease in the next pregnancy will be equal or greater in most cases (ACOG, 1996; Harrington & Fayyad, 2001). An individualized plan of care, based in part on the client's previous obstetric history, is crucial.

As stated, maternal antibody titers are assessed at the first prenatal care visit, then every two to four weeks thereafter (Harrington & Fayyad, 2002; Jackson & Branch, 2002). Each laboratory establishes its own threshold titers below which significant hemolytic disease does not occur. Once this threshold is reached, ultrasound and amniocentesis are considered to assess the possibility of hemolytic disease. Again, maternal obstetric history is crucial as hydrops has been reported in a first sensitized pregnancy, hydrops and fetal death prior to 20 weeks, and hydrops with titers as low as 1:8 (Harrington & Fayyad, 2002).

If the client has a history of a previously affected pregnancy, titers are only helpful to establish when amniocentesis or cordocentesis is needed, if at all. Invasive procedures are currently necessary to monitor a fetus because titers often remain stable in the presence of severely affected fetuses (ACOG, 1996; Harrington & Fayyad, 2002; Jackson & Branch, 2002). Invasive procedures are usually scheduled four to eight weeks prior to the point in the previously affected pregnancy that fetal morbidity was encountered (ACOG, 1996).

Amniotic fluid assays and PUBS may begin early in the second trimester, depending on the extent of disease. Bilirubin, the byproduct of red blood cell destruction, can be measured spectrophotometrically in amniotic fluid or fetal blood. The spectrophotometric value is written as ΔOD_{450} and plotted on the Liley graph. The graph is separated into three zones and management of the fetus is based upon where the ΔOD_{450} falls on the graph at a particular gestational age. Delivery or transfusion should be considered for a value that is in zone three or a rising or even horizontal titer in zone two (ACOG, 1996; Stockman, 2001). The Liley graph was developed from pregnancies of at least 28 weeks gestation. Several approaches have been taken in gestations less than 28 weeks. Some clinicians have taken the original Liley values and extrapolated backwards to 24 weeks gestation (Jackson & Branch, 2002). Queenan, Tomai, Ural, & King (1993) developed a chart of spectrophotometric measurements for earlier gestations beginning at 14 weeks and detected anemia in the presence of low ΔOD_{450} values in the second trimester. Others rely on PUBS for assessing the fetal hematocrit, using a standardized chart of appropriate hematocrit values based on gestational age (ACOG, 1996). This is appropriate management for Rh-D alloimmunization only; other antigen incompatibilities resulting in alloimmunization, such as the Kell antigen, require different management strategy. Cordocentesis is used earlier as ΔOD_{450} values and titers do not correlate with the severity of fetal anemia (Redman & Berry, 2002).

PUBS is used to monitor the fetal hematocrit, which truly determines the severity of fetal anemia, as compared to relying on amniotic fluid assays alone. Through monitoring of the bilirubin level and fetal hematocrit, the necessity and frequency of fetal transfusion can be assessed. Monitoring occurs at one to four week intervals, depending on the severity of disease (ACOG, 1996).

Research has focused on establishing sonographic markers to predict fetal anemia in order to determine the necessity for invasive testing or intervention (amniocentesis, cordocentesis, fetal transfusion, or delivery). Pleural and pericardial effusions, ascites, hepatosplenomegaly, umbilical vein distention, and placental thickness > 4 cm have been documented in the presence of fetal anemia

(ACOG, 1996; Harrington & Fayyad, 2002). However, these signs are noted when decompensation has occurred for the fetus. Mari, Detti, Oz, et al. (2002) have researched the use of the middle cerebral artery peak systolic velocity (MCA-PSV) to assess fetal hemoglobin levels to thereby determine the need for invasive procedures. Amniocentesis has been used to detect fetal anemia related to Rh-D alloimmunization for over forty years, and cordocentesis has been utilized to diagnose and manage fetal anemia for over sixteen years. While these methods have been instrumental in providing care for the fetus, possible worsening of fetal anemia and fetal loss are potential complications (Mari et al., 2002). Noninvasive, accurate assessment of fetal anemia would decrease the incidence of unnecessary invasive testing. While ultrasound has not replaced invasive testing for fetal anemia, its role will certainly continue to be refined (Harrington & Fayyad, 2002).

Nonstress tests are recommended because a hydrops-affected fetus may exhibit sinusoidal or other ominous patterns during heart rate monitoring (Neal, 2001). Diminished fetal activity, however, may precede changes detected by external monitoring. Therefore, fetal movement counts between ultrasound exams are advised to monitor an affected fetus (Neal, 2001; Vintzileos, 2000).

Treatment of Alloimmunization

Transfusions may be administered using the intraperitoneal or intravascular route, and are recommended if the fetal hematocrit is 2g/dL less than the mean for normal fetuses of the same gestational age, or a fetal hematocrit of 25 to 30 percent or less (ACOG, 1996; Cunningham et al., 2001; Harrington & Fayyad, 2002). Transfusion is at present the only method that will save a hydropic fetus if delivery is remote. Most clinicians use an intravascular route for transfusion, although combinations of intraperitoneal and intravascular routes are used in some circumstances (ACOG, 1996; Harrington & Fayyad, 2002; Stockman, 2001).

Client Teaching and Counseling

For the unsensitized client, reinforce the need for Rhogam at 28 weeks and after delivery. Support and encourage the client to be involved in her care, emphasizing the importance of prenatal care visits. A client considering home delivery needs to be aware of the importance of receiving Rhogam within 72 hours if the baby's blood type is unknown or if the infant is Rh-positive in order to prevent alloimmunization in the next pregnancy.

Some clients feel that if they miscarry early in gestation, all tissue is passed, and bleeding stops, they do not need to be evaluated in the health care setting. Stress the importance of evaluation and, at the same time, the necessity of receiving Rhogam when miscarriage occurs.

In the event of alloimmunization, carefully discuss all procedures with the client to encourage her participation and fully explain the plan of care.

ABO INCOMPATIBILITY

ABO incompatibility is not as severe because most antibodies to A and B antigens are IgM antibodies, which do not cross the placenta. Usually, the mother is blood type O, with anti-A and anti-B in her serum, and the infant is blood type A, B, or AB. Titers and amniocentesis are not required during pregnancy; however, treatment begins after delivery for the infant. Jaundice becomes clinically apparent as the infant's red blood cells are hemolyzed as a result of ABO incompatibility. The infant's bilirubin levels are monitored and phototherapy is used to treat elevated bilirubin levels. Occasionally, a transfusion is required for the infant (Cunningham et al., 2001).

Client Teaching and Counseling

Most teaching centers on information concerning the infant's condition. The mother also needs reassurance. Emphasize to the client that her infant's condition is not her fault and that she should not feel guilty about the infant undergoing treatment. Providing her with written material that explains ABO incompatibility and treatment will help. The client needs to be prepared should the infant become frankly jaundiced. Tell her that the pediatrician may change the infant's feeding schedule or type of feeding to enhance the breakdown of bilirubin. Depending on the age of the infant and the bilirubin level, phototherapy may be initiated. Traditional phototherapy involves placing the infant under a bank of fluorescent lights to lower the bilirubin level. While effective, this mode of therapy raised several issues concerning parental and familial bonding (Wong, Perry, & Hockenberry, 2002). The development of the Wallaby blanket, which wraps around the infant's torso, provides the same therapy, and reduces several adverse effects on breastfeeding, maternal attachment, and familial interaction. The low-risk infant can be discharged and therapy continued at home, thereby avoiding a longer hospital stay and disruption of the family (Kimball, 2001).

If the infant is undergoing traditional phototherapy, the mother will have less time to hold, feed, and bond with her infant. Assess this potential inability to bond and arrange to have the client provide as much care as possible. Also explain that the infant's eyes will be covered while undergoing phototherapy.

Discuss the possibility of transfusion. Discussion may assist the client in making decisions about problematic religious or cultural issues. Because transfusions can become a legal issue, every effort should be made to educate the client concerning the need for treatment. In this way, conflict may be avoided.

MATERNAL SERUM SCREENING

In the United States in the mid-1980s, maternal screening consisted of measuring maternal serum α-fetoprotein (MS-AFP) levels as a screen for neural tube defects (NTD). By the late 1980s, low levels of MS-AFP had been associated with Down syndrome, and screening was initiated for both Down syndrome and NTDs using MS-AFP. It was soon noted that a high level of β-human chorionic gonadotropin (β-hCG) and low levels of unconjugated estriol (uE3) and MS-AFP were associated with Down syndrome. Later, it was noted that low levels of β-hCG, uE3, and MS-AFP were associated with Trisomy 18—therefore, the "birth" of the triple screen. MS-AFP can be measured between 15 and 20 weeks but is most accurate from 16 to 18 weeks (ACOG, 2001b).

There is debate on the use of all three serum analytes, whether to use free versus intact beta subunits of hCG, and the possibility of using a fourth marker, dimeric inhibin-A (ACOG, 2001b; Yaran & Mashiach, 2001). There is also potential for screening in the first trimester for Down syndrome using β-hCG and pregnancy-associated plasma protein (PAPP-A) (ACOG, 2001b; Yaran & Mashiach, 2001). Clinical trials are underway to investigate first trimester versus second trimester screening for Down syndrome (Yaran & Mashiach, 2001). Currently, the standard of care is to offer maternal serum triple screen at 16 to 18 weeks to clients in the absence of risk factors (ACOG, 2001b).

Clients with a personal or family history of chromosomal anomalies or neural tube defects are offered diagnostic methods (as opposed to a screening tests) such as chorionic villus sampling or amniocentesis for assessing the fetus (ACOG, 2001b).

Currently, ACOG (2001b) states that clients older than 35 at the time of delivery (or 33 with a twin pregnancy) should be offered amniocentesis first for routine prenatal diagnosis (ACOG, 2001b). There is debate as to whether *all* women should be offered serum screening, including those women who are at a perceived increased risk due to age alone. This would potentially decrease the number of amniocenteses and thus the number of procedure-related losses. Current research using ultrasound and maternal serum markers will no doubt significantly change options available to clients desiring accurate, non-invasive screening (Egan, Benn, Borgida, et al., 2000; Rosen, Kedar, Amiel, et al., 2002; Spencer, 2002).

If clients 35 years or older or those with other risk factors request serum screening, they need to be advised of the risks and benefits of replacing a diagnostic test with a screening test and referred to specialized centers (ACOG, 2001b; DeVore & Romero, 2002).

INTERPRETATION

The levels of MS-AFP, hCG, and uE3 are reported as multiples of the median (MoM) and adjusted in the laboratory for maternal weight, presence of diabetes, gestational age, multiple gestation, and race. In a singleton pregnancy, *elevated values of MS-AFP* are greater than 2.0 to 2.5 MoM. *Low values, however, are assessed with respect to maternal age* (maternal age dependent threshold); elevated values are not. With respect to low values, normal ranges of MS-AFP are established by each laboratory based on maternal age (ACOG, 2001b; Simpson, 2002).

ETIOLOGY OF AN ABNORMAL RESULT

MS-AFP levels were initially used to screen for NTDs. However, elevated levels have also been associated with presence of undiagnosed multiple gestation, Rh alloimmunization or cystic hygroma (both of which are associated with fetal edema), anomalies other than NTDs that are associated with skin edema, and fetal death (Cunningham et al., 2001; Drugan, Weissman, & Evans, 2001; Simpson, 2002).

Low levels have been associated with incorrect gestational age, chromosomal trisomies, gestational trophoblastic disease, and fetal death (Cunningham et al., 2001).

Other factors that may not have been calculated correctly or were not taken into account are correct gestational age, maternal weight, race, and presence of diabetes (Cunningham et al., 2001; Drugan, Weissman, & Evans, 2001; Lewis, 2002; Simpson, 2002). False elevations may occur if maternal serum was drawn *after* an invasive procedure such as amniocentesis or chorionic villus sampling (Lewis, 2002).

CLINICAL MANAGEMENT

It is acceptable to repeat an elevated MS-AFP (greater than 2.0–2.5 MoM) if the value is less than 3.0 or 3.5 MoM. Values higher than 3.0 to 3.5 MoM usually indicate an increased risk for the fetus and should not be repeated; rather, a targeted ultrasound is performed alone or with amniocentesis to assess gestational age and any structural anomalies (Cunningham et al., 2001; Simpson, 2002).

If gestational age is incorrect or if another nonpathological cause of an abnormal value is noted (such as twins), the MoM is recalculated and usually found to be within normal limits. Underestimation of gestational age is the most common reason for an elevated MS-AFP. If a structural anomaly is noted, the fetus should be thoroughly assessed for other anomalies and amniocentesis offered to note genetic aberrations. If no anomaly is apparent and no other cause of an abnormal marker is found, amniocentesis is indicated (Cunningham et al., 2001).

Amniocentesis is done to assess amniotic fluid AFP (AFAFP) and perform chromosomal analysis. A positive AFAFP is validated by measuring the amount of acetylcholinesterase (AChE) in the amniotic fluid sample. AChE is present only if there is an open neural tube defect. If the elevated AFAFP level is due to contamination with fetal blood, AChE will be absent. A low level of AChE or its absence suggests something other than open neural tube defect as the etiology of the elevated AFAFP. As stated previously, a detailed ultrasonographic exam should follow the amniocentesis (Simpson, 2002).

Ninety to 95 percent of clients with abnormal MS-AFP levels have a normal level of AFAFP. Even though the AFAFP is normal, the risk for IUGR, premature labor, neonatal death, preeclampsia, fetal demise, oligohydramnios, and abruption is greater (Drugan, Weissman, & Evans, 2001). Elevated levels of β-hCG and low levels of uE3 and PAPP-A have been associated with adverse perinatal outcomes as well. The cause may be due in part to poor placental function (Krause, Christens, Wohlfahrt, et al., 2001; Smith, Stenhouse, Crossley, et al., 2002; Yaran, Cherry, Kramer, et al., 1999). Currently, ACOG does not advise heightened surveillance for abnormal levels of MS-AFP in the absence of an etiology; rather, routine obstetric care is the standard of care until a problem is identified (ACOG, 1996). A recent study by Huerta-Enochian, Katz, and Erfurth (2001) concerning the association of adverse outcome with abnormal MS-AFP also concluded that heightened surveillance did not improve pregnancy outcome; adverse outcomes were detected with routine obstetric care or were undetectable with heightened surveillance. Their opinion reflected that of ACOG that "routine pregnancy management was an acceptable method of detecting adverse outcomes when they were detectable."

Amniocentesis is not a test to determine whether to consider termination. Rather, it should be seen as a diagnostic tool. Invasive genetic testing remains the gold standard for fetal diagnosis. Diagnosis of a fetal problem allows the health care provider to supply the client with options for the pregnancy. This may be a referral to a perinatologist for further care or planning of care for the infant at delivery and beyond; termination may be considered as well. By providing information to the health care provider as well as the client, pregnancy outcome and the plan of care can be optimized. In the presence of an open neural tube defect, cesarean delivery appears to retain greater neurologic function and should be considered (Cunningham et al., 2001).

ADVANTAGES AND DISADVANTAGES

Maternal serum screening can be done in the office or clinic. If subsequent testing due to abnormal values reveals a fetal problem, treatment (if possible) may be instituted; this also enables the client to be prepared and plan care for a child with a chromosomal or structural anomaly. This certainly is an advantage for the clinician when planning fetal surveillance, as well as the mode of delivery, and the care that will be needed by the neonate after delivery. Screening and diagnosis in the second trimester also allows the client the option of choosing termination.

For those who do not wish to have an invasive procedure, triple marker screening may be an option. Diagnosis and confirmation of abnormal results, however, would require amniocentesis.

There are disadvantages. Maternal serum testing screens for abnormalities; it is not diagnostic. Further intervention is required to assess the etiology. The high rate of false positive results may increase further if certain factors, for example, race and multiple gestation, are not taken into account, and clients may proceed with amniocentesis unnecessarily (see next section).

CLIENT TEACHING AND COUNSELING

Inform the client of possible test outcomes and clinical sequence of testing that would be advised in the event of abnormal test results prior to drawing MS-AFP. Many clients can cope with having blood drawn, but the decision to do a chromosomal analysis may pose a cultural or religious dilemma for some. The sequence of events leading to diagnosis after an abnormal test result is often unanticipated. Some clients want to know if the fetus has an abnormality; others prefer not to know until the birth and may refuse further diagnostic testing. The health care provider may be caught in the middle as in the event of an abnormal MS-AFP result, wherein the fetus will be assumed to be at risk.

ULTRASONOGRAPHY

Ultrasonography uses high frequency sound waves to produce an image. A transducer directs sound waves toward an object (e.g., the fetus). When the waves interface with solid structures, energy is reflected back to the transducer, which creates electrical voltage. That voltage produces an image on screen. Real-time ultrasound differs from conventional ultrasound. Real-time ultrasound uses a multiple-pulse system of sound waves to note movement, such as fetal breathing; conventional ultrasound uses only a single pulse (Chervenak & Gabbe, 2002). Most ultrasounds are performed in two dimensions (2D). Current research is focusing upon the use of 3D ultrasound for fetal assessment (Hull, Pretorius, & Nelson, 2001; Kuno, Akiyama, Yamashioo, et al., 2001). Specialized training is needed to perform and interpret ultrasound. Abdominal ultrasound or a transvaginal probe may be used in assessment.

Ultrasound has no confirmed biologic adverse effects on the fetus (Chervenak & Gabbe, 2002). This has led many to use ultrasound indiscriminantly. Clients often want an ultrasound just to know the sex of the baby. Currently, ultrasound should be used only to the medical benefit of a mother or fetus, although most health care providers use ultrasound routinely. There is a great deal of debate about and desire for the increased use of ultrasound in the first and second trimester for the screening of genetic and congenital anomalies. Research is focusing on first trimester scanning and screening, but mainly from researchers in other countries (Timor-Tritsch, 2001)

because scanning at 11 to 14 weeks is a routine standard of care in other countries (Sen, 2001). Currently, the NIH is funding a multicenter trial known as the First- and Second-Trimester Evaluation of Risk trial, which may influence the implementation of first-trimester ultrasound use in the United States (Souter & Nyberg, 2001).

Due to a variety of reasons, routine sonography—much less transvaginal sonography—is not the rule in the United States (Timor-Trisch, 2001). Timor-Trisch advises a transvaginal ultrasound at 14 to 16 weeks and a complementary transabdominal ultrasound at 20 to 24 weeks. However, many insurance companies only reimburse for one ultrasound in uncomplicated pregnancies. With a choice of only having one ultrasound, many choose or see the need for an 18 to 22 week scan (Carvalho, Brizot, Lopes, et al., 2002; Copel, 2001; Druzin et al., 2002). There's added debate when considering the mounting research for nuchal translucency and maternal serum screening for Down syndrome in the first trimester as well as transvaginal ultrasound at 14 to 16 weeks for detection of anomalies. Developing guidelines for using maternal serum as well as ultrasound markers for detecting structural and chromosomal anomalies may dramatically decrease the unnecessary use of invasive procedures (Rosen et al., 2002).

With various changes in health care, the cost effectiveness of providing routine screening to all women remains an issue. Some studies have found benefit to routine screening, while others found no difference in perinatal outcome (ACOG, 1997b; Comstock, 2002; Goncalves et al., 2001). *Routine ultrasound examination is not currently recommended by the American College of Obstetricians and Gynecologists* (ACOG, 1997b).

Generally, ultrasonography should provide the information sought (e.g., possible source of bleeding), as well as various parameters depending on gestational age. The use of the term "level" is being phased out as it is more prudent to assess parameters that are appropriate for the gestational age. A distinction is made when a fetus is considered to be at risk for a structural anomaly, or if during a basic scan, there are questionable findings. In this case the client should be referred for a targeted ultrasound for specialized scanning (Cunningham et al., 2001; Druzin et al., 2002). The health care provider should not assume a lack of responsibility for being knowledgeable and competent when providing even a basic ultrasound, however, as most congenital anomalies occur in the absence of risk factors. The following guidelines have been developed by the American Institute of Ultrasound in Medicine (Price,

Fleischer, & Abuhamad, 2001) and will no doubt change as ultrasound becomes more refined and is utilized more for prenatal diagnosis.

Ultrasound in the first trimester should obtain the following information (Price et al., 2001).

- Presence or absence in an intrauterine gestational sac and location
- Identification of embryo or fetus
- Fetal number
- Presence or absence of fetal cardiac activity
- Crown-rump length
- Evaluation of uterus and adnexal structures

Various parameters such as fetal heart activity and the presence of a gestational sac are noted earlier, using vaginal scanning as opposed to abdominal scanning.

Ultrasound in the second and third trimester should obtain the following information (Price et al., 2001):

- Presence of fetal life, number of fetuses present, and any abnormalities of heart rate or rhythm.
- Amount of amniotic fluid.
- Location of placenta and its relationship to the cervix.
- Estimation of the gestational age, using two of the following parameters—biparietal diameter (BPD), head circumference (HC), femur length (FL), and abdominal circumference (AC). Overall, third trimester ultrasounds are not accurate assessment of GA; dating is most accurate if done before 26 weeks.
- Attempt to survey fetal anatomy (cerebral ventricles, spine, stomach, urinary bladder, umbilical cord insertion site, and renal regions). Suspected anomalies require a targeted evaluation.

INDICATIONS FOR ULTRASOUND

Gestational Age Determination

Ultrasound is used to establish gestational age (GA) throughout pregnancy; however, gestational age is most accurately assessed in the first trimester when there is minimal variation in fetal growth. GA is most accurately estimated by measuring crown-to-rump length (CRL) between 7 and 10 weeks. Based on the CRL, the gestational age can be calculated within three days 90 percent of the time (Jeanty, 2001). Other parameters are used for second and third trimester assessment of GA (see previous paragraph). As stated, third trimester ultrasounds are not accurate assessments of gestational age. The margin of error for predicting GA is greater as pregnancy advances, par-

ticularly in the third trimester. This needs to be taken into account when considering interventions on the behalf of the fetus that may be influenced by GA.

Growth Assessment

Ultrasound is indicated when a discrepancy exists between estimated gestational age and uterine size. The ultrasound is done to rule out abnormalities or to correct errors in dating. It is used serially to diagnose intrauterine growth restriction in clients at risk for decreased uteroplacental perfusion, for example, those with hypertension or a history of fetuses with intrauterine growth restriction (Manning, 2001).

Ratios of various measurements are often given to provide an index for growth. If not, they can be calculated and compared with standardized charts to determine appropriate growth for a particular gestational age.

Detection of Fetal Anomalies

Fetal anomalies can be detected with ultrasound. Assessing fetal structures for anomalies is *fetal scanning*. Ninety-eight percent of fetal structures can be assessed by transvaginal sonography by 14 weeks. Eighty percent of congenital anomalies can be detected by the second trimester (Goncalves et al., 2001). Anomalies related to a polygenic disorder cannot be diagnosed using enzyme assays or DNA at this time; therefore, ultrasound is the method of choice to assess the fetus (Simpson, 2002). Often clients present with a history of a child with structural anomalies and have a 1 to 5 percent risk of recurrence (Simpson, 2002). ACOG (2001b) recommends that clients desiring ultrasound as a method of prenatal diagnosis to avoid invasive procedures be referred to specialized centers and counseled appropriately as to the sensitivity and specificity of ultrasound.

Research continues in the area of identifying "sonographic markers" for various genetic and structural anomalies; nuchal lucency is being investigated as a marker for Down syndrome (ACOG, 2001b; Beamer, 2001; Ott & Taysi, 2001; Snijders, 2001). Diagnosis of chromosomal abnormalities requires invasive testing, however, and many clients may prefer fetal scanning to assess the fetus. Standard of care dictates referral to highly experienced clinicians (Simpson, 2002).

DeVore and Romero (2002) propose offering genetic sonography to clients 35 years and older who originally decline invasive testing; in the event sonographic abnormalities are identified, the client can choose invasive testing based on sonographic markers versus theoretical risk based on age alone. Vintzileos, Guzman, Smulian, and colleagues (2002) researched the value of combining genetic sonography and maternal serum screening in clients of advanced maternal age (35 years or greater) to assess the risk for Down syndrome. In their study, genetic sonography was defined as a targeted exam that included basic ultrasound fetal biometry but also included an assessment for the following markers: facial anomalies, hand anomalies, cardiac anomalies, short long bones, pyelectasis, nuchal fold thickening, echogenic bowel, choroid plexus cyst, echogenic intracardiac focus, clinodactyly, sandal gap, and a two-vessel cord (Vintzileos et al., 2002). In their study, no cases of Down syndrome were found in clients of advanced maternal age with normal genetic sonography (Vintzileos et al., 2002). This investigational yet rapidly evolving approach provides additional information to the client concerning fetal normalcy without increasing unnecessary risk to the fetus as is the case with traditional prenatal diagnosis.

Fetal scans are indicated for women with a family history of disorder or anomaly of the abdominal wall or central nervous, renal, cardiac, or skeletal system; exposure to any teratogen that produces structural anomalies is also an indication for ultrasound (Chervenak & Gabbe, 2002; Cunningham et al., 2001; Goncalves et al., 2001). Use and image interpretation will become more complex and diverse as technology advances.

Assessment of Amniotic Fluid Volume

Ultrasound assessment of amniotic fluid volume (AFV) has become a sensitive indicator of fetal well-being, especially when combined with other surveillance methods. The majority of amniotic fluid is produced by the fetal lungs and kidneys; fetal swallowing begins early in the second trimester and subsequently any abnormality with the gastrointestinal or genitourinary tract may be reflected in abnormal amniotic fluid volumes (Walsh, 2001).

There is a correlation of decreased AFV and placental insufficiency due to the adaptive response fetuses exhibit to hypoxemia. Known as the "brain-sparing effect," blood is shunted to the vital organs and away from the kidneys. This shunting of blood over a period of time decreases AFV because fetal urine production makes up the majority of amniotic fluid after midgestation (Bernstein, Gabbe, & Reed, 2002; Magann & Martin, 1999). Normal AFV is important for normal fetal growth, fetal move-

ment, and cushioning of the fetus, cord, and placenta (Magann & Martin, 1999).

Increased AFV has been associated with neural tube defects, gastrointestinal obstruction, immune and nonimmune hydrops, and CNS abnormalities contributing to impaired swallowing. Decreased AFV has been associated with renal abnormalities, gastrointestinal obstruction, and IUGR (Magann & Martin, 1999).

There have been several methods to measure AFV: the largest vertical pocket (LVP), two-diameter pocket measurements, and amniotic fluid index (AFI) (Magann, & Martin, 1999; Walsh, 2001). AFI appears to be the most used and the least subjective. The AFI is the sum of the deepest cord-free amniotic fluid pocket in each of the four quadrants of the uterus; at term an AFI of < 5.0 cm is indicative of oligohydramnios and an AFI of > 20 cm indicates polyhydramnios (Chervanak & Gabbe, 2002). Moore and Cayle (1990) developed a table of AFI values based on gestational age (See Table 19–1). Oligohydramnios is defined as an AFI value less than 5th percentile for a given gestational age, and polyhydramnios is an AFI greater than 95th percentile for a given gestational age. Once detected, extremes of amniotic fluid require further evaluation.

Monitoring of a Post-Term Pregnancy

Surveillance should be considered for post-term pregnancy, defined as one that lasts beyond 42 weeks. Perinatal mortality and morbidity is increased for a fetus past 41 weeks (Divon, 2002; Walsh, 2001). Many providers initiate surveillance at 41 weeks. The combination of monitoring amniotic fluid volume, the NST, biophysical profile, and fetal movement counts is used to assess the post-term fetus. Gestational age cannot be accurately determined at term (ACOG, 1999).

Monitoring an "At-Risk" Pregnancy

An example would be the serial use of ultrasound to monitor a fetus exposed to parvovirus B19. Ultrasound is used to note the development of fetal hydrops, placentomegaly, and growth disturbances. Clients should receive weekly sonographic assessment for up to ten to twelve weeks after exposure (ACOG, 2000b; McCarter-Spaulding, 2002). Ultrasound is also used in a complementary manner to diagnose and monitor the fetus who has been exposed to cytomegalovirus, varicella-zoster virus, and toxoplasmosis (ACOG, 2000b).

TABLE 19–1. Amniotic Fluid Index Percentile Values (mm)

Week	Percentile					
	2.5th	5th	50th	95th	97.5th	n
16	73	79	121	185	201	32
17	77	83	127	194	211	26
18	80	87	133	202	220	17
19	83	90	137	207	225	14
20	86	93	141	212	230	25
21	88	95	143	214	233	14
22	89	97	145	216	235	14
23	90	98	146	218	237	14
24	90	98	147	219	238	23
25	89	97	147	221	240	12
26	89	97	147	223	242	11
27	85	95	146	226	245	17
28	86	94	146	228	249	25
29	84	92	145	231	254	12
30	82	90	145	234	258	17
31	79	88	144	238	263	26
32	77	86	144	242	269	25
33	74	83	143	245	274	30
34	72	81	142	248	278	31
35	70	79	140	249	279	27
36	68	77	138	249	279	39
37	66	75	135	244	275	36
38	65	73	132	239	269	27
39	64	72	127	226	255	12
40	63	71	123	214	240	64
41	63	70	116	194	216	162
42	63	69	110	175	192	30

Reprinted with permission from Moore, T., & Cayle, J. (1990). The amniotic fluid index in normal human pregnancy. American Journal of Obstetrics and Gynecology, 162, 1168–1173.

Documentation of Fetal Viability

When fetal heart tones are inaudible by Doppler at 12 weeks or with the DeLee fetoscope at 17 to 19 weeks, or if they are absent after previous documentation, ultrasound is indicated to verify cardiac activity. A gestational sac can be seen when β-hCG is 1000 to 2000 mIU/mL. Failure to see doubling of β-hCG every 48 hours early in pregnancy may be indicative of an ectopic pregnancy or a nonviable fetus. Cardiac activity should be noted by 7 weeks with transvaginal ultrasound (ACOG, 1998a).

For women with a history of vaginal bleeding, ultrasound is needed to establish fetal viability and, if possible, to locate the origin of bleeding. Placenta previa or abruptio placentae may be diagnosed.

Detection of Ectopic Pregnancy

Ectopic pregnancy is always a possible diagnosis in the first trimester in a client with abdominal pain, vaginal bleeding, and a positive pregnancy test. Due to the inability of most extrauterine sites to maintain placental devel-

opment, β-hCG levels decrease, resulting in endometrial degeneration and vaginal bleeding (ACOG, 1998a). Abdominal ultrasound may be attempted first, depending on the protocol of the institution. If abdominal assessment is unsatisfactory, a transvaginal probe is used.

Compilation of Biophysical Profile

The biophysical profile is compiled using ultrasound (see next section).

ADVANTAGES AND DISADVANTAGES

Abdominal ultrasound is noninvasive and may promote bonding, particularly before quickening. Abdominal ultrasound presents a problem for a client experiencing nausea and vomiting during pregnancy, because she must drink approximately 1 quart of water in the hour before examination. Alternatively, the transvaginal probe does not require a full bladder. Anxiety may be increased if clients are not given information during ultrasound concerning structures seen and the well-being of the fetus. Clients' fears are lessened with positive feedback from the ultrasonographer, but due to the various levels of expertise, information may not be shared with the client until confirmed by a provider with clinical expertise in ultrasonography. Ultrasound must be performed and interpreted by a qualified individual. Depending on the test, expertise is required to collect correct data and interpret findings.

Loss of fetus or termination may be more difficult if the client has already viewed the fetus. If ultrasound has promoted bonding, a client may grieve more with demise or termination.

CLIENT TEACHING AND COUNSELING

Explain to the client what ultrasound is. Inform her that no cases of harm to a fetus have been documented. The client needs to be aware that a technician may perform the ultrasound, and, if so, that person can identify structures but cannot interpret findings. Depending on protocol, the radiologist, physician, or practitioner is responsible for discussing the results with the client.

For abdominal ultrasound, the client must drink approximately one quart of water one hour prior to procedure and therefore needs to be aware that there will be pressure on her bladder during ultrasound. If a full bladder is needed and surgery is a potential option, the bladder should be filled by catheter (usually by a technician), and the client should be informed of the need for catheterization.

For the client undergoing transvaginal ultrasound, explain that a probe will be inserted into the vagina. She can expect some pressure but should not be uncomfortable. Briefly describe the probe and reassure the client that the probe will not hurt the fetus or cause miscarriage. A full bladder is not necessary for transvaginal ultrasound.

BIOPHYSICAL PROFILE (BPP)

Real-time ultrasound allows assessment of various parameters of fetal well-being: fetal tone, breathing, motion, and amniotic fluid volume. These four parameters together with the NST constitute the biophysical profile; however, not all facilities perform NST unless other parameters of the profile are abnormal (ACOG, 1999). Man-

ning (1999) advocates using the NST only when one of the four parameters of the BPP is abnormal.

PROCEDURE

Usually the profile is compiled in an outpatient testing center within a hospital. Skilled personnel are required to perform the NST as well as to conduct and evaluate the ultrasound. Although the BPP is an advanced surveillance test, nurses with advanced training can perform the ultrasound, score the BPP, and in nonreassuring situations, initiate further assessment.

SCORING

Each component of the BPP is scored as 2 (variable normal) or 0 (variable abnormal). A total score of 10 is possible if the NST is used. Thirty minutes is allotted for testing, although fewer than 8 minutes is usually needed. The following criteria must be met to obtain a score of 2; anything less is zero (Manning, 1999).

- *Gross Body Movements.* Three or more discrete body or limb movements.
- *Fetal Tone.* One or more full extension and flexion of a limb or trunk, or opening or closing of a hand.
- *Fetal Breathing.* One or more breathing movements of at least 30 seconds' duration.
- *Amniotic Fluid Volume (AFV).* One or more pockets of fluid measuring at least 2 cm in two perpendicular planes.
- *Nonstress Test.* Performed in the event one of the first four parameters are abnormal; graded as normal (2) or abnormal (0). A normal NST is characterized by two accelerations greater than 15 bpm over baseline, each lasting at least 15 seconds within a 20-minute period. An abnormal NST characterized by fewer than two episodes of accelerations or accelerations fewer than 15 bpm above baseline within 20 minutes.

INTERPRETATION

Results of the BPP should be considered in view of the clinical history and the facilities available to care for mother and fetus. The recommendations in Table 19–2 are to be used as guidelines within an existing protocol.

Further testing, such as Doppler flow studies, may be required to validate clinical decisions. Newer ultrasound

TABLE 19–2. Interpretation of Fetal Biophysical Profile Score Results and Recommended Clinical Management

Test Score Result	Interpretation	PNM within 1 wk without Intervention	Management
10 of 10 8 of 10 (normal fluid), 8 of 8 (NST not done)	Risk of fetal asphyxia extremely rare	1 per 1000	Intervention only for obstetric and maternal factors; no indication for intervention for fetal disease
8 of 10 (abnormal fluid)	Probable chronic fetal compromise	89 per 1000[1]	Determine that there is functioning renal tissue and intact membranes; if so, deliver for fetal indications
6 of 10 (normal fluid)	Equivocal test, possible fetal asphyxia	Variable	If the fetus is mature, deliver; in the immature fetus, repeat test within 24 h; if <6/10, deliver
6 of 10 (abnormal fluid)	Probable fetal asphyxia	89 per 1000[1]	Deliver for fetal indications
4 of 10	High probability of fetal asphyxia	91 per 1000[1]	Deliver for fetal indications
2 of 10	Fetal asphyxia almost certain	125 per 1000[1]	Deliver for fetal indications
0 of 10	Fetal asphyxia certain	600 per 1000[1]	Deliver for fetal indications

PNM, perinatal mortality; NST nonstress test.

Reprinted with permission. From Manning, F. (2001a). Intrauterine growth restriction: Diagnosis, prognostication, and management based on ultrasound methods. In A. Fleischer, F. Manning, P. Jeanty, & R. Romero (Eds.), Sonography in obstetrics and gynecology *(pp. 615–632). New York: McGraw-Hill.*

machines also incorporate a Doppler system, and flow studies can be obtained at the time of the BPP (Manning, 1999).

ADVANTAGES AND DISADVANTAGES

As with ultrasound, the BPP can enhance maternal bonding and help the client recognize fetal movement. The BPP has the sensitivity to predict poor fetal outcome in high-risk pregnancies, as well as to permit assessment of amniotic fluid volume, placental characteristics, and the function of various fetal systems.

Research continues regarding questions of the effectiveness of the BPP as a screening test and the frequency with which it needs to be performed (Lyndsey, 1999). Expertise is needed to perform and assess the BPP accurately.

A modified version of the BPP, which assesses only the NST and AFI, has been utilized as well (ACOG, 1999). However, ACOG (1999) states no single antepartum fetal test can be considered superior over another.

CLIENT TEACHING AND COUNSELING

Provide information to the client about ultrasound (see preceding section), as the BPP is usually compiled through the use of abdominal ultrasound. If possible, point out the fetal anatomic structures and indicate the clinical parameters being assessed.

DOPPLER FLOW STUDIES

Doppler ultrasound velocimetry is used to obtain hemodynamic information. By transmitting an ultrasound beam across a blood vessel, the velocity of blood flow can be measured. The umbilical artery has been studied extensively, and its use in monitoring the IUGR fetus has been approved by ACOG (1999). Umbilical, aortic, cerebral, and uteroplacental circulation can be assessed as well. There is potential to measure blood flow in the fetal middle cerebral artery (MCA) to evaluate the fetus for hypoxemia and correlate the MCA value to umbilical artery (UA) flow. The brain-sparing effect is seen when comparing the two separate flow studies—UA flow demonstrates increased flow resistance, while MCA flow resistance is decreased (ACOG, 1999). Middle cerebral artery flow studies are still under investigation, however, and should be used in conjunction with umbilical arterial Doppler indices. The precise role of Doppler flow studies regarding screening, diagnosis, and management will continue to evolve (ACOG, 1999).

Because diastolic flow normally increases in relation to systolic peak throughout pregnancy, monitoring a pregnancy at risk for compromise includes noting decreased diastolic flow (Mari & Detti, 2001). Decreased diastolic flow indicates increased placental bed resistance and potential compromise for the fetus due to decreased placental perfusion. Decreased or absent diastolic flow indicates high resistance in the placenta and is often seen in pregnancies complicated by intrauterine growth retardation (ACOG, 1999). These fetuses have higher rates of morbidity and mortality. As placental insufficiency worsens, there is first a decrease in diastolic flow, then an absence, then reverse diastolic flow is seen (Mari & Detti, 2001). Absence of end-diastolic flow requires more frequent or further testing; the presence of reverse diastolic flow indicates serious fetal compromise and requires further testing and/or intervention (Mari & Detti, 2001).

Doppler assessment should be viewed with other clinical data in determining management of a compromised fetus; it should not be the sole parameter in determining fetal well-being, or the basis of clinical decisions. It is not a sensitive screening tool to predict intrauterine growth restriction among unselected populations; rather, it identifies the fetus at risk for adverse perinatal outcome because it is a test of *placental* function as opposed to an assessment of the fetus once IUGR is diagnosed (ACOG, 1999, 2000a).

Fetal Doppler echocardiography has also been used to study changes in cardiac flow related to disease states such as IUGR, maternal diabetes, fetal anemia secondary to alloimmunization, and discordant twins (Pilu, Jeanty, Perolo, & Prandstraller, 2001; Rizzo, Capponi, & Romanini, 2001).

INDICATIONS

Decreased placental perfusion caused by maternal disease or placental abnormalities is a potential indication for Doppler flow studies. As previously stated, ACOG (1999) recommends Doppler flow studies to be used once IUGR is diagnosed, and not as a screening tool for the general population; middle cerebral artery flow studies are considered investigational. However, Giles (1999) feels umbilical artery flow studies could be extended to assess the fetus in the following situations: suspected IUGR; maternal hypertension, collagen vascular disorders, and vascular disease; previous IUGR or demise. Fetal middle cerebral artery flow studies could be beneficial for suspected IUGR and Rh-D alloimmunization (Giles, 1999). Research will continue in this area.

Arrhythmias detected with auscultation or electronic fetal monitoring can be identified using M-mode echocardiography (Pilu et al., 2001).

Fetuses diagnosed with cardiac anomalies can benefit from pulsed and color Doppler ultrasonography for accurate diagnosis and cardiac function. Due to the differences in blood flow in the fetus versus the neonate, a congenital cardiac anomaly is not necessarily lethal in utero; care consists of accurate diagnosis of the abnormality, frequency of assessment, possible treatment prior to delivery, and how care will be provided to the neonate after delivery (Pilu et al., 2001).

PROCEDURE

Currently the umbilical arteries are the most widely used to assess fetal well-being with Doppler flow studies and seem to hold the greatest promise for clinical evaluation. To evaluate the umbilical artery, the blood flow is assessed during systole and diastole with a Doppler probe, thereby creating a waveform that can be plotted and measured. The systolic/diastolic (S/D) ratio is derived by dividing systolic peak by the end-diastolic component (Mari & Detti, 2001).

A pulsed wave Doppler probe is used for flow studies. The client lies supine with the uterus slightly tilted, using a wedge or cushion. After transducer gel is placed on the abdomen, the fetus is located with Doppler probe. Flow within the umbilical artery is identified, and the difference between systolic and diastolic flow is displayed. Several readings are taken, and the S/D ratio calculated (Mari & Detti, 2001).

The S/D ratio becomes irrelevant when diastolic flow is absent; therefore, other values are obtained. The pulsatility index (PI), also known as the impedance index, is the S/D ratio divided by the mean velocity; Doppler ultrasound equipment provides these values. The resistance index (RI) is the S/D ratio divided by the systolic value (ACOG, 1999).

INTERPRETATION

The PI, RI, and S/D ratio all normally decrease during pregnancy due to decreased placental resistance (Mari & Detti, 2001). Higher placental resistance is found in the presence of placental insufficiency, detected by a decrease in diastolic velocity. The values for all three indices are calculated and compared with standardized charts for fetuses of the same gestational age. Doppler indices are affected by gestational age, fetal breathing, fetal heart rate, and the location on the umbilical cord that is chosen to perform Doppler flow studies; Doppler indices are higher on the fetal end of the cord than the placental end, and this should be taken into consideration when interpreting values (Mari & Detti, 2001).

As previously stated, absence of end-diastolic flow or presence of reverse diastolic flow is correlated with adverse perinatal outcome. Recent research has noted the presence of *reverse diastolic flow* of the umbilical artery in the first trimester to be a possible predictor for poor outcome (Borrell, Martinez, Farre, et al., 2001). However, *end diastolic flow* is often absent in the first trimester and is not necessarily an ominous sign (Mari & Detti, 2001).

Reverse diastolic flow, which is caused by increased flow resistance in the placental bed, is an indication for hospitalization and evaluation for delivery. Reverse diastolic flow has been associated with poor perinatal outcome and increased perinatal mortality (ACOG, 2000a).

All abnormal results warrant further evaluation, such as fetal heart rate monitoring, biophysical profile, ultrasonography to monitor growth, or amniotic fluid indices. Delivery should be considered when other tests indicate imminent fetal danger or when reverse diastolic flow is encountered and extrauterine survival is likely (ACOG, 2000a; Giles, 1999).

ADVANTAGES AND DISADVANTAGES

Doppler has the potential to detect fetal compromise in high risk pregnancies, it is noninvasive, it has no contraindications. There are also several disadvantages. An experienced individual must perform the test; up to one hour is required for a premature fetus. To date, ACOG (1999) recommends its use in monitoring an IUGR fetus and not as a screening test for the general obstetric population. Therefore, it should be used in adjunct to other studies. Research continues to determine the indications for Doppler flow studies.

CLIENT TEACHING AND COUNSELING

Provide the same information given for ultrasound testing. The client needs to know why the test is being done, its implications, and how it complements other tests. Be sure to coordinate exams, counseling, and planning sessions; if fetal echocardiography is used due to a cardiac abnormality, be sure to coordinate exams, counseling, and planning sessions with pediatric cardiologists and neonataologists to provide continuity for the client.

AMNIOCENTESIS AND CHORIONIC VILLUS SAMPLING (CVS)

Both amniocentesis and CVS aid in the diagnosis of chromosomal abnormalities in a fetus. Cytogenetic, biochemical, and molecular testing are utilized in prenatal diagnosis. Cytogenetic testing involves the analysis of chromosomes, which is known as karyotyping. A normal female karyotype is 46,XX. Any change in the normal number of chromosomes is referred to as aneuploidy (Tinkle & Cheek, 2001). Biochemical testing is the assessment of metabolic enzymes, thereby screening for inborn errors of metabolism such as phenylketonuia. Molecular testing involves the use of DNA to diagnose disease (Tinkle & Cheek, 2001). Various methods are utilized based upon the diagnosis sought.

Generally, prenatal diagnosis is offered to clients who will be age 35 or older at delivery, because the risk of a chromosomal abnormality is equal to the risk of fetal loss associated with amniocentesis and chorionic villus sampling.

AMNIOCENTESIS

Amniotic fluid is withdrawn from the uterus, and the cells obtained are cultured to identify chromosomal and biochemical abnormalities; amniocentesis is performed at 15 to 20 weeks of gestation (ACOG, 2001b). First trimester and early second trimester amniocentesis at 11 to 14 weeks has been investigated, although it appears that first trimester amniocentesis carries a higher fetal loss rate than CVS or traditional amniocentesis; due to increased risk and amniotic fluid culture failures, many centers no longer offer early amniocentesis (ACOG, 2001b).

The majority of amniocenteses are performed to rule out chromosomal anomalies. As with CVS, ultrasound must be performed prior to the procedure to confirm gestational age and fetal viability.

Amniocentesis is done with continuous ultrasound guidance and surgical asepsis to avoid infection. A thorough ultrasound exam is performed prior to the amniocentesis to note gestational age, placental location, amount of amniotic fluid, number of fetuses, and any fetal anomalies (Drugan & Evans, 2002; Simpson, 2002). After the abdomen is cleansed, a draped sterile ultrasound transducer is used to locate an appropriate pocket of fluid. A 20 to 22 gauge, 3.5-inch-long spinal needle is inserted into the pocket of fluid. Fluid is then aspirated; a 5 mL syringe is used initially and the first 2 to 3 mL of fluid and the syringe are discarded to decrease the risk of contamination of maternal cells collected in the path of the needle. Twenty to 30 mL of amniotic fluid is then aspirated, transferred to sterile tubes, and taken to the lab for processing. Rh immunoprophylaxis is administered to Rh-negative clients (Drugan & Evans, 2002).

Indications for Invasive Prenatal Diagnosis

Increased risk of chromosomal anomalies due to advanced maternal age, previous child with chromosomal anomalies, parental balanced translocation or inversion, ultrasound diagnosis of fetal malformations, or abnormal maternal serum screening; parents are a carrier of a mendelian genetic trait; suspected fetal infection or fetal hematologic disorder (Drugan & Evans, 2002).

Although ultrasound has become more sophisticated at screening for anatomical landmarks associated with genetic anomalies, and the use of the triple screen has enhanced a noninvasive method for screening, amniocentesis remains the gold standard for fetal diagnosis of chromosomal abnormalities (Drugan & Evans, 2002).

Advantages and Disadvantages

Traditional amniocentesis is associated with a lower risk of complications than CVS, although the risk varies and is related to the experience of the clinician (ACOG, 2001b).

Amniocentesis cannot detect a closed neural tube defect and is associated with some complications. If a fetal anomaly does exist and is not detected until the second trimester with amniocentesis, the client who chooses to terminate her pregnancy is at greater risk for complications than if she had terminated the pregnancy in the first trimester (Drugan & Evans, 2002).

Complications

The fetal loss rate is approximately 0.5 percent and is influenced by operator experience; in a recent study, perinatologists had lower rates of procedure-related fetal losses compared to obstetrician-gynecologists (Blessed, Lacoste, & Welch, 2001). Minor complications include vaginal spotting, amniotic fluid leakage, and chorioamnionitis. Needle injuries have been reported, but are rare (ACOG, 2001b).

Client Teaching and Counseling

Inform the client that she may experience uncomfortable pressure during the procedure, mild cramping up to 48 hours after the procedure, and slight bruising around the insertion site. Reassure the client that fetal heartbeat will be verified after the procedure. Instruct the client to telephone if she notes bleeding, leaking fluid, severe cramping, temperature higher than 100°F, chills, as well as lack of fetal movement if fetal movement has been noted by the client already. Advise the client to avoid strenuous activity or sexual intercourse for 48 hours after the procedure.

Inform the client of the possible risks to herself and the fetus, the significance of abnormal values, and the possible consequences prior to the procedure. Be prepared to counsel the client concerning all possible options.

ASSESSING FETAL LUNG MATURITY

Amniocentesis is used in the third trimester to assess fetal lung maturity if delivery is a possibility prior to 37 weeks' gestation. The procedure is performed much in the same way as described for a second trimester amniocentesis. The fluid obtained can be analyzed through a variety of means to assess the risk of respiratory distress in the newborn. Several components are produced as the fetal lung matures, which are secreted in the tracheal fluid, and then released into amniotic fluid. This can then be assessed via amniocentesis. These components can be measured from fluid obtained from a vaginal pool, as in the case of ruptured membranes, but can give false readings on some tests due to vaginal bacteria (Lauria, 2002). Meconium and blood can alter results as well (Lauria, 2002).

The following are methods to assess lung maturity: *Lecithin-to-Sphingomyelin ratio (L/S ratio)*—Prior to 34 weeks, lecithin and sphingomyelin are found in equal amounts in amniotic fluid. At 35 weeks, the level of lecithin begins to rise. If the L/S ratio is less than 2:1, there is a greater risk of respiratory distress than if the ratio were 2:1 or greater (Cunningham et al., 2001). In the presence of a compromised fetus that could be better cared for outside the uterus, however, an L/S ratio of less than 2:1 may not weigh as significantly if the fetus is expected to deteriorate further if left in utero (Cunningham et al., 2001).

Phosphatidyglycerol (PG)—PG enhances surface-active properties that aid in prevention of alveolar collapse (Cunningham et al., 2001). PG is produced at the end of pregnancy in mature lungs, and the presence of PG is a reliable indication of pulmonary maturity. Amniostat-FLM is an immunologic semiquantitative agglutination test used to screen for PG; it is reported as either present or absent (Druzin, Gabbe, & Reed, 2002; Lauria, 2002).

Fluorescence Polarization (TDx Test—Surfactant albumin ratio)—The TDx analyzer is an automated fluorescence polarimeter and is used to assess surfactant content in amniotic fluid. A mature value is 55 mg of surfactant/g of albumin (Druzin, Gabbe, & Reed, 2002; Lauria, 2002). TDx-FLM II, a second-generation test, has been developed and found to be an excellent indicator of fetal lung maturity. Fantz, Powell, Karon, and colleagues (2002) proposed using a lower cutoff of 45 mg/g, which did not compromise sensitivity and improved specificity. Further studies are needed to confirm their results.

Foam stability index—Serial dilutions of amniotic fluid are mixed with ethanol. The highest dilution in which foam still persists is read as the FSI value. A mature value is 47 or greater (Druzin, Gabbe, & Reed, 2002; Lauria, 2002).

Lamellar body counts (LBC)—Lamellar bodies are the storage form of surfactant released by fetal pneumocytes into amniotic fluid; a value of >32,000 is usually indicative of pulmonary maturity (Druzin, Gabbe, & Reed, 2002; Lauria, 2002), although Neerhof, Dohnal, Ashwod, and colleagues (2001a) suggest a value of 50,000 for maturity, and found lamellar body counts to have the same predictive value as L/S ratios and PG analysis (Neerhof, Haney, Silver, et al., 2001b).

Each method has its own level of sensitivity, specificity, and predictive value. Not all of the above methods are utilized in every institution. The mean gestational age for lung maturity is 34 to 35 weeks, and 99 percent of fetuses will have lung maturity at 37 weeks. However, the fetus of a diabetic client is the exception, with fetal maturity usually being present by 38.5 weeks (Lauria, 2002). In complicated pregnancies, such as those with diabetes, IUGR, and Rh-D alloimmunization, the L/S ratio and presence of PG should be used to establish lung maturity (Druzin, Gabbe, & Reed, 2002; Lauria, 2002); lamellar body counts have found to be favorable in predicting fetal lung maturity in diabetics, but research is limited (Neerhof, et al., 2001a).

Corticosteroids were first used in 1972 for women who were anticipated to deliver prematurely to enhance fetal lung maturity; it was found that the incidence of early neonatal death, necrotizing enterocolitis, respiratory distress syndrome (RDS) and intraventricular hemorrhage (IVH) was decreased as well (ACOG, 1998b; NIH Consensus Panel, 1995). Based on an NIH Consensus Conference in 1994 and later with ACOG's recommendation in 1998, the following guidelines were established:

- Clients between 24 and 34 weeks who are at risk for preterm delivery are candidates for corticosteroid therapy unless delivery is imminent or there is evidence the use of corticosteroids will have an adverse effect on the client.
- A client requiring tocolytics is also a candidate for corticosteroids.
- Treatment with corticosteroids for less than 24 hours has been shown to be beneficial; therefore, corticosteroids should/be given in the presence of preterm labor unless delivery is imminent.
- Corticosteroids are given to clients less than 30 to 32 weeks gestation with premature rupture of membranes in the absence of chorioamnionitis.

However, concerns were raised regarding the long-term effects of corticosteroid use, particularly multiple doses. The NIH reconvened in August, 2000 and in summary, stated that only a single course of steroids were to be used and did not recommend repeated doses of corticosteroids, even for so-called "rescue therapy"; *only* those clients enrolled in clinical trials were to receive repeat courses of steroids (Lyons & Garite, 2002; NIH Conference Statement, 2000). ACOG (2002) supports this position as well.

The use of surfactant, given to the infant through an endotracheal tube at delivery, is decreasing the incidence of neonatal mortality related to respiratory distress syndrome (Cunningham et al., 2001). The use of corticosteroids antenatally complements surfactant therapy after delivery to reduce mortality in the infant (ACOG, 1998b; NIH Consensus Panel, 1995).

CHORIONIC VILLUS SAMPLING (CVS)

Chorionic villi are of fetal origin, and information concerning chromosome status, enzyme levels, and DNA patterns of the fetus can be obtained through analysis of these cells (Simpson, 2002; Wapner, 2001). Chorionic villi divide more rapidly than amniotic fluid cells, providing rapid chromosome analysis with preliminary results within hours and final culture results in seven to ten days (Simpson, 2002; Wapner, 2001). It is important to utilize both tests if available (both analyses are not performed in all laboratories). CVS is performed between 10 and 12 weeks, either transcervically or transabdominally; occasionally, a transvaginal route is taken in the presence of retroflexed uterus with a posterior placenta (Simpson, 2002). The reader is referred to the source (Wapner,

2001) for a detailed description for each method of sampling.

After the procedure, fetal cardiac activity is verified with ultrasound, and the fetus is monitored to note any adverse effects. In addition, Rhogam should be administered to unsensitized Rh-negative clients after the procedure (Drugan & Evans, 2002).

MS-AFP screening should be offered to all women because CVS cannot detect open neural tube defects. Amniocentesis is the preferred method of diagnosis if testing for open neural tube defects, or if tests require amniotic fluid (ACOG, 2001b).

Indications

Indications for CVS are similar to those for amniocentesis; see previous section. CVS is particularly suitable for the diagnosis of classic genetic disorders with known mutations because the amount of DNA in a few villi is greater than the amount found in 40 mL of amniotic fluid (Drugan & Evans, 2002).

Contraindications

CVS is not recommended in the alloimmunized client because CVS may worsen sensitization (Drugan & Evans, 2002). Transcervical sampling is preferred with a posterior or low-lying placenta and retroverted uterus. Transabdominal sampling is preferred with an anterior placenta and is the method of choice in clients who have active vaginal or cervical infection (Drugan & Evans, 2002).

Advantages and Disadvantages

Compared with amniocentesis, CVS permits quicker diagnosis (7 to 10 days for cell culture, depending on health care facility) and, thereby, earlier recognition of a fetal abnormality. Earlier recognition is helpful if the client must make a decision concerning termination of the pregnancy. Termination during the first trimester presents fewer risks to the client and enhances her privacy because the pregnancy is not yet obvious to others (ACOG, 2001b). Moreover, early diagnosis can be essential to recognize and treat various chromosomal anomalies (Evans et al., 2002). Although there is a risk of pregnancy loss (see Complications), very few failures occur in actually retrieving villi and performing chromosomal analysis.

One disadvantage of CVS is that currently it is only done in large facilities; not all facilities have the capability or staff with sufficient expertise. Another disadvantage is that CVS tests only for chromosomal anomalies

and cannot detect anatomic aberrations, such as open neural tube defects. Also note the complications listed.

Complications

Pregnancy loss varies depending on the center and the expertise of the provider; CVS carries a slightly higher rate of procedure failure and fetal loss than amniocentesis, but the rate has not been found to be statistically significant (Simpson, 2002). The risk of fetal loss from CVS is approximately 0.6 to 0.8 percent higher than conventional amniocentesis (ACOG, 2001b).

Fetal loss may also be coincidental. Women who are at increased risk for pregnancy loss secondary to their age or having a chromosomally abnormal fetus will have an increased rate of spontaneous abortion despite the risk of CVS or amniocentesis. (ACOG, 2001b).

Subsequent limb defects have been associated with CVS; several theories have been proposed (Simpson, 2002). ACOG recommends that CVS be performed between 10 and 12 weeks to reduce the incidence of limb defects. Limb reduction defects in the general population is 6 in 10,000 births (ACOG, 2001b; Simpson, 2002). This is approximately the same incidence as was found with CVS, particularly if CVS was performed before 9 weeks (ACOG, 2001b). Clients should be counseled that when CVS is performed between 10 and 12 weeks, the risk of limb defects is low and probably not greater than the risk to the general population (ACOG, 2001b).

Maternal cell contamination and mosaicism (the presence of one or more cell types) are potential sources of diagnostic error; interestingly, confined placental mosaicism has been associated with poor pregnancy outcome, possibly related to abnormal placental function (Drugan & Evans, 2002; Wapner, 2001). Amniocentesis is advised for confirmation if mosaicism is assessed in cell culture or direct preparation (Wapner, 2001).

Client Teaching and Counseling

Advise the client to call if she experiences moderate vaginal bleeding, severe cramping, leaking fluid, temperature higher than 100°F, or chills. Cramping may continue for up to 48 hours after CVS. The client should avoid strenuous activity and sexual intercourse for 48 hours. Discuss each step of the procedure with the client to help decrease her anxiety.

The client should be aware of the potential risks to herself and the fetus. The consequences of an abnormal result should be discussed prior to the procedure. Be aware of all options available to the client; referrals to perinatologists and pediatricians can help the client to become knowledgeable about her fetus. If the client chooses termination, counsel her appropriately and be knowledgeable about the location of centers for pregnancy termination.

PERCUTANEOUS UMBILICAL BLOOD SAMPLING (PUBS)

The terms *PUBS* and *cordocentesis* are used interchangeably in reference to the invasive sampling of fetal blood. PUBS was originally done using fetoscopy in the early 1970s. The use of ultrasound has decreased the risks of PUBS, however, and its use for a variety of indications has expanded in the last few years. PUBS not only can be a method to assess fetal well-being but can provide fetal therapy as well (Ghezzi, Romero, Maymon, et al., 2001).

PROCEDURE

PUBS can be performed at approximately 18 weeks' gestation or later as clinical indications arise (Simpson, 2002). Ultrasound is used to assess fetal viability, position, biometry, location of the placenta, and presence of fetal anomalies (Ghezzi et al., 2001). The insertion site of the umbilical cord in the placenta is identified. The maternal abdomen is cleansed and draped, just as for amniocentesis. Under ultrasound guidance, a 20- to 25-gauge needle is inserted into the amniotic cavity and into the umbilical vein; the veins can be distinguished by their size, and the direction of blood flow can be determined by using color Doppler (Ghezzi et al., 2001). Confirmation that the blood sample is of fetal origin is imperative; a number of tests are available, including the Kleihauer-Betke test and comparison of mean corpuscular volume. (Ghezzi et al., 2001).

Once the needle has been inserted into the umbilical vein, fetal blood is withdrawn into a syringe (Ghezzi et al., 2001). Samples can be evaluated for coagulation studies, blood group typing, complete blood count, karyotyping, and blood gas analysis (Ghezzi et al., 2001). Due to the risk of transplacental hemorrhage, Rh-negative clients are given Rhogam (ACOG, 1999). Intrahepatic fetal blood sampling and cardiocentesis have been researched as well, although the fetal loss rate is higher than for umbilical vein insertion (Ghezzi et al., 2001).

After the age of viability, a course of corticosteroids is advised prior to PUBS (Ghezzi et al., 2001). This is to enhance fetal lung maturity due to the risk of preterm labor or for the need for immediate delivery in the event fetal distress occurs during or after PUBS. For this reason, if the fetus is at the age of viability, PUBS should only be done in a hospital setting (as opposed to an outpatient setting) in order to deliver the fetus by cesarean section if needed (Ghezzi et al., 2001).

INDICATIONS

(Drugan & Evans, 2002; Ghezzi et al., 2001)

- Cytogenetic diagnosis: for instance, when rapid karyotype is needed, or if one or more cell types is identified (mosaicism or pseudomosaicism) at amniocentesis or CVS.
- Congenital infection: toxoplasmosis, rubella, cytomegalovirus, parvovirus, congenital syphilis.
- Congenital immunodeficiency.
- Coagulopathies.
- Platelet disorders.
- Hemoglobinopathies.
- Severe IUGR: detect etiology, assess fetal hematologic and acid-base function.
- Multiple gestation: twin to twin transfusion syndrome.
- Fetal therapy: transfusions or pharmacologic agents when transplacental passage of the drug is poor.
- Diagnosis and/or treatment: fetal anemia, nonimmune hydrops.

COMPLICATIONS

Fetal loss varies, depending on indication, operator experience, technique, and gestational age at procedure (Drugan & Evans, 2002; Simpson, 2002). Fetal complications can be hemorrhage, hematoma of the cord, placental abruption, and preterm delivery (Drugan & Evans, 2002). Maternal complications include amnionitis and transplacental hemorrhage (Simpson, 2002). Risks are higher when the client is obese, the placenta is posterior, or when PUBS is performed prior to 19 weeks (ACOG, 2001b; Drugan & Evans, 2002; Simpson, 2002).

In general, fetal loss rates due to PUBS range from 1 to 4 percent and higher depending on the indication for PUBS (ACOG, 2001b; Drugan & Evans, 2002; Simpson, 2002). With such a significant loss rate, only clients with clear indications should be offered this method of assessment. Adequate imaging of the cord is not always possible, and another method of surveillance should be chosen, or PUBS should be postponed (Ghezzi et al., 2001). Aseptic technique, and limiting the number of puncture sites will reduce complications (Simpson, 2002). Transversing the placenta may worsen alloimmunization due to intermixing of fetal and maternal blood (Drugan & Evans, 2002).

ADVANTAGES AND DISADVANTAGES

Fetal karyotype can be obtained from a culture of fetal blood in 24 to 48 hours (ACOG, 2001b). There are a number of indications for PUBS (see previous paragraph) in which the procedure is lifesaving for the fetus; while there is an increased risk of fetal loss with PUBS versus CVS or amniocentesis, fetal loss would be inevitable in some cases. The use of PUBS for fetal transfusion is lifesaving for the fetus with nonimmune hydrops fetalis if the fetus is remote from term (ACOG, 1996).

The main disadvantage is fetal loss, as well as other complications noted.

CLIENT TEACHING AND COUNSELING

The client needs to be aware of the risks involved, as well as the need for immediate intervention in the event fetal distress is noted. Other options, if applicable, should be made available to the client. Counseling and, therefore, fetal loss rates, need to be specific in regard to the indication for PUBS. Genetic studies versus transfusion for nonimmune hydrops are completely different indications and require specific counseling based on the status of the client and fetus.

POTENTIAL SCREENING METHODS FOR THE FUTURE

FETAL CELL ISOLATION FROM MATERNAL BLOOD

Fetal cells can now be obtained from a maternal blood sample, and it is possible to diagnose sex, human leukocyte antigen, Rh blood type, trisomy 13, 18, and 21, triploidy, sickle cell anemia, and thalassemia of the fetus in this manner (Wachtel et al., 2001). Fetal cells may be present in maternal circulation as early as 6 to 8 weeks of gestation, and fetal nucleated red cells seem to hold the greatest promise for research (Wachtel et al., 2001).

Research has focused on the use of polymerase chain reaction (PCR) and fluorescence in situ hybridization (FISH) in prenatal diagnosis using fetal cells extracted from maternal blood (Wachtel et al., 2001). Research will continue to explore methods of separation and enrichment of fetal cells, as well as recovering free fetal DNA

in maternal blood (Torricelli & Pescucci, 2001). It has been noted that there are an increased number of fetal cells in maternal blood in the presence of abnormal pregnancies, notably Trisomy 21, IUGR, and preeclampsia (Holzgreve & Hahn, 2001; Kitagawa, Suigiura, Omi, et al., 2002; Parano, Falcidia, Grillo, et al., 2001). This may be due to an abnormality of the placental barrier that leads to increased transfusion of fetal cells to the mother (Parano et al., 2001; Pertl & Bianchi, 2001). Combining analysis of fetal cells from a maternal blood sample with maternal serum screening may further enhance technology's ability to provide clients with noninvasive, cost-effective, yet accurate prenatal diagnosis.

FETAL FIBRONECTIN AS AN INDICATOR OF PRETERM LABOR

Current research is attempting to identify markers that would predict preterm labor; fetal fibronectin is a protein produced by fetal membranes that serves to bind the placenta and fetal membranes to the decidua (ACOG, 2001c). It is found in cervicovaginal secretions until 16 to 20 weeks (ACOG, 2001c).

It has been postulated that if fibronectin is present in cervicovaginal secretions after 20 weeks, it may be the result of a destruction of the basement membranes, possibly due to bacterial colonization. (ACOG, 2001c). There has been an association between the presence of fetal fibronectin and preterm birth, and a decreased risk of preterm birth when fetal fibronectin was not present (Witcher, 2002). The use of ultrasonography to measure cervical length, in combination with testing for fetal fibronectin, has been shown to be a strong predictor of preterm birth (ACOG, 2001c; Goering & Wilson, 2002). However, even with a reliable screening test, there still is no effective management to decrease the risk of preterm delivery (ACOG, 2001c; Goering & Wilson, 2002). It has been suggested that the absence of fetal fibronectin in the presence of symptoms of preterm labor could be useful; its absence could provide reassurance of a decreased risk of preterm birth, and therefore any unnecessary intervention could be avoided (ACOG, 2001c; Witcher, 2002).

To date, other than historic risk factors, no screening method has found to be beneficial to identify or prevent preterm birth in the general population, including the use of salivary estriol, home uterine activity monitoring, or bacterial vaginosis screening (ACOG, 2001c; Goldenberg, Klebanoff, Carey, & McPherson, 2001; Iams, Newman, Thom, et al. 2002). Cervical length assessment alone or in combination with fetal fibronectin has been useful in a high-risk population, but mainly in its negative predictive value to avoid unnecessary intervention (ACOG, 2001c; Iams et al., 2002). Research will continue to focus on fetal fibronectin, bacterial vaginosis screening and treatment, as well as cervical length assessment (Goldenberg et al., 2001; Welsh & Nicolaides, 2002).

If fibronectin is in fact related to bacterial colonization, research may focus on intervention specific to certain bacteria, or the inhibition of prostaglandin production after bacterial colonization. Research will continue in the realm of preterm birth to discover and understand the etiology, pharmacologic intervention, and ongoing surveillance needed to prevent preterm birth.

FETAL TISSUE BIOPSY

Occasionally, fetal skin sampling is utilized to diagnose disorders that cannot be diagnosed by chorionic villus sampling or amniocentesis (Simpson, 2002). Fetal skin biopsy is performed in the second trimester, at which time the majority of fetal skin tissue is differentiated (Cockell & Rodeck, 2001). Initially, this procedure was done using fetoscopy, but it is now done with ultrasound guidance (Simpson, 2002).

Fetal muscle biopsy is performed for diagnoses in which DNA analysis is not able to assess for the mutation in question, such as Duchenne muscular dystrophy. Fetal liver biopsy is also performed for rare and lethal disorders; the procedure is performed at 17 weeks or later, at which time normal liver enzyme activity has been established (Cockell & Rodeck, 2001).

Procedure-related losses following tissue biopsy are greater than those for CVS or amniocentesis—approximately 2 to 3 percent (Simpson, 2002). The severity of some disorders justifies the risk if no other method is satisfactory for diagnosis. Advances in molecular testing may make tissue sampling obsolete in the future (Simpson, 2002).

PREIMPLANTATION GENETIC DIAGNOSIS

Preimplantation genetic diagnosis (PGD) is a growing field that aims to assist couples in having a pregnancy free of an identifiable genetic disease. It is the combination of in vitro fertilization and prenatal diagnosis (Jones & Fallon, 2002). Typically, clients are carriers for an inherited disorder that they do not wish to pass on to their child; a couple may already be raising an affected child or

have experienced a miscarriage due to a genetic-related condition. They may have already had previous affected pregnancies that were terminated after prenatal diagnosis and wish to avoid termination in the future for a specific disorder (Overton, Serhal, & Davies, 2001; Simpson, 2002). In the future, potential treatment could occur prior to implantation (metabolic or gene insertion) (Simpson, 2002).

PGD is performed prior to conception (polar body biopsy) and after in vitro fertilization (blastomere biopsy—6 to 8 cell and trophectoderm biopsy); if results are negative for the disorder in question, fertilization or implantation can proceed (Jones & Fallon, 2002; Overton, Serhal, & Davies, 2001; Simpson, 2002). Monogenic disorders are diagnosed using PCR, and FISH is used to diagnose chromosomal abnormalities (Kanavakis & Traeger-Synodinos, 2002). Clients are still advised to undergo prenatal diagnosis to assess for other anomalies (Cockell & Rodeck, 2001).

Indications

Indications for PGD include many of the same for invasive prenatal diagnosis: increased risk of chromosomal anomalies due to advanced maternal age, previous child with chromosomal anomalies, parental balanced translocation or inversion, parents are a carrier of a Mendelian genetic trait (Drugan & Evans, 2002).

Couples who are referred for PGD are usually already aware they are carriers of a genetic disorder or have previously experienced an undesirable pregnancy outcome of genetic origin. Couples may also want to avoid the risk of genetic disease without the dilemma of possible termination that prenatal diagnosis raises (Cockell and Rodeck, 2001; Simpson, 2002).

Advantages and Disadvantages

Natural conception and traditional prenatal diagnosis is an imperfect yet acceptable choice for many; for others, PGD is a better option, particularly when faced with the possible decision to continue or terminate an affected pregnancy that accompanies traditional prenatal diagnosis (Jones & Fallon, 2002). For clients who have previously terminated a pregnancy due to anomalies, significant psychological repercussions occur with future pregnancies, one of which is to prepare to terminate a pregnancy again (Rillstone & Hutchinson, 2001). PGD may be a more desirable option for these clients.

PGD does have potential increased emotional, physical, and financial investment because it is the combination of IVF and prenatal diagnosis. Pregnancy rates vary, but only approximately one-third of completed cycles of PGD result in pregnancy (Kanavakis & Traeger-Synodinos, 2002). Health insurance carriers will more readily cover the cost of prenatal diagnosis versus PGD, even when the primary reason is to eliminate the transmission of an inherited disorder to a child (Jones & Fallon, 2002). The Secretary's Advisory Council on Genetic Testing is currently reviewing several issues surrounding genetic testing encompassing the issues of reimbursement, inclusion of genetic testing in a standard benefit plan, and how genetic services will be examined in light of cost versus benefit (Lewis, 2001).

The benefit is detection of specific genetic disorders prior to implantation to avoid the dilemma of possible pregnancy termination of affected fetuses. To date, evaluation of approximately 250 babies born worldwide after PGD shows no increased incidence of abnormalities in early childhood (Jones & Fallon, 2002; Kanavakis & Traeger-Synodinos, 2002). Ethical considerations have been raised concerning the use of PGD to "choose" an unaffected embryo to be implanted in order to provide stem cells at birth to treat an affected sibling, as in the case of Fanconi anemia; to provide "social" sexing for family "balancing"; and which embryos to select or discard based on the definition of what constitutes a serious genetic disorder in the realm of PGD (Damewood, 2001; ESHRE Task Force on Ethics and Law, 2001; Kanavakis & Traeger-Synodinos, 2002). As research continues, both technical and ethical issues will continue to unfold and will need to be addressed.

The author would like to thank Dr. Terry Hill for his support.

REFERENCES

Alfirevic, Z., & Neilson, J. (1995). Doppler ultrasonography in high-risk pregnancies: Systematic review with meta-analysis. *American Journal of Obstetrics and Gynecology, 172,* 1379–1387.

American Academy of Pediatrics and American College of Obstetricians and Gynecologists. (1997). *Guidelines for perinatal care* (4th ed.). Elk Grove Village, New York: American Academy of Pediatrics.

American College of Obstetricians and Gynecologists (ACOG). (1996). *Management of alloimmunization in pregnancy.* ACOG Educational Bulletin No. 227. Washington, D.C.: ACOG.

American College of Obstetricians and Gynecologists (ACOG). (1997a). *Routine storage of umbilical cord blood for potential future transplantation.* ACOG Committee Opinion No. 183. Washington, D.C.: ACOG.

American College of Obstetricians and Gynecologists (ACOG). (1997b). *Routine ultrasound in low-risk pregnancy.* ACOG Practice Patterns No. 5. Washington, D.C.: ACOG.

American College of Obstetricians and Gynecologists (ACOG). (1998a). *Medical management of a tubal pregnancy.* ACOG Practice Bulletin No. 3. Washington, D.C.: ACOG.

American College of Obstetricians and Gynecologists (ACOG). (1998b). *Antenatal corticosteroid therapy for fetal maturation.* ACOG Committee Opinion No. 210. Washington, D.C.: ACOG.

American College of Obstetricians and Gynecologists (ACOG). (1999). *Antepartum fetal surveillance.* ACOG Practice Bulletin No. 9. Washington, D.C.: ACOG.

American College of Obstetricians and Gynecologists (ACOG). (2000a). *Intrauterine growth restriction.* ACOG Practice Bulletin No. 12. Washington, D.C.: ACOG.

American College of Obstetricians and Gynecologists (ACOG). (2000b). *Perinatal viral and parasitic infections.* ACOG Practice Bulletin No. 20. Washington, D.C.: ACOG.

American College of Obstetricians and Gynecologists (ACOG). (2000c). *Macrosomia.* ACOG Practice Bulletin No. 22. Washington, D.C.: ACOG.

American College of Obstetricians and Gynecologists (ACOG). (2001a). *Fetal surgery for open neural tube defects.* ACOG Committee Opinion No. 252. Washington, D.C.: ACOG.

American College of Obstetricians and Gynecologists (ACOG). (2001b). *Prenatal diagnosis of fetal chromosomal abnormalities.* ACOG Practice Bulletin No. 27. Washington, D.C.: ACOG.

American College of Obstetricians and Gynecologists (ACOG). (2001c). *Assessment of risk factors for preterm birth.* ACOG Practice Bulletin No. 31. Washington, D.C.: ACOG.

American College of Obstetricians and Gynecologists (ACOG). (2002). *Antenatal corticosteroid therapy for fetal maturation.* ACOG Committee Opinion No. 273. Washington, D.C.: ACOG.

Baird, S., & Ruth, D. (2002). Electronic fetal monitoring of the preterm fetus. *Journal of Perinatal and Neonatal Nursing, 16,* 12–24.

Beamer, L. (2001). Fetal nuchal translucency: A prenatal screening tool. *JOGNN, 30*(4), 376–385.

Bernstein, I., Gabbe, S., & Reed, K. (2002). Intrauterine growth restriction. In S. Gabbe, J. Niebyl, & J. L. Simpson (Eds.), *Obstetrics: Normal and problem pregnancies* (pp. 869–891). New York: Churchill Livingstone.

Blessed, W., Lacoste, H., & Welch, R. (2001). Obstetrician-gynecologists performing genetic amniocentesis may be misleading themselves and their patients. *American Journal of Obstetrics and Gynecology, 184,* 1340–1344.

Borrell, A., Martinez, J., Farre, T., Azulay, M., Cararach, V., & Fortuny, A. (2001). Reversed end-diastolic flow in first-trimester umbilical artery: An ominous new sign for fetal outcome. *American Journal of Obstetrics and Gynecology, 185*, 204–207.

Bracero, L., Morgan, S., & Byrne, D. (1999). Comparison of visual and computerized interpretation of nonstress test results in a randomized controlled trial. *American Journal of Obstetrics and Gynecology, 181*(5), 1254–1258.

Carvalho, M., Brizot, M., Lopes, L., Chiba, C., Miyadahira, S., & Zugaib, M. (2002). Detection of fetal structural abnormalities at the 11–14 week ultrasound scan. *Prenatal Diagnosis, 22*, 1–4.

Chervenak, F., & Gabbe, S. (2002). Obstetric ultrasound: Assessment of fetal growth and anatomy. In S. Gabbe, J. Niebyl, & J. L. Simpson (Eds.), *Obstetrics: Normal and problem pregnancies* (pp. 251–296). New York: Churchill Livingstone.

Christensen, F., & Rayburn, W. (1999). Fetal movement counts. *Obstetric and Gynecology Clinics of North America, 26*(4), 607–621.

Cockell, A., & Rodeck, C. (2001). Prenatal diagnosis. In J. Harper, J. Delhanty, & A. Handyside (Eds.), *Preimplantation genetic diagnosis* (pp. 27–51). New York: John Wiley & Son.

Comstock, C. (2002). Universal ultrasound screening—Useful or a waste? In S. Ransom, M. Evans, M. Dombrowski, & K. Ginsburg (Eds.), *Contemporary therapy in obstetrics and gynecology* (pp. 239–242). Philadelphia: W. B. Saunders.

Copel, J. (2001). Transvaginal sonographic evaluation of fetal anatomy at 14–16 weeks. *Journal of Ultrasound in Medicine, 20*, 710–711.

Cunningham, G., Gant, N., Leveno, K., Gilstrap, L., Hauth, J., & Wenstrom, K. (2001). *Williams obstetrics* (21st ed.). New York: McGraw Hill.

Damewood, M. (2001). Ethical implications of a new application of preimplantation diagnosis. *JAMA, 285*, 3143–3144.

Devoe, L. (1999). Nonstress testing and contraction stress testing. *Obstetric and Gynecology Clinics of North America, 26*(4), 535–555.

DeVore, G., & Romero, R. (2002). Genetic sonography. *Journal of Ultrasound in Medicine, 21*, 5–13.

Divon, M. (2002). Prolonged pregnancy. In S. Gabbe, J. Niebyl, & J. L. Simpson (Eds.), *Obstetrics: Normal and problem pregnancies* (pp. 931–944). New York: Churchill Livingstone.

Drugan, A., & Evans, M. (2002). Invasive procedures for prenatal diagnosis. In S. Ransom, M. Evans, M. Dombrowski, & K. Ginsburg (Eds.), *Contemporary therapy in obstetrics and gynecology* (pp. 207–215). Philadelphia: W. B. Saunders.

Drugan, A., Weissman, A., & Evans, M. (2001). Screening for neural tube defects. *Clinics in Perinatology, 28*, 279–287.

Druzin, M., Gabbe, S., & Reed, K. (2002). Antepartum fetal evaluation. In S. Gabbe, J. Niebyl, & J. L. Simpson (Eds.), *Obstetrics: Normal and problem pregnancies* (pp. 313–352). New York: Churchill Livingstone.

Egan, J., Benn, P., Borgida, A., Rodis, J., Campbell, W., & Vintzileos, A. (2000). Efficacy of screening for fetal Down syndrome in the United States from 1974 to 1997. *Obstetrics and Gynecology, 96*, 979–85.

ESHRE Task Force on Ethics and Law. (2001). The moral status of the pre-implantation embryo. *Human Reproduction, 16*, 1046–1048.

Evans, M., Harrison, M., Flake, A., & Johnson, M. (2002). Fetal therapeutic intervention. In S. Gabbe, J. Niebyl, & J. L. Simpson (Eds.), *Obstetrics: Normal and problem pregnancies* (pp. 297–312). New York: Churchill Livingstone.

Evans, M., & Wapner, R. (2001). Future directions. *Clinics in Perinatology, 28*(2), 477–480.

Fantz, C., Powell, C., Karon, B., Parvin, C., Hankins, K., Dayal, M., Sadovsky, Y., Johari, V., Apple, F., & Gronowski, A. (2002). Assessment of the diagnostic accuracy of the TDx-FLM II to predict fetal lung maturity. *Clinical Chemistry, 48*, 761–765.

Ghezzi, F., Romero, R., Maymon, E., Redman, M., Blackwell, S., & Berry, S. (2001). Fetal blood sampling. In A. Fleischer, F. Manning, P. Jeanty, & R. Romero (Eds.), *Sonography in obstetrics and gynecology* (pp. 775–804). New York: McGraw-Hill.

Giles, W. (1999). Vascular Doppler techniques. *Obstetric and Gynecology Clinics of North America, 26*(4), 595–606.

Goering, M., & Wilson, W. (2002). Implementing preterm labor guidelines: A collaborative care improvement process. *Journal of Perinatal and Neonatal Nursing, 16*, 47–57.

Goncalves, L., Romero, R., Maymon, E., Pacora, P., Bianco, K., & Jeanty, P. (2001). Prenatal detection of anatomic congenital anomalies. In A. Fleischer, F. Manning, P. Jeanty, & R. Romero (Eds.), *Sonography in obstetrics and gynecology* (pp. 341–374). New York: McGraw-Hill

Goldenberg, R., Klebanoff, M., Carey, C., & McPherson, C. (2001). Metronidazole treatment of women with a positive fetal fibronectin test result. *American Journal of Obstetrics and Gynecology, 185*, 485–486.

Harrington, K., & Fayyad, A. (2001). Prediction of fetal anemia. *Current Opinion in Obstetrics and Gynecology, 14*, 177–185.

Hoeldtke, N., & Calhoun, B. (2001) Perinatal hospice. *American Journal of Obstetrics and Gynecology, 185*, 525–529.

Holzgreve, W., & Hahn, S. (2001). Prenatal diagnosis using fetal cells and free fetal DNA in maternal blood. *Clinics in Perinatology, 28*(2), 353–364.

Huerta-Enochian, G., Katz, V., & Erfurth, S. (2001). The association of abnormal alpha-fetoprotein and adverse pregnancy outcome: Does increased fetal surveillance affect pregnancy outcome? *American Journal of Obstetrics and Gynecology, 184*, 1549–1555.

Hull, A., Pretorius, D., & Nelson, T. (2001). Three-dimensional ultrasound in obstetrics. In A. Fleischer, F. Manning, P. Jeanty, & R. Romero (Eds.), *Sonography in obstetrics and gynecology* (pp. 1217–1224). New York: McGraw-Hill.

Iams, J., Newman, R., Thom, E., Goldenberg, R., Mueller-Heubach, E., Moawad, A., Sibai, B., Caritis, S., Miodovnik,

M., Paul, R., Dombrowski, M., & McNellis, D. (2002). Frequency of uterine contractions and the risk of spontaneous preterm delivery. *The New England Journal of Medicine, 346,* 250–255.

Jackson, M., & Branch, W. (2002). Alloimmunization in pregnancy. In S. Gabbe, J. Niebyl, & J. L. Simpson (Eds.), *Obstetrics: Normal and problem pregnancies* (pp. 893–930). New York: Churchill Livingstone.

Jeanty, P. (2001). Fetal biometry. In A. Fleischer, F. Manning, P. Jeanty, & R. Romero (Eds.), *Sonography in obstetrics and gynecology* (pp. 139–156). New York: McGraw-Hill.

Jones, S., & Fallon, L. (2002). Reproductive options for individuals at risk for transmission of a genetic disorder. *JOGGN, 31,* 193–199.

Kanavakis, E., & Traeger-Synodinos, J. (2002). Preimplantation genetic diagnosis in clinical practice. *Journal of Medical Genetics, 39,* 6–11.

Kimball, R. (2001). Healthy growth and development of the newborn/infant. In C. Green-Hernandez, J. Singleton, & D. Aronzon (Eds.), *Primary care pediatrics* (pp. 93–105). Philadelphia: Lippincott.

Kitagawa, M., Suigiura, K., Omi, H., Akiyama, Y., Kanayama, K., Shinya, M., Tanaka, T., Yura, H., & Sago, H. (2002). New techniques using galactose-specific lectin for isolation of fetal cells from maternal blood. *Prenatal Diagnosis, 22,* 17–21.

Kowalcek, I., Muhlhoff, A., Bachmann, S., & Gembruch, U. (2002). Depressive reactions and stress related to prenatal medicine procedures. *Ultrasound in Obstetrics and Gynecology, 19,* 18–23.

Krause, T., Christens, P., Wohlfahrt, J., Lei, U., Westergaard, T., Norgaard-Perdersen, B., & Melbye, M. (2001). Second-trimester maternal serum alpha-fetoprotein and the risk of adverse pregnancy outcome. *Obstetrics and Gynecology, 97,* 277–282.

Kuno, A., Akiyama, M., Yamashiro, C., Tanaka, H., Yanagihara, T., & Hata, T. (2001). Three-dimensional sonographic assessment of fetal behavior in the early second trimester of pregnancy. *Journal of Ultrasound in Medicine, 20,* 1271–1275.

Kupperman, M., Gates, E., & Washington, E. (1996). Racial-ethnic differences in prenatal diagnostic test use and outcomes: Preferences, socio-economics or client knowledge? *Obstetrics and Gynecology, 87,* 675–682.

Lauria, M. (2002). Fetal lung maturity testing. In S. Ransom, M. Evans, M. Dombrowski, & K. Ginsburg (Eds.), *Contemporary therapy in obstetrics and gynecology* (pp. 107–109). Philadelphia: W. B. Saunders.

Lewis, J. (2001) The human genome project and public policy: A nursing perspective. *JOGGN, 30,* 541–545.

Lewis, J. (2002) Genetics in perinatal nursing: Clinical applications and policy considerations. *JOGGN, 31,* 188–192.

Lyerly, A., Gates, E., Cefalo, R., & Sugarman, J. (2001). Toward the ethical evaluation and use of maternal-fetal surgery. *Obstetrics and Gynecology, 98,* 689–697.

Lyndsey, M. (1999). Intrauterine resuscitation of the compromised fetus. *Clinics in Perinatology, 26*(3), 569–582.

Lyons, C., & Garite, T. (2002). Corticosteroids and fetal pulmonary maturity. *Clinical Obstetrics and Gynecology, 45,* 35–41.

Magann, E., & Martin, J. (1999). Amniotic fluid volume assessment in singleton and twin pregnancies. *Obstetrics and Gynecology Clinics of North America, 26*(4), 579–592.

Manning, F. (1999). Fetal biophysical profile. *Obstetric and Gynecology Clinics of North America, 26*(4), 557–577.

Manning, F. (2001). Intrauterine growth restriction: Diagnosis, prognostication, and management based on ultrasound methods. In A. Fleischer, F. Manning, P. Jeanty, & R. Romero (Eds.), *Sonography in obstetrics and gynecology* (pp. 615–632). New York: McGraw-Hill.

Mari, G., & Detti, L. (2001). Doppler ultrasound: Application to fetal medicine. In A. Fleischer, F. Manning, P. Jeanty, & R. Romero (Eds.), *Sonography in obstetrics and gynecology* (pp. 615–632). New York: McGraw-Hill.

Mari, G., Detti, L., Oz, U., Zimmerman, R., Duerig, P., & Stefos, T. (2002). Accurate prediction of fetal hemoglobin by Doppler ultrasonography. *Obstetrics and Gynecology, 99,* 589–593.

McCarter-Spaulding, D. (2002). Parvovirus B19 in pregnancy. *JOGNN, 31*(1), 107–112.

Moore, T., & Cayle, J. (1990). The amniotic fluid index in normal human pregnancy. *American Journal of Obstetrics and Gynecology, 162,* 1168–1173.

National Institute of Child and Human Development (NICHD). (1997). Research Planning Workshop: Electronic fetal heart rate monitoring: research guidelines for interpretation. *American Journal of Obstetrics and Gynecology, 177,* 1385–1390.

National Institute of Health (NIH) Consensus Development Conference Statement. (2000). Antenatal corticosteroids revisited: Repeat courses. *Obstetrics and Gynecology, 98,* 144–150.

National Institute of Health (NJH) Consensus Development Panel on the Effect of Corticosteroids for Fetal Maturation on Perinatal Outcomes. (1995). Effect of corticosteroids for fetal maturation on perinatal outcomes. *JAMA, 273,* 413–417.

Neal, J. (2001). RhD alloimmunization and current management modalities. *JOGNN, 30,* 589–606.

Neerhof, M., Dohnal, J., Ashwod, E., Lee, I., & Anceschi, M. (2001a). Lamellar body counts: A consensus on protocol. *Obstetrics and Gynecology, 97,* 318–320.

Neerhof, M., Haney, E., Silver, R., Ashwod, E., Lee, I., & Piazze, J. (2001b). Lamellar body counts compared with traditional phospholipid analysis as an assay for evaluating fetal lung maturity. *Obstetrics and Gynecology, 97,* 305–309.

Oncken, C., Kranzler, H., O'Malley, P., Gendreau, P., & Campbell, W. (2002). The effect of cigarette smoking on fetal heart rate characteristics. *Obstetrics and Gynecology, 99,* 751–755.

Ott, W., & Taysi, K. (2001). Obstetric ultrasonographic findings and fetal chromosomal abnormalities: Refining the association. *American Journal of Obstetrics and Gynecology, 184,* 1414–1421.

Overton, C., Serhal, P., & Davies, M. (2001). Clinical aspects of preimplantation diagnosis. In J. Harper, J. Delhanty, & A. Handyside (Eds.), *Preimplantation genetic diagnosis* (pp. 123–140). New York: John Wiley & Son.

Parano, E., Falcidia, E., Grillo, A., Pavone, P., Cutuli, N., Takabayashi, H., Trifiletti, R., & Gilliam, C. (2001). Noninvasive prenatal diagnosis of chromosomal aneuploidies by isolation and analysis of fetal cells from maternal blood. *American Journal of Medical Genetics, 101,* 262–267.

Pertl, B., & Bianchi, D. (2001). Fetal DNA in maternal plasma: Emerging clinical applications. *Obstetrics and Gynecology, 98,* 483–90.

Pilu, G., Jeanty, P., Perolo, A., & Prandstraller, D. (2001). Prenatal diagnosis of congenital heart disease. In A. Fleischer, F. Manning, P. Jeanty, & R. Romero (Eds.), *Sonography in obstetrics and gynecology* (pp. 157–176). New York: McGraw-Hill.

Price, R., Fleischer, A., & Abuhamad, A. (2001). Sonographic instrumentation and operational concerns. In A. Fleischer, F. Manning, P. Jeanty, & R. Romero (Eds.), *Sonography in obstetrics and gynecology* (pp. 1–28), New York: McGraw-Hill.

Pryde, P., & Kay, H. (2002). Fetal macrosomia: Antenatal diagnosis and management. In S. Ransom, M. Evans, M. Dombrowski, & K. Ginsburg (Eds.), *Contemporary therapy in obstetrics and gynecology* (pp. 203–206). Philadelphia: W. B. Saunders.

Queenan, J., Tomai, T., Ural, S., & King, J. (1993). Deviation in amniotic fluid optical density at a wavelength of 450 nm in Rh-immunized pregnancies from 14–40 weeks' gestation: A proposal for clinical management. *American Journal of Obstetrics and Gynecology, 168,* 1370–1376.

Redman, M., & Berry, S. (2002). Updates in red cell isoimmunization. In S. Ransom, M. Evans, M. Dombrowski, & K. Ginsburg (Eds.), *Contemporary therapy in obstetrics and gynecology* (pp. 65–70). Philadelphia: W. B. Saunders.

Resnik, R. (2002). Intrauterine growth restriction. *Obstetrics and Gynecology, 99,* 490–496.

Rillstone, P., & Hutchinson, S. (2001). Managing the reemergence of anguish: Pregnancy after a loss due to anomalies. *JOGNN, 30,* 291–298.

Rizzo, G., Capponi, A., & Romanini, C. (2001). Fetal functional echocardiography. In A. Fleischer, F. Manning, P. Jeanty, & R. Romero (Eds.), *Sonography in obstetrics and gynecology* (pp 177–193). New York: McGraw-Hill.

Rosen, D., Kedar, I., Amiel, A., Ben-Tovim, T., Petal, Y., Kaneti, H., Tohar, M., & Fejgin, M. (2002). A negative second trimester triple test and absence of specific ultrasound markers may decrease the need for genetic amniocentesis in advanced maternal age by 60%. *Prenatal Diagnosis, 22,* 59–63.

Schechtman, K., Gray, D., Baty, J., & Rothman, S. (2002). Decision-making for termination of pregnancies with fetal anomalies: Analysis of 53,000 pregnancies. *Obstetrics and Gynecology, 99,* 216–222.

Sen, C. (2002). The use of first trimester ultrasound in routine practice. *Journal of Perinatal Medicine, 29,* 212–221.

Simpson, J. (2002). Genetic counseling and prenatal diagnosis. In S. Gabbe, J. Niebyl, & J. L. Simpson (Eds.), *Obstetrics: Normal and problem pregnancies* (pp. 187–219). New York: Churchill Livingstone.

Smith, G., Stenhouse, E., Crossley, J., Aitken, D., Cameron, A., & Connor, M. (2002). Early pregnancy levels of PAPP-A and the risk of intrauterine growth restriction, premature birth, preeclampsia and stillbirth. *Journal of Clinical Endocrinology and Metabolism, 87,* 1762–1767.

Snijders, R. (2001). First-trimester ultrasound. *Clinics in Perinatology, 28*(2), 333–350.

Souter, V., & Nyberg, D. (2001). Sonographic screening for fetal aneuploidy. *Journal of Ultrasound in Medicine, 20,* 775–790.

Spencer, K. (2002). Point-of-care screening for chromosomal anomalies in the first trimester of pregnancy. *Clinical Chemistry, 48,* 403–404.

Stockman, J. (2001). Overview of the state of the art of Rh disease: History, current clinical management and recent progress. *Journal of Pediatric Hematology and Oncology, 23,* 554–562.

Tabsh, K., & Theroux, N. (1998). Rhesus Isoimmunization. In N. Hacker & G. Moore (Eds.), *Essentials of obstetrics and gynecology* (pp. 343–350). Philadelphia: W. B. Saunders.

Timor-Tritsch, I. (2001). Transvaginal sonographic evaluation of fetal anatomy at 14–16 weeks. *Journal of Ultrasound in Medicine, 20,* 705–709.

Tinkle, M., & Cheek, D. (2001). Human genetics: Challenges and opportunities. *JOGNN, 31,* 178–187.

Torricelli, F., & Pescucci, C. (2001). Isolation of fetal cells from the maternal circulation: Prospects for the non-invasive prenatal diagnosis. *Clinical Chemistry and Laboratory Medicine, 39,* 494–500.

Touraine, J. (2001). Stem cell transplantation in utero for genetic disease. *Transplant Proceedings, 33,* 1750–1751.

Tucker, S. (2000) *Fetal monitoring and assessment.* St. Louis: Mosby.

Vintzileos, A. (2000). Antenatal assessment for the detection of fetal asphyxia. *Annals of the New York Academy of Medicine, 900,* 137–150.

Vintzileos, A., Guzman, E., Smulian, J., Yeo, L., Scorza, W., & Knuppel, R. (2002). Second-trimester genetic sonography in patients with advanced maternal age and normal triple screen. *Obstetrics and Gynecology, 99*, 993–995.

Wachtel, S., Shulman, L., & Sammons, D. (2001). Fetal cells in maternal blood. *Clinical Genetics, 59*, 74–79.

Walsh, L. (2001). *Midwifery: Community based care during the childbearing year*. Philadelphia: W. B. Saunders.

Wapner, R. (2001). Chorionic villus sampling. In A. Fleischer, F. Manning, P. Jeanty, & R. Romero (Eds.), *Sonography in obstetrics and gynecology* (pp. 721–740). New York: McGraw-Hill.

Weeks, J., Asrat, T., Morgan, M., Nageotte, M., Thomas, S., & Freeman, R. (1995). Antepartum surveillance for a history of stillbirth: When to begin? *American Journal of Obstetrics and Gynecology, 172*, 486–492.

Welsh, A., & Nicolaides, K. (2002). Cervical screening for preterm delivery. *Current Opinion in Obstetrics and Gynecology, 14*, 195–202.

Wilson, D. (2002). Prenatal evaluation for fetal surgery. *Current Opinion in Obstetrics and Gynecology, 14*, 187–193.

Witcher, P. (2002). Treatment of preterm labor. *Journal of Perinatal and Neonatal Nursing, 16*, 25–46.

Wong, D., Perry, S., & Hockenberry, M. (2002). *Maternal child nursing care*. St. Louis: Mosby.

Yaran, Y., Cherry, M., Kramer, R., O'Brien, J., Hallak, M., Johnson, M., & Evans, M. (1999). Second-trimester maternal serum marker screening: Maternal serum alpha-fetoprotein, beta-human chorionic gonadotropin, estriol and their various combinations as predictors of pregnancy outcome. *American Journal of Obstetrics and Gynecology, 181*, 968–974.

Yaran, Y. & Mashiach, R. (2001). First-trimester biochemical screening for Down syndrome. *Clinics in Perinatology, 28*(2), 321–330.

CHAPTER 20

POSTPARTUM AND LACTATION

Kathleen M. Akridge

*T*he support and experience previously provided by the extended family are not always easily accessible for today's families.

Highlights

❖ INTRODUCTION

Knowledge of the normal physiologic changes and complications of the postpartum period, parental roles, perinatal loss, and lactation is essential in managing the care of a client and her family postpartum. The health care provider must be familiar with assessment, diagnosis, management, and follow-up and know when referral is needed for further evaluation and management.

In the diagnosis and management of complications, it may be necessary to implement emergency measures until definitive care from a consulting medical professional arrives. The postpartum woman may be assessed in a hospital setting, alternative birthing site such as a birthing center, or the home.

The extended family of forty or fifty years ago has been replaced by nuclear families and such nontraditional families as single-parent and blended (two partial families joined to become one) families. The support and experience previously provided by the extended family are not easily accessible for families of today. Early hospital discharge means that many of the nurturing and infant care skills previously taught by health professionals on the second postpartum day are now crammed into a short time frame just prior to hospital discharge, when the client's attention is often focused on what awaits her at home. To meet the health needs of today's new mother, many hospitals provide follow-up telephone calls or home visits.

Many women choosing to breastfeed may be deterred when faced with engorgement, tender nipples, and nonsupportive family and friends. Women who deliver twins may believe that breastfeeding is not possible. A unique opportunity exists to make this a successful experience for the breastfeeding family.

The postpartum experience is not always joyful. Many women or couples are left to deal with the loss of the fantasized infant as they struggle with the reality of a miscarriage, deformity, or perinatal death. Knowing how to help the woman and her family and suggest appropriate referral is imperative. There is a list of support groups at the end of this chapter.

Health care during the postpartum period focuses on evaluation of the physiological and psychological changes that normally occur. Any abnormal findings or dysfunctional behavior detected during the antepartum and postpartum periods should continue to be evaluated.

THE PUERPERIUM

Postpartum, also referred to as the *puerperium*, is the period from delivery of the placenta and membranes to the return of the woman's reproductive organs to their nonpregnant state. It generally lasts about six weeks and is divided into three segments. The immediate puerperium is the first 24 hours after delivery; the early puerperium extends from the second day postpartum to the end of the first postpartum week; and the remote puerperium continues to the end of the sixth week.

IMMEDIATE POSTPARTUM

- ◆ *Uterine Involution*. This process includes shedding of the decidua and endometrium. It is monitored by assessing the amount of lochia and uterine size and tone.
  - Immediately after delivery the uterus is approximately two-thirds to three-fourths of the way between the umbilicus and the symphysis pubis; after a few hours, the uterus rises to the level of the umbilicus and remains there or one fingerbreadth below for about two days before gradually descending into the true pelvis by two weeks postpartum (Canningham et al., 2001). Any time the top of the fundus is above the umbilicus, bladder or uterine distention from blood or clots is possible.
  - Lochia is the uterine discharge during the puerperium that escapes vaginally. Lochia rubra is the earliest lochia and is red because it contains blood and decidual tissue. It begins immediately after delivery and continues the first two to three days postpartum.

- ◆ *Vagina and Perineum*. These structures are quite stretched and edematous following a vaginal delivery. The vagina gapes at the introitus; it is also smoothwalled and generally lax. Hematoma should be suspected if the woman reports excruciating pain or is unable to void, or if a tense, fluctuant mass is noted. Inspect the episiotomy for hematoma. Vulvar and rectal hemorrhoids are often present and must be observed for evidence of thrombosis. After delivery, ice bags may be applied to the perineum and hemorrhoids for 30 to 60 minutes; ice bags are removed then to prevent a secondary effect, vasodilation.

- *Vital Signs.* Blood pressure, pulse, and respirations should be stabilized to within normal limits. Fever is indicative of infection, probably in the genitourinary tract.
- *Bladder.* The bladder is edematous, hypotonic, and congested immediately postpartum. Consequently bladder distention, incomplete emptying, inability to void, and excessive urine residual may develop unless the woman is encouraged to void periodically even when she does not feel the need.
- *Breasts.* Lactation naturally begins unless a lactation suppressant has been given. Colostrum is the first fluid the infant receives from the breast. Engorgement commonly occurs 48 to 72 hours after delivery. An ice bag applied to the breasts for 15 minutes and then discontinued for 1 hour before being reapplied may give the nonlactating woman some relief from engorgement. The use of cold cabbage leaves has gained in popularity as a reliable and safe way to treat engorgement. The cold cabbage leaves are applied to the breasts, leaving just the nipples exposed. The leaves are removed in about 20 minutes when they become wilted.
- *Abdominal Muscles.* The muscles are flabby, and all have some degree of diastasis recti. If the client elected to have tubal sterilization, part of the preoperative counseling should include advising the client of a possible increase in pain or discomfort because of the abdominal surgery as well as from the postpartum afterpains. If cesarean section was performed, a dressing usually covers the incision, and it should be dry. Staples are generally used in the skin closure and are removed five to seven days postoperatively. Obviously, women undergoing a cesarean birth will experience pain.
- *Postpartum Blues and Grief.* Descriptions are provided in the sections on Psychiatric Disturbances and Perinatal Loss.

EARLY PUERPERIUM

From the second postpartum day to the end of the first postpartum week additional changes evolve.

- *Uterus.* The uterus is approximately 12 weeks size and is barely palpable just above the symphysis pubis.

- *Lochia Serosa.* The normal uterine discharge from the vagina that occurs during postpartum days 4 to 10 is lochia serosa. It contains primarily serous fluid, decidual tissue, leukocytes, and erythrocytes. Flow is decreasing. Encourage use of sanitary pads rather than tampons.
- *Vagina and Perineum.* The vagina remains smooth, and the perineum may be slightly uncomfortable. If an episiotomy was performed, the sutures will still be palpable. Attention should be given for signs of infection or hemorrhoids. Discourage douching as it may alter vaginal pH and wash out protective vaginal organisms. Bathing can soothe and cleanse the perineum. Oils and fragrances should not be used in bath water. If hemorrhoids are present, relief can be obtained with Tucks, Nupercaine ointment, dermaplast, increased fluid and fiber intake, stool softeners as needed, and warm or cool sitz baths. Urinary incontinence may indicate cystocele (see Chapter 13).
- *Breasts.* By this time, breasts contain milk for those women who are breastfeeding. Breast milk usually appears on postpartum days 3 to 5, and is a bluish white. A mother may need reassurance that the color is normal and her milk has not become "weak" (see Breastfeeding section).
- *Abdominal Muscles.* These muscles are lax, and a woman needs reassurance that it is normal. Walking and swimming may help tone muscles without exerting undue stress.
- *Diuresis and Profuse Perspiration.* These conditions are normal as long as the woman is afebrile.

LATE PUERPERIUM

From the end of the first postpartum week to the end of the sixth week maternal change continues.

- *Uterus.* The uterus returns to its nonpregnant size four to six weeks following birth.
- *Lochia Alba.* The last lochia, lochia alba, begins at about day 10 and continues until approximately day 35 postpartum. It is scant, composed primarily of leukocytes and decidual cells, and is creamy white.
- *Vagina and Perineum.* These structures begin to regain tone by 6 weeks postpartum. Rugae are normally present by that time. Atrophy, however, may still be evident in the lactating woman. Of concern are maintaining and strengthening vaginal tone, preventing pelvic relaxation, and promoting nonpainful resumption of intercourse.

♦ *Breasts.* The breasts begin to adapt to the nutritional needs of the baby, but engorgement and mastitis remain primary concerns. Assess the breastfeeding process and family support. The breasts of a nonlactating woman may contain milk for up to three months postpartum.

♦ *Renal System.* Urinary tract infection (UTI) may occur, and continuing assessment is of particular concern for clients with a history of UTI.

♦ *Abdominal Muscles.* Abdominal wall musculature becomes firmer by the end of the sixth postpartum week but may never regain its prepregnant appearance if the muscles remain weakened and stretched.

THE FOUR- TO SIX-WEEK POSTPARTUM ASSESSMENT

SUBJECTIVE DATA

Generally review the woman's systems. Specific determinations also need to be made:

♦ Number of weeks postpartum.

♦ General adaptation to motherhood; assess client's rest and sleep habits, appetite, activity level, exercise program, and nutrition.

♦ Coping ability in caring for baby and making family adjustments or living as single parent.

♦ Problems with baby (feeding, health, first exam).

♦ Family adjustments caring for baby.

♦ Sexual activity (resumption, type of contraceptive used, dyspareunia, and other concerns, including possible lack of desire, fear of discomfort or of becoming pregnant again).

♦ Family planning method desired; assess previous methods used, length of time used, satisfaction with methods, and reason for discontinuance.

Ask the client if she has called a health care provider or gone to an emergency room and whether she was admitted or readmitted. In addition, ask if she has had fever, chills, or flulike symptoms.

♦ *Breasts.* Assess for engorgement and breastfeeding concerns.

• Determine when engorgement occurred, how long it lasted, if it has been treated and how and whether it continues to be a problem or has resolved.

• If breastfeeding is discontinued, determine the length of breastfeeding and the reason for stopping.

• If the client is currently breastfeeding, ask her about concerns, frequency, nipple soreness, breast care, and enjoyment of breastfeeding.

♦ *Lochia.* In the postpartum period, assess the duration of each lochia color in sequence, presence of odor, excessive bleeding, clots, and pain.

♦ *Return of Menses.* Several factors influence the return of menses, such as contraceptive method and breastfeeding. Nonlactating women menstruate six to eight weeks following delivery, and lactating women two to eighteen months following delivery, depending on whether she is exclusively breastfeeding or if she is supplementing with formula. The first postpartum menstruation is heavier than normal menstruation and often anovulatory. Menses returns sooner in the multipara than the primipara.

OBJECTIVE DATA

Physical Examination

Generally assess the client.

♦ *General Appearance and Vital Signs.* Compare blood pressure with range before and during pregnancy. Compare weight with prepregnant weight and weight at delivery. Inquire as to rest/sleep and activity levels. Obtain 24-hour dietary recall to assess nutritional intake.

♦ *Neck.* Determine that the thyroid is nonpalpable. If thyromegaly or nodules are palpated, order thyroid function tests (TFTs) and refer client for medical evaluation (see Normal Postpartum Health Assessment).

♦ *Breasts.* Evaluation is influenced by whether the client is lactating.

• Lactating breasts should be full, without erythema, masses, or lymphadenopathy. Milk should be easily expressed.

• Nonlactating breasts are soft, without masses or lymphadenopathy. Bilateral galactorrhea may be present in nonlactating women for up to three months' postpartum; these women should return for evaluation of galactorrhea beyond three months' postpartum. Mechanical stimulation of nonlactating breasts may lead to persistence of milky discharge, but more serious causes should be ruled out.

♦ *Extremities.* Assess for varicosities and phlebitis.

♦ *Cardiovascular and Respiratory Systems.* Rate and rhythm should be regular without murmurs or extra heart sounds. Clear, equal breath sounds should be evident bilaterally. Blood volume returns to normal by approximately one week postpartum.

◆ *Abdomen and Musculoskeleton.* Assess for costovertebral angle tenderness (CVAT) and tenderness along paraspinous muscles. In addition, inspect for abdominal striae, diastasis, hernias, masses, tenderness, and lymph nodes. If she experienced a cesarean birth, assess healing. Abdominal musculature involution may require six to eight weeks.

◆ *Genitalia and Reproductive Organs.* Several structures are involved.

- External genitalia should be without edema or lesions and nontender.
- Vagina should appear rugated, except in lactating women when rugae may be decreased secondary to hypoestrogenic state. Episiotomy site should be intact, well healed, and nontender.
- Cervical internal os should be closed. If it is open, determine whether placental products have been retained. After childbirth, the cervix appears as a transverse slit. It appears stellate if severe lacerations were sustained during childbirth.
- Uterine corpus at four to six weeks postpartum is nonpregnant size. If uterine tenderness is detected, consider infection and prepare appropriate cultures (e.g., chlamydia, gonorrhea).
- Involution of ovaries and fallopian tubes is complete by six to seven weeks postpartum.
- Inspect rectum for hemorrhoids. Assess sphincter control, especially if third- or fourth-degree laceration was sustained during childbirth.

◆ *Psychological Factors.* Assess affect for mood of mother, and her interaction with infant or other indications of maternal-infant bonding. Inquire as to health of infant and whether infant has had a routine exam.

Diagnostic Tests

Various tests need to be performed.

◆ Compare antenatal and postnatal hemoglobin levels and hematocrits.

◆ Check immunity status for rubella and, if not immune (titer ≤ 1:10), confirm that rubella vaccine was given prior to hospital discharge. Nursing mothers may be vaccinated.

◆ If client is Rh-negative, check Rh status of infant and, if clinically indicated, determine whether

Rho(D) immune globulin was given to mother postpartum.

◆ Check when last Pap smear was done and results.

◆ If any sexually transmitted disease was detected during pregnancy, consider repeating tests.

PLAN

◆ *Psychosocial Intervention.* Counseling may be helpful about available social services, public health nursing, and child protective services (see Postpartum Depression Support Groups at the end of this chapter).

◆ *Family Planning.* Ask the client whether she was satisfied with previously used methods of contraception. Ask about her concerns regarding the method she wishes to use or is using now. Base your instructions about a method of contraception on the client's level of comprehension. Address safer sex as well as satisfaction with or changes in relationship with sexual partner.

◆ *Preventive Measures.* Encourage health maintenance/health promotion activities, such as breast self-examination, Kegel exercises, annual Pap examination, smoking cessation, weight reduction, and exercise. Reassure mothers of term and low-birthweight babies that it may take months for them to feel "normal" again.

FOLLOW-UP

◆ *Pap Smear.* Perform only if previously abnormal. Absence of endocervical cells on a Pap smear not uncommon in pregnant women (Jazayeri, Hefron, Harnetty, Jazayeri, & Gould, 1999).

◆ *Colposcopy.* Perform or refer if clinically indicated.

◆ *Culture.* Culture for chlamydia or gonorrhea if indicated.

◆ *Urine Testing.* Monitor for urinary tract pathology by performing dipstick. Culture urine if bacteriuria occurred during pregnancy or if physical exam warrants.

◆ *Blood Tests.* Obtain hemoglobin level, hematocrit, or complete blood count if indicated.

◆ *Immunization.* Request rubella immunization if indicated.

◆ *Intravenous Pyelogram and Urology.* Consider referring client for intravenous pyelogram and urology consultation if she has a history of pyelonephritis or hematuria of unknown etiology during pregnancy.

◆ *Glucose Testing.* Request 75 g glucola (i.e., two-hour oral glucose tolerance test) if the client was gestational diabetic. Protocols vary depending on the setting. A three-hour test may be used. Since glucose tolerance testing in the immediate postpartum period is unreliable, however, there must be a wait of at least six weeks' postpartum for a reliable testing of carbohydrate intolerance.

NORMAL POSTPARTUM HEALTH ASSESSMENT

Essential aspects of normal postpartum health assessment are pelvic musculature and breast evaluations and contraception counseling. See Chapter 14 for information on breast self-examination. Evaluation of pelvic musculature and contraception counseling are discussed here.

PELVIC MUSCULATURE

Pelvic musculature is assessed following pregnancy to evaluate involution and resumption of nonpregnant function (see Chapter 13). The general function of pelvic musculature is to support pelvic organs and assist urinary continence.

Etiology of Relaxed Pelvic Musculature

Relaxed musculature may be related to childbearing, age, obesity, or lack of exercise.

◆ Closely spaced pregnancies or large fetuses can stretch and traumatize pelvic musculature and contribute to relaxation.
◆ Aging, because of decreased estrogen production, contributes to loss of elasticity.
◆ Obesity increases intraabdominal pressure and contributes to relaxation of vaginal muscles.
◆ Failure to perform Kegel exercises permits continued relaxation.

Subjective Data

A woman may report sensations of pelvic pressure, urinary incontinence, and lack of perineal support during defecation (Sampselle & Brink, 1990). Specific information needs to be pursued.

Although urinary incontinence has been associated with vaginal delivery, a prevalence of 8.8 percent in women who have had a cesarean delivery suggests that pregnancy itself may be a risk factor for incontinence (Sampselle, Miller, Mims, et al., 1998).

◆ Involuntary loss of urine during an activity that increases intraabdominal pressure, e.g., coughing, sneezing.
◆ Age of onset and circumstances of incontinence.
◆ Increase in severity or number of pelvic symptoms, or both, such as loss of bladder control, incomplete emptying of bladder, a sensation of vaginal pressure, inability to defecate without use of counter pressure.
◆ Day and night voiding patterns.
◆ Frequency and severity of wetting.
◆ Amount of urine lost (drops, teaspoon, tablespoon, quarter of cup, layer of clothing soaked).
◆ History of and reasons for previous vaginal or urinary tract surgery.
◆ History of lower back surgery (the pudendal nerve innervates pelvic floor muscles and could have been damaged in surgery).
◆ Past history of stress urinary incontinence and method of treatment.
◆ Fluid intake.
◆ Medications, including over-the-counter, currently being used.
◆ Use of bladder irritants, such as caffeine, non-nutritive sweeteners.
◆ Number and type of deliveries (vaginal vs. cesarean) and complications (tears, lacerations, etc.).

Stress urinary incontinence (SUI) and detrusor instability should be differentiated (Adam & Preston, 2002). SUI results from an incompetent urethra. Urine is lost immediately with an event that increases intraabdominal pressure. With detrusor instability (involuntary contraction) the bladder itself is the cause of incontinence. A delay occurs between the precipitating event and urine loss; urine loss may also be sudden and without warning.

Objective Data

The physical exam should be directed toward identifying any physical or neurological conditions that could affect a woman's ability to remain continent. The examination involves abdominal, pelvic, and neurologic assessments. Assessment of the urine for evidence of infection, glycosuria, hematuria, and proteinuria should be routine, with treatment and further evaluation as indicated. The abdomen is assessed for masses, diastasis recti, organomegaly, peritonitis, and fluid collections (AWHONN, 2000a). The pelvic examination involves assessing the health of the vulva and vagina, pelvic support, and evidence of urinary leakage. The neurological evaluation assesses the vaginal strength and integrity of the sacral reflex (Adam & Preston, 2002).

Pelvic Examination. Digital measurement of pelvic muscle strength scale assesses vaginal muscles. The examiner inserts index and middle fingers 6 to 8 cm into the introitus on an anteroposterior plane and ask the client to contract her vaginal muscles around the fingers for as long as possible and as forcefully as possible. The scoring criteria are pressure, duration of pressure, and alteration in plane of examiner's fingers (Sampselle & Brink, 1990). Scores range from 1 to 4, with 4 denoting the greatest muscle strength (Table 20–1).

The next step is to assess for cystocele, urethrocele, rectocele, and enterocele. Firmly exert pressure with fingers posterior to the vaginal wall and ask the client to bear down or cough. Observe the vaginal wall to detect an anterior bulge (cystocele or urethrocele). Continue pressing posteriorly with fingers while simultaneously separating them; ask the client to cough or bear down and observe the posterior wall for a bulge (rectocele or enterocele).

Women should be examined for pelvic organ prolapse in the lithotomy, sitting, and standing positions. Examining the client only in the lithotomy position will obscure some pelvic support defects. Each organ that descends within the vaginal canal should be graded according to the maximum degree of descent. Clinical grading is as follows (ACOG, 1995).

- Grade 0—no descent
- Grade 1—descent between ischial spines and hymen
- Grade 3—descent within hymen
- Grade 4—descent through hymen

Plan

In a small study, Sampselle and colleagues (1998) found that women who did pelvic muscle exercises had less urinary incontinence at 35 weeks gestation, 6 weeks postpartum, and 6 months postpartum than women who did not do pelvic muscle exercises. They also found initial pelvic muscle strength had significant effect on pelvic muscle strength at twelve months postpartum, supporting the importance of pelvic muscle exercise.

Pelvic muscle exercise benefits women with cystocele, urethrocele, rectocele, or enterocele that bulges into the vaginal vault but not outside the introitus. It may be done in any position as long as knees are 16 to 18 inches apart. Instruct the client to contract vaginal muscles as tightly as possible for as long as possible; the goal is to hold each contraction for 5 to 10 seconds. Initially, the client should contract her pelvic muscles while slowly counting to 5, hold, and gradually release to the count of 5. The aim is 80 contractions per day (groups of 5 to 20 per session) (Sampselle & Brink, 1990).

Refer the client to a urologist or gynecologist if she has a "cele" that descends beyond the introitus (a third degree).

CONTRACEPTION COUNSELING

Assessment

Assess a woman's knowledge of and preference for available contraceptive methods (see Chapter 9). She should be instructed in her choice of a temporary or permanent method. Temporary methods include barrier, hormonal, spermicidal devices, and periodic abstinence. Permanent methods are female sterilization and male sterilization.

Reversible Contraceptive Methods

Combination Oral Contraception. If a breastfeeding mother prefers to use oral combination pills, Kennedy and Trussell (1998) and Riordan and Auerbach (2001) advise women not to begin combination oral contraceptives until at least six weeks, but preferably six months postpartum. The estrogen in the pill can decrease milk supply. If a combination pill is used, the estrogen should be ≤ 35 mcg.

Starting a breastfeeding woman on combination pills before her six-week exam increases the risk of lactation suppression (Kennedy & Trussell, 1998). If not breastfeeding, women may begin combination oral contraception three weeks postpartum (Kennedy & Trussell, 1998). Starting the combination oral contraceptive pill before

TABLE 20–1. Pelvic Muscle Strength Rating Scale

Characteristic	1	2	3	4
Pressure	None	Weak, feel pressure on fingers, but not all way around	Moderate, feel pressure all around	Strong, fingers compress override
Duration	None	< 1 s	> 1 < 3 s	> 3 s
Displacement in plane	None	Slight incline, base of fingers move up	Greater incline of fingers along total length	Fingers move up and are drawn in

From C. Sampselle & C. Brink (1990). Pelvic muscle relaxation. Journal of Nurse Midwifery, 35 (3), 130. Copyright American College of Nurse Midwives. Reprinted with permission.

2 weeks postpartum increases the risk of thromboembolic disease (Kennedy & Trussell, 1998).

Other Combination Contraceptives. Other combination contraceptives include depo-Lunelle®, NuvaRing®, and Ortho-EVRA® transdermal patch. If any of these methods are chosen, breastfeeding women should not be started on them until at least six weeks, but preferably six months, postpartum.

Progestin Only Contraceptives (POCs). Progestin only contraceptives such as the minipill, Mirena IUD®, Progestasert IUD®, and Depo-provera® are safe to use in breastfeeding women. They do not interfere with milk production and may even increase milk production. Depo-provera may be administered at the time of discharge if not lactating, and six weeks postpartum if breastfeeding.

Diaphragm. The diaphragm should be fitted at the six-week postpartum exam, as it cannot be fitted properly before that time. Episiotomies are also tender and attempting to fit a diaphragm before six weeks would only increase the client's discomfort. Fitting should also be deferred until that time because bleeding increases the risk of toxic shock syndrome.

Intrauterine Device (IUD). IUDs can be inserted immediately after the delivery of the placenta, within 48 hours postpartum, or at the six-week postpartum exam. If immediate postdelivery insertion is done, *Hatcher et al.* recommend only the Paraguard® because it has been shown to be the safest and most effective IUD for postpartum women (Kennedy & Trussell, 1998). Expulsion rates are much higher in immediate postpartum insertion than at the six-week exam (Kennedy & Trussell, 1998).

Spermicides. Because breastfeeding can cause a decrease in estrogen, spermicides may add comfort by relieving vaginal dryness during intercourse.

Lactation Amenorrhea Method (LAM). It should be stressed that breastfeeding is not an effective method of birth control but, if used solely to supply the infant with food, it is used to space pregnancies in many cultures. It can be very effective if the infant is completely breastfed without any supplements (Kennedy & Trussell, 1998). The lactation amenorrhea method is an alternative for the breastfeeding couple and can be 98 percent effective during the first six months (ACOG, 2000; Kennedy & Trussell, 1998; Mohrbacher & Stock, 1997). Criteria for LAM include: no menses (no vaginal bleeding after the 56th day after birth), *and* no supplementing regularly nor going longer than four hours between feedings during the day or longer than six hours between feedings at night,

and the baby is younger than 6 months old (Labbock, 2001; Mohrbacher & Stock, 1997; Smith & Tully, 2001).

Natural Family Planning (NFP). Women who are not exclusively breastfeeding and who do not desire pregnancy should be advised of available contraceptive options. If the woman doesn't desire medication or contraceptive devices, natural family planning should be discussed with her and her partner. Lawrence and Lawrence (1999) state that most studies show the first menses is anovulatory. Unplanned pregnancy rates rise among breastfeeding women after the onset of first menses compared with nonlactating women who use thermal or cervical mucous surveillance methods. Basal body temperature cannot be determined unless the woman has had six hours of uninterrupted sleep (Kennedy & Trussell, 1998). Lawrence and Lawrence (1999) state that studies showing changes in cervical secretions during lactation are reliable. They recommend the couple note when (1) the infant sleeps through the night, (2) the mother reduces the number of breastfeedings, (3) the infant begins solid food, (4) the infant begins other liquids or a bottle, and (5) illness occurs either in the mother or infant. They advise abstinence in any of the above situations until the situation is clear.

Cervical mucus changes may be misleading during anovulatory postpartum, as dry mucus is similar to that of preovulatory days during an ovulatory cycle; profuse, thick mucus makes identification of mucous patterns for prediction of ovulation difficult.

◆ Take basal body temperature if cervical mucus appears or the cervix opens or becomes elevated.
◆ "Infertility" of breastfeeding can be reasonably assumed if cervical mucus remains tacky for three weeks and does not become clear and stretchy (Davis, 1992). This is the strongest indicator of return to ovulation and fertility in women who are breastfeeding.
◆ With intermittent signs of cervical mucus discharge, begin BBT. When mucus lasts three or more days and its cessation is accompanied by continued low temperature, breastfeeding infertility can be assumed two days after mucus disappears (Davis, 1992; Lawrence & Lawrence, 1999). To better assess mucus, coitus should be every other day so that the presence of ejaculate and sexual lubrication does not interfere with cervical mucus.

If weaning occurs slowly after three to four months, daily BBT should be continued and cervical mucus checked for onset of ovulation. Coitus is allowed throughout a ten-day weaning period. The couple should consider themselves fertile on the eleventh day until cervical and thermal signs show ovulation has occurred (Davis, 1992). If weaning occurs naturally, the client should monitor for signs of ovulation after the sixth postpartum month (Davis, 1992; Lawrence & Lawrence, 1999).

The importance of exclusive breastfeeding, as well as the importance of continuing breastfeeding to maintain postpartum infertility, should be taught to clients and their partners. Infants are not introduced to solid foods until approximately six months old, and they may be slowly introduced to taking liquids by cup. Refer clients to breastfeeding support groups and local lactation consultants.

ASSESSMENT OF POSTOPERATIVE CESAREAN BIRTH AND STERILIZATION

Following cesarean birth, encourage ambulation to decrease risk of thrombosis and embolism. Assess for thrombophlebitis by checking the lower extremities for edema of the affected leg, positive Homan's sign, muscle pain in affected leg, tenderness, erythema, or induration along a vein in the affected leg. Give analgesics shortly before ambulation. Monitor intake and urinary output by measurement for 24 to 48 hours. Observe wound for infection. Encourage woman's contact with family and infant.

After female sterilization, clients should be aware that discomfort may be greater because of the surgical procedure, but mild analgesia, such as nonsteroidal anti-inflammatory drugs (NSAIDs), should provide relief. For women not obtaining relief with NSAIDs, medication like Tylenol #3®, Fioricet®, or Fioricet with codeine® can be used. Observe for infection, hematoma at incision site, including episiotomy (if performed). Encourage contact with infant prior to and after surgery.

TWO- TO THREE-WEEK POSTPARTUM ASSESSMENT

Subjective Data

Several points of information may be gained from the mother or from hospital records at the two- to three-week postpartum asssessment. Generally review the woman's systems, with specific attention to the following:

- Type of birth (vaginal or cesarean); amount and color of vaginal bleeding, presence of foul odor or clots; length of labor and complications during labor, delivery, postpartum.
- If cesarean birth, determine if staples removed. If episiotomy performed, assess for tears, lacerations.

- Assess for amount and frequency of pain with urination; constipation; use of medications (prescription and over-the-counter) and herbs and reason for use; effectiveness of pain medication in obtaining pain relief; hemorrhoids; fever.
- Inquire regarding problems or concerns with baby (feeding, jaundice, colic, elimination patterns, assistance in caring for baby).
- Assess family adjustments: father's role, sibling behavior, extended family.
- Support system during labor and delivery.
- Weight and sex of baby.
- Number of days in hospital, general well-being of both mother and baby.
- Allergies.
- Bladder and bowel function.
- Diet/appetite, sleep patterns/fatigue.

Review the mother's feelings about delivery. If mother experienced a cesarean birth, explore her understanding of the medical reasons.

Objective Data

Physical Examination

General Appearance, Vital Signs, Weight. Does the woman appear rested, fatigued, depressed? Does she appear neat and well groomed or ill kempt? Compare blood pressure to range during pregnancy. Compare weight to prepregnant weight and weight at delivery.

Neck. Thyroid nonpalpable or palpable, but soft and without nodules. If thyromegaly or nodules palpated, evaluate for bruits, obtain thyroid function tests (TFT), and refer for medical evaluation. (See section Postpartum Thyroiditis for further information.)

Cardiovascular and Respiratory. Regular rate and rhythm without murmurs or extra sounds. Clear, equal breath sounds bilaterally.

Breasts. (1) *Lactating:* Full, without erythema, masses, or lymphadenopathy. Milk easily expressed. (2) *Nonlactating:* Soft, without masses, lymphadenopathy. Bilateral galactorrhea may be present in nonlactating women for up to three months' postpartum.

Abdomen and Musculoskeletal. Assess for costovertebral angle tenderness (CVAT) and tenderness along paraspinous muscles. Fundus is usually nonpalpable above the symphysis and is nontender to gentle palpation. If cesarean birth or sterilization performed, the incision is well healed without exudate, and nontender. Lower extremities are inspected for redness, warmth, and pain in calves. Assess for Homan's sign (pain elicited with dorsiflexion of foot).

Genitalia/Reproductive. Inspect perineum for swelling, hemorrhoids. If episiotomy noted, assess for edema, erythema, ecchymosis, approximation of edges. Bimanual is generally deferred until six-week postpartum exam.

Psychological. Assess mother's feelings and understanding regarding labor and birth. Assess support system. Ask woman if sexual activity has been resumed. If sexual activity has been resumed, inquire as to any pain or discomfort. Inquire as to type of contraception being used or whether contraception is desired. If cesarean birth, review type of uterine incision with woman and the issue of vaginal birth after cesarean. Reassure regarding length of time to regain prepregnant weight may take one year.

Laboratory Tests. Determine rubella immunity and documentation of rubella vaccine given postpartum. For Rh-negative mothers, determine whether Rhogam® was given if infant Rh-positive.

Health Teaching. Review ways to ensure adequate rest (sleep when infant does, avoid late-night television, limit visitations by family and friends). Encourage adequate fluid intake and frequent voiding to decrease uterine "afterpains." Change perineal pads frequently. Review perineal cleansing/sitz baths/warm water soaks. Assess whether prenatal vitamins are still being taken. If history of prenatal anemia or postpartum hemorrhage, inquire whether iron supplements are being taken and dosing used. Assess for adequate rest and nutritional needs to promote tissue healing.

SIX-WEEK POSTCESAREAN BIRTH ASSESSMENT

The six-week postpartum evaluation of a woman who had a cesarean birth is the same as that of a woman who delivered vaginally, except that the abdominal incision is assessed following a cesarean birth as well as the perineum and vulva.

COMMON POSTPARTUM COMPLICATIONS

Table 20–2 summarizes the postpartum complications.

GESTATIONAL DIABETES

Gestational diabetes is carbohydrate intolerance that is induced by pregnancy (see Chapter 18).

Epidemiology

Among women with gestational diabetes, 40 percent may persist with diabetes in the postpartum; 60 percent of obese women with gestational diabetes develop diabetes later in life (Cunningham et al., 2001b).

Subjective Data

The client states she had diabetes during her pregnancy.

Objective Data

The two-hour oral glucose tolerance test has traditionally been used to detect diabetes in nonpregnant women (American Diabetes Association [ADA], 2002). In women previously diagnosed with gestational diabetes, it is administered six weeks postpartum. The test measures the rate at which a concentrated amount of glucose is removed from the bloodstream (see Chapter 21). The healthy person almost immediately produces a surge of insulin that removes a large amount of the glucose, with insulin peaking in 30 to 60 minutes. Serum glucose levels return to normal within three hours.

If the test is performed, the procedure requires that for the three days preceding the test, the client consumes a diet containing at least 150 g of carbohydrate (300 g preferred) per day. After overnight fasting (12 hours), a sample of blood is taken. The client then drinks a preparation containing 75 g of glucose. She must drink all of the solution. A blood sample is then taken two hours later.

Counsel the client regarding the purpose of the test and the need for a high carbohydrate diet during the three days prior to the test. Remind the client that overnight fasting is required. In addition, advise her not to drink alcohol and caffeine the evening prior to the test and not to smoke during the two-hour blood testing.

Differential Medical Diagnosis

Diabetes Mellitus

- *Normal Values.* Fasting, < 110 mg/dL, two-hour plasma glucose, < 140 mg/dL.
- *Impaired Glucose Tolerance.* Fasting, ≥ 110 and < 126 mg/dL and two-hour plasma glucose ≥ 140 and < 200 mg/dL after 75 g glucose load (ADA, 2002).
- *Diabetic Values.* One of the following is needed for a positive diagnosis: unequivocal elevation of plasma glucose ≥ 200 mg/dL and classic symptoms of diabetes, including polydipsia, polyuria, polyphagia,

TABLE 20–2. Summary of Postpartum Complications

Complication	Signs Symptoms	Management
Postpartum hemorrhage (early)	Soft, boggy uterus; Cool, clammy skin; Fever; Tachycardia; Vertigo; Tachypnea.	Maintain patient IV line and begin second line; Call physician; Type and cross for blood; Bimanual uterine massage if boggy uterus; Oxytocic agents; Elevate right hip; CBC and coagulation studies Meds: Oxytocin 40 units in 1000 ml of intravenous solution of lactated Ringers at 20–40 mU/min until uterus firm, then continue for 24 hours postpartum or as directed by physician. Carboprost 250 mcg intramuscularly, repeated as necessary q15–90 minutes for maximum eight doses. Preferred over methergine. Methylergonovine maleate 0.2 mg intramuscularly.
Postpartum hemorrhage (late)	Heavy lochia; Foul lochia; Fever; Opened cervical os; Pelvic or back pain; Uterine tenderness; Prolonged bleeding.	Bedrest; Physician consultation; Breastfeeding if possible. Meds: Methylergonovine maleate 0.2–0.4 mg po q6–8h for 2 days. Antibiotics if infection suspected
Subinvolution	Painless, heavy vaginal bleeding; Uterine size larger than expected; Uterine tenderness; Fever.	CBC; Endocervical cultures; Quantitative beta-HCG; Meds: Methergine 0.2 mg q3–4h × 2 days; Augmentin 500 mg qid × 7–10 days; Tetracycline 500 mg qid × 10 days. Doxycycline 100 mg bid × 10 days
Mastitis	Flulike symptoms; Malaise; Fever and chills; Erythema and swelling of affected breast with possible pitting edema.	Milk culture; Bedrest; Continue breastfeeding; Ice packs/warm packs; Increased fluid intake; Meds: First choice—Dicloxacillin sodium 250–500 mg qid × 10 days Penicillin allergy: Cephoradine (Velosef) 500 mg q6h × 10 days
Metritis with pelvic cellulitis	Unilateral/bilateral abdominal pain; Foul lochia; Fever; Parametrial tenderness; Leukocytosis.	Medical consultation; Hospitalization; Rest. Meds: (Intravenous)—Gentamicin and clindamycin are gold standard—Give until afebrile for 48 hours: Cefotetan 2 gms q12h Cefoxitin 1–2 gms q6–8h Gentamicin 3–5 mg/Kg of body weight in three divided doses q8h with clindamycin 900 mg every 8 hours. Oral: Single dose gentamicin: 5 mg/kg. Tetracycline 500 mg qid × 10 days; Augmentin 500 mg qid × 10 days; Cephalosporin 500 mg qid × 10 days.
Postpartum thyroiditis (thyrotoxicosis)	Weight loss; Increased fatigue; Palpitations; Heat intolerance; Sinus tachycardia.	Radioactive iodine uptake; Physician referral. Propranolol (40–120 mg q8h) or atenolol (25–50 mg daily) for short term.
Postpartum thyroiditis (transient hypothyroidism)	Pronounced fatigue; Continued weight gain; Coarse hair; Dry skin; Delayed reflexes; Psychologic reactions mimicking depression.	Elevated TSH; Physician consultation Meds: Thyroxine therapy—begin with 0.1 mg/day.
Urinary tract infection	Spiking fever; Costovertebral angle tenderness; Dysuria; Urgency; Oliguria.	Urinalysis with culture and sensitivity; Meds: Macrobid 100 mg q12h × 3–5 days; Sulfamethoxazole/trimethoprim q12h × 3–5 days; Trimethoprim 100 mg q12h × 3–5 days.
Appendicitis	RUQ or entire right abdominal tenderness; Positive Bryan's sign (pain elicited when enlarged uterus moved to right); Positive Alder's test (Pain elicited when clinician maintains constant pressure at area of maximal tenderness and woman rolls from supine to left position).	Endocervical and lochial cultures; CBC; UA; Medical referral; Hospitalization.

Source: ACOG (1998a & b; 2001), Cunningham et al., (2001d, 2001f, 2001h, 2001i), French & Smaill (2002), Lawrence & Lawrence (1999), Muller et al., (2001), Olson (2002).

and unexplained weight loss; fasting, $\geq$ 126 mg/dL on two occasions; two-hour plasma glucose $\geq$ 200 mg/dL after 75 g oral glucose tolerance test (ADA, 2002). Confirming the results by repeated testing on a subsequent day is recommended.

Plan

* *Postpartum Care.* In the gestational diabetic not requiring insulin (Class A_1), postpartum care is identical to that of the nondiabetic woman. Insulin requirements fall dramatically postpartum because of the decrease in placental hormones (Cunningham et al., 2001B). Insulin is no longer required postpartally in the woman with gestational diabetes requiring insulin (Class A_2). She should be advised to continue her self-monitoring of blood glucose to be sure she remains euglycemic. In the postpartum woman who had pregestational diabetes, insulin is given at approximately one-half of her prepregnancy dose.
* *Psychosocial Intervention.* Assess client's lifestyle and knowledge of diabetes and its management. If lifestyle changes are indicated, counsel the client about the specific change (e.g., diet or exercise). Provide clear, accurate information regarding nongestational diabetes and its usual signs and symptoms and management. Refer the client to support groups if indicated. Frank diabetes may develop as she ages.
* *Medication.* Medication is not usually needed after one to two days postpartum.
* *Follow-Up.* Refer client to a diabetologist if frank diabetes is revealed.

PERSISTENT HYPERTENSION

Chronic hypertension is blood pressure that remains significantly elevated in the postpartum period. It is usually indicative of chronic vascular disease. (See Chapter 21 for information about hypertension in nonpregnant women.)

Subjective Data

The client may report a family history of hypertension or a diagnosis of pregnancy-induced hypertension. She may have no specific symptoms.

Objective Data

Physical examination reveals a systolic blood pressure equal to or greater than 140, a diastolic blood pressure equal to or greater than 90, or both. No edema is evident.

Reflexes are within normal limits. Other findings are normal.

Diagnostic tests include a urine dipstick for protein, baseline electrolyte, blood urea nitrogen (BUN), and creatinine levels, urinalysis for protein urea, and baseline albumin, calcium, and phosphorus levels. More extensive testing (e.g., electrocardiogram) if indicated by extent of findings.

Differential Medical Diagnoses

Essential hypertension, hyperaldosteronism, hyperthyroidism, pheochromocytoma, renovascular disease.

Plan

* *Psychosocial Intervention.* Determine stress levels and sources of stress and counsel client regarding ways to reduce stress. Referral for support and counseling may be appropriate.
* *Medication.* The safety of medications must be considered if the client is breastfeeding.
* *Lifestyle Changes.* Provide dietary counseling to help client reduce fat, sodium, and refined sugar intake. She should maintain adequate complex carbohydrate, protein, and polyunsaturated fats. Counsel regarding exercise for aerobic health. Lactating mothers require information about specific dietary modifications and exercise. Advise mothers to stop smoking; explain cardiovascular changes that occur with smoking. In addition, advise client not to consume alcohol.
* *Follow-Up.* Postpartum follow-up should occur one week after hospital discharge; if hypertension persists, consult with a physician or refer the client for management.

POSTPARTUM ECLAMPSIA

Definitions and Pathophysiology

Eclampsia usually complicates pregnancies after 20 weeks' gestation and usually closer to term. Eclampsia normally resolves with delivery. Postpartum eclampsia may occur within 48 hours of delivery. Chames and colleagues (2002) did a multicenter analysis of data of women with eclampsia from March 1996 to February 2001 at the University of Cincinnati, the University of Tennessee (Memphis), and Central Baptist Hospital (Lexington). The study focused on women who experienced late postpartum eclampsia. The results showed that 89 women were diagnosed with eclampsia, of which 23 women had late onset (greater than 48 hours). Of these 23 women, only 5 had been previously been diagnosed with preeclampsia. More importantly, 91 percent of women with late postpartum eclampsia had at least one symptom suggestive of pre-eclampsia, but only 33 percent of the women reported the symptom to a health care provider (Chames et al., 2002). This alarming finding underscores the need for health care providers to educate all postpartum women on symptoms of pre-eclampsia. Printed instructions may be given to all postpartum women at discharge, with instructions to call their health care provider if they experience any of these symptoms. (See Chapter 18 for information about gestational hypertension.)

Subjective Data

Client may report severe and persistent occipital headaches, blurred vision, photophobia, scomata, epigastric or right upper quadrant pain, nausea or vomiting (Chames et al., 2002; Cunningham, et al., 2001e).

Objective Data

Physical Examination. Proteinuria and hypertension. Edema is no longer included in diagnostic criteria because it is so common in normal pregnancies (National Institute of Health, 2000). Hypertension is diagnosed when blood pressure is 140/90 mm Hg or greater, using Korotkoff phase V to define diastolic blood pressure (ACOG, 2002; Cunningham et al., 2001e). Assess for brisk reflexes with clonus.

Diagnostic Tests. Urinalysis, platelet count, blood urea nitrogen (BUN) LDH, ALT, AST, plasma glucose, PT, PTT), electrolytes, serum creatinine, fibrinogen. MRI of the brain with consultation. ACOG (2002) states that uric acid is only predictive of pre-eclampsia 33 percent of the time and has not proved useful.

Differential Medical Diagnoses

Cerebral venous thrombosis, intracerebral hemorrhage, hypertension, encephalopathy, pheochromocytoma, tumors of the central nervous system, metabolic disorders, epilepsy.

Plan

Medical. Refer to physician for further management and hospitalization; consider neurological consultation. Medication used is identical to management of antepartum client and consists of anticonvulsant and antihypertensive therapy (See Chapter 21).

Psychosocial. Provide emotional support; address concerns of mother regarding her own safety as well as the care of her newborn.

POSTPARTUM HEMORRHAGE

Traditionally, postpartum hemorrhage has been defined as loss of blood exceeding 500 ml within the first 24 hours after delivery (early postpartum hemorrhage) or after 24 hours but before six weeks' postpartum (ACOG, 1998a; Bukowski & Hankins, 2001; Cunningham et al., 2001f). In fact, blood loss from a vaginal delivery is about 500 to 600 ml, 1000 ml for a cesarean delivery, 1400 ml for elective cesarean hysterectomy, and 3000 to 3500 ml for emergency cesarean hysterectomy (Bukowski & Hankins, 2001; Cunningham et al., 2001f). Several authors (Brucker, 2001; Bukowski & Hankins, 2001; Cunningham et al., 2001f) report of the inaccuracy of visual measurement of postpartum blood loss, with as much as a 34 to 50 percent underestimation. ACOG (1998a) has defined postpartum hemorrhage as a "10 percent change in hematocrit between admission and the postpartum period or a need for erythrocyte transfusion." Hematocrit changes do not correlate well with the blood and RBC volume deficits that occur with postpartum hemorrhage (Bukowski & Hankins, 2001). Blood pressure may remain normal until 30 to 40 percent of blood volume is lost and may be artificially low if taken by arm cuff (Bukowski & Hankins, 2001). Even invasive hemodynamic monitoring is inaccurate, especially when the blood loss is less than 30 percent (Bukowski & Hankins, 2001). Factors contributing to hemorrhage are uterine atony, coagulopathy, birth canal trauma, and poor general health.

Early Postpartum Hemorrhage

Early hemorrhage refers to that which occurs during the first 24 hours' postpartum. Several risk factors have been identified.

- Uterine overdistention (macrosomic infant, multiple fetuses, polyhydramnios)
- Midforceps delivery, forceps rotation
- Delivery through incompletely dilated cervix
- Intrauterine manipulation
- Prolonged third stage (30–60 minutes)
- Use of drugs to induce or augment labor or of halogenated anesthetics
- History of previous postpartum hemorrhage
- Chorioamnionitis

- ◆ Retained placental tissue
- ◆ Coagulation defects
- ◆ Fibroids
- ◆ Placenta previa or abruptio placentae
- ◆ Interuterine rupture
- ◆ Uterine inversion
- ◆ Obesity
- ◆ Placenta accreta

Subjective Data

The client may report vertigo, extreme fatigue, chills, or a history of anemia.

Objective Data

Physical examination reveals cool, clammy skin; fever; rapid, thready pulse; tachypnea; pallor of nail beds and mucous membranes. Bleeding may not be massive; however, a steady seepage may continue until significant hypovolemia has occurred. If uterine atony is the cause of blood loss, uterine assessment will show that the uterus feels boggy and that clots are easily expressed with massage.

The complete blood cell count (CBC) provides a reliable measurement of blood loss.

Complete blood cell (CBC) count and clotting studies (PT, PTT, fibrinogen, and platelet count) are done to determine the nature and extent of coagulation disorders contributing to the abnormal bleeding. Consult with physician for management.

Differential Medical Diagnoses

Early postpartum hemorrhage secondary to uterine atony, early postpartum hemorrhage secondary to lacerations, hemorrhage secondary to blood coagulopathies.

Plan

Psychosocial Intervention. Provide emotional support. Inform the client in a calm tone of the procedures that are being instituted. Make instructions specific, for example, "I'm going to give you some oxygen through this mask. I want you to try to breathe normally so that the oxygen will help you." Encouraging the woman to breastfeed will help in the release of oxytocin and therefore help facilitate natural uterine contractions.

Other Interventions

- ◆ Maintain patent intravenous line and begin second intravenous line.
- ◆ Bimanual uterine massage if atonic uterus.

- ◆ If bleeding persists and uterus is firm, evaluate vagina, cervix, and uterus for lacerations.
- ◆ Elevate right hip (prevent vena cava syndrome).
- ◆ Oxygen therapy with face mask at 6 to 8 liters per minute; provide positive pressure ventilation if needed.
- ◆ Call physician and inform him or her of client's status and corrective measures already instituted.
- ◆ Assess client's response by monitoring vital signs.
- ◆ Insert Foley catheter to measure urinary output and to empty an over distended bladder.
- ◆ Record intravenous fluids infused.
- ◆ Anticipate blood transfusion and request cross-matching of blood (packed red blood cells).
- ◆ Obtain clotting studies (PT, PTT, fibrinogen, and platelet count).

Medication

Oxytocin

- ◆ *Indication.* Uterine stimulation.
- ◆ *Administration.* Diluted in intravenous fluids per hospital or agency protocol; usually 10 to 40 units in 1000 mL of normal saline or lactated Ringer's solution given at 20 to 40 mU/min (ACOG, 1998a). Oxytocin should never be given as an undiluted bolus as it can result in severe hypotension and cardiac arrythmias (Cunningham et al., 2001f).
- ◆ *Side Effects.* Hypertension, uterine tetany, nausea, vomiting, bradycardia, tachycardia, premature ventricular contractions, water intoxication.
- ◆ *Contraindication.* Hypersensitivity to oxytocin.
- ◆ *Anticipated Outcomes on Evaluation.* Decreased uterine bleeding and increased uterine tone.
- ◆ *Client Teaching.* Inform the client that she will experience increased uterine contractions, which may be quite uncomfortable.

Prostaglandins

- ◆ *Indication.* Uterine contraction.
- ◆ *Administration.* Intramuscularly—15-m PGF_{2a} (Carboprost; Prostin 15/M; Hemabate) 250 μg, repeated as necessary every 15 to 90 minutes—up to maximum of eight doses. (ACOG, 1998a; Bukowski & Hankins, 2001).

It is preferable to prostaglandin E_2, which may cause vasodilation or exacerbation of hypotension (ACOG, 1998a). Dinoprostin or prostaglandin E_2 (Cervidil, Prepidil, Prostin E_2) is preferable to carboprost for women with heart or lung disease (ACOG, 1998a). The dose is 20 mg per rectum every two hours.

♦ *Side Effects.* Mild fever, diarrhea, abdominal cramping, vomiting, hypotension, hypertension. Prostaglandins can also cause bronchostriction, pulmonary vasoconstriction, hypo- or hypertension, and arterial oxygen desaturation and should be used with great caution in clients with bronchospastic or renal disorders or arterial or pulmonary hypertension (Bukowski & Hankins, 2001).

♦ *Contraindications.* Hypersensitivity, respiratory disease.

♦ *Anticipated Outcome on Evaluation.* Decreased uterine bleeding.

♦ *Client Teaching.* Counsel the client regarding possible side effects, including abdominal cramps, low grade fever, and diarrhea.

Anesthesia/Analgesia. Choice of regional or general anesthesia depends upon client's stability, cause of hemorrhage, presence of underlying disease pathology, potential for further blood loss, need for additional surgery, and the expertise of the anesthesiologist.

Methylergonovine Maleate (Methergine)

♦ *Indications.* Uterine and vascular smooth muscle constriction.

♦ *Administration.* Intramuscularly, orally, and, in an emergency, intravenously.

   • *Intramuscular:* 0.2 mg, repeated in 2 to 4 hours (ACOG, 1998a; Cunningham et al., 2001f).

   • *Oral:* 0.2 to 0.4 mg every 6 to 8 hours, usually for 2 days.

   • *Intravenous:* Hazardous; should be reserved for emergency control of postpartum hemorrhage. If methylergonovine maleate is given intravenously, 0.2 mg is infused over 60 seconds or longer.

♦ *Side Effects.* Headache, dizziness, nausea, vomiting, chest pain, palpitation, hypertension (especially when given intravenously).

♦ *Contraindications.* Hypertension, hypersensitivity to ergot alkaloids, respiratory disease, cardiac disease, peripheral vascular disease.

♦ *Anticipated Outcome on Evaluation.* Decreased uterine bleeding.

♦ *Client Teaching.* Inform the client about possible side effects and increased uterine cramping.

Follow-Up

Advise client to eat foods high in protein and iron to aid in tissue healing and build up body iron stores. Iron sup-plements will be needed for an additional two to three months postpartum.

Late Postpartum Hemorrhage

Late hemorrhage occurs after the first 24 hours and up to one month postpartum. Its usual onset is six to ten days after delivery. Several risk factors have been identified:

♦ Retained placental tissue
♦ Uterine subinvolution
♦ Infection

Subjective Data

The client may report pelvic or back pain, uterine tenderness, or bleeding for more than two weeks.

Objective Data

Physical examination may reveal heavy lochia with a foul odor, fever, an open cervical os after the first week postpartum, and hematoma.

   A complete blood count is ordered (see Early Postpartum Hemorrhage).

Differential Medical Diagnoses

Trauma, blood coagulopathy.

Plan

♦ *Psychosocial Intervention.* Provide emotional support by assisting to calm the client and her family—speaking calmly and giving information about procedures (see Early Postpartum Hemorrhage). She may need help obtaining child or infant care.

♦ *Medication.* Methylergonovine maleate was discussed under Early Postpartum Hemorrhage. Antibiotics should be added if endomyometritis is suspected (see Endomyometritis).

♦ *Ultrasound.* Ultrasound examination is done to detect retained placental fragments.

Follow-Up

Consult with a physician to determine need for hospital admission or other management.

SUBINVOLUTION OF THE UTERUS

Subinvolution of the uterus is the arrest or prolongation of the normal involution process that occurs following pregnancy (Cunningham et al., 2001i). Complications of subinvolution include hemorrhage, pelvic peritonitis, salpingitis, and abscess formation.

Epidemiology

Several risk factors are identified in the etiology of subinvolution:

- Distended bladder
- Retained placental fragments
- Endometritis
- Cesarean birth
- Uterine myoma
- Multiparity

Subjective Data

The client may report painless, excessive vaginal bleeding; chills and fever; pelvic or back pain. Obtain sexual history from client—resumption of intercourse, use of sex toys, new partner, contraceptive used and type.

Objective Data

Physical examination of the genitalia and reproductive tract reveal whether the uterus is larger than expected for the period of puerperium and whether fundal height is normal—midway between the umbilicus and symphysis following the third stage of labor and at the level of the bony pelvis two weeks' postpartum. The uterus should return to nonpregnant size at four to six weeks' postpartum (Cunningham et al., 2001i). With subinvolution the uterus feels boggy and soft and may be tender. Uterine bleeding, excessive lochia, and leukorrhea are possible. Fever may also be present.

Diagnostic tests include serum blood tests, culture of cervical discharge, and ultrasound. Clients must be prepared for venipuncture.

- A complete blood count is performed to detect anemia and infection.
- An erythrocyte sedimentation rate (ESR) is a diagnostic evaluation for occult infective disease.
- Cervical discharge is cultured to identify a specific infective agent, such as chlamydia trachomatis or group B strep. Before a cervical specimen is obtained, the client should be informed about the use of the speculum, the testing to be done, and the reason for the test.
- Quantitative determination of the β subunit of human chorionic gonadotropin (hCG) assists the health care provider in detecting pregnancy, tro-

phoblastic tumors, and tumors that ectopically secrete hCG. Explain the rationale for requesting the test to the client.
- Pelvic ultrasound is done to evaluate whether placental fragments were retained. Instruct the client to drink four glasses of water one hour prior to the ultrasound exam. While she is supine on examining table, the transducer is placed in contact with her skin and swept over the area being studied.

Differential Medical Diagnosis

Distended bladder, ovarian cyst, pelvic adhesions, malignant uterine tumors, cystitis, gestational trophoblastic disease, anemia, uterine leiomyoma, retained placental fragments.

Plan

Psychosocial Intervention. Inform the client about the diagnosis, suspected etiology, and plan of treatment. Explain that methylergonovine may cause painful uterine contractions. Advise her of the need to rest and avoid overexertion.

Medication. For information on methylergonovine maleate, see Early Postpartum Hemorrhage. If infection is suspected, treat presumptively with antibiotics (Cunningham et al., 2001h, 2001i).

Amoxicillin Clavulanate Potassium (Augmentin)

- *Indication.* Broad spectrum antibiotic. Because augmentin contains a β-lactamase inhibitor, it is effective against bacteria that produce β-lactamase.
- *Administration.* One 500 mg tablet orally every eight hours for ten days.
- *Side Effects.* Nausea, vomiting, diarrhea, vaginitis, eosinophilia, leukopenia.
- *Contraindication.* History of penicillin allergy.
- *Anticipated Outcome on Evaluation.* Clinically decreased evidence of infection. Check culture and sensitivity report from earlier cultures to confirm effectiveness of chosen antibiotic.
- *Client Teaching.* Instruct the client to complete the ten-day medication regimen. Tell the client to telephone if side effects make compliance difficult or if no improvement in symptoms.

Tetracycline

- *Indication.* Broad spectrum antiinfective.
- *Administration.* One 500 mg tablet orally every six hours for ten days.
- *Side Effects.* Nausea, vomiting, diarrhea, increased BUN, rash, urticaria, photosensitivity, increased

pigmentation, hepatotoxicity, pseudomembranous colitis.

◆ *Contraindications.* Hypersensitivity to tetracyclines, kidney dysfunction, pregnancy, lactation.

◆ *Anticipated Outcome on Evaluation.* Decreased clinical evidence of infection. Check culture and sensitivity report to confirm organism's responsiveness to tetracycline.

◆ *Client Teaching.* Explain to the client that effects of tetracycline decrease when antacids, dairy products, or kaolin/pectin are also consumed. Advise the client to avoid sun exposure (sunscreen does not seem to decrease photosensitivity), to contact the health care provider if significant diarrhea develops, and to complete the ten-day medication regimen.

Doxycycline

◆ *Indication.* Broad spectrum antibiotic/antiinfective.

◆ *Administration.* One 100 mg tablet orally every twelve hours for ten days.

◆ *Side Effects.* Same as for tetracycline.

◆ *Contraindications.* Hypersensitivity to tetracyclines, pregnancy, lactation. Because elimination is primarily nonrenal, doxycycline, unlike tetracycline, may be used for clients with renal failure.

◆ *Anticipated Outcome on Evaluation.* Decreased clinical evidence of infection.

◆ *Client Teaching.* Emphasize the need to complete the ten-day medication regimen. Instruct the client to avoid sun exposure (sunscreen does not seem to decrease photosensitivity) and to take doxycycline with a full glass of water. Do not lie down at least one hour after administration to avoid epigastric discomfort. In addition, let the client know that the drug may be taken with meals, as its absorption is not affected by food.

Hospitalization. Hospitalization may be necessary if infection is severe, if pelvic structures in addition to the uterus are involved, or if uterine bleeding is excessive.

Follow-Up

Reassess the uterus in one to two weeks. Report signs and symptoms of hemorrhage, pelvic peritonitis, salpingitis, or abscess to physician for further evaluation and management.

MASTITIS

Mastitis, an inflammation of the breast, may be caused by tight clothing, missed infant feedings, poor drainage of duct and alveolus, or an infecting organism (*Staphylococcus aureus, Escherichia coli, Streptococcus*) (ACOG, 2000; Cunningham et al., 2001i).

Infection may be transmitted from lactiferous ducts to a secreting lobule, from a nipple fissure to periductal lymphatics, or by hematogenic means. Smith and Tully (2001), report an incidence of mastitis of 3 percent during the first seven weeks.

Subjective Data

A woman may report flulike symptoms, including malaise, fever, and chills. She may also describe a tender, hot, red, painful area or lump in the breast.

Objective Data

Physical examination is usually sufficient to diagnose mastitis. Assess vital signs. Fever is often high; tachycardia is common. Examination of the breasts reveals increased warmth, redness, tenderness, and swelling. The affected lobule is often in the outer quadrant and wedge-shaped; the nipple is cracked or abraded; and the breast distended with milk. Suspect a breast abscess if there is no resolution of symptoms after several days of antibiotic therapy (ACOG, 2000). If an abscess has formed, pitting edema is possible and fluctuation may be felt over the affected area. As an abscess usually requires both antibiotics and drainage for resolution (ACOG, 2000), the client should be referred to a physician for further management. The remainder of the exam is usually normal.

Diagnostic testing may include a culture and sensitivity, although it is seldom used. Diagnosis is generally made without culture. Culture and sensitivity identifies the causative infectious agent using an expressed sample of breast milk. Test results may not be available for 72 hours; however, antibiotic therapy needs to be started immediately.

Differential Medical Diagnoses

Clogged duct, simple breast engorgement, breast abscess, viral syndrome.

Plan

Psychosocial Intervention. Counsel the client regarding the etiology of mastitis. Unless she has been prescribed a sulfa drug (see the following), encourage her to continue breastfeeding, emphasizing that her medication is safe to use during lactation. Inform the client of the signs and symptoms of worsening mastitis and the need to call the health care provider should they develop.

Medication. Sulfa drugs should not be prescribed if the nursing infant is less than 1 month old (Lawrence & Lawrence, 1999).

Dicloxacillin Sodium (Dynapen, Dycill, Pathocil)

- *Indication.* Treatment of penicillinase-resistant organisms.
- *Administration.* 250 to 500 mg orally every six hours for ten days.
- *Side Effects.* Nausea, vomiting, diarrhea, vaginitis.
- *Contraindication.* Hypersensitivity to penicillins.
- *Anticipated Outcome on Evaluation.* Resolution of mastitis.
- *Client Teaching.* Instruct the client to complete the ten-day medication regimen even if she feels better before medication is finished; if medication is not taken for all ten days, the risk for relapse increases (Cunningham et al., 2001i; Lawrence & Lawrence, 1999). The medication is category B for pregnancy.

Cephalexin (Keflex) or Cephradine (Velosef)

- *Administration.* 500 mg every six hours for ten days; inhibits cell wall synthesis.
- *Side Effects.* Nausea, anorexia, diarrhea, maculopapular and erythematous rashes, urticaria, anaphylaxis.
- *Contraindications.* Hypersensitivity to cephalosporins.
- *Anticipated Outcome.* Resolution of mastitis
- *Client Teaching/Counseling.* Finish all medication. If medication not taken for ten days, there is an increase risk for relapse of infection.

Acetaminophen (Tylenol)

- *Indications.* Antipyretic and analgesic.
- *Administration.* 325 to 650 mg orally every four hours as needed, not to exceed 4 g per day.
- *Side Effects.* Few, if taken in therapeutic doses. Acetaminophen does not cause gastric bleeding or inhibit platelet aggregation. No relationship to Reye's syndrome has been found. Overdosage can cause hepatic necrosis.
- *Contraindication.* None is known.
- *Anticipated Outcome on Evaluation.* Decreased pain and fever.
- *Client Teaching.* Inform the client about the effects of overdosage; instruct her to take no more than 4 g per day. She should know the early symptoms of hepatic necrosis: nausea, vomiting, diarrhea, sweating, abdominal discomfort. Tell the client to telephone the

health care provider if she experiences symptoms of overdosage.

Breast Care. Ice or warm packs may be applied to the breast, whichever is more comfortable. The client should continue to nurse her infant on both breasts, but begin on the unaffected breast and thus allow the affected breast to "let down." Review breastfeeding techniques with the client.

Complications of mastitis require special breast care measures.

- Candidal invasion, described as incredible pain like "hot cords," is a fungal infection of milk ducts. Nystatin cream (Mycostatin or Mycolog) should be massaged into the nipple and areola after each feeding. Antifungal creams and ointments are not absorbed through the mucous membranes and do need to be removed before the baby breastfeeds (Riordan & Auerbach, 2001). The infant must simultaneously be given oral nystatin or the mother will be reinfected. The mother will need Fluconazole (Diflucan) 200 to 400 mg as loading dose, followed by 100 to 200 mg daily for at least two weeks (Riordan & Auerbach, 2001).

Fluid Intake. The client should increase fluid intake.

Lifestyle Changes. Bed rest, with bathroom privileges, is necessary in the treatment of mastitis to prevent the client from becoming exhausted and thereby worsening the mastitis (Lawrence & Lawrence, 1999).

Follow-Up

Referral to a breastfeeding support group or lactation consultant may be necessary (see Support Groups).

ENDOMYOMETRITIS

Endomyometritis is inflammation of the decidua, myometrium, and parametrial tissues following childbirth (Cunningham et al 2001h). Bacteria from an infected surgical incision and from a colonized cervix and vagina enter amniotic fluid during labor. Once in amniotic fluid, bacteria invade uterine tissue postpartum. Bacteria invade the remaining uterine decidua up to a few days postpartum. Endomyometritis is usually polymicrobial (French & Smaill, 2002). Anaerobic pathogens are implicated in 40 to 60 percent of endomyometritis diagnoses following cesarean section, and 25 percent of women will not respond to antibiotic therapy unless an agent giving good anaerobic coverage is also used (ACOG, 1998b). Endomyometritis that develops after vaginal delivery usually has a single pathogen as the causative agent (ACOG, 1998b).

Endomyometritis may have an early onset, generally following cesarean birth, or late onset, usually after vaginal delivery (Cunningham et al., 2001h).

Epidemiology

Risk factors include cesarean birth, membranes ruptured for longer than 24 hours, prolonged labor, numerous cervical examinations, internal fetal monitoring, cervical lacerations, bacterial infections from organisms such as chlamydia and group B streptococcus (ACOG, 1998b, Cunningham et al., 2001h).

Transmission occurs via several routes.

◆ Lymphatic transmission may be from an infected cervical laceration, uterine incision for cesarean birth, or uterine laceration.

◆ Direct invasion occurs when cervical laceration extends into connective tissue at the base of broad ligaments, providing direct access to infective organisms.

◆ Transmission may be secondary to pelvic thrombophlebitis. A thrombus may become purulent, resulting in necrosis of venous walls and pathogenic access to surrounding connective tissue.

Endomyometritis occurs among 3 to 6 percent of vaginal deliveries and 90 percent of operative deliveries done for cephalopelvic disproportion without perioperative prophylaxis (Cunningham et al., 2001h).

Subjective Data

A client may report unilateral or bilateral abdominal pain; foul-smelling lochia; fever, which is minimal if confined to decidua, but more commonly 39°C (102.2°F) or higher; malaise; and anorexia (Cunningham et al., 2001h).

Objective Data

The client appears wan and lethargic. She also appears to have pain.

◆ Vital signs show a fever of about 38°C (100.4°F); tachycardia may or may not be present.

◆ Abdominal and musculoskeletal examinations reveal significant lower abdominal pain with tenderness and rebound. Paralytic ileus may cause distention and vomiting (Cunningham et al., 2001h).

◆ Genitalia and reproductive organs have parametrial tenderness on bimanual exam. The pelvic exam may

be normal even with severe endometritis. Uterine subinvolution is possible. Discharge is increased, dark red/brown, and foul smelling. Cervical motion tenderness is also possible.

A complete blood count is ordered to detect infection or anemia. Leukocytosis (15,000 to 30,000 cells per μL) may be noted on testing of the serum sample. The client should be counseled regarding the purpose of the test and the method used to obtain the serum sample.

Cunningham and colleagues (2001h) question the appropriateness of obtaining blood or genital tract cultures prior to the initiation of antibiotics. They quote earlier studies that found pathogens in the uterine cavities of healthy postpartum women.

Chest radiography may be used to diagnose pulmonary diseases, to detect mediastinal abnormalities, and to assist in assessment of pulmonary status. Request upright anterior, posterior, and lateral views of chest. Inform the client about the test's purpose. She should be told that the radiology technician will ask her to remove her clothing to the waist, take a deep breath and exhale, and take a second deep breath and hold it while the x-ray is taken. Assure the client that the procedure takes only a few minutes, is painless, and may be safely performed during lactation.

A urine culture and sensitivity may be done to diagnose urinary tract infection. Urine is collected by sterile catheterization and placed in a sterile container.

Differential Medical Diagnoses

Endomyometritis, cystitis, pyelonephritis, mastitis, appendicitis, viral disease, septic pelvic thrombophlebitis, paralytic ileus.

Plan

Because of severe, life-threatening complications as noted previously, referral to physician for hospital admission is mandatory. Outpatient management for mild cases of late postpartum endometritis, after physician consultation, may be appropriate (Cunningham et al., 2001h). Close follow-up by telephone and returning to the office in 48 hours is mandatory.

Psychosocial Intervention. Inform the client of her diagnosis and treatment plan and inquire about her support systems.

Medication Interventions. The health care provider may choose one of the following as clinically indicated. Parenteral administration of antibiotics is mandatory in moderate to severe infections and should be continued until the client has been afebrile for 48 hours (ACOG, 1998b; French & Smaill, 2002). Oral antibiotics after parenteral treatment are not necessary and no longer recommended (ACOG, 1998b; French & Smaill, 2002).

The gold standard of treatment continues to be gentamicin 1.5 mg/kg and clindamycin 900 mg intravenously every 8 hours (Cunningham et al., 2001h; French & Smaill, 2002). Studies comparing daily with thrice-daily gentamicin found no difference in treatment failure (French & Smaill, 2002). Cunningham and colleagues (2001h) do not believe it is believe it is necessary to measure the peak and trough serum concentrations of serum gentamicin in most women.

A higher treatment failure rate occurs when an aminoglycoside and penicillin or ampicillin are used instead of the recommended aminoglycoside and clindamycin (French & Smaill, 2002). Although second- or third-generation cephalosporins, when compared to clindamycin and gentamicin, appear to be equally effective in treating endometritis, they have a higher incidence of treatment failures, (French & Smaill, 2002).

Augmentin. Augmentin is a broad spectrum antibiotic (previously discussed, p. 628) used to treat endomyometritis.

Cephalosporins. The cephalosporins, including cephradine (Velosef), cephalexin (Keflex, Keftab, Ceporex), cefaclor (Ceclor), and cefadroxil (Duricef, Ultracef), are broad-spectrum antibiotics with β-lactamase activity.

- *Administration.* Cefaclor: 500 mg orally every eight hours for ten days, not to exceed 4 g per day. Cephradine and cephalexin: 500 mg orally every six hours for ten days. Cefadroxil: initial loading dose of 1 g orally, then 1 to 2 g orally every day or every twelve hours for ten days.
- *Side Effects.* Maculopapular rash, urticaria, and gastrointestinal upset. Discontinue medication if allergy symptoms appear (urticaria, rash, hypotension, difficulty breathing).
- *Contraindication.* Hypersensitivity to cephalosporins and pencillins.
- *Anticipated Outcome on Evaluation.* Resolution of symptoms and clinical improvement.
- *Client Teaching.* Stress the importance of completing the medication regimen. Instruct the client to report signs of allergy.

Cefotetan disodium (Cefotan). 2 grams twelve hours until the client is afebrile and asymptomatic for 24–48 hours.

- *Side effects.* GI upset, rash, pruritus, local reactions, anaphylaxis, blood dyscrasias, elevated liver enzymes.
- *Precautions.* Penicillin or other allergies, renal impairment, renal or hepatic dysfunction. Monitor prothrombin time. Monitor for hemolytic anemia in prolonged use.

Cefoxitin. 1–2 grams IV every six to eight hours.

- *Side Effects.* Maculopapular and erythematous rashes, uriticaria, pseudomembranous colitis, diarrhea, transient neutropenia, hemolytic anemia, hypoprothrombinemia, anaphylaxis, pain induration sterile abscesses at IV site, phlebitis, thrombophlebitis.

Gentamicin. Gentamicin is an aminoglycoside used in the treatment of endometritis. Onset of action is immediate after IV administration, but unknown if given intramuscularly. Peak serum levels occur in 30 to 90 minutes. Gentamicin toxicity is increased when used for longer than 1 week (ACOA, 1998b). Aminoglycocide's bactericidal activity is concentration dependent, and bacterial growth is suppressed for long periods after administration. In addition, there is a phenomenon called "adaptive resistance," in which bactericidal activity of subsequent doses of an aminoglycoside is decreased by the initial dose. Clinical trials of single-dose aminoglycoside therapy apply these principles of aminoglycoside action and have proven to be as effective as conventional multiple dose regimens with less nephrotoxicity.

- *Administration.* Gentamicin: 1.5 mg/Kg of body weight in three divided doses IV every eight hours (Cunningham et al., 2001h). For single-dose therapy, 5 mg/Kg of body weight IV. If serum concentrations are monitored, obtain blood for peak gentamicin level 30 minutes to 1 hour after IV infusion; for trough levels, draw blood just before the next dose. Do not collect blood in heparinized tube as the heparin is incompatible with the aminoglycoside. Monitor renal function (output, specific gravity, urinalysis, blood urea nitrogen [BUN], and creatinine levels, creatinine clearance). Evaluate the client's hearing during therapy.
- *Side Effects.* Neuromuscular blockade; ototoxicity (tinnitus, vertigo, hearing loss); nephrotoxicity (cells or casts in the urine; oliguria; proteinuria; decreased creatinine clearance; increased BUN, nonprotein nitrogen, and serum creatinine levels).

◆ *Interactions.* Cephalothin (increased nephrotoxicity); Dimenhydrinate (may mask symptoms of ototoxicity); general anesthetics, neuromuscular blockades (may increase neuromuscular blockade); Indomethacin (may increase serum peak and trough levels of gentamicin; monitor levels closely); IV loop diuretics (increased ototoxicity); other aminoglycosides, amphotericin B, anyclovor, cisplatin, methoxyflurane, vancomycin (increased ototoxicity and nephrotoxicity); parenteral penicillins (gentamicin inactivation in vitro; do not mix together).

Clindamycin. Clindamycin is an anti-infective used in the treatment of postpartum endometritis. It is used with gentamicin.

◆ *Oral dosage.* 150 to 160 mg every six hours.
◆ *Parenteral.* IM or IV: 900 mg every eight hours (Cunningham et al., 2001h).
◆ *Side Effects.* Nausea, diarrhea, dysphagia, bloody or tarry stools, pain, anaphylaxis; sterile abscess with IM injection.

Conservative management with antibiotics usually produces a response in 48 hours. A poor response indicates abscess, retention of placental parts, or incorrect diagnosis (ACOG, 1998b; Cunningham et al., 2001h). Physician referral is mandatory.

Fluid Intake. Women with endometritis should increase fluid intake.

Lifestyle Changes. Explain to the client and her partner the client's general need for rest, as well as her need for pelvic rest (including no sexual intercourse).

Follow-Up

Medical consultation is required. In addition, telephone the client daily and schedule a return appointment 48 to 72 hours after treatment begins. Complications of endometritis can be severe.

◆ With septic pelvic thrombophlebitis, pain typically develops after the second or third postpartum day. Fever spikes continue despite antimicrobial treatment. Diagnosis is established using computerized tomography or magnetic resonance imaging (MRI) (Cunningham, 2001h). Refer the client for immediate medical treatment.
◆ Pelvic abscess is usually unilateral. Clinical presentation is one to two weeks postpartum and surgical drainage is most likely necessary, as rupture can

cause peritonitis (Cunningham, 2001h). Referral to a physician is indicated.

POSTPARTUM THYROIDITIS

Postpartum thyroiditis is a syndrome of transient or permanent thyroid dysfunction that occurs during the first postpartum year from an autoimmune inflammation of the thyroid (Muller, Drexhage, & Berghout, 2001). It may also occur after a pregnancy loss at 5 to 20 weeks gestation. It results from transient rebound of the autoimmune process following delivery or abortion. The thyroid is unable to regulate both the release of previously synthesized thyroid hormone as well as the synthesis of new thyroid hormone. It is differentiated from other forms of thyrotoxicosis by the lack of thyroid pain, its transient symptoms with spontaneous remission, and elevated serum antibodies and thyroid hormones (hyperthyroid phase) with concomitant suppression of radioactive thyroid uptake (Cunningham et al., 2001d; Muller et al., 2001; Olson, 2002).

Epidemiology

The incidence of postpartum thyroiditis is 5 to 15 percent; in women who are positive for thyroid peroxidase antibodies (TPO), 30 to 60 percent will develop postpartum thyroiditis (Muller et al., 2001). Risk factors for postpartum thyroiditis include smoking, Type 1 diabetes, and prior history of postpartum thyroiditis (Muller et al., 2001; Stagnaro-Green, 2000).

Subjective Data

A client may report symptoms of thyrotoxicosis during the first postpartum month and transient hypothyroidism with symptoms that peak after three to five months.

Thyrotoxicosis has a rapid onset in the latter half of the first postpartum month and persists for two to four months, usually resolving by the fourth postpartum month. The client reports weight loss, fatigue that occurs easily, heat intolerance, palpitations, hand tremors, nervousness, or other psychoneurotic reactions (Cunningham et al., 2001d; Olson, 2002).

In transient hypothyroidism, clinical signs peak between three and five months' postpartum. The client shows progressive and pronounced fatigue, continued weight gain in the latter months of first postpartum year, coarse hair, dry skin, and psychological reactions that mimic depression. Any complaint of fatigue, palpitations, impaired memory, depression, or loss of attention span during the first year postpartum needs to be evaluated (ACOG, 2001; Muller et al., 2001).

Objective Data

Physical examination reveals signs unique to both phases of postpartum thyroiditis. In the thyrotoxicosis phase, the client exhibits sinus tachycardia, stare or lid lag, brisk reflexes, and a firm, non-tender thyroid. Only 50 percent of women have thyroid enlargement (ACOG, 2001). The transient hypothyroidism phase involves delayed reflexes, psychomotor retardation, and psychological reactions that mimic depression.

The thyroid-stimulating hormone (TSH) test is done to diagnose primary hypothyroidism, differentiating primary from secondary hypothyroidism. If the TSH is normal, repeat it in four weeks, because a normal TSH may represent the window phase in which the shift goes from hyperthyroid to hypothyroid (Stagnaro-Green, 2000). In addition, an elevated level of serum thyroid-stimulating hormone is noted in the hypothyroid phase. The test procedure requires a blood sample. Inform the client of the venipuncture procedure and the rationale for the test and explain test results to her.

The antithyroglobulin antibody test differentiates thyroid diseases such as Hashimoto's thyroiditis and thyroid carcinoma. A blood sample is also used in this test. Inform the client of the venipuncture procedure and the purpose of the antithyroglobulin antibody test.

Thyroid peroxidase antibodies (TPO) is a diagnostic evaluation for the presence of thyroid microsomal antibodies (ACOG, 2001; Muller et al., 2001). As a blood sample is required, advise the client about the venipuncture procedure. Tell the client that high antibodies to thyroid peroxidase indicate an increased risk for developing thyroid disease in the first year postpartum (ACOG, 2001; Cunningham et al., 2001d). A TSH assay should be requested. Women with goiters and a high titer of thyroid peroxidase antibodies, but a normal TSH, should have the TSH remeasured in three to six months.

The radioactive iodine uptake test (contraindicated for pregnant or lactating women) reveals increased uptake in hyperthyroidism of Graves' disease, but decreased uptake in hyperthyroidism of thyroiditis (Muller et al., 2001; Olson, 2002). This diagnostic test evaluates the thyroid's ability to concentrate and retain iodine and is indicated in the diagnosis of thyroid disease.

The test procedure is done in conjunction with a thyroid scan and assessment of thyroid hormone levels. A fasting state is preferred. A liquid form or capsule of radioiodine is administered orally. The radioactivity of the thyroid gland is measured by scanning the gland 2, 6, and 24 hours later (Fischbach, 2001).

Provide the client with information about factors that interfere with, or lower, radioactive iodine uptake: iodized foods and iodine-containing medications (one to three weeks' duration), vitamin preparations that contain minerals (one to three weeks' duration), antithyroid medications (two to ten days' duration), thyroid medications (one to two weeks' duration), antihistamines, corticosteroids, isoniazid, thiocyanate, perchlorate, sulfonamides, orinase, Butazolidin, adrenocorticotropin, aminosalicylic acid, coumadin anticoagulant (Fischbach, 2001).

Medications and conditions that increase uptake include thyroid-stimulating hormone, pregnancy, cirrhosis, barbiturates, lithium, phenothiazine, iodine-deficient diets, and renal failure (Fischbach, 2001). Tell the client that the test is painless, but requires 24 hours to perform. Restrict iodine intake (e.g., iodized salt, seafood) for at least one week prior to the test.

Differential Medical Diagnosis

Graves' disease, postpartum depression, Sheehan's syndrome.

Plan

Psychosocial Intervention. Reassure the client regarding the validity of her symptoms. Explain to her the etiology and management of postpartum thyroiditis. Counsel the client regarding spontaneous resolution as well as possible recurrence of the condition with future births.

Medication. Levothyroxine (T4) is administered to treat hypothyroidism. Initial doses should be low, beginning with 0.1 mg/day, increasing gradually every four weeks until full replacement doses have been achieved. Replacement doses have been achieved when repeat thyroid function tests are within normal limits.

- *Side Effects.* Rare when given in therapeutic doses. Excessive doses of levothyroxine may cause thyrotoxicosis; symptoms are anxiety, insomnia, tremors, tachycardia, angina, palpitations, hyperthermia, and sweating.
- *Contraindication.* None is known.
- *Anticipated Outcomes on Evaluation.* Reversal of signs and symptoms of hypothyroidism and a decline in serum TSH levels.
- *Client Teaching.* Instruct the client to take the medication on an empty stomach to enhance absorption; morning administration decreases sleeplessness.

Medication should be kept in a light-resistant container. Advise the client to report excitability, irritability, or anxiety. Also advise her not to switch brands of levothyroxine unless approved by the health care provider.

In women with symptoms of thyrotoxicosis, a β-blocker may be used short-term until free thyroxine (FT4) levels are normal (Muller et al., 2001). Propranolol (40 to 120 mg) in divided doses every eight hours or atenolol (25 to 50 mg) daily may be used (ACOG, 2001; Muller et al., 2001; Olson, 2002).

Follow-Up

Referral to a physician is required. Regular checkups are scheduled for laboratory assessment of thyroid function. As the thyroid gland often recovers in one year, the health care provider can assess thyroid function and the need for continued thyroid replacement by halving the dose and repeating the TSH six to eight weeks later (Cunningham et al., 2001d). If the TSH continues to be normal, one can assume normal thyroid functioning and the levothyroxine can be discontinued. Yearly assessment of thyroid function is advised (Muller et al., 2001).

URINARY TRACT INFECTION

Epidemiology

Risk factors for infection, caused by bacteria in the urinary tract (see Chapter 21), include trauma to the bladder or urethra, such as that resulting from catheterization; history of urinary tract infection; sickle cell trait; diabetes mellitus, use of diaphragm, oral contraceptives, or spermicides (Carson et al., 2000). Infection is transmitted in vaginal secretions via sexual intercourse and perineal pads.

In a population-based case-control study, Schwartz and colleagues (1999) sought to find risk factors for urinary tract infection unique to postpartum women. Anemia, obesity, or diabetes were not risk factors for postpartum urinary tract infection, but women with cesarean delivery, tocolytic therapy, induction of labor, renal disease, pre-eclampsia/eclampsia, unmarried status, and longer hospital stay were at an increased risk (Schwartz et al., 1999). Their data did not identify whether these women had been catheterized, and they recommended prospective, controlled studies to look at continuous versus intermittent catheterization as risk factors for urinary tract infection.

Subjective Data

A client may report dysuria, oliguria, urinary frequency or urgency, nausea and vomiting, chills, and abdominal pain or cramping.

Objective Data

Physical examination usually reveals that general appearance and vital signs are within normal limits. Fever, however, may be present and is indicative of upper urinary tract infection (pyelonephritis). The abdomen and musculoskeletal system exam is done to detect costovertebral angle tenderness and suprapubic tenderness.

A urinalysis determines the properties of urine and abnormal products. Pyuria (white blood cells in urine), hematuria (red blood cells in urine), and positive nitrite indicate a urinary tract infection and warrant a urine culture. Nitrite test may be falsely negative if bladder bacteria have not had sufficient time to produce nitrite, the client does not eat vegetables, or uses a diuretic. Nitrite testing is also negative with some bacteria, such as *S. Saprophyticus* and *Enterococcus* (Carson et al., 2000). The test procedure for urinalysis requires a routine urine sample obtained by voiding. Instruct the client about the purpose of the test and the method of collection.

A urine culture and sensitivity is done to diagnose bacterial infection and identify offending organisms (see Endometritis for a description of the test procedure and client teaching).

Differential Medical Diagnoses

Urinary tract infection (lower or upper tracts); Chlamydia trachomatis.

Plan

Psychosocial Interventions. Provide the client with information and counsel her regarding the suspected diagnosis and pathophysiology of urinary tract infection.

Medication. One of the following drugs is administered. (Amoxicillin is no longer the first choice because many organisms causing urinary tract infections are resistant to ampicillin/amoxicillin.)

Nitrofurantoin (Macrobid)

- *Administration.* One 100 mg tablet orally every 12 hours for three to five days.
- *Side Effects.* Gastrointestinal reactions (nausea, vomiting), headache, vertigo, drowsiness.

- *Contraindications.* Hypersensitivity to the drug, glucose-6-phosphate dehydrogenase (G6PD) deficiency, renal disease.
- *Anticipated Outcomes.* Resolution of client's symptoms and negative urine culture following treatment.
- *Client Teaching.* Advise the client to complete the three- to five-day medication regimen even if symptoms disappear before that time. Medication is taken with food or milk. The client should be told to return for a followup visit if indicated.

Trimethoprim-Sulfamethoxazole (Bactrim-DS, Septra-DS, Cotrim-DS)

- *Administration.* One tablet orally every 12 hours for three to five days.
- *Side Effects.* Gastrointestinal reactions (nausea and vomiting), rash, blood dyscrasias (hemolytic anemia, leukopenia, thrombocytopenia).
- *Contraindications.* Hypersensitivity to trimethoprim or sulfonamides, G6PD deficiency, first 12 weeks or last trimester (28 to 42 weeks) of pregnancy, megaloblastic anemia.
- *Anticipated Outcomes.* Resolution of client's symptoms and negative urine culture following treatment.
- *Client Teaching.* Instruct the client to complete the three- to five-day medication regimen even if symptoms improve or disappear before that time. Medication should be taken with a full glass of water; water intake is increased to decrease crystallization in kidneys. Advise the client to avoid sunlight to prevent burns and to contact the care provider if side effects occur.

Trimethoprim

- *Administration.* One 100 mg to 200 mg tablet every 12 hours for three to five days.
- *Side Effects.* Exfoliative dermatitis, pruritus, rash, thrombocytopenia, leukopenia, nausea, vomiting, abdominal pain, increased AST (SGOT), ALT (SGPT), bilirubin, creatinine.
- *Contraindications.* Hypersensitivity, Creatinine clearance 15 ml/min, renal disease, hepatic disease, megaloblastic anemia.
- *Anticipated Outcomes.* Reduction in client's symptoms and negative urine culture following treatment.
- *Client Teaching.* Advise client to complete the course of treatment even though symptoms may disappear.

Cephalosporins

- Cephradine one 250 to 500 mg tablet every six hours for three to five days.

- Cephalex one 250 mg tablet every six hours for three to five days.

For information on cephalosporins, see Endometritis.

Quinolones (Ciprofloxin HC [Cipro])

- *Administration.* One 250 to 500 mg tablet every twelve hours for three to seven days.
- *Side effects.* Headache, tremor, drowsiness, seizures, nausea, diarrhea, dyspepsia, arthralgia, rash, photosensitivity. This drug is not recommended in lactating women due to the potential for arthropathy and other toxicity (Briggs, Freeman, & Yaffe, 2002). If Cipro is given to a lactating woman, the recommendation is that 48 hours elapse from the last dose of the medication before breastfeeding is resumed (Briggs et al., 2002).
- *Contraindications.* Avoid use with aminoglycosides, beta-lactams because of synergistic effects; antacids that contain aluminum, calcium, or magnesium may interfere with the absorption of Cipro (administer Cipro two hours before or six hours after antacids); monitor theophylline levels because of an increased risk of toxicity; avoid use with warfarin because of increased PT; iron, vitamins, minerals should be discontinued because they may interfere with ciprofloxacin absorption.
- *Anticipated outcomes.* Resolution of the urinary tract infection.
- *Client teaching.* Instruct client to finish all medication.

Levofloxacin (Levoquin, Quixin)

- *Administration.* 250 mg tablet daily for three days.
- *Side effects.* Same as for Ciprofloxacin.
- *Contraindications.* Same reaction with antacids as with Ciprofloxacin; may alter blood glucose levels of people on antidiabetic medication; increased photosensitivity; may alter PT in people on warfarin. The use of Levofloxacin, as with Ciprofloxacin, is not recommended in breastfeeding mothers.
- *Anticipated outcomes.* Resolution of urinary tract infection.
- *Client teaching.* Finish all medication.

Follow-Up

Review proper perineal hygiene with the client. In addition, reemphasize her need to increase fluid intake. (Additional follow-up is outlined in Chapter 22)

ACUTE APPENDICITIS

The appendix may become inflamed as a result of obstruction of the appendiceal lumen by hardened stool, hypertrophy of lymph follicles in the wall of the appendix, or strictures.

Epidemiology

In a pregnancy and the puerperium, the appendix is atypically positioned, as it is in obese individuals. Chronic constipation is another risk factor. Adolescents and young adults, however, are at greatest risk; the incidence of acute appendicitis is rare among pregnant and postpartum women.

Subjective Data

The client may report loss of appetite, abdominal distention, and abdominal pain.

Objective Data

Physical examination may reveal the client to be distressed, obviously in pain. Her vital signs are likely to be within normal limits; temperature may be elevated.

Abdominal muscles do not show the classic signs of appendicitis (abdominal guarding and rigidity) in early puerperium, as the appendix does not return to its usual location until involution is completed (6 to 8 weeks).

- Tenderness is common in the right upper quadrant or entire right abdomen when uterine size is twelve weeks' or greater.
- Psoas, obturator, and Rovsing's signs are not predictive of appendicitis in pregnant or postpartum women.
- Bryan's sign is positive if moving the enlarged uterus to the right elicits pain and may be a more reliable indicator of appendiceal pathology.
- Alder's test requires the health care provider to maintain constant pressure at an area of maximum tenderness while the client rolls from the supine position onto her left side. Alder's test assists in differentiating pain of uterine etiology from that of extrauterine origin; pain of uterine origin may be relieved by change in position, whereas pain of extrauterine origin will not be relieved regardless of position.

Examination of the genitalia and reproductive tract reveals that the lochia is not excessive and has no foul odor, the cervix is closed, and the uterus is nontender.

Diagnostic tests assess blood, urine, and endocervical tissue.

A complete blood count identifies anemia and specific infections. Leukocytosis is nonspecific and does not differentiate appendicitis from other inflammatory causes of abdominal pain. White blood cell (WBC) counts above 15,000/mm^3 and increased neutrophils should raise suspicion for appendicitis. A blood sample must be obtained, and the client counseled regarding the purpose of the test and the method used to obtain the sample.

The erythrocyte sedimentation rate (ESR) is used to monitor an inflammatory or malignant disease. The test also helps to detect and diagnose occult disease. A blood sample must be obtained and the client counseled regarding the purpose of the test and method of collection.

Urinalysis determines the properties of urine, including abnormal products. Pyuria (white blood cells in urine), hematuria (red blood cells in urine), and positive nitrite are indicative of urinary tract infection and warrant urine culture. (See Urinary Tract Infection for details of the test procedure and nursing implications.)

The urine culture and sensitivity is discussed under Urinary Tract Infection.

Endocervical cultures are discussed under Endometritis.

Differential Medical Diagnoses

Appendicitis; endometritis; pyelonephritis; tubo-ovarian abscess.

Plan

Counsel the client and her family about the diagnosis and assist the family to arrange for child care. Immediate referral to a surgeon is mandatory, as complications include death and appendiceal perforation.

EARLY DISCHARGE

Early discharge follows a hospital stay of 48 hours or fewer. It subjects a woman and her infant to certain risk factors. For example, physical complications may occur: discomfort at an episiotomy or cesarean incision site, endometritis, mastitis. Physiologic changes may be affected: uterine involution, increased edema and hyperemia of the bladder with possible atony, and diuresis. The client will confront other changes, such as fatigue, meeting the needs of her infant, role conflict, and adjustment within parental and family relationships (Technical Working Group, 1999).

Follow-up care in the home or by telephone should be pursued to assess the health needs (physical, psychosocial, and educational) of the mother, the family, and the infant in the early puerperium and to implement nursing plans to meet assessed needs. Criteria for prospective payment and a shorter hospital stay will need to be complied with as insurance policies may differ with both hospital stay and home visits. Referral to support groups may be helpful (see Support Groups at the end of this chapter).

A study conducted by the National Center for Health Statistics looked at risk factors for poor health and discharge timing on 9,953 women in 48 states who had a live birth. These women were cared for either by midwives or physicians. Clients of midwives who were discharged early were more likely to have either private insurance or none at all. Clients of midwives who remained in the hospital for an extra night were more likely to have not attended childbirth classes or were multiparous with birth intervals fewer than 24 months. These criteria differed from that of physicians' use of hospitalization stays for clients. Clients of physicians who were discharged early tended to have Medicaid, and had birth intervals greater than 24 months. Clients of physicians who remained in the hospital for an extra night tended to have attended childbirth classes and had more than a high school education (Margolis & Kotelchuk, 1996). As hospital stay was shortened, childbearing families and health care providers, concerned about the care dictated by managed care companies, influenced the passage of patient-protective legislation at state and federal levels (Martell, 2000). Despite the legislation passed, the needs of the woman and her newborn have not been addressed. Radmacher, Massey, and Adamkin (2002) did a retrospective chart review of well newborns to see if early discharge (< 48 hours after birth) or late discharge (> 48 hours after birth) had an effect on the rate of readmission within the first week after hospital discharge. Charts of well newborns (21,628) from January 1994 to December 1998 were reviewed. They found that late discharge infants were readmitted at almost twice the rate of early discharge infants. However, early discharge infants were readmitted for jaundice almost twice that of late discharge infants, with higher bilirubin levels. The majority of readmitted, jaundiced infants were almost always breastfed. Many visits were "worried parent–well baby," as many parents lacked the confidence to recognize normal infant behaviors from those that could indicate problems (jaundice, dehydration, infection). This lack of confidence points to a need for health care professionals to develop strategies to improve parental skills and self-confidence in caring for their newborns.

The American Academy of Pediatrics (AAP) and the American College of Obstetricians and Gynecologists (ACOG, 2002) state that the length of hospital stay should be individualized for each mother–baby dyad. The decision to discharge should be made in consultation with the family and should not be based on third-party payer policies. Although a hospital stay of less than 48 hours for healthy term infants can be done, that policy may not be appropriate for every mother–baby dyad. When no complications are present, a hospital stay of 48 hours for vaginal birth and 96 hours for cesarean birth, excluding the day of delivery, is appropriate (AAP & ACOG, 2002). If a shortened hospital stay is desired by mother and physician, the following criteria should be met (AAP & ACOG, 2002):

- Mother is afebrile, with normal rate and quality of pulse and respirations.
- Mother's blood pressure is within the normal range.
- The lochia is appropriate in amount and color for the duration of recovery.
- Pertinent laboratory results are available, including a postpartum hemoglobin or hematocrit.
- The uterine fundus is firm.
- Urinary output is adequate.
- ABO blood groups and RhD type are known, and, if indicated, appropriate amount of anti-D immune globulin has been administered.
- Any surgical wound appears to be healing without complication, with minimal edema and no evidence of infection.
- Mother is able to ambulate without difficulty.
- Mother has no abnormal physical or emotional findings.
- Mother is able to eat and drink without difficulty.
- Arrangements have been made for postpartum follow-up care.
- Mother demonstrates readiness to care for herself and infant, is aware of abnormal deviations and is able to recognize and respond to danger signs and symptoms.
- Mother had an uncomplicated vaginal delivery following a normal antepartum course and was observed after delivery for a sufficient time to ensure that her condition is stable. Pertinent laboratory data, including a postpartum hemoglobin and hematocrit, was obtained and, if appropriate, RhIg administered.
- Family or other support system should be available to the mother for the first few days following discharge.

- The mother should be aware of possible complications and how to notify the practitioner.
- Procedures for readmission of obstetric patients should be consistent with hospital policy, as well as local and state regulations.

For early infant discharge, the AAP and ACOG (1997) recommend the following criteria be met:

- Antepartum, intrapartum, and postpartum course for both mother and infant should be uncomplicated.
- Delivery was vaginal.
- The infant was a single birth at 38 to 42 weeks gestation, and birthweight is appropriate for gestational age according to appropriate intrauterine growth curves.
- The baby's vital signs are documented to be normal and stable for the 12 hours preceding discharge, including respiratory rate of fewer than 60 breaths per minute, a heart rate of 100 to 160 beats per minute, and an axillary temperature of 36.1° C (97.0–98.6° F) in an open crib with appropriate clothing.
- The infant has urinated and passed at least one stool.
- The baby has completed at least two successful feedings, and documentation has been made that the baby is able to coordinate sucking, swallowing, and breathing while feeding.
- Physical examination reveals no abnormalities that require continued hospitalization.
- The circumcision site reveals no evidence of excessive bleeding for at least two hours.
- There is no evidence of significant jaundice in the first 24 hours of life.
- The mother's (preferably both parents') knowledge, ability, and confidence to provide adequate care for the baby are documented by the fact that the following training has been received:
  - Breastfeeding or bottle feeding—The breastfeeding mother–baby dyad should be assessed by trained staff regarding nursing position, latch-on, adequacy of swallowing, and mother's knowledge of urine and stool frequency.
  - Cord, skin, and infant genital care should be reviewed.
  - The mother should be able to recognize signs of illness and common infant problems, particularly jaundice.
  - Instruction of proper infant safety (e.g., proper use of car seat and positioning for sleeping) should be provided.

- Family members or other support persons, including health care providers, such as the family pediatrician or his or her designees, who are familiar with newborn care and are knowledgeable about lactation and the recognition of jaundice and dehydration are available to the mother and the baby for the first few days after discharge.
- Laboratory data are available and have been reviewed, including the following:
  - Maternal syphilis, hepatitis B surface antigen, and HIV status
  - Cord or infant blood type and direct Coombs' test result, as clinically indicated.
- Screening tests have been done in accordance with state regulations. If a test was done before 24 hours of milk feeding, a system for repeating the test during the follow-up visit must be in place.
- Initial hepatitis B vaccine has been administered or an appointment scheduled for its administration within the first week of life.
- A physician-directed source of continuing medical care for both the mother and the baby has been identified. For newborns discharged before 48 hours after delivery, a definitive appointment has been made for the baby to be examined within 48 hours of discharge. The follow-up visit can take place in a home or clinic setting, as long as the personnel examining the neonate are competent in newborn assessment and the results of the follow-up visit are reported to the neonate's physician or designees on the day of the visit.
- Family, environmental, and social risk factors have been assessed. When risk factors are present, the discharge should be delayed until they are resolved or a plan to safeguard the infant is in place. Such factors may include, but are not limited to, the following:
  - Untreated parental substance use or positive urine toxicology results in the mother or newborn.
  - History of child abuse or neglect.
  - Mental illness in a parent who is in the home.
  - Lack of social support, particularly for single, first-time mothers.
  - No fixed income.
  - History of untreated domestic violence, particularly during this pregnancy.
  - Adolescent mother, particularly if other risk factors are present.

The AAP and ACOG (2002) recommend any newborn with a shortened hospital stay be examined by an experienced health care provider within 48 hours of discharge. They recommend the visit be considered an independent service to be reimbursed as a separate package and not as part of a global fee for labor, delivery, and routine nursery services. If this visit cannot be assured to take place, they recommend deferment of discharge until a mechanism for follow-up evaluation is identified. The follow-up visit is designed to fulfill the following functions (AAP & ACOG, 2002):

- Assess the newborn's general health, hydration, and degree of jaundice and identify any new problems.
- Review feeding pattern and technique, including observation of breastfeeding for adequacy of position, latch-on, and swallowing.
- Collect historical evidence of adequate stool and urine patterns.
- Assess quality of mother–baby interaction and details of infant behavior.
- Reinforce maternal or family education in neonatal care, particularly regarding feeding and sleep position.
- Review results of laboratory tests performed at discharge.
- Perform screening tests in accordance with state regulations and other tests that are clinically indicated.
- Identify a plan for health care maintenance, including a method for obtaining emergency services, preventive care and immunizations, periodic evaluations and physical examinations, and necessary screening.

The AAP and ACOG (2002) recommend that discharge planning for high-risk neonates should begin shortly after admission to ensure a smooth transition from hospital to home. They recommend the following criteria be met before discharge:

- The neonate be given a comprehensive physical examination to identify problems that may require ongoing close surveillance and to provide data on which to base future assessments. If preterm, the neonate was tested for anemia before discharge.
- The neonate is stable physiologically and is able to maintain body temperature without cold stress when the amount of clothing worn and the room temperature are appropriate to what the neonate will experience in the home.
- The neonate is gaining weight steadily on enteral feedings.
- The neonate is able to breastfeed or bottle feed adequately without cardiorespiratory compromise. If the

neonate is unable to feed by nipple, the parents or other care providers are competent in alternative feeding techniques.

- The neonate is free of apnea or can be monitored appropriately at home.
- The knowledge, ability, and confidence to provide adequate care for the baby's parents and/or other family members have been assessed by trained staff in the following areas:
  - Preparation, dosing accuracy, and proper storage and administration of medications.
  - Basic neonate care including bathing, cord care, temperature measurement, comforting.
  - Use of oxygen therapy or monitoring equipment, including the ability to set up and monitor oxygen delivery system or monitoring system.
  - Ability to provide appropriate nutrition to the infant, including adequate frequency and volume of feeding and the ability to mix calorically dense formulas.
  - Recognition of signs of illness and acute deterioration.
  - Basic neonatal cardiopulmonary resuscitation.
  - Proper infant safety, including car seat adaptations for infants weighing less than 2000 grams and recommended sleeping positions for premature infants.
- Appropriate immunizations have been given.
- Sensorineural screening has been accomplished or an appointment for hearing evaluation has been scheduled.
- Appropriate metabolic screening has been performed.
- Ophthalmologic assessment of neonates born at less than 27 weeks of gestational age or weighing 1250 grams or less at birth has been performed, and a follow-up appointment has been scheduled.
- A physician-directed source of continuing medical care, including periodic assessment of infant development, has been identified.
- Family, environmental, and social risk factors have been assessed and, if present, have been resolved, or a plan to safeguard the infant is in place. Factors include, but are not limited to, the following:
  - Untreated parental substance use or positive urine toxicology results in the mother or newborn.
  - History of child abuse or neglect.
  - Mental illness in a parent who is in the home.
  - Lack of social support.

- No fixed income.
- History of untreated domestic violence, particularly during this pregnancy.
- Infrequent visitation or phone inquiry during the baby's hospital stay.
- Preterm birth.
- Single parenthood.
- Adolescent motherhood.
- Closely spaced pregnancies.

HOME VISITS

Home visits are made within the first week of discharge, and should be available to any childbearing family. The family should live within a reasonable radius of the health agency. If they do not, referral to a closer agency is indicated.

FOLLOW-UP TELEPHONE CALLS

Telephone calls are made within the first week after hospital discharge to all families who elect not to have home visits.

MATERNAL ASSESSMENT

Physical inspection, psychological evaluation, and assessment of feeding technique are parts of the maternal exam and can be assessed during home visits.

Physical Examination

Focus on answering the following questions:

General Appearance and Vital Signs

- Does the client appear rested or exhausted?
- Are her blood pressure and pulse within her normal limits, based on her baseline vital signs as an inpatient (assuming no gestational hypertension)?
- Does the client complain of chills or fever? If so, determine her temperature.
- In a client with a history of gestational hypertension, how does current blood pressure compare with in-hospital blood pressure?

Breast Health and Care

- Is the client lactating?
- Are the breasts soft, or hard and painful (engorged)?
- Is the client wearing a supportive bra?
- If the client is breastfeeding, how often is the infant nursing?

- Is the client experiencing pain or nipple tenderness when she breastfeeds?
- Does the client feel comfortable with breastfeeding or insecure or worried?

Abdomen and Musculoskeletal System

- Does the client have discomfort or difficulty urinating?
- Is she constipated or does she have hemorrhoids?
- If the client had cesarean birth, how does the incision appear? Are staples present? What is the color of the skin and skin integrity? Is the incision draining? If so, what color is the drainage?
- Is there any back or neck pain or pain in the lower extremities?
- Is there swelling in the lower extremities?

Genitalia and Reproductive Organs

- What is the fundal height?
- Is there uterine tenderness?
- How much lochia is evident and what color is it? Has there been any change in these qualities?
- If an episiotomy was done, is the incision erythematous? draining? intact?

Psychological Evaluation

Assess the client's ability to cope: What is her financial status? Did she recently relocate? Are her family and significant other supportive? What is her housing situation? Is she homeless or living in overcrowded conditions?

Provide anticipatory guidance for a client concerning her neonate's behavior. Assess her and her family's knowledge of neonatal and infant development and infant cues. Assess their adjustment to the infant.

Feeding Technique

Assess feeding technique—breast or bottle—during follow-up visits or phone calls. Who is the primary provider of care for the infant? Does another person in the client's family influence infant feeding, for example, the type of milk given, the frequency of feedings, the introduction of solids?

Breastfeeding technique may be assessed by asking specific questions. How often does the infant nurse? How is the infant held when breastfed? Do her breasts feel soft after feeding? Ask the client to describe the infant's suck: Is it strong and vigorous, or does the infant frequently stop sucking and cry? How many wet diapers does the infant have in a day? Infants who are getting enough breast milk have six to eight wet diapers a day. Are supplemental feedings given? If so, ask the client the reason for supplementation.

Consider observing the mother and infant during a feeding session to assess the effectiveness of breastfeeding technique. Bottle feeding technique may also be assessed by questioning. How often is the infant fed and by whom? What type of milk is given—commercially prepared formula or table milk? How is the infant held during feeding? Is the bottle propped? Is the nipple properly positioned? Are solids given? If so, why and how is infant fed the solid food?

Environment

In children under the age of 5, 30 to 60 percent are exposed to tobacco smoke, with the greatest increase of smoking in young women (Gaffney, 2001). Smoking increases respiratory infections, invasive meningococcal disease, colic, gastroesophageal reflux, and SIDS (Bakoula, Kafritsa, Kavadias, et al., 1995; Gaffney, 2001; Klonoff-Cohen, Edelstein, Lefkowitz, et al., 1995; Peat, Keena, Harakeh, & Marks, 2001). The risk for SIDS increased three-fold when the infant was exposed to environmental tobacco smoke from a combination of the mother, father, live-in adults, or child care provider (Klonoff-Cohen et al., 1995). In a meta-analysis by Peat et al. (2001), a dose-related relationship to adverse outcomes in children was found between both the number of smokers in the home and the amount smoked.

Infant Care

Assess the client's or caregiver's knowledge of infant cues, infant sleep and wake states, and child developmental stages (see Neonatal Assessment, which follows). Inquire as to infant's position (prone, supine, side lying). In healthy infants, the American Academy of Pediatrics recommends infants no longer be placed in the prone position for sleep (AAP, 2000; AAP & ACOG, 2002). Instead, healthy infants should be placed in the supine or side-lying position (AAP, 2000; AAP & ACOG, 2002). Placing healthy infants in the supine or side-lying position is associated with a lower risk of SIDS. The supine position is also recommended for premature and low birthweight infants (AAP, 2000).

In addition to the supine position, other recommendations by the AAP (2000) to reduce the risk of SIDS includes:

- A crib that conforms to the safety standards of the Consumer Product Safety Commission and the

ASTM (American Society for Testing and Materials) for sleeping rather than a cradle, bassinet, or adult bed.
- Avoidance of soft surfaces for infant sleep, such as waterbeds, sofas, or soft mattresses; avoidance of soft materials in the infant's sleep environment, such as pillows, comforters, sheepskins, or quilts placed under the infant; loose bedding such as quilts, blankets, or sheets—if used, they should be tucked around the crib mattress to avoid covering the infant's face. Another option would be to use sleep clothing rather than blankets when putting the baby to bed.
- Avoiding bed sharing or co-sleeping. Parents who choose to bed share with their infant should not smoke or use substances such as alcohol or drugs, which may impair their arousal.
- Avoidance of overheating of the infant.
- Some tummy time should be encouraged while the infant is awake and observed to help prevent occipital flat spots and to help with developmental skills.
- Avoidance of devices that have been developed to maintain the supine sleep position, as these devices have not been tested for efficacy or safety.
- Home monitoring, while appropriate for some at-risk infants, has not been shown to decrease the incidence of SIDS.

Health Teaching

Provide the client with information about exercise and rest, nutritional needs, postpartum sexuality and fertility, health care, and the nurturing needs of the infant. (Refer to Adjustment with the Infant's Father for specific information.)

NEONATAL ASSESSMENT

Physical inspection, home safety assessment, and identification of engagement and disengagement cues are parts of the neonatal evaluation, which should be assessed during a home visit.

Physical Examination

The physical examination is directed to answering several questions.

General Appearance and Vital Signs

- Has the infant gained weight since hospital discharge? Although 5 to 10 percent of birth weight may be lost by both bottlefed and breastfed infants, the newborn should return to or exceed birthweight by the first week of life. Weigh the infant if a portable scale is available.

- Does the infant appear healthy?
- When awake, does the infant appear alert, wan, irritable?
- What color is the infant's sclera? If yellow, was bilirubin tested prior to discharge?
- When is the infant's follow-up appointment?
- Is the infant's skin clean, without lesions, bruises, or unexplained markings?

Cardiovascular and respiratory assessments include the infant's apical pulse and respiratory rate. If either is elevated, inquire regarding infant's sucking strength, frequency of feedings, and type of cry (absent, weak, vigorous). If assessment indicates possible infection, refer the client and infant for follow-up.

Abdominal assessment determines the amount and frequency of the infant's voidings and the amount and consistency of stool. Assess the abdomen for softness and tenderness.

In a male infant the circumcision site, if present, is assessed for type of discharge and evidence of healing. If circumcision was not done, instruction should be given regarding proper care: Wash external penile skin only, as foreskin of infants and young children cannot be retracted.

Genitalia of a female infant may show a small amount of vaginal blood, which is the result of maternal estrogen in utero.

Home Safety

A hazard-free environment is important. Anticipatory guidance is useful for potential safety problems at different developmental stages of the infant and child. Suggest client not leave infant unattended on bed, table, swing. If client's nails are long, suggest she trim them to keep from scratching or otherwise injuring infant. Suggest to the client, for example, that she tie knots in plastic bags before throwing them away, use child-safety gates, and select toys with no sharp edges or separable, hazardous parts. Keep loose objects from edge of table, sink, or store where a small child could reach up to grab and cause injury.

Child Development

The health care provider should observe nonverbal and verbal cues used by the infant to initiate or stop interaction with the caregiver. An infant's demonstration of dis-

engagement behaviors warrants cessation of caretaking activity and then reassessment of the infant. Evaluate the infant's sleep states (deep or light sleep) and awake states (drowsy, quiet alert, active alert, crying). An infant is most conducive to learning and taking in environmental stimuli when in an active alert state. Point out the infant's engagement and disengagement cues to the mother or care provider.

Engagement Cues

- Verbal cues are feeding sounds (sucking) and crying.
- Nonverbal cues are rooting; alerting signs; facial brightening; smooth cyclic movements of the extremities; mutual gaze; feeding posture; brow raising; and facing gaze (infant looks at parent's or caregiver's face) (Barnard, 1978).

Disengagement Cues

- Verbal cues are spitting; vomiting; hiccoughs; whimpering; crying during caregiving activity; and fussing.
- Nonverbal cues are lip compression; clenching eyes; gaze aversion; yawning; tongue show; increased foot movement; and hand-to-ear movement (Barnard, 1978).

ADJUSTING TO PARENTING

Parenting is a skill that is often learned, to varying degrees of success, by trial and error. Attachment is a process whereby affection develops between infant and parent or caregiver. The process of attachment has been defined as an emotional or affectional commitment to an individual, facilitated by positive interaction between the two and mutually satisfying experiences (Mercer, 1983). Maternal attachment begins during pregnancy as the result of fetal movement and maternal fantasies about an infant (Cranley, 1981; Cropley, 1986; Davis & Akridge, 1987).

A mother's attitudes about pregnancy may influence her feelings about the infant. Maternal grief over the loss of a fantasized perfect child may result in delayed bonding or attachment if, for example, the infant is born prematurely or with obvious birth defects. The infant's behavior can also affect maternal bonding. The infant's crying, avoidance of eye contact, refusal of breast, or withdrawal of a hand when touched is negative reinforcement for a mother.

Nursing Child Assessment Satellite Training tools have been developed to enable the health care provider to identify families that need intervention (Barnard, 1978).

BARNARD MODEL FOR ATTACHMENT AND PARENTING

Adaptation is a result of caregiver-environment-infant interaction. Kathryn Barnard noted that the infant has the tasks to produce clear clues and to respond to the caregiver. If the infant is unable (due to immaturity, illness, or other physical/neurological problems), the adaptive process is interrupted. The mother/caregiver, in turn, cannot respond to the infant's needs, resulting in feelings of maternal inadequacy. Tasks for the mother/caregiver include being able to respond to the infant's cues, to allay distress, and to provide a growth-stimulating environment. Failure interferes with the infant's ability to adapt. The infant, in turn, becomes frustrated, and learns inappropriate interaction behaviors (Barnard, 1978). The environment is also influential. For example, the family is impacted by the actual birth of the child, social deprivation, or an alternate family style, such as single parenting.

Stress or interference may cause parental insensitivity to an infant's cues, failure of the infant to give reliable cues, and failure of the infant to respond to the parent.

MERCER MODEL FOR ATTACHMENT AND PARENTING

Mercer's definition of attachment—a process affected by positive feedback through mutually enjoyable experiences—stresses "process" (progressive nature, occurring over time), "positive feedback" (social, verbal, nonverbal, real or perceived responses of one partner to another), and "mutually satisfying experience" (environment can have positive or negative impact on the mother-infant interaction) (Mercer, 1983).

Four stages of attachment are identified:

- *Anticipatory*. Mother seeks out role model.
- *Formal*. This stage begins with the birth of the child and continues for six to eight weeks; the mother's behaviors are affected primarily by the expectations of others.
- *Informal*. Mother begins to develop her own unique role behavior.
- *Personal*. Mother feels comfortable with role and others accept her role performance (Mercer, 1985, 1990).

INHIBITORS OF ATTACHMENT

Maternal Factors

Among high risk and low risk women and partners, parental competence is a major predictor of parent-infant attachment (Mercer & Ferketich, 1990). Facilitating parental competence thereby increases parent-infant attachment (Mercer & Ferketich, 1990; & Muller, 1996). Parental competence may be defined as the real or perceived ability to care for the physical and psychosocial needs of the infant.

Several factors inhibit attachment and decrease competence.

- Medication, such as narcotics, sedatives, and some forms of anesthesia.
- Physical problems from pregnancy, such as long labor, difficult delivery, or chronic illness.
- Lack of experience in caring for newborns/older infants.
- Learned maternal behaviors that have a negative influence.
- A negative self-concept.
- Lack of a positive support system.
- Grieving a significant loss.
- Anticipatory grieving over an imagined loss of infant, resulting from, for example, complicated pregnancy or postnatal problems.
- Psychological unpreparedness due to premature birth.
- Escape mechanisms, such as alcoholism and drugs.

Infant Factors

Several factors may inhibit attachment.

- Neonatal complications in full-term infants.
- Infant abnormalities.
- Immaturity resulting from premature birth.
- Multiple births.
- Feeding difficulties.

Paternal Factors

A father may exhibit behaviors that inhibit his attachment with the infant.

- Difficulty adjusting to new dependent.
- Failure to relate to newborn.
- Escape mechanisms, such as alcohol and drugs.
- Separation from mother and child because of business or military responsibilities (Mercer, 1983).

Hospital Factors

Hospital procedure may inhibit attachment.

- Separation of infant and mother immediately after birth, at night, and for long periods during day.
- Policies that discourage or inhibit unwrapping and exploring the infant, limiting mother's caretaking.
- Restrictive visiting policies.
- Hospital/intensive care environment.
- Staff behavior not supportive of mother's caretaking attempts and abilities (Baho & Hager, 1998).

PARENTS OF INFANTS WITH MALFORMATIONS

Stages of Adjustment

A wide range of change occurs during adjustment.

- Shock, irrational behavior.
- Denial.
- Grief/anger/anxiety.
- Equilibrium; lessening of anxiety and intense emotional reactions.
- Reorganization (Kennell & Klaus, 1998; Klaus & Kennell, 1983).

Long-Range Impact

Caring for a child with malformation affects all aspects of the parents' lives.

- Financial cost for surgery, medical care for chronic problems, or early stimulation, for example, physical therapy sessions.
- Guilt over time spent with affected infant compared with that spent with other child(ren).
- Social support from family and friends having adverse effect on family relationship.

Therapeutic Approach

The health care provider should realize that the infant is a complete distortion of the parents' fantasized infant and that a therapeutic approach is necessary to address their feelings.

- Parents must mourn the loss of the fantasized child before they can fully attach to the living "defective" infant.

- Guilt accompanies their mourning.
- Resentment and anger are often directed at health care personnel. Allow parents to express their feelings and take the time necessary to experience the full extent of their grief.
- The demands of the "imperfect" newborn retard mother's attempt to mourn the fantasized child.
- Mourning is asynchronous; that is, progress through the stages of mourning varies for each parent (Kennell & Klaus, 1998; Klaus & Kennell, 1983).
- Parents should not be given conflicting information concerning their infant.
- The health care provider may be a role model for parents by responding to the infant with smiles; the infant's positive features should be pointed out to parents.
- Social services may provide financial assistance, and a support group social, interpersonal, or medical support.
- Arrange for home care visit to ensure after discharge care is being implemented.

FAMILY RELATIONSHIPS

The Secundigravida

The concerns of a woman experiencing her second pregnancy are primarily for her other child and the expectation of caring for two children.

- Concern for first child may cause grieving over the dyadic relationship with the first child and her anticipation of the first child's pain.
- Managing the care of two children may cause a mother to feel overwhelmed. She may have increased expectations of the first child and may doubt her own ability to love two children equally. The temperaments of the new infant and the older sibling may be different.
- Assist the parents in developing confidence in parenting skills through parenting classes that include information about infant and child behavior, home visits, and telephone calls.
- The second pregnancy may not be as exciting or as desired as the first. The mother may not be totally engrossed in mothering her second baby as she was with the first. She may feel sad or guilty.
- Maternal self-perception changes and she sees herself as experienced. She recognizes her needs as separate from those of her role as mother.

Readjustment with the Infant's Father

A negative effect of childbirth may be the breakup of the marriage or relationship. The mother may lack support in child care and household tasks. Spouse abuse or child abuse may increase. In assessing the couple, focus on their sharing of tasks, sexual relationship, leisure activity, and financial management.

- Sharing of family tasks and responsibilities often occurs following agreement before childbirth on the division of tasks. Equal sharing of child and infant care may be agreed on, or the parents may prefer that the father be primary caregiver for the older child or children. Other parents may prefer that the father assume more household tasks and the mother have the responsibility for infant and children.
- Assess the parenting roles of the mother and father. Assess their self-expectations and their expectations of each other. Parenting behavior can be adaptive (constructive) or maladaptive (nonconstructive, harmful). The health care provider may need to identify normal infant and child behaviors and developmental tasks to the parent or caregiver. Alternative forms of discipline for an older child (e.g., "time out") may need to be discussed. Refer parent or caregiver to parenting classes through, for example, churches or March of Dimes.
- The sexual relationship may be safely resumed 2 weeks postpartum (Cunningham et al., 2001i). Physiological responses in the puerperium may cause a decrease in the intensity of the sexual experience. The decrease is due to thin vaginal walls in the hypoestrogenic state, especially during lactation; delayed congestion of the labia majora and minora until the plateau phase, and decreased strength of orgasmic contractions. Sexual activity is decreased because of fatigue, weakness, vaginal discharge or spotting, perineal pain, tight or lax vaginal muscles, breast discomfort, and decreased vaginal lubrication. Client teaching may include suggestions to enhance sexual comfort and "safer sex" behaviors and precautions.
  - Saliva (after postpartum exam) or water-soluble gel (Astroglide®, Replens®, K-Y jelly®) may be used for lubrication.
  - Lubricated condoms may provide comfort.
  - The female-superior or side-to-side positions may help control the depth of thrusting.
  - Gentle rotation of two fingers around the vagina may aid vaginal relaxation.

- Other displays of affection (holding, cuddling) are pleasurable if intercourse is not desired.
- The woman may assist partner to orgasm with masturbation or fellatio. Her partner may help her also achieve orgasm without intercourse.
- The client should perform Kegel exercises to regain vaginal tone.
- A nutritious diet will promote healing and a sense of well-being.

- Leisure time for the couple should include time alone. They may enlist the help of family and friends to watch the infant and children. Encourage communication between the couple ("I love you," "You are special to me," "Thanks for your help"). Simple gestures of affection (romantic card or flowers for him or her) provoke loving feelings.
- Management of finances may require referral to a community food bank, social services, or the Women, Infants, and Children Program (WIC).

Single Parent/Working Mother

Address the parent's child-rearing difficulties, financial insecurity, role conflict, or social isolation.

- Encourage the parent to verbalize feelings on how absence of one parent may affect parent-infant relationship or child development.
- Identify for the working mother the positive aspects of separation (daily break from infant and child care while at work).
- Stress the importance of quality rather than quantity of time spent with the infant and children.
- Assist the parent in developing confidence in parenting skills through parenting classes that include information about infant behavior, home visits, and telephone calls.
- Encourage inexpensive activities that are relaxing and enjoyable for parent and infant.
- Financial insecurity may benefit from referral to community food bank, social or legal services, or WIC. In addition, referral for housing or job training may be necessary.

A parent experiencing role conflict and uncertainty concerning responsibilities may benefit from assistance in establishing priorities and assigning appropriate tasks to older children. Referral to appropriate resources may also be necessary to develop essential skills in caretaking and home management.

Social isolation and loneliness may be eased by client's involvement in parental and social groups (apartment complex, church, extended family) and support groups (see list of Support Groups at the end of this chapter).

Lesbian Families

Such families may include legal guardian relationships, working collectives, roommates, ex-lovers now considered family members, and couples with or without children (Blackwell & Blackwell, 1999; Zeidenstein, 1990).

The health care provider should be knowledgeable regarding lesbian issues and health care concerns, comfortable providing health care to the gay population, and supportive of the lesbian family (Harvey, Carr, & Bernheine, 1989).

Lesbian concerns range from unique to common:

- Fear of custody battles require referral for legal advice on custody, because a nonbiological lesbian parent may not have a legal right to parent a child if the biological parent, her partner, dies (Bender, Jorjorian, Lynch, & Cramer, 1998; Blackwell & Blackwell, 1999; Zeidenstein, 1990).
- Fear of HIV infection is possible. An alternative insemination/unscreened donor may have been used for conception. One partner may use intravenous drugs or may have intercourse with men. The mother may receive fluid (vaginal fluid, menstrual blood) from an HIV-infected partner. One means of exchanging fluid is sharing a dildo without using a condom (Russell, Sanford, & Jobin-Leeds, 1998; Stevens & Hall, 2001). If HIV infection is a concern, counsel women regarding safer sex (see Chapter 12).
- Battering—physical, emotional, or verbal—is possible. (See page 648 for assessment tool for abuse.) Refer the woman for counseling, to a shelter, or to a support group. The woman may decide not to provide information on abuse if she is lesbian, as her sexual preference may then be included as part of her medical record and thus be subject to review by future insurers, physicians, and nurses.
- Alcoholism affects lesbian relationships and families as it does heterosexual relationships and families.
- Support may be lost from family and friends and her job (Bender et al., 1998; Zeidenstein, 1990).

A role model should be available to assist with maternal tasks.

- Determine the coparent's involvement in infant care and with partner.
- Encourage the partner's role in parenting.
- Encourage the partner's presence during health care visits.
- Referral to appropriate support groups may be helpful.

Families with Human Immunodeficiency Virus Infection

HIV-infected families are those families in which one or more persons are infected with the virus. Persons may be asymptomatic carriers or exhibit AIDS, having been diagnosed with opportunistic infections and malignancies. The epidemiology of AIDS is described in Chapter 12.

Women who have tested positive for HIV should be referred to HIV specialists during the postpartum period, so that antiretroviral therapy can be reviewed. All HIV-infected mothers should be taught how to administer ZDV syrup to their infants during the first six weeks postpartum, regardless of whether they choose to continue antiretroviral therapy after delivery (Patchen & Beal, 2001). One intramuscular injection of nevirapine may be indicated, especially if the mother did not receive antiretroviral medications during pregnancy (Patchen & Beal, 2001). Women also need to be advised that their infants need to be treated prophylactically for pneumocystic pneumonia, starting at six weeks after birth. Bactrim is usually prescribed at the six-week visit, after the ZDV syrup is discontinued (Patchen & Beal, 2001). Discussion of birth control should include the consistent use of condoms, regardless of the method chosen, to decrease the risk of acquiring other strains of HIV (Patchen & Beal, 2001). Oral contraceptives may not be as effective when women are on protease inhibitors or efavirenz (Patchen & Beal, 2001). All HIV-infected infants should be referred to a pediatric HIV specialist for antiretroviral therapy. Infants who test negatively on HIV DNA-PCR tests are usually retested at 14 days, 1 to 2 months, and 3 to 6 months (Patchen & Beal, 2001). Infants are generally ruled out to be HIV infected after two or more negative tests completed at 1 and 4 months (Patchen & Beal, 2001).

Teach clients about infection control, such as hand washing, avoiding exchange of body fluids or sharing of razors and toothbrushes, wrapping soiled peripads in sturdy plastic containers, and cleaning soiled surfaces with a dilute bleach solution of 1 part bleach to 10 parts water.

Advise clients to contact the health care provider should they note signs of infection: fever, foul smell of lochia, excessive amount of bleeding, return of bright red bleeding. Clients should also contact the health care provider if there are signs of worsening HIV infection: fatigue, anorexia, weight loss, sore throat, cough, dermatologic disorders, or unusual vaginal discharge. The infant's health care provider should be contacted if the infant exhibits fever, poor feeding, oral thrush, diarrhea, cough, or flulike symptoms.

Instruct the client on how to avoid other infection, for example, not ingesting raw meat or eggs to avoid *Salmonella* infection, not emptying cat litter to avoid the risk of toxoplasmosis, not sharing needles, and discontinuing substance abuse, including tobacco and alcohol.

Families with HIV may have several areas of concern: personal, health, and family concerns; concern for the needs of the children; financial pressures and concerns; dilemma of disclosure; and the social aspects or challenges of HIV (DeMatteo, Wells, Goldie, & King, 2002). Some of the issues of health and family concerns included a divorce, separation, or abandonment rate of one in five adults, fear of intra-family transmission through the very acts of intimacy that often bring consolation, fear of transmission through casual contact, increased stress from finances or illness, and the importance of support. Families focused on the children by attempting to maintain "normalcy" in childhood and by preparing children to become self-sufficient and independent. Parents feared that disclosure would harm the children, especially in the way others perceived them. Women dealt with disclosure in several ways. Some dealt with it by bringing the child's medication to the school rather than having it dispensed by the school nurse or by not correcting a child's false assumption for taking antiviral medication (Santacroce, Deatrick, & Ledlie, 2002). Other women with HIV dealt with their illness by "silencing" themselves by denying the importance of their own needs and feelings and put the needs of their families foremost (DeMarco, Lynch, & Board, 2002).

Families with Domestic Violence

Between two and four million women experience some form of violence each year (Kramer, 2002; Misra, 2001; Shoultz, Phillion, Noone, & Tanner, 2002). Pregnant women are twice as likely to be assaulted, and 40 percent of assaults on women occur during the first pregnancy (Humphreys & Neylan, 2001; Shoultz et al., 2002). The incidence of assaults on women with disabilities ranges from 33 to 83 percent (Kramer, 2002).

Child abuse often coexists or increases with spouse abuse (AAP, 1998; Anderson, 2002; Quillian, 1996; Synoground & Bruya, 2000). Family violence is a major factor contributing to poverty and homelessness of women (Buckner, 1998; Synoground & Bruya, 2000, Winters, 1998). Screening for domestic violence should be a routine part of history-taking and should be done when the patient is alone. Nonthreatening words and emotionally charged words (like "abused woman") should be avoided. Women from different cultures and ethnic backgrounds may respond to violence in different ways, sometimes making it more difficult for them to seek help. Shoultz et al. (2002) did a pilot study using prevention protocols that were tailored to five ethnic groups of women on two rural islands in the state of Hawaii. These women were Caucasian, Hawaiian, Filipino, Japanese, and Hispanic. The women felt that public places (schools, churches, laundromats) would be better places for obtaining information on domestic violence. The women stated that the health care provider should develop a relationship with the client and assure confidentiality. The women believed a broad, open-ended question would be more effective than using a "laundry list." The health care provider can begin with a statement like "Many women are dealing with abuse and violence in their lives, so I routinely ask about it in women" or "I am so concerned about violence that I'm asking all my clients."

Make an assessment for evidence of domestic violence, using Abuse Assessment Screen (Anderson, 2002; Kramer, 2002).

- Have you ever been emotionally or physically abused by your partner or someone important to you?
- Within the last year, have you been hit, slapped, kicked, or otherwise physically hurt by someone?
- Since you've been pregnant, were you hit, slapped, kicked, or otherwise physically hurt by someone? If yes, by whom? Total number of times.
- Were you ever forced to have sexual activities? If yes, by whom? Total number of times.
- Are you afraid of your partner or anyone you listed above?

It is also imperative to screen for child abuse. Parents who were abused as children are six times more likely to abuse their children. Kemper (1995) states the following screening questions are asked at her clinic: As a child,

1. How often did your parents ridicule you in front of friends or family?
   Frequently   Often   Occasionally
   Rarely   Never

2. How often were you hit with an object such as a hair-brush, board, stick, wire, or cord?
Frequently   Often   Occasionally
Rarely   Never

3. How often were you thrown against walls or down stairs?
Frequently   Often   Occasionally
Rarely   Never

4. Did your parents ever hurt you when they were out of control?
Yes   No

5. Do you feel you were physically abused?
Yes   No

6. Do you feel you were neglected?
Yes   No

7. Do you feel you were hurt in a sexual way?
Yes   No

8. Would you like more information about free parenting programs, parent hotlines, or respite care?
Yes   No

Once abuse has been identified, assess the potential for danger for the client. An increase in the severity or frequency of abuse, attempts at choking the woman by her partner, threats or attempts on her part to commit suicide, attempts or threats on his part to commit suicide are some indicators that the client is in danger and consideration for her safety must be undertaken. She should be encouraged to think of a safety plan that may include the following:

- Hiding money
- Hiding extra set of house or car keys
- Set up a code with family/friends
- Ask neighbor to call police if violence begins
- Remove weapons
- Have available social security numbers (his, client's, childrens'), rent and utility receipts, birth certificates (client's and childrens'), driver's license, bank account numbers, insurance policies and numbers, marriage license, valuable jewelry, important phone numbers (Anderson, 2002; Kramer, 2002; McFarlane & Parker 1994; Winters, 1998).

Offer information on available shelters, legal and criminal assistance.

When child abuse screenings are positive, it is important to follow up with open ended questions or statements. Ask the parent how the family might best address the issue. Acknowledge the individual's courage in facing and identifying problems, as well as the family's strengths. Follow-up with the family is essential.

Child or spouse abuse should be considered when a child or adult presents with an injury or symptom that is not consistent with the clinical evidence, illogical or changing explanations for an injury are given by the parent, or when there is concomitant abuse of the child's mother (AAP, 1998; Newberger, 1995). Individuals should be interviewed separately to provide privacy and convey a sense of respect for the person as an individual.

Empowering strategies to use for the survivor of abuse include acknowledging the abuse, listening, avoiding blame, exploring options, and making referrals (Anderson, 2002; Kramer, 2002).

Homeless Families.

The homeless population continues to be a health care and social concern today. Approximately 40 percent of the homeless population are families with children, with the majority most frequently headed by women (Menke, 2000; Misra, 2001; Oliveira & Goldberg, 2002; Synoground & Bruya, 2000). Single-parent, female-headed families have a 50 percent greater chance of living below the poverty line than two-parent families (Menke, 2000). Children living in poverty have more adverse outcomes, including illness, depression, behavioral problems, difficulties in school, and fear or trauma from violence (Buckner, 1998; Menke, 2000; Synoground & Bruya, 2000). The majority of homeless women cite domestic violence as the prime factor for their being homeless (Oliveira & Goldberg, 2002; Synoground & Bruya, 2000).

Health issues for homeless families are staggering.

- Social isolation
- Lack of access to health care
- Physical violence on the streets and in shelters
- Spouse abuse, child abuse, or both
- Substance abuse
- Chronic health problems
- Obesity
- Inadequate diet: insufficient iron, folic acid, calcium; low intake of dairy products, fruits, and vegetables; high intake of total fat, saturated fat, and cholesterol.
- Parasites
- Infectious diseases
- Exposure to the elements (Buckner, 1998; Menke, 2000; Oliveira & Goldberg, 2002; Synoground & Bruya, 2000).

Arrange for nursery services so that the client may attend classes in parenting skills and learn about infant behavioral cues. Identify and prevent family violence with counseling or referral. Identify and teach basic foot care: keep feet clean and dry; use proper technique for cutting toenails; use appropriate footwear; wear clean dry socks. Evaluation and care are provided at times and locations convenient to the population to be served. Assist in providing nutritional information to volunteers at soup kitchens. Refer families to community resources for lodging and job training. WIC, substance abuse programs, and domestic violence programs may also be suggested.

Discipline and Parenting Skills in Families

Parenting involves caring for children physically and emotionally in a loving manner so that they are able to become responsible, caring adults. Parenting is not an innate behavior but a learned art. For some, parenting is learned from one's own parents. One may then decide which parenting behaviors to keep and which ones to avoid. At best, this may stimulate a new parent to learn alternative parenting styles by attending parenting classes. At worst, a new parent stays with the parenting style he or she was exposed to and may have unrealistic behavior expectations of his or her child. Developing a sense of self-esteem and self-worth in the child is enhanced by discipline, provided that the discipline is supportive and develops problem solving skills. Yet many parents attempt to accomplish this task with little knowledge of normal developmental stages of infants and children leading to unrealistic expectations.

Spanking is the most common form of physical punishment, and 90 percent of U.S. families reported having spanked their children as a form of discipline (AAP, 1998; Furniss, 2000). Spanking is an ineffective means of discipline because its effectiveness decreases with subsequent use. In order to maintain its effectiveness, the intensity of the spanking needs to be increased, which can quickly escalate into abuse (AAP, 1998; Furniss, 2000). Spanking has the following consequences: an increased risk of injury when children under the age of 18 months are spanked; repeated spanking can lead to agitated, aggressive behavior in the child and physical altercation between the child and parent; spanking models an inappropriate behavior as a solution to conflict and has been associated with increased aggression in preschool and school-age children; spanking alters the relationship between parent and child, making discipline more difficult in adolescence; spanking is not effective as a long-term approach and makes other strategies (such as time out) more difficult and less effective to use; the pattern of spanking may be sustained or increased, making it more likely for the parent to use as a relief from anger (AAP, 1998).

The American Academy of Pediatrics suggests alternatives to spanking that would be more positive in changing undesired behavior in children. An effective discipline system has three vital elements: (1) a learning environment characterized by a positive, supportive parent-child relationship; (2) a strategy for teaching and strengthening desirable behaviors; and (3) a strategy for decreasing or eliminating undesirable behaviors (AAP, 1998).

A positive, supportive parent-child relationship is fostered through play and warmth and affection for the child by the parent. Parents should be encouraged to provide consistency in daily activities and interactions with the child, paying attention to the child to increase positive behavior and, conversely, ignoring and removing parental attention to decrease the frequency or intensity of undesired behaviors. Positive reinforcement can entail special time between parent and child, listening carefully to children and help them learn words to describe their feelings, allowing children to make choices whenever appropriate and helping them learn to evaluate the potential consequences, praising behaviors that are desirable, and modeling appropriate behavior and resolution strategies (AAP, 1998). Undesirable behavior can be eliminated by making clear to the child what the problem behavior is and what consequence the child can expect when this behavior occurs; being consistent in responding to the undesirable behavior when it occurs; being calm and empathetic when correcting the behavior and providing a reason for a consequence for the undesired behavior (AAP, 1998). Time out (for toddlers) or restriction of privileges (for older children) are effective ways to eliminate undesirable behavior. Rules should be fair and appropriate for the child's age.

Brazelton defines discipline as "teaching," not punishment (Brazelton 1992). Brazelton states that children sense a need for discipline, and toward the end of the second year, they will make this need known by obvious testing. He further states that self-discipline, which is the goal of discipline, comes in three stages: trying out limits, teasing to elicit a response from others as to what is and is not allowed, and internalizing these previously unknown boundaries (Brazelton, 1992).

Problem solving is one way to discipline by allowing parents and child to work together to reach a decision. Spanking and hitting are not constructive forms of discipline, are demeaning to children, and may inhibit the development of a guilty conscience (AAP, 1998). Brazelton (1992) gives the following guidelines for discipline:

- Respect a child's stage of development.
- Fit the discipline to the child's stage of development.

- Discipline must fit the child.
- When your child is with other children, try not to hover.
- Model behaviors for the child.
- After the discipline is over, help your child explain what it's all about.
- Use a time-out, but for a brief period only.
- Ask the child's advice about what might help next time.
- Physical punishment has very real disadvantages.
- Watch out for mixed messages (e.g., telling a child "Don't do that" when you really aren't sure or don't mean it).
- Stop and reevaluate whenever discipline doesn't work.
- Pick up the child to love him or her afterward.
- Remember to reinforce the child when he or she isn't teasing you by commenting on how well he or she is controlling himself or herself.

Brazelton lists behaviors exhibited by children when parents are too strict. The following behaviors should warrant closer observation of the child and family and may require intervention:

- A child who is too good or too quiet, or who doesn't dare express negative feelings.
- A child who is too sensitive to even mild criticism.
- A child who doesn't test you in age-appropriate ways.
- A child without a sense of humor and joy in life.
- A child who is irritable or anxious most of the time.
- A child who shows symptoms of pressure in other areas—feeding, sleeping, or toileting—and who may regress to an earlier kind of behavior, acting like a baby or a much smaller child.

PLAN

The plan to assist families in their adjustment to parenting should offer many alternatives to address the multitude of needs.

- *Practical Guidance.* This can include the simple suggestion to lay out clothes at night for the next day to decrease tension in the morning while dressing the infant and older child (children) for day care or school. Taking time out for both parent and child to regain self-control.
- *Child Development and Behavior.* Teaching a client about child development enables her to better under-

stand older children and the new infant; counseling should address infant's cues and states.
- *Referral.* Individual counseling may be necessary for a client who feels excessively guilty or angry about her first child's reactions to the infant. After counseling the client regarding daily nutritional needs of adults, infants, and children, referral for specific dietary needs may be helpful. Refer the client for legal assistance and domestic violence counseling and assistance if appropriate (see Parenting/Family Support Groups at end of chapter).

PSYCHIATRIC DISTURBANCES

Psychiatric disturbances occur during the puerperium. The disturbances are classified on the basis of their severity:

- *Maternity Blues or "Baby Blues."* Transient, emotional disturbances commonly occurring around the second or fourth postpartum day, lasting from a few hours to two weeks.
- *Postpartum Depression.** Characterized by lowered mood, irritability, fatigue, feelings of worthlessness, sleeping and eating changes, and subtle changes of personality.
- *Postpartum Psychosis.** Severely impaired ability to perform daily living tasks.

Epidemiology

Etiology and Risk Factors. The etiology of postpartum depression continues to be unknown. Although theories for the etiology of postpartum depression have included hormonal, neurotransmitter, genetic, and psychological factors, current evidence points to a multifactorial etiology in which the neuroendocrinologic changes of the postpartum period, placed on an individual with a vulnerability to illness, precipitates postpartum depression (Beck, 1999; Gold, 2002; Newport, Hostetter, Arnold, & Snowe, 2002).

Postpartum depression has detrimental effects on both the mother and infant in terms of parenting and developmental skills (Beck, 1999; Horowitz, Bell, Trybulski, et al., 2001). Depressed mothers interact less with their infants and experience anger and guilt over their

---

*Conditions are prolonged beyond usual period expected for "blues."

feelings of loneliness (Beck & Gable, 2001). They feel overwhelmed by the responsibility of caring for their infants. Infants of depressed mothers tend to be fussier, vocalize less, and use less positive facial expressions than infants of nondepressed mothers (Beck, 1999, 2002; Beck & Gable, 2000; Gold, 2002; Newport et al., 2002).

Maternity Blues. Maternity blues are the mildest form of depression and are usually self-limiting. They begin on the second or third postpartum day and last up to fourteen days.

Factors are unknown. Psychological factors may include the conflict caused by cultural expectations to bear children and pursue personal goals and the economic cost of childbearing and childrearing.

Postpartum Depression. Postpartum depression has a slow, insidious onset over several weeks postpartum. It usually begins within two or three weeks postpartum and may last up to a year. There is no definite etiology (Beck, 1999; Gold, 2002; Newport et al., 2002).

Risk factors for postpartum depression include history of previous depression, history of postpartum depression, prenatal depression, life stress, child care stress, prenatal anxiety, lack of social support, marital stress, and stressful life events during pregnancy or near term (Beck, 2002; Gold, 2002; Newport et al., 2002). Depression during pregnancy is one of the most important predictors of postpartum depression (Beck, 2002). Women with histories of postpartum depression are at a 50 percent higher risk of recurrent episodes in subsequent pregnancies (Gold, 2002) and 30 to 70 percent are likely to remain depressed one year or longer after delivery (Horowitz et al., 2001). Postpartum depression affects approximately 13 percent of mothers, but up to 50 percent of postpartum depression goes undiagnosed (Beck & Gable, 2001b). Studies indicate that postpartum adolescents have significantly lower rates of depression if the adolescent receives support from her mother and the infant's father (Hudson, Elek, & Campbell-Grossman, 2000). They, as did adult mothers with depression, reported more negative feeding interactions with their infants and reported less confidence in their mothering skills than adolescents without depressive symptoms (Hudson et al., 2000; Panzarine, Slater, & Sharps, 1995).

Postpartum Psychosis. Postpartum psychosis has its onset within a few weeks or, at most, three months postpartum; the affected woman is sixteen to twenty times more likely to require hospital admission in the three months postpartum than in an equivalent period preconceptionally. Of women who have had a previous episode of postpartum psychosis, 50 to 90 percent will experience another episode in subsequent pregnancy (Gold, 2002). Symptoms of postpartum psychosis closely resemble a manic or mixed manic episode and include restlessness, irritability, insomnia, a rapidly shifting mood from depressed to manic, confusion, disorientation, erratic behavior, and delusional thinking often revolving around the infant (Beck, 1999; Gold, 2002; Newport et al., 2002).

Physiological factors are theorized; there is no definite etiology. Theories involve hormonal, neurotransmitter, and genetic factors. Psychological factors reflect no definite etiology; the primary risk factor seems to be a history of bipolar disorder or unipolar disorder with psychotic features (Gold, 2002).

Incidence. Incidence varies among the three classifications. Maternity blues affect 50 to 70 percent of postpartum women. Postpartum depression affects 10 to 15 percent of women during the first three months postpartum; 25 percent of these women are likely to develop chronic, severe depression (Gold, 2002; Horowitz et al., 2001). Postpartum psychosis affects 1 to 2 per 1000 new mothers (Beck, 1999).

Subjective Data

Current Symptoms. Symptoms may be similar among the three classifications; however, distinct differences are reported by clients. It is important to identify the major problems causing the client to seek help: severe mood swings, hyperactivity, irritability, depression, obsessional thoughts, insomnia, lack of appetite, difficulty with concentration, hallucinations, delusion, inability to care for herself or child, suicidal or homicidal thoughts.

Maternity Blues. Women with maternity blues report weeping, often alternating with periods of elation; irritability; anxiety; headaches; confusion; forgetfulness; depersonalization; disturbances in sleep pattern; and fatigue (Gold, 2002; Newport et al., 2002).

Postpartum Depression. Women with postpartum depression report symptoms similar to those of maternity blues but without periods of elation. In addition, these symptoms are more intense and last longer. The client considers herself a failure as a mother; she looks for reasons for the perceived failure and associates it with real or imagined character weaknesses and questions self-worth. She experiences excessive fatigue and excessive weight gain or weight loss. Thinking and speaking may be slow. Suicide is a serious hazard and the method is often well planned (Beck & Gable, 2001b; Gold, 2002).

Postpartum Psychosis. Women with postpartum psychosis report variable symptoms. Three expressions, or phases, of psychosis are possible: manic phase, delirious state, and psychotic depression.

- Manic phase, with symptoms similar to those of the manic phase of bipolar disorder is characterized by racing thoughts, hyperactivity, and mood swings.
- Delirious state symptoms include confusion, dissociative episodes with confusion, dissociative episodes with hostility, and anxiety.
- Psychotic depression symptoms include suicidal tendencies, desire to harm the infant or others, psychomotor retardation, and prominent delusions that are often related to the infant (Gold, 2002; Newport et al., 2002).

History of Present Illness. Ask the client to describe the onset of symptoms. What symptoms were present during pregnancy or after the infant's birth? When were symptoms more severe or less severe, and how long did they last? Have symptoms caused her to make unexpected changes in lifestyle?

Past Psychiatric Condition. Ask the client if she has a history of depression, bipolar disorder, or other psychiatric illness. Were any of the illnesses related to childbearing? Did she receive any psychotropic medication? Did the medication help?

Medical-Surgical-Obstetrical History. Was the pregnancy planned or unplanned? Were there complications with this pregnancy? Have the client describe her labor and delivery. Does she have a history of medical illness (thyroid disease, other endocrinological problems)? Did the newborn have any serious health problem?

Family History. Does any family member have psychiatric problems (depression, bipolar disorder, schizophrenia, alcoholism or other substance abuse, anorexia nervosa, bulimia)? What type of help was received? Was medication received and what was the response? What was the client's childhood like? Ask her to describe her relationship with parents and her perceptions of their effectiveness as role models. Is there a history of physical or sexual abuse?

Social History. With whom does the client live? Is there someone with whom she can share the responsibility of caring for the child and house? Are there financial problems? Is she planning to work full- or part-time outside the home or full-time in the home? Is her partner emotionally supportive?

Objective Data

Physical Examination. Excessive weight loss or gain is possible. Affect may be flat; speech and thinking processes may be slow; the woman may be weepy, agitated, or irritable. She may exhibit confusion, hostility, or anxiety. The remainder of the physical examination is most likely within normal limits.

Instruments. Several instruments have been developed to identify those women at risk of postpartum depression. The *Edinburgh Postnatal Depression Scale* (EPDS) has ten statements describing depressive symptoms with four possible responses. All the items in the EPDS are similar to those in general depression scales (Beck & Gable, 2001a). Scores range from 0 to 30. A score of 12/13 indicates depression, but not its severity.

The *Postpartum Depression Screening Scale* (PDSS), based on the conceptual definition of postpartum depression, is a 35-item Likert response scale, consisting of seven dimensions, with five items in each dimension (Beck & Gable, 2001a). The woman has a choice of five responses for each question (1 = strongly disagree; 5 = strongly agree). A total score range of 35 to 59 is interpreted as normal adjustment. A total score of 60 to 79 indicates significant symptoms of postpartum depression. A total score of 80 to 175 is a positive screen for major postpartum depression, and the woman should be referred as soon as possible to a mental health team for evaluation (Beck & Gable, 2002). A sample of questions from the *Postpartum Depression Screening Scale*[†] is listed below.

Sleeping/Eating Disturbances	29. I knew I should eat but didn't.
Anxiety/Insecurity	9. I felt really overwhelmed.
Emotional Lability	17. I cried a lot for no reason.
Mental Confusion	25. I had a difficult time making even a simple decision.
Loss of Self	5. I was afraid that I would never be my normal self again.
Guilt/Shame	34. I felt like a failure as a mother.
Suicidal Thoughts	7. I have thought that death seemed like the only way out of this living nightmare.

When compared to the EPDS and the *Beck Depression Inventory-II* (BDI-II), Beck and Gable (2001a) found the PDSS had the highest combination of sensitivity and specificity (.94 and .98 respectively). When identifying women with major or minor postpartum depression, they again found the PDSS had the highest combination of sensitivity and specificity (.91 and .72 respectively).

Differential Medical Diagnoses

Maternity blues, postpartum depression, postpartum psychosis.

Plan

Psychosocial Intervention. During the antepartum period, provide the client with information related to maternal changes, such as mood swings and lifestyle changes, that could occur after birth. Suggestions should include coping strategies related to the birth:

- Get plenty of rest.
- Allow family and friends, if available, to help with household tasks and the care for older children.
- Eat a well-balanced diet that is low in salt and sugar and high in complex carbohydrates, protein, and green leafy vegetables.
- Drink plenty of fluids, especially water, and limit caffeine intake.
- Continue prenatal vitamins.
- Perform light exercise daily.
- Ensure some personal time and adult relationships.
- Avail oneself of support groups and other community resources (see Breastfeeding/Information Support Groups at the end of this chapter).

The simplest and most effective means to prevent postpartum depression would involve the major revision of current medical and insurance policies in the United States. It would involve early and frequent assessments of postpartum women the first 28 days after discharge and six to eight weeks postpartum. MacArthur, Winter, Bick, and Colleagues (2002) randomly assigned 2,064 women in the United Kingdom (UK) to a control group receiving routine postpartum care or an intervention group. The control group received the usual six to seven home visits by a midwife during the first ten to fourteen days after birth (extended to 28 days if needed), occasional general practitioner (GP) home visits, health visitor care after 28 days, and a check-up with a GP at six to eight weeks postpartum. The intervention group received an increase from midwife contact to 28 days, with an additional visit at ten

to twelve weeks' postpartum. In addition, at specific home visits, the midwife used symptom checklists and the *Edinburgh Postnatal Depression Scale* to identify and manage health problems. The findings were that women's mental health meaures were significantly improved in the intervention group (MacArthur et al., 2002) with no difference in the physical health score. Many studies (Beck, 2002) have identified history of postpartum depression, lack of support, and life stress as risk factors for postpartum depression. MacArthur and colleagues (2002) have demonstrated that mental health can be improved by addressing and managing many of these problems.

Medication Interventions. It is imperative that postpartum women be screened and treated for postpartum depression so they can function in their role as mother, providing the love so necessary in an infant's and child's life. Beck analyzed nineteen studies on postpartum depression published between 1983 and 1993. Beck's meta-analysis (1995), found that postpartum depression has a significant effect on mother-infant interaction.

Antidepressants are critical in the treatment of postpartum depression and should be continued for nine to twelve months after remission of symptoms (Gold, 2002). Conditions requiring prompt psychiatric referral include suicidal and/or homicidal ideation, evidence or concern of psychotic symptoms, severe impairment of functional capabilities, avoidance of infant or overconcern of infant's health, failure to respond to therapeutic trial of antidepressants, and comorbid substance abuse (Gold, 2002). Lithium, an antimanic, or carbamazepine, an anticonvulsant, are used to manage manic episodes. Antipsychotic drugs may be prescribed for women with postpartum psychoses who are experiencing hallucinations or other distortions of reality.

Tricyclic Antidepressants. Risks of untreated postpartum depression are significant. In addition to tragedies of suicide and infanticide, depressed mothers display a more negative interaction style with their infants; are less interactive with their infants or are more intrusive in their interaction; and experience more anxiety, panic attacks, and anger (Beck, 1999, 2002; Beck & Gable, 2000; Gold, 2002; Horowitz et al., 2001). Infants of depressed mothers tended to be fussier, made less vocalizations and positive facial expressions (Beck, 1999, 2002; Horowitz et al., 2001; Newport et al., 2002). Children over the age of 1 year were found to have impaired cognitive and emotional development (Beck & Gable, 2000; Beck, 2002; Newport et al., 2002).

Although most authorities agree that the benefits of treating postpartum depression in breastfeeding mothers outweigh any risks (Gold, 2002; Lawrence & Lawrence, 1999; Newport et al., 2002), prudent use of medication during lactation is advisable.

Tricyclic antidepressants are not the first choice in treatment because of their side effects, potential for over-dosing, drug interactions, and the need for monitoring therapeutic serum levels. The effects of tricyclics on the nursing infant are unknown, but may be of concern (AAP, 2001; Briggs, Freeman, & Yaffe, 2002). The treatment of choice is with selective serotonin reuptake inhibitors (SSRIs) (Gold, 2002).

Serotonin Reuptake Inhibitors. Selective serotonin reuptake inhibitors are also indicated to treat depression. They have fewer and less noticeable side effects and a wider margin of safety. Fluoxetine (Prozac) is administered initially, 20 mg in the morning with dosage increased according to response; it may be given in divided doses in the morning and at noon. The dosage should not exceed 80 mg per day. Fluoxetine is not recommended for breast-feeding mothers because of case reports of infant colic and fussiness and because infants receive 5 to 9 percent of maternal dose (Riordan & Auerbach, 2001; Winans, 2001).

Sertraline (Zoloft) administration begins at 50 mg orally daily. As the therapeutic response may take two to four weeks, dosage adjustments can be made after that time frame. The dosage range is 50 to 200 mg daily.

Paroxetine (Paxil) administration begins at 20 mg orally daily. Dosage may be increased in 10 mg increments up to a maximum of 50 mg daily.

Citalopram (Celexa) is not a first choice among the SSRIs for the treatment of depression in lactating women because of possible infant somnolence, weight loss, and decreased breastfeeding (Briggs, Freeman, & Yaffe, 2002). Women taking citalopram, especially in doses greater than 20 mg or in conjunction with other sedative agents, should be cautioned regarding possible toxicity in their infants, evidenced by the previous side effects of somnolence, weight loss, and decreased nursing (Briggs et al., 2002). If citalopram is used, avoiding breastfeeding from four to six hours after taking citalopram will lower infant exposure and not cause adverse effects (Winans, 2001).

Paroxetine, fluoxetine, and citalopram are listed as Category C. Sertraline is the only SSRI listed as Category B (Briggs et al., 2002). Newport and Colleagues (2002) did a detailed study of the pharmacokinetics of excretion and infant serum levels of sertraline and found the maximum calculated infant dose is typically less than 1/400th of the maternal dose.

Nefazodone (Serzone) should be avoided in preterm neonates and infants due to decreased renal and hepatic clearance of these infants (Briggs et al., 2001; Winans, 2002).

Bupropion (Wellbutrin, Zyban) may be appropriate for mothers nursing older infants less frequently, but not for neonates and young infants because of decreased hepatic clearance (Winans, 2001).

If there is concern that the nursing infant is exhibiting side effects to maternal medication, Newport and colleagues (2002) recommend suspending the medication exposure. This can be done by temporarily giving the infant formula. As the majority of SSRIs peak in breast milk in seven to nine hours after maternal dose, Newport and colleagues (2002) alternatively suggest "pumping and dumping" of this peak with the result of a 17 to 20 percent reduction in total infant daily dose (exposure). Until further information regarding formulations of generic and name brand medication is available, name brand medication should be used during pregnancy and lactation (Newport et al., 2002).

- *Side Effects.* Nervousness, anxiety, insomnia, headache, somnolence, tremor, nausea, vomiting, dry mouth, arrhythmias, dyspepsia, weight loss, rash pruritus, urticaria. Selective serotonin uptake inhibitors may prolong the half-life of diazepam. Use with tryptophan can cause agitation, gastrointestinal distress, and restlessness. Avoid use with tricyclic antidepressants because of the increased adverse effects on the central nervous system. Interaction with warfarin or other highly protein-bound drugs can increase serum level. Advise the client of the two- to four-week lag before clinical improvement of depression.
- *Contraindications.* Hypersensitivity to any of the selective serotonin reuptake inhibitors. In addition, the drug should not be used within fourteen days of cessation of MAO inhibitors. Cimetidine may increase the plasma concentration of paroxetine.
- *Anticipated Outcome on Evaluation.* Remission of symptoms of depression.
- *Client Teaching.* Include information about side effects.

Tetracyclic. Mirtazapine (Remeron) is an antidepressant chemically unrelated to the SSRIs, tricyclics, and MAOs.

It is an antagonist of 5-Ht2 and 5-Ht3 receptors, as well as H1 receptors.

It is a Category C drug for pregnancy, and it is unknown if mirtazapine is excreted in breast milk.

- *Administration.* 15 mg at bedtime, adjustments to dosing should not be made before one to two weeks of therapy. Usual dosage range is 15 to 45 mg daily.
- *Side Effects.* Somnalence, increased appetite and weight gain, dry mouth, constipation, dizziness. It can cause agranulocytosis and can cause an additive effect if taken with alcohol and CNS depressants. It should be used with caution in clients with kidney and liver impairment or a history of seizures, or if antihypertensives are used.
- *Contraindications.* Concomitant use of MAO inhibitors, alcohol, diazepam, or other CNS depressants.
- *Anticipated Outcome on Evaluation.* Abatement of depression.
- *Client Teaching.* Include information concerning side effects and contraindications.

Lithium. Lithium is indicated if antidepressant treatment precipitates a manic episode, with symptoms of racing thoughts, hyperactivity, pressured speech, increased energy, and impulsive behavior (Gold, 2002). Discontinue use of antidepressant if manic episodes occur, and begin lithium. Long-term use of lithium can induce goiter and has been associated with degenerative renal changes. Therefore, baseline thyroid function tests (T_3, T_4, thyroid stimulating hormone) and renal function tests (BUN, creatinine) should be obtained as a baseline. Thyroid stimulating hormone and renal function tests should then be done every six months. Lithium is a Category D drug for use during pregnancy, and the American Academy of Pediatrics considers lithium to be contraindicated during breastfeeding because of the potential for lithium induced toxicity in the breastfeeding infant (Briggs et al., 2002).

- *Administration.* Therapeutic range: 0.6 to 1.2 mEq/L; higher levels can produce toxicity (nausea, vomiting, diarrhea, shakiness) and extremely high levels can produce death. Subtherapeutic levels do not provide an adequate clinical response (*Nurse Practitioner's Drug Book* 2002); Serum values should be drawn eight to twelve hours after the first dose (usually before the morning dose), then weekly to monthly. Lithium is the drug of choice for clients with postpartum psychosis with manic features.
- *Side Effects.* Nausea, vomiting, diarrhea, thirst, polyuria, lethargy, slurred speech, muscle weakness,

fine hand tremor. When administered above the therapeutic range, lithium may cause headache, persistent gastrointestinal upset, confusion, hyperirritability, drowsiness, dizziness, tremors, ataxia, dry mouth, hypotension, rash, and pruritus.

- *Contraindications.* Hepatic disease, renal disease, pregnancy, lactation, severe cardiac disease and if therapy can't be monitored closely.
- *Anticipated Outcome on Evaluation.* The abatement of manic symptoms.
- *Client Teaching.* Include information related to side effects.

Antipsychotic Drugs. Antipsychotic drugs such as trifluoperazine (Stelazine), haloperidol (Haldol), and thioridazine (Mellaril) are also prescribed. See the current *Physicians' Desk Reference* (PDR) or a pharmacotherapeutic resource for detailed information. Psychiatric referral is mandatory.

Hospitalization. Because 5 percent of women with postpartum psychosis commit suicide and 4 percent commit infanticide, postpartum psychosis is a true psychiatric emergency warranting hospital admission (Gold, 2002; Newport et al., 2002).

Follow-Up

Postpartum depression poses serious sequelae for mother, infant, and family during the first postnatal year. Depressed mothers may not pick up on their infants' cues, thus failing to meet their infants' needs (Beck & Gable, 2001b).

Use of appropriate medication to alter mother's mood and enhance her sensitivity to her infant's cues will help strengthen the bond between the mother-infant dyad. Home visits, telephone calls, and psychiatric referral may be part of follow-up care.

Consider telephone calls three days after hospital discharge and a home visit seven days after discharge to assess the client's adaptation to motherhood and family responsibilities. If she is adapting well, repeat contact after another seven to ten days. On the other hand, if she is experiencing difficulty, refer her to appropriate agencies or support groups (see Breastfeeding Information/Support Groups at the end of this chapter).

- Cognitive and supportive therapies help identify and correct distorted perceptions of reality and encourage the partner or other family member(s) to assist with household and child care tasks.

◆ Concurrent marital therapy, in conjoint sessions, is especially helpful if the partner exhibits narcissistic behavior or is a substance abuser.

◆ Support groups (group therapy) complement individual therapy. They help decrease the sense of isolation.

PERINATAL LOSS

Perinatal loss involves perinatal mortality, both stillbirth and neonatal death (Cunningham et al., 2001g). A perinatal loss may also involve a perceived loss, including loss of expectation or giving one's infant up for adoption.

Stillbirth or neonatal death (death within the first 30 days of life) is obviously a loss for the mother and the family. Less obvious may be the loss felt by a woman who miscarries or elects to terminate a pregnancy. All of these losses are irrevocable.

Loss of expectation is also a real loss for some women and their families. It may be experienced in the birth of a viable infant who is premature or has congenital anomalies or deformities. Loss of expectation may also be experienced when the birthing act causes losses that precipitate maternity blues even though the infant is healthy. For example, postpartum fatigue may make daily tasks difficult to perform and contribute to postpartum blues or depression.

The woman or couple who gives up an infant for adoption experience loss, especially if they bonded with the infant before birth. Giving up the infant does not eliminate these bonds (Kennell & Klaus, 1998; Rubin, 1984).

Epidemiology

In 2001 the United States ranked 17th among other nations in infant mortality, with a rate of 10.4 per 1000 live births. Despite a decline in infant mortality to 7.0 per 1000 live births in 1999, the United States slipped to 27th place among world nations in 1997 (Brunner, 2001). Low birthweight infants are five to ten times more likely to die during their first year of life than infants of normal weight. The infant mortality rate for African Americans (14.3 per 1000 live births) remains at twice that of white infants (7.2 per 1000 live births) (U.S. Bureau of the Census, 2001).

Out of 4.0 million babies born alive in the United States, 30,000 die during the first 28 days of life from genetic disease and congenital malformations; they constitute 20 percent of total neonatal deaths (Cunningham et al., 2001c). Approximately 35 percent of stillbirths have a congenital defect (Cunningham et al., 2001c). Miscarriages occur in approximately 12–26 percent of clinically recognized pregnancies, with 80% occurring in the first 12 weeks. Approximately 50 percent of these are caused by chromosomal anomalies (Cunningham et al., 2001a).

Subjective Data

A client may report sadness, loss of appetite, inability to sleep, increased irritability or hostility toward others, preoccupation with the lost infant, inability to return to normal activities, and somatic distress (Kennell & Klaus, 1998; Kennell, Slyter, & Klaus, 1970). The client may also have feelings of guilt and preoccupation with her negligence or minor omissions (Kennell & Klaus, 1998; Kennell, Slyter, & Klaus, 1970; Rubin, 1984).

Objective Data

Data are determined concerning the client and her family's grieving by means of observation and counseling. The primary health care provider can then help them cope with their loss. If the health care provider is to assist the family through its grieving process, he or she must realize mothers and fathers grieve differently. Mothers express more grief and grieve longer than do fathers (Rillstone & Hutchinson, 2001). This difference in grieving may also lead to sexual problems. The father may desire sexual activity because he perceives coitus as a way to share and comfort as well as be comforted (Wallerstedt & Higgins, 1996). The mother may perceive this desire as callousness.

Phases of Mourning. Progression through the five stages of mourning varies among individuals and regression may occur (Williams, 2000). Perinatal grieving involves acute grief, which is most intense during the four- to six-week period following loss and less intense in the subsequent four weeks. The normal grief reaction may last from six months to two years or may never resolve. The anniversary of the loss may reactivate grief reactions.

◆ The shock and numbness stage (denial) is expressed as impaired normal functioning. The individual has difficulty making decisions and may be aloof.

◆ Searching and yearning (anger) constitute the second stage of mourning. Anger and bitterness can be transferred to other people, especially health care professionals. Restlessness and guilt feelings may also be experienced.

◆ Bargaining, which is usually a brief phase, attempts to delay loss.

◆ Disorganization (depression) is the phase when the reality of the loss occurs. Depression may occur as the full impact of loss is felt. Guilt feelings remain.

◆ Resolution may be seen as the individual begins to function better at home and at work. Self-confidence increases. The individual is able to place the loss in perspective with life (Limbo & Wheeler, 1986a; Szgalsky, 1989).

Parental Tasks. Following perinatal loss, parents must work through the loss and make it real. The parents must allow the normal grief reaction to progress. During this time, parents should meet their own needs as well as those of their other children and communicate their feelings to the children.

Multiple Gestation. Parents who experienced a multiple gestation may have an additional or more acute sense of loss from conflicting emotions. Parents need to grieve their deceased infant(s) before relating to the survivor(s). Parents may experience grief from loss of prestige as parents of twins. In addition, they may have a sense of inadequacy, as the death of one child may be perceived as the inability to raise more than one child.

Plan

Psychosocial Interventions. Measures are directed toward helping parents work through loss and make it real. Their coping abilities are assessed and, if indicated, the parents are referred to support groups for counseling.

◆ Telephone parents (especially important on what had been due date or on the anniversary of death) to reevaluate coping and readjustment. Call during the evening to involve the partner. Provide parents with the phone number of the hospital's maternity floor.

◆ Advise parents to join support groups (see Parental/Family Support Groups and Perinatal Loss Support Groups at the end of this chapter).

◆ Provide anticipatory guidance, counseling parents about the normalcy of grief, its stages, and the varying duration. Warn parents of an emotional roller coaster of "good" days and "bad" days—days when a sight, smell, or sound may bring back a flood of memories and tears. Most difficult time is two to four months after death (acute grief).

◆ Prepare parents to deal with reactions of others, especially well-meaning but insensitive comments.

◆ Advise couple that it is not uncommon for sexual intimacy to be compromised by avoidance, depression, or disinterest for up to two years after the death of a child (Wallerstedt & Higgins, 1996).

◆ Facilitate communication and expression of grief with such open ended statements as "Some fathers have said . . . . Tell me how you feel."

◆ Ask the father how he's doing—avoid expressing concern for just the mother.

◆ Recommend postponing pregnancy until both parents have worked through their grief.

◆ Provide suggestions for dealing with grief.

• Communicate with partner, family, and friends; talk about the infant or child who died.

• Eat a well-balanced diet and drink adequate fluids; avoid caffeine and alcoholic beverages.

• Exercise daily.

• Avoid tobacco as it depletes the body of vitamins, increases stomach acidity, decreases circulation, and can cause palpitations.

• Rest daily; rest at night even if unable to sleep.

• Clarify values; don't be persuaded to act or think as you think you should behave. Ignore "shoulds" (e.g., "I should be strong and not cry").

• Ease marital stress. Realize that no two people grieve the same way. Take the time to share thoughts and feelings each day and listen to what your partner is saying. Express affection for each other and other family members throughout the day.

• Recognize and respect the need for solitary time.

• Keep mementos of the baby. Some hospitals provide a picture, lock of hair, or ID bracelet.

• Read books, poems, and articles that comfort; avoid "scare" literature and technical medical bulletins.

• Keep a diary or journal of thoughts, memories, and mementos.

• Write poems or letters to the infant.

• Avoid making big decisions or changes for twenty-four months, and do not let others make decisions for you; put away baby clothes and articles when you are ready.

• Accept help from others; request help from clergy if desired (Limbo & Wheeler 1986b; Rillstone & Hutchinson, 2001; Staudacher, 1987; Williams, 2000; Workman, 2001).

Medication. Medication is not indicated.

Follow-Up

Follow-up involves continuing observation for resolution of grief. Grief is completed when an individual is able to turn outward and think of others and to formulate plans for the future. Give couple a list of resources they can turn to when they are ready. (See Resources at end of this chapter.) If grief remains unresolved, refer parents to a skilled professional counselor. Unresolved grief may be observed in several behaviors:

- Persistent yearning for recovery of lost objects.
- Overidentification with the deceased.
- Inability to cry or rage despite desire to do so.
- Misdirected anger or ambivalence toward infant.
- Lack of support group/person.
- Presence of secondary gain, e.g., increased attention to mother.

BREASTFEEDING

In 1984, 25 percent of U.S. women breastfed for six months; in 1987, the number of women breastfeeding infants at six months dropped to 21 percent, to 19.7 percent in 1992, and rose to 21.7 percent in 1996. Lawrence and Lawrence (1999) stated that in Third World countries and in acute poverty-stricken areas in the United States, an infant who is bottle fed has a greater morbidity and mortality risk within the first year than an infant who is breastfed (Lawrence & Lawrence, 1999; Smith & Tulley, 2001). Despite the increased safety of commercial infant formulas, breastfeeding has distinct advantages for both mother and infant and almost no contraindications. Human milk is physiologically compatible with the human infant's digestive tract and provides the exact balance of nutrients, electrolytes, and immunological factors necessary for optimal growth and development. Even the act of suckling employs the use of different muscles and feeding mechanism than bottle feeding (Lawrence & Lawrence, 1999). Breastfeeding is more convenient for the mother, nothing to heat or spoil, no extra bottles to transport. An emotional bond develops between mother and nursing infant that does not occur when an infant is bottle fed (Lawrence & Lawrence, 1999).

Recent research findings indicate that breastfeeding may also lower the risk for breast cancer (Beral, 2002; "Breastfeeding cuts," 2001; Labbock, 2001). The relative risk of breast cancer is decreased by almost 5 percent for every twelve months of breastfeeding in addition to a 7 percent decrease for each birth (Beral, 2002). If women breastfed for twenty-four months, there would be a two-thirds reduction in breast cancer by age 70 (from an incidence of 6.3 to 2.7 per 100 women) in developed countries (Beral, 2002).

A mother who is breastfeeding for the first time may not have the support of family and friends and needs encouragement, support, and accurate information to become self-assured about breastfeeding. Teaching should ideally begin during the pregnancy. The health care provider should help the first-time breastfeeding mother and her infant to successfully breastfeed.

TYPES OF BREASTFEEDING

Unrestricted Breastfeeding

The infant is put to breast immediately after delivery and then on demand. Breast milk is the major source of nourishment for the first year of life or longer.

The advantages of this type of breastfeeding are that less illness occurs during first year of life (Lawrence & Lawrence, 1999; Smith & Tully, 2001), the infant has mouth-nipple contact and body contact, and the breast is associated with comfort as well as food. The disadvantage is that breastfeeding requires the mother's dedication.

Token Breastfeeding

Restrictions are placed on the duration of breastfeeding and the length of each time at the breast; feedings are scheduled. The mother may pump her breasts and store the milk for others to give (e.g., daycare providers). Weaning occurs by the third month or earlier.

The advantage is that other family members can participate in feeding the infant. The disadvantages are that the milk supply may decrease, the infant is more susceptible to illnesses, and the infant learns bottle-sucking techniques, which may lead to nipple confusion.

BREAST ANATOMY

Breast tissue comprises glands, supporting connective tissue, and fatty tissue. The primary structures are skin, subcutaneous tissue, and the corpus mammae.

The skin includes the nipple, areola, and general skin. Each nipple contains fifteen to twenty-five milk ducts; each of the tubuloalveolar glands opens separately onto the nipple. The nipple also contains smooth muscle fibers, sensory nerve endings, and sebaceous and apocrine glands. Nipple erection is caused by tactile, sensory, or autonomic sympathetic stimuli. Montgomery's tubercles contain the ductular openings of sebaceous and lactiferous glands. They secrete a substance that protects and lubricates the nipple and areola during pregnancy and lactation.

Subcutaneous tissue lies just below the dermis.

The corpus mammae is divided into the parenchyma and stroma. Parenchyma includes the ductular-lobular-alveolar structures. The lactiferous ductal system connects the alveoli to the nipple. Fifteen to twenty tubuloalveolar glands are embedded in fat (Lawrence & Lawrence, 1999). They open into lactiferous ducts, which open into lactiferous sinuses, which, in turn, open onto the nipple. The stroma comprises connective tissue, fat, blood vessels, nerves, and lymphatics.

PHYSIOLOGY OF LACTATION

Lactation is hormonally controlled. The physiological changes that occur are directed toward mammogenesis, lactogenesis (milk secretion), and galactopoiesis (milk maintenance). Most milk is synthesized in the acini and smaller milk ducts during suckling (Lawrence & Lawrence, 1999).

Mammogenesis

Mammogenesis is the development of the mammary glands to their functional state.

Estrogen stimulates parenchymal proliferation and ductal growth. Luteal and placental hormones increase ductular and lobular formation; placental lactogen, prolactin, and chorionic gonadotropin accelerate mammary growth (Lawrence & Lawrence, 1999). Prolactin (from the anterior pituitary gland) stimulates glandular production of colostrum; human placental lactogen stimulates secretion of colostrum by the second trimester (Lawrence & Lawrence, 1999); and progesterone stimulates lobular growth.

Lactogenesis

Milk production by the mammary glands proceeds in two stages.

Stage I of lactogenesis begins twelve weeks before parturition and is preceded by significant increases in lactose, total proteins, and immunoglobulins and decreases in sodium and chloride (Lawrence & Lawrence, 1999). Stage II clinically begins on days 2 and 3 postpartum with copious milk secretion; mature milk is established in approximately ten days (Lawrence & Lawrence, 1999).

Galactopoiesis

Prolactin stimulates and sustains lactation (milk secretion); oxytocin stimulates milk ejection. An intact hypothalamic-pituitary axis regulates prolactin and oxytocin levels and is essential for the maintenance of milk secretion. Ejection reflex is dependent on receptors in the canalicular system of the breast. Dilation or stretching of the canalicules causes a reflex release of oxytocin. Tactile receptors for both oxytocin and reflex prolactin release are located in the nipple (Lawrence & Lawrence, 1999).

Prolactin secretion is controlled by prolactin inhibitory factor (PIF) produced by the hypothalamus. Suppression of PIF allows the anterior pituitary gland to secrete uninhibited amounts of prolactin. Catecholamine levels in the hypothalamus control PIF. Drugs and events that decrease catecholamines also decrease PIF, thereby causing an increase in prolactin (Lawrence & Lawrence, 1999). Among nonnursing mothers, prolactin levels drop to normal in two to three weeks, independent of lactation suppression therapy.

Composition of Human Milk

Milk varies with the stage of lactation, time of day, sampling time during a given feeding, maternal nutrition, and the individual. Initially, colostrum is produced. A transitional phase in production leads to secretion of mature milk.

Colostrum. A yellowish, thick fluid produced during the first postpartum week. It contains higher concentrations of sodium, potassium, and chloride than mature milk. Protein, fat-soluble vitamins, and minerals are also in larger concentration than in transitional or mature milk. This high-protein, low-fat milk meets the needs and reserves of the newborn (Lawrence & Lawrence, 1999). The mean energy value is 67 kcal/100 mL of mature milk. Colostrum facilitates the establishment of bifidus flora in the digestive tract and the passage of meconium. It contains abundant antibodies.

Transitional Milk. Secreted beginning seven to ten days postpartum and continuing until two weeks postpartum. The concentration of immunoglobulins decreases, although lactose, fat, and total caloric content increase. Water-soluble vitamins increase and fat-soluble vitamins decrease to approach the level found in mature milk (Lawrence & Lawrence, 1999).

Mature Milk. The only necessary source of nutrition for an infant's first four to six months of life and should be the primary source for the first year (Lawrence & Lawrence, 1999; Mohrbacher & Stock, 1997; Smith & Tully, 2001).

◆ Water is the major constituent. A lactating woman requires an increased water intake. If water intake is decreased, sensible and insensible water loss are decreased before water for lactation is decreased.

◆ Lipids, the second most plentiful constituent, and the most variable, provides the major portion of kilocalories. It is almost completely digestible.

◆ Proteins constitute 0.9 percent of human milk content (Lawrence & Lawrence, 1999).

◆ The predominant carbohydrate is lactose. Synthesized by the mammary gland, it is specific for newborn growth and enhances calcium absorption. Lactose appears to be critical for the prevention of rickets, as human milk is relatively low in calcium.

◆ Minerals essential to the newborn are potassium and iron.

• Potassium levels are higher than sodium in breast milk (similar to intracellular fluids). Sodium levels in cow's milk are 3.6 times greater than those in human milk (Lawrence & Lawrence, 1999).

• The concentration of exogenous elemental iron in human milk is 100 mcg/1100 mL (Lawrence & Lawrence, 1999). Normal infants need 8 to 10 mg per day in the first year of life. Prepared formulas provide 10 to 12 mg per day; infants breastfed for the first six months are not at increased risk for iron-deficiency anemia or depletion of iron stores (Griffin & Abrams, 2001; Lawrence & Lawrence, 1999; Smith & Tully, 2001). Although its concentration in human milk is low, iron is absorbed more readily than iron from other sources. Thus, infants are not at risk for iron-deficiency anemia or depletion of iron stores if they are breastfed totally during the first six months of life.

• An adequate supply of vitamins A, E, and C is present in breast milk. The amount of vitamin A in mature human milk is 280 IU and in cow's milk, 180 IU; an infant consuming 200 mL of breast milk every day obtains an adequate amount of vitamin A.

• Serum levels of vitamin E in breastfed babies rise quickly at birth and are maintained by approximately four weeks postpartum with only breast milk intake (Lawrence & Lawrence, 1999).

• Vitamin C and other water-soluble vitamins in human milk reflect maternal dietary intake (Lawrence & Lawrence, 1999). Human milk is an excellent source of these water-soluble vitamins (Lawrence & Lawrence, 1999).

Resistance Factors and Immunological Significance

Breastfeeding significantly decreases infant morbidity and mortality by protecting against enteropathogens that may contaminate other food or formula. The protective factors contained in breast milk are both cellular and humoral (Lawrence & Lawrence, 1999).

Cellular factors include macrophages, polymorphonuclear leukocytes, and lymphocytes. These cells are phagocytes and they stimulate antibody formation. The humoral factors are immunoglobulins.

◆ Immunoglobulin A (IgA) is the most important immunoglobulin in terms of biological activity, and it is the most concentrated. IgA also has antitoxin activity against *Escherichia coli* and *Vibrio cholerae* and thereby prevents diarrhea (Lawrence & Lawrence, 1999).

◆ Bifidus factor is responsible for the growth of *Bifidobacterium bifidum*, the predominant bacteria in the gut of breastfed infants. The flora of bifid bacteria inhibits pathogenic *Staphylococcus aureus, Shigella*, and *Protozoa* and encourages growth of *Lactobacillus bifidus*, which crowds out other bacteria. Lysozyme and lactoferrin act directly to inhibit pathogen growth. The resistance factor protects against *Staphylococcus* infection (Lawrence & Lawrence, 1999).

◆ Breast milk contains antibodies against poliovirus, coxsackievirus, echovirus, influenza virus, and rhinovirus and thus helps to prevent viral infections (AWHONN, 2000a; Lawrence & Lawrence, 1999).

◆ Breast milk protects against the development of allergies. An infant begins to produce antibodies to cow's milk (which is the basis of formula) within eighteen days of ingestion. Syndromes associated with cow's milk allergy include gastric enteropathy, atopic dermatitis, rhinitis, chronic pulmonary disease, eosinophilia, and failure to thrive (Lawrence & Lawrence, 1999).

CONTRAINDICATIONS

Breast Cancer

Controversy regarding the role of prolactin in the progression of mammary cancer may be a reason to contraindicate breastfeeding for pregnant women (Lawrence & Lawrence, 1999).

Hepatitis B Virus

Breastfeeding permitted in protected infants—rapid schedule of immunization (0, 1, and 2 months) of infant would be indicated. Milk donors are screened for this virus (Lawrence & Lawrence, 1999; Mohrbacher & Stock, 1997; Smith & Tully, 2001).

Cytomegalovirus

Breast milk also contains appropriate antibodies that protect the infant against cytomegalovirus. There does exist a risk for the infant who is exposed to virus but not a daily dose of antibodies, and risk for severe infection is especially great in premature infant of nonimmune mother (Lawrence & Lawrence, 1999).

Human Immunodeficiency Virus

For women in the United States who test positive for HIV, breastfeeding is contraindicated (Lawrence & Lawrence, 1999; Smith & Tully, 2001). Breastfeeding, however, remains the feeding method of choice in countries where the death rate in the first year of life is 50 percent, compared with the 18 percent risk of dying from AIDS when born to an infected mother (Lawrence & Lawrence, 1999; Smith & Tully, 2001).

Augmentation or Reduction Mammoplasty

If milk ducts were cut during mammoplasty, breastfeeding may not be possible (Lawrence & Lawrence, 1999). Incisions around the areola usually indicate that some milk ducts were cut and possible nerve damage occurred.

In women who have had implants, the ability to lactate depends on the location of the scars (Chez & Friedmann, 2000; Smith & Tully, 2001). Periareolar incisions are more apt to disrupt the ducts and the neurological innervation of the nipple. Intact innervation is necessary for the milk ejection reflex. If the periareolar incision is completely circumferential, there will be some patent ducts that will be able to secrete milk to the nipple. Where the ducts have been cut, the breast will be engorged because the milk will not be able to be secreted, and the gland will eventually undergo involution (Chez & Friedmann, 2000; Smith & Tully, 2001).

Pierced nipples are not a contraindication to breastfeeding, but jewelry should be removed before putting the baby to breast.

Active Tuberculosis

Breastfeeding is permitted if the mother's skin test is positive, and if at the same time there is no radiologic indication of disease and the client has started antituberculin medication. If the mother has a positive tuberculin skin test and positive chest film, she may breastfeed if she is taking antituberculous medication and the sputum culture is negative (Lawrence & Lawrence, 1999). The American Academy of Pediatrics considers INH, rifampin, ethambutal, and streptomycin compatible with breastfeeding (Briggs et al., 2002). If the sputum culture is positive, breastfeeding may be possible after the mother has taken medication for at least one week. Limited isolation from the mother with active disease may be required. The breastfeeding infant may be treated prophylactically by the pediatrician.

ELEMENTS OF BREASTFEEDING

Compression of Lactiferous Sinuses

Externally, the infant's mouth should cover the lactiferous sinuses, whereas internally, the correct movement of the infant's tongue provides areolar compression between the infant's tongue and palate. The lactiferous sinuses lie underneath the areola; compression of the lactiferous sinuses removes milk from the breast. Sucking may need to continue for two minutes for the full response to oxytocin release.

Number of Feedings per Day

A minimum of eight feedings are necessary in 24 hours, with each feeding providing a minimum of five to ten minutes of swallowing at each breast. The milk ejection reflex takes two to three minutes before it is effective (Lawrence & Lawrence, 1999); limiting nursing to two to three minutes does not permit the infant to obtain milk. Suck efficiency is critical to breastfeeding success.

Signs that an infant is doing well with breastfeeding include the following:

- Three or more stools every 24 hours, with meconium changing to breast milk stools by day 4.
- Six or more wet diapers every day by day 4.
- Infant is content between feedings.
- Infant awakens easily for feedings about every three hours.
- Breasts soften or feel lighter as the baby feeds.
- Nipples are healthy, not cracked or bleeding.
- Breast changes signaling lactogenesis stage II around 72 hours.

◆ Mother experiences signs of oxytocin and prolactin release—she feels drowsy, gets thirsty, and has uterine contractions/increased flow of lochia while baby is breastfeeding (Smith & Tully, 2001).

Assessment of Infant at Breast

Assessment of a breastfeeding session requires direct observation. Observe positioning and alignment, areolar grasp, sucking, mother-infant interaction, and maternal perception of infant satiety.

Positioning and Alignment. The infant should be relaxed, in a responsive state, and displaying early hunger cues—rooting and hand-to-mouth activity. Crying is a late hunger cue.

The infant's body should be flexed with the head and trunk aligned so that the head is straight on the breast, not turned laterally or hyperextended (head and body are at breast level). The infant should be brought to the breast, not the breast to the infant. Proper alignment decreases traction on the mother's nipples; the areola and nipple are more easily kept in the infant's mouth; swallowing is facilitated.

The mother's hand should cup her breast, with her fingers supporting the lower portion of the breast and her thumb resting on the upper portion. The infant should be permitted to grasp at least one-half inch of areolar tissue. This position is the "C-hold," and permits the mother to support her breast without distorting the nipple.

Areolar Grasp. The infant must have a correct mouth opening, correct lip flanging, and correct tongue placement. To elicit the grasp gently, tickle the infant's lips with the nipple to stimulate the mouth to open. When the mouth is opened wide, quickly pull the infant close to the breast and center the nipple in infant's mouth. Move the infant's head and trunk as a unit to avoid hyperflexion, hyperextension, or lateral turning of the head. Avoid holding the back of the infant's head to maneuver it onto the breast, because it does not allow the mother to feel rapid arm motion and erodes her confidence if the infant latches on. Placing a hand on the mother's arm and moving it quickly toward her breast allows the mother to feel the quick arm movement.

Breastfeeding Problems. May be determined during systematic assessment of the infant at the breast.

◆ Problems with grasping the areola may be caused by "prissily pursued" lips. The infant appears to be drinking through a straw. Only the nipple is grasped, and the mother often experiences nipple pain. The infant receives little milk because the lactiferous sinuses are not compressed. Break the suction by inserting a finger into the corner of infant's mouth and stimulate the mouth to open wide. Alternate sucking of the nipple and the areola through pursed lips will traumatize the nipple and the suck will become inefficient. Friction may abrade the mother's areolar tissue and result in ineffective sucking.

◆ Another grasping problem is negative pressure in an infant's intraoral cavity, which results in retention of the nipple and areolar tissue in the infant's mouth. This counteracts the naturally retractile nature of nipple tissue, helps to refill the lactiferous sinuses with milk from the lactiferous ducts, and conveys milk to the oropharynx. Negative pressure is achieved when an infant forms an effective seal with the border of his or her mouth.

◆ Sore nipples cause discomfort, and breastfeeding should not hurt. If the mother has sore, cracked nipples, the cause must be found: Review positioning and latch-on of the infant. A variety of measures may be tried to relieve sore nipples.

• Rule out problems such as monilia. The mother may complain of severe nipple itching or a severe pain when infant nurses. The infant may or may not show signs of thrush. The mother and infant should be treated simultaneously, the mother with Nystatin cream or Mycolog cream rubbed into the nipple after each feeding and the infant with oral Nystatin (Lawrence & Lawrence, 1999). When recurrent candidiasis is not responding to Nystatin, Lawrence and Lawrence (1999) recommend oral fluconazole (Diflucan), with a loading dose of 200 mg, then 100 mg daily for fourteen days. Although fluconazole passes through breast milk, it has a safety profile for newborns and is approved for use at 6 months of age (Lawrence & Lawrence, 1999). Lawrence and Lawrence (1999) recommend the infant be kept on Nystatin to avoid relapse and either pasteurizing or discarding breast milk of women with candida because freezing does not kill the fungus.

• Some milk may be expressed before feeding to stimulate the milk ejection reflex, thus allowing for softening of the areola before the infant latches on.

• Some milk may be expressed onto the nipples after feedings and allowed to air dry.

• The flaps of the nursing bra may be left open after feedings.

- Nursing pads with plastic liners should be avoided. Nipple shields also compound the problem by increasing nipple irritation and confusing the baby so that the baby sucks improperly and further irritates the nipple.
- Change the baby's position
- If artificial nipples (pacifiers, bottles, nipple shields) have been used, discontinue them.

Sucking. Correct sucking requires that the infant's tongue cover the mandibular-alveolar ridge on the lower gum line and curve beneath the areolar tissue.

Evaluate tongue placement by gently pulling infant's lower lip downward. Incorrect tongue placement is indicated by clicking or smacking sounds and drawing in of cheek pads with each suck, or by the loss of large amounts of milk over the infant's chin (Mohrbacher & Stock, 1997). A short tongue or one with a short lingual frenulum may not extend over the lower alveolar ridge.

Evaluate areolar compression by carefully noting the type of sucking and swallowing. A sustained slower mandibular motion indicates nutritive sucking; rapid mandibular motion indicates nonnutritive sucking. Audible swallowing is the most reliable indicator of milk intake. Documentation of an infant's breastfeeding should state: "Breastfed with audible swallowing at each breast."

Breastfeeding Positions

Whichever position (four are listed below) the mother uses to nurse her infant, she should be comfortable. Pillows should be used to help support her arm and help her hold the baby close to her breast, relaxed and without muscle strain.

- *Cradle Hold.* The mother sits up, the infant faces her, and the infant's head or arm rests on the mother's forearm or in the crook of her arm. The cradle hold is a good choice for a mother whose infant has low muscle tone; for example, an infant with Down syndrome.
- *Football Hold.* The mother sits up, the infant's head faces her breast, and the body is tucked under her arm at her side. The baby's bottom should be resting on a pillow near the mother's elbow to provide additional support for the mother and avoid muscle strain. The football hold is a good choice for a mother who recently had abdominal surgery, as the position does not put pressure on the incision.
- *Side-Lying Position.* Both the mother and infant lie on their sides, facing each other, with the infant's feet pulled in close to his or her body. Pillows under the

mother's head, behind her back, and under the knee or her upper leg may provide comfort. This position is more restful for mothers and has been found to significantly reduce fatigue among new breastfeeding mothers.
- *Slide-Over Position.* This position is especially useful with infants who refuse one breast. The mother can begin nursing the infant on the preferred side, then slide the infant over to the less preferred side once the milk ejection reflex has occurred. The infant's body position is not changed; he or she merely "slides over."

Breast Preparation

To prepare breasts for feeding, first assess them by palpating the tissue and inspecting the nipples and areolae; then teach the mother proper care of the breasts.

Palpate to detect inelastic breast tissue. Skin that is taut and firm and difficult to pick up is more prone to engorgement. Tissue can be improved by measures to prevent engorgement. (Lawrence & Lawrence, 1999).

Assess the nipples and areolae by gently compressing each areola between the thumb and forefinger. The normal nipple everts with gentle pressure; the inverted or tied nipple inverts more with gentle pressure (Lawrence & Lawrence 1999). Exercises to evert the nipple are rarely successful and can lead to premature labor (Lawrence & Lawrence 1999).

Stress the importance of avoiding soap and other drying agents on the nipples. Teach the mother to wash breasts with water only. (Lawrence & Lawrence, 1999; Mohrbacher & Stock, 1997). Routine use of ointments and creams is discouraged, as some have irritants, such as lanolin (Lawrence & Lawrence, 1999; Mohrbacher & Stock, 1997). Vitamin E or hormone creams or ointments are unsafe on the nipples unless prescribed for a specific problem, and they then should be used only in minute amounts (Lawrence & Lawrence, 1999; Mohrbacher & Stock, 1997). Sebaceous glands and tubercles of Montgomery are easily plugged by repeated application of oily substances.

Extrinsic Factors Contributing to Breastfeeding Problems

Separation at any time, delayed feedings, and introduction of bottle feedings interfere with breastfeeding.

Separation of mother and infant interferes with milk ejection reflex; the infant is not able to nurse on demand, causing a delay that contributes to milk stasis and engorgement. If, in the mother's absence, the infant learns to suck on a bottle, then sucking at the breast becomes incorrect, causing pain and trauma.

Delaying first feedings to a healthy infant—an infant is most receptive to nursing in the first 90 minutes after birth—can erode the mother's self-confidence when a sleepy infant is later brought to her to feed. Delay can also decrease the milk ejection reflex.

Limiting the frequency and duration of feedings contributes to breastfeeding problems. The milk ejection reflex occurs two to three minutes after sucking is initiated. (Lawrence & Lawrence, 1999). Limiting nursing interferes with the reflex and the infant's milk supply. The limited feedings contribute to milk stasis and engorgement and sore nipples.

Introducing bottles to an infant interferes with the milk ejection reflex by suggesting to the mother that her milk is insufficient. Bottles cause the infant to become confused as sucking at the breast differs from sucking on a commercial nipple or pacifier. An infant may reject the breast or, on the other hand, suckle frequently and for prolonged periods to be satisfied.

Breastfeeding Infants in Multiple Births

The advantages of breastfeeding infants in a multiple birth are similar to those of breastfeeding a single child: Breastfeeding provides a perfect food that is easily digested and provides immunities; the milk is easily accessible; financial savings are substantial; and a special relationship is promoted between mother and infants. A disadvantage may be that the mother finds breastfeeding multiple infants exhausting. The mother may find a support group helpful (see Support Groups and Resources).

The amount of milk produced is influenced by the size of the infants and the number of breastfeeding sessions. The mother should begin breastfeeding at the earliest possible time. An electric piston-type pump (Medela or Ameda/Egnel) may be needed if infants are unable to suckle. Optimal milk production with minimum pumping will most likely involve five pumping sessions per day, at least ten to fifteen minutes per breast. A minimum total of 100 minutes pumping over 24 hours is recommended; short, frequent sessions to express milk are more effective and stimulate more milk production than longer sessions with longer intervals. (Lawrence & Lawrence, 1999). It is not necessary for the mother to waken at night and pump (Lawrence & Lawrence, 1999).

If only one infant can feed and the other is hospitalized the mother has two options: (1) Nurse twin A while simultaneously pumping for twin B. Breast milk obtained can be taken to twin B. This schedule is rigorous and may be exhausting for the mother. (2) Begin pumping for twin B a few days prior to the infant's discharge.

Feedings may be simultaneous or individual. Simultaneous feedings are advantageous because both feedings are completed in one session. Simultaneous feedings save time and may take advantage of simultaneous letdowns. A disadvantage is that the mother loses individual time with each infant.

Individual feedings are advantageous because modified scheduling may be employed. For example, the hungrier infant sets the pace, and the second infant is awakened for feedings. A disadvantage of this type of feeding is that it is time consuming.

Simultaneous Feedings

Proper positioning is particularly important for breastfeeding two infants so that the mother does not bear the weight of the infants. Pillows should be firm and support the infants' weight. There are pillows made to assist mothers of twins.

- The double football hold is used for simultaneous feedings. The head and neck of each infant are supported by the mother's hands, with each infant's body tucked under one of the mother's arms and their feet toward her back. The infants' abdomens face up or are rotated in toward the mother's chest or side. An advantage of the double football hold is that the mother can assist with head control; the more difficult to manage infant should be placed on the side easiest for the mother to manage (Gromada & Spangler, 1998; Mohrbacher & Stock, 1997). The mother should not bend over to nurse but, instead, bring the infants close to her.
- In the combination cradle/football position, twin A is held like football and approaches the breast at 12 and 6 o'clock. Twin B is cradled across the mother's chest with her or his abdomen tucked in tightly toward the mother's abdomen and approaches the breast at 9 and 3 o'clock (Gromada & Spangler, 1998; Mohrbacher & Stock, 1997). Two advantages of this position are that it is the most inconspicuous for nursing outside the home, and it is easily mastered if one or both infants have difficulty latching onto the breast.
- In the parallel hold both infants are angled in the same direction. Twin A is cradled, held with legs behind twin B; the legs simultaneously support twin B's head. The advantage of the parallel hold is that the weight of one twin keeps the second infant attached to the breast. In addition, the mother's arms can rest comfortably on pillows (Mohrbacher & Stock, 1997).

- In the crisscross hold both infants are in cradle position, with the legs of one crossing over those of the other. The infants are in the crook of the mother's arms and are rotated toward her abdomen. The mother supports the infants by holding their buttocks. A disadvantage is that this position is difficult for infants to maintain; it requires head control (Gromada & Spangler, 1998; Mohrbacher & Stock 1997).
- "V" position is similar to crisscross. The mother is lying nearly flat on her back with pillows under her head. The infants' heads are at their mother's breasts, forming a "V," with their knees touching her upper abdomen (Gromada & Spangler, 1998; Mohrbacher & Stock 1997). This position allows the mother to rest more comfortably; it can be used for night feedings. The disadvantage is that it requires infants to have more head control and assistance in grasping the nipple.

DRUG TRANSMISSION IN BREAST MILK

Transmission of a drug in breast milk from mother to infant depends on several factors:

- Absorption of drug by mother's body: half-life or peak serum time, absorption rate, route of administration.
- Lipid solubility and plasma protein binding properties of drug.
- Movement of drug from maternal plasma to milk; cell diffusion or active transport.
- Amount of drug ingested by infant.
- Concentration of drug in milk.
- Size and relative metabolic maturity of infant.
- pH of substrate (Auerbach, 1999; Lawrence & Lawrence, 1999).

The effect of the drug can be minimized in several ways:

- Do not use a long-acting form of the drug. Infants have difficulty with excretion and detoxification usually occurs in liver; however, the infant liver is immature.
- Schedule the doses so that the least amount of the drug enters the milk: Have the mother take medication immediately after breastfeeding.
- Choose drug that passes least into milk.
- Advise the mother to take medication as directed and to watch the infant for unusual signs and symptoms or a change in feeding pattern or activity. She should

contact her health care provider if she has any concerns or questions.

The American Academy of Pediatrics (2001) recommended the following be considered before prescribing medication for the lactating woman: (1) Is the drug really necessary? (2) the safest drug should be chosen; (3) if there is a possibility that a drug may present a risk to the infant, consideration should be given to measurement of blood concentrations in the nursing infant; (4) drug exposure to the nursing infant may be minimized by having the mother take the medication just after she has breastfed the infant or just before the infant is due to have a lengthy sleep period.

Contraindications

Certain drugs are contraindicated while breastfeeding:

- Alcoholic beverages (interfere with ejection reflex).
- Chronic aspirin use may cause metabolic acidosis in infant and affect platelet function (aspirin or acetaminophen in single dose is not significantly transferred).
- Cocaine intoxication (seizures, irritability, vomiting, diarrhea).
- Chloramphenicol (potential for bone marrow toxicity).
- Cimetidine (unknown effect in nursing infant).
- Cyclosporine (possible immune suppression; unknown effect on growth or carcinogenesis) (AAP, 2001; Klonoff-Cohen et al., 1995; Mohrbacher & Stock, 1997).
- Doxorubicin (possible immune suppression; unknown effect on growth or carcinogenesis) (AAP, 2001; Klonoff-Cohen et al., 1995; Mohrbacher & Stock, 1997).
- Gold salts (rash, kidney and liver inflammation).
- Iodine (preferentially concentrated in milk with concentrations twenty to thirty times those of maternal serum).
- Lithium (infant hypotonia, lethargy).
- Methotrexate (possible immune suppression; unknown effect on growth or carcinogenesis) (AAP, 2001; Klonoff-Cohen et al., 1995; Mohrbacher & Stock, 1997).
- Minor tranquilizers (barbiturates, benzodiazepines).
- Narcotics (methadone for maintenance therapy reported safe).
- Phencyclidine (PCP).
- Thiouracil (not, however, propylthiouracil).

◆ Tobacco (smoking more than 20 cigarettes per day decreases milk supply; passive, inhaled smoke increases risks for allergies, sudden infant death syndrome, pneumonia, and bronchitis). Documented decrease in milk supply and weight gain in infant (possible immune suppression; unknown effect on growth or carcinogenesis). (AAP, 2001; Klonoff-Cohen et al., 1995; Mohrbacher & Stock, 1997).

Drugs requiring temporary interruption are radiopharmaceuticals including indium-111 and gallium-67 (AAP, 2001).

The effects of metoclopramide on nursing infants are unknown. No adverse effects have been reported; however, there is the potential for central nervous system effects (AAP, 2001).

Drugs that have caused significant effects in some nursing infants and should be used with caution include clemastine, phenobarbital, primidone, and sulfasalazine (AAP, 2001).

A mother who uses recreational drugs should not breastfeed.

Amphetamines (crack, speed, ups, uppers) are excreted in breast milk; levels in milk exceed those in maternal serum. Abstinence from amphetamines is recommended until more information is available.

Cocaine (snow, coke, crack, champagne, tool, pearl flake, blow, gold dust, dama blanca) appears to be excreted in breast milk. Cocaine intoxication has been reported in 2-week-old infants. Mothers should not apply cocaine to sore nipples.

Heroin ("H," junk, smack, China white, black tar) crosses into breast milk to cause addiction in breastfed infants, tremors, restlessness, vomiting, and poor feeding (AAP, 2001).

Hallucinogens have not been reported in breast milk. Hallucinogens include LSD (acid, lysergic diethylamide), mescaline (peyote), psilocybin (found in certain mushrooms) and Ts and blues (combination of pentazocine and tripelennamine).

Marijuana (dope, weed, herb, grass, pot, hashish, hash) has unknown long-term effects on infants; the concentration transferred into breast milk is eight times that in maternal blood (AAP, 2001).

Compatible Drugs

Certain drugs are usually compatible with breastfeeding:

◆ Acetominophen
◆ Acylovir
◆ Amoxicillin
◆ Azithromycin
◆ Cefoxitin
◆ Cimetidine
◆ Ciprofloxin
◆ Cisplatin
◆ Clindanycin
◆ Diltiazem
◆ Erythromycin
◆ Fluconazole
◆ Ibuprofen
◆ Labetalol
◆ Methyldopa
◆ Methimazole
◆ Metoprolol
◆ Mexilitine
◆ Minoxidil
◆ Piroxicam
◆ Prednisone
◆ Procainamide
◆ Progesterone
◆ Propranolol
◆ Sumatriptan
◆ Suprafen
◆ Terbutaline
◆ Ticarcillin
◆ Tolmetin
◆ Valacyclovir
◆ Verapamil
◆ Zolpidem (AAP, 2001; Lawrence & Lawrence, 1999)

BREAST PUMPS

Mothers of preterm infants or of newborns hospitalized for other reasons and mothers who work may use breast pumps. An infant's suckling, however, remains the most efficient pump. Infants suck at approximately 55 to 220 mm Hg (Biancuzzo, 1999). Pumps that match suckling stimulate the milk ejection reflex and promote milk production most effectively. The vacuum produced by a pump should not exceed the vacuum created by an infant.

Infants nurse in a burst-pause pattern. Suckling has three phases: suction, release, and relaxation. The actions are carried out approximately 40 to 50 times per minute (Biancuzzo, 1999). Infants apply suction for less than 1 second each time.

A correctly fitting flange surrounds the areola and allows the nipple to move back and forth during pumping. The flange should engulf and firmly support the breast and allow maximum nipple stretch, yet be small enough to provide gentle nipple friction.

There are different types of pumps. An electric pump obtains more milk and is easier to use than a hand-operated pump or manual expression. The double pump expresses milk most quickly and can be rented. Most pump rental stations or hiring agencies offer discounted rates for long-term rentals ($30.00 per month). An intermittent draw pump is less likely to cause trauma and provides better stimulation of the milk ejection reflex.

Manual expression of milk might be necessary in the event a part of the mechanical pump is lost or the pump is left at home. To manually express (pump) milk, the mother first washes her hands. She positions her thumb and first two fingers about 1 to 1½ inches behind her nipple, forming a "C" with her hand. She should then push straight into the chest wall and roll her thumb and fingers forward. The movement is repeated rhythmically; the thumb and fingers are rotated to milk other sinuses. She should express each breast until milk flow decreases, then gently massage the breasts to stimulate milk ejection.

Not recommended for pumping breasts is the bicycle horn pump. It cannot be sterilized, milk can be easily contaminated, and it has no collection mechanism for milk. It is difficult to clean, can damage breast tissue, and it expresses milk ineffectively.

Using a Pump

Practicing with pump before actual need for milk will facilitate successful use. A woman should become knowledgeable about the pump several weeks before milk is actually needed; she should practice putting the pump together and using it. Hands should be washed before beginning breast pumping, and manufacturer's instructions followed for cleaning the pump.

The mother moistens the breast with water (to form a seal), centers the nipple in the proper size nipple adapter, and begins pumping at the lowest setting. To stimulate the milk ejection reflex she should interrupt milk expression several times to gently massage the breast. She should switch breasts when milk flow begins to decrease.

Storing Milk

If milk is to be used within 48 to 72 hours, refrigeration is sufficient for storage. Milk should be frozen if storage will be longer than 24 hours. Do not freeze in glass containers but in rigid polyprophylene plastic containers to maintain stability of cells and immunoglobulins (Lawrence & Lawrence, 1999). Frozen milk can be stored for one month in the freezer compartment of a refrigerator or six months in a deep freeze. Methods of thawing milk can adversely affect anti-infective factors. Frozen milk should be thawed in the refrigerator and used within 24 hours. Thawing milk in warm water can cause contamination, and subjecting milk to microwave temperatures of 72° to 98°F (medium to high) can result in a marked decrease in anti-infective factors (Lawrence & Lawrence, 1999).

RETURNING TO WORK

Pumping/Expressing Milk

Advise the client to begin freezing milk for later use approximately fourteen days before returning to work. She should pump at least three times per day, after breastfeeding the infant. A formula is used to estimate the amount of milk needed per feeding:

$$\frac{\text{infant weight} \times 2.5}{\text{number of feedings}} = \text{ounces per feeding}$$

For example, for a 10-pound infant,

$$\frac{10 \times 2.5}{8} = \frac{25}{8} = \begin{array}{l} \text{approximately 3 oz of milk} \\ \text{needed per feeding} \end{array}$$

A Nuk-type nipple should be used when bottle feeding, as it most closely resembles breast.

Baby's Refusal of Bottle

Refusing to drink from a bottle occurs most often among infants approximately 3 months old. Using a bottle along with breastfeeding in the first month of life increases the likelihood of nipple confusion; poor suckling at breast results and establishment of a milk supply that meets the infant's needs is delayed (AWHONN 2000a; Lawrence & Lawrence, 1999). Someone other than mother should use a second feeding skill with the infant, for example, offering milk in a cup or spoon rather than the bottle.

Preparing for Absence

Some guidelines might help the client adapt to the challenges of breastfeeding and spending time away from the infant.

- ◆ Suggest to the client that she pack an extra bra and wear a two-piece outfit to facilitate pumping and to camouflage leakage of milk.
- ◆ Advise the client to ensure that the infant's caregiver is comfortable with the mother's desire to breastfeed and knows how to handle breast milk.

◆ Suggest to the client that she pack several diaper bags to obviate the need to return home for forgotten articles.

◆ Refer the client to a breastfeeding support group (see Breastfeeding Information/Support Groups at the end of this chapter).

BOTTLE FEEDING

Although breast milk is the perfect food for infants, not all mothers choose or are able to breastfeed their infants. Formula feedings should be given to an infant for the first year of life. If the infant is allergic to cow's milk, soy-based formulas may be used.

An amendment was passed in 1980 by Congress to the Food, Drug and Cosmetic Act specifying new regulations for commercially prepared infant formula. This act, the Infant Formula Act of 1980, gave the Food and Drug Administration (FDA) the authority to establish quality-control procedures for infant formula, to establish recall procedures, to establish and revise nutrient levels, and to regulate labeling. Manufacturers were also required to analyze each batch of formula to ensure all nutrients were present in the correct amounts, to ensure that the formula was stable over the period of recommended shelf life, and to make all records available to the FDA. The year 1986 saw the requirement for standard labeling of nutrition information and directions for preparation become mandatory.

Calories are provided to the infant in the form of carbohydrates, protein, and fat. By the end of the second week in life, full-term infants require 100–110 Kcal/kg/day of fluids to maintain cellular growth and function. Preterm infants weighing less than 2,500 grams may require 110–150 Kcal/kg/day to achieve satisfactory growth. Fluid requirements are higher than in full-term infants because of greater fluid loss. Because of the immature digestive system, premature infants will require different formula than full-term infants. (Darby & Loughead, 1996).

Teaching Bottle Feeding

◆ Point the nipple directly into the mouth and on top of the tongue, rather than toward the palate. The nipple should be full of milk at all times to avoid ingestion of air. The nipple hole should be large enough so that milk flows in drips when inverted; if it is too large, the infant can drink too fast and regurgitate or overeat.

◆ Stroke, cuddle, and talk to the infant during feedings.

◆ Never prop bottles or feed infant in totally recumbent (flat) position which can result in positional otitis media.

◆ Avoid warming bottles in a microwave oven, as milk can become too hot and burn the infant. Formula should be at room temperature.

◆ Avoid reusing milk from a previous feeding.

REFERENCES

Adam, R.A., & Preston, M.R. (2002, May). Urinary incontinence: Diagnosis and treatment. *Women's Health in Primary Care, 2*(4), 218–220, 223–230.

American Academy of Pediatrics (AAP). (1998, April). *Guidance for effective discipline (RE9740)*: Accessed May 12, 2002 from www.AAP.org.

American Academy of Pediatrics (AAP). (2000, March). *Changing concepts of sudden infant death syndrome: implications for infant sleeping environment and sleep position (RE9946)*: Accessed May 11, 2002 from www.AAP.org.

American Academy of Pediatrics (AAP). (2001, September). *The transfer of drugs and other chemicals into human milk*, 108(3): 776–789. Accessed May 18, 2002 from www.AAP.org.

American Academy of Pediatrics & American College of Obstetricians & Gynecologists (AAP & ACOG). (2002). Postpartum and follow-up care. In *Guidelines for perinatal care* (5th ed., pp. 125–161; 187–283). Elk Grove Village, IL: AAP.

American College of Obstetricians & Gynecologists (ACOG). (1995, October). Pelvic organ prolapse. (Technical Bulletin No. 214). Washington, DC: Author.

American College of Obstetricians & Gynecologists (ACOG). (1998a, January). Postpartum hemorrhage. (Educational Bulletin No. 243). Washington, DC: Author.

American College of Obstetricians & Gynecologists (ACOG). (1998b, March). *Antimicrobial therapy for obstetrical patients* (Educational Bulletin No. 245). Washington, DC: Author.

American College of Obstetricians & Gynecologists (ACOG). (2000, July). *Breastfeeding: Maternal and infant aspects* (Educational Bulletin No. 258). Washington, DC: Author.

American College of Obstetricians & Gynecologists (ACOG). (2001, November). *Thyroid disease in pregnancy* (Technical Bulletin No. 32). Washington, DC: Author.

American College of Obstetricians & Gynecologists (ACOG). (2002, January). *Diagnosis and management of preeclampsia and eclampsia* (Technical Bulletin No. 33). Washington, DC: Author.

American Diabetes Association (ADA). (2002). Clinical practice recommendations 2002. *Diabetes Care, 25* (Suppl. 1), s21–24, s5–20.

Anderson, C. (2002, April/May). Battered and pregnant: A nursing challenge. *AWHONN Lifelines, 6*(2), 95–99.

Association of Women's Health, Obstetric, and Neonatal Nurses (AWHONN). (2000a). *Continence for women* (Practice Guideline) (pp. 1–27).

Association of Women's Health, Obstetric, and Neonatal Nurses (AWHONN). (2000b). *Breastfeeding support: Prenatal care through the first year* (Monograph) (pp. 1–35). Washington, D.C: AWHONN

Auerbach, K.G. (1999, September/October). Breastfeeding and maternal medication use. *Journal of Obstetric, Gynecologic, and Neonatal Nursing, 28*(5), 554–563.

Baho, K., & Hager, J. (1998, April). Clinical focus: Keeping moms and babies together. *AWHONN Lifelines, 2*(2), 44–48.

Bakoula, C., Kafritsa, Y., Kavadias, G., Lazopoulou, D., Theodoridou, M., Maravelias, K., & Matsaniotis, N. (1995, July 25). Objective passive smoking indicators and respiratory morbidity in young children. *The Lancet, 346* (8970): 280–281.

Barnard, K. (1978). *Learning resource manual.* Seattle: University of Washington, Nursing Child Assessment Satellite Training.

Beck, C. (1995, September/October). The effects of postpartum depression on maternal-infant interaction: A meta-analysis. *Nursing Research, 44*(5), 298–304.

Beck, C.T. (1999, August/September). Postpartum depression: Stopping the thief that steals motherhood. *AWHONN Lifelines, 3*(4) 41–44.

Beck, C.T. (2002, July/August). Revision of the postpartum depression predictors inventory. *Journal of Obstetric, Gynecologic, and Neonatal Nursing, 31*(4), 394–402.

Beck, C.T., & Gable, R.K. (2000, September/October). Postpartum depression screening scale: development and psychometric testing. *Nursing Research*, 49(5): 272–282.

Beck, C.T., & Gable, R.K. (2001a, July/August). Comparative analysis of the performance of the postpartum depression screening scale with two other depression instruments. *Nursing Research, 50*(4), 242–249.

Beck, C.T., & Gable, R.K. (2001b, May/June). Further validation of the postpartum depression screening scale. *Nursing Research, 50*(3), 155–164.

Beck, C.T., & Gable, R.K. (2002). *Postpartum depression screening scale (PDSS).* Los Angeles: Western Psychological Services.

Bender, E., Jorjorian, A., Lynch, P., & Cramer, A. (1998). Relationships with women. In Boston Women's Health Book Collective, *Our bodies, ourselves for the new century* (pp. 200–228). New York: Simon & Schuster.

Beral, V. (2002, July 20). Breast cancer and breastfeeding: Collaborative reanalysis of individual data from 47 epidemiological studies in 30 countries, including 50,302 women with cancer and 96,973 women without the disease. *The Lancet, 360*(9328), 187–195.

Biancuzzo, M. (1999, July/August). Selecting pumps for breastfeeding mothers. *Journal of Obstetric, Gynecologic, and Neonatal Nursing, 28*(4), 417–426.

Blackwell, D.A., & Blackwell, J.T. (1999, October/November). Building alternative families: Helping lesbian couples find the path to parenthood. *AWHONN Lifelines, 3*(5), 45–48.

Brazelton, T.B. (1992). Discipline. In *Touchpoints* (pp. 252–260). New York: Addison-Wesley.

"Breastfeeding cuts breast cancer by 50 percent." (2001, May/June). *AWHONN Lifelines, 5*(2), 13.

Briggs, G.G., Freeman, R.K., & Yaffe, S.J. (2002). *Drugs in pregnancy and lactation* (6th ed.). Philadelphia: Lippincott Williams & Wilkins.

Brucker, M. (2001, November/December). Management of the third stage of labor: An evidence-based approach. *Journal of Midwifery and Women's Health, 46*(6), 381–392.

Brunner, B. (Ed.). (2001). *Time almanac 2002* (p. 712). Boston: Family Education Company.

Buckner, J. (1998, June). Displaced children: Meeting the health, mental health, and educational needs of immigrant, migrant, and homeless youth. *Adolescent Medicine, 9*(2), 323–334.

Bukowski, R., & Hankins, G.D.V. (2001, September). Managing postpartum hemorrhage. *Contemporary OB-GYN, 46*(9), 92–101.

Carson, C., Boggess, K., Colgan, R., Hooten, T., & Kerr, L. (2000, Fall). Current management of UTI in women. *Patient Care for the Nurse Practitioner*, 3–22.

Chames, M.C., Livingston, J.C., Ivester, T.S., Barton, J.R., & Sibai, B.M. (2002, June). Late postpartum eclampsia: A preventable disease? *American Journal of Obstetrics and Gynecology, 186*(6), 1174–7.

Chez, R.A., & Friedmann, A.K. (2000, August). Offering effective breastfeeding advice. *Contemporary OB/GYN, 45*(8), 32–33, 37–38, 43–44, 47–48, 50.

Cranley, M.S. (1981). Roots of attachment: The relationship of parents with their unborn. In March of Dimes Foundation, *Birth defects: Original article series, 17*(6): 59–82.

Cropley, C. (1986). Assessment of mothering behaviors. In S.H. Johnson (Ed.). *Nursing Assessment and strategies for the family at risk* (2nd ed., pp. 15–40). Philadelphia: Lippincott.

Cunningham, F.G., Gant, N.F., Leveno, K.J., Gilstrap, L.C., Hauth, J.C., & Wenstrom, K.D. (2001a). Abortion. In *Williams obstetrics* (21st ed., pp. 855–882). New York: McGraw-Hill.

Cunningham, F.G., Gant, N.F., Leveno, K.J., Gilstrap, L.C., Hauth, J.C., & Wenstrom, K.D. (2001b). Diabetes. In *Williams obstetrics* (21st ed., pp. 1359–1381). New York: McGraw-Hill.

Cunningham, F.G., Gant, N.F., Leveno, K.J., Gilstrap, L.C., Hauth, J.C., & Wenstrom, K.D. (2001c). Diseases and injuries of the fetus and newborn. In *Williams obstetrics* (21st ed., pp. 1039–1091). New York: McGraw-Hill.

Cunningham, F.G., Gant, N.F., Leveno, K.J., Gilstrap, L.C., Hauth, J.C., & Wenstrom, K.D. (2001d). Endocrine disorders. In *Williams obstetrics* (21st ed., pp. 1339–1358). New York: McGraw-Hill.

Cunningham, F.G., Gant, N.F., Leveno, K.J., Gilstrap, L.C., Hauth, J.C., & Wenstrom, K.D. (2001e). Hypertensive disorders in pregnancy. In *Williams obstetrics* (21st ed., pp. 567–618). New York: McGraw-Hill.

Cunningham, F.G., Gant, N.F., Leveno, K.J., Gilstrap, L.C., Hauth, J.C., & Wenstrom, K.D. (2001f). Obstetrical hemorrhage. In *Williams obstetrics* (21st ed., pp. 619–669). New York: McGraw-Hill.

Cunningham, F.G., Gant, N.F., Leveno, K.J., Gilstrap, L.C., Hauth, J.C., & Wenstrom, K.D. (2001g). Obstetrics in broad perspective. In *Williams obstetrics* (21st ed., pp. 3–13). New York: McGraw-Hill.

Cunningham, F.G., Gant, N.F., Leveno, K.J., Gilstrap, L.C., Hauth, J.C., & Wenstrom, K.D. (2001h). Puerperal infection. In *Williams obstetrics* (21st ed., pp. 671–688). New York: McGraw-Hill.

Cunningham, F.G., Gant, N.F., Leveno, K.J., Gilstrap, L.C., Hauth, J.C., & Wenstrom, K.D. (2001i). The puerperium. In *Williams obstetrics* (21st ed., pp. 403–421). New York: McGraw-Hill.

Darby, M., & Loughead, J. (1996, March/April). Neonatal nutritional requirements and formula composition: A review. *Journal of Obstetric, Gynecologic, and Neonatal Nursing, 25*(3), 209–217.

Davis, M.S. (1992). Natural family planning. In *NAACOG'S Clinical Issues in Perinatal and Women's Health Nursing, 3*(2), 280–292.

Davis, M., & Akridge, K. (1987, November/December). The effect of promoting intrauterine attachment in primiparas on postpartum attachment. *Journal of Obstetric, Gynecologic, and Neonatal Nursing, 16*(6), 430–437.

DeMarco, R., Lynch, M.M., & Board, R. (2002, April). Mothers who silence themselves: A concept with clinical implications for women living with HIV/AIDS and their children. *Journal of Pediatric Nursing, 17*(2), 89–95.

DeMatteo, D., Wells, L.M., Goldie, R.S., & King, S.M. (2002, April). The 'family' context of HIV: A need for comprehensive health and social policies. *AIDS Care, 14*(2), 261–278.

Fischbach, F. (2001). Nuclear medicine studies. In *A manual of laboratory and diagnostic tests* (5th ed., pp. 688–749). Philadelphia: Lippincott.

French, L.M., & Smaill, F.M. (2002). Antibiotic regimens for endometritis after delivery (Cochrane Review). In *The Cochrane Library, 2*. Oxford: Update Software.

Furniss, K. (2000, May/June). No child should ever be hit. *Journal of Obstetric, Gynecololgic, and Neonatal Nursing, 29*(3), 225.

Gaffney, K. (2001, Fourth Quarter). Infant exposure to environmental tobacco smoke. *Journal of Nursing Scholarship, 33*(4), 343–347.

Gold, L. (2002, March). Postpartum disorders in primary care. *Primary Care: Clinics in Office Practice, 29*(1), 27–41.

Griffin, I., & Abrams, S. (2001, April). Iron and breastfeeding. *Pediatric Clinics of North America, 48*(2), 401–413.

Gromada, K., & Spangler, A. (1998, July/August). Breastfeeding twins and high-order multiples. *Journal of Obstetric, Gynecologic, and Neonatal Nursing, 27*(4), 441–449.

Harvey, S.M., Carr, C., & Bernheine, S. (1989, May/June). Lesbian mothers: Health care experiences. *Journal of Nurse Midwifery, 34*(3), 115–119.

Horowitz, J., Bell, M., Trybulski, J., Munro, B., Moser, D., Hartz, S., et al. (2001, Fall). Promoting responsiveness between mothers with depressive symptoms and their infants. *Journal of Nursing Scholarship, 33*(4), 323–329.

Hudson, D., Elek, S., & Campbell-Grossman, C. (2000, Fall). Depression, self-esteem, loneliness, and social support among adolescent mothers participating in the new parents project. *Adolescence, 35*(139): 445–453.

Humphreys, J., & Neylan, T. (2001, June). Psychological and physical distress of sheltered battered women. *Health Care for Women International, 22*(4), 401–414.

Jazayeri, A., Heffron, J.A., Harnetty, P., Jazayeri, M., & Gould, S.F. (1999, October). Antepartum and postpartum Papanicolaou smears. Are they both necessary? *Journal of Reproductive Medicine, 44*(10), 879–882.

Kemper, K. (1995). Psychosocial screening. In S. Parker & B. Zuckerman (Eds.), *Behavioral and developmental pediatrics* (pp. 30–34). Boston: Little, Brown and Company.

Kennedy, K.I., & Trussell, J. (1998). Postpartum contraception and lactation. In *Contraceptive technology* (17th ed., pp. 589–614). New York: Ardent Media.

Kennell, J.H., & Klaus, M.H. (1998, January). Bonding: Recent observations that alter perinatal death of a newborn infant. *New England Journal of Medicine, 283*(7), 344–349.

Kennell, J., Slyter, H., & Klaus, M. (1970, August 13). The mourning responses of parents to the death of a newborn infant. *New England Journal of Medicine, 283*(7), 344–349.

Klaus, M., & Kennell, J. (1983). Adjusting to malformation. In *Bonding: The beginnings of parent-infant attachment* (pp. 140–161). St. Louis: C.V. Mosby.

Klonoff-Cohen, H., Edelstein, S., Lefkowitz, E., Srinivasan, I., Kaegi, D., Chang, J., et al. (1995, March 8). The effect of passive smoking and tobacco exposure through breast milk on sudden infant death syndrome. *JAMA, 273*(10), 795–798.

Kramer, A. (2002, March). Domestic violence: How to ask and how to listen. *Nursing Clinics of North America, 37*(1), 189–210.

Labbock, M. (2001). Effects of breastfeeding on the mother. *Pediatric Clinics of North America, 48*, 143–158.

Lawrence, R.A., & Lawrence, R.M. (1999). *Breastfeeding: A guide for the medical profession* (5th ed.). St. Louis: Mosby.

Limbo, R., & Wheeler, S.R. (1986a). Coping with unexpected outcomes. In *NAACOG Update Series: Vol. 5 (Lesson 3)*. Princeton, NJ: Continuing Professional Education Center.

Limbo, R., & Wheeler, S.R. (1986b). *When a baby dies: A handbook for healing and helping*. LaCrosse, WI: Gunderson Clinic, Ltd.

Lynch, M. (1989, March/April). Congenital defects: Parental issues and nursing supports. *Journal of Perinatal and Neonatal Nursing, 2*(4), 53–59.

MacArthur, C., Winter, H., Bick, D., Knowles, H., Lilford, R., Henderson, C., et al. (2002, February 2). Effects of redesigned community postnatal care on womens' health 4 months after birth: A cluster randomised controlled trial. *The Lancet, 359*(9304), 378–385.

Margolis, L., & Kotelchuk, M. (1996, January/February). Midwives, physicians, and the timing of maternal postpartum discharge. *Journal of Nurse Midwifery, 41*(1), 29–35.

Martell, L.K. (2000, January/February). The hospital and the postpartum experience: A historical analysis. *Journal of Obstetric, Gynecologic, and Neonatal Nursing, 29*(1), 65–72.

McFarlane, J., & Parker, B. (1994). Abuse during pregnancy: A protocol for prevention and intervention. In K. Damus & M. Freda (Eds.), *Abuse during pregnancy* (pp. 14–40). White Plains, NY: March of Dimes Foundation.

Menke, E.M. (2000, October/November). Comparison of the stressors and coping behaviors of homeless, previously homeless, and never homeless poor children. *Issues in Mental Health Nursing, 21*(7), 691–710.

Mercer, R.T. (1983). Parent-infant attachment. In L. Sonstegard, K. Kowalski, & B. Jennings (Eds.), *Women's health: Vol. II. Childbearing* (pp. 17–42). New York: Grune & Stratton.

Mercer, R.T. (1985, July/August). Process of maternal role attainment over the first year. *Nursing Research, 34*(4), 198–204.

Mercer, R. (1990). *Parents at risk*. New York: Springer Publishing Company.

Mercer, R.T., & Ferketich, S. (1990, March). Predictors of parental attachment during early parenthood. *Journal of Advanced Nursing, 153*(3), 268–280.

Misra, D. (Ed.). (2001, December). Violence against women. In *The women's health data book* (3rd ed., pp. 150–162). Washington, DC: Jacobs Institute of Women's Health and The Henry J. Kaiser Family Foundation.

Mohrbacher, N., & Stock, J. (1997). *The breastfeeding answer book*. Schaumberg, IL: La Leche League International.

Muller, A.F., Drexhage, H.A., & Bergout, A. (2001, October). Postpartum thyroiditis and autoimmune thyroiditis in women of childbearing age: Recent insights and consequences for antenatal and postnatal care. *Endocrine Reviews, 22*(5), 605–630.

Muller, M. (1996, February). Prenatal and postnatal attachment: A modest correlation. *Journal of Obstetric, Gynecologic, and Neonatal Nursing, 25*(2), 161–166.

National Institutes of Health. (2000). *Working group report on high blood pressure in pregnancy* (NIH Publication No. 00-3029). Washington, DC: U.S. Government Printing Office.

Newberger, E. (1995). Physical abuse. In S. Parker & B. Zuckerman (Eds.), *Behavioral and developmental pediatrics* (pp. 232–238). Boston: Little, Brown and Company.

Newport, D.J., Hostetter, A., Arnold, A., & Stowe, Z. (2002). The treatment of postpartum depression: Minimizing infant exposure. *Journal of Clinical Psychiatry, 63* (suppl. 7), 31–44.

Nurse Practitioner's Drug Book. (4th ed.). (2002). Philadelphia: Lippincott Williams & Wilkins.

Oliveira, N.L., & Goldberg, J.P. (2002, March/April). The nutrition status of women and children who are homeless. *Nutrition Today, 37*(2), 70–77.

Olson, G. (2002, April). Thyroid disease in pregnancy. *The Female Patient, 27*(1), 10–16.

Panzarine, S., Slater, E., & Sharps, P. (1995, August). Coping, social support, and depressive symptoms in adolescent mothers. *Journal of Adolescent Health Care, 17*(2), 113–119.

Patchen, L., & Beal, M. (2001, November/December). Preventing perinatal transmission of HIV: An evidence-based update for midwives. *Journal of Midwifery & Women's Health, 46*(6), 354–365.

Peat, J.K., Keena, V., Harakeh, Z., & Marks, G. (2001, September). Parental smoking and respiratory tract infections in children. *Paedriatic Respiratory Reviews, 2*(3), 207–213.

Quillian, J. (1996, April). Screening for spousal or partner abuse in a community health setting. *Journal of the American Academy of Nurse Practitioners, 8*(4), 155–160.

Radmacher, P., Massey, C., & Adamkin, D. (2002, January). Hidden morbidity with "successful" early discharge. *Journal of Perinatology, 22*(1), 15–20.

Rillstone, P. & Hutchinson, S. (2001, May/June). Managing the reemergence of anguish: Pregnancy after a loss due to anomalies. *Journal of Obstetric, Gynecologic, and Neonatal Nursing, 30*(3), 291–298.

Riordan, J., & Auerbach, K.G. (2001). *Pocket guide to breastfeeding and human lactation* (2nd ed.). Sudbury, MA: Jones and Bartlett.

Rubin, R. (1984). *Maternal identity and the maternal experience*. New York: Springer Publishing Company.

Russell, M., Sanford, W., & Jobin-Leeds, M. (1998). HIV, AIDS, and women. In Boston Women's Health Book Collective, *Our bodies, ourselves for the new century* (pp. 359–377). New York: Simon & Schuster.

Sampselle, C., & Brink, C. (1990, May/June). Pelvic muscle relaxation: Assessment and management. *Journal of Nurse Midwifery, 35*(3), 127–132.

Sampselle, C., Miller, J., Mims, B., DeLaney, J.O.L., Ashton-Miller, J.A., & Antonakas, C.L. (1998, March). Effect of pelvic muscle exercise and transient incontinence during pregnancy and after birth. *Obstetrics & Gynecology, 91*(3), 406–412.

Santacroce, S.J., Deatrick, J.A., & Ledlie, S.W. (2002, April). Redefining treatment: How biological mothers manage their children's treatment for perinatally acquired HIV. *AIDS Care, 14*(2), 247–260.

Schwartz, M.A., Wang, C.C., Eckert, L.O., & Critchlow, C.W. (1999, September). Risk factors for urinary tract infection in the postpartum period. *American Journal of Obstetrics and Gynecology, 181*(3), 547–553.

Shoultz, J., Phillion, N., Noone, J., & Tanner, B. (2002, July). Listening to women: Culturally tailoring the violence prevention guidelines from the "Put Prevention into Practice" program. *Journal of the American Academy of Nurse Practitioners, 14*(7), 307–315.

Smith, J.W., & Tully, M.R. (2001, November-December). Midwifery management of breastfeeding: Using the evidence. *Journal of Midwifery & Women's Health, 46*(6), 423–438.

Stagnaro-Green, A. (2000, June). Recognizing, understanding, and treating postpartum thyroiditis. *Endocrinology and Metabolism Clinics of North America, 29*(2), 417–431.

Staudacher, C. (1987). Surviving the loss of a child. In *Beyond grief: A guide for recovering from the death of a loved one* (pp. 99–126). Oakland, CA: New Harbinger.

Stevens, P., & Hall, J. (2001, July-August). Sexuality and safer sex: The issues for lesbians and bisexual women. *Journal of Obstetric, Gynecologic, and Neonatal Nursing, 30*(4), 439–447.

Synoground, G., & Bruya, M.A. (2000, May). Meeting the health needs of homeless or low-income persons: Role of the nurse practitioner. *Clinical Excellence for Nurse Practitioners, 4*(3), 138–144.

Szgalsky, J. (1989, October). Perinatal death, the family, and the role of the health professional. *Neonatal Network,* 8(2): 15–19.

Technical Working Group, World Health Organization (1999, December). Postpartum care of the mother and newborn: A practical guide. *Birth, 26*(4), 255–258.

U.S. Bureau of the Census. (2001). *Statistical abstract of the United States* (121st ed., No. 102). Washington, DC: Author.

Wallerstedt, C., & Higgins, P. (1996, June). Facilitating perinatal grieving between the mother and father. *Journal of Obstetric, Gynecologic, and Neonatal Nursing, 25*(5), 389–394.

Williams, G.B. (2000, April/May). Grief after elective abortion. *AWHONN Lifelines, 4*(2), 37–40.

Winans, E. (2001, August). Antidepressant use during lactation. *Journal of Human Lactation, 17*(3), 256–261.

Winters, M. (1998). Violence against women. In Boston Women's Health Book Collective, *Our bodies, ourselves for the new century* (pp. 158–178). New York: Simon & Schuster.

Workman, E. (2001, November/December). Guiding parents through the death of their infant. *Journal of Obstetric, Neonatal, and Gynecologic Nursing, 30*(6), 569–573.

Zeidenstein, L. (1990, January/February). Gynecological and childbearing needs of lesbians. *Journal of Nurse Midwifery, 35*(1), 10–18.

SUPPORT GROUPS AND RESOURCES

BREASTFEEDING INFORMATION/SUPPORT GROUPS

Ameda Breastfeeding Products
c/o Hollister Incorporated
2000 Hollister Dr.
Libertyville, IL 60048
(877) 992-6332 (USA)
(800) 263-7400 (Canada)
www.ameda.com

International Childbirth Educators' Assn.
P.O. Box 20048
Minneapolis, MN 55420
(952) 854-8660
www.icea.org

International Lactation Consultant Organization
4101 Lake Boone Trail, Ste 201
Raleigh, NC 27607
(919) 787-5181
www.ilca@erols.com

LaLeche League International & Breastfeeding Resource Center
1400 N. Meacham Road
P.O. Box 4079
Schaumburg, IL 60173-4808
(847) 519-7730
www.lalecheleague.org

Medela, Inc.
1101 Corporate Dr.
McHenry, IL 60050
(815) 363-1166
(800) 435-8316
www.medela.com

email: customer service@medela.com
Breast pumps, breast pump rentals (including double pumping system), breastfeeding products.

WOMEN, INFANTS, AND CHILDREN (WIC) AND FOOD STAMP PROGRAMS

Contact your local health department.

PARENTING/FAMILY SUPPORT GROUPS

Al-Anon Family Group Headquarters, Inc.
World Service Office
1600 Corporate Landing Parkway
Virginia Beach, VA 23454-5617
(757) 563-1600
(888) 425-2666 (Monday through Friday 8 A.M.–6 P.M. EST)
www.al-anon.alateen.org

Alcoholics Anonymous
Grand Central Station
P.O. Box 459
New York, NY 10163
(212) 870-3400

Association of Birth Defect Children, Inc.
Executive Director
930 Woodcock Road, Ste 225
Orlando, FL 38203
(407) 895-0802
www.birthdefects.org

Association of Maternal & Child Health Programs
1220 19th Street NW, Ste 801
Washington, DC 20036
(202) 775-0436
www.amchpl.org

AYUDA
1734 Columbia Rd.
Washington, DC 20009
(202) 387-0434
www.ayudaenaccion.org
Resource for immigrant Latina women in the Washington, DC area.

Center for Sickle Cell Disease
2121 Georgia Ave. SW
Washington, DC 20059
(202) 806-7930
www.huhosp.org/sicklecell/

Council of Families with Visual Impairment
P.O. Box 317
Watertown, MA 02471
(800) 562-6265 or
(617) 972-7441
www.spedex.com/napvi/

Custody Action for Lesbian Mothers (CALM)
P.O. Box 281
Narbeth, PA 19702
(215) 667-7508

Fragile X Program
Duke University
P.O. Box 3364
Durham, NC 27710
(919) 684-5513

Gay & Lesbian Parents Coalition International
P.O. Box 50360
Washington, DC 20091
(202) 583-8029
http://milepost1.com/~gaydad/support.groups.html

Klinefelter Syndrome & Associates
P.O. Box 119
Roseville, CA 95678-0119
(888) 999-9428
www.genetic.org/ks/

Lesbian Mothers National Defense Fund
(415) 392-6257

Little People of America, Inc. (LPA)
Box 745
Lubbock, TX 79408
(888) LPA-2001
www.lpaonline.org

Migrant Clinicians Network (MCN)
P.O. Box 164285
Austin, TX 78716
(512) 327-2017
www.migrantclinician.org
National clinical network of healthcare providers who serve migrant farm workers and other underserved mobile populations. Provides materials in English and Spanish for migrant workers; has a manual for clinicians for screening, documenting, and referring women who may be experiencing violence.

National Association of Developmental Disabilities Council (NADDC)
1234 Massachusetts Ave. NW, Ste 103
Washington, DC 20005
(202) 347-1234
www.naddc.org

National Association of Gay/Lesbian Addiction Professionals (NALGAP)
901 North Washington St. Ste. 600
Alexandria, VA 22314
(703) 465-0539
www.nalgap.org
Recovery center with services for addiction problems available to gay, lesbian, bisexual, and transsexual communities.

National Association for Sickle Cell Disease
3345 Wilshire Blvd., Ste 1106
Los Angeles, CA 90010-1880
(800) 421-8453

National Center for Lesbian Rights
870 Market St., Ste 570
San Francisco, CA 94102
(415) 392-6257
www.nclrights.org

National Center on Child Abuse and Neglect Department of Health & Human Services
U.S. Children's Bureau/NCCAN
P.O. Box 1182
Washington, DC 20013-1182
(202) 205-8586
(800) 394-3366
Information on programs in individual states, publications, and training manuals.

National Coalition against Domestic Violence (NCADV)
P.O. Box 18749
Denver, CO 80218
(303) 839-1852
Hotline (800) 799-SAFE (7233)
www.ncadv.org/contacthome.httm

National Domestic Violence Hotline
P.O. Box 161810
Austin, TX 78716
(800) 799-SAFE (7233)
(800) 787-3224 (TTY)
www.ndvh.org

National Fragile X Foundation
P.O. Box 190488
San Francisco, CA 94119-0488
(800) 688-8765
www.fragilex.org

National Gay & Lesbian Task Force (NGLTF)
1700 Kalorama Rd. NW
Washington, DC 20009-2624
(202) 332-6483
www.ngltf.org

National Information Center for Children & Youth with Disabilities
Box 1492
Washington, DC 20013-1492
(202) 884-8200 (Voice, TTY)
(800) 695-0285 (Voice, TTY)
www.nichcy.org

National Organization for Rare Disorders (NORD)
P.O. Box 8923
New Fairfield, CT 06812-8923
(203) 746-6518
(800) 999-NORD
www.rarediseases.org/cgi-bin/nord

National Organization for Victims (NOVA)
1730 Park Rd. NW
Washington, DC 20010
(202) 232-6682
(800) TRY-NOVA
www.try-nova.org

National Women's Health Information Center
8550 Arlington Blvd., Ste. 300
Fairfax, VA 22031
(800) 994-WOMAN (9662)
(888) 220-5446 (TTY)
www.4woman.gov
Health issues for women, including breastfeeding and postpartum depression.

Neurofibromatosis, Inc.
8855 Annapolis Rd., Ste.110
Lanham, MD 20706-2924
(301) 918-4600
(800) 942-6825
www.nfinc.org

Parents Anonymous, Inc.
675 W. Foothill Blvd. Ste.220
Claremont, CA 91711
(909) 621-6184
www.parentsanonymous.org

Parents of Down Syndrome Children
c/o The Arc
11600 Nebel St.
Rockville, MD 20852
(301) 984-5792
www.thearc.org

Parent Care
9041 Colgate St.
Indianapolis, IN 46268-1210
(317) 872-9913
www.familyvillage.wisc.edu/lib_prem.htm
For parents of premature and high risk infants.

Parents Helping Parents
3041 Olcott St.
Santa Clara, Ca 95054
(408) 727-5775
www.php.com

Pathways Awareness Foundation
A not-for-profit organization dedicated to education for
and about children with movement and physical challenges, and their families.
www.pathwaysawareness.org

Spina Bifida Association
4590 MacArthur Blvd., Ste. 250
Washington, DC 20007-4226
(202) 944-3285
(800) 621-3141
www.sbaa.org

Support Organization for Trisomy 18/13
2982 S. Union St.
Rochester, NY 14624
(800) 716-SOFT (7638)
www.trisomy.org

**National Organization of Mothers of Twins Clubs
(NOMOTC)**
P.O. Box 438
Thompson Station, TN 37179-0438
www.nomotc.org

POSTPARTUM DEPRESSION SUPPORT GROUPS

Depression after Delivery, Inc. (D.A.D.)
(800) 944-4PPD (4773)
www.depressionafterdelivery.com

Postpartum Support International
927 North Kellogg Ave.
Santa Barbara, CA 93111
www.postpartum.net

PERINATAL LOSS GROUPS

SIDS Alliance
1314 Bedford Ave. Ste 210
Baltimore, MD 21208
(410) 653-8226
(800) 221-SIDS (7437)
www.sidsalliance.org

The Compassionate Friends
P.O. Box 3696
Oak Brook, IL 60522-3696
(630) 990-0010
(877) 969-0010
www.compassionatefriends.org

Resolve Through Sharing
1910 South Ave.
La Crosse, WI 54601
(800) 362-9567
www.sidelines.org/loss.htm
Extensive list of loss and grief support resources.

IV ❖ Primary Care Conditions Affecting Women's Health

CHAPTER ❖ **21**

COMMON MEDICAL PROBLEMS: CARDIOVASCULAR THROUGH HEMATOLOGICAL DISORDERS

Elaine Ferrary ◆ *Rita A. Seeger Jablonski*

*C*oronary artery dis-
ease was once con-
sidered a male affliction,
although women are
now recognized to be at
equal, and in some cir-
cumstances greater, risk.
Men and women may
differ, however, in onset,
distribution, and presen-
tation of this disease.

Highlights

- Cardiovascular Disorders
- Dermatoses
- Ear, Nose, and Throat Disorders
- Endocrine Disorders
- Gastrointestinal Disorders
- Hematological Disorders

❖ INTRODUCTION

A number of disorders or medical problems are seen in practice that are clinically significant to women or are normal in any general population. It is, of course, beyond the scope of this text to touch on all medical concerns. But an effort has been made in this edition to expand and discuss subjects of interest to primary care providers. For convenience, coverage of these common concerns—listed alphabetically by organ system—has been divided into Chapters 21 and 22. In Chapter 21 cardiovascular disorders; dermatologic disorders; ear, nose, and throat disorders; endocrine disorders; gastrointestinal disorders; and hematological disorders are covered. In Chapter 22 musculoskeletal injuries, neurological disorders, ophthalmologic disorders, pulmonary disorders, and urinary tract disorders are discussed. Chapter references provide guidance in finding more in-depth information, and the index should be consulted for the location of specific problems.

The provider's level of comfort and competence in managing medical problems depends on experience, medical resources, location of practice, access to diagnostic testing, practice protocols, and scope of practice.

CARDIOVASCULAR DISORDERS

The four cardiovascular disorders considered here are coronary artery disease, hyperlipidemia, hypertension, and mitral valve prolapse.

CORONARY ARTERY DISEASE

Coronary artery disease (CAD) is caused by altered blood flow in the coronary arteries and, consequently, reduced oxygenation of the myocardium. Myocardial ischemia occurs when oxygen demand exceeds oxygen supply. The supply-demand balance may be disturbed by coronary atherosclerosis, vasospasm, thrombus formation, or cardiomyopathy.

Epidemiology

Coronary artery disease was once considered a male affliction, although women are now recognized to be at equal and, in some circumstances, greater risk. Men and women, however, may differ in the onset, distribution, and presentation of this disease (Biswas & Bastian, 2002).

The incidence of coronary artery disease is distributed throughout the population. It is the leading cause of death in women older than 50. More than 500,000 Americans die each year of heart attacks. Almost half are women. (Grady, Herrington, Bittner, et al., 2002). CAD is the most common cause of heart attacks. It is more prevalent among minorities, particularly African Americans.

Modifiable Risk Factors. Factors that may influence the development of CAD include cigarette smoking, obesity, physical inactivity, hypertension, and hyperlipidemia.

Cigarette smoking is largely responsible for cardiovascular events in premenopausal women. It increases the risk of CAD two to three times that of a nonsmoker, but the risk is reversible within a year of cessation of smoking. Smoking low-tar and low-nicotine cigarettes does not reduce the risk of cardiovascular events. With the substantial increase in the number of women smoking, the incidence of CAD is rising. Moreover, women who smoke *and* use oral contraceptives are more likely to have a heart attack (Hulley et al., 2002). In addition, the use of hormone replacement therapy by smokers may exacerbate the chance of thrombus formation.

Obesity also presents a formidable risk. Clients who are more than 30 percent overweight are more likely to develop heart disease, even if this is their only risk factor (Stampfer, Hu, Manson, Rimm & Willett, 2000).

Physical inactivity—a sedentary lifestyle—contributes to CAD by unfavorably altering serum lipid ratios.

Hypertension and hyperlipidemia and their specific contributions to risk are discussed later under Cardiac Disease.

Nonmodifiable Risk Factors. Nonmodifiable risk factors for CAD are family history, age, gender, and diabetes.

A strong family history of CAD is significant. Early sudden cardiac death of a first-degree relative warrants a more aggressive approach in controlling modifiable risk factors, even if the client is asymptomatic (Mosca, Grundy, Judelson et al., 1999).

Age and gender differences are difficult to distinguish because research studies on women and cardiovascular disease are inadequate. The average age of onset of CAD among men is between 40 and 44 years. Women tend not to develop heart problems until after menopause, most likely because of the cardioprotective effects of estrogen. After menopause the risk of CAD increases steadily. If menopause is iatrogenic (the uterus and ovaries are surgically removed), the risk of a heart attack rises more sharply than if menopause occurs naturally.

Morbidity and mortality associated with myocardial infarction are higher among women, because of the failure to identify CAD earlier in women. Anginal symptoms more likely are attributed to noncardiac causes.

Diabetes mellitus not only increases the risk of CAD but is a major predictor of mortality following a myocardial infarction.

Subjective Data

Women are likely to report chest pain (angina) as their first symptom. Men typically present with a myocardial infarction or sudden cardiac death. A thorough history includes the onset, character, location, radiation, frequency, duration, precipitating factors, relieving factors, and associated symptoms. If the client reports a clear relationship between her symptoms and physical exertion, a cardiac origin is highly suspected.

Intensity of pain does not always correlate with severity of disease (Anderson & Kessenich, 2001). Angina may be described as a minor ache or crushing chest pain. Clients may relate only associated symptoms such as dyspnea and diaphoresis with exertion. Treatment of silent ischemia is based more on objective than on subjective findings.

Objective Data

Physical Examination. May reveal nothing abnormal; however, signs of CAD may include the following:

- *General Appearance.* Obese, anxious, dyspneic.
- *Vital Signs.* High or low blood pressure, tachycardia or bradycardia, fever.
- *Skin.* Cyanosis, diaphoresis.
- *Eyes.* Arcus senilis, xanthomas, hypertensive retinopathy.
- *Neck.* Jugular venous distention, carotid bruits.
- *Lungs.* Rales, rhonchi, wheezes, or diminished breath sounds.
- *Heart.* Murmurs, gallops, rubs, clicks, irregular rhythms, displaced point of maximal impulse (PMI), heaves, and thrills.
- *Vascular System.* Absent or diminished peripheral pulses, edema, mottling.
- *Abdomen.* Hepatomegaly, bruits.

Diagnostic Tests. Laboratory testing includes a *CBC* and *renal and liver function tests to* determine underlying disease and identify risk factors.

The chest x-ray assists in differential diagnosis and in evaluating the progress of disease. It may reveal increased pulmonary markings or cardiomegaly.

Electrocardiography (ECG) permits myocardial ischemic changes to be seen in ST segment elevation or, more commonly, depression. Dysrhythmias, such as atrial fibrillation or atrial flutter, may be detected. This noninvasive test is essential to detection of myocardial ischemia; however, a normal ECG does not rule out diagnosis of infarction or ischemia. The procedure lacks specificity and sensitivity in women, particularly younger women, those with atypical chest pain and breast attenuation.

Exercise tolerance testing (ETT), a stress test, identifies the location of ischemic vessels by recording the changes that occur during exercise on an ECG. When evidence of ischemia is presented early in testing, the likelihood of multivessel involvement is increased. Approximately 40 percent of women have a false-positive reading (Hennekens, 1996; Wexler, 1991).

Nuclear perfusion studies have low false-positive rates in women when corrected for breast attenuation. Pharmacologic studies are recommended when exercise testing does not yield conclusive information or the client is deconditioned or disabled, prohibiting her from sustaining a level of exertion necessary to complete the testing. A day is usually required to complete the test.

Cardiac catheterization is the most definitive test to determine the location and extent of CAD. In experienced laboratories it is performed with low mortality (0.2 percent) or severe vascular complications (0.7 percent) (Wexler, 1991). A catheter is threaded through to the coronary vessels retrograde usually from the femoral arteries.

The client should anticipate an overnight stay and that a standard preoperative workup is done. Specific preoperative and postoperative teaching should be done by the cardiologist or designated staff member.

Echocardiography is the most sensitive, noninvasive diagnostic test used to measure cardiac size and function. It determines abnormalities in the motion of the myocardium, abnormalities in structure and ventricular function, and hypertrophy. The procedure is noninvasive. In the future, exercise echocardiograms may be more sensitive in detecting CAD than stationary echocardiograms or electrocardiograms (Hennekens, 1996; Villablanca, 1996; Wexler, 1991).

Differential Medical Diagnoses

Thoracic outlet syndrome, mitral valve prolapse, anemia, substance abuse, costochondritis, gastroesophageal reflux disorder, panic disorder.

Plan

As interventions are employed, continued surveillance of symptoms, medications, and risk factors is required.

Psychosocial Interventions. Provide anticipatory guidance about diagnostic testing and the nature of the disease. Assist clients in gaining a sense of control over the disease through risk reduction. Clients need to know the risks and benefits of all treatment options to make informed decisions about their lives and health.

Medication. Coupled with a reduction in modifiable risk factors, medication is a viable option for up to two-thirds of clients with CAD. In weighing medical against surgical intervention, the key factors are the extent and location of coronary artery occlusion.

- *Nitrates.* Nitrates may be used independently or with other medications. Nitrates are used as an antianginal agent because of their vasodilating effect.
  - *Administration.* Sublingual, topical, transdermal, and oral (long-acting or chewable tablet) forms are available. The sublingual form acts within 15 seconds and has a 15- to 30-minute duration of action. Ointments and transdermal patches may last twelve hours or longer.
  - *Side Effects.* Headaches are common. They may be relieved by changing the dosage, route of administration, or if taken with acetaminophen. Other reactions to nitrates are hypotension, dizziness, and palpitations.
  - *Contraindications.* Do not administer to clients with severe hypotension.
  - *Anticipated Outcome on Evaluation.* Anginal episodes decrease or are eliminated.
  - *Client Teaching.* Include information about all possible side effects and indications for intermittent use of nitrates as needed.
- *Aspirin.* Aspirin lowers the risk of myocardial infarctions in persons at increased risk for atherosclerosis and thrombogenesis, including persons who have had a myocardial infarction, unstable angina, or postcoronary artery bypass grafting. Aspirin inhibits platelet aggregation and prevents formation of arterial

thrombi on atherosclerotic plaques. It is recommended for men at risk for CAD or for men older than 40 with known cardiac disease; aspirin appears to have the same therapeutic benefits for women. It is considered prudent therapy for women with known cardiac disease (HSPSTF, 2002).

- *Administration.* One enteric coated 325 mg aspirin is taken daily.
- *Side Effects.* Gastrointestinal upset and bleeding.
- *Contraindications.* Do not administer to clients with gastric ulcerative disease and coagulopathies.
- *Anticipated Outcomes on Evaluation.* Progression of atherosclerotic disease slows, and the likelihood of thrombolic events decreases.
- *Client Teaching.* Include information about side effects. Aspirin needs to be used consistently to be an effective preventive measure.
- β-*Adrenergic Receptor Antagonists.* Beta blockers are indicated for hypertension and ischemic heart disease. These drugs attenuate increased blood pressure and heart rate during activity, thereby decreasing the workload of the heart. They have been shown to decrease mortality postmyocardial infarction.
  - *Administration.* The new β_1 selective agents block myocardial receptors with little effect on bronchial or smooth vascular muscle—a benefit to those with asthma or claudication.
  - *Side Effects.* Depression, impotence, peripheral vascular ischemia, and palpitations are known to occur. The beta blocker may decrease the effectiveness of other medications such as oral hyperglycemic agents.
  - *Contraindications.* Do not administer to clients with heart failure, sick sinus syndrome with atrioventricular block, bradycardia (fewer than 50 beats per minute), and asthma.
  - *Anticipated Outcomes on Evaluation.* Symptoms of angina, heart rate, and blood pressure, decrease.
  - *Client Teaching.* Plan to continue indefinitely. Review, and encourage client to report any side effects at all visits.
- *Calcium Channel Blockers.* Calcium channel blockers decrease vascular resistance, thereby increasing blood flow. They are also used for hypertension. Some calcium channel blockers are used for rate control in specific cardiac arrhythmias. Eighty percent of the dose is orally absorbed, but because of extensive hepatic metabolism, a much smaller dose reaches the systemic circulation.

- *Side Effects.* Side effects are specific to the agent and include hypotension, dizziness, constipation, headache, and peripheral edema.
- *Contraindications.* Use with caution if clients have hypotension, heart failure, and slow or altered cardiac conduction.
- *Anticipated Outcomes on Evaluation.* Episodes of angina and blood pressure decrease.
- *Client Teaching.* Make clear to the client that calcium channel blockers are more expensive than other antihypertensive medications, but are usually effective with q.d. or b.i.d. dosing and are associated with fewer side effects.

Surgical and Other Interventions. In percutaneous transluminal coronary angioplasty (PTCA), a balloon is introduced into an artery and inflated at the site of an atherosclerotic plaque. In dilating the vessel, the balloon flattens the plaque against the arterial wall, reducing its thickness. About one-third of arteries restenose. Complications include acute restenosis or vessel dissection, with the possibility of open heart surgery or death.

Coronary artery bypass grafting (CABG) is performed for select groups of clients with multivessel disease, left main coronary artery disease, or ventricular aneurysm. Generally, anginal symptoms markedly improve and improvement persists at least ten years. Surgical risks may be increased or decreased, depending on the extent of disease and the presence of other underlying medical problems at the time of surgery.

Lifestyle/Dietary Changes. Such changes can dramatically reduce morbidity and mortality. Primary prevention focuses on modifying risk factors: hypertension, hyperlipidemia, cigarette smoking, obesity, and physical inactivity (Stampfer et al., 2000). Advise the client to follow a low-cholesterol and low-fat diet (see Hyperlipidemia).

Physical activity is tailored to the individual client, considering her overall physical condition and cardiac history. Advise the client to avoid exertional activities during extreme weather conditions or after a heavy meal. The client should always carry nitroglycerin and alert the health care provider to any change in symptoms. Advise the client about cardiac rehabilitation programs, especially if she is having difficulty returning to an acceptable level of physical activity.

Cigarette smoking is a significant risk factor and should be discontinued. Involve the client in a smoking cessation program.

HYPERLIPIDEMIA

Hyperlipidemia is an increased plasma lipid concentration of cholesterol, triglycerides, or both. Water-insoluble lipids are carried in the bloodstream by lipoproteins, which are complex molecules made up partly of cholesterol and triglycerides. Lipoproteins transport both dietary and endogenous lipids from sites of absorption or synthesis to sites of storage or metabolism.

High levels of low-density lipoprotein are injurious to the vascular intima and lead to the deposition of cholesterol. This and other thrombolic events combine to form atherosclerotic plaques within the vessel, narrowing the lumen and eventually reducing blood flow to many tissues.

Classification of Lipoproteins

Four principal classes of lipoproteins have been determined (Braun & Rosenson, 2001).

- Chylomicrons are the major transporters of dietary triglycerides.
- Very low density lipoproteins (VLDLs) are responsible for the transport of endogenous triglycerides.
- Low density lipoproteins (LDLs) are the major transporter of cholesterol.
- High density lipoproteins (HDLs) collect cholesterol from the tissues to return it to the liver, thereby acquiring the pseudonym "good cholesterol."

Epidemiology

Genetic factors and lifestyle are major forces in the development of hyperlipidemia.

Risk factors are a high-fat diet, genetic predisposition, sedentary lifestyle, cigarette smoking, and underlying diseases (diabetes mellitus, hypothyroidism, chronic renal disease, liver or gastrointestinal disorders). These may all contribute to an alteration in lipid values.

Levels of LDLs and HDLs are predictors of risk (see Table 21–1). Although LDL level is a powerful predictor

TABLE 21–1. Classification of Total Cholesterol and Low Density Lipoprotein (LDL) Cholesterol

Total Cholesterol		LDL Cholesterol (mg/dL)	
		< 100	*Optimal*
< 200	Desirable	100–129	Near optimal/above optimal
200–239	Borderline High	130–159	Borderline high
≥ 240	High	160–189	High
		≥ 190	Very high

Source: NCEP (2001).

of CAD in men, HDL level appears to be a better predictor of risk for CAD in women. Even with a higher average total cholesterol and higher LDL levels, women have fewer cardiovascular events than men, possibly due to their higher HDL levels. A ratio of 4 or less is considered acceptable; a ratio of 6 or above warrants an aggressive approach. Research is almost exclusively based on men; until further studies of women are completed, it is considered clinically prudent to apply to women the same recommendations used in the care of men. Hyperlipidemia can occur in pregnant women. Treatment is usually not indicated. Follow-up at six months postpartum or at cessation of breastfeeding is recommended.

Hyperlipidemia occurs in 25 percent of the U.S. adult population.

Subjective Data

The client reports a first-degree relative with known hyperlipidemia, a family history of premature CAD, or a medical condition associated with hyperlipidemia. An extensive diet, exercise, and health belief history is key in assessing the client's current status and future teaching needs.

Objective Data

Although the physical examination may be entirely normal (see Coronary Artery Disease), physical findings that are consistent with hyperlipidemia are obesity, xanthomas, lipemia retinalis, corneal arcus, and hepatosplenomegaly.

Hyperlipidemia Screening. Diagnostic laboratory testing includes screening asymptomatic clients for hyperlipidemia every five years (see Table 21–1). It is done more often if there are additional risk factors.

The test procedure, a fasting serum lipid profile study, involves venipuncture, which is more accurate than a fingerstick. The blood sample is drawn after a minimum of eight hours of fasting. Values that classify clients as moderate to high risk are based on at least two separate studies by venipuncture, drawn two months apart. If the difference is less than 30 mg/dL, the two values are averaged. If the difference is more than 30 mg/dL, another sample is obtained and the three values are averaged.

Inform the client that she may drink water when fasting. Fasting is most important in the assessment of hypertriglyceridemia. A random (nonfasting) total cholesterol can be done as a screening measure in low-risk individuals.

The client should understand that every 1 percent decrease in a high serum cholesterol reduces her risk for coronary artery disease by 2 percent. Significantly elevated triglycerides should be treated to prevent pancreatitis.

Differential Medical Diagnoses

Diabetes mellitus; liver disease (obstructive, hepatocellular, or hepatic storage disorder), hypothyroidism, renal disease (nephrosis and renal failure), hormonal imbalance (estrogens, progestins, and androgens), hyperuricemia, acute intermittent porphyria, alcoholism.

Plan

A majority of clients with hyperlipidemia are managed by their primary care provider. Treatment must be individualized with respect to age, risk factors, clinical status, and the presence or extent of CAD (see Table 21–2).

Psychosocial Interventions. Support and encourage clients who are changing their diet and level of physical activity to reduce lipid blood levels. Clients should have realistic expectations and be given objective evidence of their efforts. If medications are indicated, reinforce the information that nonpharmacological interventions are also essential to lowering lipids. Some individuals may have a genetic predisposition to elevated serum cholesterol and, consequently, have less response to nonpharmacologic in-

TABLE 21–2. Therapeutic Approaches to LDL Cholesterol Lowering in Persons with Coronary Heart Disease (CHD) or CHD Risk Equivalents

Subcategory of LDL Cholesterol Level	LDL Cholesterol Goal	Level at Which to Initiate Dietary Therapy (TLC)	Level at Which to Initiate LDL-Lowering Drugs
≥ 130 mg/dL	< 100 mg/dL	≥ 100 mg/dL	Start drug therapy simultaneously with dietary therapy
100–129 mg/dL	< 100 mg/dL	≥ 100 mg/dL	Consider drug options*
<100 mg/dL	< 100 mg/dL	TLC & emphasize weight control and physical activity	LDL-lowering drugs not required

*Some authorities recommend use of LDL-lowering drugs in this category if an LDL cholesterol < 100 mg/dL cannot be achieved by TLC. Others prefer use of drugs that primarily modify other lipoprotein fractions, e.g., nicotinic acid and fibrate. Clinical judgment also may call for withholding drug therapy in this category.

Source: NCEP (2001).

terventions. Avoid attributing high levels to noncompliance without adequate evaluation.

Medication. Consider discontinuing medications that may adversely influence lipid levels. Medication chosen to lower lipid levels is specific to the client and the desired effect on lipid profile. Adherence to any drug regimen necessitates that the client be informed of the benefits of the drug, its potential side effects, cost, and convenience. A motivational feedback mechanism is provided by repeated serum cholesterol evaluation, which reflects the progress made.

- *Antioxidants.* Vitamin E and other antioxidants inhibit either oxidation of LDL cholesterol or its uptake into the endothelium of coronary arteries (Tribble, 1999). Reliable research data in this area are lacking. No apparent effect had been found. (Heart Outcomes Prevention Evaluation Study, 2000).
- *Psyllium.* Psyllium hydrophilic mucilloid is the active ingredient in many bulk-forming laxatives (e.g., Metamucil). It binds with cholesterol for removal via the gut. Psyllium hydrophilic mucilloid is an option for clients with mild to moderately elevated lipid levels and for whom a bulk laxative is indicated. Dosage varies with the individual: Begin with the smallest recommended dose and increase as needed. Drink sufficient fluids to avoid constipation and gas pains.
- *Bile Acid Sequestrants* (*Cholestyramine and Colestipol*). These agents reduce cholesterol by binding bile acids in the gut (National Cholesterol Education Program [NCEP], 2001).
  - *Administration.* A powder, which is mixed with a liquid, or chewable bars are taken in two to four divided doses. Usual dosage for cholestyramine is 12 to 24 g p.o.; for colestipol, 15 to 30 g.
  - *Side Effects.* Gastrointestinal complaints are common. Bile acid sequestrants may interact with fat-soluble vitamins. Triglycerides tend to increase.
  - *Contraindications.* Do not administer to pregnant women.
  - *Anticipated Outcome on Evaluation.* Both LDL and total cholesterol levels decrease.
  - *Client Teaching.* Usually lower cost than other anticholesterol agents. Require much cooperation on the client's part. Also advise the client that the preparations have a gritty quality and should be taken several hours apart from other medications.
- *Nicotinic Acid (Niacin).* Nicotinic acid reduces cholesterol by inhibiting its synthesis in the liver (NCEP, 2001).

- *Administration.* Usual drug dosage is 2 to 3 g t.i.d. in three divided doses. Start with the smallest dose and gradually increase as tolerated until the desired effect is achieved.
- *Side Effects.* Pruritus, gastrointestinal distress, and severe flushing are known side effects.
- *Contraindication.* Do not administer to clients with liver abnormalities.
- *Anticipated Outcome on Evaluation.* All lipoprotein levels are normal.
- *Client Teaching.* Advise the client that nicotinic acid is the least expensive of the medications. Flushing, a side effect, may be controlled by not drinking alcohol or warm fluids and taking one 325 mg aspirin tablet thirty minutes before the nicotinic acid, if there is no contraindication to the use of aspirin.

- *Cardiovascular disease and HRT.* A recent report from the Women's Health Initiative concluded, "Overall health risks exceeded benefits from use of combined estrogen plus progestin for an average 5.2 year follow-up among healthy post-menopausal U.S. women. All-cause mortality was not affected during the trial. The risk-benefit profile found in this trial is not consistent with the requirements for a viable intervention for primary prevention of chronic disease, and the results indicate that this regimen should not be initiated or continued for primary prevention of coronary heart disease" (WHI, 2002, p. 332).
- *Gemfibrozil (Lopid).* Gemfibrozil is a fibric acid derivative that is indicated primarily to lower plasma triglycerides. It also lowers cholesterol, but to a lesser extent, and may raise high density lipoprotein (NCEP, 2001).
  - *Administration.* Give 600 mg orally twice daily, thirty minutes prior to a meal.
  - *Side Effect.* Gastrointestinal distress is known to occur.
  - *Contraindications.* Do not administer to clients with impaired renal or hepatic function or to pregnant or breastfeeding women.
  - *Anticipated Outcome on Evaluation.* Total cholesterol decreases, with a greater effect on triglycerides.
  - *Client Teaching.* Counsel the client to be alert for drug interactions.
- *Probucol (Lorelco).* Probucol lowers serum cholesterol levels by reducing low density lipoprotein concentrations (NCEP, 2001).

- *Administration.* A 500 mg tablet is taken twice daily with meals.
- *Side Effects.* Probucol is generally well tolerated. Side effects are infrequent; however, diarrhea may occur. Ventricular arrhythmias may be a serious side effect.
- *Contraindications.* Do not administer to pregnant or breastfeeding clients. Safe use has not been established.
- *Anticipated Outcomes on Evaluation.* All cholesterol levels, including that of HDL, decrease.
- *Client Teaching.* Inform the client that a favorable decline in cholesterol levels should be seen in about two months. It is generally thought that if probucol is not effective after four months, it should be discontinued. Probucol accumulates slowly in adipose tissue and may persist six months or longer after the last dose. Advise clients to discontinue use at least six months prior to conception.

- *Hydroxymethylglutaryl Coenzyme A (HMG-CoA) Reductase Inhibitors.* These agents reduce cholesterol by inhibiting the enzyme that catalyzes the rate-limiting step in cholesterol synthesis. Slowing down the rate of cholesterol synthesis decreases the release of cholesterol into the bloodstream (NCEP, 2001).

  - *Administration.* These medications are taken once a day with the evening meal or twice daily with meals. Lovastin is usually given as 20 to 80 mg p.o. in one or two doses; Simvastatin as 40 to 80 mg p.o. in one or two doses; Pravastatin as 40 mg p.o. in one to two doses. Atorvastatin 10 to 40 mg p.o. in one dose.
  - *Side Effects.* Myalgias and elevated liver enzymes are known side effects; however, the inhibitors are generally well tolerated.
  - *Contraindication.* Consult with a physical/hepatologist when clients have known liver disease. Avoid concomittant use with potentially hepatotoxic drugs, e.g., INH.
  - *Anticipated Outcome on Evaluation.* Cholesterol levels decrease.

Surgical Intervention. None known.

Lifestyle Changes. Physical activity might include 30 minutes of aerobic exercise daily to increase HDL levels and facilitate weight loss. Cigarette smoking increases LDL levels. Encourage your client to discontinue smoking.

Dietary Interventions. Refer to the American Heart Association's progressive dietary plan for hyperlipidemia. Clients may benefit from consultation with a dietitian, especially if the diet becomes more complex with additional restrictions imposed because of other illnesses (NCEP, 2001). Dietary measures are safe and cost effective and may eliminate the need for drugs to lower cholesterol.

All family members should be involved. Meet with them collectively or at least with the primary meal provider. Emphasize the foods that can be eaten rather than those that cannot.

- *Fat* intake is reduced to 30 percent or less of the diet. A high-fat diet without cholesterol raises serum cholesterol levels by increasing bile reabsorption from the gut, which, in turn, limits the amount of cholesterol that can be excreted. Decrease saturated fats to 10 percent of caloric intake.
- *Cholesterol* is limited to no more than 300 mg per day.
- *Complex carbohydrates* include water-soluble fiber and are increased in small amounts as tolerated.
- *Weight* is maintained at ideal body weight.
- A *food diary* is recorded to target problem areas and provide feedback for the client and provider.
- A specific *food plan* is described during dietary counseling. For example, recommend mozzarella cheese made with skim milk or any dairy product with less than 1 percent fat. Recommend chicken or fish instead of beef. Offer suggestions on how to cook meat (broil, boil) to reduce fat content.

Phase II of the American Heart Association diet further restricts fat intake to 20 to 25 percent of total calories. Saturated fats are reduced to 6 to 8 percent of total fat intake and cholesterol to 150 to 200 mg per day.

Follow-Up

Ascertain whether the expectation of a 10 to 20 percent decrease in total cholesterol was reached after approximately six weeks of dietary modification. Before considering any change in the treatment plan, individuals who have no additional risk factors should continue dietary interventions for at least six months. Most medications reduce total cholesterol an average of 20 to 25 percent and triglycerides 40 to 50 percent within six weeks. Much remains to be learned concerning the management of hyperlipidemia as it relates to age and risk of CAD.

HYPERTENSION

Hypertension (HTN) is a systolic blood pressure (SBP) of 140 mm Hg or greater, a diastolic blood pressure (DBP) of 90 mm Hg or greater, or both on three separate occasions two weeks apart (see Table 21–3).

Epidemiology

Essential hypertension is idiopathic and most common. It affects approximately 50 million Americans. Risk factors are a genetic predisposition, age older than 40, minority status, alcoholism, less educated, and/or lower socioeconomic group (JNC VI, 1997). Although nicotine transiently increases blood pressure, prolonged use is not associated with an increased prevalence of hypertension. Hypertension is the leading risk factor for coronary heart disease, congestive heart failure, stroke, retinopathy, and renal disease.

Women have less hypertension before menopause, possibly due to higher levels of estrogen or lower levels of androgen or because of lower blood volume (JNC VI, 1997).

Reversible risk factors include medication, alcohol abuse, excessive dietary sodium, and obesity.

Secondary hypertension, which is uncommon, may be caused by polycystic kidneys, renovascular disease, aortic coarctation, Cushing's syndrome, and pheochromocytoma.

Subjective Data

A client with hypertension is most often asymptomatic but may complain of chest pain, headache, visual or neurological changes. She may report a family or personal medical history of hypertension, diabetes, kidney disease, hypothyroidism, cardiovascular disease, or stroke. Be alert for deviations from usual blood pressure readings or a history of elevated blood pressure. Note results and side effects of previous treatments. Identify risk factors in-

cluding recent weight gain or loss, changes in exercise or diet, increased sodium, alcohol intake, smoking or recreational drug use. Obtain a complete psychosocial history including socioeconomic status, emotional stress, coping mechanisms, and cultural habits. List all prescription and nonprescription medications that may contribute to hypertension (JNC VI, 1997).

Objective Data

Physical Examination. May include the following:

- *General.* Obesity (note pattern), pallor, sweating.
- *Fundoscopic.* Arteriovenous compression or nicking, hemorrhages, exudates, or papilledema.
- *Neck.* Thyroid abnormalities, carotid bruits, jugular/venous distention.
- *Lungs.* Wheezes, rales, or rhonchi.
- *Heart.* Murmurs, rubs, gallops, displaced PMI, regular rate and rhythm.
- *Abdomen.* Bruits, masses, hepatosplenomegaly, or enlarged kidneys.
- *Vascular.* Absent or diminished pulses.
- *Extremities.* Edema, cyanosis, clubbing.

Blood pressure findings that are abnormal are episodic elevations, discrepancies between blood pressures in contralateral arms, and decreased pressures in the lower extremities. Specific measures may be taken to ensure accurate blood pressure readings.

- Seat the client with her arm supported and positioned at the level of her heart.
- Cigarettes should not be smoked or caffeine ingested within 30 minutes of the measurement.
- Have the client rest for about 5 minutes before measuring blood pressure.
- Use appropriate cuff size. The rubber bladder should be two-thirds the size of the arm.
- Check readings in both arms. Note any discrepancies.

Diagnostic Tests. Laboratory tests include a CBC, chemistries to evaluate kidney and liver function, lipid profiles, and urinalysis. These are done to provide baseline values, for the selection and surveillance of medications, and to monitor for sequelae from hypertension.

The electrocardiogram (ECG) is used to detect left ventricular hypertrophy (LVH), the result of cardiac adaptation to increased pressure and increased afterload imposed by an elevated blood pressure. (JNC VI, 1997). Left ventricular hypertrophy is a significant independent

TABLE 21–3. Classification of Blood Pressure for Adults Age 18 and Older

Category	Systolic (mm Hg)		Diastolic (mm Hg)
Optimal	< 120	AND	< 80
Normal	< 130	AND	< 85
High-normal	130–139	OR	85–89
Hypertension			
Stage 1	140–159	OR	90–99
Stage 2	160–179	OR	100–109
Stage 3	≥ 180	OR	≥ 110

Source: JNC VI, 1997.

risk factor of cardiac dysrhythmias, congestive heart failure, and sudden death.

Differential Medical Diagnoses

Pheochromocytoma, thyroid disease, renal disease, Cushing's syndrome, primary aldosteronism, alcoholism, iatrogenic origin.

Plan

The goal of intervention is to prevent the morbidity and mortality associated with high blood pressure. The severity of hypertension, evidence of target organ damage and other risk factors for cardiovascular and cerebrovascular disease guides intervention.

Psychosocial Interventions. Involve the client in decisions concerning treatment. Acknowledge hypertension as a chronic disease that can be controlled but not cured. Contract with the client for follow-up at predetermined intervals.

Medication. Medication for moderate or severe hypertension decreases potential cardiovascular mortality and morbidity. Clients with mild hypertension benefit from medication in that it arrests the progression to a more severe condition and reduces the risk of cerebrovascular accidents. In individuals with a blood pressure persistently higher than 94 mm Hg, the benefits of drug therapy outweigh the risks (see Table 21–4) (JNC VI, 1997).

Single-dose therapies are usually a first choice to improve compliance and reduce side effects and expense. When choosing a drug, consider concomitant medical problems, e.g., beta blockers can mask hypoglycemic problems in diabetes and worsen asthma; some calcium channel blockers (nifedipine) can exacerbate migraines, even though some are used for migraine prophylaxis. Also consider race: African Americans are more likely to respond favorably when diuretics are used with calcium channel blockers (JNC VI, 1997).

- *Diuretics.* Diuretics reduce blood pressure by decreasing volume and thereby decreasing preload. They are classified by mechanism and site of action.

  Thiazides and sulfonamides are relatively contraindicated in persons with sulfa allergies. These agents may raise lithium blood levels and serum cholesterol. Concomitant administration of nonsteroidal anti-inflammatory drugs may antagonize thiazide or sulfonamide effectiveness or cause electrolyte disturbances and sexual dysfunction.

Potassium-sparing agents are used with caution with clients who are renal compromised or are using angiotensin converting enzyme inhibitors (ACEI). These agents can also potentiate the effectiveness of ACEI and calcium channel blockers.

Loop diuretics cause electrolyte disturbances. Potassium supplementation is often required.

- *Angiotensin-Converting Enzyme Inhibitors.* Angiotensin-converting enzyme (ACE) inhibitors are indicated to suppress the renin-angiotensin-aldosterone system. Structure, absorption, and duration of action differ slightly among these drugs. They are particularly effective for congestive heart failure.

  Administer ACE inhibitors once or twice daily. Although they are generally well tolerated, adverse effects may include cough (persistent and nonproductive), angioedema, hypotension, rash (most common with captopril), and hyperkalemia. Monitor renal function. Avoid potassium-containing salt substitutes (JNC VI, 1997).

- *Beta Blockers.* Beta blockers and calcium channel blockers (see Coronary Artery Disease) are also used for hypertension (see Table 21–5). Beta blockers have been shown to decrease morbidity and mortality and remain initial drugs of choice after diuretics (JNC VI, 1997).

Table 21–6 summarizes the management of care, balancing lifestyle changes and medications.

Lifestyle/Dietary Changes. Dietary modification may be an essential lifestyle change. Weight should be kept within 15 percent of desirable weight. Encourage a low-fat, low-salt diet, high in fiber. Avoid caffeine and encourage smoking cessation. Advise the client to limit alcohol intake (JNC VI, 1997).

Physical activity may include a thirty-minute aerobic exercise program at least three times a week. The program should be initiated gradually. An overall increase in physical activity is encouraged; the benefits are numerous.

- High-density lipoprotein levels increase.
- Arterial blood pressure decreases.
- Glucose intolerance improves.
- Stress decreases.

Advise the client to stop smoking. Cessation reduces the risk of coronary artery disease. The most successful strategies are those that involve both pharmacological and behavioral methods (CDC, 2001).

TABLE 21–4. Oral Antihypertensive Drugs*

Drug	Trade Name	Usual Dose Range, Total mg/day* (Frequency per Day)	Selected Side Effects and Comments*
Diuretics			Short-term: increases cholesterol and glucose levels; biochemical
(partial list)			abnormalities: decreases potassium, sodium, and magnesium levels;
			increases uric acid and calcium levels; rare: blood dyscrasias,
			photosensitivity, pancreatitis, hyponatremia
Chlorthalidone (G)†	Hygroton	12.5–50 (1)	
Hydrochlorothiazide (G)	Hydrodiuril, Microzide, Esidrix	12.5–50 (1)	
Indapamide	Lozol	1.25–5 (1)	(Less or no hypercholesterolemia)
Metolazone	Mykrox	0.5–1.0 (1)	
	Zaroxolyn	2.5–10 (1)	
Loop diuretics			
Bumetanide (G)	Bumex	0.5–4 (2–3)	(Short duration of action, no hypercalcemia)
Ethacrynic acid	Edecrin	25–100 (2–3)	(Only nonsulfonamide diuretic, ototoxicity)
Furosemide (G)	Lasix	40–240 (2–3)	(Short duration of action, no hypercalcemia)
Torsemide	Demadex	5–100 (1–2)	
Potassium-sparing agents			Hyperkalemia
Amiloride hydrochloride (G)	Midamor	5–10 (1)	
Spironolactone (G)	Aldactone	25–100 (1)	(Gynecomastia)
Triamterene (G)	Dyrenium	25–100 (1)	
Adrenergic inhibitors			
Peripheral agents			
Guanadrel	Hylorel	10–75 (2)	(Postural hypotension, diarrhea)
Guanethidine monosulfate	Ismelin	10–150 (1)	(Postural hypotension, diarrhea)
Reserpine (G)**	Serpasil	0.05–0.25 (1)	(Nasal congestion, sedation, depression, activation of peptic ulcer)
Central alpha-agonists			Sedation, dry mouth, bradycardia, withdrawal hypertension
Clonidine hydrochloride (G)	Catapres	0.2–1.2 (2–3)	(More withdrawal)
Guanabenz acetate (G)	Wytensin	8–32 (2)	
Guanfacine hydrochloride (G)	Tenex	1–3 (1)	(Less withdrawal)
Methyldopa (G)	Aldomet	500–3,000 (2)	(Hepatic and "autoimmune" disorders)
Alpha-blockers			Postural hypotension
Doxazosin mesylate	Cardura	1–16 (1)	
Prazosin hydrochloride (G)	Minipress	2–30 (2–3)	
Terazosin hydrochloride	Hytrin	1–20 (1)	
Beta-blockers			Bronchospasm, bradycardia, heart failure, may mask insulin-induced
			hypoglycemia; less serious: impaired peripheral circulation, insomnia,
			fatigue, decreased exercise tolerance, hypertriglyceridemia (except agents
			with intrinsic sympathomimetic activity)
Acebutolol§‡	Sectral	200–800 (1)	
Atenolol (G)§	Tenormin	25–100 (1–2)	
Betaxolol§	Kerlone	5–20 (1)	
Bisoprolol fumarate§	Zebeta	2.5–10 (1)	
Carteolol hydrochloride‡	Cartrol	2.5–10 (1)	
Metoprolol tartrate (G)§	Lopressor	50–300 (2)	
Metoprolol succinate§	Toprol-XL	50–300 (1)	
Nadolol (G)	Corgard	40–320 (1)	
Penbutolol sulfate‡	Levatol	10–20 (1)	
Pindolol (G)‡	Visken	10–60 (2)	
Propranolol hydrochloride (G)	Inderal	40–480 (2)	
	Inderal LA	40–480 (1)	
Timolol maleate (G)	Blocadren	20–60 (2)	
Combined alpha- and beta-blockers			Postural hypotension, bronchospasm
Carvedilol	Coreg	12.5–50 (2)	
Labetalol hydrochloride (G)	Normodyne, Trandate	200–1,200 (2)	

TABLE 21–4. (*cont.*)

Drug	Trade Name	Usual Dose Range, Total mg/day* (Frequency per Day)	Selected Side Effects and Comments*
Direct vasodilators			Headaches, fluid retention, tachycardia
Hydralazine hydrochloride (G)	Apresoline	50–300 (2)	(Lupus syndrome)
Minoxidil (G)	Loniten	5–100 (1)	(Hirsutism)
Calcium antagonists			
Nondihydropyridines			Conduction defects, worsening of systolic dysfunction, gingival hyperplasia
Diltiazem hydrochloride	Cardizem SR	120–360 (2)	(Nausea, headache)
	Cardizem CD, Dilacor XR, Tiazac	120–360 (1)	
Mibefradil dihydrochloride (T-channel calcium antagonist)	Posicor	50–100 (1)	(No worsening of systolic dysfunction; contraindicated with terfenadine [Seldane], astemizole [Hismanal], and cisapride [Propulsid])
Verapamil hydrochloride	Isoptin SR, Calan SR	90–480 (2)	(Constipation)
	Verelan, Covera HS	120–480 (1)	
Dihydropyridines			Edema of the ankle, flushing, headache, gingival hypertrophy
Amlodipine besylate	Norvasc	2.5–10 (1)	
Felodipine	Plendil	2.5–20 (1)	
Isradipine	DynaCirc	5–20 (2)	
	DynaCirc CR	5–20 (1)	
Nicardipine	Cardene SR	60–90 (2)	
Nifedipine	Procardia XL, Adalat CC	30–120 (1)	
Nisoldipine	Sular	20–60 (1)	
ACE inhibitors			Common: cough; rare: angioedema, hyperkalemia, rash, loss of taste, leukopenia
Benazepril hydrochloride	Lotensin	5–40 (1–2)	
Captopril (G)	Capoten	25–150 (2–3)	
Enalapril maleate	Vasotec	5–40 (1–2)	
Fosinopril sodium	Monopril	10–40 (1–2)	
Lisinopril	Prinivil, Zestril	5–40 (1)	
Moexipril	Univasc	7.5–15 (1–2)	
Quinapril hydrochloride	Accupril	5–80 (1–2)	
Ramipril	Altace	1.25–20 (1–2)	
Trandolapril	Mavik	1–4 (1)	
Angiotensin II receptor blockers			Angioedema (very rare), hyperkalemia
Losartan potassium	Cozaar	25–100 (1–2)	
Valsartan	Diovan	80–320 (1)	
Irbesartan	Avapro	150–300 (1)	

* These dosages may vary from those listed in the *Physicians' Desk Reference* (51st edition), which may be consulted for additional information. The listing of side effects is not all-inclusive, and side effects are for the class of drugs except where noted for individual drugs (in parentheses); clinicians are urged to refer to the package insert for a more detailed listing.

† (G) indicates generic available.

‡ Has intrinsic sympathomimetic activity.

§ Cardioselective.

** Also acts centrally.

Source: JNC VI (1997).

Biofeedback and relaxation have been demonstrated to have modest results in reducing blood pressure in selected groups and may be the most useful treatment for mild hypertension.

Follow-Up

Arrange for periodic evaluation for target organ damage and continue to reinforce the client's lifestyle modifica-

tions, educating the client that HTN is the leading cause of heart disease and stroke (JNC VI, 1997). Intervals between office visits vary and depend on the degree and lability of hypertension. Adjust medication after three to four weeks if the client's response is inadequate.

Address reasons for unresponsiveness to therapies (see Table 21–7). For clients who are following nonpharmacological therapeutic recommendations in addition to medications, a trial of step-down therapy and drug with-

TABLE 21–5. Considerations for Individualizing Antihypertensive Drug Therapy

Indication	Drug Therapy
Compelling Indications Unless Contraindicated	
Diabetes mellitus (type 1) with proteinuria	ACE I
Heart failure	ACE I, diuretics
Isolated systolic hypertension (older patients)	Diuretics (preferred), CA (long-acting DHP)
Myocardial infarction	Beta-blockers (non-ISA), ACE I (with systolic dysfunction)
May Have Favorable Effects on Comorbid Conditions[†]	
Angina	Beta-blockers, CA
Atrial tachycardia and fibrillation	Beta-blockers, CA (non-DHP)
Cyclosporine-induced hypertension (caution with the dose of cyclosporine)	CA
Diabetes mellitus (types 1 and 2) with proteinuria	ACE I (preferred), CA
Diabetes mellitus (type 2)	Low-dose diuretics
Dyslipidemia	Alpha-blockers
Essential tremor	Beta-blockers (non-CS)
Heart failure	Carvedilol, losartan potassium
Hyperthyroidism	Beta-blockers
Migraine	Beta-blockers (non-CS), CA (non-DHP)
Myocardial infarction	Diltiazem hydrochloride, verapamil hydrochloride
Osteoporosis	Thiazides
Preoperative hypertension	Beta-blockers
Prostatism (BPH)	Alpha-blockers
Renal insufficiency (caution in renovascular hypertension and creatinine ≥ 265.2 μmol/L [3 mg/dL])	ACE I
May Have Unfavorable Effects on Comorbid Conditions[†‡]	
Bronchospastic disease	Beta-blockers[§]
Depression	Beta-blockers, central alpha-agonists, reserpine[§]
Diabetes mellitus (types 1 and 2)	Beta-blockers, high-dose diuretics
Dyslipidemia	Beta-blockers (non-ISA), diuretics (high-dose)
Gout	Diuretics
2° or 3° heart block	Beta-blockers,[§] CA (non-DHP)[§]
Heart failure	Beta-blockers (except carvedilol), CA (except amlodipine besylate, felodipine)
Liver disease	Labetalol hydrochloride, methyldopa[§]
Peripheral vascular disease	Beta-blockers
Pregnancy	ACE I,[§] angiotensin II receptor blockers[§]
Renal insufficiency	Potassium-sparing agents
Renovascular disease	ACE I, angiotensin II receptor blockers

ACE I indicates angiotensin-converting enzyme inhibitors; BPH, benign prostatic hyperplasia; CA, calcium antagonists; DHP, dihydropyridine; ISA, intrinsic sympathomimetic activity; MI, myocardial infarction; and non-CS, noncardioselective.

[†] Conditions and drugs are listed in alphabetical order.

[‡] These drugs may be used with special monitoring unless contraindicated.

[§] Contraindicated.

Source: JNC VI (1997).

drawal may be considered after blood pressure has been at goal level for one year.

MITRAL VALVE PROLAPSE

Mitral valve prolapse (MVP) is a relatively benign and common disorder. Its distinguishing pathology is ventriculovalvular disproportion. The chordae tendinae, which suspend the mitral valve, are too large for the left ventricular cavity. Valve leaflets are also enlarged and thickened. The primary causative factor seems to be characteristic dysgenesis of collagenous valvular tissue (Bonow, Carabello, de Leon, Edmunds et al., 1998).

Epidemiology

Mitral valve prolapse is a genetic disorder of autosomal dominance; offspring have a 50 percent chance of being affected if one parent has the disorder. MVP occurs in several connective tissue diseases, other cardiovascular

TABLE 21–6. Risk Stratification and Treatment of Hypertensive Clients

Blood Pressure Stages (mm Hg)	Risk Group A: No risk factors, no TOD/CCD	Risk Group B: At least one risk factor, not including diabetes; no TOD/CCD	Risk Group C: TOD/CCD and/or diabetes, with or without other risk factors
High-normal (130–139/85–89)	Lifestyle modification	Lifestyle modification	Drug therapy (see Table 21–5)
Stage 1 (140–159/90–99)	Lifestyle modification, up to 12 months	Lifestyle modification, up to 12 months	Drug therapy (see Table 21–5)
Stages 2 and 3 (≥160/ ≥100)	Drug therapy (see Table 21–5)	Drug therapy (see Table 21–5)	Drug therapy (see Table 21–5)

Abbreviations: TOD = target organ damage; CCD = clinical cardiovascular disease.

Source: JNC VI, 1997.

processes, and miscellaneous muscular and thyroid abnormalities (Auten, 1996).

Studies show that MVP is the most common valvular abnormality in the United States, with about 5 percent of the general population affected (Bonow et al., 1998). Mitral valve prolapse is encountered at all ages and appears to be equally common in women and men. Prevalence varies from 2 to 40 percent, depending on the method of diagnosis (auscultation or echocardiography). The prevalence of "clinically significant" MVP is estimated to be 2 to 4 percent (Bonow et al., 1998).

Complications are mitral regurgitation, infective endocarditis, thromboembolism, and cardiac arrhythmias. They may occur, but usually are not serious and can either be prevented or treated. Sudden death is rare. The role of MVP in thromboembolic disease is less clear. It is often considered a factor in unexplained cerebral ischemic events; however, the incidence of transient ischemic attacks is quite low, at 0.02 percent. With no complications, activities and exercise are not limited.

Mitral regurgitation is caused most often by MVP, although only a very small percentage of clients with MVP progress to mitral regurgitation. Moreover, a small number within that group become hemodynamically impaired (Auten, 1996; Bonow et al., 1998).

Anxiety is not a causative factor in the development of MVP, but it can be a manifestation. Heart, hormone, and chemical disturbances may account for the symptomatology of panic disorder; however, they are not yet understood.

Subjective Data

A client with mitral valve prolapse is usually asymptomatic; however, she may report chest pain and/or palpitations. The exact etiology of pain is unknown. The chest

TABLE 21–7. Causes of Inadequate Responsiveness to Therapy

Pseudoresistance

"White-coat hypertension" or office elevations
Pseudohypertension in older patients
Use of regular cuff on very obese arm

Nonadherence to therapy

Volume overload

Excess salt intake
Progressive renal damage (nephrosclerosis)
Fluid retention from reduction of blood pressure
Inadequate diuretic therapy

Drug-related causes

Doses too low
Wrong type of diuretic
Inappropriate combinations
Rapid inactivation (e.g., hydralazine)
Drug actions and interactions
　Sympathomimetics
　Nasal decongestants
　Appetite suppressants
　Cocaine and other illicit drugs
　Caffeine
　Oral contraceptives
　Adrenal steroids
　Licorice (as may be found in chewing tobacco)
　Cyclosporine, tacrolimus
　Erythropoietin
　Antidepressants
　Nonsteroidal anti-inflammatory drugs

Associated conditions

Smoking
Increasing obesity
Sleep apnea
Insulin resistance/hyperinsulinemia
Ethanol intake of more than 1 oz (30 mL) per day
Anxiety-induced hyperventilation or panic attacks
Chronic pain
Intense vasoconstriction (arteritis)
Organic brain syndrome (e.g., memory deficit)

Source: JNC VI, 1997.

pain is atypical for angina and usually nonexertional. It may result from mechanical stress on the papillary muscle, from coronary artery spasm or embolism, left ventricular dysfunction, rate-related supply/demand imbalance, independent coronary artery disease, or extracardiac conditions. Heart palpitations are also common. Other symptoms include complaints of fast heart rate, skipped beats, lightheadedness, fatigue, weakness, dyspnea, anxiety, and postural phenomena.

Objective Data

Mitral valve prolapse is identified by means of physical examination, electrocardiogram, and echocardiogram. Laboratory tests are done to rule out other suspected medical problems.

Physical Examination. Usually normal unless MVP is associated with other conditions. Cardiac symptoms include an isolated, high-pitched, mid- to late systolic click. The client may have a late systolic murmur (late or pansystolic murmurs indicate mitral regurgitation). Chest auscultation is best done with the diaphragm over the cardiac apex. Examine the client in the supine and left lateral recumbent positions. The click is heard earlier and occupies much of systole when sitting or standing. Postural auscultation is the key to diagnosis. If the client is squatting, the click may be closer to S2. Murmur often disappears during pregnancy because of expanding blood volume and the subsequent increase in left ventricular cavity size.

Diagnostic Tests. See Coronary Artery Disease and Hypertension sections for tests done to rule out medical problems that may be associated with MVP.

Electrocardiogram abnormalities are present in up to 50 percent of clients, but do not usually account for subjective complaints.

The echocardiogram confirms the diagnosis and extent of disease. It is recommended to determine whether mitral valve leaflets have hypertrophied, which increases the risk of infective endocarditis and progression to mitral regurgitation. Obtaining an echocardiogram to confirm MVP is not universally accepted.

Differential Medical Diagnoses

Marfan's syndrome, rheumatic fever, trauma, hypertrophic cardiomyopathy, atrial septal defect, anorexia nervosa, pectus excavatum, connective tissue disorders, anxiety or depressive disorders.

Plan

Psychosocial Interventions. Educate the client about her common, benign condition. The valve functions properly, and usually no treatment is needed. Mitral valve prolapse does not appear to alter the course of pregnancy. Periodic auscultatory examinations are necessary to note any changes.

Medication. Although not usually required, medications may be prescribed.

β-*Adrenergic or calcium channel blockers* are usually effective in controlling symptoms (palpitations) (Bonow et al., 1998). Their use is described under Coronary Artery Disease.

Anxiolytic drugs are recommended **only** if there is an underlying anxiety disorder.

Anticoagulants and antiplatelet medications are a possible therapeutic intervention for those at high risk for thromboembolic disease. Their effectiveness in terms of primary prevention remains unknown.

Antimicrobial prophylaxis is recommended for clients with mitral valve prolapse **and** mitral regurgitation or those who have MVP associated with thickening and redundancy of the valve leaflets. Prophylaxis is **not** recommended for prolapse without valvular regurgitation (see Table 21–8). Prophylaxis may prevent risk of endocarditis in clients with valvular disease who must undergo procedures that may cause transient bacteremia, although bacterial endocarditis may occur despite preventive measures. Guidelines for administration have been established and are considered standard practice; however, controlled clinical trials are inadequate. Bacteremia should be considered if a client experiences unexplained malaise or fever following a surgical or dental procedure. Poor dental hygiene or periodontal infections may produce bacteremia in the absence of dental procedures.

Surgical Interventions. Valve repair or replacement is indicated for symptomatic and hemodynamically signifi-

TABLE 21–8. Recommended Prophylaxis for Dental, Oral, or Upper Respiratory Tract Procedures in Patients Who Have Mitral Valve Regurgitation[a]

Drug	Dosing Regimen
Amoxicillin[b]	3.0 g orally 1 hour before procedure; then half the dose 6 hours after initial dose
In Amoxicillin/Penicillin-Allergic Patients	
Erythromycin[c]	Erythromycin ethylsuccinate (E.E.S.) 800 mg or erythromycin stearate (Erythromycin Stearate Filmtab) 1.0 g orally 2 hours before procedure; then half the dose 6 hours after initial dose
or	
Clindamycin (Cleocin)	300 mg orally 1 hour before procedure; then half the dose 6 hours after initial dose

[a]Prolapse alone does not warrant medication.
[b]The antibiotics amoxicillin, ampicillin, and penicillin V are equally effective in vitro against beta hemolytic streptococci (the most common cause of endocarditis following dental procedures); however, amoxicillin is now recommended because it is better absorbed from the gastrointestinal tract and provides higher and more sustained serum levels.
[c]These forms of erythromycin are recommended because of more rapid and reliable absorption.

Source: Auten (1996), Bonow et al. (1998).

cant mitral regurgitation. The procedure depends on the extent and etiology of disease.

Follow-Up

Recommend follow-up in two to five years for asymptomatic clients without murmurs.

DERMATOSES

Skin problems account for many primary care visits. Rashes or lesions may appear on exposed areas of the body or on the face and may cause the client embarrassment and concern. She is likely to seek attention promptly and may expect rapid resolution. The provider needs to be a "derm detective," taking a thorough history and using observational skills. Knowing the correct term to describe the lesion and looking at the pattern of distribution often lead to the correct diagnosis (see Table 21–9).

SCALING MACULES, PATCHES, AND PLAQUES

Superficial Fungal Infections

Superficial mycotic infections of the skin are identified according to the area of the body affected. There are two main classes of organisms, Tinea and Candida. The lesions are varied in appearance, but almost all caused by Tinea have a scaly appearance. These scales may be scraped and examined for hyphae under a microscope using KOH.

Epidemiology. Tinea and candidal dermatophyte infections are common in adults and children and in hot, humid climates. Diabetics, the obese, and women who exercise to the point of profuse sweating may be especially prone to recurrent candidal infections. Exposure to infected pets, may precede ringworm (Aly, Forney, & Bayles, 2001; Hooper & Goldman, 1999; Martin & Elewski, 2002; O'Dell, 1998).

Subjective/Objective Data and Associated Findings, and Differential Diagnoses for Specific Disorders. See Table 21–10.

Diagnostic Tests. Tinea versicolor, Tinea corporis (ringworm), and *Tinea pedis* are usually diagnosed on the basis of history and characteristic appearance/distribution. Scales on the lesion may be scraped onto a slide, covered with KOH, and examined under the microscope for hyphae if diagnosis in doubt. *Tinea capitis* (scalp ring-

TABLE 21–9. Dermatologic Terminology

Lesion: general term for a single small area of affected skin
Rash: collective term for many lesions that may occur singly, in clusters, or are confluent

Primary Lesions

Macule: small flat area of color change no larger than 2 cm; usually smooth but may have fine scale
Patch: macule larger than 2 cm, usually arising from enlarging macules
Papule: small palpable mass less than 1.5 cm, usually elevated; may be skin colored or pigmented
Plaque: flat-topped palpable lesion larger than 1.5 cm; a papule that has enlarged in length and width
Nodule: papule that has enlarged in three dimensions, length, width, and depth and is larger than 1.5 cm
Wheal: pale pink slightly elevated fluid filled papule
Vesicle: fluid-filled papule; small blister
Bulla: vesicle larger than 1 cm; may represent coalescence of vesicles
Pustule: vesicle containing polymorphonuclear leukocytes; therefore, appears white; does not by itself signify infection
Purpura: microvascular disruption characterized by hemorrhage into the skin producing ecchymoses (> 3 mm) or petechiae (< 3 mm)

Secondary Lesions

Scale: loose fragments of keratin; appears on a rapidly proliferating epithelium
Crust: dried exudate that develops when the epithelium has been disrupted and plasma exudes to the surface
Erosion and Ulcer: represent epithelial and dermal disruption, respectively; may have a soft base or crust
Excoriation: scratch marks
Lichenification: thickening of skin from chronic rubbing

Using these terms along with a description of the distribution, color, and associated findings make an algorithmic approach to diagnosis possible.
Subjective Data. Key questions to ask for all common dermatoses:
   What did the rash look like when it first appeared?
   Has the rash spread?
   What past or current treatment? Results?
   Previous occurrence?
   Pruritic? Painful?
   Any other household members with similar rash?
   Recent history of new medication or cosmetic?
   Any other symptom or medical problem?

Source: Hooper & Goldman (1999), Whitmore (1999).

worm) and *Tinea unguium* (nail fungus) are diagnosed by fungus culture before treatment is begun (Aly et al., 2001; Elewski, 1999a; Hooper & Goldman, 1999; Johnson & Nunley, 2000a; Martin & Elewski, 2002; O'Dell, 1998; Rodgers & Bassler, 2001).

Plan

Psychosocial. Fungal infections may cause body image disturbance and concern regarding contagion. Nail infections may require months of treatment before resolution. Reassurance about self-limited nature of most common

TABLE 21–10. Scaling Macules, Patches, and Plaques

Diagnosis	Subjective Data	Objective Data Distribution	Differential DX
Tinea versicolor	Mildly pruritic	Pale macules that do not tan Fine scale when scraped (KOH +) Young adults *Mainly on trunk*	Vitiligo (no pigmentation) Lyme disease
Tinea corporis (ringworm)	Mildly pruritic May have cat	Annular lesion with scaly border and central clearing or scaly patches with distinct border *Exposed areas*	Psoriasis (on knees, elbows) Secondary Syphilis (on palms, soles) Pityriasis rosea (more lesions)
Tinea capitis (scalp ringworm)	Usually asymptomatic May have asymptomatic carrier in family	Scaly plaque of alopecia or broken hairs Kerion formation may occur (inflamed, boggy nodule) Cervical adenopathy Diagnosis on basis of fungal culture *Scalp*	Seborrheic dermatitis (oily scales) Impetigo (more inflamed, honey colored crust) Psoriasis
Tinea pedis (athlete's foot)	May have intense itching and burning	Scaling and fissuring of toe webs or scaling, thickening and cracking of skin of heel and sole KOH positive *Feet, toes*	Contact dermatitis (appears on dorsum of foot) Dyshidrosis (KOH neg., vesicles) Eczema, pitted keratolysis
Tinea unguium	Usually asymptomatic Often history of Tinea pedis	Thickened, yellow crumbly nails Keratin and debris under nail Diagnosis by fungal culture *Finger and toenails*	Psoriasis (pitting of nails) Candidiasis (no debris)
Pityriasis rosea	Occasional pruritis History of larger lesion preceding eruption	Fawn-colored, oval scaly macules or papules in Christmas tree pattern on back Spring and fall Young adults female more than male *Trunk distribution*	Secondary syphilis (nonpruritic on palms and soles, RPR +) T. corporis (fewer lesions)
Eczema and nummular eczema	Pruritic History of atopy (asthma, allergy)	In flare, weepy, inflamed, lichenified skin Often Dennie's lines (infraorbital fold) and nasal crease May have secondary impetigination *Distribution eczema—face, sides of neck, flexural aspects of knees, elbows, wrists* *Nummular: Backs of hands, fingers, extensor aspects of forearms, legs*	Contact dermatitis (differentiated by history and distribution) Psoriasis (silvery scales)
Seborrheic dermatitis	Pruritis in hairy areas Chronic	Yellow, grayish greasy scales in irregular patches Dandruff on scalp *Seborrheic areas of body: scalp, eyebrows, nasolabial folds, presternal and public regions*	Psoriasis (red plaques with silvery scales) Tinea capitis (positive fungal culture)
Psoriasis	May or may not be pruritic Family history First eruption 12–20 yrs old	Begins as pink macules covered by fine silver scale Enlarges to coalesce to well-demarcated plaques that are raised from the surrounding skin Pinpoint bleeding with removal of large scale (Auspitz's sign) Pitting of nails *Characteristic distribution: knees, elbows (extensor surface) scalp, lumbosacral area, and often gluteal folds*	Seborrheic dermatitis (see previous) Nummular eczema (see previous)
Cutaneous Lupus Erythematosus	Asymptomatic Onset in 40s	Red, scaly round or oval plaques 5–20mm diameter with well-defined border Scales are tacklike May result in alopecia and scarring with hypoor hyperpigmentation *Characteristic butterfly pattern on face, also on scalp, hairline, ears*	Seborrheic dermatitis (scales greasy)

Source: Goldstein et al. (2000); Hooper & Goldman (1999); Hsu, Le, & Khoshevis (2001); Lee & Simpkins (2000); Martin & Elewski (2002); Noble, Forbes, & Stamm (1998); Sontheimer & Kovalchick (1998); Weinstein & Berman (2002); Werth (2001); Whitmore (1999); Youngquist & Usatine, (2001).

dermatoses is helpful to the client. Be open to these issues.

Tinea Versicolor

Medication Administration. Topical agents comprise first-line therapies for *Tinea versicolor.* For two weeks, zinc pyrithione, econazole, ketoconazole, or selenium sulfide 2.5% shampoo to trunk, arms, and legs (to knees). Leave it in place for ten minutes and then shower off (Aly et al., 2001; Martin & Elewski, 2002). If this strategy is unrealistic, apply any imidazole cream (ketoconazole, bifonazole, clotrimazole, etc.), naftifine, ciclopirox, or terinafine to the same areas twice a day for two weeks (Aly et al., 2001; Martin & Elewski, 2002). In the case of severe *Tinea versicolor* that is unresponsive to topical treatments, oral ketoconazole 400 mg may be used.

- *Administration.* Take medication with an acidic beverage, such as orange juice or soda, then engage in a sweat-producing activity because ketoconazole is delivered in sweat to the skin. Let the perspiration air-dry and to wait 8 to 12 hours before showering or bathing. May repeat in one week or one month. If this regimen is ineffective, take ketoconazole 200 mg daily for seven days (Aly et al., 2001).
- *Adverse Effects.* Ketoconazole may cause disulfram reaction with alcohol ingestion. Other adverse effects include headache, nausea, vomiting, elevation of liver enzymes, pruritis.
- *Contraindications.* Ketoconazole can be hepatoxic. Assess for history of liver disease. Draw baseline liver enzymes.
- *Interactions.* Decreased absorption with antacids and H2 blockers. May alter levels of dilantin and increase effects of hypoglycemic agents and coumadin.

Follow-up. Advise client to call to schedule appointment if no response after three weeks of treatment. Prior to initiating another wave of treatment or using an alternative medication, verify continued presence of scales or hypahe using KOH (Aly et al., 2001). Advise client that it may take months for pigment to return to previous shade.

Using selenium sulfide, econazole, or ketoconazole lather weekly may prevent recurrences. Apply shampoo to skin for 10 minutes prior to bathing (Aly et al., 2001). Also, instruct her to avoid using products such as bath or massage oils, which can increase the risk of reinfection because of the lipophilic properties of the organism responsible for tinea versicolor (Malassezia furfur) (Goldstein, Smith, Ives, & Goldstein, 2000).

Tinea Corporis (Body Ringworm)

Plan

Medication. Topical antifungals such as Miconazole 2 percent or Clotrimazole cream, available over the counter.

- *Administration.* Advise client to apply lotion as directed on label, usually one to two times daily. Apply the cream to affected area and include a border of healthy skin 2 cm past affected areas. Continue application one week after the skin has cleared (Weinstein & Berman, 2002).
- *Adverse Effects.* Pruritic rash, irritation.
- *Contraindication.* Known sensitivity to Azole products.

Diet/Lifestyle. Advise client that household pet may be source of infection. Follow-up with veterinarian is suggested.

Follow-Up. Advise her to schedule appointment if no response to therapy after one week treatment.

Tinea Capitis (Scalp Ringworm)

Note: Organism should be identified by fungal culture before therapy is begun. Topical antifungals will not eradicate infection but twice weekly shampooing with Selenium 2.5 percent will decrease shedding of spores.

Plan

Medication. Oral griseofulvin remains the medication of choice.

- *Administration.* Griseofulvin ultramicrosize 250 mg b.i.d. for one to two months. Should be taken with meal having highest fat content to minimize GI distress and enhance absorption (Hooper & Goldman, 1999).
- *Adverse Effects.* Headache (usually resolves within a week), nausea, vomiting, rash, photosensitivity, granulocytopenia, hepatotoxicity. Draw baseline complete blood count (CBC) with differential and liver enzymes before initiation of therapy and four weeks later. Can potentiate the effects of alcohol.
- *Contraindications.* Known hypersensitivity, liver failure, porphyria. Use caution if allergic to penicillin (griseofulvin produced by *Penicillium*).
- *Expected Outcome.* It may require three months to eradicate infection.

Diet/Lifestyle. Griseofulvin has slightly metallic taste. Encourage client to maintain adequate nutrition as sense of taste may be altered. Stress importance of adherence to daily dose to prevent relapse. Advise client to avoid over-exposure to sunlight. Alcohol should be avoided during treatment. Stress importance of personal hygiene and scalp care, not sharing combs, brushes, hats, towels. Tinea capitis can be spread by asymptomatic carriers. All members of the client's household should use selenium sulfide shampoo or 2% ketoconazole shampoo three times weekly until the client is cured. The shampoos need to remain on the scalp for five minutes prior to rinsing (Aly et al., 2001; Elewski, 1999b; Goldstein et al., 2000; Martin & Elewski, 2002).

Griseofulvin has multiple drug interactions and should be prescribed carefully. Other antifungal agents with fewer side effects are also effective against tinea capitis:

- *Terbinafine.* Administer 250 mg daily for four weeks; some studies have demonstrated efficacy in two weeks. Common side effects include GI disturbances, taste disturbances, and rashes. If terbinafine will be used for more than six weeks (see tinea unguium, below), baseline liver function tests should be obtained and repeated at six-week intervals during therapy (Aly, et al., 2001; Elewski, 1999b; Goldstein et al., 2000; Hooper & Goldman, 1999; Martin & Elewski, 2002). Consult a pharmacology text for more information.
- *Itriconazole.* Administer 100 mg b.i.d. daily for four weeks. Common side effects include GI disturbances and headaches. If itriconazole will be used for more than six weeks (see tinuea unguium, below), baseline liver function tests should be obtained and repeated at six-week intervals during therapy (Aly et al. 2001; Elewski, 1999b; Goldstein et al., 2000; Hooper & Goldman, 1999; Martin & Elewski, 2002). Itriconazole interacts with multiple medications; consult a pharmacology text for more information.

Follow-Up. Evaluate after one month for response to therapy. Refer to physician or dermatologist if abnormal test results or if condition not improved or worse.

Tinea Pedis (Athlete's Foot)

Plan

Medication. Topical antifungal such as miconazole 2 percent or terbinafine (available over the counter).

- *Administration.* Apply as directed after feet are washed and dried completely. Continue to use for seven to ten days after lesions disappear. If macerated tissue between toes, advise client to apply aluminum subacetate (Domeboro) soaks for twenty

minutes two to three times a day to help dry lesions before applying miconazole.
- *Adverse Effects.* Contraindications, see Tinea Corporis.
- *Expected Outcome.* May take several weeks to eradicate infection. Advise client infection may recur. Some become chronically affected and may need systemic therapy such as griseofulyin 500 mg po daily for one month (see previous discussion), itraconazole 200 mg po b.i.d. for one week (see discussion below), terbinafine 250 mg po daily for four weeks (see previous discussion) (Aly et al., 2001; Goldstein et al., 2000; Martin & Elewski, 2002). Fluconazole is another option:
  - *Fluconazole.* Administer 150 to 200 mg once weekly for four weeks. Side effects include nausea, vomiting, diarrhea, headache, and rash. May be administered without regard to meals. If drug will be used for more than six weeks (see tinea unguium, below), baseline liver function tests should be obtained and repeated at six-week intervals during therapy (Aly et al., 2001; Elewski, 1999b; Goldstein et al., 2000; Hooper & Goldman, 1999; Martin & Elewski, 2002). Fluconazole interacts with multiple medications; consult a pharmacology text for more information.

Diet/Lifestyle. Educate client regarding conditions that lead to infection, e.g., trapped moisture between toes, going barefoot in community showers and bathing places. Advise client to wear cotton socks, change several times a day if profuse sweating of feet, dry between toes thoroughly.

Follow-Up. Evaluate response to therapy in one week. Refer to physician if no improvement or if secondary infection.

Tinea Unguium

Note: Must establish diagnosis by fungal culture before beginning treatment.

Plan

Medication. Griseofulvin and ketoconazole have been superceded by terbinafine and itraconazole, the treatments of choice (Gupta, 2000). Terbinafine is administered 250 mg once daily for six weeks (fingernail onychomycosis) or twelve weeks (toenail onychomycosis). Itraconazole can be administered in a traditional or in a "pulsed" fashion.

◆ *Administration.* Itraconazole 200 mg po daily for six weeks (fingernails) or twelve weeks (toenails); 200 mg po b.i.d. for seven days, repeat in monthly intervals for a total of two monthly doses (fingernails) or three monthly doses (toenails) (Aly et al., 2001; Kirchner, 2001; Rand, 2000).

◆ *Adverse Effects.* Nausea, vomiting, headache, rash, elevated liver enzymes.

◆ *Interactions.* Coadministration with terfenadine, astemizole, cisapride may cause serious cardiac arrhythmias and even death. Coadministration with midazolam or triazolam may potentiate sedative effects. May enhance anticoagulant effect of coumadin; may enhance hypoglycemic effect of oral hypoglycemic agents. Contraindicated for concurrent use with 3-hydroxy-3 mtheylglutaryl coenzyme A (HMG-CoA), reductase inhibitors (e.g., atorvastatin) because of the risk for rhabdomyolysis (Aly et al., 2001; Kirchner, 2001; Rodgers & Bassler, 2001).

◆ *Contraindications.* Hepatic disease, pregnancy or women at risk for pregnancy, nursing mothers.

◆ *Expected Outcome.* Mean time to complete cure ten months but may clear after three to four months. Often recurrent.

Recently, ciclopirox solution 8%, a topical nail lacquer, has been approved for the treatment of onychomycosis. The lacquer should be applied daily to the affected nail for forty-eight weeks. This treatment may be preferred if unable to tolerate the oral regimens (Gupta, 2000).

Diet/Lifestyle. Advise client to file nails daily. In clients who acquired infection from artificial nails, advise them infection may recur if artificial nails are worn again.

Toenail onychomycosis usually occurs with tinea pedis. Will need to treat tinea pedis in order to minimize reoccurrence of onychomycosis.

Follow-Up. Evaluate client after one month. Repeat liver enzyme tests. Refer to physician or dermatologist if not responding to therapy in expected time frame or if condition worsens.

PITYRIASIS ROSEA

The cause of pityriasis is unknown. Because it is generally a disease of children and young adults, does not recur, and often follows an upper respiratory infection, a viral etiology is possible. It could also be a postviral immunological reaction. (Hsu et al., 2001; Youngquist & Usatine, 2001).

Epidemiology

Most common in young adults and slightly more common in females. Usually occurs in fall or spring. There may be an association between pityriasis and familial histories of asthma and atopic dermatitis (Hooper & Goldman, 1999; Hsu et al., 2001; Youngquist & Usatine, 2001).

Subjective/Objective Data, Associated Findings, and Differential Diagnoses

See Table 21–9.

Diagnostic Tests. Pityriasis resembles the rash of secondary syphilis but is usually differentiated by distribution and lack of palm or sole involvement. An RPR titer should be drawn if diagnosis is in doubt or if client is at risk for syphilis.

Plan

Psychosocial Interventions. Reassure the client that this is a self-limited problem and is not thought to be contagious. Lesions may remain hyperpigmented in Asian, Latino, and African American clients; may persist for several weeks.

Medication. Pityriasis resolves spontaneously in one to three months without treatment. Management is mostly symptomatic; if pruritis is present, antihistamines such as diphenhydramine 25 mg to 50 mg at bedtime may reduce discomfort and promote sleep. Topical steroid creams may also eliminate the discomfort but will not reduce the duration of the disease. Use low- to mid-potency preparations (e.g., 1 percent hydrocortisone, triamcinolone 0.1 percent), depending on degree of inflammation, applied two to three times daily in thin film (see Table 21–10) (Hooper & Goldman, 1999; Hsu et al., 2001; Youngquist & Usatine, 2001).

Colloidal oatmeal baths (Aveeno) may provide relief from pruritis. Packets may be purchased without prescription for nominal cost. Advise client to mix with tepid water and soak two to three times per day for ten to fifteen minutes.

◆ *Adverse Effects.* See Table 21–10.

◆ *Contraindication.* Sensitivity to steroid cream. Use cautiously if possibility of fungal or bacterial skin lesion, if impaired circulation (may increase risk of skin ulceration).

◆ *Expected Outcome.* Advise client rash may take one to three months to clear.

Follow-Up

Advise client to call or schedule visit if rash worsens or if persists more than three months.

ATOPIC DERMATOSES: ECZEMA AND NUMMULAR ECZEMA

Atopic dermatitis is a chronic disease with exacerbations and remissions throughout the lifetime of the client. It is usually diagnosed in infancy. Its most prominent feature is uncontrolled scratching that seems to arise spontaneously. This is known as the itch-scratch cycle, the more the skin is rubbed or scratched, the more highly pruritic it becomes. Nighttime scratching to the point of excoriation of the skin can occur.

Nummular eczema appears most commonly as coin-shaped lesions on the extensor surfaces of forearms and legs. Eczema in adults affects mainly the flexural aspects of elbows, wrists and knees. The epidemiology and treatment is the same for both. See Eczema and Nummular Eczema.

Epidemiology

Most clients with eczema note flares in times of stress and fatigue. Serum IgE levels are often elevated in individuals with severe disease. They may also have asthma and/or hay fever. Nummular eczema is more common in young adult women and elderly men (Hooper & Goldman, 1999; Whitmore, 1999).

Subjective/Objective Data and Differential Diagnoses

See Table 21–10, Eczema and Nummular eczema.

Plan

Psychosocial Interventions. Stress management and helping the client get restful, restorative sleep are key. An exercise and fitness program and courses in meditation, yoga, or biofeedback may be necessary. Since this is more often than not a lifetime problem with unexplained recurrences, the client may experience a feeling of helplessness. She may also have body image concerns. Use of makeup may have to be limited. It is important to be sensitive to these issues and to provide support.

Medications. Steroid creams and/or ointments are the cornerstone of treatment. See Table 21–10 for list. Potency of steroid is determined by severity of presentation. Start with midpotency if possible but may initially require high potency topical steroid for two to three weeks twice a day, then taper to every other day, then to weekends only. As soon as inflammation subsides, have client switch to emollients, such as Eucerin or Aquaphor. Tapering steroid use is important to minimize rebound flares. See Pityriasis roseae and Table 21–10 for discussion of topical steroids.

Severe or extensive outbreak may require oral prednisone taper. Start with 40 mg, then taper down by 10 mg amounts every two to three days over a period of ten to fourteen days.

- ◆ *Administration.* Take indicated dose in A.M.
- ◆ *Adverse Effects.* Insomnia, headache, nervousness, hypertension, acne, delayed healing, thrush, fluid retention, weight gain, hyperglycemia, hypokalemia, muscle weakness.
- ◆ *Contraindications.* Presence of systemic fungal infection, known hypersensitivity to prednisone. Use with caution if GI ulceration, renal disease, hypertension, diabetes, osteoporosis, congestive heart failure, tuberculosis, glaucoma, cirrhosis of the liver, hypothyroidism, and psychotic tendencies as it may exacerbate these conditions.
- ◆ *Client Teaching.* Advise client to take in A.M. to avoid sleep disturbance, not to discontinue abruptly. Advise client on adverse effects, reassure that these are temporary and resolve after completing taper.

Acute weeping lesions may be treated with aluminum subacetate solution (Domeboro soaks) or colloidal oatmeal (Aveeno) in tepid baths or as wet dressings for ten to fifteen minutes two to three times a day. Skin is rinsed, patted dry, and topical steroid is applied after bathing or soaking.

If yellow, honey-colored crusts or pustules appear, secondary impetigination may have occurred. Antistaphylococcal medications such as dicloxacillin 250 mg q.i.d. or erythromycin 250 mg q.i.d. (if allergic to penicillin) may be prescribed for seven days.

Adverse effects of both antibiotics include nausea, vomiting, diarrhea. Contraindicated in those clients with known hypersensitivity.

Systemic antihistamines, such as hydroyzine 25 mg may help to control pruritis especially at night. It may be taken every six hours.

Adverse effects include drowsiness, dry mouth, blurred vision, constipation, and urinary retention (Clark et al., 2000).

- ◆ *Contraindications.* Known hypersensitivity. Use with caution in pregnancy and in clients with glaucoma or urinary retention.

◆ *Client Teaching.* May potentiate effects of barbiturates, alcohol, tranquilizers, or other central nervous system depressants.

Lifestyle Modifications. See prior discussion of psychosocial interventions. It may be helpful for the client to keep a symptom diary including cosmetic use, foods eaten, stressful events when she first notes flare-up to increase insight and sense of control. Modifications in skin care such as use of moisturizers or emollients such as Eucerin or Aquaphor several times a day, avoidance of prolonged hot water baths and of wool clothing next to skin are helpful. She should keep her fingernails trimmed and filed. Lowering of the thermostat in winter prevents overheating and perspiring, especially at night. Prompt showering after workouts helps eliminate irritative properties of perspiration.

Follow-Up

During flare-ups, evaluate client every week for response to therapy. Telephone contact is also helpful to provide support. Have client call at first signs of flare.

SEBORRHEIC DERMATITIS

Seborrheic dermatitis is a more localized form of chronic atopic dermatitis that is usually confined to the scalp. It may spread to the forehead and eyebrows. On the body it may appear in the groin, axillae, and the presternal region. The hallmark of seborrhea is greasy yellow or grayish scales overlying irregular reddish patches of skin. Blepharitis is a complication of seborrheic dermatitis. (See discussion in Common Ophthalmologic Problems in Chapter 22.)

Epidemiology

Genetic predisposition that begins in puberty and persists. More common in men. Flares occur in cold weather months, when the air is dry. Clients with Parkinson's disease or HIV infection may be more at risk (Johnson & Nunley, 2000a; Martin & Elewski, 2002).

Subjective Data/Objective Data/Differential Diagnoses

See Table 21–10, Seborrheic dermatitis.

Plan

Psychosocial Interventions. Due to scalp and face involvement, may be source of great distress to client. It is highly visible and often gives appearance of poor hygiene. Client will need reassurance and prompt resolution. Like eczema, condition may be exacerbated by emotional stress, food allergies, and fatigue.

Medication. Shampoo daily or every other day with products containing 2.5% selenium sulfide or 1 to 2% pyrithione zinc (such as Head & Shoulders®). The shampoo must remain on the scalp for ten minutes prior to rinsing. If flakes are difficult to remove, try applying warm olive oil or mineral oil to her scalp, allowing it to soak in for several hours, and shampooing with dishwasher liquid or tar shampoo. If the daily use of the selenium or pyrithione shampoos are damaging her hair, advise following these products with a moisturizer (Johnson & Nunley, 2000a). Advise that shampoos may cause pruritis. Topical application of low potency steroid lotion or cream in small amounts may be used on areas of marked inflammation after shampooing (see Table 21–11). Advise client to avoid fluorinated steroids on face.

Treatment of the scalp may improve affected areas of the face. On intertriginous areas, shampoos may be used but avoid greasy ointments. Advise client to avoid using ketoconazole shampoo on genital area.

Lid margins may be cleaned with baby shampoo (Johnson & Johnson) applied undiluted with a cotton swab at night.

Diet/Lifestyle. Once the seborrhea is controlled, the client may reduce the use of medicated shampoos to twice a week or as needed. Advise client that hygiene and environment play a role in exacerbations. Sweat retention tends to make it worse as well as lapses in daily shampoo routine. Stress reduction, adequate rest, nutrition, and hydration promote healthy skin and scalp.

Follow-Up

Have client telephone or schedule visit to discuss response to therapy after one to two weeks, depending on severity of presentation.

PSORIASIS

Psoriasis, like eczema, is a lifelong, chronic disease (with acute flares) whose course is unpredictable. It is characterized by red plaques that are covered with silvery or white scales. Its cause is unknown but there is mounting evidence that at least one gene on chromosome 17 is responsible for familial psoriasis (Linden & Weinstein, 1999). Immunologic factors may also play a role. Clients with psoriasis

TABLE 21–11. Topical Corticosteroids

Generic Name (Brand Name)	Potency Class	Indications and Comments
Hydrocortisone 0.5 & 1.0% cream and lotion	Low	Seborrhea, mild eczema, mild contact dermatitis Available over the counter
Desonide 0.05% (Tridesilon)	Low	As for hydrocortisone, but more efficacious, especially for lesions on face By prescription Expensive
Triamcinolone acetonide 0.1% ointment, cream, lotion (Kenalog, Aristocort)	Medium	Eczema and nummular eczema, pityriasis rosea, psoriasis, contact/allergic dermatitis, dyshydrosis Use lotion on scalp
Mometasone furoate 0.1% cream and lotion (Elocon)	Medium	Same as Triamcinolone
Fluocinolone acetonide 0.025% cream and ointment (Lidex)	Medium	Same as Triamcinolone
Betamethasone dipropionate 0.05% cream and lotion (Diprosone, Maxivate)	High	Psoriasis, cutaneous lupus erythematosis Eczema, severe contact/allergic dermatitis
Amcinonide 0.1% ointment, cream, lotion (Cyclocort)	High	Same as Betamethasone
Fluocinonide 0.05% gel, ointment, cream, and lotion (Lidex)	High	Same as Betamethasone
Clobetasol propionate 0.05% cream, ointment (Temovate)	Ultra	Limit use to two continuous weeks Cannot occlude
Halobetasol propionate 0.05% cream, ointment (Ultravate)	Ultra	Slightly more effective in psoriasis than Clobetasol Same as Clobetasol

*Note fluorinated

NOTE: Vehicle choice depends on distribution, extent, area of body, and cosmetic consideration.

Ointment: Use where additional moisturizing desired
   Use if client reports stinging with cream
   Can be occlusive, for given strength more efficacious than creams
   Can cause maceration, acne
   May not be suitable for cosmetic reasons
Cream: Usually best vehicle choice
   Mild emollient
   Can be comedogenic

Lotion: Use for hairy areas or where large areas involved
   May be drying to the skin
   Short exposure time, may rub off before absorbed
Gel: Use when drying effect desired, good for scalp

Size of dispenser usually small (15 grams) and large (60 grams). For an adult of average size, it takes 20–30 grams to cover body once. One arm is covered by about 3 grams in one application. One palm requires about 0.5 grams in one application.

Adverse effects. Topical steroids may cause local irritation, overgrowth of bacteria or fungus, acneiform eruption, hypopigmentation, striae, miliaria. Advise client to use sparingly and never on mucous membranes or in genital area. Can be systemically absorbed if not used carefully. Midpotency to high potency steroids on face can cause hypopigmentation, rosacealike rash. Striae formation in the genital-groin area can occur with fluorinated topical steroids; therefore, only hydrocortisone should be used in these areas.

Source: Clark, Queener, & Karb (2000); Hooper & Goldman (1999); Johnson & Nunley (2000a).

have an increased incidence of HLA antigens (Elder, Nair, Henseler, et al., 2001).

Epidemiology

Onset is often in young adulthood, but may also appear initially in children or older adults. It is not uncommon, and 2 percent of the U.S. population may be affected. Ten to 15 percent of clients with psoriasis may also have psoriatic arthritis with polyarticular involvement (Hooper & Goldman, 1999; Pardasani, Feldman, & Clark, 2000).

Subjective/Objective Data, Associated Findings/Differential Diagnoses

See Table 21–10, Psoriasis.

Plan

Psychosocial Interventions. Because psoriasis typically affects exposed areas of the body, it can have a huge impact psychologically. Early onset appears to have the greatest negative effect on the quality of life, impacting both social and occupational sectors.

Medication. Mid- to high potency topical steroids are most often used (see Table 21–11).

- *Administration.* Use twice daily for two to three weeks. Greater penetration may be achieved by removal of the superficial scale by soaking or by use of a keratolytic agent such as salicylic acid. (See discussion of salicylic acid use in section on warts.) Switch to lower potency steroid combined with nightly application of tar gel product such as Estar or Psorigel. Warn client that tar is messy to apply and will stain clothes and sheets.

Because topical corticosteroids do not produce long-term remission and may make psoriasis more difficult to treat in the long run, they are usually combined with other agents. One such agent is topical calcipotriene, a vitamin D$_3$ analog that is available as a cream, ointment, and solution. A multiphasic approach combining calcipotriene and a topical corticosteroid is usually best. First, the client should apply the topical steroid and calcipotriene twice daily until the plaques are flat, about four weeks. Calcipotriene is then solely applied to the lesions twice daily, saving the topical steroid for "pulse" therapy: that is, twice daily for only two days a week. Once the lesions have progressed from bright red to pink, the calcipotriene is used alone and the topical steroid is discontinued (Pardasani et al., 2000).

Calcipotriene cannot be used on the face. Side effects include skin irritation (15% of patients) and hypercalcemia if more than 100 grams of it is used weekly. Use cautiously in clients with impaired renal function or a history of kidney stones (Pardasani et al., 2000).

Oral steroids are seldom used by the primary practitioner due to frequent rebound flares and worsening of the condition. Scalp lesions may be treated with tar shampoos (Neutrogena T/Gel) used daily or 2 percent ketoconazole (Nizoral) shampoo by prescription used twice weekly.

If psoriasis affects more than 30 percent of the body, refer to a dermatologist for light therapy with UVB three times a week for PUVA (psoralen plus UVA). PUVA may increase the risk of cataract formation and skin cancer.

Other therapies used by dermatologists include methotrexate, cyclosporine, and synthetic retinoids. Refer to pharmacology text for further information on these agents. (Lebwohl, Drake, Menter, et al., 2001; Pardasani et al., 2000).

Oral antihistamines at bedtime such as hydroxyzine (Atarax) 25 mg may be helpful if pruritis is severe or interferes with rest.

- *Expected Outcome.* Advise client psoriasis is a chronic condition with periods of flare and remission.

Diet/Lifestyle. Some clients may find exposure to sunlight is beneficial but warn them about harmful effects of prolonged exposure such as skin cancer and premature aging of the skin. Sunscreen should always be worn. Advise client to try to avoid trauma to affected areas and to resist rubbing and scratching in order to avoid secondary infection. Arthritis associated with psoriasis often improves with successful skin treatment.

Daily use of emollients may help prevent flares. Avoid emollients containing lactic acid or alpha-hydroxy acids because they can be irritating (Pardasani et al., 2000).

Follow-Up

Follow weekly during flares. If client referred to dermatologist, request treatment plan to ensure continuity of care.

CUTANEOUS LUPUS ERYTHEMATOSUS (CLE)

Cutaneous lupus erythematosus is an umbrella term that refers to fifteen different clinical manifestations of lupus erythematosus (see Chapter 22). Some of the skin conditions represent a limited presentation of systemic lupus (SE), while others are associated with greater systemic involvement. Lupus-like lesions may also occur in the absence of systemic disease as a side effect of medications such as penicillamine, glyburide, calcium channel blockers, and thiazide diuretics (Sontheimer & Kovalchick, 1998; Werth, 2001).

There are three categories of cutaneous lupus erythematosus (CLE): acute cutaneous lupus erythematosus, subacute cutaneous lupus erythematosus, and chronic cutaneous lupus erythematosus. Acute cutaneous lupus erythematosus is the "butterfly rash" or malar rash commonly associated with lupus erythematosus, although the macular rashes may appear on sun-exposed areas of the body: V-area of the neck, forearms and calfs, and trunk (Sontheimer & Kovalchick, 1998). Most clients with acute cutaneous lupus erythematosus have concurrent symptoms of systemic lupus erythematosus. Subacute cutaneous lupus erythematosus presents with nonscarring, well-defined, red annular lesions, red scaly plaques, or a papularsquamous rash (Hsu et al., 2001). Ten percent of clients with acute cutaneous lupus erythematosus proceed to develop severe forms of systemic lupus erythematosus, often with kidney and central nervous system involvement (Sontheimer & Kovalchick, 1998). Chronic cutaneous lupus erythematosus comprises several chronic skin diseases specific to lupus erythematosus. The most commonly seen subcategory of chronic cutaneous lupus erythematosus is discoid lupus erythematosus. Localized discoid lupus erythematosus presents as lesions on the face and scalp that cause scarring. Between 25 and 40 percent of clients experience spontaneous remission and only 5 percent of afflicted persons will develop full-blown systemic lupus erythematosus (Werth, 2001). If the scarring lesions are not limited to the head and scalp, then the woman has generalized discoid lupus erythematosus and her risk of progressing to full-blown systemic erythematosus is greater (Sontheimer & Kovalchick, 1998).

Epidemiology

CLE first appears in young adults with equal frequency in men and women. A familial pattern has been observed. It is a lifelong disease with exacerbations occurring after sun exposure (Sontheimer & Kovalchick, 1998; Werth, 2001).

Subjective/Objective Data/Associated Signs/Differential Diagnosis

See Table 21–10, Discoid lupus.

Plan

Clients should be referred to the dermatologist for biopsy. The examination should include a substantive history, CBC, sedimentation rate, ANA, and urinalysis.

Psychosocial Interventions. Discoid lupus can cause scarring, patchy alopecia, and loss of pigment (especially in darker complexioned individuals). The cosmetic results can be devastating. Aggressive and early treatment may help avoid scarring and permanent alopecia. Be supportive and alert to the need for psychological counseling.

Medications. High-potency topical steroids are the initial treatment (see Table 21–11). As the skin lesions improve, titrate the potency of the topical steroids downward until she is using a low-potency preparation (Werth, 2001). Dermatologist may inject triamcinolone 2.5 to 10 mg/ml once a month into lesions before advancing to systemic medications such as antimalarials.

- *Expected Outcome.* Lesions usually respond to triamcinolone injection.
- *Client Teaching.* Client should be aware of medications that can increase sensitivity to sunlight including doxycycline, thiazides, and piroxicam.
- *Lifestyle.* The client should avoid outdoor activities during times of the day when sunlight is strongest (10 A.M.–3 P.M.). Advise use of sunscreen with high SPF always. Protective clothing should be worn.

Follow-Up

Request visit notes and treatment plan from dermatologist. Some clients may be managed by primary care provider after initial referral.

VESICULAR DERMATOSES

Contact Dermatitis

Contact dermatoses can be classified into two main types: irritant and allergic. Eighty percent are due to exposure to common universal irritants, such as soap, solvents, and detergents. The most common contact allergens include poison ivy, poison oak, nickel, latex, hair dye, topical medications, perfumes, cosmetics, and adhesive tape. Allergy to an antibiotic may cause dermatitis. The presentation of contact dermatoses may be acute as in poison ivy or subacute if repeated exposure has occurred and sensitization has developed over time.

Epidemiology. The elderly may be more prone to contact dermatitis due to thinning of the skin and loss of protective moisture. Certain occupations, especially those requiring contact with irritants and allergens cited previously, are at increased risk (Hooper & Goldman, 1999; Whitmore, 1999).

Subjective/Objective Data, Associated Features, Differential Diagnosis. See Table 21–12, Contact or allergic dermatitis.

Plan. The first step in treatment is to remove the offending agent. Client may have to be referred to dermatologist for patch testing if diagnosis of agent unclear.

TABLE 21–12. Vesicular Dermatoses

Diagnosis	Subjective Data	Objective Data Distribution	Differential DX
Contact or allergic dermatitis	Pruritic Burning History of trigger	Weeping, encrusted vesicles and bullae in acute stage May have linear streaking pattern *Distribution asymmetric and pattern may be diagnostic* *Look for site of contact*	Impetigo (positive culture) Scabies (location, no weeping)
Scabies	Pruritis especially at night History of contagion, overcrowded living	Excoriations and vesiculopapular lesions and burrows *Distribution is diagnostic; webs of fingers. toes; heels of palms, buttocks, breasts, elbows, axillae* *Rarely on face* *Early in course lesions isolated*	Eczema (distribution, scaling, history)
Herpes simplex labialis	Burning, tingling often precedes eruption Recurrent Triggered by stress, sunlight	Small grouped vesicles on erythematous base Blisters fragile and may present as erosion *Distribution: vermillion border of lip, rarely in mouth*	Aphthous ulcers (ulcers only on oral mucosa or gingiva)
Herpes zoster	Very painful Usually not recurrent	Grouped, tense vesicles in linear pattern *Distribution: typically only face or trunk spreading over 1–2 dermatomes*	Poison ivy, oak (vesicles confluent not grouped)
Dyshidrosis	Very pruritic Recurrent Triggered by stress Common in young adults	Tapioca vesicles 1–2 mm that may coalesce to form blisters that dry and become scaly or fissured *Distribution is characteristic: palms, fingers, soles of feet*	Tinea pedis (between toes) Secondary syphilis (+RPR, not vesicular) HSV if immunocompromised

Source: Callahan, Adal, & Tomecki (2000); Elgart (2002); Hooper & Goldman (1999); McCrary, Severson, & Tyring (1999); Schmader (2001); Stankus, Dlugopolski, & Packer (2000); Venna, Fleischer, & Feldman (2001); Whitley & Gnann (1999); Yeung-Yue, Brentjens, Lee, & Tyring (2002).

Psychosocial Interventions. This is usually a self-limited problem, which is resolved in two to three weeks once the offending agent is removed. Practitioner should be aware, however, that removal of the offender may cause distress, by necessitating a change in lifestyle, occupation, or grooming.

Medications. If lesions are weeping, apply wet dressings of Burow's solution (5% aluminum acetate solution) or a 1:10 dilution of vinegar and water for 20 to 30 minutes every four to six hours. Pruritic and inflammatory lesions respond well to topical steroids. If the lesion is on the face or in intertriginous areas, use midpotency steroids for no more than two weeks. If the lesion is on the remainder of the body, use a high-potency topical steroid for no more than two weeks. Ointments are more soothing than creams but also a little messier. If the client is experiencing an acute, severe reaction with extensive skin involvement, she may require a single intramuscular injection of triamcinolone 40 mg and betamethasone 6 mg

or a three-week course of systemic steroids such as prednisone: 60 mg every morning for one week, 40 mg every morning for the second week, and then 20 mg every morning for the third week (Hooper & Goldman, 1999).

Oral antihistamines such as hydroxyzine or diphenhydramine 25 to 50 mg by mouth three to four times daily are effective against pruritis. Since these agents are sedating, the woman may opt to take them at bedtime or to use a nonsedating antihistamine such as loratadine or cetirizine 10 mg orally once a day (Hooper & Goldman, 1999).

- ◆ *Expected Outcome.* Usually resolves in two to three weeks.
- ◆ *Lifestyle.* As noted, may require client to change or modify work, grooming, or hobby, depending on offending agent. Prevention is key.

Follow-Up. Evaluate client after one week of treatment for response. Refer to dermatologist if not responding to treatment or if patch testing indicated.

Scabies

Scabies is an intensely pruritic dermatitis caused by infestation with the mite Sarcoptes scabei. The female mite burrows under the skin and deposits eggs, which hatch and mature over a three-week incubation period, causing intense pruritis. It can be passed on by person-to-person contact or through bedding and clothes. It spreads on the skin by fingernail contamination.

Epidemiology. All ages affected and all socioeconomic groups. Outbreaks occur in nursing homes and hospitals (Venna et al., 2001).

Subjective/Objective Data/Differential Diagnoses. See Table 21–12, Scabies.

Diagnostic Tests. Usually diagnosed on basis of history and appearance of burrows in characteristic locations, webs of fingers, genitalia. Burrows can be opened with scalpel blade at the end or dark point, and mite can be placed on slide and examined under oil immersion for confirmation.

Plan

Psychosocial Interventions. May cause embarrassment to client due to concern over hygiene. Client education important concerning mode of transmission, occurrence in all socioeconomic groups.

Advise her that partner may be infected (common site is penile shaft and glans) and should be treated.

Medication. Permethrin Cream (Elimite) 5 percent. Applied neck to toes, with special care to include webs of fingers and toes, axillary, gluteal folds, under breasts. Advise client not to wash hands after application, should be left on overnight eight to twelve hours then rinsed. Single application is usually effective.

- ◆ *Adverse Effects.* Usually mild stinging, pruritis.
- ◆ *Contraindications.* Known sensitivity to permethrin or chrysanthemums.
- ◆ *Expected Outcome.* Single application usually effective if applied thoroughly and as directed. Pruritis may persist especially if atopic history, but client is no longer contagious after 24 hours of treatment completion. Topical low- to midpotency steroid cream may be used after treatment if inflammation and pruritis persist. Oral antihistamines such as 25 mg hydroxyzine (Atarax) taken at bedtime may relieve pruritis (see Table 21–11).

Lifestyle Modification. Instruct client to wash all bedding, clothes, and towels in hot soapy water and dry on hottest dryer setting. Nonwashable items may be placed in airtight plastic bag for two weeks or sent to dry cleaner. Advise client of possibility of reinfection if partner is not treated. Advise her she may spread infestation to others up to 24 hours after completion of treatment. No special attention is needed for furniture or inanimate objects.

Follow-Up. Advise client to call to schedule visit if treatment is not effective.

Herpes Simplex

Herpes simplex (cold sore or herpes labialis) is a recurrent infection caused by the virus Herpesvirus hominis. It appears as tightly clustered vesicles on the vermillion border of the lips, but may appear on other areas of the face. The blisters are fragile, and most common presentation is a secondary erosion that forms a crust. Following the initial infection, the virus remains dormant in the dorsal root ganglia and reactivates during times of stress, trauma, head colds, fever, and exposure to sunlight. The first episode may be asymptomatic.

Epidemiology. Herpes simplex infection is transmitted by exposure to a clinically infected person, an asymptomatic virus shedder, or reactivation of a latent infection. Appearance of the vesicle occurs three to five days after exposure and lasts five to ten days. Contagion is possible during the first few days of vesicle appearance. Vesicles usually appear in the same site with recurrent infections. Lesions may not clear in immunocompromised individuals. (Hooper & Goldman, 1999; Yeung-Yue et al., 2002).

Subjective/Objective Data/Differential Diagnoses. See Table 21–12, Herpes simplex.

Diagnostic Tests. Usually diagnosed on basis of prior history but can be confirmed by opening vesicle dome with small needle, swabbing fluid exudate with sterile swab, and sending for viral culture.

Plan

Psychosocial Interventions. Client may be concerned about appearance and about contagion. Discuss importance of frequent handwashing to prevent autoinoculation and refraining from oral sex. Advise her that lesion usually resolves in a week. Be sensitive to issues of possible sexual transmission and address them accordingly. Client education very important to clear up misconceptions between Type I and Type II Herpes. See discussion of HSV in chapter on Vaginitis and Sexually Transmitted Disease.

Medication. Orolabial herpes responds better to penciclovir cream 1% every two hours for four days. Acyclovir is an older drug that was the first used to treat herpes simplex outbreaks: 200 mg five times a day for ten days. This antiviral reduced the duration of the symptoms and viral shedding. Newer drugs include famciclovir, 250 mg b.i.d. for five days or valacyclovir 400 mg three times a day for seven to ten days (Hooper & Goldman, 1999; Yeung-Yue et al., 2002). Benefits are more modest for recurring episodes and treatment must be initiated at the earliest sign of a lesion.

Warm compresses may be applied to lesions for comfort and removal of exudate. Advise client to discard after use to prevent spread of virus. Topical over-the-counter preparations such as Blistex may be beneficial to keep lesion moist and prevent painful cracking and fissuring.

Lifestyle. Advise client to apply sunscreen before exposure to sunlight. May also apply warm, moist cloths, but advise client these may contain virus and should not be handled by other household members. Careful and frequent handwashing is the key to prevent spreading to vulnerable contacts such as the elderly and infants.

Follow-Up. Advise client to call to schedule visit if not cleared in seven to ten days.

Herpes Zoster

Shingles or herpes zoster is a painful vesicular eruption along a dermatome. It is caused by reactivation of the varicella-zoster virus whose first appearance causes chicken pox.

Epidemiology. In younger adults, thoracic dermatomes are most often affected. In older adults, the area of distribution of the trigeminal nerve is frequently involved. If more than two dermatomes are affected, individual may be immunocompromised.

Postherpetic neuralgia is an excruciatingly painful complication, especially if the trigeminal nerve is involved. The infection may also spread to the eye and cause a dendritic pattern conjunctivitis. Disseminated zoster in immunocompromised individuals may be life threatening. (Lee & Simpkins, 2000; Schmader, 2001).

Subjective/Objective Data/Differential Diagnoses. See Table 21–12, Herpes zoster.

Diagnostic Tests. History and appearance are usually diagnostic, but a viral culture will confirm diagnosis. (See previous discussion on herpes simplex for method of culture.) Confirmation by culture is especially important if

vesicles cross several dermatomes. If this is the case and the culture is positive for herpes zoster, client should be evaluated for immunocompromise.

Plan. Refer immediately to ophthalmologist if eye appears to be involved. Refer to physician if appears to be disseminated, involves more than two dermatomes, or appears on face or scalp.

Psychosocial Interventions. Facial appearance may cause body image disturbance. Reassure client that infection usually resolves in two to three weeks and does not recur (unless immunocompromised).

Medication. Oral Acyclovir 800 mg five times a day for seven days if started within the first 72 hours may accelerate clearing and reduce pain. (See discussion of acyclovir in chapter on Vaginitis and Sexually Transmitted Disease.) Valacyclovir 1 gram orally three times daily for 7 days and famciclovir 500 mg by mouth three times daily for 7 days are also effective, but must be started within 72 hours of the appearance of the zoster rash (Lee & Simpkins, 2000; Schmader, 2001; Stankus et al., 2000).

No method of treatment has been effective in reducing incidence of postherpetic neuralgia. Clients 60 years old and older and immunocompromised clients are at greatest risk for this painful condition (Lee & Simpkins, 2000).

Colloidal oatmeal soaks (Aveeno) or calamine lotion may be soothing to the skin.

Follow-Up. Evaluate client in one week for response. Refer to physician immediately if condition does not improve.

DYSHIDROSIS (DYSHIDROTIC ECZEMA)

Dyshidrosis or pompholyx is a very common eczematous dermatitis of the hands and feet. It has the characteristic appearance of tapioca grains on the sides of the fingers. It is intensely pruritic.

Epidemiology

First appearance is usually in young adulthood and in times of stress. Its course and recurrence is unpredictable, but episodes tend to decrease in late adulthood. Often associated with atopy and nickel allergy (Hooper & Goldman, 1999).

Subjective/Objective Data/Differential Diagnoses

See Table 21–12, Dyshidrosis.

Diagnostic Tests. Diagnosis is usually made on the basis of history and characteristic appearance. Because of its appearance on palms and soles, an RPR to rule out secondary syphillis is suggested. May coexist with tinea pedis (athlete's foot) so KOH prep may be indicated.

Plan

Psychosocial Interventions. Clients who internalize stress to a great degree or who are obsessive-compulsive may need referral for psychological counseling. Fissuring and chapping of the skin may be disfiguring. Advise client prevention of flares is key. See lifestyle measures following.

Medication. Mid- to high-potency steroid cream or ointment may be helpful to decrease pruritis and to treat peeling and fissuring, which occur after vesicular stage. If weepy and eczematous, advise application of cool, moist compresses or Burow's soaks (Domeboro) twice a day for fifteen minutes to dry, debride, and reduce swelling before application of topical steroid (see Table 21–11). Oral steroids are generally not used because of chronicity of condition.

Advise client that dyshidrosis may not respond well to topical steroids, except for relief of pruritis and inflammation. Acute flares usually resolve within two to three weeks.

Lifestyle. Avoiding irritants is the key to preventing flares. Advise client to wear cotton gloves inside latex or plastic gloves when hands are immersed in water. Always use hand cream after washing hands, especially those creams containing emollients, such as Eucerin and Aquaphor.

Follow-Up

Evaluate client after seven to ten days of therapy for response.

PUSTULAR AND NODULAR DERMATOSES

Acne Vulgaris

Acne is a common skin condition under the influence of hormonal and genetic factors. It usually starts with stimulation of the sebaceous glands by androgen; therefore, its appearance coincides with puberty. Sebaceous glands in-

crease in size, and output of sebum rises to a point where plugging of the follicle occurs.

Bacteria, mainly *Propionibacterium* acnes, causes breakdown of the sebum, disruption of the follicle wall into the dermis, and subsequent inflammation (Johnson & Nunley, 2000b; Thiboutot, 2000).

Epidemiology. First appears in mid- to late adolescence and usually wanes in severity in 20s but can persist in women into their 40s. Begins with oily skin and plugged follicles known as whiteheads (closed comedones) and blackheads (open comedones) over the nose and forehead. The sebum inside the plugged duct may cause irritation to adjacent skin and produce inflammatory lesions, nodules, and pustules. Severe cystic acne is more common in males and is rarely found in women. Women often find acne worsens just before menses and may improve (or become worse) with pregnancy. Its course during a lifetime is unpredictable but appearance of cysts and family history of scarring are bad prognosticators (Johnson & Nunley, 2000b; Thiboutot, 2000).

Subjective/Objective Data/Differential Diagnoses. See Table 21–13, Acne vulgaris.

Diagnostic Tests. Diagnosis is made on basis of history and appearance. Pustular lesions resistant to treatment may have to have exudate sent for culture and sensitivity.

Plan

Psychosocial Interventions. Acne is an overwhelming concern to adolescents and young adults. Depending on its severity, it can lead to depression and social isolation. The practitioner must be alert to these concerns and anticipate any need for psychological counseling. Be supportive of appropriate coping mechanisms (Johnson & Nunley, 2000b; Thiboutot, 2000).

Medications. Treatment is directed to predominant type of lesion. The aim is to prevent scarring. Be sure to ask the client about efficacy of past and present treatments. Advise her to avoid astringents unless skin is very oily and use only on oily spots.

Choice of vehicle for topical agents depends on appearance of skin. Creams and lotions moisturize, but creams are heavier and may be more appropriate for very dry or irritated skin. Gels and solutions are alcohol-based and tend to dry the skin. Client preference should also be taken into consideration.

For the comedonal stage, over-the-counter products that contain salicylic acid (Stridex), resorcinol, and/or sulfur (Sulforcin), benzoyl peroxide (Fostex, Clearasil

TABLE 21–13. Pustular and Nodular Dermatoses

Diagnosis	Subjective Data	Objective Data Distribution	Differential DX
Acne vulgaris	Usually onset at puberty May have mild pain, itching May have history of topical or oral steroid use	Inflammatory, open and closed comedones, papules and pustules nodules, and cysts with scarring but hallmark is comedone *Distribution: face, neck, upper back, chest, shoulders*	Folliculitis (hairy areas, rare on face)
Rosacea	Middle-aged onset History of flushing, burning, esp. with hot food and drink	Inflammatory papules, flushing, telangiectases Comedones absent Often associated with seborrhea and blepharitis *Distribution: only on face*	Acne vulgaris (comedones prominent)
Impetigo	Pruritis	Pustules (may have macules and vesicles also) Honey-colored crust When crust removed, leaves denuded area *Distribution: often on face*	Contact dermatitis (trigger, linear pattern)
Folliculitis	Itching and burning History of hot tub use, diabetes, excessive sweating	Pustules at base of hair follicle May have erythema of surrounding skin *Distribution: hairy areas of body*	Acne (see above) Impetigo (see above) Pseudofolliculitis (pustules at side not in follicle, caused by ingrown hair)
Furuncles and carbuncles	Painful Common in diabetics, obese with oily skin, staph carriers	Abscess of hair follicle with enlarging, conical shape May coalesce to form carbuncle Becomes flocculent with purulent discharge *Distribution: most common sites are hairy areas exposed to irritation, friction, moisture as face, neck, axillae, buttocks, groin, upper back*	Inflamed epidermal cyst (history of cyst, cheesy exudate) Acne (not in follicle)
Warts	No symptoms unless on sole of foot (painful)	Flesh-colored papule or nodule 1–10 mm that may form mosaic Surface is rough, verrucated (sawtoothed), or flat May be pedunculated or have cauliflowerlike appearance Plantar warts resemble corns or calluses *Distribution: anywhere on body but commonly on hands, face, neck, upper trunk, soles of feet, genital area*	Squamous cell cancer (biopsy always if in doubt)

Source: Elgart (2002); Higgins & Du Vivier (1999); Hooper & Goldman (1999); Johnson & Nunley (2000b); O'Dell (1998); Rhody (2000); Thiboutot (2000).

Maximum Strength) are fairly effective if used on a regular basis. Alpha-hydroxy acids loosen follicular plugging.

♦ *Administration.* Dab directly on individual lesions twice daily after washing and drying skin.
♦ *Adverse Effects.* May sting or burn.

The most effective agent is topical tretinoin (Retin-A) because it unplugs comedones and prevents new ones from forming. It is considered appropriate for almost all acne.

♦ *Administration.* Start with lowest concentration 0.025 percent gel or cream applied once daily at bedtime after washing and drying skin to remove dirt and makeup. Choice of vehicle depends on whether client's skin is dry (cream preferred) or oily (gel is drying). May be used every other day if used in combination with antibiotic (see following).
♦ *Adverse Effects.* Include burning, peeling, and redness.
♦ *Contraindications.* Include known sensitivity to Vitamin A/retinoic acid.
♦ *Client Teaching.* Warn client to avoid contact with eyes and mucous membranes. Apply sparingly, total amount used should be equivalent to size of one or two peas. Do not dot on lesions but lightly spread on skin. Advise her it may initially cause exacerbation of inflammatory lesions seven to ten days after starting but resolves over several weeks. Avoid prolonged exposure to sunlight and always wear sunscreen SPF 15 or higher. Concentration can be increased if needed to 0.05 percent or 0.1 percent gel or cream.

If client is able to tolerate, benzoyl peroxide can be used in the morning and tretinoin at night. Benzoyl peroxide (concentrations 2.5% gel and liquid, 5% and 10% gel, liquid and cream) is effective against *Propionibacterium* acnes and inflammation, and tretinoin speeds cell turnover and prevents new comedones.

- *Administration.* Advise her to start with application of medications on alternate nights until she has adjusted to irritating effects of each, then proceed to use of benzoyl peroxide in morning and tretinoin at night.
- *Adverse Effects.* Local stinging and burning.
- *Contraindications.* Known sensitivity to either agent.
- *Client Teaching.* Avoid eyes, mouth, angles of nose, mucous membranes. Wash hands after using each.

This can be a very effective treatment and can result in dramatic clearing after six to eight weeks (Hooper & Goldman, 1999; Thiboutot, 2000).

Topical antibiotics such as clindamycin (Cleocin T) available 10 mg/ml as gel, lotion, or cream and erythromycin (A/T/S, Erycette) 2% gel, ointment, or solution may be used in combination with tretinoin.

- *Administration.* Antibiotic is applied twice a day and tretinoin at night. When used simultaneously, apply antibiotic first, allow to dry, then apply tretinoin.
- *Adverse Effects.* Local irritation, stinging, burning.
- *Contraindication.* Known sensitivity to ingredients.
- *Client Teaching.* See aforementioned. If rash appears, discontinue at once and call provider.

    In more difficult cases, a benzoyl peroxide-erythromycin gel combination (Erythromycin/BP gel) can be used in the morning with tretinoin at night. Initially, start using each on alternating nights until adjustment to irritating effects. Contraindication is known sensitivity to any ingredients.
- *Expected Outcome.* Advise client it may take at least four weeks to achieve desirable results.

If papules and pustules predominate and there is scarring, consider adding an oral antibiotic, such as erythromycin 250 mg q.i.d., tetracycline 500 mg po b.i.d., or minocycline 100 mg b.i.d. Minocycline is the least photosensitizing of the tetracyclines, is somewhat more effective than tetracycline, and can be taken with food (Johnson & Nunley, 2000b; Thiboutot, 2000).

- *Adverse Effects.* Include lightheadedness, change in skin pigmentation if taken over long periods of time, development of vaginal yeast infection.

- *Contraindications.* Known sensitivity to tetracyclines and pregnancy (teratogenic) (Johnson & Nunley, 2000b; Thiboutot, 2000).

Topical antibiotic preparations may be used such as erythromycin gel or clindamycin (Cleocin T) but be aware that *Propionibacterium* acnes can develop resistance to both these preparations. Use erythromycin gel in combination with benzoyl peroxide as discussed previously (Johnson & Nunley, 2000b; Thiboutot, 2000).

If acne does not respond to any of the aforementioned therapies, the client may be a candidate for isotretinoin. Isotretinoin is administered orally, 2 mg/kg/day for twenty weeks. Side effects are numerous and include chelitis, raised liver enzymes and lipid levels, photosensitivity, joint pain, visual changes, and severe headaches. *Because of its teratogenicity, extreme care must be taken if used by clients of childbearing age.* The client should have a negative pregnancy test on record and begin taking the isotretinoin on the first day of menses. Advise her to use two forms of birth control (Hooper & Goldman, 1999; Johnson & Nunley, 2000b).

Note: If client is taking oral contraceptives, switch her to a lower androgen formulation. The U.S. Food and Drug Administration (FDA) labels Ortho Tri-Cyclen, a triphasic combination of norgestimate and ethinyl estradiol, for the treatment of acne in adolescent girls and women (Johnson & Nunley, 2000b).

Diet/Lifestyle. There is no evidence that chocolate or fatty foods make acne worse. Nor does vigorous scrubbing or sun tanning make it better. Gentle cleansers, such as Dove, Basis, or Neutrogena are recommended. Advise client never to pick or squeeze pimples; this can lead to scarring. Review current cosmetic products. Changing to oil-free makeup can lessen comedone formation. Reassure client best results come from adherence to agreed upon treatment plan and patience, may take four to six weeks to see improvement.

Follow-Up. Refer clients with severe or cystic acne to dermatologist. After one week of treatment plan, evaluate client, then again at one month.

Rosacea

Rosacea is a chronic skin condition that develops in middle age. It may progress through four stages:

Stage I: Prerosacea—transient flushing and erythema of the face and neck
Stage II: Vascular rosacea—persistent erythema and telangiactasia

Stage III: Inflammatory rosacea—multiple inflammatory papules and pustules

Stage IV: Glandular hyperplastic rosacea—(usually in men) lymphedema and hypertrophy of connective tissue (Higgins & du Vivier, 1999; Hooper & Goldman, 1999)

Epidemiology. Rosacea affects women three times more than men. Onset is between ages 30 and 50. Fair-skinned individuals are predisposed to rosacea, which is thought to be a reactionary flush to specific precipitating factors, including alcohol, sunlight, stress, vasodilating drugs, and hot/spicy foods (Higgins & duVivier, 1999; Hooper & Goldman, 1999).

Subjective Data/Objective Data/Differential Diagnoses. See Table 21–13, Rosacea.

Diagnostic Tests. Diagnosis is usually made on the basis of history and appearance. If lupus or cutaneous sarcoidosis is suspected, diagnosis is made by biopsy and client should be referred to dermatologist.

Plan

Psychosocial Interventions. Rosacea is a chronic disease, and treatment is continuous. Reassure client that early intervention and prevention of flares help. Body image concerns and embarrassment should be addressed. A glandular, hyperplastic stage (usually seen in men) may cause rhinophyma in which nose appears enlarged and bright red or violaceous. Client may be suspected of being a heavy drinker because of flushed appearance of skin.

Medications. Metronidazole (MetroGel 0.75%, Metrocreme 1%) is the topical treatment of choice (Hooper & Goldman, 1999). If rosacea is severe, oral antibiotics may be used concurrently with topical treatment.

- *Administration.* Applied twice daily.
- *Adverse Effects.* Transient redness, burning, irritation.
- *Contraindications.* Allergy to metronidazole or its component ingredients. Use cautiously if history of blood dyscrasias; may potentiate oral anticoagulants.
- *Client Teaching.* Avoid contact with eyes.
- *Oral Antibiotic.* Tetracycline 500 mg b.i.d. or if gastric upset, Minocycline 50 to 100 mg b.i.d.
- *Administration.* Twice a day for six to eight weeks. Advise client not to take with food. May taper dose down to maintenance dose of Tetracycline 250 to 500 mg or Minocycline 50 mg every other day.
- *Adverse Effects.* Photosensitivity, light-headedness, dizziness, diarrhea, anorexia.
- *Contraindications.* Pregnancy, known sensitivity.

Isotretinoin 1–2 mg/kg/day used over three to six months may cause a remission of rosacea. In some cases, low-dose chronic use (10 mg every other day) may help treat rhinophyma (Hooper & Goldman, 1999). Please see discussion of isotretinoin in acne vulgaris section.

Diet/Lifestyle. Discuss triggers of flushing and erythema such as excessive cold, wind, heat, alcohol, and spicy foods.

Follow-Up. Evaluate client in one week for tolerance of therapy, then again at one month. Refer to dermatologist if condition worsens or rhinophyma (enlarged red nose) (Higgins & du Vivier, 1999; Hooper & Goldman, 1999).

Impetigo

Impetigo is a contagious infection of the skin that is caused by *Staphylococcus aureus* coagulase positive and/or group A beta hemolytic *Streptococcus*. Most cases of impetigo today are due to *Staphylococcus*. The lesions may be vesicles, pustules, and/or bullae, but the diagnostic feature is honey-colored crust (Elgart, 2002; O'Dell, 1998).

Epidemiology. Most common in childhood, especially on the face around the nares, but in adults can occur on any exposed surface. It can spread to others. Secondary impetigination can occur with eczema or other vesiculobullous dermatoses and is treated as impetigo (Elgart, 2002; O'Dell, 1998).

Subjective Data/Objective Data/Differential Diagnoses. See Table 21–13, Impetigo.

Diagnostic Tests. Diagnosis is usually based on history and appearance. Treatment is empiric with broad spectrum antibiotic covering staph and strep, but culture and sensitivity of exudate may be helpful if resistant organisms in community are a concern.

Plan

Psychosocial Interventions. Reassure client impetigo responds very quickly to oral antibiotics.

Medication. Dicloxacillin 250 mg po q.i.d. for seven days or, if allergic to penicillin, erythromycin 250 mg q.i.d. for seven days. (See previous discussion of Dicloxacillin under Mastitis, chapter on Postpartum and Lactation. Erythromycin discussed earlier under Eczema.)

In areas where erythromycin resistant staphylococcus, Ciprofloxacin 250 mg po b.i.d. for seven days is a reasonable but expensive alternative. (Hooper & Goldman, 1999).

Adverse effects include GI upset, headache, dizziness, nightmares.

Contraindicated in known sensitivity, nursing mothers.

If impetigo is localized to small area, mupirocin 2 percent ointment (Bactroban) may be used topically three times a day. (O'Dell, 1998).

- *Adverse Effects.* May cause local stinging. If no response in three days, switch to oral antibiotics and culture.
- *Expected Outcome.* Rapid resolution of infection.

Lifestyle. Warm, moist compresses may be used to soften and remove crusts. Advise client to separate washcloths and towels from other household members.

Follow-Up. Advise client to call or to schedule visit if not resolved in five to seven days.

Folliculitis

Folliculitis is an infection or inflammation of the hair follicle caused by *Staphylococcus aureus* (or if arises after use of hot tub, *Pseudomonas aeruginosa folliculitis*), by a fungal dermatophyte, by oils (industrial or cosmetic), or perspiration. The causative agent can be differentiated on the basis of history, location of the pustules, bacterial culture, KOH preparation and fungal culture, and lack of response to antibacterial therapy.

Epidemiology. Bacterial folliculitis is more prevalent in diabetics. Common sites are the groin and exposed areas of the arms and legs. Folliculitis may appear during the first week of oral steroid therapy (steroid acne) or may flare when dose is tapered. Hot tub folliculitis appears in one to four days after use of a contaminated tub. The rash is tender and pruritic. (Elgart, 2002; Hooper & Goldman, 1999).

Fungal folliculitis is characterized by the clustering of the follicular pustules, commonly on the hands, arms, legs, and scalp. In women, infection often occurs when the dermatophyte from tinea pedis is spread to the legs when shaving. The follicles cluster on the lower legs. Fungal folliculitis can also arise from misdiagnosed tinea corporis that is treated with steroids. Pustular follicles then arise on the face and dorsum of the hand (O'Dell, 1998; Rhody, 2000).

Pseudofolliculitis is caused by ingrowing hairs. Pustules and papules are located beside the follicle but not in the follicle. (Hooper & Goldman, 1999).

Subjective Data/Objective Data/Differential Diagnoses. See previous discussion and Table 21–13, Folliculitis.

Diagnostic Tests. Bacterial culture and sensitivity, fungal culture and/or KOH prep are ordered as appropriate. Often empiric treatment is started based on history and appearance while waiting for culture result.

Plan

Psychosocial Interventions. Because pustules appear on exposed areas, client may have body image concerns.

Medication. If bacterial in origin dicloxacillin 250 mg q.i.d. for fourteen days (see discussion under Impetigo). Small areas may be treated with muciprocin 2 percent ointment (see discussion under Impetigo).

Fungal folliculitis usually responds only to oral antifungals such as griseofulvin (see Tinea Pedis). Confirm by fungal culture before starting therapy.

Folliculitis on the back, which has been diagnosed as acne and does not respond to acne treatment, may be due to *Pityrosporum orbiculare*, which is treated with topical 2.5 percent selenium sulfide applied for 15 minutes daily for three weeks.

Medication is not indicated for irritant folliculitis, except for use of drying soaks such as Burow's or benzoyl peroxide.

Aluminum subacetate (Burow's) soaks or compresses twice a day for 15 minutes provide soothing relief to skin, especially if exudative.

Lifestyle. Control of blood sugars is helpful in diabetics. Advise women who acquire infection as a result of shaving legs to use depilatory until resolved or use disposable shavers. Treat water in hot tubs with appropriate chemicals. If irritant folliculitis is caused by occupational exposure to oil, suggest client wear protective clothing and gloves. She may need to switch to oil-free makeup.

If excessive perspiration is the cause, suggest client shower promptly after exercise, avoid tight, occlusive clothing, lose weight if indicated.

Follow-Up. Evaluate client in seven days for response to therapy. Culture if not responding and consider referral to dermatologist if immunocompromised.

Furuncles and Carbuncles

A furuncle (abscess or boil) is an infection of the hair follicle. It is more extensive and deep-seated than folliculitis and involves the adjacent tissue. Furuncles develop acutely with sudden onset of pain and tenderness. If the furuncles enlarge and coalesce, they may form a carbuncle (Rhody, 2000).

Epidemiology. Furuncles are caused by *Staphylococcus aureus*. Heat and moisture favor their development, especially where trauma has occurred. Immunocompromised individuals are at higher risk for development. At risk for recurrent infections are chronic nose and throat carriers of Staph.

Subjective Data/Objective Data/Differential Diagnoses. See Table 21–13, Furuncles and carbuncles.

Diagnostic Tests. Bacterial culture of exudate after incision and drainage is recommended. Treatment is started immediately and is modified if needed based on sensitivity.

Plan

Psychosocial Interventions. Furuncles often develop in the axillae and the anogenital area causing pain and embarrassment. Be alert also to hygiene and body image concerns.

Medications. Dicloxacillin 250 to 500 mg four times a day for ten to fourteen days. If sensitive to penicillin, erythromycin 250 mg four times a day or Azithromycin 250 mg two capsules on day 1 and one capsule daily for the next four days (Hooper & Goldman, 1999). (See previous discussions of these agents in sections on Folliculitis, Impetigo.)

If client is chronic carrier, application of 2 percent muciprocin (Bactroban) ointment to nares, anogenital area, and axillae may help eliminate carrier state (O'Dell, 1998).

Local Measures. Warm soaks applied for 20 to 30 minutes three times a day may help immobilize lesions and prevent spread. Advise client not to manipulate furuncles to minimize risk of much deeper and even systemic infection. Floculant lesions may have to be incised, drained, and packed.

Lifestyle. Because furuncles may develop in moist, warm areas, advise client to wear loose clothing and fabrics that allow perspiration to evaporate and to avoid use of petroleum, oil-based cosmetics and lotions.

Follow-Up. Evaluate client in one week for response to therapy. If furuncle incised and drained, schedule client for daily evaluation to change packing, irrigate. Refer to physician if infection recurs. Client or intimate contacts may be staph carriers.

Warts (Human Papillomavirus)

Warts are benign tumors of the skin caused by the human papillomavirus. There are more than 63 types of HPV and some have premalignant potential. Cutaneous warts fall into three broad classifications:

Common warts
Plantar warts of the foot
Flat warts

They can occur on any part of the body including the hands, face, feet. Mucosal warts arise on mucous membranes such as the conjunctiva, oral mucosa, larynx, and the anogenital area (Elgart, 2002; Hooper & Goldman, 1999). (See discussion of genital warts in chapter on sexually transmitted disease.)

Epidemiology. Warts often arise in childhood and regress spontaneously, usually in one to two years. In adults, they are less likely to regress. They are caused by a virus and have an incubation period of two to eighteen months. Warts are contagious by fomites, by autoinoculation from one area to another, and from person to person. Warm, moist environments subjected to trauma or friction favor the growth. A single very small papule may grow to 5 to 10 mm, and new warts may cluster around to form a mosaic of 3 cm. (Elgart, 2002; Hooper & Goldman, 1999).

Subjective/Objective Data/Differential Diagnoses. See Table 21–13, Warts.

Diagnostic Tests. Usually diagnosed on basis of appearance. Biopsy indicated if located on sun-damaged skin; if large, chronic wart in elderly; if color, border change; if long-standing wart of finger (high potential for squamous cell cancer).

Plan

Psychosocial Interventions. Concern about appearance leads many women to seek treatment. Depending on location, warts may also interfere with work, hobbies, or activities of daily living. Reassure client that, even though common cutaneous warts are benign, you appreciate her concern regarding possible malignancy or skin cancer. Give client realistic expectations of successful treatment. It may take several visits to eradicate lesions. Give client option of no treatment by pointing out possibility of spontaneous regression, possibility of skin damage, scarring from treatment.

Treatment. Any suspicion of squamous cell carcinoma must be biopsied. Any mucosal wart should be excised immediately and sent to the pathologist.

There are three mainstays of treatment for cutaneous warts: salicylic acid, cantharidin, and liquid nitrogen cryotherapy.

Salicylic acid is available over the counter under various trade names (Compound W, Wart-Off, Freezone).

- *Administration.* Apply to the entire area after bathing and soaking the wart for several minutes. Pat dry and use applicator to cover the wart. Adjacent skin should be avoided, may use petrolatum to protect. Use every night and rinse off in morning. For warts on soles of feet (plantar warts), may cover with occlusive dressing or salicylic plaster. Apply daily. Remove dead skin by filing off with pumice stone. Frequency of treatment is dependent on tenderness and results.
- *Adverse Effects.* Warn client about local irritation. Contraindicated if allergic to aspirin.
- *Client Teaching.* May require repeated treatments, less effective than cathardin but less painful.

   Cantharidin (Cantharone) is not available at all pharmacies. It is a blistering agent that must be formulated from its ingredients by the pharmacist and is for office use only.
- *Administration.* Solution is applied to wart with a wooden applicator and left on for 24 hours under an occlusive dressing. It is applied in the office. Solution is removed with mild soap and water the next day. It is reapplied weekly depending on results.
- *Adverse Effects.* Moderate to severe pain may develop 12 to 24 hours after treatment (Hooper & Goldman, 1999).
- *Contraindications.* Known sensitivity to agent. Use with caution if client is diabetic, or has impaired circulation.

See Chapter 11 (Vaginitis and Sexually Transmitted Diseases) for discussion of liquid nitrogen cryotherapy.

Lifestyle. Advise client that warts are contagious and may be spread to other areas of the body or to other close contacts after a break in the skin or maceration. A single wart may contain millions of infectious virions (Hooper & Goldman, 1999). Treatment of plantar warts may require client to stay off feet or use crutches. Assess effect on occupation and activities of daily living.

Follow-Up. Evaluate response to therapy after one week. Advise client to call if significant pain develops after office treatment. Refer insulin dependent diabetics, those who do not respond to treatment, to dermatologist.

ANOGENITAL PRURITIS

Anogenital pruritis is a diagnosis of exclusion after all other causes of pruritis have been ruled, such as viral or bacterial infection, infestation, sensitivity to soaps or chemicals, psoriasis, or atrophic vaginitis. Poor hygiene may be at fault.

Epidemiology

Pruritis vulvae is not uncommon in women. It does not involve the anal area in most cases.

Subjective Data

Intense pruritis, especially at night. Client may report scant white discharge.

Objective Data

Absence of physical findings is the rule. May see excoriations, erythema, and/or fissuring.

Differential Diagnoses

Candidiasis, pediculosis, contact or allergic dermatitis, psoriasis, seborrhea, atrophic vaginitis, human papilloma virus.

Plan

Psychosocial Interventions. Condition may be extremely embarrassing to client and may lead to social isolation in extreme cases.

Medication. Pramoxine cream or lotion or hydrocortisone-pramoxine 1 percent cream, lotion or ointment applied three to four times a day for up to four weeks. Wash hands after use and avoid contact with eyes.

- *Adverse Effects.* May burn or sting.
- *Contraindications.* Known sensitivity.
- *Client Teaching.* Scrupulous hygiene.

Diet/Lifestyle. If constipation present, may be exacerbating pruritis. Follow high-fiber diet, drink plenty of fluids. Advise cleaning skin after every bowel movement with moistened soft cloth. Sitz baths may also relieve discomfort.

Follow-Up

Reevaluate after seven to ten days for response to therapy.

CELLULITIS

Cellulitis is an infection of the skin and subcutaneous tissue without purulent formation.

Epidemiology

Cellulitis may follow superficial injury to the skin, folliculitis, stasis ulcer. Often the initial insult may be inapparent. It is caused primarily by gram positive cocci, such as *Staphylococcus* or *Streptococcus.*

Subjective Data

Client complains of pain and tenderness.

Objective Data

Diffuse border of warm, red skin.

Diagnostic Tests. Diagnosed on basis of appearance. Bacterial culture from injection and aspiration of saline rarely yield valuable results and may further spread cellulitis.

Differential Diagnoses

Severe contact dermatitis may resemble cellulitis but is pruritic and not as painful.

Plan

Psychosocial Interventions. Reassure client that with prompt treatment and adherence to treatment plan, cellulitis resolves promptly.

Medications. See prior discussion of Impetigo.

Diet/Lifestyle. Advise client to apply warm soaks at least three times a day, elevate extremity. If legs or feet affected, limit ambulation as much as possible.

Follow-Up

Mark area affected and evaluate within one to two days by telephone contact or office visit. Close follow-up needed for frail and/or elderly client, client with hand or anogenital involvement.

DERMATOLOGICAL CONDITIONS NEEDING REFERRAL

Erysipelas

Erypsipelas is a superficial cellulitis of the upper dermis found commonly on the legs, feet, and face (Callahan et al., 2000). Over a period of a few days, it spreads rapidly to form a smooth, erythematous hot area. It is caused by beta-hemolytic streptococcus. The client may appear toxic on presentation with chills, fever, and pain. If erysipelas is not treated immediately, it can spread systemically and be fatal (Callahan et al., 2000; Hooper & Goldman 1999).

Epidemiology. Can occur at any age. Older clients and those who are immunocompromised are at greatest risk. Occurs after break in skin or trauma (Callahan et al., 2000; Hooper & Goldman, 1999).

Subjective Data. Client may report first appeared as small papule near nose and spread rapidly. May complain of chills, fever, and malaise.

Objective Data. Edematous, sharply marginated hot red area that may have vesicles or bullae on surface. May pit to finger pressure.

Diagnostic Tests. White count and erythrocyte sedimentation rate are elevated. Blood culture may be positive for strep.

Differential Diagnoses. Urticaria following insect bite (resolves over next 24 hours). Cellulitis has less definite margin (Callahan et al., 2000).

Plan. Refer to physician immediately. Client is put on bed rest with affected body part elevated (Callahan et al., 2000). Usually treated with Dicloxacillin 250 mg orally four times a day or penicillin with clavulanate potassium 500 mg orally twice a day. For clients allergic to penicillin, clindamycin 300 mg orally four times a day for ten to fourteen days is an alternative (Hooper & Goldman, 1999).

If the woman is frail or immunocompromised, she may require hospitalization and intravenous antibiotics.

Erythema Nodosum

The lesions of erythema nodosum are large 4 to 10 cm red, painful slope-shouldered or flat-topped plaques that appear on the anterior lower legs and less commonly on the thigh. The most common causes of this inflammatory vascular reaction include reactions to medications such as sulfa, penicillin, progestins; infections such as streptococcus, deep mycoses, tuberculosis, hepatitis B, and syphilis; autoimmune disease and malignancies such as sarcoidosis, leukemia, and inflammatory bowel disease (Whitmore, 1999).

Epidemiology. More common in women. May appear in pregnancy.

Subjective Data. Client may report fever, malaise, and joint pain before appearance of nodules.

Objective Data. Usually bilateral distribution on anterior lower leg or around ankle. Warm to touch, 4 to 10 cm in size, tender.

Differential Diagnoses. Cellulitis does not appear as multiple lesions. Erythema multiforme has a more general distribution.

Plan

Psychosocial Interventions. Erythema nodosum may be the presenting sign of a chronic, serious disease. Psychosocial support for such a diagnosis should be anticipated.

Treatment is based on underlying cause. Consult with the physician regarding further workup. Comfort measures include nonsteroidal anti-inflammatory agents and, in some cases, bed rest.

Palpable Purpura

Purpura arises from the escape of the red blood cells into the skin due to an immune complex mechanism or trauma. It has two forms, petechiae (3 mm or less) and ecchymoses (larger than 3 mm). Purpura do not blanch with pressure. Nonpalpable purpura are caused by platelet abnormalities, actinic purpuras, and use of steroids. The most common cause of nontraumatic palpable purpura is a cutaneous vasculitis secondary to infection, connective tissue disease, or medication sensitivity. Noninflammatory etiologies include subacute bacterial endocarditis, amyloidosis, and embolic disease. Some palpable purpura are idiopathic. Serious causes and any underlying blood dyscrasia must be ruled out (Hooper & Goldman, 1999; Whitmore, 1999; Zieve, 2000).

Epidemiology. Depends on underlying cause.

Subjective Data. A careful history will often lead to diagnosis. Key items are recent onset of pharmacotherapy, fever, history of collagen vascular disease, malignancy, sexually transmitted disease, travel history, and insecticide exposure.

Objective Data. Careful examination of the skin, heart, lungs, abdomen, joints, and genitalia. Laboratory tests may include CBC, ESR, blood cultures, ANA, rheumatoid factor, BUN, creatinine, and urinalysis. Range of tests depends on likely etiology and client's presentation. Skin biopsy may be needed if cause is not self-limited such as drug reaction or infection.

Differential Diagnoses. Cutaneous vasculitis, bacteremia, Rocky Mountain spotted fever, subacute bacterial endo-

carditis, amyloidosis, trauma, cholesterol emboli, disseminated intravascular coagulation, pseudo-purpura such as Kaposi's sarcoma, Sweet's syndrome (fever, rash on upper body five to ten days after upper respiratory infection; may be marker of leukemia) (Hooper & Goldman, 1999; Whitmore, 1999; Zieve, 2000).

Plan. Consultation with physician to outline diagnostic tests and possible further referral.

Skin Cancer

Skin cancer is the most common type of cancer in the United States. Its incidence has increased dramatically in the last ten years, over 65 percent for nonmelanoma cancers.

The three most common types are basal cell cancer, squamous cell cancer, and malignant melanoma. Basal and squamous cell cancers are more common; however, malignant melanoma accounts for almost all the deaths. Women, because of their sun bathing, are particularly at risk.

The United States Public Health Service's Healthy People 2000 program recommends annual skin examinations for adults over 50 years old with risk factors for skin cancer.

Basal Cell Skin Cancer. Basal cell cancer (BCC) arises from basal keratinocytes. It grows by direct extension and destruction of surrounding tissue. Metastasis is uncommon (Whitmore, 1999).

Epidemiology. Risk factors are similar for all types of skin cancer (Goldstein & Goldstein, 2001; Sachs, Marghoob, & Halpern, 2001).

- Fair skin that burns easily and tans poorly (see Table 21–14)
- Substantial time spent outdoors, particularly occupational, for example, farmers and sailors
- History of childhood sunburns
- Family history of skin cancer
- X-ray, radiation burn sites, UV light therapy, chronic venous stasis ulcers
- Arsenic ingestion (rare)
- Immunosuppression

Fair skin and sun exposure are the key risk factors. More than 90 percent of basal cell cancer occurs on sun exposed areas of the head and neck but are rare on the back of the hand. The cancer may occur at sites of previous trauma, such as in thermal burns and scars. Basal cell cancer has many clinical forms that vary in appearance and malignant potential.

TABLE 21–14. Skin Cancer Prevention Guidelines

1. *Avoid sun exposure*
   - Skin types I-IV are especially susceptible.
   - Protect infants and children. Children cannot protect themselves and significant increased risk may be associated with exposure in first decade.
   - Use caution with sun-sensitizing medications: tetracycline, tricyclics, antihistamines, antipsychotics, hypoglycemics, diuretics, antieoplastics, retin A.

2. *Avoid tanning salons. Artificial sunlight is no safer than sunlight.*

3. *When you must be in the sun, protect yourself*
   - Avoid peak times for ultraviolet B: 10 A.M. to 2 P.M.
   - Wear protective clothing: hats, especially broad-brimmed; light-colored clothing.
   - Beware of reflective surfaces: snow and cement.
   - **Use sunscreen or sun block whenever going outdoors:** Choose strong enough sun protective factor (SPF). Apply adequate amounts of sunscreen; manufacturer's directions are more than most people use. Apply lotion 30 to 60 minutes before expected sun exposure, as it takes time for *para*-aminobenzoic acid (PABA) to bind in the stratum corneum. Reapply at least every 40 to 80 minutes and more frequently if swimming or perspiring.

4. *Types of sunscreens/sunblocks*
   - Chemical sunscreens
     - PABA and PABA esters are the first choice because they effectively block ultraviolet B (UVG), which is associated with skin cancers.
     - Non-PABA sunscreens include benzophenones and cinnamates, which weakly block UVB; use if allergic to PABA.
   - Physical sunblocks: zinc oxide and titanium dioxide; opaque and often cosmetically unacceptable.

5. *Skin type and choice of sun protection factor (SPF)*

Skin Type	Skin Color and Sunburn History	SPF
I	Very fair: always burns, never tans	≥15
II	Fair: burns easily, tans minimally	≥15 or more
III	Light brown: burns moderately, tans gradually and uniformly	10–15
IV	Moderate brown: burns minimally, always tans well	6–15
V	Dark brown: rarely burns, tans profusely	6–15
VI	Deeply pigmented: never burns	Low

Sources: Goldstein & Goldstein (2001); Hooper & Goldman (1999); Jerant, Johnson, Sheridan, & Caffrey (2000).

It is estimated that one in seven Americans will develop basal cell cancer. It is the most common type of skin cancer in the United States. Basal cell cancer is common among Caucasians and rare among African Americans. It may occur at any age. The incidence markedly increases after age 40 but basal cell carcinomas are becoming increasingly common in 20- to 30-year-olds (Sachs, Marghoob, & Halpern, 2001; Whitmore, 1999).

Subjective Data. Basal cell cancer is primarily asymptomatic; its course is unpredictable. The lesion may remain small with almost no perceptible growth for years or it may grow rapidly. Symptoms such as enlargement, change in color, pain, itching, and bleeding should be investigated. If a client is uncertain about how long a crust lesion has been present, have her return for follow-up in two weeks. If the suspicious lesion remains unchanged, refer her for biopsy (Goldstein & Goldstein, 2001; Jerant et al., 2000).

Objective Data. Because the early stages of skin cancer are primarily asymptomatic, screening is crucial. A complete

physical exam reveals more than six times the pathology revealed by exams limited to normally exposed sites.

Physical examination should employ a magnifying lens and good lighting to observe suspicious lesions. It is helpful to wet the lesion with oil or an alcohol swab and stretch the lesion between two fingers to check for color patterns. Look for signs of dysplastic nevus syndrome (see Table 21–15). In addition to good visualizations, careful palpation for lymphadenopathy is necessary.

Basal cell cancer usually begins as a small shiny papule that enlarges over months and develops telangiectasias and a pearly border. After time, it develops a central ulcer that recurrently crusts and bleeds. Less common forms of basal cell cancer appear as flat plaques. Keep in mind that the lesion may take many forms. A basal cell carcinoma of the eyelid may have the appearance of a sty that recurs on the lower lid (Hooper & Goldman, 1999).

Diagnostic tests may be performed by a dermatologist following referral. A suspicious lesion is evaluated and skin biopsy may be necessary.

Differential Medical Diagnoses. See Table 21–16.

TABLE 21–15. Differential Diagnoses of Dysplastic Nevi

Sign	Common Mole	Dysplastic Nevi
Shape	Round or oval	Irregular
Margins	Sharp, well circumscribed	Hazy, indistinct
Color	Light brown to black, uniform pigmentation	Variegated tan, dark brown on pink background
Topography	Flat or smooth dome shape	"Fried egg" shape, papular center with macular periphery or pebble contour
Size	Usually < 6 mm	Usually > 5mm, up to 12 mm
Number	Usually 12 to 25	One or many, often > 100
Location	Usually face and upper extremities	Mostly on covered areas: buttocks, scalp, and female breasts
Age of onset	Few appear after early adulthood	Continue to appear after age 35

Sources: Hooper & Goldman (1999); Kanzler & Mraz-Gernhard (2001).

Plan

PSYCHOSOCIAL INTERVENTIONS. Help the client to understand the importance of compliance with referrals and treatment regimens. Reassure her that prompt referral and treatment results in a high rate of cure, about 90 to 95 percent.

The following organizations provide materials for client and health care education on skin cancer:

National Cancer Institute
Cancer Information Service
31 Center Drive (MSC 2580)
Bldg. 31, Room 10A07
Bethesda, MD 20892-2580
Phone: (800)4-CANCER (422-6237)

Skin Cancer Foundation
245 Fifth Avenue, Suite 2402
New York, NY 10016
Phone: (212) 725-5176 or 1-800-SKIN-490

MEDICATION. None is administered.

TABLE 21–16. Differential Diagnosis of Skin Cancer

Benign skin lesions	Nevi, seborrheic keratosis, cysts, skin tags, dermatofibromas, keloids
Dermatoses	Seborrhea, eczema, psoriasis, human papilloma virus, fungi
Lesions with premalignant potential	Actinic keratosis, leukoplakia, dysplastic nevus syndrome
Skin cancers	Basal cell cancer, squamous cell cancer (Bowen's, Paget's), malignant melanoma, mycosis fungoides (rare T-cell lymphoma that originates in skin)
Cutaneous metastasis	3–5% of those with metastatic disease develop secondary skin cancers

Sources: Goldstein & Goldstein (2001); Hooper & Goldman (1999); Jerant et al. (2000); Kanzler & Mraz-Gernhard (2001); Whitmore (1999).

SURGICAL INTERVENTIONS. Surgical excision may be recommended following skin biopsy.

LIFESTYLE CHANGES. There is no safe tan. Sun exposure accelerates photoaging (Hooper & Goldman, 1999). Convincing young women to avoid sun tanning is *very* difficult because of cultural norms and feelings of invulnerability. In prevention education, an emphasis on photoaging may be more effective. All people wrinkle; the question is how much and how soon. Have the woman look at how smooth and soft the skin of her upper inner arm is and compare it with that on the back of her hand. This demonstrates photoaging. Encourage all women to follow the skin cancer prevention guidelines in Table 21–13.

Also encourage the client to stop smoking.

Follow-Up. Referral to a dermatologist is necessary after identification of a suspicious lesion.

Squamous Cell Cancer. Squamous cell cancer (SCC) arises in the epithelium. Like basal cell cancer, squamous cell cancer is most common on areas exposed to the sun; however, distribution is somewhat different. SCC is commonly found on the scalp, the back of the hand, the ear and the lower lip. It often arises from a precursor lesion called *actinic keratosis*. Actinic keratosis, a premalignant skin condition of the elderly, may appear as flat tan or brown spots with adherent scales and mild surrounding erythema. These often feel rough. Induration, inflammation, and oozing suggest degeneration into malignancy. Squamous cell cancer arising from actinic keratoses is not aggressive but can eventually metastasize (Garner & Rodney, 2000; Sachs et al., 2001).

Squamous cell cancers that arise at thermal burn sites or sites of chronic inflammation have a higher metastatic potential than squamous cell cancers evolving from actinic keratoses (Garner & Rodney, 2000; Sachs et al., 2001).

Epidemiology. The etiology of squamous cell cancer differs somewhat depending on the type; however, all of these cancers usually appear on sun-exposed areas of fair-skinned persons. These types (simplified here) and their locations include Bowen's disease, on the trunk and extremities; Paget's disease, on the areola, nipple, and vulva; and extramammary Paget's disease, on the anogenital region, axilla, external ear canal, and eyelids.

Paget's disease of the areola manifests as a sharply demarcated area of erythema and scaling, often with oozing and crusting. It is associated with breast cancer, but easily confused with eczema. By contrast, eczema is bilateral and resolves with treatment; Paget's lesions are mostly unilateral and progressive.

Squamous cell cancer is common in the oral cavity of women who smoke and drink, often on the posterior lateral borders of the tongue. Leukoplakia, a white opaque patch found on the lips, oral mucosa, and vulva, is a precursor lesion that may degenerate into squamous cell cancer.

Incidence reports show that squamous cell cancer is the second most common skin cancer among the general population. It is the most common among African Americans, especially those with a history of a scarring process, such as a burn or leg ulcer (Garner & Rodney, 2000; Sachs et al., 2001).

Subjective Data. Squamous cell cancer is primarily asymptomatic, but a client may report itching, irritation, bleeding, or a change in skin appearance.

Objective Data. See Objective Data under Basal Cell Cancer.

Physical examination reveals a variable appearance among clients, but the lesions usually begins as a reddish papule or plaque with a scaly or crusted surface. It may mimic dermatitis. Later, the lesion may appear nodular or warty. Eventually, it ulcerates and invades underlying tissue.

Lesions on the lower lip may start with a thickened, dry, scaly surface on the vermillion border. Later it may progress to a nodule. Lesions of the lower lip, especially those on the inside mucous membrane, are very aggressive and demand prompt referral for treatment (Garner & Rodney, 2000).

Diagnostic evaluation and management are carried out by a dermatologist.

Differential Medical Diagnoses. See Table 21–15.

Plan

PSYCHOSOCIAL INTERVENTIONS. Emphasize the importance of skin cancer prevention (see Table 21–13). Some actinic keratoses may regress if the client avoids sun exposure. Stress the importance of the treatment regimen

outlined by the specialist. Refer her to the resources listed for basal cell cancer.

MEDICATION. Methotrexate or 5-fluorouracil (Efudex) may be injected by the dermatologist after biopsy for certain selected types of lesions. Failure to respond necessitates excision of the lesion (Garner & Rodney, 2000).

SURGICAL INTERVENTIONS. Excision, cryosurgery, or electrodesiccation and curettage may be performed depending on the extent of the lesion.

LIFESTYLE CHANGES. See those recommended for clients with basal cell cancer.

Follow-Up. Continue to monitor the client for new lesions every three months and teach her how to perform monthly self-examinations of the skin.

Malignant Melanoma. Malignant melanoma (MM) arises from melanocytes. It is associated primarily with sun exposure. Because most malignant melanomas arise from pigmented moles, any change in a mole is always of concern. Removal of benign moles does not decrease the risk for malignant melanoma. It may develop anywhere there are melanocytes or pigmented skin, such as mucous membranes, eyes, and the central nervous system. Malignant melanoma may arise de novo, that is, from sites where no mole is visible.

Malignant melanoma is deadly. Early identification and prompt surgical excision offer the only change for cure. The radial growth phase is a "window of opportunity" during the first several months to years of a malignant melanoma. A mole removed while it is less than 0.76 mm deep is associated with a 93 percent cure rate. Excision of vertical growths greater than 4 mm results in only 50 percent survival at five years (Padgett & Hendrix, 2001).

Dysplastic nevus syndrome (DNS), also known as familial atypical mole and melanoma (FAMM) syndrome, is a familial syndrome found in 2 to 5 percent of the population. Individuals with dysplastic nevus syndrome have at least 6 percent lifetime risk for malignant melanoma. Clients exhibit large asymmetric and irregularly pigmented nevi. If they have two close family members with malignant melanoma, their lifetime risk for developing malignant melanoma is over 50 percent and may approach 100 percent (Kanzler & Mraz-Gernhard, 2001; Whitmore, 1999).

Epidemiology. An epidemic of skin cancers has occurred since the 1920s when tans became "fashionable." More than 500,000 new skin cancers are diagnosed each year in the United States. Malignant melanoma accounts for only

3 percent of these cancers, yet it is responsible for three-quarters of the deaths from skin cancer (Jerant et al., 2000; Padgett & Hendrix, 2001).

The most important risk factor for melanoma is skin color. It is rare in African Americans. In nonblacks major risk factors include number of moles, tendency to freckle, tendency to burn in sunlight, past history of sunburns (especially in childhood), family history of atypical nevi, family history of malignant melanoma. Immune dysfunction may also be a risk factor. Research indicates that immunocompromise may allow transformation of dysplastic nevi into malignant melanoma (Jerant et al., 2000; Padgett & Hendrix, 2001).

Subjective Data. Four major symptoms are enlargement, color change, pain (sometimes itch), and bleeding. Most clients present with only one symptom, and any symptom warrants referral for evaluation. Refer to a dermatologist all women with a family history of dysplastic nevus syndrome, especially if they also have a family history of melanoma.

Objective Data. A physical examination will help identify suspicious changes. The ABCDs (asymmetry, border, color, diameter, surface/sensation) can assist practitioners, as well as clients, in performing skin exams (see Table 21–17).

Physical examination focuses on sun exposed areas (back, head, and neck) where most malignant melanomas occur. Acrolentiginous melanoma is a rare, but rapidly fatal lesion, occurring most often among African Americans on their palmar, plantar, or nail bed surfaces. Each of the several types of melanoma has its own particular idiosyncrasies and growth patterns. Be suspicious of variegated color, irregular borders and surfaces, and an increase in size (see Table 21–17).

Small dysplastic nevi may be difficult to differentiate from common moles on physical exam. If the client has a family history of dysplastic nevus syndrome and any questionable lesion, refer her to a dermatologist.

Diagnostic tests are conducted by a dermatologist. Refer any suspicious lesion for evaluation and probable biopsy.

Differential Medical Diagnoses. See Table 21–15.

Plan

PSYCHOSOCIAL INTERVENTIONS. Educate the client about moles and reassure her that not all moles are harmful. In general, people are born without moles. Small, flat, tan "common" moles develop in childhood and increase in size and number after puberty. They may become smooth domes. By early adulthood, individuals average 12 to 25 moles. In individuals who live long lives, the moles recede and disappear before death.

MEDICATION. Refer to dermatologist.

SURGICAL INTERVENTION. Surgical excision may be performed.

LIFESTYLE CHANGES. Encourage the client to follow skin cancer prevention guidelines (see Table 21–14). She should also perform monthly self-exams of the skin and stop smoking.

Follow-Up. Refer a client with any suspicious lesion to a dermatologist. If dysplastic nevus syndrome is suspected, refer the client. With numerous dysplastic nevi, baseline photographs and perhaps serial photodocumentation are needed.

Immunocompromised clients may be seen every three to four months by the dermatologist. Family members of clients with dysplastic nevus syndrome must be screened; often an early operable melanoma is found in a distant relative. All women should be taught the ABCDs of melanoma (see Table 21–17). A complete skin exam should be conducted at the time of the client's annual physical. Encourage women to examine their skin monthly at home.

EAR, NOSE, AND THROAT DISORDERS

These disorders are frequently encountered in primary care; the most common—the common cold, otitis media, acute sinusitis, and pharyngitis—will be addressed here.

THE COMMON COLD

The common cold is a mild, self-limited condition caused by a viral infection of the upper respiratory mucosa. The nasal mucosa is prominently involved.

TABLE 21–17. ABCDs of Skin Cancer

A	Asymmetry	One half shaped unlike the other
B	Border	Irregular, notched, or scalloped
C	Color	Haphazard shades of brown, red, blue, gray
D	Diameter	Greater than 6 mm (size of the tip of a pencil eraser)
S	Surface or sensation	Surface distortion may be subtle or obvious, assess by focusing light at side of lesion; sensation refers to itch, burn, or pain

Epidemiology

Studies of the common cold demonstrate that age and environmental contacts are the two major factors influencing the extent of illness. Numerous groups and hundreds of viral strains cause "cold" symptoms. Rhinoviruses are the most common group. Others include coronaviruses, respiratory syncytial virus, adenovirus, echovirus, coxsackievirus, and parainfluenza virus.

Transmission is primarily via direct contact with infected secretions, usually hand-to-hand and subsequent hand-to-face contact. It is evident that good handwashing is crucial in breaking the chain of transmission. Less often, transmission occurs via respiratory droplets from coughs or sneezes. Crowds and poor ventilation promote transmission. The incubation period is usually 48 to 72 hours.

Incidence of the common cold among average adults is two to four colds per year; the average child has six to twelve colds per year; parents of small children have about six colds per year. People seek primary care most often for viral upper respiratory conditions. The vast majority of these illnesses are benign and self-limited; however, they have a major social and financial impact. They are responsible for more absences from work and school than any other type of illness.

Subjective Data

The client's chief complaints are malaise, rhinorrhea, and a "scratchy" throat. Nasal secretions are usually clear and copious at onset, changing to mucoid appearance later in the illness. Mucopurulent secretions *do not* necessarily indicate a secondary bacterial infection. Fever is rare in adults. Symptoms peak in two to four days, then gradually resolve. The total course of the illness is usually five to ten days. When nasal symptoms last longer than ten to fourteen days, the client needs to be evaluated for sinusitis or allergies (Meltzer, 2002).

Objective Data

Physical examination reveals a benign general appearance. Fever is either low grade or absent. Nasal mucosa is often edematous with clear discharge.

The pharynx appears to have mild erythema. Lymphoid hyperplasia of the posterior pharynx is more common than tonsillar enlargement. Lymph nodes are usually nonpalpable, but small anterior cervical nodes may be palpable. Lungs are clear.

Differential Medical Diagnoses

Bacterial infections (*Mycoplasma pneumoniae, Chlamydia psittaci,* group A beta hemolytic streptococcus); viral syndromes (Epstein-Barr or mononucleosis, cytomegalovirus); allergic rhinitis (seasonal, associated itching and copious clear nasal discharge) (Meltzer, 2002). Colds resolve in a few days; other syndromes are more severe and/or long lasting.

Plan

A large part of intervention is helping the client care for herself.

Psychosocial Interventions. Educate the client on the expected course of her illness and the need for self-care. Empower her to pursue self-care when appropriate. Provide information about viral and bacterial infections.

Medication. See Table 21–18.

Lifestyle Changes. Lifestyle changes may help prevent the spread of colds. Advise clients to practice good handwashing and to avoid hand-to-face contact. Increasing fluid intake helps keep secretions loose and moving. Physical activity may be carried out as tolerated.

Strongly encourage cessation of smoking, as it increases the risk for secondary bacterial infections affecting ears, sinuses, and the lungs.

TABLE 21–18. Overview of Oral Medication Types Used for the Common Cold[a]

Class	Indications	Side Effects	Contraindications
Decongestants	Shrink swollen nasal mucosa	Neurologic agitation, increased blood pressure	Avoid with hypertension
Antihistamines	Dry up mucous membrane secretions	Drowsiness (no effect on blood pressure)	Avoid with asthma and history of asthma "flair" with use of antihistamines; Avoid giving with sedating medications or alcohol
Antipyretics/analgesic	Relieve discomfort or fever	Gastrointestinal irritation with nonsteroidal anti-inflammatory drugs	Aspirin is associated with Reye's syndrome; use acetaminophen, especially in clients under age 18

[a]Numerous drugs are included in each class. See specific pharmacotherapeutics texts for details.

Source: Brunton (2002). American Family Physician (2002).

Follow-Up

Teach clients to look for pain (in ear, face, or chest), fever (fever higher than 102°F or fever that recurs after initial few days), and distressing cough that is associated with dyspnea, fever, or localized chest pain, or that is persistent and progressive.

OTITIS MEDIA

Otitis media (OM) is an acute infection of the middle ear. The majority of infections are caused by eustachian tube dysfunction, which in adults is caused primarily by edema from viral upper respiratory infections and allergies. Barotrauma (flying/scuba diving) and cancer can also impair eustachian tube function. Chronic negative pressure in the middle ear leads to serious effusion and overgrowth of respiratory tract bacteria, with subsequent purulent discharge and inflammation (Pichichero, 2000).

Epidemiology

Studies indicate that otitis media is a bacterial disease of the respiratory tract mucosa. The three primary pathogens are *Streptococcus pneumoniae, Hemophilus influenzae,* and *Moraxella catarrhalis* (previously *Branhamella catarrhalis*). Resistant strains of *M. catarrhalis* and *H. influenzae* can produce β-lactamase, which inactivates penicillin and amoxicillin (Tigges, 2000).

Otitis media is most often a secondary bacterial infection following a viral upper respiratory tract infection or problems with allergies.

Incidence reports show otitis media most common among children; however, at least 4.4 percent of the adult population has one episode per year (Tigges, 2000).

Subjective Data

Usually the client reports a history of viral respiratory infections, allergies, or barotrauma. She describes unilateral or bilateral ear pain associated with decreased hearing. Systemic symptoms are uncommon in adults. New onset of recurrent otitis media with no preceding history of upper respiratory infections or allergies may be indicative of cancer, especially in women who smoke and drink alcohol.

Objective Data

Data are gathered primarily from physical examination of the ears.

Physical examination reveals a general benign appearance. Vital signs are usually normal, fever rare. The external canal of the ear should appear normal, with no tragus or mastoid tenderness. Otoscopy is used to evaluate five parameters of tympanic membrane appearance:

Otoscopic Exam

- *Color.* Erythema is consistent with acute infection.
- *Contour.* The membrane may be bulging in acute suppurative otitis media, and retracted in serous otitis.
- *Translucence.* The membrane may be thick and opaque in chronic otitis.
- *Structural Changes.* An irregular light reflex or blisters indicate infection.
- *Mobility.* A light reflex should move with insufflation; immobility is consistent with infection.

- *Mastoid.* Should not be tender.
- *Nasal Cavity.* Turbinate may be erythematous, gray, and boggy. A clear discharge may be present.
- *Oropharynx.* May be benign or changes are consistent with allergic rhinitis or pharyngitis.
- *Neck.* Nodes may be present.

If the canal is obscured by copious purulent drainage and the possibility of rupture exists, do not instill anything into the ear or attempt to clean it out.

Diagnostic tests are not usually indicated. An audiogram may be helpful in assessing hearing, and tympanometry may help assess mobility.

Differential Medical Diagnosis

Several conditions of a serious nature should be considered.

External otitis is also called "swimmer's ear." The canal is usually swollen with exudate and tender with external manipulation of the ear. *Treatment with otic drops, usually Cortisporin otic suspension, is required.*

Serous otitis media is characterized by a retracted tympanic membrane, possibly an air-fluid level, and often decreased hearing. There is no erythema, and the condition is common with allergies and upper respiratory infections.

Mastoiditis is a life-threatening condition caused by the spread of infection from the middle ear to the air cells of the mastoid process. Any tenderness over the mastoid should lead to suspicion of mastoiditis. Refer the client immediately for hospitalization.

Meningitis usually causes the client to appear toxic; severe neck pain occurs with flexion.

Malignant otitis externa is associated with a 50 percent fatality rate and is seen in diabetics and in those immunocompromised with external otitis. Refer the client to a physician immediately (Tigges, 2000).

Plan

Medication. Use of antibiotics and other medication is debatable. In European countries, such as The Netherlands, antibiotics are not prescribed because improvement is seen in ten days regardless of treatment. In this country, however, it is felt that the risk of suppurative complications is too great, supporting aggressive treatment with antibiotics (Tigges, 2000, Pichichero, 2000).

In general, the first choice is amoxicillin (Polymox) 250 or 500 mg orally three times daily for ten days; the second choice is trimethoprim-sulfamethoxazole double-strength tablets (Bactrim DS) twice daily for ten days. Third-choice antibiotics include cefaclor (Ceclor), amoxicillin/clavulanate potassium (Augmentin), Azithromycin (Zithromax), and Clarithromycin (Biaxin) can also be used. For analgesia, acetaminophen and NSAIDs usually suffice. Decongestants have never been proven to shorten the course of otitis media and are used only symptomatically for nasal congestion. Refer to a pharmacotherapeutics text for details.

Tympanostomy (myringotomy) is not usually required for adults. Refer the client to an ear, nose, and throat specialist if she does not improve after two or three ten-day treatment regimens.

Lifestyle Changes. Advise the client to avoid vigorous nose blowing and to increase fluid intake. Encourage the client to stop smoking, as smoking increases the risk of otitis media.

For fluid behind the ear, teach the client to carry out gentle autoinsufflation: She manipulates the posterior pharynx (swallowing, chewing gum, yawning) to speed drainage of fluid from the middle ear.

Follow-Up

Ask the client to return to the clinic if acute symptoms, such as pain, are not improved in 48 hours or if she is not asymptomatic in ten days.

ACUTE SINUSITIS

Acute sinusitis is infection of one of the four sinuses: maxillary, frontal, ethmoid, and sphenoid. The mucosal lining becomes swollen and occludes air exchange and mucous drainage, resulting in inflammation, bacterial replication, and purulent discharge.

Epidemiology

Studies reveal that numerous conditions can predispose an individual to acute sinusitis. The most common risk factors are viral upper respiratory infections, allergic rhinitis, and dental extraction and abscesses. Barotrauma (flying or diving), foreign bodies, tumors, and polyps are less common but they can block the ostia (or openings) to the sinuses (Chrostowski & Pongracic, 2002).

The primary organisms causing acute sinusitis are *Streptococcus pneumoniae, Haemophilus influenzae, Moraxella catarrhalis,* group A streptococci, and staphylococci. Organisms involved in chronic infections include those already listed as well as mixed anaerobes, which are often difficult to treat (Chrostowski & Pongracic, 2002).

Incidence reports show acute sinusitis as a common condition; it complicates about 0.5 percent of all upper respiratory infections.

Subjective Data

Taking a detailed history is imperative, as a physical exam is of limited use in making the diagnosis. The classic history is a preceding upper respiratory infection lasting five days or longer, with subsequent development of copious yellow-green nasal discharge and intense, localized facial pain, worse on forward bending. Discomfort is often intense and constant. Depending on which sinus is infected, the pain may be referred to the teeth or palate (maxillary), the eyebrow area (frontal), or behind the eyes or at the top of the head (ethmoid and sphenoid). Note whether symptoms are unilateral or bilateral. Some infections present with only a history of purulent nasal discharge and fatigue, with no associated face pain.

Infection can be acute (1 day to 3 weeks), subacute (3 weeks to 3 months), or chronic (more than 3 months). The time frame is important to ascertain, and then treat the infection aggressively, as chronic infection is more difficult to treat and at times can require surgical intervention (Chrostowski & Pongracic, 2002).

Objective Data

Physical Examination. Reveals a benign general appearance. Vital signs are usually normal; fever is rare. If fever is high, consider referral. (Caution: Clients are in pain and may be taking analgesics that mask fever; ask if they have taken any acetaminophen, aspirin, or NSAIDs in the previous 4 hours.)

Abnormal eye movements, facial edema, and erythema around the eyes suggest spreading cellulitis; immediate referral is necessary.

A purulent nasal discharge and edematous turbinates may be noted, as may a purulent postnasal drip.

Sinuses are difficult to assess; percussion for tenderness and transillumination are often unreliable.

Diagnostic Tests. Since plain films of the sinus offer only low specificity and sensitivity, more clinicians are using computed tomography (CT) scans (without contrast) when such tests are indicated. CT scans offer good visualization of the ostiomeatal complex, the openings of the anterior ethmoid maxillary, and frontal sinuses. Nasal endoscopy allows direct visualization of the anatomic and pathologic features of the nose.

Differential Medical Diagnosis

Viral upper respiratory infections, allergic rhinitis, rebound medicamentosa from topical decongestants, dental extractions and abscesses, nasal polyps and tumors (Chrostowski & Pongracic, 2002).

Plan

Psychosocial Interventions. Encourage the client to comply with the antibiotic regimen. Educate her about the warning signs and symptoms of complications: facial swelling, visual problems, high fever, increased pain.

Medication. Antibiotics, decongestants, and analgesics may be helpful.

The *antibiotic* of first choice is amoxicillin, 500 mg orally three times daily for twenty-one days. An alternative is trimethoprim-sulfamethoxazole double strength (Bactrim DS) twice daily for twenty-one days.

Decongestants may help to shrink tissue and drain infection. Monitor hypertensive clients closely.

Analgesics include NSAIDs, which help to ease the pain and edema.

Antihistamines are usually avoided, as they may dry mucous membranes and impair ciliary movement to clear sinuses.

Surgical Interventions. Surgical management may be recommended by an ear, nose, and throat specialist if the client's symptoms do not improve.

Lifestyle Changes. Use of a room humidifier, hot showers, and nasal saline nose drops may keep mucous membranes moist and draining. Application of warm packs to the affected area may provide comfort. Increasing fluid intake also helps to keep secretions loose. Advise physical activity as tolerated, and discourage smoking.

Follow-Up

Consider the potentially lethal complications of acute sinusitis, including periorbital cellulitis and abscess leading to meningitis, osteomyelitis, or cavernous sinus thrombosis. Refer clients to a physician if they appear toxic, have a high fever, or exhibit redness or swelling around the eyes, difficulty moving the eyes, or double vision.

Symptoms should improve greatly 48 hours after starting antibiotics. If not, refer the client to a physician. All symptoms should resolve before completion of medications. If not, or if they recur, refer the client to a physician. Rule out tumors and polyps if acute episodes recur or if symptoms persist with treatment. Assess for and treat allergic rhinitis after acute symptoms resolve.

PHARYNGITIS

Pharyngitis, an inflammatory condition of the pharynx, has numerous causes. Three causes discussed here in depth are group A beta hemolytic streptococci (GABHS), infectious mononucleosis, and *Neisseria gonorrhoeae* (see Table 21–19).

Epidemiology

Identification of GABHS necessitates immediate treatment, because these organisms can cause rheumatic fever if untreated and if associated with local suppurative complications such as tonsillar abscess (Martin, & Horan, 2000). Infectious mononucleosis is acute infection with the Epstein-Barr virus. Although pharyngitis caused by mononucleosis cannot be treated, it should be identified so that the client can be monitored for potentially lethal complications, such as airway compromise and splenic rupture. Pharyngitis caused by *N. gonorrhoeae* may be confused with pharyngitis caused by GABHS or mononucleosis, but it must be identified so that sexual partners can be treated (Martin & Horan, 2000).

Transmission of GABHS (scarlet fever) occurs primarily among children of school age or people living under crowded living conditions, such as college dormitories and military barracks. Mononucleosis is primarily a disease of the young passed through mucous membrane secretions. Gonorrheal pharyngitis is most commonly seen among homosexual males, but should be considered in any sexually active adult with a sore throat who fails to respond to treatment (Martin & Horan, 2000).

Incidence reports show that GABHS are responsible for about one-third of the sore throats seen in primary care. GABHS commonly occur among children between

TABLE 21–19. Differential Diagnosis of Pharyngitis

Bacterial Diseases	Viral Diseases	Other Diseases
GABHS[a] Large tonsils beefy red ± exudate Fever (>101 °F) Nodes anterior and very tender Rash, scarlatina sandpaperlike Often headache Often vomit once No cough	**Mononucleosis** Large tonsils, palatine petechiae ± exudate Fever may or may not occur Nodes posterior or generalized Rash, faint, maculopapular Headache may or may not occur Persistent anorexia/fatigue Rare cough 30% splenomegaly 10% hepatomegaly	**Mycoplasma** Rarely diagnosed in absence of bronchitis/pneumonia **Candida** "Thrush," rule out AIDS, cancer, and diabetes
Gonorrhea 1% of sore throats in adults ± exudate History of oral sex	**Common cold** URI caused by rhinovirus, etc. usually nasal symptoms may be hoarse	**Allergies** Consider if "cold lasts >3 weeks," worse in morning and nighttime, postnasal drip
Diphtheria Pseudomembrane Unimmunized population	**Herpes simplex** Ulcers on gums, hard palate tissue and lips	**Spirochetes** Syphilis Acute necrotizing ulcerative gingivitis Ulcers on gums "Trench mouth"
Haemophilus influenzae Rare in adults Epiglottis in children	**Coxsackievirus** Ulcers on soft palate and tonsillar pillars	**Dehydration**
Group D and C streptococci Rarely cause suppurative complications, therefore not treated	**Cytomegalovirus** Mononucleosis-like syndrome may be asymptomatic or quite ill, will shed virus, dangerous to pregnant women with no immunity	**Irritant gases** **Trauma** **Foreign body** **Neoplasm**
Tuberculosis	**Measles, mumps, rubella, varicella**	

[a]GABHS, group A beta hemolytic streptococci; URI, upper respiratory infection.

Sources: (Lang & Towers, 2001, Martin & Horan, 2000).

3 and 15 years of age; however, these organisms cause 5 to 20 percent of sore throats among persons older than 15 (Lang & Towers, 2001). Ninety percent of the population has had mononucleosis by age 40. Most adults are not aware that they had it in childhood. The infection tends to be more severe if contracted as an adult (Martin & Horan, 2000).

Gonorrhea is responsible for about 1 percent of pharyngitis infections among adults treated in primary care.

Subjective Data

Histories reported by women vary, depending on the etiology of pharyngitis. Pharyngitis caused by GABHS is associated with a classic history of sudden onset of malaise, fever (usually higher than 101°F), tender anterior cervical nodes, headache, and a severe sore (not "scratchy") throat. Nasal symptoms are infrequent and cough is rare. Often a woman has been exposed to small children. If an abscess is present, the client may experience excruciating unilateral pain and may report drooling or spitting saliva, rather than swallowing it. Ask the client about a history of abscesses, as recurrence is common.

Infectious mononucleosis in adults usually presents with a history of gradual onset of fatigue that becomes severe (sleeping 12 to 14 hours per day). Appetite decreases. Sore throat begins, and the client complains of "aches" around the neck caused by prominent neck adenopathy. Fever is variable; temperature may be normal to greater than 103°F. Side tenderness and jaundice may be caused by hepatosplenomegaly. Symptoms are most prominent in the first two weeks, and gradual full recovery usually occurs in six weeks (Lang & Towers, 2001).

Gonorrheal pharyngitis may be mild or severe. The diagnosis is suspected if a client reports a new sexual partner and oral sex. The diagnosis is primarily suspected if persistent sore throat is not cured by usual management (Martin & Horan, 2000).

Objective Data

Because physical examination cannot differentiate between viral and bacterial causes of pharyngitis, specific laboratory tests are required for diagnosis.

Physical Examination. Findings depend on the etiology (see Table 21–20). The client may be flushed, appear sick

TABLE 21–20. Differential Diagnosis of Infectious Pharyngitis: Exudative Versus Nonexudative

Exudative	Nonexudative
Group A beta hemolytic streptococci	Rhinovirus
Mononucleosis	Coronavirus
Adenovirus	Respiratory syncytial virus
Neisseria gonorrhoeae	Influenza virus
Mixed anaerobic bacteria	Parainfluenza virus
Herpes simplex virus	

Source: Martin & Horan (2000).

and have fever. A fine, red, sandpaper-like rash is consistent with GABHS (scarlet fever). A maculopapular rash is consistent with mononucleosis and hemorrhagic pustules with gonorrhea. Jaundice can occur in mononucleosis.

Nasal congestion and a hoarse voice are primarily of viral origin and are rare in pharyngitis caused by GABHS, mononucleosis, or gonorrhea. "Hot potato" voice and drooling are red flags and may indicate an abscess. In pharyngitis caused by GABHS, tonsils are often large and beefy red with a thick white exudate. Suspect an abscess or peritonsillar cellulitis if the soft palate shows unilateral bulging, the uvula is deviated or edematous, or if the client will not open her mouth because of pain (Lang & Towers, 2001). Never force a client's mouth open; if epiglottis is present, it may cause spasm and occlusion of the airway.

Neck adenopathy is nonspecific. As a rule, however, large, very tender anterior nodes are consistent with pharyngitis caused by GABHS or gonorrhea; posterior cervical nodes and generalized adenopathy are more consistent with pharyngitis caused by mononucleosis.

The lungs should be clear. Abdominal examination may reveal side tenderness, indicating hepatosplenomegaly from mononucleosis or the mononucleosis-like cytomegalovirus.

Genitalia are examined only if gonorrhea is suspected.

Diagnostic Tests. Specific for bacterial and viral infections. For pharyngitis caused by GABHS, in-office rapid strep tests or cultures are helpful. The white blood cell count may be slightly elevated in streptococcal pharyngitis, but may be greater than 15,000 if an abscess exists.

For infectious mononucleosis, the mononucleus spot test (or heterophile antibody test) often does not turn positive for five to twelve days or longer after onset of illness. The CBC is usually normal or shows a slightly decreased white blood cell count with a predominance of lymphocytes and monocytes. The diagnosis may be made

with a blood smear showing 20 percent atypical lymphocytes. If the client exhibits the classic clinical picture of mononucleosis but the monospot remains negative, consider ordering a battery of tests to rule out cytomegalovirus, toxoplasmosis, and histoplasmosis.

For gonorrheal pharyngitis, order a throat culture; use calcium alginate swabs, plate on Thayer Martin medium, and incubate.

Differential Medical Diagnoses

See Tables 21–19 and 21–20.

Plan

Psychosocial Interventions. Explain to the client her condition or the differential diagnoses being considered if tests were inconclusive. Inform her about the course of treatment to expect and the red flag symptoms that should prompt her to call the health care provider.

Medication. Refer to a current pharmacotherapeutics text for details.

For pharyngitis caused by GABHS, penicillin V (Betapen-VK) 250 to 500 mg orally four times daily for ten days (administer erythromycin if the client is allergic to penicillin V).

NOTE: Although amoxicillin is effective against GABHS, do not give it when the strep test is negative and mononucleosis cannot be ruled out as cause of exudative pharyngitis. Clients with mononucleosis develop a total body maculopapular rash if given amoxicillin (Lang & Towers, 2001).

For pharyngitis caused by infectious mononucleosis, analgesics such as ibuprofen may be given. Steroids may be used if tonsillar enlargement threatens the airway (Martin & Horan, 2000).

For gonorrheal pharyngitis, if uncomplicated, inject ceftriaxone sodium (Rocephin) 125 to 250 mg (by weight) intramuscularly (see Chapter 11 for recommendations). Also administer oral doxycycline (Vibramycin) or tetracycline (Achromycin) to treat the possibility of concurrent chlamydial infection.

Surgical Interventions. Surgery may be needed if abscess is present. Refer the client for needle aspiration and possible incision and drainage.

Lifestyle Changes. If pharyngitis-caused mononucleosis is diagnosed, encourage the client to listen to her body and to rest when she feels tired. She should avoid vigorous activity for about six weeks and protect her sides because of the risk of rupturing the spleen (Martin & Horan,

2000). Otherwise, activity is as tolerated. Warn the client to avoid hepatotoxins, such as alcohol. The client may use warm saline gargles and lozenges if she feels they help.

If gonorrheal pharyngitis is diagnosed, education about safer sex practices should be discussed and all sex partners should be tested and treated.

If pharyngitis caused by GABHS is diagnosed, decreased activity and alcohol avoidance are recommended. In general, encourage clients to increase fluids and nutrition. Discourage smoking.

Follow-Up

Follow-up is specific to the condition.

Pharyngitis caused by GABHS should improve greatly in 48 hours; otherwise have the client return to rule out abscess or other infection.

Clients with pharyngitis caused by mononucleosis are sickest on about days 4 to 8 of illness and should be followed on the basis of the clinical picture. Observe for airway obstruction, hepatitis, and splenic enlargement.

Clients with gonorrheal pharyngitis are at risk for numerous complications, such as disseminated gonococcal infection with bacteremia and purulent arthritis. Ensure that all sexual contacts are treated.

ENDOCRINE DISORDERS

The four most commonly occurring endocrine disorders discussed in this chapter are hypothyroidism, hyperthyroidism, thyroid nodules, and diabetes.

HYPOTHYROIDISM

Hypothyroidism is a clinical syndrome associated with subnormal levels of circulating thyroid hormones. A client may be asymptomatic; the condition may be mild to severe. Myxedema is the advanced form of hypothyroidism characterized by proteinaceous infiltration of the skin and subcutaneous tissues with multiple organ system involvement (Cooper, 2001; Klein & Ojamaa, 2001).

Epidemiology

The cause differs among the four types of hypothyroidism: primary, secondary, goitrous, and transient.

Primary hypothyroidism is characterized by atrophy or destruction of thyroid tissue due to an autoimmune response. Primary hypothyroidism accounts for more than 90 percent of hypothyroid disease. Primary hypothy-

roidism may also be iatrogenic (following radioiodine therapy or thyroidectomy for hyperthyroidism), idiopathic, or the result of a congenital disorder (cretinism) (Cooper, 2001; Toft, 2001).

Secondary hypothyroidism results from insufficient stimulation of an intrinsically normal gland. It may occur in primary disorders of the pituitary or hypothalamus, which result in deficiencies of thyroid-stimulating hormone (TSH) or thyrotropin-releasing hormone (TRH).

Goitrous hypothyroidism is due to defective thyroid hormone synthesis and is characterized by development of a goiter. Goitrous disorders include Hashimoto's thyroiditis; iodine deficiency; acquired hypothyroidism, caused by the use of goitrogens (propylthiouracil, methimazole, lithium, or iodine); peripheral resistance to thyroid hormone; and infiltrative disorders (amyloidosis, sarcoidosis, lymphoma, or malignancy). *Transient hypothyroidism* can occur as the result of pregnancy or significant illness (Arafah, 2001). It usually resolves within six months of onset, and close monitoring is all that is required (Klein & Ojamaa, 2001).

Routine screening of asymptomatic adults is not recommended. It may be clinically prudent, however, to screen those at increased risk, namely, elderly women, newborns, those with a strong family history of thyroid disorders, postpartum women four to eight weeks after delivery, and clients with autoimmune disease (Cooper, 2001; Toft 2001).

The onset of hypothyroidism is most common in women between 30 and 60 years of age. It develops in both men and women. It is a common disorder of the elderly. The prevalence of thyroid disease in clients more than 60 years of age is about 4 percent, eight times higher than in the general population (Cooper, 2001; Toft, 2001).

Subjective Data

Hypothyroidism is easily misdiagnosed because its presentation is nonspecific and it involves multiple organ systems. Less than one-third of the elderly manifest typical symptoms: cold intolerance; weight gain; dry skin; weakness; fatigue; hoarseness; inattention or difficulty concentrating; dizziness; constipation; arthralgias; muscle cramps; menstrual irregularities, particularly menorrhagia; galactorrhea and depression.

Objective Data

Physical Presentation. Depends on the progression of disease from a subclinical one to a medical emergency, such as that which often precedes myxedema coma.

Physical Examination

- *General Appearance.* Flat affect; low pitched, slow speech.
- *Vital Signs.* Bradycardia, hypertension.
- *Skin.* Thin, brittle nails with transverse grooves; dry, scaly cool skin with a diffuse wavy pallor.
- *Head.* Coarse, dry, brittle hair with alopecia; facial edema; enlarged tongue; thinning or absence of the lateral eyebrows.
- *Neck.* Normal, enlarged, small, or absent thyroid; thyroid nodules; tracheal deviation.
- *Chest.* Exertional dyspnea, pleural effusions.
- *Heart.* Cardiomegaly, arrhythmias.
- *Abdomen.* Gastrointestinal hypomotility, ascites.
- *Neurologic Exam.* Cerebellar dysfunction, delayed deep tendon reflexes, parathesias, peripheral neuropathies.
- *Endocrine System.* Galactorrhea.

Diagnostic Laboratory Tests. Reveal levels of circulating thyroid hormones. The active thyroid hormones are tetraiodothyronine (thyroxine or T4) and triiodothyronine (T3). Both T3 and T4 circulate in the serum, bound to three proteins: thyroxine-binding globulin (TBG), thyroxine-binding prealbumin (TBPA), and albumin. The small fractions of T3 and T4 that circulate free (not bound to protein) are the active forms. Alterations in TBG (e.g., with pregnancy, estrogen replacement, or the use of oral contraceptives) may change total circulating T3 and T4 levels but do not affect free unbound forms.

Primary hypothyroidism is confirmed by a high level of thyroid-stimulating hormone (TSH) and a low level of free T4. A serum TSH is the most sensitive test; it is elevated in more than 95 percent of clients with hypothyroidism (Cooper, 2001; Toft, 2001, Weetman, 2000).

Secondary hypothyroidism is differentiated from primary hypothyroidism by the thyrotropin-releasing hormone (TRH) test of pituitary-thyroid regulation. If secondary hypothyroidism is suspected, the client should be referred to an endocrinologist.

Differential Medical Diagnoses

Cardiac disorders, renal disorders, neuromuscular disorders, and depression are common diagnostic considerations.

Plan

Psychosocial Interventions. It may be necessary to address acute anxiety reactions, which are often among the manifestations of this multisystem disorder. Reassure the client that her symptoms will gradually abate with treatment. Depressed clients may benefit from short-term counseling.

Medication. Levothyroxine (Levoxine, Synthroid), a synthetic T4 hormonal replacement, is the medication of choice.

- *Administration.* Begin with levothyroxine 25 to 50 mcg daily and increase by 25 mcg every six weeks according to TSH levels. Dosages need to be adjusted with caution in the elderly and in clients with cardiac disease.
- *Side Effects.* Palpitations and dysrhythmias are known to occur, particularly in clients with cardiac disease.
- *Contraindications.* Contraindications are outweighed by the risk of not treating the hypothyroidism. Use caution, however, in clients with cardiac disease and the elderly.
- *Evaluation of Drug Action.* To ensure equilibrium, measure serum TSH values no sooner than every six weeks after initiating therapy and again three to four months after a maintenance dose is reached. Annual TSH values are done to monitor therapy, as needs may change with time.
- *Client Teaching.* Review with the client signs and symptoms of hypothyroidism and hyperthyroidism, which may indicate the need for medication change.

The decision to treat subclinical hypothyroidism must be evaluated on an individual basis. If the client is symptomatic, a trial of levothyroxine may be indicated. If the client has coexisting medical problems, a referral to an endocrinologist is indicated (Cooper, 2001).

Lifestyle Changes. The daily medication regimen and chronic condition may cause the client to alter her self-perception. Encourage positive, affirming activities. Diet and exercise are not restricted.

Follow-Up

Once the maintenance dose has been established, annual visits are all that may be required to check the TSH level and reinforce client teaching.

HYPERTHYROIDISM (THYROTOXICOSIS)

Thyrotoxicosis is a hypermetabolic state that results from an excess of circulating thyroid hormone. Excessive thyroid hormone does not always result from thyroid gland hyperactivity; thus thyrotoxicosis, not hyperthyroidism, is the preferred term.

The most common condition is Graves' disease, an autoimmune disorder. Thyroid-stimulating immunoglobulin (TSIs) binds to thyroid cell receptors and stimulates overproduction of thyroid hormones T4 and T3. The cause of TSI production is unknown. Graves' disease is characterized by diffuse thyroid enlargement (goiter), hyperthyroidism, ophthalmopathy, and occasionally pretibial myxedema (Toft, 2001; Weetman, 2000).

Other causes of thyrotoxicosis include toxic multinodular goiter, toxic adenoma, subacute thyroiditis, autoimmune thyroiditis, and excessive exogenous thyroid hormone (Weetman, 2000).

Epidemiology

Graves' disease, which accounts for up to 90 percent of all cases of thyrotoxicosis, appears to be familial in origin. Family history also shows an increased incidence of other autoimmune disorders. Toxic multinodular goiter is usually seen after age 50 in individuals with preexisting nontoxic goiter. Silent thyroiditis occurs fairly frequently in postpartal women.

Graves' disease occurs predominantly among women 20 to 40 years old. Up to 2 percent of women are affected. Either sex at any age may be affected (Toft, 2001).

Subjective Data

Clients may report tremulousness; palpitations; heat intolerance; increased perspiration; eye irritation, excessive lacrimation, photophobia, and diplopia; dyspnea; unexplained weight loss, despite increased appetite; frequent bowel movements; fatigue; weakness, especially of the proximal muscles; and decreased menstrual flow or amenorrhea.

Objective Data

Symptoms are related to excessive sympathomimetic activity and increased catabolic activity. The elderly do not usually present with classic symptoms. Cardiac symptoms, including atrial fibrillation, are more common among the elderly, whereas goiter and eye symptoms may be absent.

Physical Examination

- *General Appearance.* Rapid, rambling, anxious speech.
- *Vital Signs.* Tachycardia, systolic hypertension, widened pulse pressure.

- *Skin.* Warm, smooth, moist skin and onycholysis.
- *Eyes.* Exophthalmus, proptosis, upper lid retraction, periorbital swelling.
- *Neck.* Enlarged, soft thyroid gland, nodules, thyroid bruits.
- *Chest.* Tachypnea.
- *Heart.* Atrial fibrillation, hyperdynamic apical impulse, systolic flows murmur.
- *Vascular System.* Bounding peripheral pulses.
- *Abdomen.* Hyperactive bowel sounds.
- *Musculoskeletal System.* Myopathy, especially in the proximal lower extremities.
- *Central Nervous System.* Fine tremor, hyperreflexia.

Diagnostic Laboratory Tests. Show an elevated serum free T4 and a low TSH. If results are normal yet suspicion remains high, refer the client to an endocrinologist for further evaluation. Additional studies might include a serum T3 or thyrotropin-releasing hormone test. Dopamine hydrochloride and corticosteroids can suppress TSH levels (Cooper, 2001; Toft, 2001; Weetman, 2000).

Differential Medical Diagnoses

Amphetamine or cocaine abuse, anxiety states/panic disorder, chronic obstructive pulmonary disease, pheochromocytoma, myeloproliferative disease, diabetes.

Plan

Treatment must be individualized with consideration to the etiology and severity of disease, client's age, concomitant disease, and risks and benefits of therapeutic modalities (Klein & Ojamaa, 2001).

Psychosocial Interventions. Reassure the client that her condition is not a malignant process and can be treated quite effectively.

Medication. Antithyroid drugs, beta blockers, and radioactive iodine are used.

Antithyroid Drugs. Antithyroid drugs are not without significant side effects; in rare cases potentially fatal reactions can occur. The client should be referred to an endocrinologist for treatment. Methmazole (Tapazole) 5 to 20 mg/day initially; 5 to 20 mg/day maintenance; thought to be the more potent than PTU; may be given in one daily dose. Propylthiouracil (PTU) 300 to 600 mg/day initially; 50 to 200 mg/day maintenance; must be given in three equally divided doses because of its shorter half-life; PTU is the drug of choice in pregnancy as it is more highly protein bound and crosses the placenta less readily. The medication may be reduced by half when the client's symptoms have resolved, the goiter has decreased, and the T4 has normalized. It is not useful to check labs more often than every four to eight weeks. Drug therapy is maintained for one year. Approximately 50 to 60 percent of clients will experience a relapse (Cooper, 2001; Toft, 2001; Weetman, 2000).

- ◆ *Side Effects.* The most frequent side effects are rash, malaise, fever, urticaria, arthralgia, gastrointestinal disturbances, and loss of taste. Transient leukopenia occurs in approximately 12 percent of adults.
- ◆ *Contraindication.* Do not administer antithyroid drugs to clients with cardiac disease.
- ◆ *Anticipated Outcome on Evaluation.* Level of circulating thyroid hormone decreases as evidenced by a return to normal TSH level.
- ◆ *Client Teaching.* Inform the client that although the duration of therapy is controversial, it is rarely longer than two years.

Beta Blockers. Beta blockers are indicated to alleviate symptoms of thyrotoxicosis: tachycardia, palpitations, hypertension, tremor, heat intolerance, and anxiety. Beta blockers are used as an adjunct to radioactive iodine until its therapeutic effect is achieved. Propranolol (Inderal) is the most commonly used beta blocker. The goal is to titrate the dose to maintain a heartrate between 70 and 90 and decrease other symptoms. The usual dose is 160 mg/day in either divided doses or long-acting preparation. See section on hypertension for further discussion of beta blockers.

Radioactive Iodine. Radioactive iodine is the treatment of choice for clients over age 40. The client is referred to an endocrinologist for administration.

- ◆ *Administration.* The tracer dose of radioactive iodine in tablet form is administered and followed by irradiation.
- ◆ *Side Effects.* Within the first year, hypothyroidism occurs in 10 percent of those treated. The likelihood of hypothyroidism developing increases by 5 percent each subsequent year over the next twenty years.
- ◆ *Contraindication.* Radioactive iodine is never administered to pregnant women.
- ◆ *Anticipated Outcome on Evaluation.* If an adequate dose of RAI is given, it will be 100 percent effective. Approximately 20 percent of clients require a second dose. Complete resolution of symptoms occurs within six months of treatment.

- ◆ *Client Teaching.* Inform the client that RAI is inexpensive and effective. Many clients then exhibit hypothyroidism and require T4 replacement. Periodic testing for hypothyroidism (TSH level) should be done indefinitely. The amount of radiation received is comparable to the amount necessary to perform a barium enema. Clients should not become pregnant for six months after treatment.
- ◆ *Surgical Interventions.* Surgical intervention is limited and controversial. It may be an option for pregnant women or for those who do not respond to antithyroid medications.

Follow-Up

The treatment will dictate the follow-up. Educate the client about the symptoms of hyper- and hypothyroidism.

THYROID NODULES

A thyroid nodule is a mass that presents as a single palpable nodule or as a part of a multinodular gland. The diagnostic challenge is to distinguish a benign nodule from a malignancy.

Epidemiology

Studies often reveal a history of radiation exposure. The period of latency ranges from five to thirty-five years, with an average of twenty years. A family history of thyroid malignancies or endocrine tumors is common. About 20 to 30 percent of persons exposed to ionizing radiation develop palpable thyroid abnormalities; 50 percent have nodules. Of those nodules, 30 to 50 percent are malignant. Single nodules are more likely to be malignant than is a multinodular gland (Hermus & Huysmans, 1998).

Incidence reports reveal that about 4 percent of the adult population has thyroid nodules; the incidence increases to 5 percent among individuals older than 60 years. Nodules are four times more common in women than men; however, malignant nodules are more common in men. At least 95 percent of all palpable nodules are benign (Hermus & Huysmans, 1998).

Thyroid cancer is rare, and deaths from thyroid cancer are even rarer.

Subjective Data

A client may report a medical history of thyroid disorders, endocrine tumors, and/or head or neck irradiation. Although most women are asymptomatic, a client may have hoarseness, vocal cord paralysis, and dysphagia.

Objective Data

Physical Examination. May be unremarkable or reveal symptoms of hypo- or hyperthyroidism. Nodules range from barely palpable to visible; their physical characteristics do not secure a diagnosis of benign or malignant. Although nodules may be tender, most are nontender. Thyroid malignancy is suggested by a solitary firm nodule with associated nontender cervical lymphadenopathy.

Diagnostic Methods. These include thyroid function tests, biopsy, and imaging. Laboratory tests usually show normal thyroid function (Hermus & Huysmans, 1998).

A fine-needle aspiration biopsy is the most reliable diagnostic method. If the aspirate shows malignancy, the probability is that it is 95 percent correct. If suspicious, a 45 percent chance of malignancy is probable. Biopsy determines which nodules will be surgically excised; biopsy is the only definitive evaluation and surgery the definitive treatment.

The test procedure requires an experienced cytologist. It is safe, inexpensive, and accurate. A fine-needle aspiration biopsy followed by a thyroid scan for suspicious lesions seems to be the most cost effective approach.

Ultrasonography determines consistency but does not define benign versus malignant disease. It is used as a guide for fine-needle aspiration.

Radionuclide imaging classifies nodules as "hot" or "cold." A malignant lesion incorporates less iodine than normal thyroid tissue; therefore, it should appear "cold." This technique is not sensitive; although a "hot" nodule reduces the likelihood of malignancy, it does not exclude the possibility (Hermus & Huysmans, 1998).

Thyroid suppression is controversial and logistically difficult to interpret because of clinical limitations in sizing nodules.

Differential Medical Diagnoses

Hemorrhagic cysts, Hashimoto's thyroiditis.

Plan

Psychosocial Interventions. Inform the client that although it is rare for a nodule to be malignant, the risk is real.

Surgical Interventions. Surgical management of thyroid cancer is controversial. It is generally agreed that the nodule be removed and suppressive therapy utilized. The amount of thyroid to be removed (one lobe or total thyroidectomy) and the method of follow-up may vary.

Follow-Up

Refer all clients with thyroid nodules to an endocrinologist who will manage treatment.

DIABETES MELLITUS

Diabetes mellitus is a chronic disorder that is characterized by hyperglycemia; associated with major abnormalities in carbohydrate, fat, and protein metabolism; accompanied by a marked propensity to develop relatively specific forms of renal, ocular, neurologic, and premature cardiovascular diseases (American Diabetes Association [ADA], 2002a, 2002b).

Diabetes is diagnosed by clinical signs and symptoms of polyuria, polydipsia, polyphagia, weight loss, and/or blurred vision with persistent hyperglycemia; fasting plasma glucose levels exceed 110 and/or random plasma glucose levels exceed 126 on at least three separate occasions (ADA 2002b, 2002c).

The causes of diabetes are unknown, although current thought includes genetic predisposition, unknown precipitating events, progressive autoimmune destruction of pancreatic beta cells, and obesity (ADA 2002a, 2002c; Hu, et al., 2001).

Epidemiology

The majority of diabetes can be classified into two types: type I or insulin-dependent diabetes and type II or noninsulin-dependent diabetes. Other types of diabetes can be associated with other specific conditions or syndromes (pancreatic, endocrine, medications) and are beyond the scope of this book.

Type I (Insulin-Dependent) Diabetes. Type I diabetes accounts for 3 percent of all new cases of diabetes diagnosed each year in the United States. Its annual incidence rate in the under 20 age group is 15 per 100,000. Type I can develop at any age, although generally most cases are diagnosed when the client is under 30 (ADA, 2002b).

Clients with type I are insulinopenic. Insulin therapy is essential to prevent rapid and severe dehydration, catabolism, ketoacidosis, and death. They are usually lean and often have experienced significant weight loss, polyuria, and polydipsia before presentation.

Type II (Noninsulin-Dependent) Diabetes. Type II diabetes is characterized by fasting hyperglycemia and insulin resistance. It is usually diagnosed after age 40 but can occur at any age. It affects an estimated 85 to 90 percent of the 16 million Americans diagnosed with diabetes. Because type II diabetes is a slowly progressive disease, the number of individuals with undiagnosed DM is thought to be nearly the same as the number diagnosed (Warren-Boulton, Greenberg, Lising, Gallivan, 1999).

The likelihood of developing type II is approximately equal by sex but is greater in African Americans, Hispanics, and Native Americans. Obesity (more than 20 percent over ideal body weight), a family history of diabetes, age 40 or over, hypertension, hypercholesterolemia, gestational diabetes, or having one or more infants weighing more than 9 pounds at birth are major risk factors (ADA, 2002c; Hsu et al., 2001; Yanovski & Yanovski, 2002).

Type II diabetes is characterized by insulin resistance and is present in the majority of all clients with fasting blood sugars (FBS) greater than 110. Sites of insulin resistance include hepatic and peripheral tissues. Postbinding abnormalities are primarily responsible for insulin resistance. Impaired binding may be secondary to associated obesity and hyperinsulinemia but may also contribute to impaired tissue insulin sensitivity. Diet recall may reveal high fats, sweets, and starches. There is evidence that weight reduction, exercise, and diet change are beneficial in primary and secondary prevention of NIDDM (ADA 2002b, 2002c; Expert Committee, 2002).

The American Diabetes Association recommends screening adults with one or more risk factors every three years.

Impaired Glucose Tolerance. Impaired glucose tolerance is characterized by a fasting plasma glucose level of >110 mg/dl and <126 mg/dl on two separate occasions. These clients may develop type II diabetes and should be monitored closely.

Subjective Data

The client may report a history of weight loss, polydipsia, polyuria, polyphagia, blurred vision, endocrine disorders, alcoholism, pancreatitis, gestational diabetes, medications (e.g., steroids, thiazide, diuretic), frequent urinary tract infections, yeast vaginitis, poor healing wounds, or a family history of diabetes.

Objective Data

- *General.* Recent weight gains or losses.
- *Eyes.* Fundoscopic-diabetic retinopathy.
- *Mouth/Throat.* Candidiasis.
- *Gastrointestinal.* Diminished bowel sounds. Right upper quadrant tenderness (pancreatitis).
- *Genitourinary.* Vulvo-vaginal candidiasis.

- *Neurological.* Decreased sensation peripherally, gait disturbances, carpal tunnel syndrome.
- *Extremities.* Decreased pulses, poor healing wounds, temperature or color changes.
- *Diagnostic.* Fasting blood sugar >110 mg/dl on two separate occasions or random BS over 200. Glycosolated Hemoglobin greater than 8. Oral glucose tolerance testing is useful to confirm the diagnosis of gestational diabetes and evaluate clients with complications suggestive of diabetes (background retinopathy, neuropathy).
- *Other Lab.* Elevated amylase (pancreatitis) or cholesterol (especially triglycerides).

Differential Medical Diagnoses

Medication induced diabetes (steroids, thiazide, diuretics), hypothyroidism, hyperthyroidism, human immunodeficiency virus (HIV), substance abuse.

Plan

The goals are to achieve normal metabolic control, reduce the potential for development of complications, promote a reasonable body weight, and encourage healthy eating habits. The Diabetes Control and Complications Trial (DCCT) (ADA 2002a, 2002c) showed an overall reduction in potential complication when these goals are achieved. Before treating, assess the client's self-care attitudes, abilities, and priorities.

Treatment modalities include dietary modifications, increased physical activity, pharmacologic intervention, and intensive and continued client education (ADA, 2002c).

Psychosocial Interventions. The diagnosis of diabetes is a lifelong, life altering one. Explore the client's perception of her self-image, her health beliefs, and her perception of diabetes. Consider a referral to a diabetes support group.

Dietary Interventions. The client should be encouraged to follow a low-fat, no-added-salt diet and to avoid sweets. Consider a referral to a nutritionist and the local chapter of the American Diabetes Association or the local diabetes educators in your community.

Physical Activity. Encourage the client to develop a regular exercise plan based on her current fitness level. Establish fitness goals and follow-up at regular visits.

Pharmacologic Intervention. The Type I diabetic is essentially insulinopenic and requires exogenous insulin. The type II or NIDDM diabetic will require pharmacologic intervention when diet modification and increased physical activity fails to control glucose levels alone. The physiologic abnormalities of NIDDM progress gradually over time and then lose efficacy. Five years of success on a given treatment is what may reasonably be expected.

Oral Agent Therapy

- ♦ *Sulfonylureas.* All sulfonylureas act by increasing the secretion of insulin in response to fasting blood glucose levels. They reduce the fasting hyperglycemia but have little effect on postprandial glucose. In choosing a sulfonylurea (or any agent), expense, ease of dosing, and comorbid conditions, must be considered. See Table 21–21.
- ♦ *Acarbose (Precose).* Acarbose, taken at the beginning of a meal, interferes with hydrolysis of dietary disaccharides and complex carbohydrates, delaying absorption of glucose and other monosaccharides. It can be helpful in lowering postprandial plasma glucose concentrations.
  - *Administration.* Acarbose is taken at the beginning of a meal. The recommended starting dose is 25 mg t.i.d. and increasing at four- to eight-week intervals, depending on postprandial blood glucose concentrations and tolerance, up to 50 mg t.i.d. for clients weighing fewer than 60 kg, or 100 mg t.i.d. for heavier clients.

TABLE 21–21. Diabetes Oral Agent Therapy

Agent	Dose Range	Doses/Day
First-Generation Sulfonylureas		
tolbultamide	500–3000	b.i.d. or t.i.d.
tolazamide	100–1000	qd or b.i.d.
chlorproamide	100–500	qd
Second-Generation Sulfonylureas		
glipizide	2.5–40	qd or b.i.d.
glyburide	5–20	qd
micronized glyburide	0.75–12	qd
gliperamide	1–4	qd
Other Agents		
acarbose	25–50	t.i.d. with meals
metformin	100–2550	b.i.d. or t.i.d.
pioglitazone	15–30	qd
rosiglitazone	2–8	b.i.d.
repaglinide	0.5–4	30 min. before meals
nateglinide	60–120	30 min. before meals

Source: Ahmann & Riddle (2002); Hsu et al. (2001); Warren-Boulton et al. (1999).

TABLE 21–22. Insulin Therapy

	Onset of Action	Peak	Duration
Short Acting			
Regular	30–45 minutes	2–3 hours	5–6 hours
Insulin aspart	30 minutes	1–3 hours	3–5 hours
Insulin lispro	30 minutes	30 minutes–3 hours	2–6 hours
Intermediate Acting			
NPH	2–3 hours	6–9 hours	12–14 hours
Lente	2–3 hours	6–9 hours	12–14 hours
Long Acting			
Ultralente	4–10 hours	8–20 hours	18–28 hours
Insulin glargine	5 hours	*	18–28 hours

*Has no pronounced peak.

Source: Ahmann & Riddle (2002); American Pharmaceutical Assoc. (2001); Warren-Boulton et al. (1999).

- *Adverse Effects.* Unabsorbed carbohydrates undergo fermentation in the colon, leading to gastrointestinal distress, which may diminish with time. Acarbose may decrease intestinal absorption of iron and cause anemia.
- *Interactions.* Acarbose may increase the risk of hypoglycemia when taken with other hypoglycemic agents. Oral treatment of hypoglycemia must be with glucose because sucrose may not be adequately hydrolyzed and absorbed. Acarbose may decrease the bioavailability of metformin, and their gastrointestinal adverse effects may be additive; concurrent use should probably be avoided.
- ♦ *Metformin (Glucophage).* A biguanide hypoglycemic agent for treatment of clients with NIDDM not adequately controlled by diet alone. Metformin is absorbed from the gastrointestinal tract over approximately six hours and excreted by the kidneys without being metabolized. It decreases glucose production in the liver and increases glucose uptake but does not cause clinical hypoglycemia. It has no effect on pancreatic insulin secretion and requires the presence of insulin to be effective. It is used to overcome insulin resistance. In a study by DeFronzo et al. (1995), the substitution of metformin for glyburide resulted in little benefit.
  - *Administration.* Metformin is available in 500 mg and 850 mg tablets. The starting dose is 500 mg b.i.d. with the morning and evening meal. The

usual dosage is 850 mg b.i.d., and the maximum is 850 mg t.i.d.

- *Adverse Effects.* Metformin can cause a metallic taste, diarrhea, nausea, vomiting, and anorexia. Most of these symptoms diminish or disappear with a decreased dose or discontinuance of the drug.
- *Lactic Acidosis.* All biguanides inhibit lactate metabolism, and increased concentrations of the drug associated with renal impairment can cause lactic acidosis. Even a temporary reduction in renal function, such as occurs after angiography, can cause lactic acidosis. The drug should be discontinued two days before such procedures and restarted only after renal function returns to normal. Increased alcohol intake, conditions associated with hypoxemia (heart failure, shock, hepatic failure), or surgery are indication for stopping metformin (ADA, 2002c).

Combination Therapy. The combination of *metformin* and *glyburide* was found superior to treatment with either drug alone (ADA, 2002c). This has been shown to lower plasma glucose and glycosylated hemoglobin values in clients with NIDDM who had poor responses to maximal doses of a sulfonylurea. It is recommended to start with either a sulfonylurea or metformin, increase as indicated and add the second agent when the maximum dosage has been reached. Due to the progressive nature of diabetes in some clients, oral agents will fail and insulin should be started. For most, this will mean a permanent commitment to insulin.

The combination of a *sulfonylurea* and *insulin* has been used as a traditional step between management by oral agents and aggressive insulin therapy. The combination recommended by the American Diabetes Association is half the dose of the oral agent in the morning and 0.2 units/kg at bedtime. See Tables 21–21 and 21–22.

Insulin Therapy

INSULIN-DEPENDENT DIABETES (TYPE I). In these clients, the production of insulin by the beta cell is lost and the client becomes dependent on the use of exogenous insulin. Understanding the actions of the various insulins is crucial to designing an insulin program that will mimic the body's own insulin release.

Intensive insulin therapy in three or more injections a day, with home glucose monitoring, will provide ideal control. The basal dose of insulin is given as either a long-acting or intermediate-acting insulin. A bolus dose is given premeal to mimic the endogenous release of insulin at mealtimes. Before adjusting doses, confirm diet and exercise patterns, recent illnesses or stressors, any hypoglycemia or hyperglycemia events, or other medication changes.

NON-INSULIN-DEPENDENT DIABETES (TYPE II). These clients may require exogenous insulin to supplement decreased endogenous production or decreased insulin response. The starting dose in NIDDM is 0.5 per kilogram of an intermediate-acting insulin in a single or two doses. It is best to match the peak action of insulin to the rise in glucose that occurs in the early morning hours between 3 and 8 A.M. Therefore the P.M. dose would be administered at bedtime (ADA, 2002a; Stoller, 2002).

Follow-Up

Follow-up should be individualized based on the client's current needs. Perform regular screening for microvascular and macrovascular complications (ADA, 2002). Regular review of the client's home glucose monitoring diary and technique as well as reinforcement of dietary and exercise recommendations is advised. If diabetes is difficult to control, consider other medications as the cause—thiazide diuretics and beta blockers can cause hyperglycemia. Beta blockers can also mask the signs and symptoms of hypoglycemia.

GASTROINTESTINAL DISORDERS

This section covers the following disorders: gastroesophageal reflux disease, peptic ulcer disease, gallbladder disease, irritable bowel syndrome, anal fissures, and hepatitis.

GASTROESOPHAGEAL REFLUX DISEASE

Gastroesophageal reflux disease (GERD) is a clinical syndrome characterized by heartburn, a burning sensation resulting from the backward flow of gastric contents into the esophagus. The most common form is idiopathic lower esophageal sphincter incompetence. It is primarily a motility disorder. Contributing factors include gastric hyperacidity, impaired esophageal clearance, increased volume of gastric contents, and altered mucosal resistance (Hubbard, 2002; Ray, Secrest, Chien, & Corey, 2002).

Etiology reveals that hiatal hernias predispose to GERD, but are not pathognomonic. Pregnancy and obesity may exacerbate symptoms. Cigarette smoking, chocolate, fatty foods, caffeine, alcohol, and some medications (tetracycline, doxycycline, quinidine, slow-release potassium supplements, iron, calcium channel blockers, and nonsteroidal anti-inflammatory drugs) also aggravate GERD. Delayed gastric or esophageal emptying and prolonged exposure to gastric acid increase the frequency and severity of symptoms, complications, and recurrence of gastroesophageal reflux (Hubbard, 2002, Ray et al., 2002).

Epidemiology

GERD is common at all ages, but more prevalent among persons 60 to 70 years old. Incidence is reported to be as high as 20 percent in the general population and accounts for almost half of all noncardiac chest pain (Hubbard, 2002; Ray et al., 2002). GERD is reported in 46 percent of all asthmatics. The higher incidence of GERD among asthmatics may be related to medications.

Early diagnosis and appropriate treatment can prevent secondary complications, such as esophageal strictures, ulcers, Barrett's esophagus, bleeding, pulmonary disease, and hoarseness.

Subjective Data

The client describes a burning sensation or pain underneath the sternum followed by a bitter taste. It may be related to certain foods. Intensity varies, but the sensation usually increases after eating, with forward bending, when supine, or with vigorous exercise. Less common symptoms that may be reported are odynophagia, dysphagia, and pulmonary manifestations, such as nocturnal coughing, wheezing, and hoarseness.

Objective Data

Physical examination is usually benign.

Endoscopy. The most definitive approach to diagnosis. It allows direct visualization and biopsy. Endoscopy is usually performed under conscious sedation.

Advise the client of the risks and benefits of the procedure. It is associated with increased risks for clients who have cardiopulmonary disease, are elderly, or otherwise debilitated.

Upper Gastrointestinal X-ray. Determines the extent of damage to esophageal mucosa. It detects ulcers, strictures, hiatal hernias, and masses. Double-contrast studies are more sensitive and specific than single-contrast studies. They have a sensitivity of 80 to 90 percent, which

decreases with ulcers less than 5 mm in diameter. Barium is used as contrast in x-rays of the upper gastrointestinal tract.

A 24-Hour pH Monitor (a portable unit). Useful in determining the total acid exposure and identifying episodes of nocturnal reflux. The pH probe is manually placed in the esophagus; reflux is defined by a distal esophageal pH less than 4.

The Bernstein Test. Used to demonstrate the relationship of symptoms to pain. Symptoms are simulated: hydrochloric acid and normal saline are alternately infused into the esophagus, while the patient's response is recorded. The test is potentially uncomfortable for clients.

Esophageal Manometry. Indicated for clients who are not responding to conventional medical therapy or for whom surgery is being considered. Lower esophageal pressure is measured, and esophageal peristalsis and the competence of the lower esophageal sphincter are assessed. Normal lower esophageal sphincter pressure ranges between 10 and 25 mm Hg. A pressure of 6 mm Hg or less or inappropriate sphincter relaxation is also highly diagnostic.

Differential Medical Diagnoses

Peptic ulcer disease, esophageal strictures, Barrett's esophagus, angina, pancreatic disease, esophageal candidiasis, Zollinger-Ellison syndrome, respiratory disease (Ray et al., 2002).

Plan

In determining the management of symptoms, consider their severity, the cost of procedures, the risk-benefit of diagnostic testing, the age and health status of the client, and the cost of medications.

Psychosocial Interventions. Involve the client as an active partner in management. She should know that the condition is chronic but manageable.

Medication. Medications are not corrective but protect the mucosa from chronic insult. They suppress and neutralize acid and are cytoprotective.

Antacids neutralize gastric acid.

Alginic acid (Gaviscon) forms a foamy coating over gastric contents, protecting the esophageal mucosa during regurgitation.

H2 receptor agonists block parietal cell actions and thereby decrease gastric acid formation. Few side effects are noted; however, close observation for drug interactions is important.

The *dopamine antagonist/protokinetic agent metoclopramide hydrochloride* (Reglan) increases esophageal sphincter pressure and enhances gastric emptying. It is associated with central nervous system, and other side effects. It may be given in conjunction with an H2 blocker.

The *"acid proton pump" inhibitor omeprazole* (Prilosec) inactivates the hydrogen-potassium ATPase enzyme that drives the proton pump of the parietal cell. It is indicated for intractable reflux esophagitis, Zollinger-Ellison syndrome, and hyperhistaminic states.

Cholinergic drugs (e.g., bethanecol hydrochloride) increase lower esophageal sphincter pressure.

Anticholinergic agents reduce acid secretion but are rarely used because of their adverse effects.

Sucralfate (Carafate tablets) binds bile salts and pepsin, aids mucosal regeneration, and enhances prostaglandin synthesis, making it cytoprotective.

Misoprostol (Cytotec), a synthetic prostaglandin analog, reduces mucosal injury related to use of nonsteroidal anti-inflammatory drugs. Diarrhea may preclude prolonged use.

Surgical Interventions. Surgery may be indicated for clients who have evidence of reflux and failed a six-month trial of medical management (Hubbard, 2002). Surgery is reserved for those who have not responded to simple therapeutic maneuvers or medications, or have advanced disease or complications, such as esophageal stricture, severe bleeding, and pulmonary aspiration. A hiatal hernia is not an indication for surgery. Surgery is effective in 90 percent of cases; the Nissen fundoplication procedure restores sphincter competence.

Lifestyle/Dietary Changes. Lifestyle and dietary changes may be effective initial and adjunctive therapies (Ray et al., 2002). Controlled studies, however, show their benefits are limited.

The diet should not include offending foods (spicy foods, high-fat foods, citrus juices, chocolate, peppermint, onions, and caffeine). Ideal body weight should be maintained and alcohol eliminated. Advise the client to take the following measures:

- Avoid recumbent positions within three hours of a meal.
- Elevate the head of the bed on four- to six-inch blocks or on a bed wedge.
- Avoid bending forward.
- Discontinue cigarette smoking and use of all nicotine products.

- Avoid constricting clothing.

Follow-Up. Follow-up to determine response to therapy, to reinforce nonpharmacologic measures, and to assess for respiratory symptoms.

PEPTIC ULCER DISEASE

Peptic ulcers are small sores, or lesions, in the lower end of the esophagus or the lining of the stomach, duodenum, or jejunum. The two main types of peptic ulcer disease (PUD) are duodenal and gastric.

Pepsin, the chief enzyme of gastric juices, combines with hydrochloric acid to digest food in the stomach. Normally, the lining of the stomach resists corrosion, but for unclear reasons, resistance can break down and an ulcer develops. Because most clients with these ulcers demonstrate normal acid production, research is directed toward mucosal defense mechanisms (Alsace & Maradiegue, 2000).

Epidemiology

Peptic ulcer disease affects approximately 4 million Americans a year. It occurs more frequently in men (Alsace & Maradiegue, 2000).

Risk factors include cigarette smoking, medical or family history, and medication. Nonsteroidal anti-inflammatory drugs (NSAIDs)/aspirin or steroids in high doses or used long term can contribute to the development of PUD, particularly among women older than 65 years. The risk is the same for plain or buffered aspirin but less if it is enteric-coated, because with the coating the tablet dissolves in the small intestine.

Medical conditions predisposing individuals to PUD are hyperparathyroidism (secondary to increased calcium, which increases gastric secretion), cirrhosis, renal failure and chronic steroid use. The evidence that increased stress causes or activates ulcer formation is not conclusive.

In clients older than 50, it is necessary to rule out gastric cancer as an etiology, especially if symptoms have a recent onset or are persistent despite treatment.

Transmission may involve *Helicobacter pylori* (*Campylobacter pyloris*), although its role in the pathogenesis of ulcers is unclear. Investigators believe that gastroduodenal mucosa infected with the organism is more likely to undergo ulceration. It is agreed that it is the causative organism in type B antral gastritis (Alsace & Maradiegue, 2000).

Subjective Data

Less than half of clients with PUD present typically. Clinical features in the elderly are often vague or may be absent until a complication occurs.

Gnawing, burning, epigastric, or upper abdominal pain radiating to the back may awaken clients in the night or early morning. Typically, symptoms of a peptic ulcer are brought on by an empty stomach and may be relieved by eating.

On the other hand, gastric ulcers are usually aggravated by eating. Pain begins almost immediately after eating. It is not uncommon for months or years to pass without pain. Associated symptoms include dyspepsia, heartburn, and nausea or may be more severe with vomiting and weight loss. Bowel habits generally remain unaltered.

Objective Data

Diagnostic tests and other procedures are the sources of objective data. Physical examination rarely helps in diagnosis. Epigastric tenderness is neither specific nor sensitive. Rectal exam may be hemocult positive. The sensitivity is 10 to 70 percent (Alsace & Maradiegue, 2000).

Diagnostic laboratory tests are used to evaluate a client for complications, such as bleeding, or indications of malabsorption. Blood is drawn for CBC and chemistries.

The upper gastrointestinal series and endoscopy are explained under Gastroesophageal Reflux Disease.

H. pylori is diagnosed by endoscopic biopsy, serum IGG or by breath test.

Differential Medical Diagnoses

Esophageal stricture, Barrett's esophagus, angina, respiratory disease, gallbladder disease, gastroesophageal reflux disease.

Plan

Psychosocial Interventions. Provide information and support concerning diet and possibly long-term medications. The role of stress is controversial.

Medication. See Gastroesophageal Reflux. If *H. pylori* is diagnosed, a two-week course of clarithromycin (Biaxin) and omeprazole (Prilosec) 20 mg qd should relieve symptoms. Less expensive courses are often for longer periods of time and require t.i.d. and q.i.d. dosing (Alsace & Maradiegue, 2000).

Ulcer recurrence may be prevented with chronic H2 blockers at half the initial therapeutic dose among persons at high risk for recurrence (asthmatics, cigarette smokers, and diabetics) or clients at high risk for complications (renal transplant recipients and clients with systemic disease) (Alsace & Maradiegue, 2000) (see Table 21–23).

Dietary Interventions. Have the client eliminate from her diet any offending foods and alcohol. Frequent, small bland meals with milk were encouraged for years; however, there is no evidence this will promote healing. Milk may exacerbate symptoms as it stimulates acid secretion.

Follow-Up

Follow-up differs for gastric and duodenal ulcers. Gastric ulcers take longer to heal and require a full eight weeks of treatment. Duodenal ulcers may heal more quickly but recur in about 80 percent of clients within one year and are more likely to be a chronic condition. Refer clients with ulcers that are unresponsive (persistent symptoms) to a GI specialist.

GALLBLADDER DISEASE

The two gallbladder diseases discussed in this chapter are cholecystitis and cholelithiasis.

Cholecystitis is acute inflammation of the gallbladder, usually caused by a gallstone blocking the outlet of the gallbladder or cystic duct. Edema, infection, and ulceration result. If this process continues, necrosis, perforation, and peritonitis may result.

TABLE 21–23. Management of Peptic Ulcer Disease

Symptoms consistent with peptic ulcer disease
+
Absence of complications[a]
+
Age < 50 years

↓

Avoid exacerbating agents, e.g., aspirin, alcohol, smoking

Treat empirically with H2 blocker ⟶ Symptoms persist/worsen

↓   ↓

Therapeutic response at 2-week   Endoscopy/x-ray
  follow-up   If biopsy needed, refer
Continued for total of 6–8 weeks   to GI specialist

[a]History of GI/peptic ulcer disease, bleeding, weight loss, persistent pain, vomiting.

Source: Alsace & Maradiegue (2000).

Cholelithiasis is the presence or formation of gallstones. Generally, gallstones form whenever cholesterol is oversaturated. Gallstones are classified by composition (Greenberger & Paumgartner, 2001).

Cholesterol stones constitute 80 percent of all gallstones in the United States and contain, in addition to cholesterol, bile acids, calcium salts, proteins, and phospholipids.

Pigment stones are black or brown. Black pigment is more common in the United States, brown among native Asians.

Epidemiology

The incidence of gallstones in the United States is approximately 10 percent. Eighty percent of stones are thought to be the cholesterol type (Alsace & Maradiegue, 2000).

Risk factors are multiparity, use of estrogens (including oral contraceptives), obesity, rapid weight loss, high-fat diet. Crohn's disease (involving the ileum or ileal resection), regional enteritis, cirrhosis, diabetes, a family history of gallbladder disease, total parenteral nutrition, and solid organ transplant. There is a 50 percent chance of recurrence with a previous history of gallbladder disease (Alsace & Maradiegue, 2000).

Gallbladder disease occurs primarily among overweight women 40 to 65 years of age. The incidence among women is almost three times that among men and increases with age (Alsace & Maradiegue, 2000).

Subjective Data

Initially, a client reports diffuse, intermittent right upper quadrant pain, an ache or pressure that occurs at night or early in the morning. It progresses to a continuous, more severe pain and may radiate to the epigastrium or right shoulder. Onset of pain may be sudden and last from 20 minutes to five or six hours; it may continue as a dull ache for 24 hours or longer. Intervals between episodes vary considerably, from weeks to years. Pain may be accompanied by nausea, vomiting, constipation, or fever (Greenberger & Paumgartner, 2001).

Objective Data

Physical examination during the acute phase of disease maybe helpful along with diagnostic tests.

Physical Examination. Not helpful in the nonacute phase. During the acute symptom phase, specific changes may be observed:

- ◆ *General.* Restless, fever, jaundice.
- ◆ *Eyes.* Icteric.
- ◆ *Chest.* Clear to auscultation, splinting with respiration.
- ◆ *Abdomen.* RUQ tenderness; Murphy's sign; a palpable globular mass may be found behind the lower border of the liver.

Diagnostic Laboratory Tests. May reveal elevations of serum transaminases, alkaline phosphatase (due to obstructed biliary tract), or serum lipase or amylase (gallstone pancreatitis). An increase in white blood cells with a left shift denotes cholecystitis or cholangitis.

Ultrasonography is used to diagnose gallstones. It is a quick and inexpensive way to evaluate the liver, pancreas, and other abdominal organs. It is now the diagnostic test of choice.

Endoscopic retrograde cholangiopancreatography (ERCP) aids in the diagnosis of common duct calculi, biliary dilatation, cystic duct obstruction, and cancer.

An *oral cholecystogram* is a diagnostic evaluation for cholelithiasis. The client takes iopanic or tyropanoic acid tablets the night before the exam. The dye concentrates in the gallbladder and permits its visualization the following day. The method is well tolerated. It is 90 to 95 percent accurate in detecting stones.

Differential Medical Diagnoses

Angina, peptic ulcer disease, esophageal spasm, appendicitis, intestinal obstruction, gastroesophageal disease, pancreatitis, myocardial ischemia, pyelonephritis.

Plan

Psychosocial Interventions. Discuss with the client that surveillance of recurrence alone may be suitable management for infrequent symptoms and little disability.

Medication. Medication is limited to comfort measures. A client who has asymptomatic gallstones can be monitored and will not necessarily require intervention. Use of oral bile salts is limited to clients with small radiolucent stones (indicating cholesterol composition) and a functioning gallbladder and to clients with mild or infrequent symptoms. Oral salts are also given to clients who refuse surgery or who are poor surgical candidates. The medication is taken daily for six months to two years. Treatment requires follow-up visits and ultrasound examination. Medication is expensive (Alsace & Maradiegue, 2000; Greenberger & Paumgartner, 2001).

Bile salts alter the ratio of bile acids to cholesterol and lecithin as well as reduce HMG-COA reductase activity, thereby reducing hepatic cholesterol synthesis.

Surgical Interventions. The laparoscopic approach to cholecystectomy is the treatment method of choice. It reduces postoperative pain as well as hospitalization and at-home recovery time.

Lithotripsy, extracorporeal shock-wave therapy of gallstones, is gaining popularity but its use is limited. Its distinct advantage is that it is non-invasive. More research is needed to determine the rate of recurrence, adverse sequelae, and cost effectiveness.

Follow-Up

Refer clients with acute cholecystitis to a collaborating physician, gastrointestinal specialist, or surgeon for evaluation and treatment. Acute cholecystitis can be a life-threatening emergency. Major complications are perforation of the gallbladder with resultant peritonitis and internal biliary fistula. Fever, severe pain, and elevated white blood cell counts are indications for prompt surgical referral. The size, number, and location of gallstones influence the decision to treat aggressively versus conservatively. A more aggressive approach will likely be based on greater pain and disability from biliary attacks.

IRRITABLE BOWEL SYNDROME

The etiology of irritable bowel syndrome (IBS) is probably multifactorial. Contraction of colonic smooth muscle is controlled by cyclic alterations of smooth muscle membrane potential. In IBS, the normally orderly movement of colonic contents is altered. The entire gut, particularly the colon, is affected (Owyang, 2001).

Epidemiology

Etiology reveals a threefold increase in psychiatric illnesses (anxiety, hysteria, and depression) among persons with irritable bowel syndrome. When psychiatric illness is a cofactor, clients are more often middle-aged (Alsace & Maradiegue, 2000).

Irritable bowel syndrome occurs most often among women between the ages of 20 and 50 years, but it may develop at any age. It is one of the most common reasons for referral to gastrointestinal specialists. About 30 percent of the general population may have symptoms, but only 14 percent seek medical attention.

Subjective Data

A careful history is the key to diagnosis. Acute stressful events, such as acute illness, job demands or loss of job, financial pressures, and illness or death of a close friend or relative, seem to precipitate attacks. Poor dietary habits may also be influential. About 50 percent of clients report nausea, heartburn, and dyspeptic symptoms. Colic abdominal pain varies in intensity. It may be precipitated by eating, but is typically relieved by a bowel movement. A client may experience diarrhea, constipation, or both. In addition, she may report abdominal distention, increased amounts of rectal mucus, and a feeling of incomplete evacuation. The condition does *not*, however, awaken clients from sleep, does *not* usually result in any appreciable weight loss (if any, it is less than 10 percent of body weight) and does *not* cause rectal bleeding (Owyang, 2001).

Objective Data

Diagnosis is often made only after other gastrointestinal disorders have been excluded. Consequently, expensive and unnecessary testing may occur. A detailed history guides the workup.

Physical Examination. May reveal diffuse abdominal tenderness. A rectal exam is essential. Hemorrhoids and anal fissures are evaluated.

Diagnostic Laboratory Tests. CBC, chemistries, urinalysis, and examination of stools for ova and parasites (particularly Giardia). Stools for culture, white blood cells, red blood cells. An erythrocyte sedimentation rate is done to rule out inflammatory bowel disease. A lactose tolerance/hydrogen breath test may be done.

Flexible sigmoidoscopy is used to rule out polyps, malignancy, and inflammatory bowel disease. The procedure is usually well tolerated. In the absence of organic lesions, irritable bowel syndrome is strongly suspect.

A colonoscopy is indicated for clients older than 40 years or with a strong family history of colon cancer. The test rules out polyps and malignancy. The client is given a cathartic 24 hours prior to procedure to evaluate bowel debris. Usually the procedure is performed utilizing conscious sedation.

Differential Medical Diagnoses

Laxative abuse, lactose intolerance, Crohn's disease, ulcerative colitis, colon cancer, parasitic infestation, sorbitol intolerance, thyroid disorders, diabetes, eating disorders.

Plan

Psychosocial Interventions. Although symptoms can be stress related, overemphasizing the role of stress can induce confusion and guilt in the client. She should know that irritable bowel syndrome is a chronic condition that can be managed. Reassure her that her condition is not cancer and will not progress to inflammatory bowel disease. Symptoms are controllable, although it may take time and a trial-and-error approach to find the right therapeutic management for an individual. A plan should focus on diet and lifestyle. Discuss stress reduction techniques.

Medication. Medications that may be used address a variety of symptoms (Owyang, 2001).

Psyllium is a bulk laxative that improves regularity and is the main pharmacotherapeutic intervention.

Calcium channel blockers decrease smooth muscle response to neurohumoral stimulation.

Nitrates stimulate production of cyclic guanosine monophosphate within the cell, inhibiting smooth muscle contractions.

Anxiolytics are nonspecific in their action and reserved for underlying anxiety disorders.

Lopraumide HCl, 4 mg initially followed by 2 mg after each unformed stool will control diarrhea.

Antispasmodic agents such as dicyclomine hydrochloride (Bentyl) are used for abdominal pain and cramping.

A tricyclic antidepressant or *selective serotonin reuptake inhibitor* is used when depression, with or without anxiety, is present.

Lifestyle/Dietary Changes. These changes include modifications in diet, exercise, and elimination.

A low-residue diet is recommended for diarrhea and a high-fiber diet for constipation. Advise the client to avoid gas-producing foods (e.g., cabbage and beans) and to eat at regular hours; to chew food thoroughly; and to increase intake of fluids, especially fruit juices and water.

Daily exercise is helpful. Also advise the client to avoid straining at bowel movements; the urge to defecate should be promptly followed by elimination.

Follow-Up

A diagnosis of irritable bowel syndrome does not require frequent x-rays or colonscopic examinations. The frequency of follow-up visits depends on the severity of the client's symptoms. Systems are reviewed, the effectiveness of intervention assessed, and a physical examination done. Encourage the client to return should her symptoms exacerbate or change. Irritable bowel syndrome is a chronic illness that requires support and reinforcement of the prescribed therapeutic regimen.

ANAL FISSURES

An anal fissure is a linear ulcer on the margin of the anus.

Epidemiology

Anal fissures are a secondary irritation from diarrhea or straining related to constipation, laxative overuse, or trauma. Their exact incidence is unknown.

Subjective Data

A client may report bleeding and pain with and often after defecation. Pain may be severe and last 30 minutes or more following bowel movement. Pruritis ani may occur (Alsace & Maradiegue, 2000).

Objective Data

Internal hemorrhoids may be found. Lateral traction on buttocks should expose the fissure. If not, inspection with an anoscope should aid in visualization. In the acute stage, tissues are erythematous and inflamed. Chronic fissures may erode the anoderm and expose the base of the internal sphincter.

Differential Medical Diagnoses

Primary lesion of syphilis, tuberculosis ulcerations, herpes, malignant epithelioma, abscesses, anorectal fistulas, cancer, Crohn's disease.

Plan

Psychosocial Interventions. Address the client's acute fear of cancer that may be aroused by her pain or bleeding. Reassure her that symptoms will resolve and can be prevented.

Medication. Stool softeners and lubricating anesthetic ointments (short-term) are used for severe pain. Avoid laxatives and suppositories.

Surgical Interventions. An internal sphincterotomy is usually performed to decrease the pressure of chronic fissures in the anal canal. A short two- to three-day hospital stay is required, the wound heals quickly, and the procedure is curative in 90 to 95 percent of cases.

Lifestyle/Dietary Changes. Advise the client to follow a high-fiber diet and increase fluids. Sitz baths are of no proven value.

Follow-Up

Most symptoms resolve within two to four weeks. If, however, no improvement occurs, refer the client to a surgeon.

HEPATITIS

Hepatitis is an inflammation of the liver caused by any one of several viruses or other factors. Five different viruses—hepatitis A, B, C, D, and E are responsible for most liver infections. Some lead to chronic hepatitis, a disease that can lead to cirrhosis, hepatic cancer, and death. Hepatitis A is the most common form. It does not produce long-term complications, and recovery is usually complete in one to two months. Hepatitis A is spread through a fecal-oral route and is most contagious in the late incubation period before symptoms develop. Infected individuals do not remain carriers.

Hepatitis B is spread through blood and body fluids. It can develop into chronic hepatitis in approximately 6 to 10 percent of those infected, which can lead to cirrhosis or hepatocellular carcinoma. (Dienstag & Isselbacher, 2001). Symptoms are similar to hepatitis A, although fever is less likely.

Hepatitis C is spread through contaminated needles, blood transfusions (especially prior to 1992) and possibly sexual contact. Fifty to 80 percent or greater of those with acute infection progress to chronic disease, with 20 to 30 percent advancing to cirrhosis (Iosue, 2002; Lauer & Walker, 2001). Liver cancer is also possible. Symptoms are similar to hepatitis B. No vaccine has been developed (Lauer & Walker, 2001).

Hepatitis D occurs in conjunction with hepatitis B. Transmission is from contaminated needles; sexual contact is less likely. There is no vaccine for hepatitis D, although vaccination against hepatitis B is protective (Dienstag & Isselbacher, 2001).

Hepatitis E is a virus spread similarly to hepatitis A. No cases have been reported in the United States. A vaccine has not been developed (Dienstag & Isselbacher, 2001).

Epidemiology

It is estimated that 200,000 to 300,000 persons become infected with HBV each year in the United States, with the greatest number of cases in the 20 to 39 age group.

Approximately 1.0 to 1.25 million people have chronic, asymptomatic HBV infection. Fifty to 67 percent of acute HBV infections are asymptomatic. Routine screening for hepatitis B virus (HBV) infection in the general population is not recommended (Alsace & Maradiegue, 2000). Certain high-risk groups may be screened to assess eligibility for vaccination. High-risk groups include IV drug users, heterosexual contact with HBV-infected individuals, heterosexual contact with at risk individuals (IV drug users), multiple sexual partners, and male homosexual activity.

The number of cases of hepatitis A each year is unknown. Approximately half of all reported hepatitis cases in the United States are attributable to hepatitis A, with the greatest number of cases in the 20 to 39 age group.

Four million Americans are estimated to have hepatitis C (AHRQ, 2002).

Subjective Data

The client may complain of fatigue, lack of appetite, nausea and vomiting, muscle and joint aches, low grade fever, rash, and jaundice.

Objective Data

Exam may be normal in acute phase

- *General.* Client may be ill-appearing and/or jaundiced.
- *Eyes.* Icteric in acutely ill.
- *Oropharynx.* Pharyngitis may be present in hepatitis A.
- *Lungs.* Rhonchi and/or wheezing.
- *Heart.* Sinus tachycardia associated with fever.
- *Abdomen.* Striae, decreased bowel sounds, diffuse or right upper quadrant tenderness, hepatomegaly, and possibly splenomegaly.
- *Extremities.* Joint tenderness and possibly joint swelling.

Diagnostic Tests. Most laboratories offer acute and convalescent hepatitis panels that include hepatitis A and B. Polymerase chain reaction (PCR) is used to detect hepatitis C (Lauer & Walker, 2001). Anyone who received a blood transfusion before 1992 needs to be tested for hepatitis C, according to August 1997 Public Health Service advisory committee.

The screening test for HBV infection is the identification of HbsAg. The immunoassays have a sensitivity and specificity of greater than 98 percent.

Chemistry panels to assess electrolyte and liver function, complete blood count to assess for anemia, platelet counts and coagulation screen to assess clotting abilities and liver function.

Differential Medical Diagnoses

Drug-induced hepatitis, gallbladder disease, other viral syndromes, and metastatic cancer.

Plan

Treatment is supportive. Encourage small frequent meals earlier in the day. Nausea progresses throughout the day. Clients unable to tolerate PO fluids will require IV fluids and anti-emetics. No specific drug therapy is available for uncomplicated hepatitis. Avoid exposure to hepatotoxic drugs.

Psychosocial. Counseling concerning high risk behaviors and the possibility of transmission. Encourage client to have sexual partner(s) tested if indicated. If possible, the client should avoid sex as long as HBsAg is in the serum.

Medication

Vaccines. The hepatitis B vaccine has an 85 to 95 percent protective efficacy when administered in three intramuscular doses (Alsace & Maradiegue, 2000). Injection into the deltoid muscle is recommended because injection into the buttocks has been associated with a suboptimal response. Soreness at the injection site is the most common side effect. RecombivaxHB and Engerix-B are the vaccines licensed for use in the United States. They may be used interchangeably at any point in the vaccination schedule. Both are given in a three-dose series, with the second and third doses administered one and six months after the first dose. The recommended dose is 1 mL. Pregnancy and lactation are not contraindications (Alsace & Maradiegue, 2000). Preexposure prophylaxis is recommended in health care workers, male homosexuals, dialysis clients, neonates, and children (Alsace & Maradiegue, 2000).

The hepatitis A vaccine has been proven efficacious in children; clinical trial in adults have not been performed. The vaccine produces seroconversion rates of 90 to 100 percent after one dose and 99 to 100 percent after two doses in healthy adult volunteers. Immune globulin with the first dose may be necessary for high risk individuals (Alsace & Maradiegue, 2000).

HBIG is used in postexposure situations (e.g., sexual contacts, needle sticks). The adult dose is 0.06 ml per kg intramuscularly. Ideally, it is given within two days of exposure and again one month later. It is not useful after one week post-exposure.

Follow-Up

Follow-up to provide continued support, check for resolution of acute symptoms, and follow liver enzymes and coagulation panels one to two times a week. As symptoms resolve, the interval between visits may be lengthened. Recheck liver function studies, hepatitis convalescent panels, and coagulation studies six months after resolution of acute symptoms. Refer clients with evidence of chronic disease to a hematologist. Chronic carriers and their families need to be counseled to avoid transmission risks, anxiety and/or depression related to the diagnosis.

HEMATOLOGICAL DISORDERS

The last section of this chapter covers most of the common and a few of the rarer disorders of the blood. It begins with an overview of anemia and then differentiates among iron deficiency anemia, thalassemia, anemia of chronic diseases, and finally less common anemias: glucose-6-phosphate dehydrogenase deficiency; sickle cell anemia, and sickle trait; anemia caused by vitamin B_{12} deficiency; and folate deficiency.

OVERVIEW OF ANEMIA

Anemia is a *sign* of an *underlying* problem; it is not a diagnosis. Identifying anemia is the beginning of a workup, much as identifying a fever is the start of a diagnostic workup. Correcting the anemia may be of little importance compared with finding its cause.

In general, anemia is defined either as a reduction in red blood cell (RBC) volume measured by hematocrit (Hct) or a decrease in the percent concentration of hemoglobin (Hgb) in the peripheral blood. In women, hemoglobin concentrations below 12 g/100 mL or hemotocrit values less than 37 percent are indicative of anemia (Waterbury, 1999). Clinical practice sites and laboratories may vary in their parameters.

Laboratory values may be affected by age, sex, altitude, smoking, and hydration state. Beware of "spurious anemia" caused by hemodilution during pregnancy and congestive heart failure. Look at the individual's clinical picture (Adamson & Longo, 2001; Waterbury, 1999). All blood cell types (RBCs, white blood cells [WBCs], and platelets) are derived from the pluripotent stem cells in the marrow. Pancytopenia, or a decrease in all cell types—WBCs (leukopenia), RBCs (anemia), and platelets (thrombocytopenia)—requires referral to a hematologist (Waterbury, 1999).

Three mechanisms cause anemia: blood loss; decreased red cell production, usually as a result of insufficient building supplies such as iron, vitamin B_{12}, and folate; and increased red cell destruction (hemolysis). To determine the mechanism, ask the following three questions.

What Is the Mean Corpuscular Volume? Mean corpuscular volume (MCV) is one of three RBC indices and indicates blood cell size. Normal MCV is approximately 80 to 100 fL. According to the MCV, anemias are categorized as microcytic, normocytic, or macrocytic (see Table 21–24).

What Is the Reticulocyte Count? Reticulocytes are immature RBCs that retain nuclear particles for 24 hours after leaving the marrow. Normally, reticulocytes constitute about 1 to 1.5 percent of circulating RBCs. Increased reticulocyte count (> 3 percent) may be an indication of rapid bleeding or hemolysis as the body attempts to replenish lost RBCs. Reticulocyte counts less than 1 percent may indicate nutritional deficiencies or marrow dysfunction (Adamson & Longo, 2001; Waterbury, 1999).

What Is the Clinical Picture? Based on the client's demographic characteristics and problem list, certain types of anemia would be suspected (see Table 21–25).

Among the many types of anemia (most of them rare), three account for approximately 90 percent of the anemias in the United States. They are iron-deficiency anemia (IDA), thalassemia, and the anemia of chronic diseases (ACD) (Adamson, 2001; Adamson & Longo, 2001; Benz, 2001; Waterbury, 1999).

TABLE 21–25. Differential Diagnosis Suggested by Clinical Picture

Female	Iron deficiency
Race	
Blacks	G6PD,[a] thalassemia, hemoglobinopathies
Mediterranean origin	G6PD, thalassemia
Southeast Asians	Hemoglobinopathies (e.g., HgB E)
Infections	G6PD, immune hemolysis
Thyroid disease	IDA, pernicious anemia
Alcoholism	Bleeding, folate deficiency, IDA, sideroblastic anemia, hemolysis, hypersplenism
Renal failure	Decreased production, hemolysis, bleeding
Connective tissue disorders	Anemia of chronic diseases, IDA, hemolysis
Cancer	Anemia of chronic diseases, hemolysis
Lead exposure	Sideroblastic anemias, IDA
Drugs	
Sulfa	G6PD
Dilantin	Megaloblastic anemia (folate), pure red cell aplasia
Antitubercular drugs	Sideroblastic anemia
Gold	Aplastic anemia

[a]G6PD, glucose-6-phosphate dehydrogenase deficiency; IDA, iron-deficiency anemia.

Sources: Adamson (2001); Adamson & Longo (2001); Astor et al., (2002); Babior & Bunn (2001); Benz (2001); Waterbury (1999).

IRON-DEFICIENCY ANEMIA

Iron-deficiency anemia can be caused by inadequate dietary intake of iron or by loss of iron through bleeding. Because the body aggressively recycles iron, adults with reasonable nutrition do not experience deficits. Nutritional inadequacies occur primarily in infants, children,

TABLE 21–24. Differential Diagnoses of Anemia by Erythrocyte Morphology

Microcytic Anemia (MCV[a] < 80)	Macrocytic Anemia (MCV > 100)	Normocytic Anemia (MCV 80–100)
Iron deficiency	B_{12} deficiency	Anemia of chronic disease[b]
Thalassemias	Folate deficiency	Endocrinopathy
Anemia of chronic disease[a]	Liver disease	Hemolysis
Sideroblastic	Alcoholism	Myeloma
Aluminum toxicity	Myelodysplastic syndromes	Renal disease
	Marked reticulocytosis	Sideroblastic[a] anemia
	Spurious anemia	Bleeding
		Aplastic anemia

[a]Mean corpuscular volume.
[b]Some overlap can occur depending on stage of disease.

Sources: Adamson & Longo (2001); Astor, Muntner, Levin, Eustace, & Coresh (2002); Babior & Bunn (2001); Benz (2001); Waterbury (1999).

and pregnant women. In a woman who is not pregnant, blood loss is assumed to be the cause of iron-deficiency anemia. In premenopausal women, menstruation is the primary cause of blood loss. In postmenopausal women and in men, IDA is presumed to result from occult gastrointestinal blood loss (rule out colon cancer) until proven otherwise (Adamson, 2001; Waterbury, 1999).

Epidemiology

Studies reveal that IDA among pregnant women is caused by nutritional deficits and among nonpregnant women, primarily by blood loss. Risk factors for bleeding include frequent heavy menses, miscarriages, abortions, deliveries, and surgeries. On average, women lose about 50 mL of blood per month as a result of menses; women with heavy menses may lose five times this amount. Oral contraceptive use decreases menstrual blood flow 30 to 60 percent and thus protects against IDA. Progestin-containing contraceptive methods may also decrease blood loss. Risk factors for occult bleeding include GI disorders (Crohn's diverticulosis) and a family history of colon cancer or hemolytic anemias (Adamson, 2001; Waterbury, 1999).

Incidence reports show that IDA is the most common nutritional disorder in the world. It is seen primarily in children; however, it is estimated to occur in 20 percent of adult women, 50 percent of pregnant women, and 3 percent of adult men (Adamson, 2001; Waterbury, 1999).

Subjective Data

Subjective data vary for premenopausal and postmenopausal women. Premenopausal women report heavy or frequent menses. Acute loss of large volumes of blood may cause the sudden onset of shortness of breath, faintness, thirst, weakness, and rapid pulse. More commonly, however, blood loss is slow and subtle, especially in postmenopausal women. In that manner, the body is able to adjust to the gradual decrease in RBCs; no symptoms develop until the hemoglobin is 6 to 8 g/dL. In severe chronic cases, symptoms may include fatigue, dysphagia, sore tongue or mouth, and pica.

History-taking should focus on sources of blood loss or hemolysis. Ask about blood donations, recent surgeries, epigastric burning or pain, melena (rectal bleeding), family history of colon cancer, medications, diet, smoking, alcohol use, NSAID use, previous anemia, and splenectomy (Adamson, 2001; Waterbury, 1999).

Objective Data

Physical Examination. May reveal nothing abnormal. Occasionally, however, signs of anemia may be detected.

- *General Appearance.* Fatigue, tachypnea.
- *Vital Signs.* Increased pulse and respirations; may be orthostatic, with decreased blood pressure on standing.
- *Skin.* Pallor, tenting, pale palpebral conjunctiva, nails with spooning, separation, and ridges.
- *Mouth.* Angular stomatitis (sores at corners of mouth), cheilosis (red, sore lips), glossitis (beefy red tongue consistent with vitamin B_{12} deficiency).
- *Chest.* Rapid respiratory rate, rales.
- *Heart.* Flow murmurs, tachycardia.
- *Abdomen.* Splenomegaly (hemolysis), hepatomegaly (liver disease, alcoholism), masses (colon cancer), epigastric tenderness (gastritis).
- *Pelvic Exam.* Rule out mass.
- *Rectal Exam.* Rule out mass, guaiac stool.
- *Central Nervous System.* Altered mental status (rule out lead poisoning and vitamin B_{12} dementia), paresthesia (pernicious anemia) (Adamson, 2001; Waterbury, 1999).

Diagnostic Tests. Performed in stages; avoid the expensive shotgun approach to ordering tests.

Initial laboratory tests include a baseline complete blood cell count (CBC) with indices (MCV, mean corpuscular hemoglobin [MCH], mean corpuscular hemoglobin concentration [MCHC]) and reticulocyte count. A fecal test for occult blood is done on the basis of the clinical picture.

Initial findings are evaluated. If data reveal microcytic (MCV <80), hypochromic anemia with a low reticulocyte count, the diagnosis is most likely IDA. Confirm the diagnosis prior to treatment by ordering an iron panel, which usually comprises a serum iron, total iron binding capacity (TIBC), and percent saturation. Also order a serum ferritin test. (*Note:* Iron-deficiency anemia usually occurs gradually. Consequently, laboratory values change slowly over time. The continuum of change begins with decreased serum ferritin and progresses to decreased serum iron, increased TIBC with decreased percent saturation, and finally to decreased MCV and hemoglobin [indices usually are normal until hemoglobin is 10 g/dL].) (Adamson, 2001; Waterbury, 1999).

Consult the physician if laboratory data are not consistent with the clinical picture or the hematocrit is less than 25 percent/dL. Also plan consultation if the client has a positive stool guaiac, history of bleeding, family history or a family history of colon cancer.

Follow-up tests are crucial to ensure that the diagnosis is correct and that anemia is resolving with treatment. At one week, the reticulocyte count should increase 5 to 10 percent; at one month, the hemoglobin should increase 2 points; at two to three months, all normal levels should be reached. Iron is continued another three months or more (Adamson, 2001; Adamson & Longo, 2001; Waterbury, 1999).

Differential Medical Diagnoses

See Tables 21–24 and 21–25.

Plan

Psychosocial Interventions. Reassure the client with iron-deficiency anemia secondary to menses or pregnancy that her condition is common. Advise her that it takes at least six months to completely refill iron stores. Stress the importance of follow-up laboratory tests to confirm the diagnosis. Encourage compliance with oral iron and dietary measures. If the client is postmenopausal, explain the need for further testing to locate the source of blood loss.

Medication. Ferrous sulfate is given once iron-deficiency anemia has been documented, confirmed by laboratory tests, and the underlying cause has been diagnosed and treated.

- *Administration.* A 325 mg tablet is taken three times a day, with 500 mg vitamin C (to aid absorption), for a minimum of 6 months (Adamson, 2001; Adamson & Longo, 2001; Waterbury, 1999). Also see Chapter 5, Menstruation and Related Problems and Concerns.
- *Side Effects.* The most frequent are gastrointestinal: nausea, constipation, and black stools. The difficulty tolerating iron may be minimized if the client consumes the dose with food, starting slowly with one tablet per day, increases her fluid intake, and increases her dietary fiber. Increase the dose as tolerated.
- *Contraindications.* Do not administer iron if a deficiency has not been documented by laboratory tests. Iron overload can be fatal and hard to reverse. Mistakenly treating other types of anemia, such as sideroblastic anemia and anemia of chronic diseases, with iron can lead to overload and death (Adamson, 2001; Adamson & Longo, 2001; Waterbury, 1999).

- *Client Teaching.* After diagnosis, explain to the client that follow-up and treatment will continue for about six months. Stress the importance of obtaining follow-up laboratory tests at one and three months and continuing medications as ordered. Advise the client to keep iron out of the reach of children.

Dietary Interventions. The diet should include foods high in iron: lean meats, egg yolk, shellfish, leafy greens, raisins, and dried apricots and peaches. Advise the client to avoid taking iron with tea, antacids, or dairy products.

The iron supplement contained in multivitamins (18 mg iron) will not correct iron-deficiency anemia but will help prevent recurrences of the problem in menstruating women. The average U.S. diet contains 10 to 15 mg of iron per day; only about 1 to 2 mg per day is absorbed. Dietary measures alone are usually insufficient to correct the iron losses from heavy menstruation. Generic once-daily multivitamins with iron are a reasonable approach to avoiding IDA in otherwise healthy women, but will not correct an anemia (Adamson, 2001; Adamson & Longo, 2001; Waterbury, 1999).

Follow-Up

All clients should be retested to confirm the IDA diagnosis and to determine if the anemia is improving. (As stated earlier, after one month with adequate treatment the hemoglobin should increase 2 points; at two to three months the ultimate goal of the hemoglobin within normal range should be reached. Iron supplementation is continued for three months thereafter.) If the client is compliant, yet no improvement occurs, reconsider the diagnosis.

THALASSEMIA

Thalassemia encompasses a group of hereditary anemias in which synthesis of one or both chains of the hemoglobin molecule (α and β) is defective. A low hemoglobin level and a microcytic, hypochromic anemia result. Individuals who are heterozygous for α- or β-thalassemia have *thalassemia minor;* those who are homozygous have *thalassemia major.* β-Thalassemia major (Cooley's anemia) is a fatal condition. The most severe form of α-thalassemia major results in hydrops fetalis syndrome.

Epidemiology

In the United States, β-thalassemia minor occurs primarily among African Americans and persons of Mediterranean descent. α-Thalassemia occurs primarily among

Southeast Asians. Its transmission is genetic. β-Thalassemia minor is a silent "carrier" state in which the individual fails to produce a β hemoglobin chain. The body compensates by selectively producing hemoglobin A_2, which does not require a β chain (Benz, 2001; Waterbury, 1999). α-Thalassemia minor is a more benign state and more difficult to diagnose, as hemoglobin A_2 does not increase and other confirmatory tests are not readily available for adults. β-Thalassemia affects fewer than 1000 Americans (Benz, 2001; Waterbury, 1999).

Subjective Data

Thalassemia minor is an asymptomatic condition, diagnosed inadvertently primarily by abnormal laboratory findings.

Objective Data

Physical examination reveals nothing abnormal.

A routine CBC will indicate a combined extremely low MCV (usually less than 65 fL) and only a slightly decreased hemoglobin (usually between 10 and 12 g/dL) (Benz, 2001; Waterbury, 1999).

Hemoglobin electrophoresis can confirm a diagnosis of β-thalassemia because of the increased level of hemoglobin A_2; the test cannot confirm α-thalassemia. The clinical picture and other laboratory results must be evaluated.

The test for α-thalassemia is not easily available. If, however, a client has a clinical picture consistent with β-thalassemia trait (very low MCV and mild anemia) yet hemoglobin electrophoresis does not show an increase in hemoglobin A_2, suspect the α-thalassemia trait. Refer the client for genetic counseling.

Differential Medical Diagnoses

See Table 21–24.

Plan

Psychosocial Interventions. Make the appropriate genetic counseling referral and support the client as she makes decisions regarding childbearing. Reassure her that she is not "sick" and does not need lifelong treatment for anemia.

Medication. None is required. Caution the client that blindly and constantly supplementing her diet with iron tablets is dangerous and a needless expense (Benz, 2001; Waterbury, 1999).

ANEMIA OF CHRONIC DISEASES

Anemia of chronic diseases (ACD) is a common but poorly understood condition. It is seen in clients with cancer or chronic inflammatory disorders, such as lupus and rheumatoid arthritis. Despite adequate iron supplies, the body cannot use its stored iron. Red blood cells may be normocytic or microcytic; no uniform hematologic picture can be outlined (Benz, 2001; Waterbury, 1999).

Epidemiology

The cause of anemia of chronic diseases is unknown, although it is associated with chronic inflammatory conditions.

Subjective Data

The condition is usually asymptomatic. When anemia becomes severe, symptoms relative to the coexisting chronic disease may exacerbate. In addition, symptoms of anemia, such as fatigue and shortness of breath, may be present.

Objective Data

For information on the physical examination, see Iron Deficiency Anemia.

No specific diagnostic tests are conclusive; the anemia is primarily a diagnosis of exclusion. A CBC may reveal normocytic or microcytic anemia; however, no consistent pattern is found in other tests. The serum ferritin is usually adequate. For diagnosis, refer to a physician.

Differential Medical Diagnoses

See Table 21–24.

Plan

Psychosocial Interventions. Support the client in dealing with chronic illness.

Medication. None is required. Caution the client to avoid taking iron unless prescribed: excess intake may cause iron overload (Benz, 2001; Waterbury, 1999). Ask the client if she is taking a nonsteroidal anti-inflammatory drug. Gastrointestinal bleeding and subsequent iron deficiency may confuse the clinical picture.

Follow-Up

Consultation with a physician is necessary for all clients with ACD. If anemia is severe, refer the client to a hematologist.

LESS COMMON ANEMIAS

These rarer but still prevalent anemias are usually caused by dietary deficiencies and/or genetic inheritance.

Glucose-6-Phosphate Dehydrogenase Deficiency

Glucose-6-Phosphate Dehydrogenase Deficiency (G6PD deficiency), which is inherited, causes a hemolytic anemia. The enzyme protects RBCs against breakdown by free oxygen. Until an acute hemolytic episode is triggered, the client remains asymptomatic. Hemolysis can be precipitated by viral or bacterial infections or by certain oxidizing drugs.

Glucose-6-phosphate dehydrogenase deficiency is usually discovered accidentally; for example, a pregnant woman who is followed with serial hematocrits may be diagnosed when a marked anemia develops after treatment with an antibiotic, such as sulfa. If hemolysis is severe, she is referred to a hematologist. The woman is instructed to avoid aspirin, sulfa, nitrofurantoin, primaquine, phenacetin, and some vitamin K derivatives (Bunn & Rosse, 2001).

Glucose-6-phosphate dehydrogenase deficiency is seen primarily in African Americans and persons of Mediterranean descent (Bunn & Rosse, 2001).

Sickle Cell Anemia

Sickle cell anemia is an inherited disease seen primarily in clients of African descent. People with *sickle cell trait* have erythrocytes containing 20 to 40 percent hemoglobin S, with the remaining hemoglobin appearing as normal adult.

Epidemiology. Sickle cell anemia and sickle cell trait are caused by various genetic defects in hemoglobin chains. Roughly 8 percent of the African American population in the United States possess the sickle cell gene (Waterbury, 1999). Occasionally, sickle cell trait occurs in persons of Mediterranean, Arabian, or East Indian descent (Waterbury, 1999).

Subjective Data. Most often persons with sickle cell trait are asymptomatic; occasionally, however, episodes of hematuria, increased bacteriuria, and pyelonephritis during pregnancy are associated with this trait. Clients with sickle cell anemia will report frequent painful crises.

Objective Data. Examination is usually benign in sickle cell trait and between sickle cell disease crises. See Tables 21–24 and 21–25 for differential diagnoses.

Plan. Management consists primarily of documenting the condition, encouraging genetic counseling, and reassuring the client that sickle cell trait is benign. Clients in acute crisis should be referred for emergency management.

Vitamin B$_{12}$ Deficiency

Anemia caused by vitamin B$_{12}$ deficiency is megaloblastic, most often caused by pernicious anemia and occasionally by gastrointestinal disorders that result in gastrectomy. Lack of dietary vitamin B$_{12}$ is rarely a problem, as body stores last three to five years. Vitamin B$_{12}$ absorption, however, may be affected. It requires the intrinsic factor produced by the stomach lining and an intact ileum, where absorption actually occurs. Pernicious anemia is an autoimmune disorder that usually becomes symptomatic around age 60 when the stomach is unable to produce intrinsic factor; as a result, the small intestine is unable to absorb vitamin B$_{12}$. The "classic triad" of vitamin B$_{12}$ deficiency includes weakness, sore tongue, and paresthesias (particularly loss of vibratory sense). The Schilling test is used for diagnosis. Treatment involves monthly vitamin B$_{12}$ injections (Babior & Bunn, 2001).

Folate Deficiency

Folate deficiency, related primarily to inadequate nutrition, may cause a megaloblastic anemia. Folate does not accumulate in the body; therefore, the anemia is more common than that caused by vitamin B$_{12}$ deficiency. Folate deficiency most commonly occurs during pregnancy and among alcoholics. Lab work reveals a megaloblastic anemia (MCV > 100) and a decreased folate level. Diagnosis is confirmed by an appropriate clinical response to administration of folic acid, usually 1 mg per day. Management should also address the underlying condition, such as alcoholism. Sources of folic acid (leafy vegetables, fruits, nuts, and liver) should be increased in the diet. Certain drugs, for example, dilantin and trimethoprim, inhibit folate absorption (Babior & Bunn, 2001). It is interesting to note that the macrocytic anemias caused by vitamin B$_{12}$ and folate deficiency can cause false-positive Pap smears. Abnormal Pap smears should be repeated after adequate treatment with vitamin B_{12} or folic acid (Babior & Bunn, 2001).

REFERENCES

Adamson, J. W. (2001). Iron deficiency and other hypoproliferative anemias. In E. Braunwald, S. L. Hauser, A. S. Fauci, D. L. Longo, D. L. Kasper, & J. L. Jameson (Eds.), *Harrison's principles of internal medicine* (15th ed., pp. 660–666). New York: McGraw-Hill.

Adamson, J. W., & Longo, D. L. (2001). Anemia and polycythemia. In E. Braunwald, S. L. Hauser, A. S. Fauci, D. L. Longo, D. L. Kasper, & J. L. Jameson (Eds.), *Harrison's principles of internal medicine* (15th ed., pp. 348–353). New York: McGraw-Hill.

Agency for Healthcare Policy and Research Smoking Cessation Clinical Practice Guideline. (1996). *Journal of the American Medical Association, 275,* 1270–1280.

Agency for Healthcare Research and Quality [AHRQ]. (2002). *Management of chronic hepatitis C* (Rep. No. 60). Washington, DC: U.S. Department of Health and Human Services.

Ahmann, A. J., & Riddle, M. C. (2002). Current oral agents for Type 2 diabetes. *Postgraduate Medicine, 111,* 32–46.

Alsace, N. H., & Maradiegue, A. H. (2000). Gastrointestinal health. In P. V. Meredith & N. M. Horan (Eds.), *Adult primary care* (pp. 380–430). Philadelphia: Saunders.

Aly, R., Forney, R., & Bayles, C. (2001). Treatments for common superficial fungal infections. *Dermatology Nursing, 13,* 91–94.

American Diabetes Association (ADA). (2002a). Position statement: Standards of care for patients with diabetes mellitus. *Diabetes Care, 25,* S33–S49.

American Diabetes Association (ADA). (2002b). Position statement: Screening for diabetes. *Diabetes Care, 25,* S21–S24.

American Diabetes Association (ADA). (2002c). Standards of medical care for patients with diabetes mellitus. *Diabetes Care, 25,* S33–S49.

American Diabetes Association (ADA). (2002d). Insulin administration. *Diabetes Care, 25,* S112–S115.

Anderson, J., & Kessenich, C. R. (2001). Women and coronary heart disease. *Nurse Practitioner, 26,* 12–30.

Appropriate use of common OTC analgesics and cough and cold medications. (2002). American Family Physician [Online]. Available: http://www.aafp.org/afp/otcmonograph/. Accessed: June 18, 2002

Arafah, B. M. (2001). Increased need for thyroxine in women with hypothyroidism during estrogen therapy. *New England Journal of Medicine, 344,* 1743–1749.

Astor, B. C., Muntner, P., Levin, A., Eustace, J. A., & Coresh, J. (2002). Association of kidney function with anemia: The third National Health and Nutritional Examination Survey (1988–1994). *Archives of Internal Medicine, 162,* 1401–1408.

Auten, G. (1996). Endocarditis: Current guidelines on prophylaxis, diagnosis, and treatment. *Consultant,* 973–993.

Babior, B. M., & Bunn, H. F. (2001). Megaloblastic anemias. In E. Braunwald, S. L. Hauser, A. S. Fauci, D. L. Longo, D. L. Kasper, & J. L. Jameson (Eds.), *Harrison's principles of internal medicine* (15th ed., pp. 676–680). New York: McGraw-Hill.

Benz, E. J. (2001). Hemoglobinopathies. In E. Braunwald, S. L. Hauser, A. S. Fauci, D. L. Longo, D. L. Kasper, & J. L. Jameson (Eds.), *Harrison's principles of internal medicine* (15th ed., pp. 666–674). New York: McGraw-Hill.

Biswas, M. S., & Bastian, L. A. (2002). Risk factors for heart disease among women: Communicating probabilities of disease. *JCOM, 9,* 333–340.

Bonow, R. O., Carabello, B. de Leon, A., Jr., Edmunds, L. H., Jr., Fedderly, B. J., Freed, M. D., et al. (1998). Guidelines for the management of patients with valvular heart disease: Executive summary. A report of the American College of Cardiology/American Heart Association Task Force on Practice Guidelines (Committee on Management of Patients with Valvular Heart Disease). *Circulation, 98,* 1949–1984.

Braun, L. T., & Rosenson, R. S. (2001). Assessing coronary heart disease risk and managing lipids. *Nurse Practitioner, 26,* 30–37.

Brunton, S. (2002). Allergy management strategies: An update. *Patient Care, Spring,* 16–25.

Bunn, H. F., & Rosse, W. (2001). Hemolytic anemias and acute blood loss. In E. Braunwald, S. L. Hauser, A. S. Fauci, D. L. Longo, D. L. Kasper, & J. L. Jameson (Eds.), *Harrison's principles of internal medicine* (15th ed., pp. 681–692). New York: McGraw-Hill.

Callahan, E. F., Adal, K. A., & Tomecki, K. J. (2000). Cutaneous (non-HIV) infections. *Dermatologic Clinics, 18,* 497–508.

Centers for Diesease Control and Prevention (CDC). (2001). *Women and smoking: A report of the Surgeon General-2001.* Center for Disease Control and Prevention [Online]. Available: http://www.cdc.gov/tobacco/sgr/sgr_forwomen/factsheet_outcomes.htm. Accessed: June 11, 2002.

Chrostowski, D., & Pongracic, J. (2002). Control of chronic nasal symptoms. *Postgraduate Medicine, 111,* 77–95.

Clark, J. B. F., Queener, S. F., & Karb, V. B. (2000). *Pharmacological basis of nursing practice* (6th ed.) St. Louis: Mosby.

Cooper, D. S. (2001). Subclinical hypothyroidism. *New England Journal of Medicine, 345,* 260–265.

DeFronzo, R., et al. (1995). Efficiency of metformin in patients with non-insulin-dependent diabetes mellitus. *New England Journal of Medicine, 333,* 541–549.

Dienstag, J. L., & Isselbacher, K. J. (2001). Chronic hepatitis. In E. Braunwald, S. L. Hauser, A. S. Fauci, D. L. Longo, D. L.

Kasper, & J. L. Jameson (Eds.), *Harrison's principles of internal medicine* (15th ed., pp. 1742–1752). New York: McGraw-Hill.

Elder, J. T., Nair, R. P., Henseler, T., Jenisch, S., Stuart, P., Chia, N., Christophers, E., & Voorhees, J. J. (2001). The genetics of psoriasis 2001: The odyssey continues. *Archives of Dermatology, 137,* 1447–1454.

Elewski, B. E. (1999a). Tinea capitis: A current perspective. *Journal of the American Academy of Dermatology, 42,* 1–20.

Elewski, B. E. (1999b). Treatment of tinea capitis: Beyond griseofulvin. *Journal of the American Academy of Dermatology, 40,* S27–S30.

Elgart, M. L. (2002). Skin infections and infestations in geriatric patients. *Clinics in Geriatric Medicine, 18,* 89–101.

Expert Committee on the Diagnosis and Classification of Diabetes Mellitus (2002). Report of the Expert Committee on the diagnosis and classification of diabetes mellitus. *Diabetes Care, 25,* S5–S20.

Garner, K. L., & Rodney, W. M. (2000). Basal and squamous cell carcinoma. *Primary Care; Clinics in Office Practice, 27,* 447–458.

Goldstein, A. O., Smith, K. M., Ives, T. J., & Goldstein, B. (2000). Mycotic infections. Effective management of conditions involving the skin, hair, and nails. *Geriatrics, 55,* 40–42.

Goldstein, B. G. & Goldstein, A. O. (2001). Diagnosis and management of malignant melanoma. *American Family Physician, 63,* 1359–1368.

Grady, D., Herrington, D., Bittner, V., Blumenthal, R., Davidson, M., Hlatky, M., Hsia, J., Hulley, S., Herd, A., Khan, S., Newby, L. K., Waters, D., Vittinghoff, E., & Wenger, N. (2002). Cadiovascular disease outcomes during 6.8 years of hormone therapy. *Journal of American Medical Association, 288,* 49–57.

Greenberger, N. J., & Paumgartner, G. (2001). Diseases of the gallbladder and bile ducts. In E. Braunwald, S. L. Hauser, A. S. Fauci, D. L. Longo, D. L. Kasper, & J. L. Jameson (Eds.), *Harrison's principles of internal medicine* (15th ed., pp. 1776–1788). New York: McGraw-Hill.

Gupta, A. K. (2000). Ciclopirox nail lacquer: The first prescription topical therapy for onychomycosis. *Journal of the American Academy of Dermatology, 43,* S81–S85.

Heart Outcomes Prevention Evaluation Study Investigators (2000). Vitamin E supplementation and cardiovascular events in high-risk patients. *The New England Journal of Medicine, 342,* 154–160.

Hennekens, C. (1996). Coronary disease: The leading killer. *Patient Care,* 116–141.

Hermus, A. R., & Huysmans, D. A. (1998). Treatment of benign nodular thyroid disease. *New England Journal of Medicine, 338,* 1438–1447.

Higgins, E. & du Vivier, A. (1999). Alcohol intake and other skin disorders. *Clinics in Dermatology, 17,* 437–441.

Hooper, B. J., & Goldman, M. P. (1999). *Primary dermatologic care.* St. Louis, MO: Mosby.

Hsu, S., Le, E. H., & Khoshevis, M. R. (2001). Differential diagnosis of annular lesions. *American Family Physician, 64,* 289–296.

Hu, F. B., Manson, J. E., Stampfer, M. J., Colditz, G., Liu, S., Solomon, C. G., & Willett, W. C. (2001). Diet, lifestyle, and the risk of Type 2 diabetes mellitus in women. *New England Journal of Medicine, 345,* 790–797.

Hubbard, P. M. (2002). Update on gastroesophageal reflux disease. *American Journal for Nurse Practitioners, 3,* 9–18.

Hulley, S., Furberg, C., Barret-Connor, E., Cauley, J., Grady, D., Haskell, W., Knopp, R., Lowery, M., Satterfield, S., Schrott, H., Vittinghoff, E., & Hunningshake, D. (2002). Noncardiovascular disease outcomes during 6.8 years of hormone therapy. *Journal of American Medical Association, 288,* 58–65.

Iosue, K. (2002). Chronic hepatitis C: Latest treatment options. *Nurse Practitioner, 27,* 32–49.

Jerant, A. F., Johnson, J. T., Sheridan, C. D., & Caffrey, T. J. (2000). Early detection and treatment of skin cancer. *American Family Physician, 62,* 357–368.

Johnson, B. A., & Nunley, J. R. (2000a). Treatment of seborrheic dermatitis. *American Family Physician, 61,* 2703–2710.

Johnson, B. A., & Nunley, J. R. (2000b). Use of systemic agents in the treatment of acne vulgaris. *American Family Physician, 62,* 1823–1830.

Kanzler, M. H., & Mraz-Gernhard, S. (2001). Primary cutaneous malignant melanoma and its precursor lesions: Diagnostic and therapeutic overview. *Journal of the American Academy of Dermatology, 45,* 260–276.

Kirchner, J. T. (2001). Oral therapy for the treatment of onychomycosis. *American Family Physician, 63,* 345.

Klein, I., & Ojamaa, K. (2001). Thyroid hormone and the cardiovascular system. *New England Journal of Medicine, 344,* 501–509.

Lang, M. M., & Towers, C. (2001). Identifying poststreptococcal glomerulonepthritis. *Nurse Practitioner, 26,* 34–47.

Lauer, G. M., & Walker, B. D. (2001). Hepatitis C virus infection. *New England Journal of Medicine, 345,* 41–52.

Lebwohl, M., Drake, L., Menter, A., Koo, J., Gottlieb, A. B., Zanolli, M., Young, M., & McClelland, P. (2001). Consensus conference: Acitretin in combination with UVB or PUVA in the treatment of psoriasis. *Journal of the American Academy of Dermatology, 45,* 544–553.

Lee, V. K., & Simpkins, L. (2000). Herpes zoster and postherpetic neuralgia in the elderly. *Geriatric Nursing, 21,* 132–135.

Linden, K. G., & Weinstein, G. D. (1999). Psoriasis: Current perspectives with an emphasis on treatment. *American Journal of Medicine, 107,* 595–605.

Martin, E. S., & Elewski, B. E. (2002). Geriatric dermatology, Part II: Cutaneous fungal infections in the elderly. *Clinics in Geriatric Medicine, 18,* 59–75.

Martin, J. H., & Horan, N. M. (2000). Eye, ear, nose, and throat health. In P. V. Meredith & N. M. Horan (Eds.), *Adult primary care* (pp. 232–266). Philadelphia: Saunders.

McCrary, M. L., Severson, J., & Tyring, S. K. (1999). Varicella zoster virus. *Journal of the American Academy of Dermatology, 41,* 1–14.

Meltzer, E. O. (2002 Spring). Allergic rhinitis: A systemic inflammatory process. *Patient Care,* 7–15.

Mosca, L., Grundy, S. M., Judelson, D., King, K., Limacher, M., Oparil, S., Paternak, R., Pearson, T. A., Redberg, R. F., Smith, S. C., Winston, M., & Zinburg, S. (1999). Guide to preventive cardiology for women. *Circulation, 99,* 2480–2484.

National Cholesterol Education Program (NCEP). (2001). Executive summary of the third report of the National Cholesterol Education Program (NCEP) Expert Panel on detection, evaluation, and treatment of high blood cholesterol in adults (Adult Treatment Panel III). *Journal of the American Medical Association, 285,* 2486–2497.

Noble, S. L., Forbes, R. C., & Stamm, P. L. (1998). Diagnosis and management of common tinea infections. *American Family Physician, 58,* 163–177.

New Therapeutics Bulletin: Lantus (Insulin glargine). 2001. Washington, DC: American Pharmaceutical Association.

O'Dell, M. L. (1998), Skin and wound infections: An overview. *American Family Physician, 57,* 2424–2432.

Owyang, C. (2001). Irritable bowel syndrome. In E. Braunwald, S. L. Hauser, A. S. Fauci, D. L. Longo, D. L. Kasper, & J. L. Jameson (Eds.), *Harrison's principles of internal medicine* (15th ed., pp. 1692–1695). New York: McGraw-Hill.

Padgett, J. K., & Hendrix, J. D., Jr. (2001). Cutaneous malignancies and their management. *Otolaryngologic Clinics of North America, 34,* 523–553.

Pardasani, A. G., Feldman, S. R., & Clark, A. R. (2000). Treatment of psoriasis: An algorithm-based approach for primary care physicians. *American Family Physician, 61,* 725–733.

Pichichero, M. E. (2000). Acute otitis media: Part 1. Improving diagnostic accuracy. *American Family Physician, 61,* 2051–2056.

Rand, S. (2000). Overview: The treatment of dermatophytosis. *Journal of the American Academy of Dermatology, 43,* S104–S112.

Ray, S. W., Secrest, J., Chien, A. P. Y., & Corey, R. S. (2002). Managing gastroesophageal reflux disease. *Nurse Practitioner, 27,* 36–53.

Rhody, C. (2000). Bacterial infections of the skin. *Primary Care; Clinics in Office Practice, 27,* 37–42.

Rodgers, P. & Bassler, M. (2001). Treating onychomycosis. *American Family Physician, 63,* 663–672.

Sachs, D. L., Marghoob, A. A., & Halpern, A. (2001). Skin cancer in the elderly. *Clinics in Geriatric Medicine, 17,* 715–738.

Schmader, K. (2001). Herpes zoster in older adults. *Clinical Infectious Diseases, 32,* 1481–1486.

The Sixth Report of the Joint National Committee on Prevention, Detection, Evaluation, and Treatment of High Blood Pressure (JNC VI). (1997). *Archives of Internal Medicine, 157,* 2413–2446.

Sontheimer, R. D., & Kovalchick, P. (1998). Cutaneous manifestations of rheumatic diseases: Lupus erythematosus, dermatomyositis, scleroderma. *Dermatology Nursing, 10,* 81–97.

Stampfer, M. J., Hu, F. B., Manson, J. E., Rimm, E. B., & Willett, W. C. (2000). Primary prevention of coronary heart disease in women through diet and lifestyle. *New England Journal of Medicine, 343,* 16–22.

Stankus, S. J., Dlugopolski, M., & Packer, D. (2000). Management of herpes zoster (shingles) and postherpetic neuralgia. *American Family Physician, 61,* 2437–2444.

Stoller, W. A. (2002). Individualizing insulin management. *Postgraduate Medicine, 111,* 51–66.

Thiboutot, D. (2000). New treatments and therapeutic strategies for acne. *Archives of Family Medicine, 9,* 179–187.

Tigges, B. B. (2000). Acute otitis media and pneumococcal resistance: Making judicious management decisions. *The Nurse Practitioner, 25,* 69–85.

Toft, A. D. (2001). Subclinical hyperthyroidism. *New England Journal of Medicine, 345,* 512–516.

Tribble, D. L. (1999). Antioxidant consumption and risk of coronary heart disease: Emphasis on vitamin C, vitamin E, and beta-carotene. *Circulation, 99,* 591–595.

United States Preventive Services Task Force (2002). Aspirin for the primary prevention of cardiovascular events: Recommendations and rationale. *American Family Physician, 65,* 2107–2110.

Venna, S., Fleischer, A. B., Jr., & Feldman, S. R. (2001). Scabies and lice: Review of the clinical features and management principles. *Dermatology Nursing, 13,* 257–262.

Villablanca, A. (1996). Coronary heart disease in women: Gender differences and effect of menopause. *Postgraduate Medicine, 100,* 191–202.

Warren-Boulton, E., Greenberg, R., Lising, M., & Gallivan, J. (1999). An update of primary care management of Type 2 diabetes. *Nurse Practitioner, 24,* 14–31.

Waterbury, L. (1999). Anemia. In L. R. Barker, J. R. Burton, & P. D. Zieve (Eds.), *Principles of ambulatory medicine* (5th ed., pp. 619–633). Philadelphia: Lippincott, Williams, and Wilkins.

Weetman, A. P. (2000). Graves' disease. *New England Journal of Medicine, 343,* 1236–1248.

Weinstein, A., & Berman, B. (2002). Topical treatment of common superficial tinea infections. *American Family Physician, 65,* 2095–2102.

Werth, V. (2001). Current treatment of cutaneous lupus erythematosus. *Dermatology Online Journal, 7*, 2.

Wexler, A. (1991). Differences in use of procedures between women and men hospitalized for CAD. *New England Journal of Medicine, 325*, 221–230.

Whitley, R. J., & Gnann, J. W. (1999). Herpes zoster: Focus on treatment in older adults. *Antiviral Research, 44*, 145–154.

Whitmore, S. E. (1999). Common problems of the skin. In L. R. Barker, J. R. Burton, & P. D. Zieve (Eds.), *Principles of ambulatory medicine* (5th ed., pp. 1499–1539). Philadelphia: Lippincott, Williams, and Wilkins.

Women's Health Initiative (WHI). (2002). Risks and benefits of estrogen plus progestin in healthy postmenopausal women. *Journal of American Medical Association, 288*, 321–332.

Yanovski, S. Z., & Yanovski, J. A. (2002). Obesity. *The New England Journal of Medicine, 346*, 591–602.

Yeung-Yue, K. A., Brentjens, M. H., Lee, P. C., & Tyring, S. K. (2002). The management of herpes simplex virus infections. *Current Opinion in Infectious Diseases, 15*, 115–122.

Youngquist, S., & Usatine, R. (2001). It's beginning to look a lot like Christmas. *Western Journal of Medicine, 175*, 227–228.

Zieve, P. D. (2000). Disorders of hemostasis. In L. R. Barker, J. R. Burton, & P. D. Zieve (Eds.), *Principles of ambulatory medicine* (5th ed., pp. 634–642). Philadelphia: Lippincott, Williams, and Wilkins.

CHAPTER 22

COMMON MEDICAL PROBLEMS: MUSCULOSKELETAL INJURIES THROUGH URINARY TRACT DISORDERS

Rita A. Seeger Jablonski ◆ *Elaine Ferrary*

*S*ixty to 90 percent of the population will experience low back pain during their lifetime. It is second only to the common cold in lost days of work and is the leading cause of disability in those under 45 years of age.

Highlights

- Musculoskeletal Conditions
- Neurological Disorders
- Ophthalmologic Disorders
- Pulmonary Disorders
- Urinary Tract Disorders

❖ INTRODUCTION

This chapter continues the coverage of usual medical problems found in the general primary care practice. Chapter references provide guidance for finding more in-depth information.

MUSCULOSKELETAL CONDITIONS

Whether physically active or sedentary, clients often visit a primary care setting complaining of aches in muscles, back, arms, wrists, legs. This section discusses the following: ankle sprain and knee sprain, acute low back pain, carpal tunnel syndrome, bursitis, fibromyalgia, gout, osteoarthritis, rheumatoid arthritis, and systemic lupus erythematosus.

ANKLE SPRAIN AND KNEE SPRAIN

Ankle sprain and knee sprain are the two most common sports-related injuries. The lateral ligaments of the ankle are most often involved in a sprain. Knee sprain typically involves the medial or lateral collateral ligament or the meniscus.

Epidemiology

The majority of all sports-related injuries involve the ankle (Liu & Nguyen, 1999). Once an ankle injury has occurred, the ankle is four times as likely to be injured again (Liu & Nguyen, 1999). Activities that involve running and jumping, such as basketball, volleyball, and dance, place the female athlete at risk for ankle sprain. Knee injuries occur in sports where the leg is planted and the body pivots, such as basketball, skiing, tennis, ice skating, and dance (Safran, Benedetti, Bartolozzi, & Mandelbaum, 1999).

Subjective Data

Ask the client to describe in detail the circumstances of the injury. Most ankle sprains occur when the foot is plantar-flexed and inverted. Eversion injuries are usually more severe and may involve fracture of the ankle mortise joint. The client may have continued her activities and noted pain and swelling only after several hours. Any report of a popping noise or sensation of tearing at the time of injury is significant for extensive ligament tear and disruption in both knee and ankle injuries. Ask about treatment following trauma (ice, elevation, medication) and any history of previous injuries.

Objective Data: Ankle Sprain

Physical Examination. Observe for deformity, ecchymosis, and swelling. Observe gait if client is able to bear weight.

Range of Motion. Move the joint through its range of motion if possible (the client may have to be distracted). In assessing the ankle, cradle it in your hand and palpate the medial and lateral malleoli and the fifth metatarsal. Flex and extend the ankle. Assess resistance to anterior and varus stress.

Grade I sprain: Mild pain and tenderness; little or no swelling

Grade II sprain: Slight to moderate instability; moderate pain and tenderness; moderate swelling and ecchymosis

Grade III sprain: Significant instability; marked pain and tenderness; marked swelling and ecchymosis. Grade III sprains must be referred to orthopedist.

Diagnostic Tests. Films are indicated if the client has point tenderness of the medial or lateral malleolus and if she is unable to bear weight right after the injury. X-ray the foot if there is tenderness at the base of the fifth metatarsal.

Differential Medical Diagnoses

Ankle fracture (x-ray confirms), fracture of the fifth metatarsal (x-ray confirms), gout (not associated with trauma).

Plan

Psychosocial Interventions. If client is a competitive athlete or dancer, injury may cause great anxiety and possibly loss of income. Reassure her that with rest and careful rehabilitation, recovery is usually complete.

Medication. Nonsteroidal anti-inflammatory drugs such as Ibuprofen 600 mg orally three times a day for seven to ten days (see Table 22–1). If NSAIDs are contraindicated,

TABLE 22–1. Classification of Nonsteroidal Anti-Inflammatory Drugs

Classification	Recommended Dosages	Advantages	Disadvantages
I. Salicylate Preparations			
Aspirin	650 mg q 4 hours Max: 4 g/24 hours	Inexpensive OTC	High incidence of GI distress Increased bleeding time Tinnitus Bronchospasm Frequent dosing
Diflunisal (Dolobid)	250–500 mg b.i.d. Max: 1g/day	Twice daily dosing Less effect on kidney function, beta blockers, diuretics, ACE-I	GI distress May potentiate warfarin Headache Tinnitus Moderately expensive
Salsalate (Disalcid)	1500 mg b.i.d. Max: 3 g/day	Less GI distress than aspirin	Weaker anti-inflammatory properties compared to aspirin Does not affect platelet aggregation–no cardiac protection
II. Propionic Acid Derivatives			
Ibuprofen (Motrin)	200–800 mg t.i.d. or q.i.d. Max: 3.2 g/day	Effective first line drug Inexpensive Available OTC in 200 mg tablets	GI effects Fluid retention May induce meningitis in clients with SLE
Naproxen (Naprosyn)	250–500 mg b.i.d. Max: 1 g/day	Available OTC in 275 mg tablets	GI effects Fluid retention May increase LFTs
Ketoprofen (Orudis)	50 mg q.i.d. or 75 mg b.i.d. Max: 300 mg/day	Available OTC in 125 mg tablets	GI effects Tinnitus Dizziness
Oxaprozin (Daypro)	600–1200 mg/day Max: 1200 mg/day or 1800 mg/day if used for RA	Once daily dosing Useful in RA, OA	GI effects Moderately expensive but available in cheaper generic form
III. Acetic Acids			
Indomethacin (Indocin)	50 mg t.i.d./q.i.d. 75 mg SR b.i.d. Max: 400 mg/day	Useful in gout Inexpensive	GI effects Headache Agranulocytosis Anemia Potentiates warfarin Increases lithium levels
Sulindac (Clinoril)	150–200 mg b.i.d. Max: 400 mg/day	Least effect on kidney function Useful for RA, acute gout, bursitis	GI distress Potentiates warfarin May cause hepatitis Moderately expensive but available in cheaper generic form Does not affect platelet aggregation
Diclofenac (Voltaren)	50 mg q.i.d. or 75 mg b.i.d. Max: 150 mg/day	Useful in ankylosing spondylitis, RA, OA	GI distress May cause hepatitis
Nabumetone (Relafen)	1000–2000 mg/day Max: 2000 mg/day	Once daily dosing Decreased incidence of GI effects	Moderately expensive
Etodolac (Lodine)	200–400 mg t.i.d. Max: 1200 mg/day Extended release: 400–1000 mg/day	Does not lower prostagalandins, therefore fewer GI effects	Both forms moderately expensive but the shorter-acting one is available in cheaper generic form

TABLE 22–1. (*cont.*)

Classification	Recommended Dosages	Advantages	Disadvantages
IV. Oxicams			
Piroxicam (Feldene)	20–40 mg qid	Available in seneric form (inexpensive)	Avoid in elderly Increased incidence of GI effects Potentiates warfarin
V: Selective COX-2 Inhibitors			
Celecoxib (Celebrex)	100–200 mg b.i.d. Max: 400 mg/day	May have lower incidences of GI bleeding than traditional NSAIDs	Most common side effects are diarrhea, nausea, headache, lower extremity edema, and hypertension Derived from benzenesulfonamide; do not use in clients with an allergy to sulfonamides No effect on platelet aggregation Expensive
Rofecoxib (Vioxx)	12.5 to 50 mg once daily Max: 50 mg/day	May have lower incidences of GI bleeding than traditional NSAIDs Approved for OA, acute pain, dysmenorrhea	Most common side effects are diarrhea, nausea, dyspepsia, abdominal pain, peripheral edema Expensive Not recommended for acute pain > 5 days
Meloxicam (Mobic)	7.5 mg/daily Max: 15 mg/daily	Newly approved for OA Some risk of GI bleeding	Avoid using with aspirin, ACEIs, furosemide, thiazides, lithium, warfarin Expensive
Valdecoxib (Bextra)	10 mg q/day [OA, RA] 20 mg b.i.d. prn [dysmenorrhea] Max: 40 mg/day	Newly approved for OA, RA, dysmenorrhea May have lower incidences of GI bleeding than traditional NSAIDs	Most common side effects are diarrhea, nausea, headache, lower extremity edema, and hypertension Avoid using with aspirin, warfarin No effect on platelet aggregation Expensive

Abbreviations: Angiotensin converting enzyme inhibitors (ACEI); twice a day (b.i.d.); Cyclooxygenase (COX); maximum (MAX); osteoarthritis (OA); four times a day (q.i.d.); rheumatoid arthritis (RA); slow release (SR); three times a day (t.i.d.); systemic lupus erythematosus (SLE); over the counter (OTC); liver function tests (LFTs).

Sources: Ables (2002); Allen (2002); Burson (2002); Clark, Queener, & Karb (2000); Kehoe, (2002); Matsumoto & Wigley (1999); Palacioz (2002).

acetaminophen may be used for pain control. If sprain is severe, short-term use of narcotic analgesics may be indicated. Consult physician.

Lifestyle. Rest, ice, compression, and elevation (RICE) are ordered for the first 48 to 72 hours postinjury to reduce swelling and pain. If the sprain is grade II, nonweight bearing is advised for 72 hours. Begin gentle range of motion exercises after 48 hours. Start strengthening exercises as soon as pain and swelling subside. Begin with calf and peroneal muscle stretches. Pool exercises may help if pain and stiffness prevent full stretches. Cross training by cycling and stationary cross country ski machines increases all-over muscle tone and endurance. Encourage client to recondition slowly and not overdo. Advise her that pain of reinjury may be masked by analgesics.

Wrapping with elastic bandage is not considered effective support when client is returning to previous level of activity. If used in combination with high-top shoes, efficacy is increased. Taping is often used but may lose

support capability during exercise. Lace-up supports and semirigid stirrup supports have been shown to prevent reinjury (Liu & Nguyen, 1999).

Follow-Up

Evaluate after 72 hours. Clients with grade I injuries may be able to start rehabilitation at this point. Grade II sprains should be examined for compartment syndrome, manifested by increased swelling, pain, and restriction of movement. Reassess grade II sprains at seven days postinjury for possible return to weight bearing and rehabilitation or, if indicated, referral to orthopedics/physical therapy.

Objective Data: Knee Sprain

Physical Examination

♦ *Range of Motion.* Ask the client to flex and extend the knee. Typically, she will not be able to extend fully. If the patella was dislocated at the time of trauma (common in women), it will relocate on extension.

- *Palpation.* Client will complain of intense pain when the patella is pushed laterally. Palpate the knee for tenderness and effusion. (See discussion of technique in section on bursitis.) Large effusions appear just above the patella and are obvious. Small effusions can be detected by applying pressure to the lateral patella and observing for a bulge medially. Assess for instability during varus and valgus stress, with the ankle held under the elbow of the examiner and with the client supine. Joint laxity indicates injury to the medial and/or lateral collateral ligaments (Byank & Beattie, 1999).

The most reliable and accurate test for instability of the anterior cruciate ligament is Lachman's test. The client is supine and flexes the knee 15 to 20 degrees. The examiner places one hand on the proximal tibia and one hand on the distal femur. She or he shifts the tibial plateau anteriorly while holding the femur stationary. A soft end point to the maneuver or anterior translation indicates a tear of the anterior cruciate ligament.

Diagnostic Tests. X-ray the knee only if there was direct trauma to the patella and if a fracture or avulsion injury is suspected. For soft tissue injuries with high suspicion of cruciate ligament tear, MRI is indicated.

Differential Medical Diagnoses

Knee fracture (x-ray confirms), bursitis (palpable swelling and warmth on the patella, may not have history of trauma), meniscal tear (swelling and pain along joint line, locking or popping with varus/valgus stress) cruciate ligament tear (laxity with full extension on Drawer sign test and Lachman's maneuver).

Plan

Refer client with patellar fracture and cruciate and collateral ligament tears to orthopedist immediately.

Psychosocial Interventions. See section under Ankle Sprain.

Medication. See Ankle Sprain.

Lifestyle. RICE for first 72 hours. Knee immobilizer more effective than elastic bandage. Continue immobilizer or wrap until ligament tenderness and swelling have resolved (may take two to six weeks). Weight bearing as tolerated. Isometric quadriceps exercises with tensing of the quadriceps muscle ten times every hour. Gradual rehabilitation lasting about twice as long as the period of immobilization. Advise client to start with straight leg raising ten repetitions three times a day; may add handweight held on the quadriceps as tolerated (avoid ankle weights). Taping 6 inches above and below the joint line or use of short padded knee brace may be indicated when client resumes previous activity to prevent reinjury (Byank & Beattie, 1999).

Follow-Up

Evaluate in 72 hours for decrease in swelling and pain. If range of motion has decreased and pain has increased refer to physician for possible referral to orthopedics. Meniscal tears that do not respond may require arthroscopy.

ACUTE LOW BACK PAIN

Acute low back pain is a very common, usually benign and self-limited disorder. It may arise as a result of myofascial strain, degenerative change, or injury to the spine with or without nerve impingement. It may also accompany a serious underlying systemic disorder.

Epidemiology

Sixty to 90 percent of the population will experience low back pain during their lifetime (Philadelphia Panel, 2001). Fifty percent of those of working age will report back problems each year. It is second only to the common cold in lost days of work and is the leading cause of disability in those under 45 years of age.

Subjective Data

The health history is key to rule out more serious underlying disorders. Important information includes age, provocative event, onset, character and radiation of pain, previous history of cancer or other serious medical condition, unexplained weight loss, pain that is worse at rest, response to self-care or previous therapy, history of intravenous drug use, history of urinary disorder. Only 2 percent of acute low back pain is due to non-mechanical causes, such as systemic disease or infection.

Typically the client reports onset after physical activity such as heavy lifting. It is made worse by twisting or bending. The pain may be localized to the lumbarsacral spine or may extend down the posterior thigh to the knee. Disc herniation with sciatic impingement causes unilateral radiation below the knee with numbness or weakness. Cauda equina compression, a surgical emergency, causes saddle anesthesia, bilateral leg weakness, and loss of bladder and/or bowel control. The client is referred immediately to a neurosurgeon.

Other elements to elicit in the health history include occupational history, present work status, any pending litigation or compensation issues, previous rehabilitation for back problems, substance abuse, and depression.

Objective Data

Physical Examination

- *General Appearance.* Observe posture, gait; ask client to walk on toes, on heels, balance on one foot.
- *Spine.* Inspect for deformity. Observe range of motion for limitation. Palpate for tenderness.
- *Lower Extremities.* Observe for quadriceps wasting. If there are lower extremity symptoms or signs, test deep tendon reflexes and great toe dorsiflexion strength.

    Palpate the spine for tenderness.

    The straight leg raising test is positive if the nerve root is irritated. It has low specificity but high sensitivity for herniation at the L4-5 and L5-S1 level. The client is supine, and the examiner raises the leg. It is positive if radicular pain is elicited before the leg reaches 60 degrees or fewer.
- *Abdomen.* Examine for tenderness and auscultate for abdominal bruit.

Diagnostic Tests. Radiologic studies are not routinely ordered unless pathological fracture, infection, tumor, or traumatic injury is suspected. In the latter case, imaging may be important if litigation is a possibility. Anteroposterior and lateral lumbar films are the selected views.

MRI in clients with nerve root impingement signs is usually ordered only if results would change the course of therapy or if surgery is being considered.

Radionuclide bone scan is ordered only if high suspicion for osteomyelitis or metastasis.

Complete blood count may be indicated if infection is suspected (Department of Veterans Affairs, 1999).

Differential Medical Diagnoses

Myofascial strain, herniated disk, compression fracture, fibromyalgia, osteoarthritis, spondylolisthesis, ankylosing spondylitis (rare in women), osteomyelitis, iatrogenic (from excessive bed rest or inactivity), pyelonephritis, bleeding aortic aneurysm, cancer of the pancreas, PID, tumor of the pelvis, multiple myeloma, various psychosocial factors such as mood disorder, drug-seeking behavior, interpersonal or occupational stress.

Plan

Psychosocial Interventions. Reassure the client that acute low back pain is in most cases a self-limited problem. In 90 percent of the cases, it resolves within six weeks, no matter what interventions are used (Della-Giustina, 1998). The drug-seeking client and the client with depression, should be referred appropriately.

Medication. NSAIDs and analgesics such as acetaminophen are used to manage pain. They can be used singularly or concurrently. If used concurrently, explain to the client that she should alternate the NSAID and the other analgesic. One regimen, for example, is 500 mg Naprosyn (naproxen) twice daily, with 650 mg acetaminophen (Tylenol) every four to six hours (Della-Giustina, 1998). See previous discussion of these medications.

Muscle Relaxants. If muscle spasms are present, muscle relaxants may be used for two to three days.

Cyclobenzaprine (Flexeril) 10 mg

- *Administration.* One tablet orally four times a day.
- *Contraindications.* Hyperthyroidism, congestive heart failure, cardiac disease, use of monoamine oxidase inhibitors.
- *Adverse Effects.* Drowsiness, dizziness, tachycardia, hypotension, dyspepsia.

Methocarbamol (Robaxin) 750 mg

- *Administration.* Two tablets orally four times a day.
- *Contraindication.* Known hypersensitivity.
- *Adverse Effects.* Drowsiness, dizziness, bradycardia, hypotension, gastrointestinal upset.

NOTE: Warn client not to use these medications with alcohol.

Benzodiazepines. Sciatic pain from nerve root impingement may not respond to above drugs, and a brief course of a benzodiazepine such as diazepam and bed rest with hips and knees slightly flexed may offer the only relief. These are controlled substances and must be used with caution. Refer to a pharmacology text for further information.

Nonpharmacological Interventions. The Philadelphia Panel (2001) developed evidence-based clinical practice guidelines based on a rigorous review of current research studies. The panel concluded that continuation of normal activities as tolerated was the sole beneficial intervention for women with acute low back pain (Philadelphia Panel, 2001).

Local application of ice for 15 to 30 minutes four times a day may be beneficial. Heat is not indicated early in the course of treatment because it may exacerbate the pain.

Bed rest with bathroom privileges for more than three days may lead to more disability from deconditioning (Philadelphia Panel, 2001). Exercises are not indicated during the acute phase of pain and muscle spasm, but passive flexion and extension of the spine may provide relief. It is recommended to do these for 5 minutes every hour as tolerated.

Diet/Lifestyle. The working client should return to work within four to seven days. If her job involves heavy lifting, a review of proper body mechanics is indicated. Referral to a physical therapist may be necessary for a program of exercises and work conditioning. The obese client will benefit from weight loss. Strengthening of the abdominal muscles is indicated for all clients with chronic low back pain. Swimming pool exercises such as walking with water resistance against the trunk are helpful when weightbearing exercises are not well tolerated due to lower extremity weakness.

Follow-Up

Reevaluate the client after two weeks for response to therapy and return to normal activities. Refer to a physician those who complain of no improvement or a worsening of symptoms.

CARPAL TUNNEL SYNDROME

Carpal tunnel syndrome (CTS) is the most common entrapment neuropathy and is caused by compression of the medial nerve at the wrist. Although some consider CTS to be a work-related repetitive use disorder, research studies have not consistently reached that conclusion (Clarke Stevens, Witt, Smith, & Weaver, 2001; England, 1999; Olney, 2001; Szabo, 1998).

Epidemiology

Carpal tunnel syndrome afflicts nearly one million adults in the United States and women comprise almost 80% of the cases. The average age of onset is 51 for women (Szabo, 1998). Total medical costs and indirect costs,

such as wages lost from work, range from $5,000 to $100,000 per CTS case (Olney, 2001; Szabo, 1998).

Diabetes, rheumatoid arthritis, collagen vascular disorders, pregnancy, menopause, obesity, and hypothyroidism are medical conditions associated with CPS (Clarke Stevens et al., 2001; England, 1999; Olney, 2001; Szabo, 1998).

Subjective Data

The client complains of numbness, tingling, and pain in the hand that may radiate to the wrist and distal arm. The diagnostic hallmark is numbness and pain that wakes her up at night. Pain also occurs with activities that involve flexion or extension of the wrist. Fine motor coordination may be affected, causing her to drop things. The numbness and tingling is relieved by shaking the wrist in the manner of shaking down a mercury thermometer. When asked to pinpoint the areas of the hand most affected, she will identify the thumb, index, and middle fingers. She may not have pain.

Objective Data

Physical Examination. Examine base of thumb for thenar atrophy.

Tinel's and Phalen's tests are sensitive and specific in the diagnosis.

Phalen's sign is positive when flexing the wrist 90 degrees for 30 to 60 seconds causes numbness and tingling in thumb and first two or three fingers.

Tinel's sign is positive when tingling symptoms are reproduced by tapping with fingers or reflex hammer over the carpal tunnel.

Assess grip and pinch strength and sensitivity to touch. Assess for associated medical conditions such as rheumatoid arthritis, hypothyroidism, and diabetes.

Diagnostic Tests. Electromyography and nerve conduction studies will confirm the diagnosis. In most primary care settings, this is not ordered unless other complicating factors such as cervical disc disease or possible work compensation is at issue. Diabetics may also require more extensive studies and referral to a neurologist if there is a question of peripheral neuropathy.

Differential Medical Diagnoses

Cervical radiculopathy (pain above the shoulder, numbness and tingling occurs with cough, sneeze). Ulnar neuropathy (pain in ulnar nerve distribution). Thoracic outlet syndrome (weakness of hand muscles, sensory loss over ulnar region of hand and forearm). Peripheral neuropathy of diabetes (history, numbness not position dependent).

Plan

Psychosocial Interventions. The diagnosis of CTS may have serious implications for the client's occupational or recreational activities. It is important to be sensitive to these issues and provide reassurance and support. Early intervention and ergonomics are key.

Medication. Nonsteroidal anti-inflammatory drugs may help in early disease and during acute flares. See Table 22–1. Steroid injections of the wrist by an experienced practitioner thoroughly familiar with the carpal tunnel may relieve pain and numbness for weeks to years. Usual dose is triamcinolone 20 to 40 mg. See discussion of steroid injections under Bursitis.

Vitamin B_6 (pyridoxine) has no therapeutic effect in documented clinical trials. In large doses, it can be neurotoxic. Those who do report decrease in symptoms may have underlying peripheral neuropathy.

Diet/Lifestyle. Ergonomic interventions such as positioning keyboards to minimize wrist flexion, wearing wrist support during provocative activities will usually help. Wrist splinted in neutral position with palmar support worn at night is useful in early disease.

Follow-Up

Reevaluate client in ten to fourteen days. If no improvement is noted or if client has long standing history, refer to orthopedic surgeon. Age of 50 years, duration of disease more than ten months, and unrelenting numbness and tingling are poor prognosticators for success of conservative management. The client with probable co-existing morbidity as indicated by positive rheumatoid factor or antinuclear antibody is referred to a rheumatologist.

BURSITIS

Bursitis is an inflammation of the bursa, the fibrous sac that lies between some tendons and bones and acts as a cushion. The bursa is lined with a membrane that secretes synovial fluid. The most common causes of bursitis include trauma (acute and repetitive injury), infection, and arthritic conditions. The shoulder, the elbow, the hip, the knee, and the ankle are affected sites.

Epidemiology

At least 150 bursal sacs exist in the body. The number is not fixed, and bursae may develop in areas of structural friction (Hellmann, 1999). Clients of all ages and levels of activity are affected; the daily jogger, the dance student, the golfer or softball player, the client with osteo- or rheumatoid arthritis, the child care provider who spends a lot of time on her knees. Essentially, any client who participates in activities that place continuous, repetitive stress on joints and muscles is at risk for bursitis.

Subjective Data

The client notes an abrupt onset of swelling and localized point tenderness over the affected bursa. There is usually an aching pain and pain on range of motion, but inflammation of the olecranon bursal sac (resembling a goose egg at the tip of the elbow) may cause no pain. The client typically has a history of repeated minor trauma or overuse.

Be sure to ask her about any recent unexplained fever, history of rheumatoid arthritis, systemic lupus erythematosus, or gout, past medical history, surgical history, occupational and recreational activities.

Objective Data

Physical Examination. Inspect the affected site for swelling, erythema. Observe the client's moving the adjacent joint through active range of motion for limitations.

Shoulder Pain. Shoulder pain is assessed by having the client perform a series of movements. First, ask her to raise her arms up over her head, or as high as possible. Note the height of the arm raise and the presence of pain, if any. Have the client reach across her chest to touch the opposite shoulder and reach behind her neck to touch the opposite superior scapula (abduction and external rotation). Ask the client to place her arm and hand behind her back and reach for the opposite inferior scapula (adduction and internal rotation). The examiner should also assess passive range of motion and resisted movements (Kern, 1999). In the case of olecranon bursitis, the examiner will examine the olecranon process of the ulna for swelling and painless passive extension and flexion of the elbow ("student's" or "miner's elbow") (Hellmann, 1999).

Knee. To evaluate the knee, ballotte the patella. This is done by milking the fluid into the space between the patella and the femur. Start about 15 cm above the superior margin of the knee and slide index finger and thumb along the sides of the femur. While maintaining pressure on the kneecap, tap the patella. An effusion is present if the fingers on either side of the patella feel the tap. In bursitis no effusion is present, and the fluid cannot be milked into the space beneath the patella.

Hip. The evaluation of the hip for trochanteric or ischial bursitis includes full active and passive range of motion of the hip and palpation of the greater trochanter and ischial tuberosity for point tenderness.

All Affected Joints. Observe for erythema. Palpate the site for crepitus, tenderness, warmth. Note degree of range of motion if possible for comparison on follow-up. Test extremity for strength and pain at extremes of range of motion. If bursitis is chronic, supporting muscles may have atrophied from underuse and weakness.

Diagnostic Tests

Arthrocentesis. If infection is suspected, aspirate fluid must be sent for analysis: cell count, appearance, culture, microscopy (presence of crystals), gram stain.

Complete Blood Count. To rule out infection.

Other Tests. May include an erythrocyte sedimentation rate, antinuclear antibody, rheumatoid factor, and/or uric acid based on differential diagnosis.

Radiographs. Usually not necessary unless there was acute trauma that preceded the pain, obvious deformity, instability, or conservative treatment for two to three weeks has failed.

MRI. Indicated only when surgery is considered.

Bone Scan. In the case of lower extremity pain if the diagnosis is in doubt and the management would be changed, a bone scan may be indicated to rule out stress fracture, avascular necrosis, osteomyelitis.

Differential Medical Diagnoses

Osteoarthritis, rheumatoid arthritis, gout (see discussions of these conditions for defining features).

Upper extremity pain: fracture, shoulder dislocation, rotator cuff tear, adhesive capsulitis; referred pain from neck injury, Pancoast tumor of the lung, pneumonia or pleural effusion.

Lower extremity pain: sciatica, lumbar disc disease, avascular necrosis of the femoral head, pelvic stress fracture, pelvic tumor, meniscal tear, thrombophlebitis, ligamentous injury or tear, achilles tendinitis, Reiter's syndrome.

Plan

Psychosocial Interventions. If occupational or recreational factors have contributed to development of bursitis, the client may have concerns about future disability. Advise her that with rest, medication, and following suggested rehabilitation, bursitis can be managed and controlled without permanent damage.

Medication. NSAIDs are the first line medications for control of pain and reduction of inflammation. The usual course of treatment is for four to six weeks if the symptoms have been present for fewer than three weeks and there is no significant loss of motion in the joint (see Table 22-1).

Infectious Bursitis

ANTIBIOTICS. In the case of infectious bursitis, consult with a physician. If outpatient treatment, start patient immediately on antibiotic that covers staphylococcus, such as dicloxacillin 500 mg Q.I.D. or cephalexin 500 mg Q.I.D., pending culture result. Continue antibiotics for fourteen days. Consult pharmacology text for further information on these medications.

Chronic Bursitis

STEROID INJECTION. In chronic bursitis or when conservative management fails, injection of a corticosteroid such as betamethasone 6 mg or triamcinolone 20 to 40 mg mixed with 3 cc of lidocaine into the bursa at the point of maximal tenderness provides rapid pain relief. Only those practitioners experienced in the procedure should attempt this.

- *Adverse Effects.* Complications include infection, tendon rupture, fat atrophy, skin pigment change, hyperglycemia. Client must be informed of possible adverse effects before the procedure.

   Injections can be repeated in two weeks. If there is no improvement after the second injection, the client must be referred. In many cases, referral to a rheumatologist is helpful in order to rule out any associated diseases (Hellmann, 1999).

Nonpharmacological Treatment. The acronym PRICEMM is helpful to guide the treatment of bursitis (protection, relative rest, ice, compression, elevation, medication, and modalities) (Butcher, Salzman, & Lilligard, 1996; Byank & Beatie, 1999).

- *Protection.* For heel and knee bursitis, foam padding or bracing of the site can protect from friction injury. Retrocalcaneal bursitis often results from poorly fitting shoes or worn heel counters. Ice skaters and distance runners are groups at risk.

Bursitis of the hip, especially ischiogluteal bursitis (Weaver's Bottom), is aggravated by prolonged sitting and is distinguished by pain in the gluteal region. Client may benefit from sitting on a foam pad or "doughnut" cushion.

Clients with bursitis of the shoulder may use a sling to support the weight of the arm, but this must be removed three or four times a day to prevent adhesive capsulitis.

◆ *Relative Rest.* Encourage the client to engage in alternative exercise activities such as swimming.

In the case of shoulder bursitis, the client should perform pendulum circles with the affected arm three times a day. Later, advance to more frequent light resistance range of motion exercises using a towel or elastic bands. Do these for ten minutes twice a day.

For bursitis of the knee, strengthening the quadriceps and the hamstring muscles is important.

◆ *Ice.* Place ice on affected site for ten minutes twice a day or more, especially before aggravating activities.

◆ *Compression and Elevation.* Ace bandage is applied and extremity is elevated.

◆ *Modalities* may include ultrasound and/or high voltage electrical stimulation under the direction of a physical therapist. Also if muscle weakness or loss of range of motion, refer for physical therapy (Butcher, et al., 1996; Byank & Beatie, 1999).

Diet/Lifestyle. If the client is obese, weight loss and exercise are encouraged to prevent future exacerbations or progression to chronic bursitis. Dedicated athletes should cross train in activities that do not stress the affected site and may benefit from referral to sports medicine clinician. Clients whose occupation aggravates the bursa, such as workers who must raise the arm over the head repetitively, should implement a program to strengthen surrounding muscle groups.

Follow-Up

Reevaluate in seven days or in two weeks if steroid injection. Continue therapy for fourteen more days if response noted. If no improvement noted, consult with physician for further workup, need for steroid injections, or referral.

FIBROMYALGIA

Fibromyalgia (also called fibrositis) is a common, often underdiagnosed, pain syndrome characterized by generalized migratory pain and fatigue. It is considered a soft tissue rheumatic disease. It is defined by tender points on the axial skeleton in all four body quadrants. There are several other syndromes often associated with fibromyalgia, including migraine headaches, irritable bowel syndrome, and affective disorders. Low cortisol levels, elevation of substance P (a neurotransmitter involved in pain perception), and altered serotonin levels are thought to contribute to the symptoms seen in fibromyalgia (Clark & Odell, 2000; Millea & Holloway, 2000).

Epidemiology

Fibromyalgia is thought to affect as many as 6 million people in the United States. At least 10 percent of clients seen in primary care may have the disorder, which affects 3.4 percent of all women but only 0.5 percent of all men (Clark & Odell, 2000; Millea & Holloway, 2000).

Subjective Data

The client's history supplies important clues to the diagnosis. The usual presenting complaints are widespread "joint" pain and overwhelming fatigue. The client may have visited several other providers and/or the emergency room to find an explanation for her condition. She may have been prescribed nonsteroidal anti-inflammatory drugs, which did not provide lasting pain relief.

It is important to review all systems because a constellation of other disorders has been associated with fibromyalgia. Their presence is not required for diagnosis but strongly suggests it.

Neurological. Higher incidence of migraine and tension headaches; fleeting parasthesias; difficulty concentrating; short-term memory difficulty; sensitivity to loud noise.

Cardiopulmonary. Noncardiac chest pain, palpitations, mitral valve prolapse; higher incidence of multiple chemical and environmental sensitivities, rhinitis, nasal congestion.

Gastrointestinal. Irritable bowel syndrome, heartburn, esophageal dysmotility.

Genitourinary. Dysmenorrhea, urinary frequency, urgency, interstitial cystitis.

Psychologic. Higher incidence of depression and somatization.

Objective Data

Physical Examination

Criteria for Diagnosis. History of pain for at least three months in all four quadrants of the axial skeleton.

Pain in 11 of 18 paired tender points elicited by 4 kg (about 9 pounds) of firm digital palpation pressure:

Occiput
Cervical spine C5–C7
Trapezius muscle
Supraspinatus muscle
Second rib at costochondral junction
Lateral epicondyle
Upper outer gluteal muscle
Greater trochanter
Knees at medial fat pad

Examine all joints identified as painful for swelling, warmth, synovitis, instability, and deformity.

Diagnostic Tests. There is no specific laboratory or diagnostic test to establish the diagnosis. Diagnosis is based on history, presence of tender points, and absence of inflammation. A few screening tests are helpful including complete blood count, erythrocyte sedimentation rate, blood chemistry panel, and thyroid panel. Imaging studies are usually not necessary or helpful.

Differential Medical Diagnoses

Rheumatoid arthritis, systemic lupus erythematosus (joint inflammation, elevated sedimentation rate); hypothyroidism (high TSH); polymyalgia rheumatica (shoulder and girdle pain and weakness, anemia, high sedimentation rate, age greater than 50); polymyositis (weakness), myofascial pain syndrome (pain arises from pressure to trigger points, which also causes twitching in the taut muscle and may feel nodular to the examiner) (Millea & Holloway, 2000).

Plan

Psychosocial Interventions. The client may feel overwhelming relief that a diagnosis has been made. Reassure her that although fibromyalgia is a chronic disease for which there is no cure, it is not progressive. She can make an enormous difference in the quality of her life by adopting healthy lifestyle measures. Encourage her to take an active role in devising the plan of care.

Medication *Amitryptiline.* 10 mg orally one to two hours before bed-time. Dosage may be increased by 10 mg qhs per week to a maximum of 70 to 80 mg qhs.

- *Mechanism of Action.* Amitryptiline is a tricyclic antidepressant that affects serotonin activity and is thought to potentiate endogenous opioids (endorphins). These two mechanisms may account for amitryptiline's analgesic effect in chronic pain syndromes (Clark & Odell, 2000; Millea & Holloway, 2000).

- *Adverse Effects.* Include vivid dreams or nightmares for the first few nights, hungover feeling in the morning. Other adverse effects include dry mouth, constipation, nausea.

  Contraindicated in those who are hypersensitive to tricyclic antidepressants. Also in recovery phase of myocardial infarction (may induce arrhythmias).

- *Expected Outcome.* Client will note improved and more restful sleep. Advise her it may take several weeks and some titration of the medication to achieve maximal effect.

- *Client Teaching.* Advise client to keep sleep diary and note dosage at which sound sleep with minimal hangover is achieved. Advise her of additive effects of alcohol, antihistamines, sedatives, and tranquilizers.

Cyclobenzaprine (Flexeril). 10 mg taken at bedtime may be prescribed if client unable to tolerate amitriptyline. Titrate to maximum dose of 40 mg. Contraindications, adverse effects, client teaching similar to amitryptiline.

NSAIDs. Research has suggested that acetaminophen (Tylenol) is more effective than NSAIDs in pain management (Clark & Odell, 2000; Millea & Holloway, 2000). The effect of newer NSAIDs, such as the COX-2 inhibitors, has not been well studied.

Antidepressents. Low doses of fluoxetine (Prozac) singly or combined with amitryptiline may prove helpful in improving sleep quality and functional status (Clark & Odell, 2000; Millea & Holloway, 2000). Low doses of other SSRIs may be beneficial to the client. See discussion of SSRIs in the chapter on Psychosocial Health Concerns.

Narcotic Analgesic. Should be avoided.

Lifestyle/Diet. The cornerstone of treatment is promotion of adequate rest and appropriate exercise. Advise client to avoid caffeine and alcohol before bedtime. Encourage her to start a daily program of low impact aerobic and stretching exercises. Examples include water exercises, stationary cycling, cross country skiing machines. Acupuncture and massage therapy may also be effective. Advise client results do not occur overnight, may take several weeks or months before significant difference is appreciated.

Follow-Up

Regularly scheduled visits during flares are recommended, at one- to two-week intervals. During each visit, focus on self-help strategies such as time management to ensure adequate sleep and daily exercise routine. Encourage client to keep diary of activities and symptom occurrence.

GOUT

Gout is first and foremost a disease of abnormal uric acid metabolism. It is characterized by increased production or reduced excretion of uric acid from the blood stream. The excess uric acid is converted to sodium urate crystals that precipitate and become deposited in joints or other tissue.

There are four stages of gout: asymptomatic hyperuricemia, acute gouty arthritis, symptom-free periods between attacks, and chronic tophaceous gouty arthritis, (Townes, 1999).

Epidemiology

Gout is more common in men than in women. In women, the onset is after menopause. There is primary gout, which is due to an inborn error of metabolism, and secondary gout, which may have a genetic predisposition. It is an acquired hyperuricemia from diuretic use, myeloproliferative disorders, chronic renal disease, hypothyroidism, alcoholism, and psoriasis. Transplant recipients may have decreased renal function and take medication that decreases uric acid excretion (especially cyclosporine). They are at high risk of developing gout.

Subjective Data

In the first stage of gout, the client will be asymptomatic. Hyperuricemia is detected during routine blood and urine screening.

In the acute attack, the client will complain of sudden onset of severe monarticular pain with swelling and erythema. She may report a low grade fever and malaise. The joints most commonly affected are the first metatarsophalangeal joint, the ankle, the elbow, and the knee. The attack may have followed an episode of excessive alcohol intake, high purine diet, initiation of diuretic therapy for hypertension, renal dysfunction, surgery, or infection. Typically, the initial attack is followed by a period of remission of months to years.

If the client reports a history of gout, she may present with polyarticular symptoms that may be indistinguishable from rheumatoid arthritis.

Be sure to include thorough sexual history, illicit drug use, surgical history (especially joint replacement), and risk of immunocompromise.

Objective Data

Physical Examination

- *General Appearance.* Typically, the initial attack is monoarticular and affects the great toe (podagra).
- *Inspection.* The affected joint will be quite swollen and perhaps dusky red.
- *Palpation.* Joint is warm or even hot to touch and exquisitely tender. The client may not be able to tolerate anything touching the site, such as sheets, socks, or other articles of clothing.

    Tophi, nodular deposits of monosodium urate monohydrate crystals, may be found on the helix of the ear, the ulnar aspect of the forearm, achilles tendon, and olecranon bursa.
- *Range of Motion.* It may not be possible to move the joint through its range of motion due to pain.

Diagnostic Tests

Arthrocentesis. Diagnosis is confirmed by aspiration of the joint and microscopic inspection for crystals. If a reliable history of recurrent gouty attacks is given, it may not be necessary to tap the joint.

Serum Uric Acid Level, CBC, ESR. May be drawn, but these tests do not confirm diagnosis. Serum uric acid is almost always elevated > 6.0 mg/dl in women.

X-rays. Generally not indicated for the acute attack but in later disease may show punched out areas in the bone due to radiolucent urate tophi.

Differential Medical Diagnoses

Cellulitis (client able to move joint through range of motion, pain is superficial), septic joint (differentiated by arthrocentesis), pseudogout (crystals in aspirate are calcium pyrophosphate, uric acid level is normal), rheumatoid arthritis (differentiated by aspirate) (Kwoh, Anderson, Greene, et al., 2002; Lee & Weinblatt, 2001).

Plan

Psychosocial Interventions. If the client has a high alcohol intake, advise her that alcohol may precipitate gouty attacks and should be used with caution. If she is unable to control her intake, refer for substance abuse counseling. The transplant recipient who develops gout as a result of her medication may be coping with anger and despair.

Medication. Pharmacological intervention is based on stage of illness.

Asymptomatic Hyperuricemia. Asymptomatic hyperuricemia requires no medication. See following for diet and lifestyle management. If client is taking diuretic, it may contribute to hyperuricemia.

Acute Gout. The acute attack is treated with an NSAID, often indomethacin 25 to 50 mg TID continued until the attack resolves (5 to 10 days). In clients unable to take NSAIDs (e.g., transplant recipients) intraarticular injection of triamcinolone 10 to 40 mg (depending on the size of the joint) is effective and provides relief in 6 to 12 hours. Joint aspiration is required, however, to rule out the septic joint.

Colchicine. May also be used in the acute attack, but it has fallen out of favor due to the high incidence (80 percent) of significant and often serious gastrointestinal symptoms, such as nausea, vomiting, diarrhea, and abdominal cramping. It is most effective if taken early in the attack (first few hours).

- *Administration.* 0.5 to 0.6 mg po every hour until pain is relieved or until nausea or diarrhea. Not to exceed 8 mg total dose. See following for discussion of colchicine.

Chronic Gout. Repeated attacks are treated with colchicine 0.6 mg b.i.d. Specific indications are mild hyperuricemia and frequent attacks (Townes, 1999).

- Exact mechanism of action of colchicine is unknown but may involve leukocyte migration and reduction of lactic acid produced by leukocytes, resulting in decreased deposition of uric acid.
- *Adverse Effects.* Vomiting, diarrhea, abdominal pain, nephrotoxicity, myopathy, confusion, peripheral neuritis, bone marrow depression.
- *Contraindications.* Serious renal, hepatic, and cardiac disease. Also those with blood dyscrasias or inflammatory bowel disease.
- *Expected Outcome.* Suppression of acute attacks.
- *Client Teaching.* Advise client to report any adverse effects, e.g., dysphagia (sore throat), rash, unusual bleeding, weakness, numbness.

Uric Acid–Lowering Agent. Uric acid lowering agent such as *allopurinol* may be indicated if serum uric acid levels remain high (8.5 to 9.0 mg/dl) after diet modification and alcohol avoidance. Monitor CBC, serum uric acid levels, hepatic and renal function at onset of treatment and periodically thereafter.

- *Dosage* is 100 to 300 mg orally per day.

- *Mechanism of Action.* Allopurinol is a xanthine oxidase inhibitor that reduces uric acid production.
- *Adverse Effects.* Headache, sleepiness, rash, Stevens-Johnson syndrome, nausea, vomiting, diarrhea, metallic taste, agranulocytosis, anemia, bone marrow depression, elevated liver enzymes.
- *Contraindications.* Known hypersensitivity, hemochromatosis. Use with caution in pregnancy, breastfeeding, renal impairment, bone marrow depression.
- *Client Teaching.* Advise client to discontinue medication immediately at first sign of rash (occurs most often in those taking diuretics or those with renal impairment). Advise client to drink ten to twelve glasses of water per day to maintain urine output.

Triamcinolone. If client is unable to take NSAIDs, steroid injection of triamcinolone 10 to 40 mg, depending on the size of the joint, may provide relief. Before injection, joint aspiration for gram stain and microscopic examination for crystals should be done to rule out sepsis (see discussion under bursitis).

Prednisone. Oral prednisone 40 to 60 mg/day, tapered over a week, if several joints are affected (see discussion under asthma for information on steroid taper).

Diet/Lifestyle. The obese client should be advised on weight loss. Stress the importance of avoiding liquid fad diets or fasts. Hyperuricemia is associated with obesity and hyperlipidemia. Dietary sources of purines do not cause gouty attacks, but a low cholesterol diet is important in maintaining health. A high liquid intake is important to aid urate excretion and minimize formation of urate stones in the kidney. Bed rest is important in the acute attack. Cold compresses and elevation of the extremity may increase comfort.

Follow-Up

Evaluate the client in seven to ten days. After the initial attack if a second attack occurs within six months, refer to a rheumatologist.

OSTEOARTHRITIS

Osteoarthritis (OA), or degenerative joint disease, usually becomes symptomatic at age 40 to 50 years. The onset is insidious, the changes in joints slowly progressive. It begins with joint space narrowing followed by osteophyte formation. Virtually all individuals over the age of 70 are affected.

Epidemiology

Of all the arthritic conditions in the United States, OA is the most common (Altman, Hochberg, Moskowitz, & Schnitzer, 2000; Felson & Nevitt, 1999). Between 10 and 15 percent of the adult population aged 30 or older has symptoms of OA in at least one joint. The most commonly affected joints are the knees and hips. Although OA is more prevalent among men initially, by the age of 50 the disease affects women more than men (Felson & Nevitt, 1999).

Subjective Data

Important areas to cover in the symptom history include onset, nature and duration of the pain. Be sure to include issues of lifestyle, obesity, and/or occupational factors that may contribute to the condition.

The client complains of increased pain with use. Although she may find pain is more severe in the knee or the hip, the hands and feet are the most common sites of early arthritic changes. She may also note morning stiffness. This usually lasts fewer than 30 minutes. Going up or down stairs, bending, or kneeling may have become increasingly difficult. A family history of arthritis or a previous injury to the affected joint may exist. Ask her about former or current activities, such as jogging, weight or fitness training, or dancing.

Objective Data

Physical Examination. The physical exam focuses on the affected joint(s).

Gait. Observe the client's gait for antalgia.

Inspect for erythema, deformity, muscle atrophy, or swelling.

Palpate the joint for warmth, swelling, tenderness. *Inflammation* manifested by warmth, swelling, or effusion requires further evaluation to rule out infection, inflammatory processes such as rheumatoid arthritis or gout, or autoimmune disease (see following Differential Medical Diagnoses).

Range of Motion. Move the joint through its active and passive range of motion, noting limitation, crepitus, and client's expression of pain.

Diagnostic Tests. The most important question to answer before ordering a specific test or an x-ray is whether the outcome of the test will alter the plan of care or the prognosis of the client. If the pain is recent in onset (i.e., within last few weeks) and the joint does not appear inflamed or unstable, no further diagnostic tests are indicated.

Radiographic Evaluation. Indicated if the pain has persisted despite conservative management, if trauma preceded the pain, or the joint appears unstable.

Laboratory Tests. Erythrocyte sedimentation rate (ESR), antinuclear antibody titer (ANA), serum uric acid, and/or rheumatoid factor should be drawn if a high suspicion of rheumatoid arthritis, gout, or systemic lupus erythematosus is raised. These tests should not be used to screen because of their low specificity.

Arthrocentesis. Fluid aspirate must be tested to rule out infection if the joint is warm, an effusion is present, and the client reports a history of fever, recent unprotected sex, or sexually transmitted disease.

Differential Medical Diagnoses

See Table 22–2.

Diagnosis is usually based on physical exam, lack of systemic or constitutional symptoms such as malaise or fever, and minimal joint inflammation.

TABLE 22–2. Comparison of Osteoarthritis and Rheumatoid Arthritis

	Osteoarthritis	Rheumatoid Arthritis
Onset	Age 50–55 years old (men often earlier)	Age 20–60 yrs old
M/F ratio	Men = Women	Women two to three times more than men
Constitutional symptoms	Absent	Present
Joints affected	Hips, knees, spine, DIP, PIP, MTP	Wrists, MCP, PIP, MTP
Pattern	Asymmetrical, often monoarticular in weightbearing joints	Symmetrical, often polyarticular
Other signs	Crepitus	Swelling, warmth, tenderness
	Heberden's nodes on dorsum of DIP	Deformities such as swan's neck and boutonniere of fingers
	Osteophyte formation and joint space narrowing on x-ray	Rheumatoid nodules on bony prominence especially elbows
Laboratory tests	None indicated	Elevated sedimentation rate +Rheumatoid factor

Key: DIP = Distal interphalangeal joint; PIP = Proximal interphalangeal joint; MTP = Metatarsophalangeal joint; MCP = Metacarpophalangeal joint.

Source: Altman et al. (2000); Ignatavicius (2001); Kwoh et al. (2002); Lee & Weinblatt (2001).

Rheumatoid arthritis presents with the warm spongy joint enlargement of synovitis as opposed to the bony hard and cool enlargement in osteoarthritis.

Systemic lupus erythematosus usually features discoid skin lesions or malar rash and complaints of extreme fatigue, anorexia, and weight loss.

Gout has an acute onset usually with monarticular involvement, especially the first metatarsophalangeal joint.

Other bone diseases: Always be alert to the possibility that pain, especially back pain, may be due to other bone diseases such as osteoporosis, metastatic neoplasia, or multiple myeloma. Suspicion is raised by history and lack of response to conservative therapy.

Plan

Psychosocial Interventions. A diagnosis of arthritis for a woman in her 30s or 40s is distressing in view of the chronicity and progressive character of the disease process. Reassure her that with pharmacological management of her pain and with promotion of overall fitness and control of body weight, arthritis need not significantly alter her lifestyle.

Medication. Analgesics such as acetaminophen and nonsteroidal anti-inflammatory drugs are the cornerstones of pain management.

Acetaminophen. 325 to 650 mg po every 4 hours not to exceed 4 grams per day for one month or 2.6 grams daily for long-term use.

- *Adverse Effects.* Usually mild but may include nausea, abdominal pain, mental changes, difficulty in urination, rash.

  Contraindicated with known allergy to medication, active liver or kidney disease.
- *Client Teaching.* Advise that many OTC medications contain acetaminophen. Include the amounts in calculation of daily dose. Warn of risk of liver damage if history of heavy or binge drinking, liver disease.

  NOTE: Acetaminophen does not have antiinflammatory properties. Several studies have shown, however, that it may be as effective as an NSAID in relieving pain of osteoarthritis (Altman et al., 2000).

Nonsteroidal Anti-inflammatory Drugs. See Table 22–1 for dosage and comments.

- *Adverse Effects.* Predominantly GI distress, GI bleeding, peptic ulcer formation. Also headache, peripheral edema, tinnitus, prolonged bleeding time, bronchospasm.

- *Contraindications.* Known sensitivity or allergy to NSAID or aspirin. Active GI, liver disease or kidney disease, diabetes with renal insufficiency, asthmatics who experience bronchospasm with aspirin or NSAID.
- *Client Teaching.* Advise client she may take acetaminophen 325 to 650 mg po in intervals between NSAID dosages (if 8–24 hours) to manage acute flare-ups. Always advise to take with food, to stop medication if GI distress. If client on antihypertensive agent, NSAID may lower its effectiveness. May potentiate anticoagulants, hypoglycemic effects of insulin and oral hypoglycemics.

NOTE: NSAIDs carry a risk of GI bleeding. Before the advent of COX-2 inhibitors, providers often combined NSAIDs with 200 mcg of misoprostol three to four times a day. Diarrhea and flatulence are the most common side effects of misoprostol (Altman et al., 2000). Several COX-2 inhibitors have been approved for use by clients with OA and are listed in Table 22–1.

Intra-articular injection of steroids is usually not indicated unless there is an associated synovitis caused by accumulation of intra-articular debris, evidence of tendinitis, or trochanteric bursitis. Steroid injection is difficult and should be attempted only by the skilled practitioner after consultation with physician and appropriate radiologic studies.

Diet/Lifestyle. Modest weight loss, even as little as 10 percent of body weight, may dramatically improve OA symptoms in weight-bearing joints. Exercise programs consisting of aerobic and muscle-strengthening activities can reduce pain and improve function. If the client is unable to tolerate traditional low-impact aerobics and weight training, refer her to an aquatic program. Many community pools and health clubs offer a full range of water aerobic and weight-training programs. The buoyancy and resistance offered by the water reduces jarring of joints but allows for full range of motion. One documented advantage of aerobic and weight-training programs is better proprioception and reduced sensory dysfunction in knee joints (Altman et al., 2000). This may lead to fewer knee injuries or falls.

Specific exercises that strengthen supporting muscles such as the quadriceps are beneficial. Clients can be shown how to do these exercises while sitting down. Non-weight-bearing exercises such as swimming and stretching promote and maintain flexibility. Canes and walkers can reduce joint load and improve mobility in those with advanced disease. Client teaching on proper body mechanics in the use of assistive devices is required. Referral to a physical or occupational therapist may be indicated, especially if limitations in activities of daily living are noted. This service is often covered by insurance.

Alternating heat for 15 minutes followed by ice for 15 minutes may relieve pain and muscle spasm. Advise client with co-existing diabetes or peripheral vascular disease not to exceed exposure times. Various over-the-counter heat generating creams such as capsaicin cream (Zostrix) are also available. Advise client it may be helpful to use cream, apply ice, or take medication before aggravating activity such as shopping or housework.

Glucosamine and chondroitin are two popular supplements purported to reduce the pain and destruction of OA. Existing research studies using these agents are difficult to interpret because of different outcome measurement tools, varying dosage levels, and design flaws. However, these studies suggest that glucosamine and chondroitin may offer mild improvement in OA symptoms (McAlindon, LaValley, Gulin, & Felson, 2000). Glucosamine and chondroitin are available in pill form and as gelatin-based powdered drink mixtures.

Follow-Up

Follow-up at one to two weeks for evaluation of therapy and any adverse effects of medications. If high risk for GI bleed, obtain baseline CBC. Monitor renal function, liver function and CBCs at three-month intervals if on daily medication. Refer to orthopedic surgeon if pain is intolerable with medication or if significant loss of movement and disability.

RHEUMATOID ARTHRITIS

Rheumatoid arthritis (RA) is a chronic inflammatory disease of the joints affecting the synovial membrane and tendon sheath. There is no known cause. Although RA has systemic manifestations, the hallmark of the disease is synovitis of the peripheral joints in a symmetric distribution. This usually results in cartilage destruction, erosion of the bone, and joint deformities. The course is unpredictable. Some individuals have mild disease with little joint damage, while others experience crippling disease and nerve compression syndromes.

Epidemiology

Rheumatoid arthritis affects 1 percent of the adult population and is responsible for 9 million office visits annually. Women are affected more than men, in a 2.5:1 ratio.

It is a disease of middle age, commonly noted among 40- to 70-year-olds (Kwoh et al., 2002; Lee & Weinblatt, 2001).

Subjective Data

The client commonly reports a prodrome of extreme fatigue, anorexia, weight loss, weakness, and mild musculoskeletal pain. She may have a history of low grade fever. Inflammatory changes of swelling and erythema in several joints such as the hands, wrists, and knees appear in a symmetric pattern. These changes may emerge gradually over a period of weeks or months. The defining features of rheumatoid arthritis are morning stiffness lasting more than one hour and symmetric peripheral joint swelling and pain.

Objective Data

Physical Examination. Inspection of the affected sites reveals swelling and often erythema. Palpation elicits tenderness, and the joint is warm to touch. Range of motion may be limited due to accumulation of synovial fluid and pain. If disease is in later stages, soft tissue contractures can result in deformities. Examples of these are radial deviation of the wrist with ulnar deviation of the fingers, swan neck and boutonniere deformities of the digits involving the PIP and DIP joints. Deformities can also develop in the feet.

Extraarticular manifestations of disease process include rheumatoid nodules on extensor surfaces, especially the elbow and lower arm, the achilles tendon and the occiput; muscle atrophy; rheumatoid vasculitis; pleuropulmonary inflammation; scleritis; osteoporosis.

Diagnostic Tests. Results of diagnostic tests may be misleading, and no test is specific for diagnosis. The American Rheumatism Society's revised criteria for diagnosis include morning stiffness, arthritis of three or more joints, arthritis of hand joints, symmetric pattern, rheumatoid nodules, presence of rheumatoid factor, and radiographic changes. Four of the seven criteria must be present for diagnosis. (Matsumoto & Wigley, 1999).

Seventy to 90 percent of persons with RA test positive for rheumatoid factor (RF). If the client is tested early in her disease, she may have a negative RF test. Retest in six months. In healthy older clients, RF may be present in 10 to 25 percent of persons older than 70 who do not have the disease (Matsumoto & Wigley, 1999). There is no correlation between RF levels and extent of disease. Other disease entities with similar presentation may generate rheumatoid factor, such as systemic lupus erythematosus, sarcoidosis, mononucleosis, hepatitis B. Therefore, rheumatoid factor is not useful as a screening test but can confirm diagnosis.

Complete Blood Count. May reveal a normochromic normocytic anemia. Erythrocyte sedimentation rate is increased in active disease.

Radiographic Evaluation. Radiographs of the hands and feet are recommended because these are the joints frequently affected. Radiographs of other affected joints are also recommended. These radiographs can serve as baseline indicators for future comparisons. Also, active disease may cause insidious joint damage not noted during the examination, so periodic radiographs help monitor the success of treatment in preventing or slowing joint damage (Kwoh et al., 2002).

Differential Medical Diagnoses

Osteoarthritis has minimal joint inflammation, lacks constitutional symptoms, and affects weight-bearing joints (see Table 22–2).

Systemic lupus erythematosus has a similar presentation and age of onset and may be differentiated by malar rash or characteristic discoid lesions, positive antinuclear antibody, and antibody to double stranded DNA.

Gout is monarticular, more common in men.

Plan

Psychosocial Interventions. Diagnosis of a chronic disease with an unpredictable course is a major life stressor in addition to the pain and fatigue that accompany it. Reassure the client that the goals of therapy include pain management, preservation of function, and control of destructive processes. Be alert for signs of depression that may necessitate referral for counseling. Encourage the client to join a support group. Reassure her that even though you may refer her to a rheumatologist and/or physical therapist, you will continue to provide primary care and case management.

Medication. The goal of treatment is to control RA because it cannot be cured. Preservation of joint function is important. Disease-modifying antirheumatic drugs (DMARDs) are the first-line treatment for RA. DMARDs include D-penicillamine, gold, hydroxychloroquine, minocycline, etanercept, and infliximab (Ignatavicius, 2001). Methotrexate is one of the oldest DMARDs and is usually administered orally once a week (7.5 to 25 mg). Onset of medication is four to eight weeks. Side effects (alopecia, stomatitis, GI intolerance, anemia) can be minimized by adding folic acid (1 mg/day) or folinic acid (5 mg/week) (Lee & Weinblatt, 2001). NSAIDs can be added for pain management (see Table 22–1), and low-dose systemic steroids may be used as well.

Nonpharmacological Interventions. Include referral to a licensed physical therapist for pain management, physical conditioning, and preservation of function. The therapist can provide a home therapy routine as well as adaptive devices to assist with activities of daily living. (Ignatavicius, 2001; Kwoh et al., 2002; Lee & Weinblatt, 2001).

Lifestyle/Diet. Although diet claims for relief and even cure of arthritis abound, there is no scientific basis for these claims. Advise that a sensible diet that includes a wide variety of foods and a program of physical conditioning and overall health maintenance assures the best outcome. Encourage adequate rest periods to decrease joint inflammation.

Follow-Up

Once the initial diagnosis is made, follow-up is based on disease progression. All clients should be reevaluated in four to eight weeks for response to therapy. If treatment is not successful within the first three months, refer to a physician or rheumatologist for combination therapy and more aggressive management (Kwoh et al., 2002). Most clients have a disease pattern of periodic exacerbations with periods of remission. About 15 percent have remission after an initial flare without major deformity developing. Predictors of future disability include age, female sex, radiologic pathology, increased titers of rheumatoid factor. (Lee & Weinblatt, 2001).

SYSTEMIC LUPUS ERYTHEMATOSUS

Systemic lupus erythematosus (SLE) is a disorder of unknown etiology that can affect almost any organ system. It is characterized by damage to cells and tissue caused by immune complexes and pathogenic autoantibodies.

Epidemiology

SLE is generally a disease of women in their childbearing years; 90 percent of all cases fall into this category. It is more common in African Americans. Approximately 500,000 people in the United States suffer from SLE (Wallace & Linker-Israeli, 1999). There appears to be a genetic predisposition (McAlindon, 2000).

Subjective Data

The client may present with only a malar or discoid rash, or she may complain of generalized joint pain and malaise. Most experience arthralgias, myalgias, and intermittent arthritis as the earliest manifestation. Multiple system involvement may also be indicated by chest pain and nonspecific gastrointestinal complaints (anorexia, weight loss, nausea). Be sure to ask about medication use. Several drugs cause a syndrome resembling lupus, especially procainamide and hydralazine. Other drugs that have been implicated more rarely include isoniazid, chlorpromazine, d-penicillamine, methyldopa, and oral contraceptives. Discontinuation of the offending drug usually resolves clinical symptoms in a few weeks. (Clark et al., 2000).

Objective Data

Vital Signs. Temperature may be slightly elevated.

Physical Examination. If suspicion of SLE is high, a thorough head to toe physical exam is indicated, including weight.

- *Skin.* The rash of SLE is more often malar in a butterfly shape than discoid (as in discoid lupus). It is flat or slightly raised, erythematous, appearing over the cheeks and the bridge of the nose but can extend to the chin, ears, or any sun-exposed area. Client may also have aphthous ulcers in the buccal mucosa and vasculitic skin lesions such as purpura, infarcts (splinter hemorrhages) of skin, digits, or nails and leg ulcers. Twenty percent of those with SLE have discoid lupus lesions. (See discussion of discoid lupus in dermatology section.) The client may have patchy alopecia. (Klippel & Arayssi, 2000).
- *Eyes.* The eye and retina should be examined for episcleritis, conjuctivitis, swelling of the optic disc, and vascular abnormalities.
- *Heart.* Cardiac involvement is indicated by the presence of a pericardial friction rub, gallop rhythm, or new onset of murmur.
- *Lungs.* Pulmonary manifestations include adventitious lung sounds, pleural rub, and increased respiratory rate.
- *Abdomen.* Palpate the abdomen for tenderness and note any guarding. Clients with SLE are at risk for peritonitis and pancreatitis.
- *Musculoskeletal Exam.* Musculoskeletal manifestations include joint swelling, especially the proximal intraphalangeal (PIP), metacarpophalangeal (MCP) joints of the hands, the wrists, and knees. The client may have only hand and feet puffiness and tenosynovitis.
- *Neurological Exam.* Perform a thorough neurological examination, concentrating on cognitive function, cranial nerves for palsy, and cerebellar dysfunction.

Diagnostic Tests *Urine pregnancy test* for all women of child-bearing age.

Routine urinalysis to detect proteinurea, hematuria.

Antibody to double stranded DNA (most specific test to detect SLE).

Antinuclear antibody (ANA, most sensitive test to detect SLE). Antinuclear antibody titer may remain positive for years.

Chest x-ray if indicated to detect effusion.

ECG, echocardiogram if indicated to detect pericarditis, endocarditis, valvular abnormality.

Flat plate of the abdomen if ascites, liver enlargement.

Complete blood count to detect anemia.

Serum chemistries to assess renal and hepatic function.

Differential Medical Diagnoses

Rheumatoid arthritis; skin disorders such as urticaria, erythema multiform, rosacea; scleroderma; multiple sclerosis. Always consider drug-induced lupus, from procainamide, hydralazine, and less frequently isoniazid, chlorpromazide, d-penicillamine, methyldopa, oral contraceptives (Clark et al., 2000).

If client is diagnosed with SLE, she is referred to a physician for further management.

She may be followed by a rheumatologist, nephrologist, cardiologist, pulmonologist, or neurologist based upon the stage and manifestation of disease.

Plan

Psychosocial Interventions. SLE is a chronic disease with no known cure. Its course is unpredictable with emissions and flares. The overall survival rate is about 85 percent over ten years (Trager & Ward, 2001).

The client will need a high degree of support and empathy from the provider. She may go through denial, anger, despair. If pregnant, she will need information and counseling on how the pregnancy may affect the course of her disease. She may have to consider terminating the pregnancy. Assure her that even though she is seen by various specialists, you are available for support and education.

Medication. Drug therapy based on systemic manifestations of disease.

Anti-Inflammatory Agents. Most clients with mild SLE are treated with nonsteroidal anti-inflammatory drugs and topical corticosteroids for joint pain and skin rashes.

Systemic Steroids. Those with complications of disease such as thrombocytopenic purpura, hemolytic anemia, myocarditis, pericarditis, and nephritis are treated with glucocorticoids. During acute exacerbations, doses may be given every 8 to 12 hours. When disease is controlled, one morning dose of prednisone or other short-acting glucocorticoid is given and tapered down to the lowest dose that suppresses acute flare (Clark et al., 2000).

Azothioprine. Cytotoxic agents such as azathioprine in cases of lupus nephritis may prevent renal failure, but their use is controversial and may cause serious side effects.

NOTE: See previous discussion of oral steroids and pharmacologic text for further information on above medications.

Experimental Therapy. Newer experimental treatment modalities include plasmapheresis, total lymph node irradiation, intravenous gamma globulin, and cyclosporine. (Wallace & Linker-Israeli, 1999).

Diet/Lifestyle. The practitioner can be a very important resource for the client in promoting healthy diet and lifestyle to retard disease progression. Infection and renal disease are the major causes of death in those with SLE. Adequate rest and nutrition, a positive outlook, protection of joints, regular exercise as tolerated, use of sunscreen on skin are key to maintaining optimum health in the presence of illness.

Follow-Up

The practitioner should continue to follow the client for routine health care including an annual well-woman exam, mammogram, and treatment of episodic illness.

NEUROLOGICAL DISORDERS

The term *neurological disorders* casts a broader net than one might first suppose, since within its boundaries can be found everything from the common headache to seizures and Parkinsonism. This section encompasses information on headache, fever, dizziness and vertigo, Bell's palsy, two alterations in consciousness—syncope and seizures—and Parkinsonism and essential tremor.

HEADACHE

Headache is one of the most common complaints leading to office and emergency room visits. It accounts for many lost work days and disruptions in family relationships. This section focuses on the two most common types: tension and migraine. Most experts agree that tension and migraine headaches are on a continuum, with some overlap and shared characteristics and etiologies.

Prior to discussing the common and more benign headaches, it is best to understand less common headache variants and potentially more dangerous headaches requiring referral and further diagnostic testing.

Some headaches are due to organic causes such as brain tumors, bleeding, or meningitis. These headaches usually present with some of the "red flags" listed in Table 22–3. If these red flags are present, prompt imaging and consultation with a neurologist is necessary (C.J. Johnson, 1999; G.D. Johnson, 1998).

Uncommon Headache Variants

Several uncommon headache variants must be considered in diagnosis: cluster headaches, complex migraines, and headaches caused by pseudotumor cerebri, temporal (giant cell) arteritis, and subarachnoid hemorrhage.

Keep in mind that systemic illnesses can affect headaches and that anxiety about the cause of the headache may magnify or distort the clinical features. Look at the total picture including the possibility of referred pain from sinus infections or dental infections.

Cluster Headaches. Cluster headaches are an uncommon variant type of migraine. Reports show that 90 percent occur among men. Attacks usually begin between ages 20 and 40 and occur in "clusters," usually nightly in

TABLE 22–3. Red Flag Symptoms for Dangerous Headaches

No recognizable benign pattern for headaches
Client description: "Worst headache ever"
Onset of headache with exertion (cough, strain, Valsalva maneuver)
Vomiting without nausea
Personality changes (decreased alertness or cognition)

Any abnormality on physical exam
   Neck not supple, pain with flexion
   Fever
   Focal neurological signs

Seizure(s)
Sudden change in headache pattern especially in those over age 50
Progression of symptoms

six-week cycles. The pain often begins 1 to 2 hours after falling asleep and wakes the client up. Excruciating pain lasts about 1 hour and is described as "boring" around one eye. Tearing and nasal congestion often occur on the affected side. In contrast to migraine, those affected are restless, often getting out of bed and pacing. Cluster headaches are frequently triggered by alcohol of histamine. Refer the client to a neurologist (C.J. Johnson, 1999).

Complex Migraine Headaches. Complex migraines are associated with focal neurological signs, which may continue after the prodrome and into or past the headache phase. They may be confused with stroke. Always refer the client to a neurologist.

An unusual variation in young people is the basilar migraine. The client may complain of vertigo, double vision, numbness and may have an ataxic gait, visual field changes, and changes in level of consciousness (C.J. Johnson, 1999).

Pseudotumor Cerebri. Headaches may be caused by pseudotumor cerebri (benign intracranial hypertension). The intracranial hypertension, often of unknown etiology, is most often seen among children or obese young women. It has been associated with use of tetracycline, vitamin A, corticosteroids, and oral contraceptives as well as pulmonary disease and endocrine disturbances. A client is in no apparent distress. She may report "mild headache"; papilledema is noted on the physical exam. Partial or complete visual loss may occur if not treated. Refer the client to a neurologist immediately.

Temporal Arteritis. Headaches may also result from temporal (giant cell) arteritis. The arteritis is of unknown etiology and occurs primarily after age 50. Clients may have associated fever, malaise, and muscle aches, especially in the shoulders and hips. Clients usually, although not always, have a headache. Visual symptoms such as diplopia occur among 50 percent. Temporal arteritis is also associated with proximal muscle weakness (polymyalgia rheumatica). Tenderness over the temporal artery and rarely the occipital artery may be elicited. The erythrocyte sedimentation rate is dramatically elevated, often greater than 100 mm per hour. Refer the client to a neurologist immediately. Treatment with steroids is initiated to prevent blindness.

Subarachnoid Hemorrhage. Subarachnoid hemorrhage may be reported as a sudden onset of the "worst headache of my life."

This may be followed by nausea, vomiting, and a decreasing level of consciousness. The hemorrhage is usually secondary to trauma, a ruptured aneurysm or congenital arteriovenous malformation. Subarachnoid hemorrhage is most common between ages 25 and 50. The individual may collapse and lose consciousness. Neck stiffness and neurological signs almost always occur. Refer the client to a neurologist immediately or an emergency room for an emergent CT scan.

Tension Headaches

The pathophysiology of tension headaches is poorly understood. Although once referred to as muscle contraction headaches, current research indicates that muscle contraction is not always present with this type of headache. Stress or tension is almost always involved, but the exact pathophysiology is unknown. Tension headaches can be episodic or chronic daily headaches.

Epidemiology. Studies reveal that tension headaches are the most prevalent of all headache types. They are more common in women than in men and decrease in frequency with age (C.J. Johnson, 1999). Episodic tension headaches are the classic stress-related headaches. Chronic daily headaches, on the other hand, are often associated with depression that requires treatment.

Subjective Data. A headache history, taken with interest and concern, is the key to the diagnosis. Patterns should be established (see Table 22–4). Rule out a history of trauma, neurological signs, and concurrent disorders.

Have the client keep a headache diary. She should record the day and time of the headache and surrounding events, such as diet, physical activity, and menstrual cycle. She should note aggravating and relieving factors. Have her record the time and dose of any medication taken, both prescribed and over the counter.

When taking a history, it is important to have a client identify different types of headaches, as she may easily have more than one. Ask her to describe specific symptoms (see Table 22–4).

Objective Data. Data are based on a complete physical examination and, in some instances, diagnostic tests. Physical examination includes examination of the nervous system and eyes, nose, and throat (see Table 22–5).

Usually no diagnostic tests are indicated for tension headaches. For any patient older than 40 with a new type of headache, order a CBC and erythrocyte sedimentation rate to rule out temporal arteritis.

TABLE 22–4. Headache Symptom Patterns in History

Symptom	Migraine Headache	Tension Headache
Onset	10% have aura; may awake with headache	Gradual; often begin during times of stress
Duration	Usually 8–12 hours; range 3 hours to rarely 3 days	Usually 8–12 hours; may last days, weeks, months
Frequency	Usually one or two per month or fewer with pain free periods; rarely one per week	Wide range (daily to rarely)
Pain location	Approximately 60% unilateral; may switch side or become bilateral	Approximately 90% bilateral; frontal area, "hat band" area, or back of neck
Pain quality	Throbbing; moderate to severe	Constant; nagging to severe
Associated symptoms	Nausea, vomiting photophobia, phonophobia	Varied from mild intolerance to light and noise to nausea and anorexia
Triggers	Stress; menses; alcohol; food; "letdown" after stress	Stress
Relieving factors	Rest in dark room; sleep	Relaxation exercise; Tylenol/NSAID[a]

[a]Nonsteroidal anti-inflammatory drug.

Differential Medical Diagnoses. Temporomandibular joint syndrome, chronic myositis, cervical OA, migraines, perimenstrual headache, cluster headache, cranial masses (tumors, edema), sinusitis, tooth abscess, temporal arteritis, pseudotumor cerebri.

Plan

Psychosocial Interventions. It is crucial to reassure the client that tension-type headaches are usually not associated with any severely negative consequences. A thorough physical exam can greatly decrease the woman's anxiety level. Once reassured, she can better focus on lifestyle changes and stress management techniques that might help to decrease the frequency of headaches.

Medication. Nonsteroidal anti-inflammatory drugs (NSAIDs) are very helpful for tension headaches as well as migraine and perimenstrual headaches. Ibuprofen is the first choice; naproxen sodium is helpful for perimenopausal headaches. Refer to the previous discussion of NSAIDs in section on Musculoskeletal Disorders.

- *Side Effects.* Gastrointestinal distress and bleeding may occur.
- *Contraindications.* Do not administer to those clients with a history of peptic ulcer disease, bleeding disorders, pregnancy, kidney problems, or allergic reactions to NSAIDs.
- *Anticipated Outcome on Evaluation.* Headache is relieved.
- *Client Teaching.* Advise the client that NSAIDs are most effective when taken at onset of pain. Encourage her to break the pain cycle and give adequate amounts of medication. Narcotics should not be given for this diagnosis, as clients may become physically dependent and experience withdrawal and rebound headaches.

NOTE: Chronic daily headaches are often drug-rebound headaches caused by overuse of analgesics, especially narcotics, acetaminophen, and ibuprofen. Anyone taking these medications more than four times a week is at risk.

Lifestyle/Dietary Changes. The client may require support in evaluating current life situation and stressors. Help her to prioritize activities and to let go of unnecessary tasks and difficulties. Teach general stress management principles and coping mechanisms. Refer the client for counseling if indicated.

Dietary changes are not applicable unless over- or undereating is a source of tension or stress.

Exercise or other physical activity is an effective stress reducer. Encourage and support lifestyle changes that incorporate 30 minutes of aerobic exercise at least five days a week.

Follow-Up. Plan a follow-up visit two weeks after the initial visit to support and reassess the client. If headaches have not significantly improved or if the client has experienced any new symptoms, such as those listed in Table 22–4, refer her to a neurologist. Headache may be an indicator of other psychological problems such as depression. One study found a significant correlation between a history of childhood sexual assault and headaches in adulthood in women (Golding, 1999).

Migraine Headaches

Migraine headaches are recurrent episodic accompanied by nausea and/or vomiting and photophobia. According to the IHS classification at least two of the following features must also be present: unilateral location, pulsating

TABLE 22–5. Physical Exam for Headache

General appearance: Note affect, photophobia.
Vital signs: Blood pressure and temperature must be charted.
    Blood pressure—Hypertension (HTN) rarely causes headaches; pain with diastolic > 120–140. HTN may aggravate migraine.
    Temperature—Fever, rule out meningitis, arteritis, sinusitis, abscess.
Mental Status: Usually assessed within framework of interview.

Cranial Nerves[a]	Head, Eyes, Ears, and Throat
(If normal, efficient charting states "cranial nerves II–XII intact.")	
I. Olfactory: usually not done	
II. Optic: visual acuity, visual fields by confrontation	Disc flat (rule out papilledema)
III,IV,VI. Oculomotor, trochlear, abducens	
PERRLA,[b] EOMs, note ptosis of upper lids	
V. Trigeminal	Palpate "click" from temporomandibular joint
Motor—palpate masseter, open and close jaw	Palpate temporal area (rule out arteritis)
Sensory—touch forehead, cheek, jaw	
VII. Facial	Check tenderness over sinuses (rule out sinusitis)
Observe facial symmetry	
Raise eyebrows, frown	
Close eyes, resist opening	
Smile, puff out cheeks	
VIII. Acoustic: hearing watch tick	Look at tympanic membrane
IX,X. Glossopharyngeal, vagus	Check teeth
Symmetrical movement soft palate	
XI. Spinal accessory	Check nodes
Atrophy, shrug upward against hands	Check neck stiffness
Turn head against your hands	Bruits
	Tender neck muscles
XII. Hypoglossal	
Tongue movement, fasciculations	

Screening motor and cerebellar function
  Walk: note gait, heel/toe walk
  Hop on one foot, Romberg
  Deep knee bend, check arms pronator drift
  Finger to nose
Screening sensory
  Pain and vibration (tuning fork), hands and feet
  Stereognosis
Reflexes
  Check deep tendon reflexes, Babinski, and other systems if indicated by history

[a] For efficiency, examine cranial nerves and head, eyes, ears, nose, and throat system simultaneously.
[b] PERRLA, pupils equal, round, reactive to light and accommodation; EOM, extraocular movement.

quality, moderate to severe intensity, and aggravated by physical activity. (C.J. Johnson, 1999; Silberstein, 2000).

The pathogenesis of migraine is thought to be composed of three phases. The first phase begins in the brainstem. The second phase involves vasomotor activation (constriction and dilatation) of arteries both inside and outside the brain. The third phase starts with activation of the brain's head and face pain processing center and the subsequent release of neuropeptides. Pain can be generated during any one of these phases. Most studies of the etiology of migraine pain now focus on disturbances in serotonergic mechanisms as the primary cause. (G.D. Johnson, 1998).

In migraines with an aura, previously called "classic migraines," focal neurological symptoms usually precede the headache and may last up to about 20 minutes. Auras are often visual; they may include visual field deficits, a scintillating scotoma (a luminous patch with irregular outline in the visual field), or a fortification spectrum (a dark patch with zigzag outline). Other neurological auras, such as aphasia and hemiplegia, occur occasionally. When the aura fades, the headache usually begins.

Migraines without an aura, previously called "common migraines," have the features of classic migraines, such as throbbing pain, nausea, vomiting, photophobia, and phonophobia, but no aura.

Perimenstrual headaches occur either two to three days before onset of menses or during the first days of flow. They are frequently severe, usually without aura, and accompanied by nausea and vomiting. It is hypothesized that they are related to fluctuations in estrogen and serotonin levels. Many women consider them as part of premenstrual syndrome (PMS) and may fail to report them (Boyle, 1999).

Epidemiology. The overall incidence of migraine is 18 percent in women and 6 percent in men (Silberstein, 2000). There is usually a strong positive family history. It is more common in women than in men by a ratio of 3:1. Onset is often in childhood, usually at the time of puberty, generally decreasing in frequency after menopause. Pregnancy may relieve or intensify migraine. (C.J. Johnson, 1999; Silberstein, 2000). The use of oral contraceptives may be a risk factor for more frequent, more intense migraines; on the other hand, oral contraceptives may make migraines better. Women with neurological symptoms accompanying the headache (other than visual aura) should not take oral contraceptives. Those on hormone replacement with estrogen who report new onset of migraine or an increase in incidence may need an adjustment in dosage or a change from conjugated to pure estrogen. (Boyle, 1999).

Subjective Data. Obtaining a complete history is essential (see Table 22–4). The history is used to differentiate between migraines and tension headaches because their treatments differ. The criteria for migraine without an aura include a recurring idiopathic headache with at least two of the following: nausea (with or without vomiting), unilateral pain, throbbing, photophobia or phonophobia, association with menstrual cycle, positive family history.

Objective Data. A physical examination is done (see Table 22–5). For recurrent migraines, no diagnostic workup is necessary. For an initial diagnosis, a CBC and chemistries may be helpful. Anemia, electrolyte imbalance, and increased calcium can aggravate migraines.

Differential Medical Diagnoses. See section on Tension Headaches.

Plan

Psychosocial Interventions. Psychosocial intervention is critical, especially for a client who has migraines with an

TABLE 22–6. Overview of Medications for Migraines[a]

Abortive Measures: Appropriate for clients experiencing occasional headaches, not more than one a month.

NSAIDs[b]: Very effective, especially if taken early because they block the sterile inflammation of migraines. Any NSAID may be tried. Naproxen sodium (Naproxyn, 550 mg p.o. b.i.d.) helpful for women suffering with perimenstrual vascular headaches.

Antiemetics: Oral or per rectum. Prochlorperazine (Compazine) suppositories are an example. Help nausea and aid client in "sleeping off" the headache.

Serotonin agonist: Sumatriptan (Imitrex) 6 mg subcutaneously or 100 mg orally. May repeat dose in 1 hour if headache not relieved or if it recurs. Maximum dose is 12 mg s.q. or 300 mg po in 24 hours.

  Caution. Not to be used within 24 hours of an ergot preparation. First dose should be given under observation by health care provider due to adverse effects of general feelings of heaviness and sensation of chest tightness and pressure. Should not be given to those with coronary artery disease or at high risk of unrecognized cardiovascular disease, e.g., post menopausal women, women with hypertension, obesity, diabetes, strong family history, or smokers.

Ergots: Potent vasoconstrictors. May be given intramuscularly, orally, sublingually, by inhalation, or rectally. Most helpful if client has "aura" and can take immediately. Example: Ergotamine tartrate SL (Ergostat) 2 mg at onset and 1 mg every 30 minutes until headache is relieved or to a maximum of 6 mg per day, 12 mg per week.

  A widely recognized, effective treatment for acute migraine is dihydroergotamine mesylate (D.H.E. 45 injection) given 1 mg IM. Give antiemetic first or concurrently.

  Caution. Be familiar with doses of medications used. Overuse can lead to "ergotism" (prolonged vasoconstriction that can cause tissue ischemia and gangrene). Beta blockers increase the risk for ergotism; simultaneous use is contraindicated.

Preventive Measures: Indicated for three or more attacks per month or one prolonged attack per month. Give adequate trial of 3 to 6 months of therapy.

Beta blockers: Numerous types (propranolol, long-acting preparation increases compliance). Effective in 50 percent of cases.

  Caution. Contraindicated with such conditions as asthma and congestive heart failure.

Tricyclics: Numerous types (amitriptyline [Elavil] often used, starting with a 25 mg dose at bedtime, increasing as necessary).

NSAIDs: Ibuprofen, naproxen sodium, aspirin. Observe for gastrointestinal side effects.

Calcium channel blockers: Numerous types (verapamil [Calan, Isoptin] po 240–360 mg per day). Usually ordered by neurologist.

Methylsergide (Sansert): **Last choice.** Ordered only by a neurologist. Can cause fibrosis of heart valves and peritoneum if given longer than six months.

[a] Please consult a current pharmacotherapeutics text for details.
[b] Nonsteroidal anti-inflammatory drugs.

Source: C.J. Johnson (1999); Silberstein (2000).

aura, as these can be very frightening. Reassure the client that she is not having a stroke and involve her as an active participant in measures to prevent and abort attacks.

Medication. See Table 22–6.

Lifestyle/Dietary Changes. Focus primarily on what triggers the migraine. Often there is a "let-down" trigger; for example, the headache starts Saturday morning following a stressful week. Counsel the client to readjust her lifestyle and help her with stress management.

Diet may be a factor in the occurrence of migraines. The most common triggers are chocolate, alcohol, and aged cheeses. Ask the client to keep a diary of foods eaten and to avoid foods associated with the onset of migraine. Encourage her to eat at regularly scheduled intervals; a drop in blood sugar level may trigger a headache.

Advise the client that physical activity, including aerobic exercise for 30 minutes three to five times a week, helps to reduce stress.

Follow-Up. Teach the client the warning signs of headaches with serious underlying causes (see Table 22–3). If such a warning sign occurs, refer her to a neurologist immediately. Otherwise, arrange to see the client about every four to six weeks until the migraines improve. If no improvement is seen in eight weeks or the migraines worsen, refer her to a neurologist.

FEVER

Body temperature is regulated between 97 to 99 degrees Fahrenheit (36 to 37.2 degrees Centigrade). When heat production exceeds heat dissipation, for example during vigorous exercise, the core body temperature may rise above this range until regulatory mechanisms such as sweating, hyperventilation, and vasodilatation promote heat loss and return the body temperature to normal. A sustained elevation of body temperature is called fever and represents a regulated rise to a new set point. (Pierce, 1999). Fever of unknown origin (FUO) is a temperature greater than 101°F (38.2°C) that occurs on several occasions during a three-week period in a person whose diagnosis is not apparent after one week or more of study. (Pierce, 1999). It should be noted that in the vast majority of occurrences the diagnosis is either readily apparent after a history and physical exam or becomes evident within a few days.

Epidemiology

The febrile response in children is greater than in adults; in the elderly it may be absent even in bacterial illnesses (Pierce, 1999).

The setting in which the fever occurs is also important. Acute fever in a traveler to southeast Asia or Africa may be due to malaria or an insect-borne virus. A college student with fever is likely to have a viral infection or mononucleosis. An elderly person recently hospitalized may have urinary tract infection (UTI), pneumonia, phlebitis, or wound infection. Someone with an immune disorder may have an infection caused by an opportunistic agent (Pierce, 1999).

Subjective Data

A symptom history may suggest the cause of fever, especially upper respiratory congestion, myalgias, gastrointestinal upset, ear pain, cough, painful or frequent urination, or rash.

In the absence of these symptoms, inquire about recent use of major tranquilizers such as haloperidol and fluphenazine or antibiotic use. Neuroleptic malignant syndrome is a rare but potentially life-threatening reaction to these drugs. Serum sickness may follow antibiotic treatment and is usually accompanied by rash and arthralgias. Also inquire about illicit drug use and possible occupational exposures to infected animals or chemicals.

Elderly patients may report no other symptom than fever but suspect tuberculosis (TB), occult neoplasm, or urinary tract infection.

Objective Data

Physical Examination. A thorough head to toe exam of all organ systems is necessary if the etiology of the fever is not elicited by the history. If the fever is high (greater than or equal to 102°F or 39°C) with few systemic complaints, look for a bacterial infection of the chest, throat, or abdomen. If there is a low grade fever (less than or equal to 101.5°F or 38.6°C) associated with systemic complaints and few focal findings, think virus.

Do not neglect the dental exam. Abscessed devitalized teeth may cause fever without pain.

Fever after an upper respiratory infection suggests sinusitis. Shaking chills suggest pyelonephritis or pneumonia.

Diagnostic Tests. Laboratory studies are indicated by the results of the history and physical. These may include complete blood count with differential, urinalysis; monospot (detects mononucleosis); erythrocyte sedimentation rate (elevated in inflammatory condition such as rheumatoid arthritis, inflammatory bowel disease); liver function tests (elevated in hepatitis); antistreptolysin; titers (elevated in recent streptococcal infection); Lyme titer; and cultures of blood, stool, urine, and throat.

Radiographic Studies. A chest x-ray or flat plate of the abdomen may also be useful.

If endocarditis is suspected, order an ECG (electrocardiogram) and possibly an echocardiogram if valvular involvement is likely.

Tuberculosis skin test with controls should be placed when appropriate and especially if no obvious etiology is found.

Human immunodeficiency virus (HIV) test is indicated if high-risk behaviors elicited by history.

Differential Medical Diagnoses

See Table 22–7.

Plan

Psychosocial Interventions. Reassure the client that you will continue to follow her closely and inform her of all test results. Answer all questions as fully and candidly as possible and provide an office telephone number.

Medication. Antipyretics such as acetaminophen or ibuprofen may be taken for comfort and are best given on a regular schedule every 6 hours as opposed to as needed. The etiology of the fever will guide the prescription of other medications.

Lifestyle/Diet Changes. Tepid water baths and plenty of fluids (at least 8 ounces of water or juice every hour while awake) will promote comfort and prevent dehydration. Ask client to keep temperature diary by checking body temperature at least three times a day before taking antipyretic medications.

Follow-Up

Telephone follow-up within two to three days. Schedule appointment in one week to review findings and assess response to any medications prescribed. If no obvious

TABLE 22–7. Differential Diagnosis of Fever

Etiology	Symptoms and Associated Factors	Physical Findings
Upper Respiratory Infection:		
Viral	Mild fever Temp 101.5°F (38.6°C) Sore throat, rhinitis, ear fullness Systemic symptoms	Cough, oropharynx injected (no exudate)
Bacterial	High fever—Temp 102°F (39°C) More common in children Pronounced localized symptoms	Tonsillar exudate Bulging tympanic membrane
Other Viral Syndromes (influenza gastroenteritis)	Mild fever Muscle aches, nausea, vomiting, diarrhea	Minimal physical findings
Drug Reaction	Often high fever Occasionally rash Use of OTC or prescription drug	Fever abates when drug stopped
Urinary Tract Infection	Often high fever and chills, backache, urinary frequency and urgency Often hematuria	Costovertebral angle and suprapubic tenderness
Chronic Hepatitis	Intravenous drug use Low grade fever Fatigue, anorexia	Right upper quadrant tenderness Hepatomegaly Jaundice
Tuberculosis	Low grade fever Weight loss Night sweats May have been incarcerated	Chest findings + skin test for purified protein derivative (PPD)
Infectious Mononucleosis	Young adult Low grade fever Fatigue	Pharyngitis Adenopathy Splenomegaly
Chronic Fatigue Syndrome	Debilitating fatigue lasting more than 6 months Mild recurrent or persistent low grade fever for 6 months Sore throat, muscle weakness, myalgia, migratory arthralgia without swelling or redness Neuropsychologic complaints	Nonexudative pharyngitis Posterior or anterior cervical adenopathy 2 cm or more Low grade fever on 2 separate occasions

Source: Pierce (1999); Waterbury & Zieve, (1999).

cause is found after completion of initial diagnostic testing, consult with physician.

DIZZINESS/VERTIGO

Dizziness is a sensation of disequilibrium or altered orientation in relation to one's surroundings. Dizziness as lightheadedness must be distinguished from vertigo. Dizziness may be a sensation of generalized weakness (presyncopal light-headedness) or an inability to maintain balance (disequilibrium). Vertigo is a hallucination of movement. With objective vertigo, the client has the sensation of the room spinning; with subjective vertigo, she has the feeling of her own body spinning when the eyes are closed. (Hasso, Drayer, Anderson, et al., 1999; Sisson & Kramer, 1999).

Epidemiology

Dizziness as a chief complaint accounts for 1 percent of office visits per year. Up to one-third are diagnosed as vestibular in origin, one-fifth are attributed to hyperventilation, and the remainder to neurologic, psychiatric, and cardiovascular etiologies. It is a frequent complaint of the elderly and may be a predictor of risk for falling, morbidity, and/or functional decline. (Hasso et al., 1999; Sisson & Kramer, 1999).

The key to differentiating self-limiting versus more serious causes of dizziness is to obtain a thorough history and perform a careful examination.

Subjective Data

The client may have difficulty clarifying what she means by "feeling dizzy." Important questions include the following: Are you spinning? Is the room spinning? Is the dizziness most noticeable when you first stand, sit up, or turn your head? Did the dizziness start suddenly or has it gone on for a while? How long does the feeling last? What makes the dizziness decrease? What kind of medicines are you taking and for how long?

Significant associated symptoms will assist in the correct diagnosis, especially nausea, tinnitus, ear fullness, one-sided weakness, double vision, facial numbness, numbness or tingling of the extremities. It is also important to ask if the dizziness has been followed by loss of consciousness or seizure activity. If pregnancy is a possibility, a sexual history and evaluation of contraceptive measures are needed.

Objective Data

Physical Examination

◆ *Vital signs.* Postural blood pressure readings.
◆ *Head and neck.* Auscultate for carotid bruit. Examine ear canal and tympanic membrane. Test hearing acuity with 512 Hz tuning fork.
◆ *Full neurological exam,* including evaluation of the cranial nerves (sensory and motor), assessment of cerebellar function, and sensory/motor function. Observe gait for spasticity, ataxia, antalgia, and foot drop.
◆ *Specific provocative tests and maneuvers* may also aid in correct diagnosis. Having the client hyperventilate for a minute or two may reproduce symptoms if no focal abnormalities are found on exam. The Dix-Hallpike maneuver is done on clients with positional vertigo (those whose vertigo disappears at rest). It involves rapid change from the sitting position to lying down with the head turned to one side and the neck extended over the end of the exam table 30 to 45 degrees. A diagnosis of paroxysmal positional vertigo can be established with any of the following findings:

• *Subjective vertigo.*
• *Nystagmus* preceded by a latent period of several seconds after completion of the Dix-Hallpike maneuver. Care should be used in doing this maneuver and should not be performed on frail patients or those with atherosclerotic disease. (Sisson & Kramer, 1999).

Diagnostic Tests. If a cardiovascular cause of dizziness is suspected, a 12-lead electrocardiogram (ECG) is appropriate to rule out arrhythmias and conduction disorders.

If focal neurological deficits are found during the physical exam, computed tomography (CT) of the head and/or audiogram may be ordered to rule out hemorrhage or tumor.

Pregnancy test, beta human chorionic gonadotropin (HCG), is ordered as needed for women of reproductive age.

Differential Medical Diagnoses of Dizziness/Lightheadedness and Vertigo

Many physical and psychological maladies have symptoms that include dizziness or vertigo. Otitis media, reactive hypoglycemia, migraine headaches, and orthostatic blood pressure may cause sensations of dizziness or lightheadedness. Many medications, especially antihypertensives, are responsible for symptoms of dizziness or lightheadedness. Afflictions of the inner ear structures, such as Ménière's disease, labryinthitis, and acoustic neuroma cause vertigo. Anxiety and associated hyperventilation cause lightheadedness. Sick sinus syndrome results in recurrent episodes of dizziness. Consult with a physician if cardiac etiology is suspected or if focal neurologic deficits are noted.

Psychosocial Interventions. If a benign or self-limiting etiology is found, client reassurance is most important. The elderly may need family support with medication use. Emphasize importance of making the home environment safer to prevent falls. If referral to a cardiologist, neurologist or ear, nose, throat (ENT) surgeon is indicated, reassure the client that you will be available for her other health needs and as a resource.

Medication. Positional vertigo: Meclizine HCL 25 mg, one po every 6 hours as needed for dizziness.

- *Adverse Effects.* Drowsiness, dry mouth, blurred vision, nausea, constipation, diarrhea.
- *Contraindications.* Known hypersensitivity. Use with caution in elderly due to sensitivity to antihistamine effects; may increase dizziness, cause sedation or hyperexcitability. Use with caution in glaucoma, asthma.
- *Client Teaching.* May potentiate effects of alcohol or other central nervous system (CNS) depressants.

If otitis media is diagnosed, appropriate antibiotics are given (see discussion of otitis media in Respiratory Infections).

Ménière's disease is treated with diuretics, such as hydrochlorothiazide 50 to 100 mg daily (see previous discussion of diuretics under hypertension) and a low salt diet.

Lifestyle Changes. If vertigo is acute, bedrest and a low salt diet are helpful. Advise the client to use care in movement. Driving may have to be curtailed until the symptoms resolve. Provocative head maneuvers such as the Dix-Hallpike (five repetitions performed twice a day) may habituate the vestibular response of positional vertigo.

Follow-Up

Refer those with labyrinthine, cardiovascular, psychiatric, and neurologic disorders to a physician. Telephone follow-up to assess alleviation of acute symptoms may be warranted. Anyone who is not referred should be seen within seven to ten days.

BELL'S PALSY

Bell's palsy is an idiopathic facial paralysis of the seventh cranial nerve. Its pathogenesis is unknown. There is no evidence to support the theory that it is related to reactivation of the herpes simplex virus, but the benefits of acyclovir treatment lend credence to the possibility that Bell's palsy may have a viral etiology (Grogan & Gronseth, 2001).

Epidemiology

Bell's palsy has an annual incidence of 20 per 100,000. Eighty percent recover with full or near-normal function, but 8,000 persons per year retain permanent facial weakness (Grogan & Gronseth, 2001).

Subjective Data

The client may report a sudden onset of pain behind the ear that precedes the paralysis by a day or two. Taste sensation may be diminished or absent. She may also find that her sense of hearing is heightened. She may complain of tearing and inability to close the eye on the affected side. Eating may be difficult.

Objective Data

Physical Examination. The affected side of the face is expressionless with smoothing of forehead wrinkles and flattening of the nasolabial fold. The corner of the mouth sags on the affected side, and the mouth is drawn to the unaffected side. The ipsilateral eyebrow may be raised or lowered. The client will be unable to wink, but on attempt, the eye will rotate upward. There may be a pooling of tears in the lower eyelid. Either side of the face can be affected and the extent of paralysis can range from mild to complete.

A complete neurological exam to determine if other neurological deficits are present is necessary. The ear and surrounding area should also be evaluated.

Differential Medical Diagnoses

Herpes zoster may also produce a facial palsy, but a vesicular eruption is present. Acoustic neuromas can produce palsy, but hearing loss accompanies this disorder. Bilateral palsy, facial weakness that progresses slowly over several weeks and/or persists more than six months, focal neurological signs discovered during the physical exam suggest other more serious diagnoses, such as stroke or infarct, tumor, or multiple sclerosis.

Plan

Psychosocial Interventions. Client reassurance of good recovery in several weeks to months is important. Eighty percent have full recovery in a few months (Grogan & Gronseth, 2001). Incomplete paralysis in the first week is the most favorable prognostic sign. Body image may suffer as client waits for resolution.

Medication. Research supports the early use of prednisone, 1 mg/kg (maximum: 70 mg) in two divided doses for six days, followed by a four-day taper. Symptoms also responded to combined treatment with acyclovir (800 mg po five times a day for seven to ten days) (Grogan & Gronseth, 2001). Many subjects in research studies experienced spontaneous improvement without treatment, leaving the examiner to conclude that medications may not be necessary. Aside from emotional support to the woman and possible placebo affects, the steroids may at least reduce any discomfort present with Bell's palsy.

Lifestyle/Comfort Measures. Liquid tears may protect the eye from excessive drying, and an eye patch should be worn at night.

Follow-Up

Telephone follow-up is suggested within two weeks. The client should return for office evaluation in six to eight weeks. Consult with physician if residual paralysis.

ALTERATIONS IN CONSCIOUSNESS

Syncope

Syncope is sudden loss of consciousness and postural tone that resolves rapidly and spontaneously. It arises from an interruption in the flow of blood to the brain. If cerebral tissue is deprived of glucose or oxygen for more than 5 seconds, syncope can occur. If the event lasts more than 15 seconds, tonic movements can occur that may resemble seizure activity. (Sisson & Kramer, 1999). The challenge to the provider is to determine if syncope is due to underlying cardiovascular disease or another serious cause.

Epidemiology. Syncope is a relatively common complaint and may account for 3 percent of emergency room visits and up to 6 percent of hospital admissions. Most studies show that in at least 40 percent of individuals with syncope, no cause will be identified. (Sisson & Kramer, 1999). Up to half of all adults will experience a syncopal episode during their lives. In the elderly, the incidence is increased because of decreased blood flow to the brain, a result of the aging process. (Sisson & Kramer, 1999).

Subjective Data A complete history including a detailed account of the syncopal episode, premonitory symptoms, and postsyncopal recover period is crucial to identifying a potential cause. Other factors to note are associated symptoms such as angina, palpitations, nausea, visual changes, numbness in the face or extremities.

Ask if the event was preceded by exertion, heat exhaustion, dehydration, or emotional stress. Tachyarrhythmias usually have an abrupt onset with no warning and lead to a fall, which may result in injury. Neurogenic syncope or seizure may be preceded by an aura and followed by confusion, drowsiness, and incontinence. Often the event is not witnessed and details may not be provided.

Ask the client about her medications purchased over the counter.

Past medical history may elicit key factors such as history of myocardial infarction or seizure disorder.

Objective Data

Physical Examination. Thorough cardiac and neurologic exams are key.

CARDIOVASCULAR. Blood pressure readings in both arms sitting, supine, and standing must be obtained. The client's blood pressure is measured in both arms 5 minutes after she has stood up from a supine position. A fall of 30 mmHg in the systolic blood pressure is significant for orthostatic hypotension. Important parts of the exams to differentiate cardiac from noncardiac causes include heartrate and rhythm to detect arrhythmia, presence of bruit or murmur, character of peripheral pulses, presence of edema or adventitious lung sounds indicating congestive heart failure.

NEUROLOGICAL. Includes evaluation of gait, presence of nystagmus, assessment of cranial nerves, cerebellar function, mental and/or emotional status.

Diagnostic Tests

12-LEAD ECG. The single most important diagnostic test to differentiate cardiac from noncardiac causes of syncope is the 12-lead ECG. If the office ECG is normal and a cardiac cause is strongly suspected, ambulatory ECG (Holter monitoring), may be necessary.

ECHOCARDIOGRAM. If a murmur is auscultated and the syncopal event occurred with exertion, an echocardiogram may detect left ventricular outflow tract abnormality.

Carotid dopplers are indicated if a carotid bruit is detected.

Routine blood tests are usually not helpful unless anemia, hypoglycemia, or electrolyte abnormality is strongly suspected.

Head CTs are not helpful in diagnosis unless focal neurological findings are present; likewise electroencephalograms (EEG) are generally not diagnostic.

Differential Medical Diagnoses. Cardiac causes of syncope can be due to obstruction, ischemia, or arrhythmia. Clients with obstructive causes often report syncope with exertion. This occurs when cardiac output is fixed by aortic stenosis or hypertrophic obstructive cardiomyopathy. Pulmonary hypertension can also cause exertional syncope.

Bradyarrhythmias from complete heart block or other high grade atrioventricular block can present with syncope unrelated to posture. Sick sinus syndrome (characterized by sinus bradycardia and sinus pause that is preceded by supraventricular tachycardia) is suspected in the client who complains of palpitations just prior to the syncope.

Tachyarrhythmias, especially self-terminating ventricular tachycardia, are common in clients with coronary artery disease and reduced left ventricular function. It can be life threatening if the rhythm converts to ventricular fibrillation. Torsades de Pointes, an arrhythmia associated with prolongation of the QT interval, is a cause of syncope. It may result from certain medications such as antiarrhythmic agents, antidepressants; the interactions of common drugs such as terfenadine with erythromycin; from metabolic abnormalities (hypokalemia, hypomagnesemia, hypocalcemia); and drug use (cocaine, sympathomimetics).

Wolf-Parkinson-White syndrome, a supraventricular tachycardia, can be diagnosed by 12-lead ECG.

Ischemic events such as acute angina and infarct can present as syncope. The client may have not have had any preceding chest pain.

Consider cardiac origin of syncope in any client with organic heart disease, especially the elderly and in those with no premonitory symptoms who collapse abruptly.

Cerebrovascular disease causing temporary interruption of blood flow to the vertebral or basilar arteries is detected by neurological exam. Focal findings may include vertigo, cranial nerve abnormalities, and bilateral sensory motor abnormalities.

Noncardiac causes include vasovagal syncope, which is the most common type in healthy young women. It is often preceded by pain, fear, emotional stress. It may be accompanied by tonic clonic movements or muscle twitches and may be mistaken for seizures. Rapid recovery and lack of confusion or drowsiness differentiate it from seizure activity.

Situational syncope is also mediated by autonomic reflex mechanisms. Examples include cough, micturition, and defecation syncope.

Drug-related syncope can be caused by diuretics, antihypertensives, antiarrhythmics, cocaine or alcohol.

Clients with frequent syncopal episodes of unknown origin may have underlying psychiatric problems. (Sisson & Kramer, 1999).

Plan. Consult with physician for further diagnostic workup and referral of any client with cardiac or neurological causes of syncope.

Psychosocial Interventions. Reassurance is offered to the client with noncardiac, nonneurologic syncope. If an underlying psychiatric disorder is suspected, suggest referral for counseling.

Medication. The client who is referred to cardiology or neurology may be placed on a variety of medications, depending on the underlying etiology of the syncope. The practitioner should become familiar with these agents and provide medication teaching if needed. Be especially alert for interactions with other medications the client may be prescribed or take as over-the-counter remedies.

If the cause of the syncope is a result of medications the client was taking at the time of the event, adjustment in dosage or stopping the medication may be necessary.

Lifestyle Changes. If substance abuse is present, advise the client of the consequences of continued abuse and refer to appropriate drug treatment program. Recommend stress reduction measures. In the elderly or frail client who is at risk for recurrence, fall precautions are needed. Some clients may have to stop driving.

Follow-Up. Telephone or office follow-up in seven to ten days is recommended for those not scheduled for further workup. Alert them that recurrent syncope requires further diagnostic testing.

Seizures

A seizure is a paroxysmal, transient change in neurologic function caused by a disturbance in the electrical activity of the brain. Chronic, recurrent seizures are diagnosed as epilepsy. Seizures are classified as simple, complex partial, absence, and generalized tonic-clonic seizures. The seizure may entail a brief lapse of attention or a period of several minutes of loss of consciousness with abnormal movements.

Epidemiology. Epilepsy is usually diagnosed between 5 and 20 years of age but can start later in life as a result of trauma or disease. Epilepsy affects about 0.5 percent to 2 percent of the population of the United States (Kaplan, 1999). The incidence of seizures rises sharply in the older population, approaching 140 per 100,000 in persons aged 80 and up (Rowan, 1998).

Subjective Data. First ask the client whether she has ever been diagnosed with a seizure disorder and if she is still taking anticonvulsant medication. If the answer is no, then a detailed account of events or sensations that preceded and followed the seizure is key. A febrile illness, headache, or mental confusion suggest an acute infection. Headache with vomiting and a neurological deficit point to a tumor or an intracranial bleed. Recent heavy use of alcohol or barbiturates with sudden withdrawal can trigger seizures. It is also important to ask about prior history of head trauma, kidney disease, or cardio-vascular disease. Assess risk factors for human immunodeficiency virus (HIV). In the elderly patient, Alzheimer's disease may be a cause.

Some clients may have a prodrome or premonition of an impending seizure but memory of this may be lost in the postictal state.

Prodromal symptoms include headache, mood change, fatigue, and myoclonic jerking. These precede the seizure by several hours and are not considered part of the aura that immediately precedes the seizure.

If the seizure was witnessed, ask for a description. Partial seizures affect only part of the brain. Simple partial seizures may be characterized by focal motor symptoms such as convulsive jerking or altered sensation such as parasthesias or tingling that spread to other parts of the extremity or body. Consciousness is not impaired. Complex partial seizures are characterized by impairment of consciousness along with the symptoms and signs of simple seizures.

Generalized seizures involve the whole brain. Absence seizures have an abrupt onset of unresponsiveness to external stimuli that may be very brief. Typically, they begin in childhood. Myoclonic seizures are distinguished by single or multiple myoclonic jerks. Tonic-clonic seizures (grand mal) are characterized by sudden loss of consciousness, rigidity (tonic phase) lasting about a

minute followed by clonic jerking of the muscles lasting 2 to 3 minutes. Immediately after the seizure, the client may recover consciousness, fall asleep, or have another seizure. The postictal state is characterized by stupor or confusion. Often the client is incontinent during the seizure or may have suffered injury from a fall or from tongue biting (Kaplan, 1999).

Objective Data

Physical Examination. A complete neurological and cardiovascular exam may reveal no abnormalities, especially in younger women.

Note body temperature. Assess for nuchal rigidity.

Examine the skin for signs of alcohol or drug abuse (jaundice, needle marks). Subcutaneous nodules and cafe au lait spots may indicate the presence of neurofibromatosis.

Perform a complete cardiovascular examination to distinguish seizure from syncope. (See previous section on syncope.)

A thorough neurological examination may reveal focal neurological deficits that point to a space occupying lesion, such as tumor or abscess, chronic subdural hematoma, or to arteriovenous malformation. Assess mental status, especially in the elderly, for signs of Alzheimer's disease.

Diagnostic Tests. Diagnostic tests are selected on the basis of prior history and physical exam. Blood chemistries that measure liver and kidney function, blood glucose, and anticonvulsant medication levels may be indicated as well as a complete blood count. In high risk populations, an HIV test may be appropriate. If cardiovascular cause suspected, an ECG is needed to complete the workup.

Any woman with a new onset seizure needs an EEG and a CT scan with and without contrast or magnetic resonance image (MRI).

Differential Medical Diagnoses

- *Syncope.* See previous section on syncope.
- *Transient Ischemic Attacks.* These last longer than seizures and are accompanied by weakness or numbness, not by abnormal motor activity.
- *Migraine headache* can present with aura preceding the headache that can make it difficult to distinguish from partial seizures. There are also migraine equivalents, which may be characterized by hemiparesis, numbness, and/or aphasia without headache. Usually the symptoms and signs develop more slowly (over several minutes) and the time factor helps distinguish from seizure activity.

◆ *Panic Attacks.* These may be harder to distinguish from absence or simple seizures but psychiatric history may provide clues.

◆ *Orthostatic Syncope.* Usually occurs after a change in posture, lasts a few seconds, and is followed by prompt recovery as opposed to postictal confusion.

◆ *Pseudoseizures.* May be hysterical conversion reaction or malingering. They are usually neither preceded by a tonic phase nor followed by postictal behavior. The EEG is usually normal.

◆ *Generalized Tonic-Clonic Seizures.* May occur 48 hours after withdrawal from alcohol in the client with a history of chronic or high intake. Treatment with anticonvulsants is generally not required unless status epilepticus occurs. As long as the client abstains from alcohol, seizure should not recur.

Plan

Referral. Refer to a physician any client who is suspected to have had a seizure. MRI, CT scan, and/or EEG may be ordered before referral to a neurologist. If the underlying cause is infection, admission to the hospital may be indicated. If the underlying etiology is cardiovascular, refer to a cardiologist for further workup. The client with an alcohol withdrawal seizure should be referred for detoxification and rehabilitation.

Medication. Anticonvulsant medication is selected by the neurologist, based on the type of seizure. Once stabilized on a dose, she usually returns to the care of the primary care provider.

The practitioner should be familiar with the more commonly prescribed anticonvulsant medications discussed subsequently. For more complete information, consult a pharmacology reference.

The drugs of choice for simple and complex partial and tonic-clonic seizures are phenytoin and carbemazeine.

PHENYTOIN. 300 to 400 mg po per day as single dose or divided t.i.d.

◆ *Administration.* It takes five to ten days to reach a state drug level. Client may be admitted to the hospital for loading until a steady state is achieved and seizures are controlled. Optimum serum drug level is 10 to 20 mcg/ml.

◆ *Adverse Effects.* Gingival hyperplasia, hirsutism, skin rash, ataxia, slurred speech, nystagmus, hypotension, nausea, vomiting, hepatic toxicity, and blood dyscrasias.

Toxicity signs include drowsiness, nausea, vomiting, nystagmus, slurred speech, ataxia, and tremors.

Overdose can be lethal due to respiratory and circulatory collapse.

◆ *Contraindications.* Known hypersensitivity, sinus bradycardia, and heart block. Use with caution in hepatic, renal dysfunction, and in the elderly.

Phenytoin has potentially serious interactions with many other medications. Consult a pharmacology reference for further information.

◆ *Client Teaching.* Emphasize adherence to prescribed doses of medication, signs of toxicity, interactions with other medications and over-the-counter drugs. Advise client not to drink alcohol while taking medication; it will decrease effectiveness and may increase adverse CNS effects. Advise client on oral contraceptives that phenytoin may decrease contraceptive effects, and discuss alternative methods. Medication should be taken with food to minimize GI effects. Encourage client to wear Medic Alert tag.

CARBAMAZEPINE. 600 to 1,200 mg po in divided doses (usually twice a day).

◆ *Administration.* Steady state levels achieved in three to four days. Therapeutic range is 4 to 12 mcg/ml in serum.

◆ *Adverse Effects.* Diplopia, nystagmus, dysarthria, ataxia, drowsiness, nausea, blood dyscrasias, hepatotoxicity.

Signs of toxicity include impaired breathing, respiratory depression, tachycardia, shock, arrhythmias, impaired consciousness, psychomotor disturbances, nausea, vomiting, oliguria, or anuria.

◆ *Contraindications.* Known hypersensitivity to carbamazepine and to tricyclic antidepressants; past or present history of bone marrow depression; use of monoamine oxidase inhibitors within the last fourteen days (can cause hypertensive crisis). Use with caution if hepatic, cardiac, or renal dysfunction; increased intraocular pressure; elderly (may cause agitation, confusion, activate latent psychosis).

Consult pharmacology reference for interactions with other medications.

◆ *Client Teaching.* See discussion of phenytoin.

VALPROIC ACID. For absence seizures, myoclonic seizures, and certain tonic-clonic seizures.

◆ *Administration.* Usual dose is 750 to 1,250 mg in three doses. It takes two to four days to reach the steady state. Therapeutic range is 50 to 100 mcg/ml.

- *Adverse Effects.* Weight gain, hair loss, tremor, drowsiness, nausea, vomiting, diarrhea, hepatic toxicity, thrombocytopenia. Toxicity is indicated by somnolence and coma.
- *Contraindications.* Known hypersensitivity and hepatic dysfunction. Use with caution in clients on anticoagulants.
- *Interactions.* Valproic acid may potentiate the effects of monoamine oxidase inhibitors, anti-depressants, and anticoagulants. May cause absence seizures if used with clonazepam.
- *Client Teaching.* Teach client importance of taking as prescribed. Advise client of adverse effects. Take with food to minimize GI effects. Swallow—do not chew—to avoid mucosal irritation and unpleasant taste. Encourage client to wear Medic Alert tag.

Newer anticonvulsants such as felbamate, gamapentin, and lamotrigine are approved for adjunctive therapy for partial and secondarily generalized seizures. Some neurologists are using gabapentin and lamotrigine as first-line medications in older adults because of fewer side effects and medication interactions than the older AEDs (Rowan, 1998). Consult a pharmacology text for further information.

Diet/Lifestyle. The client with well-controlled seizure disorder is capable of leading a normal life, including work, school, and driving (depending on state laws). She should be counseled regarding the importance of healthy eating and rest patterns to maintain optimal health. Confront possible alcohol and illicit drug use openly and advise client of risks. Preconception counseling and consultation with the neurologist before pregnancy is advisable.

Follow-Up. For the person with an isolated seizure and no further workup scheduled, telephone follow-up in seven days is suggested. Follow-up office visit in three months is warranted as well as immediate follow-up should the seizure recur. Telephone follow-up is advised after client is seen by neurologist or other specialist to become familiar with treatment plan. Request written plan from consultant.

PARKINSONISM AND ESSENTIAL TREMOR

Tremor is a purposeless, rhythmic movement resulting from the involuntary alternating contraction and relaxation of opposing groups of skeletal muscles. Essential or familial tremor is usually inherited and has no other associated features. Parkinsonism is a movement disorder characterized by tremor, rigidity, and bradykinesia. It is slowly progressive and caused by an imbalance of the neurotransmitters dopamine and acetylcholine.

Epidemiology

Essential tremor and Parkinsonism are common disorders. Familial essential tremor is often inherited in an autosomal dominant pattern. It can appear at any age. Parkinsonism affects 1 in 100 adults over 50 years of age. It can be found in equal numbers of males and females and occurs in all ethnic groups (Olanow, Watts, & Koller, 2001).

Subjective Data

Important questions to ask the client: What parts of the body are involved? Does the tremor occur with movement (intentional tremor) or at rest? Does the tremor only affect one side of the body or is it symmetrical? Does any other member of the family have a similar disorder? Does emotional stress make the tremor worse and does alcohol make it less noticeable? Are there any other associated complaints such as hoarseness, dysphagia, drooling, depression, nightmares, slowed movement, problems cutting food, turning in bed, and buttoning clothing? Do you use caffeine, stimulant drugs, drink alcohol, take theophylline, anticonvulsants?

Objective Data

Physical Examination. A complete neurological exam is performed, including assessment for cognitive impairment.

Begin with observation of the client's gait, posture, and facial expression. The client with Parkinson's disease takes small, shuffling steps, with little swinging of the arms. The posture is stooped. She may have difficulty stopping and turning around. The facial expression may be fixed with little blinking. Examine the skin for signs of seborrhea of the scalp and face (common in Parkinson's disease).

Examine the mouth and lips for tremor and drooling.

Assess the extremities for strength and deep tendon reflexes. There is usually no weakness and no alteration of deep tendon reflexes.

Observe the tremor. The benign essential tremor will involve one or both hands and/or the head. It persists at rest but worsens with use of the affected hand. No other abnormalities are noted during the exam.

The tremor of Parkinson's disease often becomes less apparent with activity. In early disease, it is confined to one limb or one side of the body. Emotional stress may exacerbate it.

Assess for rigidity. The client with Parkinsonism exhibits increased resistance to passive movement. She may have difficulty arising from a sitting position.

Assessment of cognitive function may be incorporated into the rest of the exam. If deficits are found, more in depth testing may be needed such as the Folstein Mini-Mental Status Examination. (See Table 22–8).

Diagnostic Tests. Selected on basis of examination findings but may include rapid plasma reagent (RPR), vitamin B-12 and folate levels, complete blood count (CBC), blood chemistries for electrolyte levels and liver function, thyroid stimulating hormone (TSH).

Differential Medical Diagnoses

Huntington's disease involves rigidity and bradykinesia but is distinguished by choreic movements, which are irregular and jerky, as opposed to tremor, which is rhythmic. It is an inherited disease.

Depression may present with expressionless face and slowed movement. It can be difficult to distinguish from early Parkinson's disease and may coexist at the time of diagnosis.

Progressive supranuclear palsy (PSP) and multiple system atrophy (MSA) appear clinically similar to PD.

PSP can be differentiated from PD by the woman's inability to move her eyes in vertical planes, especially downward. Clients with consistent orthostatic hypotension that cannot be attributed to other causes (e.g., dehydration, medications) may have MSA (Olanow et al., 2001).

Plan

Consult with the physician if Parkinsonism is suspected. Initial management may be at the primary care level.

Psychosocial Interventions. Reassure the client with essential tremor that though the tremor may become progressively worse with age, no other functional abnormalities are associated with this disorder. Provide emotional support to the client and her family affected with Parkinsonism. This is a progressive, debilitating illness. Not only does it affect motor function, 15 to 30 percent of clients develop dementia (Kaye, 1998). Anticipatory guidance is key to the plan. Refer family to support and information groups, such as the Parkinson's Disease Foundation, the National Parkinson's Foundation, the American Parkinson's Disease Association, Inc.

Medication. Essential tremor is treated with propranolol starting dose 60 mg po titrating up for effect to maximum dose of 240 mg. See previous discussion of beta blockers in section on hypertension.

Pharmacologic intervention for Parkinsonism is based on restoring dopaminergic function through the use

TABLE 22–8. Folstein Mini-Mental State Examination

Maximum Score	Client Score	Questions
5		"What is the (year) (season) (date) (day) (month)?"
5		"Where are we?" Name of (state) (county) (city or town) (place, such as hospital or clinic) (specific location, such as floor or room).
3		The examiner names three unrelated objects clearly and slowly, then asks the client to name all three of them. The client's response is used for scoring. The examiner repeats them until client learns all of them if possible.
5		"Begin with 100 and count backwards by subtracting 7." Stop at 65 (5 responses).
3		If the client learned the three objects above, ask her to recall them now.
2		The examiner shows the client two simple objects, such as a wrist watch and pencil, and asks her to name them.
1		"Repeat the phrase, 'No ifs, and, or buts.' "
3		The examiner gives the client a piece of blank paper and asks her to follow the three-step command: "Take the paper in your right hand, fold it in half, and put it on the floor."
1		On a blank piece of paper, the examiner prints the command "Close your eyes," in letters large enough for the client to see clearly, then asks her to read it and follow the command.
1		"Make up and write a sentence about anything." This sentence must contain a noun and a verb.
1		The examiner gives the client a blank piece of paper and asks her to draw a symbol (two interlocking pentagons). All 10 angles must be present and 2 must intersect.
Total Possible = 30	Client's Total =	(If total score is 23 or below, further evaluation may be indicated)

Source: Folstein, Folstein, & McHugh (1995).

of levodopa (which is metabolized to dopamine) combined with carbodopa (a dopa-decarboxylase inhibitor), which inhibits levodopa metabolism outside the brain (Olanow et al., 2001).

Current management guidelines offered by neurologists suggest using dopamine agonists such as ropinirole, pramipexole, and cabergoline as first-line therapy for clients less than age 70 with PD (Olanow et al., 2001). Clients treated with levodopa for seven to ten years develop complications such as dyskinesias and treatment fluctuations (periods of motor control ["on"] and periods of motor inhibition ["off"]). Early treatment with dopamine agonists delay the need for levodopa, and these agonists may have neuroprotective functions (Jankovic, 2000). Refer to a pharmacology text for further discussion and current research on these medications.

Parkinsonism Medication

CARBODOPA-LEVODOPA (SINEMET OR SINEMET CR)

- ◆ *Administration.* Available in several dosage combinations and as an immediate release and a controlled release form. Consult with physician regarding preferred form. Dosage will depend on stage of disease and diurnal progression of symptoms. See pharmacology text for further discussion on adjusting dosage.
- ◆ *Adverse Effects.* Worsening of Parkinsonism symptoms, dyskinesias, cardiac rhythm irregularities, orthostatic hypotension, spasm or closing of eyelids, severe nausea and vomiting. In clients with dementia, may cause hallucinations and psychosis.
- ◆ *Contraindications.* Known hypersensitivity, asthma, emphysema, severe cardiovascular disease, narrow-angle glaucoma, malignant melanoma, history of myocardial infarction.
- ◆ *Expected Outcome.* Improvement in ability to perform activities of daily living.
- ◆ *Client Teaching.* Adverse effects, signs of toxicity (muscle twitching and blepharospasm are early signs).

Selegiline, a monamine oxidase-B inhibitor, has been tested for potential neuroprotective properties. Some neurologists advocate the use of selegiline prior to treatment with levodopa (Olanow et al., 2001). Researchers have found that selegiline improves the symptoms of PD initially and may initially delay the need for levodopa therapy. This drug, however, does not slow or prevent the development of levodopa complications once levodopa is begun (Jankovic, 2000). Refer to a pharmacology text for further information.

Other medications may be added based on associated symptoms and progression of disease. These are best initiated in consultation with neurologist.

Lifestyle/Diet. Clients with essential tremor should be advised to avoid self-medication with alcohol. If tremor is not well controlled with medication, client may have problems with handwriting and other manual skills. Be sensitive to impact on social and professional life.

Help with activities of daily living in the form of assistive devices may help client with Parkinsonism maintain independence. These measures may include rails and banisters in the home, eating utensils with large handles, nonskid mats for table and bath, communication devices to enhance speech. Client may need special texturized diet if swallowing difficulties are present.

Occupational and physical therapy referrals may be appropriate.

Follow-Up

The client diagnosed with essential tremor should be seen in two weeks for response to medication and possible adjustment of dosage.

Client with Parkinsonism should be seen within two to three days of initiation of carbodopalevodopa to assess response and to observe for toxicity. If referred to neurology, request copy of plan. Continue to provide primary care services.

DEMENTIA/ALZHEIMER'S DISEASE

Dementia is a progressive organic mental disorder with characteristic behaviors and cognitive decline. The hallmark is short-term memory loss, but associated features may include impaired judgment, impaired abstract thinking, language or motor function disturbance, and/or personality change. It must be distinguished from delirium or acute confusional state, which are usually reversible when the underlying cause is corrected. A major irreversible cause of primary dementia in the elderly is Alzheimer's disease. Other causes of dementia are listed in Table 22–9.

Epidemiology

Dementia affects one in ten U.S. adults over the age of 65. It is probably the most feared problem of aging. Alzheimer's accounts for 60 percent to 70 percent of irreversible dementia. It is age related, has an insidious onset, and may follow a familial pattern. Recent studies indicate that women who take estrogen long after menopause (a

TABLE 22–9. Causes of Dementia

Probably Irreversible Causes
Alzheimer's disease
Multi-infarct dementia
Alcohol
Parkinson's disease
Huntington's disease
Mixed (Alzheimer's and multiinfarct)
Trauma
Anoxia

Potentially Reversible Causes
Depression
Normal-pressure hydrocephalus
Drugs
Neoplasm
Metabolic
Infections
Subdural hematoma

Source: Friedland & Wilcock (2000); Rockwood (2000).

decade or more) may be less likely to develop Alzheimer's disease (Friedland & Wilcock, 2000; Hebert, Beckett, Scherr, & Evans, 2001).

Multi-infarct dementia accounts for 15 to 20 percent of dementias, is more common in men, and is associated with hypertension and transient ischemic attacks (TIAs). According to recent studies, about 11 percent of dementias are reversible or partially reversible. The clients more likely to have a reversible dementia are those with recent acute onset, rapid deterioration, atypical presentation, multiple drug use or polypharmacy, history of depression, and onset younger than 60 to 70 years old (Friedland & Wilcock, 2000; Rockwood, 2000).

Subjective Data

The first symptom noted is forgetfulness or loss of short-term memory. This must be distinguished from the benign senescent forgetfulness that sometimes accompanies aging and from depression. Progression of symptoms differentiates benign senescent forgetfulness from the short-term memory loss of Alzheimer's. The family may begin to note increasing difficulty with daily activities such as balancing the checkbook, dressing appropriately, cooking. The client may have some loss of expressive and comprehensive language including word finding difficulty. She may have undergone a personality change, becoming more irritable and impatient; she may be paranoid

in her thinking at times. At this point, the family may bring the client in for evaluation. The client herself may have no specific complaint but may become agitated when asked simple questions that she is unable to answer. It is important to review prescription and nonprescription medications taken and alcohol intake.

Objective Data

Physical Examination

- *General Appearance.* Begin with careful observation of the client, paying special attention to gait, affect and facial expression, initiation or fluency of speech. Physical appearance may resemble Parkinsonism with stooped gait, mask-like face, and slowed movement.
- A *complete cardiovascular exam* focuses on blood pressure and the presence of carotid bruits.
- The *neurological exam* focuses on motor, sensory, hearing, vision, cranial nerves, tremor, reflexes, and cerebellar function.

The client in the early stages of Alzheimer's may have an essentially normal exam up to this point.

Diagnostic Tests. A Folstein or other Standard Mini-Mental Test (see Table 22–8) to assess cognitive function will aid in the diagnosis, but be aware that educational and cultural differences may make scoring difficult.

Standard lab tests to order include CBC, B_{12} and folate, thyroid function, biochemical profile. Consider an RPR or HIV test if high risk for syphilis or acquired immunodeficiency syndrome (AIDS) dementia.

Order CT or MRI if tumor, subdural hematoma, stroke, hydrocephalus, or multi-infarct dementia is suspected. There is no imaging modality available to definitively diagnose Alzheimer's disease.

Differential Medical Diagnoses

The client with normal pressure hydrocephalus may have gait disturbance (broad-based stance) and incontinence.

Creutzfeldt-Jacob disease is a rare, rapidly progressive fatal neurological disease characterized by behavior change, myoclonus, and rigidity.

Parkinson's disease may manifest with early symptoms of dementia when neuromuscular features are not prominent.

Huntington's disease is diagnosed on basis of family history and the accompanying movement disorder. Onset is 20 to 50 years of age.

Korsakoff's syndrome due to chronic alcohol use involves memory loss and some impairment of cognitive function. It is associated with thiamine deficiency and has a sudden onset.

Tumor, multi-infarct, subdural hematoma are differentiated on the basis of the imaging modality used.

Plan

Psychosocial Interventions. The practitioner must approach the client and her family with tact and understanding. First, the diagnosis must be made clear. The practitioner should emphasize that maintaining optimal health status for the client will improve the quality of life for both family and client. The practitioner should provide the client and family with resources to help educate them about AD; the Alzheimer's Association [www.alz.org, (800) 272-3900] is a good place to start. The practitioner will need to convey to the family/caregivers the importance of establishing proxy decision makers for future financial and health concerns. It is usually easier to enlist the client's cooperation during the early stages of AD than in later stages, when paranoia may prove to be an obstacle. Attorneys, financial planners, and other professionals are good resources for help in managing her affairs.

Family members may be overwhelmed with the task of caring for a person with dementia. At every visit, take time to talk to caregivers and be alert for caregiver stress or possible elder abuse. Reiterate the importance of maintaining a safe environment. A bracelet with the client's name, address, and phone number is a must especially if she wanders off. Attempts to keep the client oriented, such as repeatedly telling the client, "No, you are not in your house, you are living with me now," may only serve to increase agitation. Refer family members to respite services; respite services range from a few hours during an afternoon to entire weekends. Some nursing homes and assisted living facilities offer varying degrees of respite and adult day programs for cognitively impaired elders.

Medication

Donepezil HCL (Aricept)

- *Mechanism of Action.* Cholinesterase inhibitor that has shown some benefit in enhancing cognitive function in those with mild to moderate Alzheimer's.
- *Administration.* Starting dose is 5 mg once a day in the evening. May increase to 10 mg each evening after four to six weeks of therapy.
- *Adverse Effects.* Nausea, vomiting, diarrhea, muscle cramps, fatigue, anorexia, insomnia.

- *Contraindications.* Known sensitivity to donepezil or piperidine derivative. Cautious use if other serious medical conditions such as sick sinus syndrome, ulcers, asthma, urinary or intestinal obstruction.

Tacrine (THA)

- *Mechanism of Action.* A centrally acting anticholinesterase inhibitor may improve cognition in early Alzheimer's.
- *Administration.* Starting dose 10 mg q.i.d. (taken between meals if tolerated). Increase in 40 mg/d increments no sooner than every six weeks to maximum dose 160 mg/d.
- *Adverse Effects.* May cause hepatic failure (dose-related), vomiting, diarrhea, agitation, confusion, dizziness, insomnia, somnolence, hallucinations, purpura.
- *Contraindications.* Hepatic disease, inability to adhere to weekly monitoring of liver function. Cautious use if other serious medical conditions such as sick sinus syndrome, ulcers, asthma, urinary or intestinal obstruction.
- *Expected Outcome.* May improve cognitive function in early disease.
- *Client/Family Teaching.* Prepare client and family that they may see no improvement. Only about one-third of clients respond. Very expensive. Must have liver function test levels drawn every week for first eighteen weeks of therapy, then every three months. Must have weekly levels when dose increased. Advise family to monitor urine output (may cause outflow obstruction). Advise family abrupt discontinuation can cause acute degeneration of cognitive function.

Antidepressants, such as secondary amine *tricyclic antidepressants* (nortriptyline and desipramine) or one of the selective serotonin reuptake inhibitors, may improve quality of life significantly in early disease. See chapter on Psychosocial Health Concerns for further information on these medications.

Diet/Lifestyle. A healthy and varied diet, adequate rest, maintenance of regular elimination, and skin hygiene are vitally important areas for the client, especially when she is unable to provide these for herself. Advise family to avoid using antihistamines for sleep problems. These medications have a high potential to cause confusion. Instead suggest limiting chocolate, colas, tea, and coffee that contain caffeine. Providing a safe environment is key as well as including client in family or community activities as much as possible.

Follow-Up

Once the diagnosis is made, a follow-up visit in two weeks is suggested to ascertain how the client and her family are adjusting to the diagnosis. Consult with physician if signs of psychosis appear or if increasing agitation and behavioral disturbances. Regularly scheduled visits every three months or more often based on the client's status (Friedland & Wilcock, 2000).

OPHTHALMOLOGICAL DISORDERS

CONJUNCTIVITIS

The most common eye problem encountered in primary care is a red eye. The redness is caused by injection of the conjunctival, episcleral, or ciliary blood vessels. In evaluating the client, it is important to remember that common problems are common; that is, that conjunctivitis caused by a virus, bacteria, or allergen is usually the diagnosis. It is imperative, however, to rule out other more serious disorders. As always, a good history and physical exam are keys to diagnosis.

Epidemiology

Several species of bacteria normally colonize the conjunctival sac, most commonly *Staphylococcus albus* and *aureus, Corynebacterium,* and *Streptococcus.* Acute bacterial conjunctivitis may be caused by an overgrowth of *Staphylococcus aureus.* It may also be caused by pneumococcal infection, especially in colder weather, and by *Haemophilus* in warmer regions of the United States. In younger individuals, *Haemophilus* is more often the causative organism than *Staphylococcus aureus.* Other bacteria implicated in acute conjunctivitis include *Neisseria gonorrhoeae, Neisseria meningitidis, Escherichia coli,* and *Proteus* species. Chronic bacterial conjunctivitis is usually caused by *Staphylococcus aureus* or *epidermidis* or by *Streptococcus pyogenes.* It is often associated with blepharitis.

Sexually active young adults are at risk for inclusion conjunctivitis caused by *Chlamydia* contamination of the eye after sexual contact and at risk for the hyperacute conjunctivitis caused by *Neisseria gonorrhoeae.* Alcoholics and other individuals with nutritional deficiencies are at risk for all types of infectious conjunctivitis.

Viruses are the causative organism in most cases of infectious conjunctivitis. Most commonly implicated are the adenoviruses. A more serious form of viral keratoconjunctivitis is caused by the Herpes simplex virus that may spread to the eye after contact with genital lesions. Herpes zoster may also spread to the eye (Schachat, 1999c).

Seasonal conjunctivitis is a recurrent, transient, and self-limiting allergic conjunctivitis associated with a particular time of year and allergen (Quinn, Mathews, Noyes, et al., 1999). Vernal conjunctivitis, on the other hand, is a much more severe inflammation associated with dry, warm climates. It is more in young males (< 20 years of age) of African descent and usually lasts four years. It may exhibit a seasonal pattern in more temperate climates (Quinn et al., 1999).

Subjective Data

Important questions to ask:

Do you wear contact lenses? Contact lens wearers are at higher risk for infectious conjunctivitis, especially bacterial. Often they continue to wear the lens and are at risk for infection by anaerobes and for corneal ulceration.

When did the redness first appear? Which eye? The onset of viral and acute bacterial conjunctivitis as well as inclusion conjunctivitis is abrupt, often affecting one eye and after several days spreading to the other eye by autoinoculation. Irritant conjunctivitis follows contact with a trigger such as a chemical.

Is there any change or loss of vision? Blurred vision may occur with inclusion conjunctivitis. Epidemic keratoconjunctivitis caused by several *adenovirus* types may be associated with formation of a pseudomembrane that reduces vision. *Herpes* infection of the eye may also cause decreased visual acuity especially if not treated promptly.

Any discharge? Copious, thick exudate is the hallmark of gonococcal conjunctivitis. Mucopurulent to mucoid discharge accompanies other forms of infectious conjunctivitis. Allergic conjunctivitis causes tearing.

Any pain? Foreign body sensation? Pruritis? Gonococcal conjunctivitis is accompanied by discomfort, swelling of the eyelid, and tenderness. Chronic bacterial conjunctivitis and *Herpes* virus keratoconjunctivitis may cause a foreign body sensation. If treatment of *Chlamydial* conjunctivitis is delayed, iritis may develop resulting in photophobia. Allergic conjunctivitis is characterized by often intense pruritis.

Previous eye injury, head trauma, infection, or surgery? Viral conjunctivitis often follows an upper respiratory infection. Previous eye surgery may put client at risk for bacterial conjunctivitis. Eye injury puts client at risk for subsequent iritis and corneal abrasion (which must be differentiated from the red eye of conjunctivitis).

Any contact with infected genital secretions? Always retain high suspicion of sexually transmitted etiology of conjunctivitis in sexually active client. *Gonococcal, Chlamydial,* and *Herpes* virus conjunctivitis require prompt diagnosis and referral to an ophthalmologist to prevent serious consequences including loss of vision.

Any chronic disease? Medications taken routinely? Immunocompromised individuals are at higher risk for infectious conjunctivitis. Clients with psoriasis or seborrhea are more prone to chronic conjunctivitis. Conditions associated with increased risk of iritis include Herpes zoster, Herpes simplex infections, Lyme disease, tuberculosis, syphilis, and autoimmune disease such as inflammatory bowel disease and sarcoidosis.

Any association with occupation or hobby? Welders who do not wear protective eyeglasses are at risk for a punctate keratitis (arc welder's eye), which presents with redness and photophobia. Irritant or allergic conjunctivitis may follow accidental exposure to chemical used in a hobby or craft.

Any family member with similar problem? Viral conjunctivitis is highly contagious.

Objective Data

Physical Examination. Appearance of the eye and lids. Conjunctival (bulbar and palpebral) injection is the hallmark of conjunctivitis. Lids may be very swollen in gonococcal conjunctivitis, erythematous in chronic bacterial conjunctivitis with crusting at the base of the eyelash (see Table 22–10).

Chlamydial inclusion conjunctivitis produces follicles on the palpebral conjunctiva, especially on the lower lid. Marked swelling of the conjunctiva occurs in allergic conjunctivitis. Examine for exudate. The exudate of gonococcal conjunctivitis is thick, copious and accumulates in the lashes. Acute bacterial conjunctivitis is characterized by thinner mucopurulent discharge. The exudate of viral and allergic conjunctivitis is watery.

Compare pupils for equality of size, important in differentiating conjunctivitis from iritis and glaucoma. Conjunctivitis causes no inequality. In iritis, pupil is small and unequal.

Examine for swelling of preauricular nodes present in viral conjunctivitis, including Herpes keratoconjunctivitis.

Evert eyelid to examine for foreign body that may have triggered injection of the conjunctiva.

Evaluate extraocular movements, test pupillary reaction, visual fields.

Direct ophthalmoscopy of fundus and disc. Flashlight examination of anterior chamber.

Diagnostic Tests

Visual Acuity. It is imperative to assess visual acuity. If this is not done, a serious mistake in diagnosis may occur, placing the practitioner at risk for negligence. If the client has forgotten or lost her corrective lenses, a pinhole disk may be used to optimize acuity.

Client with chemical conjunctivitis caused by acid or alkali needs pH measurement of conjunctival secretion after initial irrigation with large amounts (one to two liters) of normal saline or water. If pH is less than or greater than 6.8 to 7.0, continue to irrigate to prevent permanent damage and refer immediately to the ophthalmologist.

TABLE 22–10. Objective Findings in Conjunctivitis

	Viral	Bacterial	Chlamydia	Allergic
Exudate	Serous	Copious mucopurulent or mucoid NOTE: Gonococcal conjunctivitis drainage is copious and purulent	Thin, serous	Watery profuse
Unilateral vs. Bilateral	Bilateral NOTE: HSV unilateral	Unilateral	Often unilateral	Bilateral
Associated Features	Enlarged preauricular nodes Pharyngitis Abrupt onset Palpebral conjunctiva injected HSV: Dendritic pattern if fluorescein stained	Blepharitis Hordeolum Eyelids stuck together	Urethritis Prominent follicles upper and lower lids Nontender preauricular node May have mild keratitis	Asthma Atopy Itchy eyes Swollen eyelids Chemosis (edema) of cornea and conjunctiva

HSV: Herpes Simplex Virus

Source: Quinn et al., (1999); Schachat, (1999a, 1999c).

Fluorescein Staining. Fluorescein staining of conjunctiva and examination by slit lamp or Wood's Lamp for epithelial staining defect if corneal injury suspected. Fluorescein staining assists in the diagnosis of Herpes keratoconjunctivitis, which has a characteristic dendritic appearance.

If gonococcal or Chlamydial is infection suspected, confirmation by stained smear and culture is needed. Prompt diagnosis and treatment prevent blindness.

Acute bacterial conjunctivitis and chronic conjunctivitis are usually diagnosed by examination and history; however, if there is doubt about the causative organism a culture and sensitivity should be obtained.

Differential Medical Diagnoses

Iritis presents with intense photophobia, redness localized around the cornea, and smaller unequal pupil of the affected eye (see Table 22–11).

Acute angle closure glaucoma causes diminished vision, hazy or steamy cornea, dilated unequal pupil in the affected eye, with redness around the cornea.

Scleritis, an inflammatory condition of the deeper vessels of the sclera, is characterized by pain, no exudate, and a localized redness, often most intense in the superior globe of the eye.

Corneal abrasion and foreign body are diagnosed by history, foreign body sensation, and epithelial staining defect on staining and slit lamp or Wood's Lamp examination.

Plan

The client with acute angle closure glaucoma, foreign body that has penetrated the cornea or is not removed by irrigation, iritis, scleritis, or keratoconjunctivitis caused by Herpes virus or arc welding is referred immediately to an ophthalmologist.

Psychosocial Interventions. Reassure client eye tissue heals very quickly; with adherence to treatment regimen, good outcome is expected. Client may be sensitive about appearance, especially if exudate present. She should avoid mascara and eyeliner until conjunctivitis resolved. She may need a work excuse if she works in health care setting, food service, or child care. If conjunctivitis is due to sexually transmitted disease, advise client that partner(s) need treatment.

Medication

Viral Conjunctivitis

NORMAL SALINE EYE DROPS

- *Administration.* Two drops each eye every 2 to 3 hours for as long as needed.
- *Side Effects.* May experience transient stinging of eyes.
- *Contraindication.* None.
- *Expected Outcome.* Advise the client it may take seven to ten days before conjunctiva clear.

NOTE: Ophthalmologists recommend that antibiotic eye drops not be used for the treatment of viral conjunctivitis due to the potential for allergic response. Agents such as sodium sulfacetamide and erythromycin have low potential; gentamicin, neomycin, and tobramycin have high potential. If it is difficult to distinguish whether conjunctivitis is due to virus or bacteria. If client is at risk for bacterial superinfection, treat with low potential agent and evaluate after three to five days for response.

Allergic Conjunctivitis

NAPHAZOLINE HYDROCHLORIDE. Ophthalmic solution 0.1 percent.

- *Administration.* Instill 1 to 2 drops each eye every three to four hours for relief of itching and redness.

TABLE 22–11. Differential Diagnoses of Red Eye

	Conjunctivitis	Corneal Abrasion	Iritis	Acute Glaucoma
Signs and Symptoms				
Pain	Mild	Moderate to severe	Moderate to severe	Severe (often with nausea and vomiting)
Foreign Body Sensation	Mild	Moderate to severe	None	None
Vision	Normal	Blurred	Blurred with photophobia	Greatly reduced
Pupil Size	Normal	Normal	Small and fixed in affected eye	Dilated
Other Information	May follow upper respiratory infection	Hx important for foreign body, abrasion, contact lens wear, use of arc welding equipment	"Ciliary flush" redness from iritis extends into cornea. Urgent referral to opthalmologist needed.	Anterior chamber shallow

Source: Quinn et al. (1999); Schachat, (1999b, 1999c).

♦ *Adverse Effects.* Transient stinging, pupillary dilation, hyperemia, increased or decreased intraocular pressure.

♦ *Contraindications.* Sensitivity to ingredients, history of glaucoma.

♦ *Expected Outcome.* May be recurrent problem, but medication should relieve symptoms.

♦ *Client Teaching.* Advise client to report blurred vision, eye pain, lid swelling and discontinue use if occurs. Use of cool compresses as needed for added comfort. May add oral antihistamine such as Benadryl if severe itching.

Chemical Conjunctivitis. Cool compresses for 15 to 20 minutes several times a day and use of topical vasoconstrictor solution such as naphazoline hydrochloride solution (see prior information).

NOTE: If chemical trigger is acid or alkali, immediately irrigate eye with normal saline or water, measure pH. When neutral pH achieved, examine fluorescein-stained eye with slit lamp and/or refer to physician.

Acute Bacterial Conjunctivitis

SODIUM SULFACETAMIDE. (Sulamyd—10 percent) solution.

♦ *Administration.* Two drops in the eye every 3 hours while awake for five to seven days.

♦ *Adverse Effects.* Blurred vision, transient burning and stinging. Hypersensitivity, intense itching and/or burning.

♦ *Contraindication.* Known sensitivity to sulfonamides.

♦ *Expected Outcome.* Symptoms usually resolve in a couple of days.

♦ *Client Teaching.* Advise client not to let dropper touch eye, remove exudate with warm, clean cloth before instilling drops. Teach signs/symptoms of sensitivity and advise client to discontinue use immediately and call practitioner if sensitivity develops. Wait 10 minutes before using another eye preparation.

Hyperacute Bacterial Conjunctivitis. Hyperacute bacterial conjunctivitis due to *Neisseria gonorrhoeae* must be referred to ophthalmologist for topical and systemic antibiotic therapy to prevent corneal damage and systemic spread.

NOTE: If client allergic to sulfonamides, erythromycin ophthalmic ointment may be used four times a day for the same duration of time. See following for adverse effects and client teaching.

Chronic Bacterial Conjunctivitis

ERYTHROMYCIN OPHTHALMIC OINTMENT

♦ *Administration.* Apply to lower lid inner canthus to outer canthus four times a day for at least two weeks.

♦ *Adverse Effects.* Blurred vision, transient burning and stinging.

♦ *Contraindication.* Known sensitivity to erythromycin.

♦ *Expected Outcome.* Reduces bacterial count but may recur.

♦ *Client Teaching.* Advise client to clean eyelashes with neutral soap such as baby shampoo (see Blepharitis for details) before applying ointment. Advise client scrupulous hygiene may help prevent recurrence.

Inclusion Conjunctivitis (Chlamydial Conjunctivitis). Requires referral to ophthalmologist for systemic therapy and confirmation of diagnosis. If there is any doubt about the diagnosis, refer. Sexually active women may have no associated symptoms, such as vaginal discharge. Diagnosis is based on suspicion, prominent follicles on lower palpebral conjunctival sac, and confirmation by Giemsa-stained conjunctival scraping. Treatment is with Doxycycline 100 mg twice a day for three to five weeks.

Lifestyle. Clients with infectious conjunctivitis should avoid spread by not sharing towels, washcloths, makeup. Advise client to discard any eye makeup used at time of onset of symptoms.

Frequent handwashing is emphasized, and always after touching eyes. May not return to work until exudate resolved if employed in health care, child care, or food service.

Clients with allergic conjunctivitis should try to determine trigger(s) and avoid as much as possible.

If conjunctivitis is associated with sexually transmitted disease, advise client on other risks of unprotected sex such as pelvic inflammatory disease, sterility, HIV infection.

CORNEAL ABRASION

Corneal abrasion is caused by disruption of the epithelial covering of the cornea. It may follow trauma, any superficial contact such as with dust, debris, or prolonged exposure to ultraviolet light such as sunlight, sunlamp, or welder's arc.

Epidemiology

Contact lens wearers are at higher risk for abrasion (and ulceration) not only because insertion of the lens may result in abrasion but because the cornea over time may become less sensitive to insult and treatment may be delayed. Clients in occupations involving prolonged exposure to dirt, dust, debris, sunlight, and wind are also at higher risk for corneal abrasion.

Subjective Data

Client reports history of trauma, severe pain, foreign body sensation, and photophobia.

Objective Data

Physical Examination. Diffuse or localized redness. May have profuse tearing. Client may be unable to open eye for examination if pain severe. Oblique illumination of the cornea by penlight may reveal irregular area on corneal surface. Always evert eyelid to examine for foreign body.

Diagnostic Tests

Visual Acuity. Is recorded. (Practitioner may have to instill one to two drops topical ophthalmic anesthetic such as procainamide before starting examination.)

Fluorescein Staining. Fluorescein strip is dampened with sterile normal saline and lightly touched to the conjunctival surface of lower lid. After stain is blinked into surface of eye, cornea is examined with slit lamp or Wood's lamp. Epithelial staining defect appears as deep green with cobalt blue filter.

Differential Medical Diagnoses

Herpes simplex keratitis. Suspect if previous history of herpes keratitis, coexisting fever blister or herpes genitalis, vague or absent history of trauma, dendritic corneal stain pattern.

Ultraviolet keratitis. History of exposure to sunlight, snow, sunlamp, or welder's arc without adequate eye protection. Symptoms occur 6 to 12 hours after exposure. Client complains of intense pain and photophobia and may be unable to open eyes. Staining reveals diffuse punctate pattern of both corneas.

Plan

Refer immediately any client with herpes keratoconjunctivitis or ultraviolet keratitis to physician and/or ophthalmologist. Consult with physician if corneal abrasion. Deep or extensive abrasions, corneal ulceration, contact lens wearers should always be referred for follow-up with ophthalmologist.

Psychosocial Interventions. Reassure client that cornea heals very rapidly but emphasize strict adherence to treatment plan to prevent complications such as ulceration and infection.

Medication

Erythromycin Ophthalmic Ointment. Is used to prevent infection.

- *Administration.* Apply to lower lid and with firm pressure place sterile dry dressing over eye to prevent lid movement. Tape is placed from cheek to forehead to secure bandage.
- *Adverse Effects.* Transient stinging of eye.
- *Contraindication.* Sensitivity to erythromycin (rare).
- *Expected Outcome.* Superficial abrasion usually heals within 24 to 48 hours without complication.
- *Client Teaching.* Advise patient not to drive. She should rest at home, not remove bandage, and keep unaffected eye closed as much as possible. She should be seen the next day by the practitioner (if skilled in using slit lamp) or referred to an ophthalmologist (always if contact lens wearer).

Lifestyle Changes. If the client is a contact lens wearer and has recurrent episodes of conjunctivitis, irritation, or abrasion, advise her to return to ophthalmologist or optometrist who originally prescribed lenses for further evaluation.

Follow-Up

Client is always examined the next day using slit lamp or Wood's lamp after fluorescein staining. If staining defect remains or if client continues to complain of foreign body sensation or pain, consult with physician immediately. Request copy of visit note and treatment plan if referred to ophthalmologist in order to assure continuity of care.

DISORDERS OF THE EYELID

Hordeolum and Chalazion

A hordeolum is an abscess of the meibomian gland (internal hordeolum) or the gland at the base of the lash (external hordeolum or sty). It can occur on the upper or the lower lid. It is caused by *Staphylococcus*. If the abscess is internal, it can press on the conjunctiva and cause a cellulitis of the lid.

A chalazion is a granulomatous inflammation of the meibomian gland that is caused by an internal hordeolum.

Epidemiology. Both conditions are common in children and adults. Clients with compromised immunity such as diabetics may be more prone to develop hordeolum.

Subjective Data. The client with hordeolum may complain of pain in proportion to the degree of swelling. If a chalazion is large, it may press on the eyeball and cause pain, conjunctival injection, or even blurring of vision.

Objective Data. Hordeolum causes a red, tender swelling of the lid, usually arising from the skin surface. If the hordeolum is internal (less common), it is larger and can press on the conjunctiva. If the entire lid becomes swollen, it can progress to a cellulitis. Chalazion is a small nontender nodule that can be palpated within the upper or lower eyelid. If the lid is everted, a corresponding area of redness is seen. A chalazion may become infected, and the presentation would be similar to a hordeolum with painful swelling.

Physical Examination. Inspection of the eyelid and everting the lid usually confirm the diagnosis. If the hordeolum is internal, the cornea should be examined for abrasion (see previous section on corneal abrasion).

Diagnostic Test. None is indicated.

Differential Medical Diagnoses. Chalazion and hordeolum are often confused. Chalazion tend to be smaller and chronic; they are usually not painful unless they are quite large. Hordeolum presents with pain and localized redness.

Blepharitis (see following) involves the whole eyelid and is usually accompanied by scaling, itching, and burning.

Plan

Psychosocial Interventions. Both hordeolum and chalazion can be disfiguring and cause body image concerns. Reassure the client that if conservative measures do not resolve the conditions, prompt referral to the ophthalmologist will follow.

Medication and Treatment

HORDEOLUM

- Bacitracin or erythromycin ophthalmic ointment instilled into the conjunctival sac every 3 hours. (See above discussion of erythromycin ointment in section on conjunctivitis.)

SODIUM SULFACETIMIDE SOLUTION (SULAMYD-10)

- If drops preferred and client not allergic to sulfa, may be prescribed, two drops in affected eye every 3 hours while awake. (See previous discussion in section on conjunctivitis.)
- Warm compresses applied for 15 minutes to the affected eye three or four times a day are also helpful to reduce swelling. If the acute stage is not resolved

within 48 hours, refer to an ophthalmologist for incision and drainage.

CHALAZION

- Erythromycin ophthalmic ointment. If the chalazion is large or if it appears to be infected, inflamed, or affects vision, treat with erythromycin ophthalmic ointment and refer to an ophthalmologist.
- Small chalazion may be treated with warm compresses as above.

Lifestyle. Ophthalmic ointment may cause blurred vision and impair driving and close work. Advise client not to rub, scratch or touch eye, wash hands before and after applying medication or compresses.

Follow-Up. If hordeola recur, client may have a chronic Staphylococcal infection of the eyelid. In addition, recurrent eyelid lesions may be basal cell carcinoma. Refer to the ophthalmologist.

Blepharitis

Blepharitis is an inflammation of the lid margins that is usually chronic. There may be acute exacerbations and infectious flare-ups.

There are two types of blepharitis, anterior and posterior. Anterior blepharitis involves the eyelid skin, lashes, and glands. It may be chronic with swelling of the lids along the lash line and scaling of the skin. It is often associated with seborrhea and dandruff. There can be acute flare-ups of anterior blepharitis caused by *Staphylococci*.

Posterior blepharitis is an inflammatory condition of the eyelids caused by dysfunction of the meibomian glands.

Epidemiology. Blepharitis is the most common disorder of the eyelids. The client often has associated seborrhea, dandruff, and/or acne rosacea.

Subjective Data. The client usually complains of burning, itching, and irritation. She may also have noted mucous discharge if the meibomian glands are inflamed.

Objective Data

Physical Examination. In anterior blepharitis, the client's eyes are red-rimmed and the conjunctiva may be injected. Scales may be seen clinging to the eyebrows and eyelids. If there is an acute flare, there may be a loss of lashes. The redness and crusting will be more pronounced.

In posterior blepharitis, telangiectasias can be seen on the lid margins. The openings of the meibomian glands may be plugged, inflamed, and exudative. Associated tears may be greasy. There may be mild entropion of the lid margin.

Diagnostic Test. Usually not indicated. Physical exam confirms the diagnosis.

Differential Medical Diagnoses. See previous section on hordeolum and chalazion.

Plan

Psychosocial Interventions. Reassure the client that even though this is a chronic condition, flare-ups can be minimized with meticulous hygiene and self-care. Body image concerns should be explored because of the scaling and redness of the lids.

Medication and Treatment

ANTERIOR BLEPHARITIS

- If the client has frequent exacerbations, nightly application of erythromycin or bacitracin ophthalmic ointment applied with a cotton swab to the lid margin may be indicated. (See previous discussion of these medications in section on conjunctivitis.)
- Tar or selenium shampoo daily controls scaling of the scalp.
- Acute flare of anterior blepharitis is treated with sodium sulfacetamide (Sulamyd-10) drops every 2 to 3 hours while awake or erythromycin ointment applied four times a day. (See previous discussion of these medications in section on conjunctivitis.)
- The cornerstone of treatment is scrupulous hygiene of the scalp, eyebrows, and lid margins. Scales should be removed from the lashes and eyebrows with a damp cotton applicator dipped in baby shampoo twice a day. Advise the client to pull the lower lid down so that lash margins are thoroughly scrubbed. Follow with warm water cloth to rinse. If scales adhere to lashes, advise client to apply warm compresses for several minutes before swabbing with baby shampoo to loosen scales.

POSTERIOR BLEPHARITIS

- Inflammatory flares may require systemic therapy with erythromycin 250 mg four times a day or tetracycline 250 mg twice a day. (See previous discussion of these medications under common dermatological conditions.)
- Consult with physician regarding use of topical steroid drops.
- Mild posterior blepharitis may only require daily expression of meibomian glands by gentle pressure to

lids followed by cleansing regimen as described previously.

- Client with associated entropion may require referral to ophthalmologist for surgery if lashes rub on cornea.

Lifestyle Modifications. Advise the client to use hypoallergenic cosmetics and not to share eye makeup. She should avoid rubbing the eyes and wash hands often especially after touching eye area.

Follow-Up. During acute flares evaluate for response to therapy in one week. Encourage client to call if inflammation starts in order to initiate therapy promptly.

UVEITIS

Uveitis is an inflammation of the uveal tract of the eye, which includes the iris, ciliary body, and choroid. Uveitis is most often confined to the anterior structures of the iris and ciliary body. Posterior uveitis is rare and usually does not present with a painful red eye but with complaint of decreased vision and spots in the visual field (Schachat, 1999c).

Epidemiology

In the client without accompanying systemic illness, the most common cause of acute anterior uveitis is trauma. Systemic disorders associated with anterior uveitis include the HLA-B27 complexes (sarcoidosis, psoriasis, inflammatory bowel disease, ankylosing spondylitis, Reiter's syndrome). Herpes simplex and herpes zoster may also cause anterior uveitis. Posterior uveitis may be caused by sarcoidosis (usually bilateral involvement), tuberculosis, syphilis, toxoplasmosis, leprosy. In many cases of anterior uveitis, no underlying cause is determined (Perez & Foster, 2001).

Subjective Data

In anterior uveitis, the client complains of eye pain, redness, photophobia, and blurred vision. She may deny history of trauma or coexisting illness. In posterior uveitis, the client presents with complaint of gradual diminution of vision, spots appearing in the visual field, and no inflammation or pain.

Objective Data

Physical Examination. In acute anterior uveitis, the affected pupil is small and may be irregular. The conjunctiva is injected around the limbus. Profuse tearing may be present. In posterior uveitis, the eye appears normal or quiet.

Diagnostic Tests

Visual Acuity. Always record visual acuity. If client has forgotten or lost corrective lenses, a pinhole disk may be used to optimize acuity. Acuity in the affected eye is diminished from baseline.

Slit Lamp Examination. Slit lamp examination of the anterior chamber reveals inflammatory cells and flare.

NOTE: Practitioner who is not skilled in the use of a slit lamp should not attempt to examine the client without confirmation of findings made by physician.

Plan

Refer immediately to ophthalmologist. Treatment involves use of topical mydriatic and cycloplegic agents that dilate the pupil and paralyze the ocular muscles of accommodation and use of topical corticosteroids to suppress inflammation.

GLAUCOMA

Glaucoma is a condition of abnormally elevated pressure within the eye caused by an obstruction of outflow of the aqueous humor. Acute (angle-closure) glaucoma occurs when the obstruction arises from the iris and blocks the exit of aqueous humor from the anterior chamber. It is acute in onset, occurring with pupillary dilatation, and is an ophthalmology emergency. The client must be referred immediately to prevent vision loss and damage to the optic nerve. Open angle glaucoma develops slowly from an obstruction within the canal of Schlemm. Over time it too can cause optical nerve damage and blindness if not detected and treated appropriately.

Epidemiology

Glaucoma is the second most common cause of irreversible blindness in the United States. There are two major types of glaucoma, primary and secondary. Primary open angle and primary acute angle closure (angle-closure glaucoma) are seen most commonly in primary care. Primary open angle glaucoma is the most common cause of glaucoma in the United States and is responsible for 20 percent of blindness (Schachat, 1999b).

Open angle glaucoma is more common among African Americans with earlier onset and more severe damage at time of diagnosis. The risk of glaucoma increases with age and has an hereditary pattern. Risk factors for damage to the optic nerve due to open angle glaucoma include the following: elevated intraocular pressure; enlargement of the optic cup; vascular abnormalities, e.g., hypertension, diabetes, migraine; myopia; and use of steroids (Schachat, 1999b).

Subjective Data

Acute angle closure glaucoma presents with sudden onset of extreme pain and blurred vision. Client may associate onset with sitting in darkened theater, time of stress, or having pupil dilated during ophthalmoscopic examination. She may experience nausea and abdominal pain.

Open angle glaucoma has an insidious onset and there are no symptoms in the early stages. Later the client may note constriction of the visual field with central vision preserved. She may note haloes around lights if the intraocular pressure is markedly elevated.

Objective Data

Physical Examination. Acute angle closure glaucoma causes a red eye, steamy-appearing cornea, and a moderately dilated pupil that is nonreactive to light. The globe feels hard when lightly touched. The client with open angle glaucoma has a normal-appearing eye. The nurse practitioner in primary practice may not be skilled in tonometric measurement to assess intraocular pressure but she or he can perform the most useful method of screening, ophthalmoscopic examination of the optic disk. The average cup to disk ratio is 0.3 and is equal bilaterally. Examine disk for narrow rim and hemorrhage. An enlarged cup or an asymmetric cup-to-disk ratio is grounds for referral to an ophthalmologist for visual field and tonometric analysis (Schachat, 1999b).

Assessment of visual fields by confrontation may be done but may not be reliable. Constriction of vision is gradual and subtle. Thorough examination is done with specialized equipment usually not found in primary practice and requires 10 to 20 minutes per eye.

Diagnostic Tests

Visual Acuity. Central vision is usually preserved, but every good eye exam begins with acuity.

Visual Fields by Confrontation. Detects tunnel vision through use of special instrument used by trained personnel in optometrist or ophthalmologist's office.

Tonometry. Examination of intraocular pressure using tonometry is not recommended for the primary care provider, because common handheld devices alone are not sensitive or specific enough to accurately assess intraocular pressure. Instead, visualization of the optic disc through a dilated lens, measurement of intraocular pressure, and visual field assessment by an optometrist or ophthalmologist result in better screening outcomes for glaucoma. Clients who are at high risk (African American age 40 or older, all adults age 65 or older) should receive glaucoma screening every year or two (Schachat, 1999b).

Differential Medical Diagnoses

See Table 22–11.

- *Acute Angle Closure Glaucoma.* Client complains of intense pain and photophobia, pupils are unequal, cornea has steamy appearance.
- *Optic Neuritis.* Sudden loss of vision, pain especially with eye movement, usually central vision lost. Associated with underlying disorder as multiple sclerosis, sarcoidosis, systemic lupus erythematosus.

Plan

The client with acute angle closure glaucoma is referred immediately to a physician. It is an ocular emergency and is usually treated by laser iridotomy to reduce pressure. Subsequent treatment is the same as open angle glaucoma.

If open angle glaucoma is suspected, the client is referred for outpatient ophthalmologic evaluation as soon as possible.

Psychosocial Interventions. A diagnosis that carries with it the risk of blindness is very frightening. Reassure the client that with early diagnosis, treatment, and careful follow-up, glaucoma can be managed. A high level of compliance is necessary and the medications can be very expensive. Assessment of the client's support system and social situation is important to promote a favorable outcome.

Medication. Treatment for open angle glaucoma usually begins with a topical beta adrenergic blocker such as timolol or betaxolol. The mechanism of action is to reduce production of aqueous humor.

Topical Beta Adrenergic Blocker

- *Administration.* One drop to the conjunctival sac twice a day. Advise client to press on the lacrimal sac after instillation to decrease systemic absorption.
- *Side Effects.* Bronchospasm, exacerbation of congestive heart failure, cardiac condition disturbance, depression, confusion, hypotension.

- *Contraindications.* Known hypersensitivity, severe bradycardia, overt cardiac failure, second and third degree heart block, asthma, severe chronic obstructive pulmonary disease.
- *Expected Outcome.* Ophthalmologist will monitor response to therapy and adjust dosage until maintenance drug regimen is determined. The practitioner should assess adherence and barriers to the treatment plan. He or she should examine the optic disc during periodic screenings between eye doctor visits for any changes.
- *Client Teaching.* Inform the client that glaucoma can be managed but not cured. Therefore, adherence to dosage and administration of eye drops is crucial. Inform client to report any adverse effects promptly.

Miotics Pilocarpine. This is the most widely used agent. It lowers intraocular pressure through contraction of the sphincter muscle of the iris, resulting in pupil constriction.

- *Administration.* One or two drops in the eye four times per day.
- *Side Effects.* Blurred vision, increased bronchial secretions, nausea, vomiting, diarrhea.
- *Contraindications.* Known hypersensitivity, overt congestive heart failure.
- *Expected Outcome.* See aforementioned.
- *Client Teaching.* See prior information. Warn patient about blurred vision and driving or operating equipment.
- *Surgical Interventions.* Argon laser trabeculectomy may be performed on those for whom optimal pressure has not been achieved with topical medications or who are unable to tolerate these agents. It is done on an outpatient basis under topical anesthesia. Glaucoma filtration surgery is reserved for those clients who have failed all other methods. It involves establishing an alternative exit for aqueous humor. It can be done on an outpatient basis (Schachat, 1999b).

Follow-Up

Request notification from ophthalmologist of any change in treatment regimen and timing of follow-up visits. Assess client adherence to plan of care.

CATARACTS

A cataract is an opacity of the lens of the eye. Because lens fibers are produced throughout a lifetime and none is lost, the density of the lens increases with age. A cataract may or may not be associated with visual impairment. The specific changes in vision that result are loss of contrast sensitivity and glare.

Epidemiology

Incidence of cataract increases with age after the age of 50. It is estimated from several studies that the prevalence is close to 50 percent in individuals over 75 years old. Risk factors associated with development include exposure to ultraviolet-B radiation, diabetes, smoking, heavy alcohol use, history of trauma, retinal detachment, prolonged systemic steroid therapy, and certain systemic illnesses such as diabetes, myotonic dystrophy, and atopic dermatitis (Schachat, 1999a).

Subjective Data

The client may complain of impaired vision, "like a fog over my eyes." The location of the opacity often determines whether near vision or far vision is affected. The client with a central opacity complains of glare because pupillary constriction causes light to enter the area most opacified. She may report that she sees better in low light than in well-lighted rooms. She may have stopped driving at night due to the glare from oncoming head-lights. Color vision may be impaired. There is no complaint of pain or redness.

Objective Data

Physical Examination. Conjunctiva are clear.

- *Funduscopic Examination.* As the cataract becomes denser, the retina becomes harder to visualize.

Diagnostic Tests

- *Visual Acuity.* May or may not be affected depending on location of opacity.

Differential Medical Diagnoses

Glaucoma, retinal vascular occlusive disorders, macular degeneration.

Plan

Refer client to an ophthalmologist for further evaluation. Other retinal disorders may be present.

Psychosocial Interventions. Reassure the client that early detection and regular follow-up with an ophthalmologist improves outcome. Advise client surgery may not be indicated immediately.

Medication. None.

Nonsurgical Measures. Changing eyeglass prescription as needed, especially when myopia is induced by the cataract. Bifocals, magnifying lenses, and appropriate lighting may be helpful until surgery is performed.

Surgery. The decision to perform surgery is based on clinical judgment and visual acuity, usually when acuity is reduced to 20/50 or less (based on state driving laws requiring better vision to drive). The latest technique involves ultrasonic fragmentation of the lens nucleus with implantation of an intraocular lens. Postoperative complications include risk of infection, glaucoma, retinal detachment, hemorrhage, posterior capsular opacification. In 95 percent of cases acuity is improved. (Schachat, 1999a).

Lifestyle. Before surgery client may have curtailed some activities such as night driving, hobbies, reading. She may experience the loss of independence or income.

Follow-Up

Usually followed by ophthalmologist for six to eight weeks after surgery. The practitioner should continue to monitor vision and perform functional assessments at each visit after release from the surgeon. Be alert for posterior capsular pacification, which can develop several months to several years after removal of the lens. Signs and symptoms same as for cataracts.

PULMONARY DISORDERS

This section on disorders associated with the lung covers asthma and influenza as well as the lower respiratory tract infections, pneumonia and acute bronchitis.

ASTHMA

Asthma is a chronic inflammatory disorder of the airways. Chronic inflammation is responsible for increased airway hyperresponsiveness to a variety of stimuli, for recurrent symptoms, airway narrowing, and respiratory symptoms. Inflammation is responsible for acute bronchoconstriction, swelling of the airway wall, chronic mucus plug formation, and airway wall remodeling. Asthma can begin in response to sensitizing agents and the development of atopy later in life. Atopy is considered to be the strongest risk factor for the development of asthma (Jablonski, 2000).

It is important to understand that any client with asthma, regardless of severity, may develop an acute severe asthma exacerbation. The clients most at risk are those with a history of multiple hospital admissions, past intubation, multiple psych/social problems, a recent decrease in corticosteroids, and noncompliance with lifestyle modifications and medications.

Effective management of asthma relies on four integral components: measurement of lung function to assess and monitor the client's asthma, pharmacologic therapy, environmental measures to control allergens and irritants, and client education (DHHS, 2001a; NIH, 2002).

An acute asthma exacerbation has an early and late phase response. The early/bronchoconstrictive phase is characterized by the rapid development of reversible airway obstruction in response to a stimulus, usually within minutes but may occur up to 2 hours later.

The late phase response can occur 6 to 12 hours later. It is an inflammatory response less likely to respond to bronchodilators.

Epidemiology

Asthma morbidity and mortality are on the rise. The prevalence of asthma rose from 30.7 per 1000 population in 1980 to a two-year average of 53.8 per 1000 in 1993/1994. This represents an increase of 75 percent. The estimated direct and indirect monetary costs for this disease totaled $11.3 billion in 1998 (NHLBI, 1999). Asthma is associated with predisposing and causal factors and can vary in severity (see Table 22–12).

Subjective Data

The client may report a history of any of the following: chest tightness, shortness of breath, dyspnea on exertion, or a nonproductive cough. The symptoms may occur with exercise, exposure to animals with fur, smoke, pollen, changes in temperature, strong emotional expression, aerosol chemicals, and dust mites. Many clients will have a history of childhood asthma, a history of seasonal allergies, and/or a family history of asthma.

Objective Data

Physical Examination. The physical examination between exacerbations may be normal.

Evaluate the client for signs of atopy: eczema, allergic conjunctivitis, rhinitis, coughing, sneezing.

During an exacerbation, the client may exhibit signs of acute respiratory distress such as wheezing, coughing, tachycardia, and anxiety.

Diagnostic Tests. In clients with mild to moderate asthma, all laboratory tests may be normal. Well-controlled asthma blood gases will be normal. During an exacerbation, mild to moderate hypoxia and hypocapnia with a

respiratory alkalosis may be present. During a severe exacerbation, respiratory acidosis may be present.

Measurement of lung function for diagnosing asthma is analogous to measurement in other chronic disease. For most, peak expiratory flow (PEF) correlates well with FEV1 (NHLBI, 1999). Regular home monitoring can help clients detect early signs of deterioration.

Differential Medical Diagnoses

Cardiac disorders, allergic rhinitis/sinusitis, sarcoidosis, chronic obstructive pulmonary disease, airway obstruction, cystic fibrosis pulmonary embolism, gastroesophageal disorders, cough associated with angiotensin converting enzyme inhibitors, obesity.

Plan

Treatment must be individualized with consideration to medication, risk reduction, and severity of disease.

Psychosocial Intervention. Clients with asthma frequently have poor recognition of their symptoms and poor perception of severity, especially if their asthma is severe and long standing. Clients frequently are concerned with lost time from work and decreased productivity. The client may also need to consider a job change away from triggering agents.

Medication. Medication choice focuses on airway inflammation associated with both acute and chronic asthma. The trend is to focus on preventive use of avoidance strategies and anti-inflammatory drugs to treat the underlying disease process rather than only the acute consequences. See Tables 22–13, 22–14, 22–15 and 22–16. Clients with asthma are at risk for flus and pneumonia; consider influenza and pneumovax vaccines.

Client Education. Stress avoidance of known triggers, proper use of metered dose inhalers, and use of peak flow monitors, and smoking cessation.

Follow-Up

Follow-up of acute exacerbations should be individualized based on severity and client comfort and reliability.

Asymptomatic clients should be followed on an as-needed basis with emphasis placed on continued client education.

INFLUENZA

Influenza, an acute, usually self-limiting, upper respiratory infection, may be caused by influenza A, B, or C virus. Strains of the A virus are the most common and

TABLE 22–12. Agents Causing Asthma in Selected Occupations

Occupation or Occupational Field	Agent
laboratory animal worker, veterinarian	dander and urine proteins
food processing	shellfish, egg proteins, pancreatic enzymes, papain, amylase
dairy farmer	storage mites
poultry farmer	poultry mites, droppings and feathers
grainery worker	storage mites, aspergillus, indoor ragweed, and grass pollen
research worker	locusts
fish food manufacturing	midges
detergent manufacturing	*Bacillus subtilis* enzymes
silk worker	silkworm moths and larvas
baker	flour, amylase
food processing	coffee bean dust, meat tenderizer (papain), tea
farmer	soybean dust
shipping workers	grain dust (molds, insects, grain)
laxative manufacturing	ispaghula, psyllium
sawmill workers, carpenters	wood dust (western red cedar, oak, mahogany, zebrawood, redwood, Lebanon cedar, African maple, eastern white cedar)
electric soldering	colophony (pine resin)
cotton textile workers	cotton dust
nurse	psyllium, latex
	Inorganic Chemicals:
refinery worker	platinum salts, vandium
plating	nickel salts
diamond polishing	cobalt salts
manufacturing	aluminum fluoride
beauty shop	persulfate
welding	stainless steel fumes, chromium salts
	Organic Chemicals:
manufacturing	antibiotics, piperazine, methyldopa, salbutamol, cimetidine
hospital worker	disinfectants (sulfathiazole, chloramine, formaldehyde, glutaraldehyde)
anesthesiology	enflurane
poultry worker	aprolium
fur dyeing	paraphenylene diamine
rubber processing	formaldehyde, ethylene diamine, phthalic anhydride
plastics industry	toluene diisocyanate, hexamethyl diisocyanate, dephenylmethyl isocyanate, phthalic anhydride, triethylene tetramines, trimellitic anhydride, hexamethyl tetramine
automobile painting	dimethyl ethanolamine diisocyanates
foundry worker	reaction product of furan binder

Source: International Census Report on Diagnoses and Treatment of Asthma. (1992). (NIH Publication No. 92–3091).

most virulent. B virus infection has some increased association with Reye's syndrome. C virus infection is a mild illness, usually not significant or identified clinically.

Epidemiology

Etiology of the influenza virus reveals the unique ability to vary antigenically from year to year, hence the terms antigenic drift (minor variations) and antigenic shift (major variations). Prior exposure provides limited immunity. Epidemics occur every two to three years; about every ten years, the strains vary dramatically and produce a "pandemic" (Prisco, 2002).

Transmission is primarily through aerosolized particles from a cough or sneeze, although the virus can be spread by clothing or hand contact. The incubation period is about 18 to 72 hours. Infectious viral shedding occurs for ten days but is most prominent in the first 48 hours of illness.

In an epidemic year, 20 to 30 percent of the population may contract influenza. Deaths are usually due to pneumonia (influenza pneumonia is the sixth leading cause of death in the United States) or to cardiovascular decompensation related to the influenza (Couch, 2000).

Groups at risk for influenza complications include persons over 65, persons with chronic cardiac or pulmonary disorders, persons with chronic metabolic disor-

TABLE 22–13. Tolerance of Nonsteroidal Anti-Inflammatory Drugs in Aspirin-Induced Asthma

Precipitate Asthma Exacerbations	Well Tolerated (Cause no bronchoconstriction)
Salicylates	Sodium salicylate
Aspirin	Choline salicylate
Diflunisal	Choline magnesium
Salesate (salicylsalicylic acid)	Salicylamide
Polycyclic acids	Dextropropoxyphene
Acetic acids	Azapropazone
Incomethacin	Benzydamine
Suliudac	Chloroquine
Tolmetin	Paracetamol*
Arylaliphatic acids	
Naproxen	
Diclofanac	
Fenoprofen	
Ibuprofen	
Ketoprofen	
Tiaprofenic acid, Fluribrofen	
Enolic acids	
Piroxicam	
Fenamates	
Mefanamic acid	
Flufenamic acid	
Cyclofenamic acid	
Pyrazolones	
Aminopyrine	
Noramaidopyrine	
Sulfinpyrazone	
Phenylbutazone	

*When beginning therapy, give half a tablet of paracetamol and observe patient 2 to 3 hours for symptoms that occur in no more than 5 percent of patients.

Source: Clark, et al. (2000). NHLBI (1999).

ders (e.g., diabetes mellitus), renal dysfunction, immunosuppression, and nursing home residents (Couch, 2000).

Subjective Data

History reveals the four hallmarks of influenza: headache, myalgias, especially in the legs and back; fever, often to 102°F to 104°F for three to four days or longer; and nonproductive cough, which usually is not prominent at the beginning of illness but increases over time. Watery eyes and dry throat may be present, but nasal symptoms are usually absent.

Objective Data

Physical Examination. The client may be flushed and sweating. She appears ill. High fever is common, usually greater than 102° F, but rarely 106° F or higher. Heart and respiratory rates are increased.

The eyes, ears, nose, and throat usually appear normal. The lungs are clear. If crackles or rhonchi are heard, obtain a chest x-ray to rule out influenza pneumonia.

Monitor the heart to assess cardiovascular status. Influenza may precipitate cardiovascular failure in cardiac clients.

Diagnostic Tests. Usually not required unless the fever lasts longer than four days, in which case a white blood cell count should be ordered. If the WBC is greater than 12,000, suspect pneumonia and order a chest x-ray.

Differential Medical Diagnoses

Parainfluenza virus, respiratory syncytial virus, adenovirus, other viral syndromes. In the absence of an epidemic, it is difficult to identify influenza from many other viral syndromes. Note that influenza is always associated with cough.

Plan

Psychosocial Interventions. Inform the client about the expected course of disease, and teach the warning signs of influenza pneumonia and cardiac complications. Reassure her that taking acetaminophen is permitted. Aspirin, however, should be avoided because of its association with Reye's syndrome. Comfort will be increased and myalgia decreased if fever is controlled.

Medication. Medication is administered for prophylaxis and treatment.

Antiviral Drugs. Amantadine and Rimantadine are both approved for prophylaxis and treatment in influenza A; they not effective against influenza B.

♦ *Administration.* For prophylaxis, administer for two weeks with a late vaccine in the midst of an outbreak. For treatment amantadine must be given within 24 to 48 hours of the onset of symptoms.

The usual adult dose for those 65 years or younger is 200 mg b.i.d. for ten to fourteen days.
♦ *Side Effects.* Side effects are infrequent and cease when medication is stopped. The client may experience central nervous system symptoms, including nervousness, dizziness, and insomnia.
♦ *Contraindications.* Do not administer to any client with renal compromise or clients older than 65 years.
♦ *Expected Outcomes.* When used for treatment, amantadine should decrease the severity and duration of illness.
♦ *Client Teaching.* When amantadine is given for prophylaxis, inform the client that it is 70 to 90 percent

TABLE 22–14. Stepwise Approach for Managing Asthma in Adults and Children Older Than 5 Years of Age: Treatment

Classify Severity: Clinical Features Before Treatment or Adequate Control			Medications Required To Maintain Long-Term Control
	$\dfrac{\text{Symptoms}/\text{Day}}{\text{Symptoms}/\text{Night}}$	*PEF or FEV$_1$* *PEF Variability*	*Daily Medications*
Step 4 Severe Persistent	$\dfrac{\text{Continual}}{\text{Frequent}}$	$\dfrac{\leq 60\%}{> 30\%}$	• Preferred treatment –High-dose inhaled corticosteroids AND –Long-acting inhaled β$_2$-agonists AND, if needed, –Corticosteroid tablets or syrup long term (2 mg/kg/day, generally do not exceed 60 mg per day). Make repeat attempts to reduce systemic corticosteroids and maintain control with high-dose inhaled corticosteroids.
Step 3 Moderate Persistent	$\dfrac{\text{Daily}}{>1 \text{ night}/\text{week}}$	$\dfrac{> 60\% \; - \; < 80\%}{> 30\%}$	• Preferred treatment –Low-to-medium dose inhaled corticosteroids and long-acting inhaled β$_2$-agonists. • Alternative treatment –Increase inhaled corticosteroids within medium-dose range OR –Low-to-medium dose inhaled corticosteroids and either leukotriene modifier or theophylline. If needed (particularly in patients with recurring severe exacerbations): • Preferred treatment –Increase inhaled corticosteroids within medium-dose range, and add long-acting inhaled β$_2$-agonists. • Alternative treatment –Increase inhaled corticosteroids in medium-dose range, and add either leukotriene modifier or theophylline.
Step 2 Mild Persistent	$\dfrac{> 2/\text{week but} < 1\text{x}/\text{day}}{> 2 \text{ nights}/\text{month}}$	$\dfrac{\geq 80\%}{20-30\%}$	• Preferred treatment –Low-dose inhaled corticosteroids. • Alternative treatment (listed alphabetically): cromolyn, leukotriene modifier, nedocromil, OR sustained release theophylline to serum concentration of 5–15 mcg/mL.
Step 1 Mild Intermittent	$\dfrac{\leq 2 \text{ days}/\text{week}}{\leq 2 \text{ nights}/\text{month}}$	$\dfrac{\geq 80\%}{< 20\%}$	• No daily medication needed. • Severe exacerbations may occur, separated by long periods of normal lung function and no symptoms. A course of systemic corticosteroids is recommended.

All Patients

• Short-acting bronchodilator: 2–4 puffs short-acting inhaled β$_2$-agonists as needed for symptoms.
• Intensity of treatment will depend on severity of exacerbation; up to 3 treatments at 20-minute intervals or a single nebulizer treatment as needed. Course of systemic corticosteroids may be needed.

• Use of short-acting inhaled β$_2$-agonists on a daily basis, or increasing use, indicates the need to initiate or increase long-term control therapy.

Step Down

Review treatment every 1 to 6 months; a gradual stepwise reduction in treatment may be possible.

Step Up

If control is not maintained, consider step up. First, review patient medication technique, adherence, and environmental control.

TABLE 22–14. (*cont.*)

- Minimal or no chronic symptoms day or night
- Minimal or no exacerbations
- No limitations on activities; no school/work missed
- PEF > 80% of personal best
- Minimal use of inhaled short-acting β_2-agonist (< 1x per day, < 1 canister/month)
- Minimal or no adverse effects from medications

Note

- The stepwise approach is meant to assist, not replace, the clinical decision making required to meet individual patient needs.
- Classify severity: Assign patient to most severe step in which any feature occurs (PEF is % of personal best; FEV_1 is % predicted).
- Gain control as quickly as possible (consider a short course of systemic corticosteroids); then step down to the least medication necessary to maintain control.
- Provide education on self-management and controlling environmental factors that make asthma worse (e.g., allergens and irritants).
- Refer to an asthma specialist if there are difficulties controlling asthma or if step 4 care is required. Referral may be considered if step 3 care is required.

Source: DHHS (2001a).

effective in preventing influenza A and it is only protective for the duration of therapy. It does not replace the vaccine as it fails to work against influenza B.

Influenza Trivalent Vaccine. The high risk groups for whom annual administration of vaccine is currently recommended are persons with congenital or acquired heart disease, chronic lung disease, chronic renal disease, chronic severe anemia, and immunocompromising illness (diabetes, cancer). Others for whom the vaccine is indicated are persons over 60, those living in chronic care/nursing homes, family members of high risk groups and health care workers.

- *Administration.* Influenza trivalent vaccine (two strains of A and one of B) is administered annually beginning in September. Vaccinations begin protection in 2 weeks; protection peaks in 1 to 2 months and gradually declines over time. Vaccines may be given anytime after an outbreak begins but should be supplemented with 2 weeks of amantadine treatment until the vaccine can induce a response.
- *Side Effects.* Side effects are rare with modern inactivated vaccines. Less than 5 percent of recipients develop a febrile reaction; some local soreness may be noted.
- *Contraindications.* Those with an egg allergy or febrile illness.
- *Expected Outcome.* The vaccine will be 80 percent effective in preventing disease. If the disease is contracted, the course of illness will be less severe.
- *Contraindications.* There are no contraindications to administering the vaccine in combination with other childhood and adult vaccines provided they are given at separate sites.
- *Client Teaching.* Encourage the client to obtain the vaccine annually in September rather than waiting

for symptoms to appear. Stress that influenza is contagious.

Lifestyle Changes. Encourage the client to increase intake of fluids to prevent dehydration, to get adequate bed rest, to avoid contact with others; discourage smoking.

Follow-Up

Influenza pneumonia occurs approximately one week after the onset of influenza symptoms. It is characterized by severe dyspnea, cyanosis, and often scanty blood-tinged sputum. The lungs may sound clear, evaluation by chest x-ray and pulse oximetry will assist in determining severity of illness. Pneumonia, which can occur at any age, accounts for one-half of the deaths associated with influenza. If you suspect pneumonia, refer the client for possible hospital admission.

Preventing influenza is crucial. Only 20 percent of the high risk population is vaccinated against this deadly disease, and amantadine is underused in epidemics. To facilitate implementation of a vaccination program in an office setting, one staff member should be designated to head the effort each fall. During that season, charts of high risk clients should be flagged and posters placed in waiting and exam rooms. Consider becoming involved in a community-wide education effort.

LOWER RESPIRATORY TRACT INFECTIONS: PNEUMONIA AND ACUTE BRONCHITIS

Pneumonia is defined as an acute infection of the alveolar spaces or interstitial tissues (or both) of the lung. There are four classifications of pneumonia: typical, or classic bacterial, pneumonia; atypical pneumonia; aspiration pneumonia; and hematogenous pneumonia. This section

TABLE 22–15. Usual Dosage for Long-Term-Control Medication

Medication	Dosage Form	Adult Dose	Child Dose*
Inhaled Corticosteroids *(See Estimated Comparative Daily Dosages for Inhaled Corticosteroids.)*			
Systemic Corticosteroids *(Applies to all three corticosteroids.)*			
Methylprednisolone	2, 4, 8, 16, 32 mg tablets	• 7.5–60 mg daily in a single dose in a.m. or qod as needed for control	• 0.25–2 mg/kg daily in single dose in a.m. or qod as needed for control
Prednisolone	5 mg tablets, 5 mg/5 cc, 15 mg/5 cc		
Prednisone	1, 2.5, 5, 10, 20, 50 mg tablets; 5 mg/cc, 5 mg/5 cc	• Short-course "burst" to achieve control: 40–60 mg per day as single or 2 divided doses for 3–10 days	• Short-course "burst": 1–2 mg/kg/day, maximum 60 mg/day for 3–10 days
Cromolyn and Nedocromil			
Cromolyn	MDI 1 mg/puff	2–4 puffs tid-qid	1–2 puffs tid-qid
	Nebulizer; 20 mg/ampule	1 ampule tid-qid	1 ampule tid-qid
Nedocromil	MDI 1.75 mg/puff	2–4 puffs bid-qid	1–2 puffs bid-qid
Inhaled Long-Acting β_2-Agonists *(Should not be used for symptom relief or for exacerbations. Use with inhaled corticosteroids.)*			
Salmeterol	MDI 21 mcg/puff	2 puffs q 12 hours	1–2 puffs q 12 hours
	DPI 50 mcg/blister	1 blister q 12 hours	1 blister q 12 hours
Formoterol	DPI: 12 mcg/single-use capsule	1 capsule q 12 hours	1 capsule q 12 hours
Combined Medication			
Fluticasone/Salmeterol DPI	100, 250, or 500 mcg/50 mcg	1 inhalation bid; dose depends on severity of asthma	1 inhalation bid; dose depends on severity of asthma
Leukotriene Modifiers			
Montelukast	4 or 5 mg chewable tablet 10 mg tablet	10 mg qhs	4 mg qhs (2–5 yrs) 5 mg qhs (6–14 yrs) 10 mg qhs (> 14 yrs)
Zafirlukast	10 or 20 mg tablet	40 mg daily (20 mg tablet bid)	20 mg daily (7–11 yrs) (10 mg tablet bid)
Zileuton	300 or 600 mg tablet	2400 mg daily (give tablets qid)	
Methylxanthines *(Serum monitoring is important [serum concentration of 5–15 mcg/mL at steady state]).*			
Theophylline	Liquids, sustained-release tablets, and capsules	Starting dose 10 mg/kg/day up to 300 mg max; usual max 800 mg/day	Starting dose 10 mg/kg/day; usual max: • < 1 year of age: 0.2 (age in weeks) + 5 = mg/kg/day • ≥ 1 year of age: 16 mg/kg/day

Source: DHHS (2001a).

focuses on the two types seen most often in primary care, typical and atypical.

Acute bronchitis has been defined as an acute, usually transient, inflammation of the tracheobronchial tree. It most often occurs in response to a viral infection, to a noxious stimulus, or to the use of certain medications, such as angiotensin-converting enzyme inhibitors. Secondary bacterial bronchitis can be a complication of a viral respiratory infection. Invaders include the usual respiratory pathogens, such as Streptococcus pneumonia, Hemophilus influenza, Chlamydia pneumonia, and Mycoplasma pneumonia (see Table 22–17).

Epidemiology

Studies show more than 10 million cases of pneumonia are diagnosed annually; of these approximately 500,000 require hospitalization (Boldt & Kiresuk, 2001). It is the most common cause of infectious death in the United States. The very young, the very old, and the immuno-compromised are most at risk. Acute bronchitis is more common; a large percentage of cases are caused by viral pathogens or atypical pathogens.

Subjective Data

The symptoms reported by clients with pneumonia and acute bronchitis are compared in Table 22–18.

Pneumococcal pneumonia has a classic history of a sudden onset of rigor and fever of 101°F to 106°F. Clients report a rusty-colored or purulent sputum, chest pain, and shortness of breath.

Mycoplasma pneumonia, on the other hand, has a less dramatic clinical picture and history. The cough is paroxysmal and may be nonproductive. Fatigue and shortness of breath are common.

Questions to ask include the following: How long has the cough lasted? Was the cough preceded by a URI?

TABLE 22–16. Estimated Comparative Daily Dosages for Inhaled Corticosteroids

Drug	Low Daily Dose		Medium Daily Dose		High Daily Dose	
	Adult	Child*	Adult	Child*	Adult	Child*
Beclomethasone CFC 42 or 84 mcg/puff	168–504 mcg	84–336 mcg	504–840 mcg	336–672 mcg	> 840 mcg	> 672 mcg
Beclomethasone HFA 40 or 80 mcg/puff	80–240 mcg	80–160 mcg	240–480 mcg	160–320 mcg	> 480 mcg	> 320 mcg
Budesonide DPI 200 mcg/inhalation	200–600 mcg	200–400 mcg	600–1200 mcg	400–800 mcg	> 1200 mcg	> 800 mcg
Inhalation suspension for nebulization (child dose)		0.5 mg		1.0 mg		2.0 mg
Flunisolide 250 mcg/puff	500–1000 mcg	500–750 mcg	1000–2000 mcg	1000–1250 mcg	> 2000 mcg	> 1250 mcg
Fluticasone MDI: 44, 110, or 220 mcg/puff	88–264 mcg	88–176 mcg	264–660 mcg	176–440 mcg	> 660 mcg	> 440 mcg
DPI: 50, 100, or 250 mcg/inhalation	100–300 mcg	100–200 mcg	300–600 mcg	200–400 mcg	> 600 mcg	> 400 mcg
Triamcinolone acetonide 100 mcg/puff	400–1000 mcg	400–800 mcg	1000–2000 mcg	800–1200 mcg	> 2000 mcg	> 1200 mcg

* Children 12 years of age and younger

Source: DHHS (2001a).

Have you missed work or school? Do you have an underlying respiratory disorder? Did the cough begin abruptly? Did the cough begin after the initiation of a new medication?

Objective Data

Physical Examination. Positive findings on exam can be found in Table 22–18.

Diagnostic Tests

Labwork. Is ordered only if pneumonia is suspected. The serum white blood count is often higher than 12,000 in pneumonia and normal in bronchitis. Cold agglutinins are found in 75 percent of cases of Mycoplasma pneumonia

TABLE 22–17. Pneumonia Pathogens Observed in Primary Care

Classic	Atypical
Common	
Streptococcus pneumoniae (also called pneumococcal)	Mycoplasma pneumoniae Viral
Uncommon	
Haemophilus influenzae Staphylococcus aureus Klebsiella pneumoniae	Legionella pneumophila Chlamydia psittaci Francisella tularensis

Source: Bartlett, Davell, & Mandell (2000); Boldt & Kiresuk (2001).

(titer of 1:64 or greater). Arterial blood gases can be useful in determining severity of illness.

Chest X-ray. Is indicated if pneumonia is suspected and will guide treatment and follow-up. Lobar or segmental consolidation is strongly suggestive of Pneumococcal pneumonia. The chest x-ray may be false negative if the client is dehydrated.

Gram Stain. A gram stain of sputum may be helpful if an adequate sample is obtained. Good smears have fewer than 10 squamous epithelial cells and more than 25 neutrophils per high power field. These results can guide empirical therapy if one organism predominates. Gram-positive diplococci suggests Streptoccus pneumonia; gram-negative coccobacilli suggests Haemophilus influenzae; absence of a predominant bacterium with neutrophils suggests Mycoplasma pneumoniae.

A sputum culture, if carefully obtained, will confirm the diagnosis and is critical for immunocompromised clients.

Differential Medical Diagnoses

Asthma, exposure to noxious substances, allergic rhinitis, gastroesophageal reflux disorder, medication induced, aspiration, other infectious causes, pulmonary edema and foreign body.

TABLE 22–18. History and Examination to Differentiate Pneumonia and Acute Bronchitis

Symptoms/Signs	Bronchitis	Pneumonia
History		
Onset	Gradual, over 5–10 days, usually preceded by URI*	Acute onset, ± preceding URI
Fever	Mild or absent	Usually 101–106° F
Chills	Mild, recurring, or intermittent	True "rigor," teethratting chill
Chest pain	Vague "tightness" or chest congestion	Intense, pleuritic, localized
Sputum	Scant to copious	"Rusty" colored in pneumococcal or mucopurulent
Dyspnea	Rare	Common
Examination		
General appearance	Not toxic, no apparent distress	Often toxic, weak, may use accessory muscles
Vital signs	Often normal	Often tachycardia, tachypnea, fever
HEENT*	Heart	Normal or findings consistent with URI
Lungs		Crackles, won't clear with cough; signs of consolidation (E to A changes, dull to percussion) ± rub
Heart	At normal baseline	Tachycardia

* URI, Upper respiratory infection: HEENT, head, eyes, ears, nose and throat.

Source: American Thoracic Society (2001); Bark, Curhan & Rimm (2000); Bartlett et al., (2000).

Plan

Psychosocial Interventions. Reassure the client and teach her the warning signs of potential complications. In addition, advise her to notify the health care provider immediately if symptoms of complications develop (see Table 22–19).

Medication. Antibiotics and metered-dose inhalers (MDIs) are used in treatment. Pneumonococcal vaccine is used in prevention.

Antibiotics. See Table 22–20. There is great debate in the literature concerning the use of antibiotics in bronchitis. Most literature is advocating a watch and wait approach. If the client develops symptoms of complications or shows no improvement in three days, the use of antibiotics should be considered. When considering the use of extended spectrum antibiotics such as clarithromycin or azithromycin, consider the cost as well as efficacy.

- *Metered-Dose Inhalers.* MDIs can be useful in treating the cough associated with acute bronchitis. (See Table 22–16).

TABLE 22–19. Criteria for Outpatient Management of Pneumonia*

1. Able to take fluids and oral medications.
2. Not toxic, no respiratory distress, only single lobe involvement.
3. No underlying chronic disease, such as chronic obstructive pulmonary disease or diabetes.
4. Pneumonia not related to aspiration (alcoholism or sedation, for example).
5. Adequate support system at home to provide care, observation, and immediate transportation to hospital if condition worsens.

* Client must meet the following criteria.

Source: American Thoracic Society (2001); Bark et al., (2000); Bartlett et al. (2000).

- *Pneumococcal Polysaccharide Vaccine.* It is recommended for healthy adults over 65; anyone with heart, lung, liver, or renal disease; diabetics; alcoholics; immunocompromised adults (including clients with HIV and splenectomized clients); and children older than 2 years who have risk factors such as sickle cell disease, HIV, and nephrotic syndrome.

  Recent recommendations are to revaccinate after 6 years individuals at highest risk and to revaccinate without waiting those individuals who are highest risk who have received the 14-valent vaccine. Refer to a current pharmacotherapeutics text.
- *Administration.* The vaccine is given in a single intramuscular dose.
- *Side Effects.* Side effects are minor and local. Fifty percent of clients experience pain or redness at the site of injection; 1 percent have a fever or rash.

TABLE 22–20. Antibiotics for Lower Respiratory Infections*

Pneumococcal pneumonia	Penicillin V (betapen) levofloxacin 250–500 qd × 7 days
Mycoplasma pneumonia	Doxycycline 100 mg b.i.d. × 7–14 days
Bronchitis	Usually of viral origin; no antibiotics indicated. If mycoplasma bronchitis or secondary bacterial bronchitis is suspected, erythromycin 250 mg p.o. q.i.d. × 10 days is treatment of choice. Smokers are highly likely to develop a secondary bacterial bronchitis. Trimethoprim-sulfameth oxazole or amoxicillin may be administered to treat mixed organisms or *Haemophilus influenzae*.

* For details see a current pharmacotherapeutics text.

Source: Bartlett, et al., (2000).

♦ *Contraindication.* Do not administer to any client who has had a known reaction to the vaccine or an egg allergy.
♦ *Expected Outcome.* Overall, the vaccine has a protective effect in 64 percent of recipients.
♦ *Client Teaching.* Encourage the client to receive the vaccine if she is in a high risk category. Emphasize that more than 500,000 cases of pneumonia occur every year with a 5 percent mortality rate. Discuss the side effects with the client.

Lifestyle Changes. Advise the client to humidify the environment if possible, to increase the intake of fluids, to get proper nutrition, and to rest. Cough suppressants are used only if the cough is excessive and disrupts rest. Discourage smoking.

Follow-Up

Any client with pneumonia should be reevaluated every 24 hours. Most clients with pneumonia should be afebrile in 72 hours. Refer for hospitalization any client who does not rapidly improve. Possible complications of pneumonia include pleural effusion, emphysema (suspect a lung abscess if fever persists), disseminated intravascular coagulation, and nephritis.

Clients with bronchitis should gradually improve and the cough resolve over the course of several weeks. Any client with a cough lasting more than six weeks requires a chest x-ray to rule out other conditions such as lung cancer, lymphoma, tuberculosis, and pulmonary edema. If the x-ray is negative, consider asthma.

CHRONIC OBSTRUCTIVE PULMONARY DISEASE

Chronic obstructive pulmonary disease (COPD) refers to several pulmonary disorders with airway obstruction as the common denominator. The two most common disorders, emphysema and chronic bronchitis, will be addressed here. Chronic bronchitis is characterized by cough and hypersecretion (phlegm production) for at least three months of the year for two consecutive years with airway obstruction documented by spirometry. Emphysema is characterized by abnormal permanent enlargement of the airspaces distal to the terminal bronchiole, destruction of their walls, without obvious fibrosis. Most clients with COPD demonstrate features of coexistent chronic bronchitis (pink puffer) and emphysema (blue bloater). Pure forms of chronic bronchitis and emphysema are rare (Barnes, 2001).

Cigarette smoking is the single most important risk factor for the development of COPD. Clients with COPD may exhibit signs of bronchial hyperresponsiveness with episodes of wheezing in addition to their baseline airway obstruction (Doherty, 2002).

Epidemiology

COPD is the fourth leading cause of death in the United States; more than half of patients with COPD die within ten years of diagnosis. Cigarette smoking is the most common cause of COPD. Cigar and pipe smoking also increase risk but to a lesser extent. Host susceptibility is a key factor since approximately 15 percent of smokers develop COPD. Males are affected more often than females, but this is changing as more females continue to smoke. Chronic exposure to coal, cement, grain dusts, or acid fumes could result in chronic bronchitis (Barnes, 2001; Blanchard, 2002; CDC, 2001; Rennard, 2002).

Subjective Data

The client will give a history of smoking or chronic occupational exposure. She will usually be over 50 but may be significantly younger relative to the age of onset and number of cigarettes per day.

Chronic bronchitis is characterized by cough, phlegm production (white/gray, worse in the morning), and dyspnea. Clients with emphysema will complain of dyspnea and little productive cough.

Objective Data

Physical Examination

♦ *General.* Normal body weight with chronic bronchitis. Weight loss with emphysema.
♦ *Skin.* Cyanosis with advanced disease.
♦ *Neck.* Jugular venous distention.
♦ *Lungs.* Tachypnea, accessory muscle use, pursed lip breathing, wheezing, rhonchi that shift with cough, decreased breath sounds.
♦ *Heart.* Positive S-3 or S-4 with advanced disease.
♦ *Abdomen.* Accessory muscle use. Enlarged liver with advanced disease.
♦ *Extremities.* Lower extremity edema with advanced disease.

Diagnostic Tests. Pulmonary function tests (PFTs) to assess for obstruction. Arterial blood gases to assess oxygenation. An oxygenation saturation of less than 88 percent and a PaO_2 of less than 55 is indicative of severe hypoxemia requiring supplemental oxygen (Blanchard, 2002). A complete blood count (CBC) may demonstrate polycythemia. A chest x-ray may demonstrate overdistended lungs.

Differential Medical Diagnoses

Asthma, congestive heart failure, sarcoidosis, interstitial lung disease, cystic fibrosis, sleep apnea, and cardiac disease.

Plan

Encourage smoking cessation. Studies show a significant improvement in lung function and slowing of the rate of decline in FEV1.

Psychosocial Interventions. Involve the client in decisions concerning treatment. Acknowledge COPD is a chronic debilitating disease that can be treated and quality of life can be improved. Discuss the possibility of progression of the disease. Discuss with the client and her significant others advanced directive wishes.

Depression, fear, and chronic fatigue are common occurrences in clients with COPD and are frequently related to the client's emotional state, not pulmonary dysfunction. Inability to carry out activities of daily living can lead to low self-esteem. Assess the client's emotional state at frequent intervals.

Medication

Bronchodilators. Beta-agonists (e.g., albuterol) are effective in hyperreactive clients. They have a rapid onset of action. Caution must be used in clients with cardiac disease (Barnes, 2000; Doherty, 2002).

Anticholinergics (ipratropium). In stable COPD, ipratropium is a more potent bronchodilator than albuterol.

Methylxanthines. Theophylline has a narrow therapeutic range and can have potentially life-threatening interactions with other drugs. Long-acting preparations can have a positive effect on nocturnal symptoms. Caution must be used in clients with cardiac and/or hepatic disorders.

Corticosteroids. The efficacy of corticosteroids in COPD has not been established. Inhaled corticosteroids are beneficial in clients with underlying hyperreactive/inflammatory processes. See Table 22–16.

Combination Therapy. Strong evidence from clinical trials consistently indicates that use of long-acting inhaled beta-agonists added to low-to-medium doses of inhaled corticosteroids leads to improvements in lung function and symptoms and reduced supplemental beta-agonist use. Adding a leukotriene modifier or theophylline to in-

haled corticosteroids, or doubling the dose of inhaled corticosteroids, also improves outcomes but the evidence is not substantial (Jansen & Lazarus, 2002).

Other Medications. Encourage the client to receive the influenza vaccination annually. The client should receive amantadine for any high risk exposures (see Influenza section).

The client should receive a Pneumovax injection at the time of diagnosis and every six years after. These injections will decrease the risk of further lung damage and possible progression of COPD.

Oxygen. Home oxygen therapy has been documented to increase the life span and improve quality of life in hypoxemic clients. Oxygen is indicated when the PaO_2 reaches 55 or below and/or the O_2 saturation reaches 88 percent or below. The dosage of oxygen should be the liters per minute needed to attain a PaO_2 between 65 and 80 mm Hg. The usual dose is 2 liters per minute.

Lifestyle/Dietary Changes. Encourage the client to increase her hydration to two to four liters in 24 hours to thin secretions and facilitate expectoration. The client with COPD has increased nutritional needs at a time when her disease may make her feel anorexic secondary to increased work of breathing, diaphragm pressure. Encourage the client to eat small, frequent, high-calorie meals. A nutrition consult may be helpful. Encourage frequent regular exercise. The American Lung Association and local hospitals frequently offer support groups.

Follow-Up

Regular follow-up to assess for progression of disease, nutritional status, psychosocial status, medication usage, and polycythemia. Annual pulmonary function tests and arterial blood gases to assess the client's current status, or they may be required to document the continued need for oxygen therapy.

URINARY TRACT DISORDERS

This section discusses three common disturbances: urinary tract infection, interstitial cystitis, and urinary incontinence.

URINARY TRACT INFECTION

Urinary tract infection (UTI) denotes the presence of microorganisms anywhere from the kidney (acute pyelonephritis), to the bladder (cystitis), to the distal urethra (urethritis). Urine is sterile, with the possible exception that the normal urethra may be colonized by diphtheroids, lactobacillus, and alpha hemolytic streptococci. Ascent of pathogenic bacteria typically begins with the rectal flora moving upward to the vaginal introitus, distal urethra, bladder, and finally, occasionally, the kidney.

With repeated infections, it is important to differentiate between reinfection and relapse. In relapse, subsequent infections are caused by the same organism and serotype responsible for the initial infection. Relapse usually occurs within six weeks of treatment (Murphy, 1999). Reinfection, on the other hand, results from infection from a different organism and serotype.

Epidemiology

Etiology. In a bladder infection, a combination of specific host and pathogen factors are involved. In healthy women, a few serotypes of *Escherichia coli* are responsible for more than 85 percent of bladder infections, yet these serotypes constitute only 1 percent of rectal flora. A specific interrelationship between bacterial adhesion and epithelial cell receptors in women may predispose them to infection (Eriksen, 1999; Madersbacher, Thalhammer, & Marberger, 2000).

Periurethral cells in infection-prone women more readily bind *E. coli* cells than do periurethral cells in women who are not prone to infection. In women with recurrent UTIs, periurethral tissue is laden with pathogenic bacteria. Any additional factor, such as the motion of sexual intercourse, may cause these women to develop infection. Surface mucin that coats the bladder helps prevent bacterial attachment. That lining may decrease with age and falling estrogen levels, however (Eriksen, 1999; Madersbacher et al., 2000).

Sexual activity places women at risk for all types of UTIs. The risk for cystitis is highest with vaginal intercourse. Any manipulation of the urethra, however, such as oral sex and masturbation, has some associated risk. Voiding prior to intercourse has not been shown to decrease risk of infection; however, voiding after intercourse decreases infection rates (Madersbacher et al., 2000; Murphy, 1999). Diaphragm and spermicide use greatly increases risk. Recent studies suggest that diaphragms spermicides may predispose women to UTIs by altering vaginal flora (Eriksen, 1999; Madersbacher et al., 2000; Murphy, 1999).

Transmission. Most often women serve as their own reservoir for pathogenic bacteria. Bacterial growth in the urinary tract of women is primarily related to urethral manipulation, most often as a result of intercourse. Residual urine, blockage of urine flow, or decreased voiding due to dehydration can also promote bacterial growth. Common pathogenic organisms in the urinary tract of women are listed in Table 22–21.

Urethritis may be caused by sexually transmitted diseases, primarily gonorrhea, chlamydia, and herpes. Urethritis and dysuria in males are usually secondary to sexually transmitted diseases; therefore, male partners with suspected urinary tract infections should be carefully assessed and treated for sexually transmitted diseases as appropriate. Some men develop dysuria in the presence of *Ureaplasma urealyticum,* which is not currently considered a cause of sexually transmitted disease.

Incidence. Approximately 20 percent of women will experience a lower urinary tract infection. Among women with a UTI, 25 percent with an acute uncomplicated infection will have a recurrence (Madersbacher et al., 2000; Schwartz, Wang, Eckert, & Critchlow, 1999) UTIs may occur at any time in the life span, but are more common with increasing age. The high prevalence rate with increased age is associated with falling estrogen levels, bladder emptying problems, an increase in chronic systemic problems, concurrent diseases, bowel incontinence, overuse of catheters, and poor nutrition (Eriksen, 1999; Nicolle, 2000).

Subjective Data

After data are collected, the primary care provider must discern whether symptoms are vaginal or urinary (see Table 22–22) and whether the upper urinary tract is

TABLE 22–21. Common Pathogenic Organisms in Women

Gram-Negative Pathogens	Gram-Positive Pathogens
Escherichia coli (responsible for >85% of UTIs)[a]	*Staphylococcus saprophyticus* (previously thought not to be a pathogen; now second most common cause of UTI in women)
Proteus mirabilis (a urea-splitting organism, associated with stone formation)	*Staphylococcus aureus*
Klebsiella species	Group A beta hemolytic streptococci
	Enterococci

[a] Urinary tract infections.
Source: Madersbacher et al. (2000); Murphy (1999).

TABLE 22–22. Historical Clues to Dysuria

Cystitis	Vaginitis	Urethritis
Abrupt onset	Gradual onset	Gradual onset
Internal dysuria	External dysuria	Internal dysuria
Change in voiding: frequency, urgency, small volumes, possibly nocturia and/or incontinence	No change in voiding pattern	May have some change in voiding pattern, no nocturia
Symptoms aggravated by voiding	Symptoms more continuous	Symptoms primarily associated with voiding
May have grossly bloody or odorous urine	No change in urine appearance	No change in urine appearance
No vaginal discharge	Vaginal discharge odor, itch, or irritation	May or may not have vaginal discharge or bleeding
10% complain of suprapubic tenderness	No abdominal symptoms	Abdominal pain if associated with pelvic inflammatory disease

involved (see Table 22–23). It is important to review a woman's history of UTIs or urinary problems and any recent medications; antibiotics will yield negative urine findings, and medications such as pyridium can make urine orange or green. Be sure to ask about over-the-counter medications such as those containing phenylpropanolamine or pseudoephedrine, which may impair bladder emptying (Clark et al., 2000; Murphy, 1999).

An accurate sexual history is crucial. Women do not always volunteer important information such as having vaginal discharge or a new sex partner and, consequently, need to be questioned carefully. Women can usually discern whether dysuria is internal or an external burning as the urine passes over the labia. Vaginal infections, such as *Trichomonas, Candida,* bacterial vaginosis, and herpes simplex, may cause external dysuria.

Most often, urethritis in women is caused by *Chlamydia trachomatis,* the most prevalent bacterial sexually transmitted disease in the United States. Infrequent infections of the urethra may include *Neiserria gonorrhoeae, Trichomonas,* herpes simplex, and *Candida.*

Dysuria occurring gradually over five to seven days is more characteristic of urethritis and acute pyelonephritis than cystitis, which usually has an abrupt onset. Urethritis symptoms, such as dysuria, with no recognized pathogens and no pyuria may be secondary to trauma or postmenopausal estrogen deficiency (Murphy, 1999).

TABLE 22–23. Differentiation of Upper and Lower Urinary Tract Infections by means of History and Physical Examination

Lower UTI[a] (Cystitis)	Upper UTI (Acute Pyelonephritis)
Usually sudden onset	Often gradual onset over >5 days
Dysuria and voiding symptoms	± Voiding symptoms
No systemic symptoms	Fever, chills, nausea, vomiting
No costovertebral angle tenderness	Often costovertebral angle tenderness
Serum WBC count normal	Serum WBC count often elevated
No WBC casts	May have WBC casts

[a] UTI, urinary tract infection; WBC, white blood cell.

Accurate discrimination between upper and lower UTIs by means of a history or physical exam is difficult. Because pyelonephritis can cause permanent renal damage or death, if untreated, it is crucial to try to make the correct diagnosis using a history (see Table 22–23). Differences may distinguish lower UTI (cystitis) from upper UTI (acute pyelonephritis). The typical presentation of acute pyelonephritis is abrupt onset of fever and flank pain; it may also be associated with generalized symptoms, such as nausea, vomiting, and chills. Pain may be perceived as low back or abdominal. Women with acute pyelonephritis may have no symptoms of dysuria or other common bladder symptoms.

History must confirm the presence or absence of any systemic symptoms: fever, chills, nausea, vomiting, diarrhea, headache, or malaise. Be sure to ask about any previous history of pyelonephritis or kidney stones. Cystitis is rarely associated with fever or systemic symptoms; therefore, the presence of fever or systemic symptoms is strongly suspicious of pyelonephritis. Risk factors for upper UTIs also need to be assessed.

Objective Data

Physical Examination. The client is generally assessed; occasionally a pelvic exam is necessary.

- *General Appearance.* A client with acute pyelonephritis may appear toxic.
- *Vital Signs.* Blood pressure and temperature are elevated.
- *Costovertebral Angle Tenderness.* Determine whether it is present.
- *Abdomen.* Check for suprapubic tenderness; a more extensive exam is done if the abdomen is very tender or if the bladder is palpable from distention.
- *Pelvic Exam.* A pelvic exam may or may not be indicated based on the history and results of lab tests. When it is done, examine Skene's and periurethral

glands. A pelvic exam may be necessary if the client has a history of external dysuria or gradual-onset dysuria especially with vaginal discharge or other vaginal symptoms; new or multiple sex partners; or internal dysuria (but the urinalysis appears benign with no pyuria).

Diagnostic Tests. Methods of testing include urine dipstick urinalysis, urine culture and sensitivity, vaginal wet mounts, and various cultures. The leukocyte esterase dipstick detects pyuria associated with infection. A positive reading on the leukocyte esterase dipstick correlates with ten or more WBCs per cubic millimeter (Sacher & McPherson, 2000).

Urinalysis is the cornerstone of diagnosis. It is important to teach women how to collect a urine specimen* and to examine urine within one hour of collection, because bacteria multiply (see Table 22–24)

Although a urine culture and sensitivity test is beneficial in determining the type of bacteria and its sensitivity to antibiotics, a urine culture and sensitivity test is not routinely done unless the client does not improve with treatment or the clinical picture is unclear. There is increasing evidence of bacterial resistance to trimethoprim-sulfamethoxazole (Bactrim) (Schaeffer & Stuppy, 1999). In cases of treatment failures, a culture and sensitivity test may be warranted to identify the causative organism and prescribe the best antibiotic.

With uncomplicated cystitis, urine pretreatment cultures are not recommended unless the diagnosis is in question. The purpose of posttreatment cultures is to rule out relapses or untreated foci of infection.

Pretreatment urine cultures are recommended in specific circumstances.

- All complicated urinary tract infections, including suspected pyelonephritis, history of structural abnormalities, and history of frequent urinary problems/infections
- Uncertain diagnosis
- Symptoms present longer than seven days
- History of UTI within preceding three weeks (possible relapse)

- History of recent catheterization or urologic surgery
- Pregnancy or suspected pregnancy
- Diabetes or other immunocompromising disorders

Posttreatment cultures are recommended in the following circumstances.

- Failure to improve with treatment
- Diagnosis of acute pyelonephritis
- Presence of complications

Vaginal wet (KOH and saline) mounts are used to rule out *Trichomonas, Candida,* and *bacterial vaginosis* (see Chapter 11).

STD cultures are done to rule out gonorrhea and chlamydia.

Differential Medical Diagnoses

Primary differential diagnoses are urethritis cystitis, and pyelonephritis (see Tables 22–22 and 22–23). Differential diagnoses also include asymptomatic bacteriuria, interstitial cystitis, and renal calculi.

Asymptomatic Bacteriuria. Asymptomatic bacteriuria is defined as bacteria in the urine with no symptoms of urinary tract infection. Whether to treat is debatable. Current recommendations are to treat pregnant women as if the condition were a urinary tract infection. Elderly women who have a high incidence of bacteriuria have not been harmed by asymptomatic bacteriuria nor do they benefit from treatment. In fact, treatment is expensive and may cause drug toxicity (Murphy, 1999).

Interstitial Cystitis. Interstitial cystitis is a syndrome of painful bladder without infection, characterized by urinary frequency, urgency, nocturia, and bladder pressure sensations that are often relieved by voiding. The urologist diagnoses interstitial cystitis by excluding other causes of painful bladder (cancer, tuberculosis, cystitis, herpes). Diagnosis is supported when cystoscopy reveals mucosal bleeding after distention of the bladder. Etiology is uncertain. (See Interstitial Cystitis in this chapter.)

Renal Calculi. Renal calculi, called kidney stones, may cause intermittent flank pain or pain that radiates around to the abdomen. They are associated with hematuria. Clients may develop superimposed urinary tract infections. Most calculi are composed of calcium oxalate and phosphate and can be visualized on x-ray of the kidney, ureter, and bladder. Uric acid stones, on the other hand, do not show up on x-rays and are associated with urea-

*Studies reported in the *Journal of Pediatrics, American Journal of Medicine,* and *New England Journal of Medicine* have shown that the procedure to obtain a clean catch urine specimen does not reduce bacterial contamination of urine cultures. A study of 100 women was reported in 1993 by the University of Virginia Health Sciences Center. It confirmed that to obtain a good urine sample for culture, it is not necessary to first clean the urinary meatus or to hold the labia apart while voiding.

TABLE 22–24. Urinalysis Findings Altered by Urinary Tract Infections[a]

Color/appearance	Often dark, turbid with foul smell; may be grossly bloody (hemorrhagic cystitis)
Dipstick	
Specific gravity	If too dilute, may be false-negative reading (i.e., low count of WBCs RBCs, bacteria).
pH	If very high pH, may be associated with urea stone-forming *Klebsiella;* low pH retards bacterial growth
Nitrites	Confirms presence of bacteria that convert nitrates to nitrites (does not always mean infection if asymptomatic; see asymptomatic bacteriuria section)
Protein	May have 1+ or 2+ protein with lower UTI; however, 3+ or 4+ urine deserves special attention and follow up to rule out kidney damage.
	Vaginal secretions may contaminate urine and give false positive for some protein; deserves follow-up
Leukocyte esterases	Quick way to determine pyuria, not as accurate as microscopic.
Microscopic Exam	Usually performed on spun urine; in women, normal urinary sediment may contain one or two RBCs and up to 4 WBCs per high-power field
RBCs	40–60% of women with cystitis have some microscopic hematuria; most common cause of hematuria is infection; also seen with stones, glomerulonephritis, neoplasm, tuberculosis
WBCs	May come from any part of urinary tract; "clumping" may be seen in infection; presence of 5–10 WBCs per high-power field is suspicious for UTI, although false positives are common in women
Bacteria	Usually visible in true infection
Casts	RBC and/or WBC casts indicate kidney involvement
Epithelial cells and mucous	Large amounts of either suspicious for vaginal contamination

[a] WBC, white blood cell; RBC, red blood cell; UTI, urinary tract infection.

splitting bacteria, such as *Proteus mirabilis.* UTIs with *Proteus* must be evaluated to rule out calculi (Spector, 1999).

Plan

Psychosocial Interventions. Discuss pain/discomfort management with the client and explain the mechanisms of urinary tract infections. Reassure her that a UTI is not a sexually transmitted disease, although intercourse may be mechanically related to the condition. Inform the woman so that she can identify her own precipitating factors and use appropriate preventive measures.

Medication. Table 22–25 lists the management options for cystitis and Table 22–26 describes outpatient management of acute pyelonephritis.

Surgical Interventions. Women with recurrent cystitis rarely have anatomic abnormalities that require surgical intervention. Referral to a urologist, however, is suggested for women with recurrent problems who have a history of childhood infections, more than one episode of acute pyelonephritis, possible nephrolithiasis, relapsing infections, infections caused by *Proteus mirabilis,* or

painless hematuria. Prolapse of the bladder, uterus, or rectum in older women may cause bladder outlet obstruction and impaired emptying resulting in urine stasis and increasing the risk of infection. These women may benefit from referral for urodynamic studies (Murphy, 1999).

Lifestyle Changes. Teach the client healthy voiding practices: void at first urge, void after intercourse. Encourage the client to make these practices routine. Advise her to maintain adequate hydration and to avoid use of contraceptive methods associated with increased UTI risk, such as a diaphragm.

Older women may benefit from use of estrogen cream therapy, 2 grams intravaginally twice a week. A recent trial demonstrated the efficacy of an estradiol-releasing ring on reducing UTIs in postmenopausal women. The silicone ring, containing 2 mg of estradiol, remains in the vagina for twelve weeks, during which time a steady amount of hormone is released. The subjects used the ring for 36 weeks. The investigator discovered that 80 percent of the control group and 51 percent of the experimental group developed UTIs during the study. Vaginal atrophy and irritation was significantly reduced in the experimental group (Eriksen, 1999). This

TABLE 22–25. Treatment Options for Uncomplicated and Recurrent Cystitis[a]

Uncomplicated Cystititis: Rare or Infrequent Episodes of Cystitis	
First-Line Medications	
1. Single-dose therapy	No longer recommended due to low rates of cure.
2. Three-day treatment	
Advantages	New area of study that combines decreased cost and decreased side effects.
Disadvantages	Twice the side effect rates as single dose; more research on effectiveness needed.
Medications of choice	TMP/SMX[b] double-strength tablets b.i.d. $\times$ 3 days or nitrofurantoin (Macrodantin) 50–100 mg q.i.d. $\times$ 3 days.
Client teaching	Call to return to clinic quickly if not improved or symptoms reappear.
3. Traditional 7- to 10-day treatment	
Advantages	Only a 5% failure rate; most research done with this approach.
Disadvantage	Twice the side effect rate of single dose, increased cost, decreased compliance.
Medication of choice	TMP/SMX DS b.i.d. $\times$ 7 days or nitrofurantoin 50 mg q.i.d. $\times$ 7 days.
Client teaching	Encourage finishing medication as ordered; if side effects occur, stop medications and telephone primary health care provider.

Second-Line Medications
Several new, expensive medications are now available for urinary tract infections. They should be reserved for clients with allergies or with resistant organisms, e.g., ciprofloxacin (Cipro) 250 or 500 mg b.i.d. $\times$ 7 days or norfloxacin (Noroxin) 400 mg b.i.d. $\times$ 7 days.

Recurrent Cystititis: Arbitrarily Defined as Three or More Episodes of Cystitis Per Year	
1. Postcoital prophylaxis	
Indications	Highly effective for the 85% of women who have onset of symptoms 24 to 48 hours after intercourse; intercourse does not occur as frequently as daily.
Medications	Oral antibiotic is taken just prior to or just after intercourse.
Options	50 mg nitrofuraniton, 250 mg cephalosporin, half single-strength TMX/SMX.
2. Intermittent self-start therapy	Client must be motivated and reliable about following directions.
Indications	Home dipslide cultures are prepared by client at onset of symptoms and the client self-starts traditional first-line antibiotics as prescribed; dip slides are inexpensive and save cost of two office visits; client must demonstrate a clear knowledge of the procedures and the signs of relapse and pyelonephritis.
	3-day course of traditional antibiotics
Medications	TMP/SMX double strength b.i.d. $\times$ 3 days or nitrofurantoin 50–100 mg q.i.d. $\times$ 3 days p.o.
3. Low-dose continuous prophylaxis	
Indications	Method of choice with high or daily sexual frequency; absence of any infection must be documented by urine culture prior to start.
Medications	Cephalexin (Keflex) 250 mg, trimethoprim 100 mg, TMP/SMX 1/2 tablet single strength. Given daily at bedtime or three times weekly; nitrofurantoin avoided, as long-term exposure may cause hypersensitivity reactions in the lung and kidney maybe an option during pregnancy; breakthrough infections treated with the full traditional 7-day therapy as indicated.

[a] See a current pharmacotherapeutics text for details.
[b] TMP/SMX, trimethoprim—sulfamethoxazole (Bactrim).

Source: Madersbacher et al. (2000); Murphy (1999); Schaeffer & Stuppy (1999).

may be a treatment option in the future for women who would prefer an alternate to current estrogen-delivery methods.

Follow-Up

Women should feel much improved within 24 to 48 hours of starting medication; if not, they should be instructed to telephone or return to the clinic. Teach clients the warning signs and symptoms of pyelonephritis and instruct them to telephone immediately if any of the symptoms develop.

For management of urethritis and vaginitis, see Chapter 11. For pregnant women, aggressive screening for urinary tract infection and treatment is recommended. UTIs and asymptomatic bacteriuria in preg-nancy are associated with increased fetal and maternal morbidity.

INTERSTITIAL CYSTITIS

Interstitial cystitis (IC) is a chronic, painful bladder disorder whose course is unpredictable. It is characterized by urinary frequency, urgency, nocturia, and suprapubic pain in the absence of urinary pathogens. The etiology is unknown, but most accepted theories involve an initial insult to the bladder wall by toxin, allergen, or immunologic agent that causes an inflammatory response.

Interstitial cystitis is frequently misdiagnosed as psychogenic in origin or goes undiagnosed for years. It can profoundly affect the client's ability to work and to

TABLE 22–26. Acute Pyelonephritis: Outpatient Management[a]

Criteria for Outpatient Management [b]
1. Diagnosis is secure (consult with physician)
2. No underlying, complicating disease, such as diabetes
3. Not pregnant
4. No history of recent urinary tract instrumentation
5. Not toxic, must be able to tolerate oral therapy and fluids
6. Follow-up must be easily accessible in 24 hours
7. Culture and sensitivity must be sent the day treatment is initiated

Medications
1. Must be broad spectrum (ampicillin and first-generation cephalosporins should not be used) trimethoprim—sulfamethoxazole (Bactrim) double strength b.i.d. or ciprofloxacin hydrochloride (Cipro) 500 mg b.i.d. for 14 days
2. Addition of a stat dose of intramuscular gentamicin (dose based on weight) or ceftriaxone 1 GM, IM used by some clinicians
3. Client should improve substantially in the first 24 hours; consult/refer if not improved.

[a] Consult a pharmacotherapeutics text for details.
[b] Woman must meet these criteria to attempt outpatient management.

maintain a home, family, and satisfying sexual relationship. There is no uniformly effective treatment; however, an individualized management plan that actively involves the client helps prevent permanent disability (Moldwin & Sant, 2002).

Epidemiology

Interstitial cystitis is thought to affect almost half a million people in the United States. It is often overlooked or misdiagnosed, resulting in lower documented numbers of persons with the disorder. Presently, 20,000 to 40,000 persons carry a diagnosis of interstitial cystitis. Ninety percent of IC sufferers are female, and the majority of them are between the ages of 40 and 60 (Henderson, 2000). Persons with IC may spend four to seven years and visit five physicians before receiving the appropriate diagnosis (Henderson, 2000; Parsons, 2002).

Theories of Etiology. Currently accepted theories of the origin of IC include epithelial cell dysfunction, mast cells, neurogenic causes, infection, and genetics.

Glycosaminoglycans provide a protective coating to the bladder urothelium, preventing the urine from leaking through and damaging nerves and muscles. It is hypothesized that the glycosaminoglycan layer is more permeable in persons with IC and that the leaking urine irritates nerves and creates the symptoms associated with IC (Henderson, 2000; Parsons, 2002; Warren & Keay, 2002). Several studies have shown that the instillation of solutions into the bladders of persons with IC resulted in either absorption of solutes into the bloodstream from the bladder (which did not occur in healthy controls without

IC) or irritation of the bladder (which did not occur in healthy controls without IC) (Chai, 2002; Parsons, 2002; Warren & Keay, 2002).

Mast cells are thought to be involved in the etiology of IC, but their role remains elusive. These cells may interact with existing nerve cells in the bladder lining, resulting in an up-regulation of nerve cells and thus increased pain pathways. Substance P, a small chain peptide, is also thought to play a part in IC (Parsons, 2002; Warren & Keay, 2002). Because some individuals with IC have responded to treatment with antibiotics, investigators believe that an organism or organisms may be responsible for IC (Warren & Keay, 2002). On the other hand, the occurrence of IC in identical twins and the relative lack of IC in fraternal twins points to a possible genetic predisposition (Warren & Keay, 2002). Finally, like many diseases, IC may be the result of multiple pathologies (Moldwin & Sant, 2002).

Subjective Data

The client may have consulted several health care providers in the past several months or years without getting relief from her symptoms. She will report urgency, frequency, and acute suprapubic pain. She may have to void every hour while awake and several times at night. She may complain of painful intercourse. Because of these disruptions in her life, she may be sleep deprived, anxious, depressed, and suffer from social isolation. She may describe periods of flare in symptoms right before her menses, at menopause, with certain foods, and/or at times of stress.

Be sure to ask about coexisting conditions such as migraine headaches, irritable bowel syndrome, fibromyalgia, chronic fatigue syndrome, allergies, and hypersensitivities to foods and medications. Review gynecologic history for previous urinary tract infections, pelvic inflammatory disease, vaginal infections, bladder instrumentation, hysterectomy, laporoscopic procedures. Ask her about both traditional and nontraditional treatments she has tried and the outcomes.

Objective Data

Physical Examination. The physical exam focuses on the abdomen and pelvis.

- *General Appearance.* The client may seem anxious. Her gait may be slow and measured to avoid jarring pain.
- *Vital Signs.* Afebrile.

- Palpate the back for costovertebral angle and lower back tenderness.
- Percuss the abdomen for bladder distension and palpate for suprapubic tenderness and masses.
- *Pelvic Exam.* Because interstitial cystitis is a diagnosis of exclusion, a complete pelvic exam is indicated to rule out infection, pelvic inflammatory disease, uterine and adnexal masses. Be sure to examine the urethra, Bartholin's and Skene's glands.

Diagnostic Tests. Urinalysis to detect infection, hematuria. Urinanalysis will be normal with interstitial cystitis.

Pregnancy test, wet prep, gonorrhea, and/or chlamydia cultures as indicated by exam.

Differential Medical Diagnoses

- *Cystitis.* Presence of white blood cells and bacteria in urine sediment.
- *Renal Calculi.* Presence of hematuria, colicky flank pain.
- *Pelvic or vaginal infection* indicated by exam, wet prep, cultures.
- *Pelvic masses* such as fibroid tumor, ovarian cyst detected by examination, history.
- *Genital herpes* indicated by history and presence of lesions.
- *Tubercular cystitis* and bladder detected on cystoscopy (see following).

Plan

Diagnosis/Management. The client is referred to the urologist for cystoscopy under general anesthesia. Diagnosis is made on the basis of presence of fissures, hemorrhage, and/or ulcers in the bladder wall and biopsy showing inflammatory process (presence of mast cells).

Psychosocial Interventions. Reassurance and support of the client are the first steps in alleviating some of her discomfort. She may feel overwhelming relief that her pain is considered real and not "all in her head." Actively involve her in the plan of care. Ask her to keep a diary of voiding patterns, symptoms, and flares with pain scales and associated conditions such as onset of menses, periods of high stress. When the diagnosis is confirmed by a urologist, refer her to the Interstitial Cystitis Association, a nonprofit organization that provides information and support and funds research.

The Interstitial Cystitis Association
P.O. Box 1553
New York, NY 10159–1553
www.ichel.org

Medication. There is no definitive medical treatment for interstitial cystitis. Occasionally, the dilatation of the bladder during diagnostic cystoscopy results in relief of symptoms.

Pentosan Polysulfate Sodium (Elmiron). This polysaccharide is structurally similar to heparin but with one-fifteenth of its anticoagulant properties. The drug is taken orally, 100 mg three times a day (Moldwin & Sant, 2002). Studies have shown that up to 900 mg in three divided doses may be needed for control of symptoms (Parsons, 2002). Common side effects include dyspepsia, reversible alopecia, and increased bruising. Please consult a pharmacology text for additional information.

Amitriptyline. 10 mg to 75 mg po at night is used for its analgesic and anticholinergic properties (Moldwin & Sant, 2002). See previous discussion of amitriptyline in section on fibromyalgia.

Hydroxyzine (Atarax). 25 to 50 mg po at night may be prescribed for its anticholinergic property of inhibiting mast cell production (Moldwin & Sant, 2002). See previous discussion of hydroxyzine in section on common dermatoses.

Dimethylsulfoxide (DMSO Solution). One of the experimental modalities of treatment uses dimethylsulfoxide (DMSO solution) a solvent thought to have anti-inflammatory properties. A urologist instills 30 to 50 cc into the bladder at weekly intervals. Results have not been consistent in relieving symptoms, and the client often relapses when installations are stopped.

Lifestyle Changes. Because no medication appears to show consistent relief of symptoms, an individualized approach to the client involving a self-care regimen is recommended.

The most effective plans include the following:

- *Dietary Modifications.* Avoidance of high acid foods and fluids that contain high fat and low carbohydrates. See Table 22–27. Obviously, eliminating all of the food in Table 22–27 would be impossible. Some persons with IC have no food sensitivities. Advise the client to begin with a bland diet and slowly add foods, paying attention to any symptoms that

TABLE 22–27. Dietary Modifications For Interstitial Cystitis

Foods to Avoid	
Chocolate	Alcoholic beverages
Soy sauce	Hot, spicy foods
Fruits, especially citrus or foods with citric acid	Coffee, tea, all caffeine
	Carbonated soft drinks
Artificial sweeteners	Avocado
Brewer's yeast	Cheese (especially aged)
Chicken liver	Corned beef
Fava and lima beans	Mayonnaise
Pickled herring	Onions (small amount for flavoring
Rye bread and rye products	acceptable)
Yogurt	Vitamins with aspartate, yeast, synthetic
Sour cream	vitamin D
High animal protein meals	Fermented foods
Vinegar and vinegar products	Tap water
Sprouts of any kind	Foods with molds
Foods with chemical additives	Fried foods
Hydrogenated fats including margarine or shortening	Smoked foods

Note: There are no controlled studies suggesting that dietary changes can relieve symptoms; however, many clients identify acid foods or fluids with exacerbation of symptoms.

Source: Moldwin & Sant (2002).

begin within 30 minutes to 6 hours after ingestion (Moldwin & Sant, 2002). If symptoms occur, have her eliminate that food until symptoms lessen, then proceed with more additions. Including high fiber foods may also be helpful. Encourage the client to drink 64 ounces of water daily. Many IC sufferers restrict their fluid intake, thinking that this will minimize their symptoms. Instead, water restriction results in concentrated urine, which may aggravate their symptoms (Moldwin & Sant, 2002). Eating several small meals per day instead of large meals.

- *Nutritional Supplements.* Vitamins A, B_6, and C may have protective effects on the bladder. Vitamin E is a natural vasodilator. Magnesium may have antianxiety properties.
- *Stress Reduction.* Stress is the most significant factor for flare of symptoms. Adequate rest, exercise, participation in support group, and relaxation techniques such as yoga and deep-breathing are recommended.
- *Bladder Retraining.* Used when pain is absent or at lower level. Method is to increase time between voids in intervals, for instance, 10 to 15 minutes longer each time.

Set goal with client for target time between voids based on voiding pattern before treatment began. Teach her how to do Kegel's exercises (Moldwin & Sant, 2002)

(See discussion in section that follows on urinary incontinence.)

Follow-Up

Continue to follow for primary health care. As with other pain syndromes, it is better to schedule client for regular visits to assess response to therapy. A suggested interval may be every two weeks at the beginning of the treatment plan and then monthly. Maintain close communication with urologist.

URINARY INCONTINENCE

Urinary incontinence (UI) is the involuntary loss of urine that is demonstrable and that is sufficient to be a social or hygienic problem (Luft & Vriheas-Nichols, 1998). It is a common and costly problem in younger and older women. It has significant psychosocial and economic impact on the individual, her caregivers, and society. It is estimated that less than half the individuals with UI consult health care providers about the problem. This may be due to its acceptance as a natural condition of aging, the availability of absorbent products (minipads and Depends), and lack of information on treatment options and benefits (DuBeau, 2000; Luft & Vriheas-Nichols, 1998).

Appropriate management can result in significant improvement. Development of an effective treatment plan depends on accurate identification of the subtype of urinary incontinence.

Subtypes

Control of bladder function is maintained by voluntary and involuntary mechanisms. The detrusor muscles of bladder and internal urethral sphincter are under autonomic nervous system control, which may be modulated by cerebral cortex connections. The external urethral sphincter and pelvic floor muscles are under voluntary control.

Other factors that contribute to urinary continence include adequate estrogen, which may help maintain bladder sphincter tone; adequate bladder capacity, elasticity, and smooth muscle tone; maintenance of an acute posterior urethravesicular angle to support the bladder neck and urethra.

Subtypes of urinary incontinence are based on compromise of aforementioned mechanisms.

Urge incontinence is the involuntary loss of urine associated with a strong desire to void. It is caused by *detrusor instability* due to involuntary detrusor contractions. These involuntary contractions may be caused by a neurological disorder such as stroke or multiple sclerosis, or occur as part of the aging process.

Stress urinary incontinence (SUI) is involuntary loss of urine during coughing, sneezing, laughing, or other physical activities that increase intraabdominal pressure. The most common cause of SUI in women is urethral hypermobility or significant displacement of the urethra and bladder when intraabdominal pressure is increased. Other causes include intrinsic urethral sphincter weakness, which may be congenital or acquired after trauma or radiation therapy, multiple incontinence surgical procedures, spinal cord lesion, or hypoestrogenism.

In older women UI is most often a combination of urge and stress incontinence. It is important to identify which component is most bothersome in order to target treatment.

Overflow incontinence is the result of overdistention of the bladder. It usually presents with frequent or constant dribbling or urge/stress incontinence symptoms. It is caused by under-active or a contractile detrusor or by bladder outlet obstruction. Medications (diuretics, anticholinergics, psychotropics, alpha-adrenergic blockers), neurologic conditions such as diabetic neuropathy, spinal cord injury, or radical pelvic surgery causing prolapse of pelvic organs may impair or alter the innervation of the detrusor muscle. Overflow incontinence secondary to outlet obstruction is rare in women.

Other types of incontinence include functional incontinence caused by factors outside the urinary tract such as chronic physical or cognitive impairment and unconscious or reflex incontinence common in paraplegics (Finucane, 1999).

Epidemiology

Urinary incontinence (UI) affects 13 million persons in the United States, predominantly women. The prevalence increases with age and is one of the major reasons for institutionalization (DuBeau, 2000; Finucane, 1999).

Risk factors for development of UI in women include increasing age, increased parity, immobility, impaired cognition, obesity, medications (diuretics, anticholinergic agents, psychotropics, narcotic analgesics, alpha-adrenergic blockers), hysterectomy, smoking, alcohol use, fecal impaction, estrogen depletion, pelvic muscle weakness, and childhood nocturnal enuresis. Of these factors that are modifiable, obesity and hysterectomy may have the most impact on prevention of daily incontinence (DuBeau, 2000; Finucane, 1999; Luft & Vriheas-Nichols, 1998).

Subjective Data

Information should include a focused medical, neurologic, and genitourinary history that includes the above cited risk factors and a review of medication use, both prescribed and over the counter.

Ask detailed questions about the associated symptoms and factors of her incontinent episodes including the following:

- ◆ Duration and characteristics (stress, urge, dribbling)
  - What symptoms are most bothersome to the client
  - Frequency, timing, and amount of continent and incontinent voids, e.g., dribbles in underpants vs soaking through clothing
  - Triggers of incontinence (cough, exercise, surgery, trauma, new medication)
  - Other lower urinary tract symptoms such as nocturia, dysuria, hesitancy, weak and/or thin stream, hematuria, suprapubic pain
  - Fluid intake, especially coffee or other caffeine containing foods and fluids
  - Alterations in bowel, sexual function
  - Previous treatment and outcome
  - Amount of absorbent pads, briefs (Depends) used
  - Expectations of treatment
  - Psychosocial evaluation of mental status, mobility, living environment

Objective Data

Physical Examination

- ◆ Vital signs for hypertension, elevated temperature.
- ◆ Gait for mobility.
- ◆ Neuromuscular assessment to detect abnormalities that suggest multiple sclerosis, stroke, spinal cord lesion, and to assess cognition, strength, and manual dexterity.
- ◆ Cardiovascular status for presence of edema that may contribute to nocturia.
- ◆ Lungs for crackles or wheezes that may indicate congestive heart failure, chronic obstructive pulmonary disease, asthma that may contribute to cough.
- ◆ Abdominal examination to assess for organomegaly, masses, diastesis recti, bladder distension, or other factors that may affect intraabdominal pressure.

◆ Rectal examination to assess sphincter tone, presence of fecal impaction, rectal mass.
◆ Pelvic examination to assess perineal skin, genital atrophy, pelvic organ prolapse (cystocele, rectocele, uterine prolapse), pelvic mass. Palpate anterior vaginal wall for discharge from urethra or tenderness, which suggests diverticulum, carcinoma, or inflammation of the urethra.

Diagnostic Tests Urinalysis to detect hematuria (infection, cancer, stone), glucosuria (polyuria), pyuria, and bacteria.

Cough Stress Test. Test is done when bladder is full but before urge to void is strong. Done in lithotomy position. Examiner observes for urine loss from urethra while client coughs vigorously. If instant loss, SUI likely. If leakage delayed or persists after cough, detrusor instability may be cause of UI. If no leakage and symptoms suggest SUI, perform test in upright posture.

Postvoid Residual (PVR). Can be done by catheterization or pelvic ultrasound. Observation of urine stream can be noted for hesitancy, straining, slow or interrupted stream. Measure postvoid residual within a few minutes after voiding. It is generally accepted that PVRs fewer than 50 cc are normal. If repetitive PVRs range from 100 to 200cc, then inadequate emptying. One measure of PVR may not be sufficient.

If transient, reversible, or modifiable causes of UI have been detected, client may need no further evaluation and may be treated with trial of medications and behavioral modalities described subsequently.

Plan

Those who should be referred to a urogynecologic specialist include the following:

◆ Those whose UI persists after initial therapeutic trial
◆ Uncertain diagnosis (lack of correlation between symptoms and findings)
◆ Consideration of surgical referral especially if failure of previous surgery
◆ Hematuria without infection
◆ Comorbid conditions such as incontinence with recurrent symptoms of urinary tract infection, persistent difficulty emptying bladder, history of radical pelvic surgery, symp-tomatic pelvic prolapse, abnormal PVR, neurological condition (Finucane, 1999).

Psychosocial Interventions. Because urinary incontinence is so common and underreported, it is suggested that questions about bladder function be a routine part of the annual gynecologic exam for women of all ages. Not only can this lead to prompt treatment of reversible causes of UI but also can relieve client hesitancy in bringing the subject up.

Client education about causes and initial therapy are important in order to reassure her that certain modalities may relieve or resolve her incontinence. Be realistic. In some clients, incontinence may never be cured but may only be manageable. Advise client that corrective surgery or bladder tuck may not cure incontinence. Be sure to refer her to support groups such as

National Association for Continence
(formerly Help for Incontinent People)
PO Box 8310
Spartanburg, SC 29305
(800) BLADDER or (800) 252-3337

Medication

Stress Urinary Incontinence

ESTROGEN. Postmenopausal women in whom stress incontinence is related to intrinsic sphincter atrophy may benefit from estrogen replacement as the initial therapy. (See hormone replacement therapy in Chapter 15.) The estrogen may be administered orally, transdermally, or transvaginally. Some reports suggest topical estrogen may bring faster relief by local effect. Remember women with intact uteri should be given a progestin.

◆ *Expected Outcome.* Advise her that beneficial effects may not occur earlier than six to twelve weeks after initiation of treatment.

IMIPRAMINE. Alternative is imipramine (Tofranil). An anticholinergic and alpha-adrenergic agonist. May be of benefit. No large scale studies to support its use.

◆ *Administration.* 75 mg p.o. daily if first-line medications fail or are contraindicated. Nighttime dose may be used to avoid daytime drowsiness.
◆ *Adverse Effects.* Nausea, drowsiness or insomnia, weakness, fatigue, postural hypotension.
◆ *Contraindications.* Known hypersensitivity to tricyclic antidepressants, recovery phase of myocardial infarction. Caution in cardiovascular disease.

Urge Incontinence with Detrusor Instability

ANTICHOLINERGIC AGENTS. First-line medications are anticholinergic agents that work by blocking bladder contractions and relaxing sphincter muscle.

OXYBUTYNIN. (Ditropan) 2.5 to 5.0 po three times a day. Also available in a controlled-release formula (Ditropan XL).

- *Adverse Effects.* Dry skin, dry mouth, blurred vision, change in mental status, nausea, constipation.
- *Contraindications.* Known hypersensitivity, narrow angle glaucoma (not wide angle), gastrointestinal or urinary obstruction, myasthenia gravis.
- *Expected Outcome.* Advise improvement usually modest.

TOLTERODINE TARTRATE (DETROL). 2 mg twice daily, with or without food.

- *Mode of Action.* Muscarinic receptor antagonist, decreases bladder contractions. Has more specificity for bladder than oxybutynin.
- *Adverse Effects.* Dry mouth, headache, vertigo/dizziness, abdominal pain, fatigue, constipation, dyspepsia, and urinary retention.
- *Contraindications.* Urinary retention, gastric retention, uncontrolled narrow angle glaucoma. Use with caution in clients being treated for narrow angle glaucoma.
- *Expected Outcome.* Advise improvement may be modest (Baker, 2002).

PROPANTHELINE. Second-line anticholinergic is Propantheline (Pro-Banthine) 7.5 to 30 mg po three to five times a day.

- *Adverse Effects.* Urinary retention, blurred vision, dry mouth, nausea, constipation, tachycardia, drowsiness, confusion.
- *Contraindications.* Known hypersensitivity, narrow angle glaucoma, urinary or gastrointestinal obstruction, myasthenia gravis.
- *Expected Outcome.* Advise degree of improvement may be modest.

Both the aforementioned medications should be used only in conjunction with voiding schedule or behavioral interventions as discussed subsequently. Client must be carefully monitored for urinary retention.

TRICYCLIC ANTIDEPRESSANTS. Tricyclic antidepressants such as Imipramine (see prior discussion) as smooth muscle relaxant may also be effective.

Overflow Incontinence Due to Detrusor Hypomobility (When Obstruction Is Ruled Out). Is usually the result of neurological disorders such as diabetic neuropathy. Anticholinergics and tricyclic antidepressants should be avoided. Pharmacologic intervention is usually ineffective except for Bethanecol.

BETHANECOL. (Urecholine) 10 to 25 mg three to four times a day (Clark et al., 2000).

- *Mode of Action.* Cholinergic agonist that stimulates muscarinic receptors of parasympathetic nervous system. Increases tone of detrusor muscle resulting in contraction, decreased bladder capacity, and subsequent urination.
- *Adverse Effects.* Abdominal pain, diarrhea, bradycardia, hypotension, bronchoconstriction.
- *Contraindications.* Known hypersensitivity, coronary artery disease, peptic ulcer, Parkinsonism, asthma.
- *Expected Outcome.* Advise client may be ineffective. Check postvoid residual urine volumes before and after treatment to assess efficacy.

Behavioral Interventions

- *Habit training* is targeting scheduled voids to match client's voiding habits as observed by caregiver. It can achieve good results with those who are homebound and have a caregiver.
- *Bladder training* is recommended for management of urge incontinence and mixed stress and urge incontinence. Client is advised to resist urge to void or postpone voiding and urinate on a fixed schedule. Initial goal is usually set for 2 to 3 hours between voids while awake. Adjustment of fluid intake may be needed. Goal is to increase intervals over a period of several months.
- *Pelvic muscle exercises* are especially useful for stress urinary incontinence and urge incontinence. The first step is to make the client more aware of muscle function. The examiner teaches the woman how to do the exercises by inserting the gloved finger into vagina and instructs client to tighten muscles around finger. Client is advised to sustain contraction for at least 2 to 4 seconds followed by an equal period of relaxation. She is instructed to perform these exercises with five repetitions every half-hour during the day, or alternatively, for 10 minutes twice a day. The key is consistency. Advise her to contract these muscles before and during situations when leaking occurs (e.g., cough, sneeze, laughter, exercise).

Other behavioral modalities that may be of benefit include biofeedback, vaginal weight training, and pelvic floor electrical stimulation. These may be used in conjunction with pelvic muscle exercises. Consult physician or urogynecologist for referral.

Diet/Lifestyle. Client education regarding factors that may impact incontinence include the following:

- Avoiding excessive alcohol and caffeine.
- Use of fiber and stool softeners to avoid constipation.
- Medications that may have adverse effects on incontinence including diuretics, psychotropic agents, narcotic analgesics, over-the-counter products for appetite control and colds, calcium channel blockers.
- Control of blood sugar to prevent polyuria.
- If prescribed diuretics are part of treatment for co-existing medical conditions, edema dosages may be minimized by use of nonpharmacologic interventions such as use of support stockings, leg elevation, and sodium restriction.
- Barriers to reaching toilet and environmental alterations such as bedside commode.

Follow-Up

Telephone follow-up in one week to assess adherence and barriers to treatment plan. Office visit in two weeks. Try initial treatment for four to six weeks. If no improvement, refer to physician or urogynecologist for further urodynamic studies.

REFERENCES

Ables, J. C. (2002). New drug: Mobic (Meloxicam). *Prescriber's Letter* [On-line]. Available: *www.prescribersletter.com Detail-Document#: 160610.* Accessed June 18, 2002.

Allen, J. (2002). New drug: Celecoxib (Celebrex, formerly Celebra). *Prescriber's Letter* [On-line]. Available: *www.prescribersletter.com Detail-Document#: 150125.* Accessed June 18, 2002.

Altman, R. D., Hochberg, M. C., Moskowitz, R., & Schnitzer, T. J. (2000). Recommendations for the medical management of osteoarthritis of the hip and knee: American College of Rheumatology Subcommittee on Osteoarthritis Guidelines. *Arthritis & Rheumatism, 43,* 1905–1915.

American Thoracic Society. (2001). Guidelines for the management of adults with community-acquired pneumonia. *American Journal of Respiratory and Critical Care Medicine, 163,* 1730–1754.

Baker, D. E. (2002). Tolterodine tartrate (Detrol). *Prescriber's Letter* [On-line]. Available: *www.prescribersletter.com Detail-Document#: 140508.* Accessed June 26, 2002.

Bark, J., Curhan, G. C., & Rimm, E. B. (2000). A prospective study of age and lifestyle factors in relation to community-acquired pneumonia in U.S. men and women. *Archives of Internal Medicine, 160,* 3082–3088.

Barnes, P. J. (2001). Chronic obstructive pulmonary disease. *New England Journal of Medicine, 343,* 269–280.

Bartlett, J. G., Davell, S. F., & Mandell, L. A. (2000). Guidelines for the management of community acquired pneumonia in adults. *Clinical Infectious Disease, 31,* 347–382.

Blanchard, A. R. (2002). Treatment of COPD exacerbations. *Postgraduate Medicine, 111,* 65–75.

Boldt, M. D., & Kiresuk, T. (2001). Community-acquired pneumonia in adults. *Nurse Practitioner, 26,* 14–23.

Boyle, C. A. (1999). Management of menstrual migraine. *Neurology, 53,* S14–S18.

Burson, S. C. (2002). Rofecoxib (Vioxx). *Prescriber's Letter* [On-line]. Available: *www.prescribersletter.com Detail-Document#: 150602.* Accessed June 18, 2002.

Butcher, J., Salzman, K., & Lilligard, W. (1996). Lower extremity bursitis. *American Family Physician, 53,* 2317–2324.

Byank, R. P., & Beatie, W. E. (1999). Exercise-related musculoskeletal problems. In L. R. Barker, J. R. Burton, & P. D. Zieve (Eds.), *Principles of ambulatory medicine* (5th ed., pp. 939–959). Philadelphia: Lippincott, Williams, & Wilkins.

Centers for Disease Control and Prevention (CDC). (2001). *Women and smoking: A report of the surgeon general—2001.* Center for Disease Control and Prevention [On-line]. Available: *http://www.cdc.gov/tobacco/sgr/sgr_forwomen/factsheet_outcomes.htm.* Accessed: June 11, 2002.

Chai, T. C. (2002). Diagnosis of the painful bladder syndrome: Current approaches to diagnosis. *Clinical Obstetrics & Gynecology, 45,* 250–258.

Clark, J. B. F., Queener, S. F., & Karb, V. B. (2000). *Pharmacological basis of nursing practice* (6th ed.) St. Louis: Mosby.

Clark, S. & Odell, L. (2000). Fibromyalgia syndrome: Common, real and treatable. *Clinician Reviews, 10,* 57–64.

Clarke Stevens, J., Witt, J. C., Smith, B. E., & Weaver, A. L. (2001). The frequency of carpal tunnel syndrome in computer users at a medical facility. *Neurology, 56,* 1568–1570.

Couch, R. B. (2000). Prevention and treatment of influenza. *New England Journal of Medicine, 343,* 1778–1787.

Della-Giustina, D. (1998). Guidelines for treating common—and uncommon—back pain syndromes. *Consultant, 38,* 1528–1537.

Department of Health and Human Services (DHHS). (2001a). Executive summary. Department of Health and Human Services [On-line]. Available: *http://aspe.hhs.gov/sp/asthma/overview.htm.* Accessed: June 11, 2002.

Department of Veterans Affairs. (1999). *Low back pain or sciatica in the primary care setting.* Bethesda, MD: Department of Veterans Affairs.

Doherty, D. E. (2002). Early detection and management of COPD. *Postgraduate Medicine, 111,* 41–60.

DuBeau, C. E. (2000). Urinary incontinence. In J. G. Evans, T. F. Williams, B. L. Beattie, J. P. Michel, & G. K. Wilcock (Eds.), *Oxford textbook of geriatric medicine* (2nd ed., pp. 677–689). Oxford: Oxford University Press.

England, J. D. (1999). Entrapment neuropathies. *Current Opinion in Neurology, 12,* 597–602.

Eriksen, B. (1999). A randomized, open, parallel-group study on the preventive effect of an estradiol-releasing vaginal ring (Estring) on recurrent urinary tract infections in postmenopausal women. *American Journal of Obstetrics & Gynecology, 180,* 1072–1079.

Felson, D. T., & Nevitt, M. C. (1999). Estrogen and osteoarthritis: How do we explain conflicting study results? *Preventive Medicine, 28,* 445–448.

Finucane, T. E. (1999). Geriatric medicine: Special considerations. In L. R. Barker, J. R. Burton, & P. D. Zieve (Eds.), *Principles of ambulatory medicine* (5th ed., pp. 82–98). Philadelphia: Lippincott, Williams, & Wilkins.

Folstein, M. J., Folstein, S., & McHugh, P. R. (1975). Mini-mental state: A practical method for grading the cognitive status of patients for the clinician. *Journal of Psychiatric Research, 12,* 189–198.

Friedland, R. P., & Wilcock, G. K. (2000). Dementia. In J. G. Evans, T. F. Williams, B. L. Beattie, J. P. Michel, & G. K. Wilcock (Eds.), *Oxford textbook of geriatric medicine* (2nd ed., pp. 922–932). Oxford: Oxford University Press.

Golding, J. M. (1999). Sexual assault history and headache: Five general population studies. *Journal of Nervous & Mental Disease, 187,* 624–629.

Grogan, P. M., & Gronseth, G. S. (2001). Practice parameter: Steroids, acyclovir, and surgery for Bell's palsy (an evidence-based review): Report of the Quality Standards Subcommittee of the American Academy of Neurology. *Neurology, 56,* 830–836.

Hasso, A. N., Drayer, B. P., Anderson, R. E., Braffman, B., Davis, P. C., Deck, M. D. F., Johnson, B. A., Masaryk, T., Pomeranz, S. J., Seidenwurm, D., Tanenbaum, L., & Masdeu, J. C. (1999). *American College of Radiology appropriateness criteria: Vertigo and hearing loss.* American College of Radiology [On-line]. Available: *http://www.acr.org.* Accessed June 6, 2002.

Hebert, L. E., Beckett, L. A., Scherr, P. A., & Evans, D. A. (2001). Annual incidence of Alzheimer disease in the United States projected to the years 2000 through 2050. *Alzheimer Disease & Associated Disorders, 15,* 169–173.

Hellmann, D. B. (1999). Nonarticular rheumatic disorders. In L. R. Barker, J. R. Burton, & P. D. Zieve (Eds.), *Principles of ambulatory medicine* (5th ed., 928–938 Philadelphia:) Lippincott, Williams, & Wilkins.

Henderson, L. J. (2000). Diagnosis, treatment, and lifestyle changes of interstitial cystitis. *AORN Journal, 71,* 525–530.

International Consensus report on diagnosis and treatment of asthma. (1992). (NIH Publication No. 92-3091).

Ignatavicius, D. D. (2001). Rheumatoid arthritis and the older adult. *Geriatric Nursing, 22,* 139–142.

Jablonski, R. A. S. (2000). Discovering asthma in the older adult. *Nurse Practitioner, 25,* 14–39.

Jankovic, J. (2000). Parkinson's disease therapy: Tailoring choices for early and late disease, young and old patients. *Clinical Neuropharmacology, 23,* 252–261.

Janson, S., & Lazarus, S. C. (2002). Where do leukotriene modifiers fit in asthma management? *Nurse Practitioner, 27,* 19–29.

Johnson, C. J. (1999). Headaches and facial pain. In L. R. Barker, J. R. Burton, & P. D. Zieve (Eds.), *Principles of ambulatory medicine* (5th ed., pp. 1214–1229). Philadelphia: Lippincott, Williams, & Wilkins.

Johnson, G. D. (1998). Medical management of migraine-related dizziness and vertigo. *Laryngoscope, 108,* 1–28.

Kaplan, P. W. (1999). Seizure disorders. In L. R. Barker, J. R. Burton, & P. D. Zieve (Eds.), *Principles of ambulatory medicine* (5th ed., pp. 1230–1251). Philadelphia: Lippincott, Williams, & Wilkins.

Kaye, J. A. (1998). Diagnostic challenges in dementia. *Neurology, 51,* S45–S52.

Kehoe, W. A. (2002). New drug: Valdecoxib (Bextra). *Prescriber's Letter* [On-line]. Available: *www.prescribersletter.com Detail-Document#: 180102.* Accessed June 18, 2002.

Kern, D. E. (1999). Shoulder pain. In L. R. Barker, J. R. Burton, & P. D. Zieve (Eds.), *Principles of ambulatory medicine* (5th ed., pp. 891–905). Philadelphia: Lippincott, Williams, & Wilkins.

Klippel, J. H., & Arayssi, T. (2000). Connective tissue disorders. In J. G. Evans, T. F. Williams, B. L. Beattie, J. P. Michel, & G. K. Wilcock (Eds.), *Oxford textbook of geriatric medicine* (2nd ed., pp. 585–593). Oxford: Oxford University Press.

Kwoh, C. K., Anderson, L. G., Greene, J. M., Johnson, D. A., O'Dell, J. R., Robbins, M. L., Roberts, W. N., Simms, R. W., & Yood, R. A. (2002). Guidelines for the management of rheumatoid arthritis: American College of Rheumatology Subcommittee on Rheumatoid Arthritis Guidelines. *Arthritis & Rheumatism, 45,* 328–346.

Lee, D. M., & Weinblatt, M. E. (2001). Rheumatoid arthritis. *Lancet, 358,* 903–911.

Liu, S. H., & Nguyen, T. M. (1999). Ankle sprains and other soft tissue injuries. *Current Opinion in Rheumatology, 11,* 132–135.

Luft, J., & Vriheas-Nichols, A. A. (1998). Identifying the risk factors for developing incontinence: Can we modify individual risk? *Geriatric Nursing, 19,* 66–70.

Madersbacher, S., Thalhammer, F., & Marberger, M. (2000). Pathogenesis and management of recurrent urinary tract infection in women. *Current Opinion in Urology, 10,* 29–33.

Matsumoto, A. K., & Wigley, F. M. (1999). Rheumatoid arthritis. In L. R. Barker, J. R. Burton, & P. D. Zieve (Eds.), *Principles of ambulatory medicine* (5th ed., pp. 988–1010). Philadelphia: Lippincott, Williams, & Wilkins.

McAlindon, T. (2000). Update on the epidemiology of systemic lupus erythematosus: New spins on old ideas. *Current Opinion in Rheumatology, 12,* 104–112.

McAlindon, T. E., LaValley, M. P., Gulin, J. P., & Felson, D. T. (2000). Glucosamine and chondroitin for treatment of osteoarthritis: A systematic quality assessment and meta-analysis. *JAMA, 283,* 1469–1475.

Millea, P. J., & Holloway, R. L. (2000). Treating fibromyalgia. *American Family Physician, 62,* 1575–1587.

Moldwin, R. M., & Sant, G. R. (2002). Interstitial cystitis: A pathophysiology and treatment update. *Clinical Obstetrics & Gynecology, 45,* 259–272.

Murphy, P. A. (1999). Genitourinary infections. In L. R. Barker, J. R. Burton, & P. D. Zieve (Eds.), *Principles of ambulatory medicine* (5th ed., pp. 331–341). Philadelphia: Lippincott, Williams, & Wilkins.

National Heart, Lung and Blood Institute (NHLBI). (1999). *Data fact sheet: Asthma statistics.* Bethesda, MD: U.S. Department of Health and Human Services.

National Institutes of Health (2002). *Guidelines for the diagnosis and management of asthma—update on selected topics 2002.* (NIH Publication No. 02-5075). Bethesda, Maryland.

Nicolle, L. E. (2000). Urinary tract infection. In J. G. Evans, T. F. Williams, B. L. Beattie, J. P. Michel, & G. K. Wilcock (Eds.), *Oxford textbook of geriatric medicine* (2nd ed., pp. 700–712). Oxford: Oxford University Press.

Olanow, C. W., Watts, R. L., & Koller, W. C. (2001). An algorithm (decision tree) for the management of Parkinson's disease: Treatment guidelines. *Neurology, 56,* S1–S88.

Olney, R. K. (2001). Carpal tunnel syndrome: Complex issues with a "simple" condition. *Neurology, 56,* 1431–1432.

Palacioz, K. (2002). Choosing NSAIDs. *Prescriber's Letter* [On-line]. Available: *www.prescribersletter.com Detail-Document#: 161017.* Accessed June 18, 2002.

Parsons, C. L. (2002). Interstitial cystitis: Epidemiology and clinical presentation. *Clinical Obstetrics & Gynecology, 45,* 242–249.

Perez, V. L., & Foster, C. S. (2001). Uveitis with neurological manifestations. *International Ophthalmology Clinics, 41,* 41–59.

Philadelphia Panel. (2001). Philadelphia Panel evidence-based clinical practice guidelines on selected rehabilitation interventions for low back pain. *Physical Therapy, 8,* 1641–1675.

Pierce, N. F. (1999). Undifferentiated acute febrile illness. In L. R. Barker, J. R. Burton, & P. D. Zieve (Eds.), *Principles of ambulatory medicine* (5th ed., pp. 307–311). Philadelphia: Lippincott, Williams, & Wilkins.

Prisco, M. K. (2002). Update your understanding of influenza. *Nurse Practitioner, 27,* 32–38.

Quinn, C. J., Mathews, D. E., Noyes, R. F., Oliver, G. E., Thimons, J. J., & Thomas, R. K. (1999). *Optometric clinical practice guideline: Care of the patient with conjunctivitis.* St. Louis, MO: American Optometric Association.

Rennard, S. I. (2002). Overview of causes of COPD. *Postgraduate Medicine, 111,* 28–38.

Rockwood, K. (2000). Disordered levels of consciousness and acute confusional states. In J. G. Evans, T. F. Williams, B. L. Beattie, J. P. Michel, & G. K. Wilcock (Eds.), *Oxford textbook of geriatric medicine* (2nd ed., pp. 932–937). Oxford: Oxford University Press.

Rowan, A. J. (1998). Reflections on the treatment of seizures in the elderly population. *Neurology, 51,* S28–S33.

Sacher, R. A., & McPherson, R. A. (2000). *Widman's clinical interpretation of laboratory tests* (11th ed.) Philadelphia: F. A. Davis.

Safran, M. R., Benedetti, R. S., Bartolozzi, A. R., & Mandelbaum, B. R. (1999). Lateral ankle sprains: A comprehensive review. Part 1: etiology, pathoanatomy, histopathogenesis, and diagnosis. *Medicine and Science in Sports and Exercise, 31,* S429–S437.

Schachat, A. P. (1999a). Common problems associated with impaired vision: Cataracts and age-related macular degeneration. In L. R. Barker, J. R. Burton, & P. D. Zieve (Eds.), *Principles of ambulatory medicine* (5th ed., pp. 1473–1480). Philadelphia: Lippincott, Williams, & Wilkins.

Schachat, A. P. (1999b). Glaucoma. In L. R. Barker, J. R. Burton, & P. D. Zieve (Eds.), *Principles of ambulatory medicine* (5th ed., pp. 1481–1487). Philadelphia: Lippincott, Williams, & Wilkins.

Schachat, A. P. (1999c). The red eye. In L. R. Barker, J. R. Burton, & P. D. Zieve (Eds.), *Principles of ambulatory medicine* (5th ed., pp. 1488–1498). Philadelphia: Lippincott, Williams, & Wilkins.

Schaeffer, A. J., & Stuppy, B. A. (1999). Efficacy and safety of self-start therapy in women with recurrent urinary tract infections. *Journal of Urology, 161,* 207–211.

Schwartz, M. A., Wang, C. C., Eckert, L. O., & Critchlow, C. W. (1999). Risk factors for urinary tract infection in the postpartum period. *American Journal of Obstetrics & Gynecology, 181,* 547–553.

Silberstein, S. D. (2000). Practice parameter: Evidence-based guidelines for migraine headache (an evidence-based review): Report of the Quality Standards Subcommittee of the American Academy of Neurology. *Neurology, 55,* 754–762.

Sisson, S. D., & Kramer, P. D. (1999). Dizziness, vertigo, motion sickness, syncope and near syncope, and disequilibrium. In L. R. Barker, J. R. Burton, & P. D. Zieve (Eds.), *Principles of ambulatory medicine* (5th ed., pp. 1252–1273). Philadelphia: Lippincott, Williams, and Wilkins.

Spector, D. A. (1999). Urinary stones. In L. R. Barker, J. R. Burton, & P. D. Zieve (Eds.), *Principles of ambulatory medicine* (5th ed., pp. 565–576). Philadelphia: Lippincott, Williams, & Wilkins.

Szabo, R. (1998). Carpal tunnel syndrome as a repetitive motion disorder. *Clinical Orthopaedics and Related Research, 351,* 78–79.

Townes, A. S. (1999). Crystal-induced arthritis. In L. R. Barker, J. R. Burton, & P. D. Zieve (Eds.), *Principles of ambulatory medicine* (5th ed., pp. 974–988). Philadelphia: Lippincott, Williams, & Wilkins.

Trager, J., & Ward, M. M. (2001). Mortality and causes of death in systemic lupus erythematosus. *Current Opinion in Rheumatology, 13,* 345–351.

Wallace, D. J., & Linker-Israeli, M. (1999). It's not the same old lupus or Sjogren's any more: One hundred new insights, approaches, and options since 1990. *Current Opinion in Rheumatology, 11,* 321–329.

Warren, J. W., & Keay, S. K. (2002). Interstitial cystitis. *Current Opinion in Urology, 12,* 69–74.

Waterbury, L., & Zieve, P. D. (1999). Selected illnesses affecting lymphocytes: Mononucleosis, chronic lymphocytic leukemia, and the undiagnosed patient with lymphadenopathy. In L. R. Barker, J. R. Burton, & P. D. Zieve (Eds.), *Principles of ambulatory medicine* (5th ed., pp. 651–656). Philadelphia: Lippincott, Williams, & Wilkins.

CHAPTER 23

PSYCHOSOCIAL HEALTH CONCERNS

Angela Carter Martin

*F*or a woman to achieve changes for herself and her family, she must acknowledge her self-worth. The health care provider can play a vital supporting role.

Highlights

- Stress
- Abuse of Women
    Sexual Harassment
    Violence
    Sexual Abuse
- Substance Abuse
    Smoking Cessation
- Mental Health Problems
    Depression
    Anxiety
    Post-Traumatic Stress Disorder
    Anorexia Nervosa
    Bulimia
    Binge-Eating Disorder
- Homelessness

❖ INTRODUCTION

In the last forty years, women have striven to legitimately and fully participate in the social, political, and economic systems in our country. Technological advances, improved living conditions, and decreased mortality related to pregnancy and childbirth have contributed to a life expectancy at birth for a woman to 79.5 years (CDC, 2001).

Women have achieved these advances despite prejudice, oppression, lower incomes, and the perpetuation of harmful myths and stereotypes, including those inflicted by the medical establishment. They are naturally hardy, and their inherent strengths contribute to their ability to adapt and use effective coping. This chapter is written from a philosophy of empowerment and acceptance of the right for individual expression for all women; however, women, as well as men, do suffer from the effects of psychological stress and disability from psychological concerns and disorders. Despite recent criticism of psychiatry as attempting to socially control woman and participating in the medicalization of unhappiness (Wright & Owen, 2000), others have argued that to focus on one gender over the other only further distorts rather than clarifies an understanding of mental health issues (Busfield, 1996). Instead, authors have encouraged health care professionals to focus on gender relations as a way of understanding gender differences in psychiatric diagnoses. Crowe (2000) also criticizes the use of the DSM-IV as a way for the medical establishment to construct normality rather than describing the experience of psychological dysfunction in a way that is helpful to patients and their providers. The author also supports this view; however, the DSM-IV is the text that is used by a variety of health care professionals to classify and identify patients with certain problems. In the spirit of promoting communication among disciplines, the traditional DSM-IV nomenclature is used in this chapter. All health care providers are encouraged to look for cultural and gender biases inherent in traditional references and to take those into consideration when working with all patients. Despite these advances, women do experience excessive stress and mental health problems that are associated with alienation, powerlessness, and poverty (Barnes, Pase, & VanLeeuwen, 1999; Kenney & Bhattacharjee, 2000; Thomas, 1997).

To thoroughly address women's health, the primary care provider (PCP) must consider the potential psychosocial problems that women face. Women experience higher rates of selected mood and anxiety disorders than do men (Narrow, 1998). Historically, women were often diagnosed with mental health problems, while men received a medical diagnosis and treatment that fell outside the practice of psychiatry. How often this occurs today is not known. Since society has come to accept the existence of legitimate psychological problems, so too have the numbers of men willing to be treated for such problems increased. The author hopes that a balance between overdiagnosis and pathologizing human behavior, recognizing human suffering and pain, and providing effective interventions can be struck in the clinical area.

Other specific problems are sexual harassment, physical and verbal abuse, and sexual assault; unwanted pregnancy; substance abuse; and eating disorders. Identifying women at risk for these health problems and managing their care are important roles for primary care providers.

Prevention of these complex psychosocial problems requires that women, and society as a whole, acknowledge their existence (Murry & Lopez, 1996). Community education, referrals, support systems, and counseling offer women the opportunity to learn new skills and behaviors that can reduce the incidence of psychosocial problems and their associated mortality and morbidity. With resources available in the community, primary care providers can support women in their efforts to prevent or reduce the numbers of complex psychosocial problems they face. For a woman to achieve changes for herself and her family, she must believe in her selfworth. The primary care provider can play a vital supporting role.

STRESS

Stress is a unique and individual expression in response to any number of events. It occurs when the adaptive or coping mechanism is overwhelmed by events. An event is not always negative; it may be positive, such as marriage or a promotion.

Stress is the result of an intertwining of forces: stressors, perceptions of those stressors, emotional and physiological responses to those perceptions, and efforts to cope. The degree to which a certain stressor causes stress is determined by the perception of that stressor. Stressors may include interpersonal problems, time demands, and internal conflicts.

Stress had been implicated in the pathophysiology of atherosclerotic processes, heart disease, hypertension, and stroke (Kopp, 1999). While direct evidence that stress causes cardiovascular dysfunction or disease is not always conclusive (Institute of Medicine, 2001), there is enough evidence for health care providers to be concerned about stress levels in patients and to make recommendations for stress reduction.

Risk factors are poor support systems, ineffective coping skills, and psychopathological conditions. No precise data are available about the incidence of stress; however, all individuals experience it to some degree.

Health is not just a biological phenomenon, but also reflects a woman's adaptation to sociocultural factors in her life. Health care providers who strive to promote women's wellness, vitality, and overall well-being will help clients improve their quality of life. Stress assessment and reduction are important interventions.

SUBJECTIVE DATA

A woman may react to stress by becoming anxious or depressed, developing physical symptoms, or using substances. Women who are victims of violence or abuse often display signs of excessive stress early in the abuse or in reaction to acts of violence. See Abuse of Women, Sexual Abuse or Rape, Anxiety, Depression, and Substance Abuse sections.

OBJECTIVE DATA

See Abuse of Women, Sexual Abuse or Rape, Anxiety, Depression, and Substance Abuse sections.

DIFFERENTIAL MEDICAL DIAGNOSES

Coronary heart disease, chronic pain, headaches, hypertension, asthma, rheumatoid arthritis, irritable bowel syndrome, ulcers, eczema, anxiety, depression, muscular tension, insomnia, fatigue.

PLAN

Psychosocial Intervention

Discuss with the client ways to avoid a stressful situation. If a stressful situation is unavoidable, discuss ways to minimize stress by altering the stressor. If a stressor is unavoidable, the client needs to develop coping skills to deal with it. Coping is achieved through a healthy lifestyle (sleep, balanced nutrition, exercise, relaxation (Martin, 2002). Help the client to identify self-induced stress caused by unrealistic expectations and to correct the stress-producing thoughts. Encourage the client to develop a relaxation program; it might include progressive muscle relaxation, meditation, and breathing exercises. Time management and assertiveness training may also be helpful. Kenney and Bhattacharjee (2000) report women with medium or high stressors and low assertiveness, low hardiness, or the inability to express feelings were more likely to report physical symptoms than women who were stronger in these traits, suggesting an interactive model.

Follow-Up

If physical causes for the client's symptoms do not exist, refer the client to a mental health specialist for a complete psychological evaluation.

ABUSE OF WOMEN

SEXUAL HARASSMENT

Sexual harassment encompasses unwelcome sexual advances, requests for sexual favors, and other oral or physical conduct or written communications of an intimidating, hostile, or offensive nature or action taken in retaliation for reporting such behavior regardless of where such conduct might occur (U.S. Equal Opportunities Commission, 2002). Sexual harassment is a common experience for women of all ages, occurring most often among women working in a male-dominated profession. However, it may occur in any work environment (ANA, 2002). Few women file complaints against the perpetrator. It is thought that women frequently fail to report sexual harassment because they prefer to have the abuse stopped rather than to see the perpetrator punished (Kilpatrick & White, 2000).

Subjective Data

A woman may express an inability to concentrate, reduction in confidence, decreased motivation that affects her job, tension, nervousness, anger, fear, or helplessness (Malamut & Offermann, 2001). These feelings may or may not carry over into her life outside of home. Physical complaints may include nausea, loss of appetite, headaches, chest pain, and chronic fatigue, which may lead to use or abuse of alcohol, prescriptive drugs, or nonprescriptive drugs to reduce stress-related symptoms.

The history includes several specific points of information.

- *Chief complaint,* with brief description in chronological order of present problem, document dates when harassment began, and what action, if any, the client has taken to stop the harassment.
- *Medical history,* noting childhood illnesses; injuries (be observant for injuries that are not consistent with explanation); hospitalizations and surgeries; previous major illnesses; allergies; habits (start with less offensive), including caffeine, tobacco, alcohol, and illicit drugs; and medications, prescriptive and nonprescriptive.
- *Family medical history,* noting substance abuse and any mental health problems.
- *Social history,* noting family relationships (married/separated/divorced/single), support system, occupational history (time at present job, recent loss of job or job change), and economic status.
- *Subjective psychological functioning,* with cognitive abilities (orientation to present, memory, history of psychiatric illness) and cultural implications, evaluate for anxiety and depressive symptoms.
- *Lifestyle history,* noting nutrition and rest and exercise patterns.

Objective Data

A thorough physical examination and wide range of diagnostic tests complete the diagnostic process.

Physical Examination

- *General Appearance.* The client may appear disheveled or be well groomed, may be over- or underweight, and may appear anxious or nervous.
- *Eyes.* Circles may be visible under eyes. Eyes may be red and puffy from lack of sleep or crying.
- *Neck.* Neck muscles may be tense and tender from stress or tension.
- *Skin.* Observe for bruising, lacerations, burns, dryness, or cold and clamminess.
- *Nails and Hair.* The nails and hair may be dull and brittle.
- *Chest.* Note any increase in respiratory rate.
- *Vascular System.* Note any increase in blood pressure and heartrate.
- *Abdomen.* Bowel sounds may be hypoactive or hyperactive. Abdomen may be tender on palpation.
- *Musculoskeletal System.* Examination may reveal bruising, redness, edema, joint pain or swelling, poor posture, tense muscles, or limited range of motion.
- *Nervous System.* Poor coordination, unsteady gait, abnormal cranial nerve evaluation, sluggish speech, flight of ideas, inability to concentrate, and poor memory are possible findings.
- *Genitalia.* If indicated. See Sexual Abuse.

Diagnostic Tests (depending on the clinical presentation)

- Electrocardiogram
- Electroencephalogram
- Complete blood count to rule out anemia and infection
- Thyroid panel to rule out thyroid disease
- Other lab tests as necessary for health promotion/maintenance and/or to evaluate symptoms

Nursing Implications

Throughout the physical examination, validate all normal findings and reassure the client. Before laboratory tests, explain the test, review what the process involves and why the test is being done. Explain any abnormal findings completely.

Differential Medical Diagnoses

Depression, chronic fatigue syndrome, gastroenteritis, dyspepsia/ulcers, migraine or cluster headaches, panic/anxiety attacks, stress.

Plan

Psychosocial Intervention. Listen carefully to the client's description of the harassment. Provide information about the emotional, physical, economic, and family effects of harassment. Validate the connection between physical and emotional symptoms and the harassment. Explore the impact of harassment on marital and family life. Validate the client's experience and help her resist devaluing herself. Discuss options and their ramifications. Encourage assertiveness training and stress management and review existing coping skills. Help refine coping skills as needed. Often feelings of empowerment will alleviate symptoms of depression and anxiety (Jorqenson & Wahl, 2000).

Follow-Up

Refer the client to a psychotherapist or other mental health professional for individual or group counseling. Referral for legal counsel may also be appropriate.

VIOLENCE

The abuse occurs in many forms, from forceful physical abuse to less obviously damaging verbal abuse. Intent to hurt the victim ranges from slapping, beating, pushing, biting, and threatening to attack with a weapon. Psychological aggression and abuse not only refer to verbal abuse, such as insults, constant negative feedback, screaming, and swearing, but may include depriving a woman of sleep and food. This violence often involves a combination of abusive acts. Violence against women is primarily partner violence (Tjaden & Thomas, 1998; US-DHHSS, 2001). However, less than half of women who reported incidents of violence committed by intimates to authorities obtained final court orders (Zoellner, Feeny, Albarez, Watlington, et al., 2000).

Epidemiology

Etiology. Violence and abuse are often the result of inefficient coping and stress-reducing skills. Frequently, the abuser's behavior is the result of learning; the abuser may have witnessed abuse or been abused (Burgess, 2002).

Walker (1984) describes the battering cycle, or cycle of violence, as characterized by tension-building incidents. Tension builds with acts of intimidation and initial, though lesser, physical abuse (shoving, pushing, name calling). As it escalates, the woman first tries to placate her partner. When this does not work, she withdraws to prevent a confrontation. During this time, the woman's repressed anger can contribute to her sense of guilt and low self-esteem. The partner may become more aggressive as she withdraws.

Explosion occurs following mounting tension with physical and verbal attack and subsequent injury. The woman often feels she was at fault and the outburst was justified. The explosive phase usually lasts 24 hours or fewer, which allows the abuser to release tension.

During the honeymoon that follows the explosion, the abuser repents and promises never to abuse again. The abused woman wants to believe that the abuse will stop and stays in the relationship.

In the repetitive cycle, abuse does not stop with one incident, but increases in frequency and severity (Mahoney, Williams, & West, 2001). Learned helplessness, low self-esteem, feelings of guilt, lack of resources, and anticipatory fear eventually immobilize a woman to the point where she feels there is no way to escape. The abused woman usually has a small social network with whom she can confide but probably will not because of her shame and guilt. She is usually dependent on her abuser, both emotionally and financially, and makes excuses for the abuser's behavior. The abused woman is caught between maintaining the relationship, economic survival, and the well-being of her partner and children on the one side, and her own physical and emotional well-being on the other (Draucker, 2002).

Risk Factors. History of abuse as a child, poor self-esteem, substance abuse or dependence, limited resources, absence of support persons, and pregnancy are risk factors (McNutt, Carlson, Gagen, & Winterbauer, 1999).

Incidence. A national survey conducted from November 1995 to May 1996 estimated that approximately 1.5 million females and 834,700 males are raped and/or physically assaulted by an intimate partner annually in the United States (Tjaden & Thomas, 1998). Minority women are particularly at risk for such abuse (Raj, Silverman, Wingood, & DiClemente, 1999). In a study of prevalence of violence against women in a primary care setting, 53.6 percent of women respondents had ever experienced any type of violence. Nurse researchers have found that 22 to 35 percent of women who seek treatment at hospital emergency departments present because of injuries caused by domestic violence (Campbell, Pliska, Taylor, & Sheridan, 1994).

Subjective Data

All women should be screened for domestic violence (Yeager & Seid, 2002). Few women who seek medical care will state the cause of their injuries. Health care providers seeing nonacutely ill women in an office setting may not be confronted with any specific sign or symptom suggestive of battering.

Vague symptoms may present during the tension building phase secondary to increased stress. Symptoms may include backaches, headaches, fatigue, anxiety, stress, insomnia, anorexia, indigestion, hypertension, allergic skin reactions palpitations, hyperventilation, chest pain, choking sensation, claustrophobic feelings, and pelvic pain (Campbell, 1998; Warshaw & Ganier, 1998).

In relating her history, a client may be hesitant, embarrassed, or evasive. She can look depressed, abuse alcohol and medications, and have a history of suicide attempts. Gathering a complete social history—including substance use and abuse, family situation, and support systems—is important. If the client reports abuse, documentation of all details is important. Explore any history of prior episodes of abuse with the client (Griffin & Koss, 2002).

Indicators of possible battering include change in appointment pattern (increased or frequently missed appointments), complaints of problems at home or with partner (partner jealous, possessive), making excuses for partner's behavior, and ambivalent statements about battering or signs of fear when discussing it. Provide the client with privacy while interviewing. If the abuser is with her, try to speak to her alone without raising the abuser's suspicion.

Objective Data

Do a complete physical exam and carefully document the findings. Assure the client that the assault was not her fault. Explicitly document the extent and types of abuse and note if the client's explanation is not consistent with her injuries. Encourage the client to respond to questions; however, if she becomes upset, explain concern and describe the cycle of violence, emphasizing its repetitive and escalating nature.

In the physical examination, a body map documenting the current injuries, healing injuries, and scars will be helpful in describing the client's presentation in the future. Take photographs if written consent given. Try to photograph the client's face or attach some type of identifying information, e.g., driver's license when taking photographs.

- *General Appearance.* The client may appear well groomed or chaotic with torn clothes. She may be nervous and emotional or calm and collected. There may be injuries that require immediate attention or no visible signs of injury.
- *Head, Face, and Throat.* These are the most typical locations of injury.
- *Skin.* Note any lacerations, burns, and bruises of the skin, both old and new. Be sure to examine all areas covered by clothing. If the patient has not changed clothes, inspect clothes for evidence of violence.

- *Chest.* Chest exam may reveal difficulty breathing because of pain from fractured ribs.
- *Vascular System.* Look for elevated blood pressure and heartrate.
- *Abdomen.* Abdominal pain may be evident with palpation. In pregnant women, the breast and abdomen are targets of assault.
- *Genitalia.* See the section on Sexual Abuse.
- *Musculoskeletal System.* Look for fractures of the extremities, ribs, and skull; pain with palpation, redness, swelling, and bruising.

All primary care providers should be knowledgeable about specific legal guidelines in their state. Notify police when the law requires it or if a client requests legal assistance (Warshaw & Ganley, 1998).

Differential Medical Diagnoses

Trauma not related to abuse, suicide attempt, self-mutilation.

Plan

Because of their potential for early contact with victims, primary care providers are in an excellent position to intervene in the cycle of domestic and/or family violence (McAllister, 2000).

Psychosocial Intervention. Ideally, intervention should begin during the tension-building phase or immediately after an abusive incident.

Identification of the Problem

Many primary care providers fail to recognize the signs and symptoms of abuse. Explore all suspicions of abuse, even at the risk that the abuse does not exist (Waalen, Goodwin, Spitz, Petersen, & Saltzman, 2000).

- Support the client in acknowledging a problem.
- Affirm that abusive behavior is unacceptable.
- Assist the woman to gain access to available community resources, such as housing, counseling, legal services (The provider does not, however, initiate contact).
- Help the client to identify options, as she may believe she has none.
- Assist the client to develop an escape plan if she plans to stay in the abusive situation. (This includes placing clothes, money, and copies of necessary documents in an easily accessible, secret, and secure place.) (Warshaw & Ganley, 1998)

Follow-Up

Counseling is essential; also, encourage clients to consider asking for professional help. Often, however the client is not ready to seek assistance. Providers respect the client's decision. Abused women will often leave and return several times to an abusive relationship before deciding that the relationship should be ended. Pursue treatment of all injuries and order x-rays as needed. Additional information regarding assessment and treatment can be reviewed in an on-line course offered by Web Trainer. This course has been developed by the American Medical Women's Association (2002) and can be accessed via the Internet.

SEXUAL ABUSE OR RAPE

Sexual abuse or rape is forced sexual intercourse perpetrated against the will of a victim. Force may be employed by physical violence, coercion, or threat of harm. Acquaintance rape usually occurs in a dating situation and is perpetrated by someone the woman knows and trusts. Sexual assault involves actions other than rape: sodomy, forced anal intercourse; oral copulation, forced copulation of mouth of one person with sexual organ or anus of another; rape with a foreign object, forced penetration of genital or anal openings with a foreign object; and sexual battery, unwanted touching of an intimate part for sexual arousal. Health care providers may be required to report assault-related injuries to law enforcement agencies (Houry, Sachs, Feldhaus, & Linden, 2002).

Epidemiology

Etiology. Rape challenges a woman's ability to maintain her defenses and arouses feelings of guilt, anxiety, and inadequacy. The overwhelming experience heightens her sense of helplessness and intensifies her conflict about dependence and independence. The survivor's response is determined by her stage in life, her defensive structures, and her coping ability.

Rape trauma syndrome comprises the sequential reactions of the survivor in dealing with her experience. The syndrome, described as a two- or three-stage process, helps explain how rape victims respond to the traumatic experience of rape (Stenchever, Mishell, Herbst, & Droegemueller, 2001).

The immediate response, or acute phase, occurs immediately after the assault or the disclosure of assault. The survivor's lifestyle is completely disrupted and reac-

tions are tearfulness and agitation or a relaxed calm. This stage can last as long as three to six months, with typical symptoms being anxiety, fears and phobias, suspiciousness, major depressive symptoms, feelings of inferiority, inability to think clearly, and difficulty functioning at home, work, or school. In addition, feelings of guilt, shame, embarrassment, and self-blame are common. Psychophysiological disturbances affect eating, sleeping, gastrointestinal function, and sexual intimacy. Ensuring safety and regaining control over her life are the survivor's main emotional needs during this time. Medical attention is important. In a study of 1,076 victims, general body trauma was reported in 67 percent of the sample (Riggs, Houry, Long, Markovchick, & Feldhaus, 2000).

The middle phase, or readjustment stage, is a period of transition when the survivor rationalizes that she could have prevented the assault and develops unrealistic plans to avoid another.

The final stage, or reorganization phase, may last two years or longer and is difficult and painful. During this stage, the survivor begins to deal with the reality of her victimization and may make changes in lifestyle, relationship, and work.

Along with a two- or three-stage model of recovery, other authors discuss recovery within the broader content of post-traumatic stress disorder (PTSD) as described in the *Diagnostic and Statistical Manual of Mental Disorders* (American Psychiatric Association, 2000). (See section on Post-Traumatic Stress Disorder for a complete discussion.) Another mental health disorder that may occur as an outcome of rape is acute stress disorder, differentiated from post-traumatic stress disorder by the time symptoms are exhibited. The symptoms last for at least two days but do not persist longer than four weeks after the traumatic event (APA, 2000).

Risk Factors. Any woman is at risk; however, dating situations, unfamiliar partners, alcohol and drug use, and miscommunication create additional risk.

Incidence. Rape is one of the most frequently committed and underreported violent crimes in the United States. In one recent study of an emergency department population, the lifetime prevalence rate of sexual assault was 39 percent with only 46 percent of the women reporting the crime to police. They were also more likely to report the attack to the police if the assailant was a stranger versus if a partner (Feldhaus, Houry, & Kaminsky, 2000). Certain female populations may be at an increased risk for sexual assault. Rickert and Wiemann (1998) reported a lifetime rate of sexual assault among adolescents up to 68 percent.

Subjective Data

A client may report various physical and psychological problems. Explore a history of sexual abuse in any woman who presents with multiple physical complaints, even if associated with functional limitations.

Careful recording of the details of the assault, along with the client's gynecological, sexual, and social histories, is essential. If the assault occurred within the last 72 hours, refer the client to a designated sexual assault center with trained sexual assault examiners for the completion of the assessment. The following information is for educational purposes of nonexpert examiners and for the assessment of victims who report the assault later. Detailed forms are available for the documentation of such an assessment.

Symptoms may include headaches, sleep disturbance, loss of appetite with weight loss or gain, eating disorders (Medscape, 2002), nausea, vomiting, constipation, diarrhea, sexual dysfunction, menstrual irregularities, abnormal vaginal discharge, and urinary dysfunction. The client may report difficulty in relationships with others and in functioning at home, work, or school.

The history of assault will include date, time, location, description, use of a weapon, and type of weapon; the part of the body penetrated, the object used to penetrate (body part or foreign object); occurrence of ejaculation; and involvement of alcohol or other drugs. Record any information about the assailant. Question the client about her activities after the assault: Did she shower, change clothes, urinate, or defecate?

The past medical history includes dates of immunizations, especially tetanus and hepatitis. Prior HIV titer or status if known.

The obstetric and gynecologic history includes the date of the client's previous menstrual period, pregnancies, abortions, and miscarriages; contraceptive methods used; and history of sexually transmitted infections.

The sexual history includes information about the client's sexual activity; Was she sexually active within one week before or after assault? Has she been the victim of past sexual assaults (give dates)? Does she have any HIV high risk sexual contact? Providers should use neutral language that includes the possibility of homosexual, bisexual, or heterosexual activity when asking about sexual partners.

The social history includes information about whether the survivor lives alone, has a support system, wants someone notified, needs social service assistance, or wants police notified if they are not aware of assault.

Objective Data

Forensic evaluation refers to documentation of injuries, collection and preservation of evidence and, with additional training, interpretation of injuries observed (Ryan & Houry, 2000). Health care providers, especially in rural areas, are often the first point of contact for the women who have been raped, and therefore, should be prepared to conduct evaluation. Document findings from the physical examination and any forensic tests conducted (Patel & Minshall, 2001).

Complete a thorough physical examination and sexually transmitted disease (STD) testing after treating major injuries, no matter how much time has elapsed since the assault. If the woman has not showered or changed clothes since the assault, have her disrobe while standing on a sheet to collect any evidence. Then, give her a gown. Place any clothes that may contain evidence in a labeled paper bag. A comprehensive review of assessment and treatment is presented by McConkey, Sole, and Holcomb (2001).

Physical Examination

- *General Appearance.* The survivor may be calm and relaxed or tearful and emotional. Notice torn and stained clothes; injuries may be visible.
- *Head, Face, and Throat.* There may be lacerations, abrasions, and bruising. Dried secretions may be present on the face, mouth, or ears. The client may complain of headaches.
- *Chest.* There may be bruising, lacerations, and abrasions and tenderness on palpation. Note any increased respiration, difficulty breathing, or hyperventilation.
- *Abdomen.* Bruising, lacerations, abrasions, and tenderness may be evident, indicating potential internal injuries.
- *Musculoskeletal System.* Look for potential fractures by examining skin for lacerations, abrasions, bruising, and the back and extremities for tenderness.
- *Gastrointestinal.* Symptoms may include anorexia, nausea, vomiting, and abdominal or rectal pain.
- *Genitalia and Reproductive Tract.* The perineum, rectal area, and vagina may have bruises, lacerations,

and abrasions. Bartholin's and Skene's glands and the urethral meatus may be tender. Uterine size, shape, and consistency may be abnormal. Note any tenderness with cervical motion and uterine and adnexal palpation. Watch for tears or pain on rectovaginal examination as suggestive of internal pelvic trauma.

◆ *Psychiatric.* The client may report symptoms of anxiety, depression, suicidal ideation, mood swings, phobias, sexual difficulties, uncontrollable memories or flashbacks, substance abuse, detachment from others or dissociative symptoms.

Use a body map to document all injuries, including their size, location, and coloration. Photographs of abrasions, with some form of identification appearing on the photographs, may be helpful if the victim plans legal action. Obtain written consent.

Diagnostic Tests. Complete within 24 to 72 hours of the assault. Forensic specimen collection is best when done by an experienced practitioner (Stenchever, et al., 2001). All laboratory findings are documented in the medical record. Use a Wood's light to check the perineum and thighs for blood or semen.

Obtain gonorrhea and chlamydia cultures from the endocervix, vaginal vault, rectum, and oropharynx, as indicated by history or evidence of penetration.

Collect urine for microscopic examination. A serum pregnancy test is preferred, if available. A urine pregnancy test is an alternative, if an enzyme-linked immunosorbent assay (ELISA); immunometric test is used. Sensitivity for urine beta HCG is 25 mIU/mL as compared to a quantitative serum test where results can be obtained with a beta subunit radio immunoassay HCG level as little as 5 mIU/mL (Bailey, 1998). Obtain cervical and rectal swabs for evidence of herpes simplex virus. Determine HIV status at this time.

Wet mount specimens can show trichomonas, clue cells, and motile sperm for up to 72 hours. Include the pH of vaginal discharge and presence of positive whiff test.

Collect a vaginal smear to detect sperm and p30 prostate specific antigen; considered more reliable than phosphatase determination.

Bloodwork includes blood type/Rh, hepatitis antigen, rapid plasma reagin (RPR), and HIV antibody titer serum.

Collect fingernail scrapings from each hand and save in separately labeled bag.

Collect hair samples by combing both head and pubic hair; specimens placed in labeled bags.

Blood and dried fluids found on the survivor's body and clothing collected and labeled for DNA fingerprinting. Saliva is collected for blood group antigen testing.

Nursing Implications

In caring for a victim of sexual abuse or rape, it is important to understand that evaluation and treatment of the survivor require a multidisciplinary approach. If possible, a rape counselor who is present during the entire evaluation process can be helpful to provide client support.

If a woman calls and reports rape, instruct her to avoid showering or changing her clothes. Encourage her to go to the emergency room nearest her or to the health care provider's office.

Before taking a complete history, explain the process and that the information will help in her medical management as well as for forensic use (Stenchever, et al., 2001). Determination of rape occurs in a court of law; therefore, the wording in the history should reflect only the client's report of the incident. It is important to record, sign, and date all information. Ask the client to sign a consent form and release of information form. Reassure the woman that answers to questions, especially those covering her sexual history, will ensure proper medical treatment. Throughout her visit, explain each procedure and why it is being done and restore her sense of control. Give her options and seek consent with each procedure. Reinforce that rape was not her fault. Provide information about available social services, including a crisis hotline. Assist her to decide whether to report the crime and encourage her to seek follow-up care.

Differential Medical Diagnoses

Trauma not related to sexual assault.

Plan

Psychosocial Intervention. Refer the client for counseling. Women who do not deal realistically with rape and resolutions of issues may develop severe, long-term sequelae, such as depression, substance abuse, anxiety disorder, and suicide. If the woman desires legal action, assist the woman in contacting the proper authorities.

Medication. Offer medication for sexually transmitted diseases or possible pregnancy.

Treatment for STDs (antibiotic prophylaxis) should be offered because of increased risk of sexually transmitted diseases: chlamydia trachomatis, neisseria gonorrhea, treponema pallidum, and trichomonas vaginalis

(Stenchever et al., 2001). See Chapter 11 for treatment guidelines. Review the risks and benefits of both treatment and observation. If the client refuses prophylactic antibiotics, then do follow-up cultures at the six-week visit. If the client consents to prophylactic antibiotics, then treat her according to current Centers for Disease Control (CDC) guidelines for chlamydia, gonorrhea, syphilis, and trichomoniasis.

Offer postcoital contraceptive (PCC) medication to the client unless pregnancy exists or suspected. Holmes et al. (1996) estimates the national rape-related pregnancy rate at 5 percent and states that among adult women, 32,101 pregnancies result from rape annually in the United States. Many of these pregnancies could be prevented. Emergency contraception reduces the risk of pregnancy by 75 percent. PCC is a safe, effective tool in avoiding unintended pregnancy. It is offered at the time of assault, regardless of the cycle phase.

A number of options are now available for emergency contraception. The FDA has approved several specific methods (ACOG, 2001). (See Chapter 9, Emergency Contraception, for a review of this treatment.) Perform a pregnancy test before any administration of medication. A history of thrombosis or perhaps of hypertension would be potential contraindications for some methods, especially if combination estrogen-progestin oral contraceptive options are used. Significantly less side effects and risks are seen with Plan B. Review side effects of whichever method is provided with the client. Offer hepatitis B and tetanus vaccination if indicated.

Follow-Up

A telephone call or return office visit within 24 to 48 hours of initial treatment allows for ongoing evaluation of problems and concerns. Schedule an appointment for one week after initial treatment to evaluate physical and emotional status. If the client has no complaints, defer the physical exam. Review all laboratory findings with the client. Inquire about counseling. If the client does not participate in counseling, encourage her to begin and provide a referral. Schedule the last visit at four to six weeks. At that time, complete a repeat physical exam, collect specimens for repeat cultures for STDs, rapid plasma reagin, and HIV antibody. Repeat HIV testing in three-month intervals up to one year following exposure. Perform a pregnancy test as needed.

Golding (1996) found that a sexual assault history with physical symptoms often correlate with impaired functioning and personal and social costs to the woman. In following women with a history of assault, the re-

searcher points to the importance of primary care provider's role in helping affected women recover from the assault. If the trauma remains unresolved and/or the abuse is chronic, referral to community services and mental health care is necessary.

SUBSTANCE ABUSE

ALCOHOL, COCAINE, SEDATIVES-HYPNOTICS, CANNABIS, OPIATES, AND TOBACCO

The DSM-IV-TR makes a distinction between substance abuse and substance dependence. Primary care providers will regularly see clients with both conditions. Substance abuse will be the primary focus of this section. Information on treating substance dependence is available from any psychiatric textbook or substance treatment manual. A maladaptive pattern of psychoactive substance use is indicated by at least one of the following: The client continues to use a psychoactive or potentially addicting substance despite her awareness of persistent or recurrent social, occupational, psychological, or physical problems that are caused or exacerbated by its use; the client continues to use the substance in situations where use is physically hazardous; some symptoms of disturbance occur within a twelve-month period; the client does not fulfill criteria for psychoactive substance dependence (APA, 2000). Substance abuse is multidimensional with interacting factors that predispose the client to addictive use. Gender, age, race, physiology, and genetics all contribute to development of addictive disease (APA, 2000). Women are particularly susceptible to substance abuse and dependence if they have other psychiatric diagnoses, such as a history of sexual or other violent assault, depression, anxiety, or eating disorders (Becker & Walton-Moss, 2001).

Epidemiology

Etiology. Substance abuse and the risk factors for addiction are in many instances predictable. Clients who have a family history of addiction are at risk for addiction to drugs and compulsive behaviors (APA, 2000).

Female physiology may be influential. Women develop adverse health consequences from the use and abuse of alcohol and other drugs over shorter time periods and with lower consumption than men. Studies have documented that women have a physiological response to alcohol that is significantly different from men. Women enter substance abuse treatment at generally the same ages as men, but with shorter histories of substance use and more severe consequences (Brady & Randall, 1999). One recent study indicates that alcoholic women showed deterioration of muscles, including the heart muscle, equal to that of men even though the women's lifetime dose of alcohol was 60 percent that of men (Urbano-Marquez, Estruch, Fernandez-Sola, et al., 1995).

Psychological factors are influential. Psychopathology and psychological conflicts place women at risk for substance abuse. Traditional patterns of women's socialization include the belief that the needs of spouse, children, and others come first and that the expression of such feelings as anger and competition is unfeminine. Women may attempt to deal with their negative feelings through pharmacological suppression or drinking (Brady & Randall, 1999).

Associated Factors. Specific risk factors exist.

- An addictive parent
- Divorce or separation
- Living alone with children
- Lesbian lifestyle
- Reliance on pharmacological agents or alcohol to relax, sleep, feel more comfortable in social settings, or control unpleasant feelings
- Adolescent smoking

Incidence. Heavy drinking was reported by 5.6 percent of the population aged 12 and older, or 12.6 million people (SAMHSA, 2001). Although men have higher rates of alcoholism and other substance abuse, alcohol abuse is a significant problem for women. Among younger women in the general population, the proportion of drinkers is beginning to approximate that of men. In addition, rates of substance abuse in women may be underreported. Though older women drink less and have fewer drinking problems than older men, their use of prescribed psychoactive drugs is thought to cause more problems.

In 2000, approximately 14 million Americans reported that they currently used illegal drugs (SAMHSA, 2001). Women used virtually the same types of illegal drugs as did men, but they used them less frequently than men did (5 percent versus 7.7 percent in 1993) (SAMHSA, 2001). Among youth aged 12 to 17 in 2000, the rate of current illicit drug use was similar for boys (9.8 percent) and girls (9.5 percent). Illicit drug use included marijuana, cocaine, heroin, hallucinogens, and inhalants, and nonmedical use of prescription-type pain relievers, tranquilizers, stimulants, and sedatives. The drug "ecstacy" (MDAA) was included under hallucinogens. This drug is a growing problem, especially in adolescent

women with serious health consequences. In 2000, an estimated 6.4 million persons had tried ecstasy at least once in their lifetime (SAMHSA, 2001).

Marijuana is the most commonly used illicit drug. Of the 5.7 million users of illicit drugs other than marijuana, 3.8 million were using psychotherapeutics nonmedically. Psychotherapeutics include pain relievers (2.8 million users), tranquilizers (1.0 million users), stimulants (0.8 million users), and sedatives (0.2 million users) (SAMHSA, 2001).

Among pregnant women aged 15 to 44 years, 3.3 percent reported using illicit drugs in the month prior to the survey (based on the combined 1999 and 2000 NHSDA samples). Although this rate is significantly lower than the rate among nonpregnant women aged 15 to 44 years (7.7 percent), among pregnant women aged 15 to 17 years, the rate of use was 12.9 percent, nearly equal to the rate for nonpregnant women of the same age (13.5 percent) (SAMHSA, 2001). While all pregnant women should be screened for illicit drug use, adolescent and pregnant women may need specific interventions geared to reducing drug use.

In addition, cigarette smokers are more likely to use other tobacco products, illicit drugs, and alcohol than are nonsmokers. Among past month smokers in 2000, 39.4 percent were heavy alcohol users. Among nonsmokers, 14.4 percent were binge alcohol users and 3.0 percent were heavy alcohol users. Only 3.2 percent of nonsmokers were current illicit drug users, compared with 15.6 percent of smokers (SAMHSA, 2001). Tobacco addiction causes a number of preventable deaths in the United States. While the prevalence of smoking has declined to nearly 29.3 percent of the U.S. population and the health risks associated with smoking are widely known, millions of Americans continue to smoke (SAMHSA, 2001). Rates for women who smoked in 2000 remain at approximately 14.1 percent (SAMHSA, 2001).

Subjective Data

Careful observation and listening may reveal symptoms of abuse of a specific substance. Histories are also essential. Symptoms of abuse are often specific to a particular substance.

Alcohol abusers often report gastritis, vomiting, and diarrhea. They may lose or gain weight. In addition, a client may report nervousness, anxiety, depression, sleep disturbances, pelvic pain, abnormal vaginal discharge, infertility, or sexual dysfunction.

Cocaine abuse may lead to sinusitis and upper respiratory infection, allergic rhinitis, nasal congestion, and epistaxis. Weight loss may be experienced. Abstinence from cocaine may produce anxiety, fatigue, depression, irritability, and sleep disturbances.

Abuse of sedatives-hypnotics (benzodiazepines) may cause headaches, nausea, paranoia, and sleep disturbances. Withdrawal may cause insomnia and irritability. When used with alcohol, sedatives-hypnotics increase central nervous system depressant effects.

Cannabis (marijuana) abuse may provoke fatigue, decreased motivation, panic attacks, anxiety, and paranoia. Hallucinogens can cause mood swings, memory loss, hyperactivity, and even death. Ecstasy can increase heart rate and blood and heart oxygen consumption without increasing the heart's ejection fraction, putting users at risk for a heart event such as a myocardial infarction (Lester, Baggott, Welam, Schiller, et al., 2000).

Abuse of opiates produces an initial sense of euphoria, followed by a sense of tranquility and then sleepiness. Tolerance and dependence develop requiring higher doses to maintain the desired level of euphoria. Opiates do not directly cause serious organ damage.

Use of tobacco causes many effects on the body. Chronic cough, wheezing, dyspnea, sore throat, and bad breath are rarely mentioned as complaints by clients. Clients do become concerned, however, about chronic obstructive pulmonary disease, asthma, cardiovascular disease, lung cancer, and other potentially fatal illnesses, all of which have been associated with tobacco use. Tobacco products also contain nicotine, which is known to cause addiction and withdrawal.

Histories are the best indicators of early substance abuse. Screening for substance abuse focuses on adverse consequences (e.g., family or marital problems, seizures or withdrawal symptoms) rather than on physical or laboratory findings. An alcohol history may use a screening questionnaire such as the CAGE questionnaire, which looks at patterns and consequences, or the *Short Michigan Alcoholism Screening Test* (SMAST), which deals with consequences. Diagnosis should not rest solely on the questionnaire; rather, the questionnaire is used to determine the index of suspicion for abuse. Clients will often describe starting out experimenting with a substance, like tobacco, to go on to using more and more to achieve the same effects.

The health care provider should always approach the client in a nonbiased manner. When questioning about abuse *always* begin with questions about less sensitive substances: How many cups of coffee do you drink per day? How much tobacco do you use per day? How many drinks per day? Then ask about tolerance (How many drinks does it take for you to feel high?) and the occurrence of blackouts. Inability to remember what happened when drinking is a probable sign of alcoholism.

The drug history includes information about prescription medication, over-the-counter medication, and illicit drugs (substance abuse may progress from alcohol, to cannabis, to cocaine, etc.). Inquire if one drug is taken in conjunction with another or with alcohol. Previous treatment for substance abuse should be noted. Has the client tried to quit smoking in the past? If so, how did she quit and how long did she maintain nonuse of the substance.

The social history includes information about marital or family problems, job or promotion loss due to poor performance or absenteeism, financial difficulties, and multiple arrests for disorderly conduct or driving under influence of a drug. Inquire about behavior changes, such as termination of old friendships and loss of interest in favorite pastimes.

Past medical histories include questions about accidental injuries and illnesses related to abuse. For example, individuals who abuse cocaine have frequent urinary tract infections, sinusitis, nosebleeds, and burns if the drug is smoked; alcohol abuse may cause gastroenteritis, ulcers, hepatitis, and pneumonia; and cannabis frequently causes urinary tract infections. Smoking causes increased rates of upper respiratory and lung infections. A history of pneumonia or chronic bronchitis may be elicited.

The reproductive system and sexual history includes questions about pregnancies, abortions, sexually transmitted infections, pelvic inflammatory disease, abnormal Pap smears, menstrual irregularities, sexual dysfunction, and STD and HIV risk factors. Substance use and abuse decrease inhibitions. Consequently, a woman is more likely to engage in sexual intercourse, which may increase the risk of sexual abuse. Substance abuse may lead to frequent partners if sex is exchanged for substance; intravenous drug use increases the risk of hepatitis B and HIV infection.

Family medical history includes information about mental illness, dysfunctional family, and substance abuse. Exposure to second-hand smoke should be noted.

Objective Data

Although histories and observation are important investigative tools, diagnosis is rarely made without laboratory tests and physical examination.

Alcohol. Alcoholism may be diagnosed with the use of physical examination and a variety of diagnostic tests: blood, liver, electrolyte, thyroid, glucose, and stool (Snow, 2000).

Physical Examination

- *Skin.* Hair loss, cigarette burns, seborrheic dermatitis, palmar erythema, infections, thrombosed and spider veins (particularly on the chest) may be evident.
- *Head and Eyes.* Poor dentition is likely, with possible lesions on the posterior lateral tongue (increased risk for oropharyngeal cancer with alcohol and tobacco abuse) and alcohol odor to the breath. The face may be red and puffy; signs and symptoms of sinusitis present; the nose enlarged with prominent veins; the eyes puffy with erythematous conjunctiva, yellow sclera, or dilated pupils; the voice hoarse with or without cough; and the parotid gland enlarged.
- *Chest.* The client may complain of a chronic cough. Auscultation of egophony "E" to "A" changes indicate possible pneumonia. Point tenderness may be caused by ribs fractured during falls. Symptoms of chronic bronchitis, asthma, tuberculosis, noncardiogenic pulmonary edema may be noted.
- *Vascular System.* Examination may reveal cardiac arrhythmia, tachycardia, and hypertension. Symptoms may be suggestive of mitral value disease.
- *Abdomen.* The liver is palpable and tender in hepatitis. The spleen may be enlarged. Ascites may be present. Abdominal pain suggests gastritis, ulcers, duodenitis, esophagitis, ileitis, irritable bowel syndrome, or pancreatitis.
- *Musculoskeletal System.* Bruises or fractures indicate trauma. An abnormal gait and decreased muscle strength are related to myopathy. Gout causes red, tender, and edematous joints.
- *Genitalia and Reproductive Tract.* Menstrual irregularities, unplanned pregnancy, abnormal vaginal discharge, and pelvic pain with adnexal and cervical motion tenderness are possible findings.
- *Nervous System.* Examination may reveal abnormal cranial nerve findings, ataxia, positive Romberg, peripheral neuropathy, cerebral degeneration, myopathy, optic neuropathy, and presence of tremors or seizures.

Diagnostic Tests

- *Blood Tests.* Blood alcohol level may be elevated, positive toxicology screen for multiple substances; hemoglobin and hematocrit decreased (anemia); mean corpuscular volume increased (common finding in alcohol abuse); prothrombin time prolonged; platelets decreased (clotting disorder); elevated uric acid.
- *Liver Function Tests.* Serum g-glutamyltransferase (SGGT) (most sensitive), alanine aminotransferase (ALT), aspartate aminotransferase (AST), lactate dehydrogenase (LDH), amylase, alkaline phosphatase, total bilirubin, cholesterol, and triglycerides all increased (indicative of alcoholic liver disease).
- *Electrolytes.* Serum magnesium, calcium, phosphorus, and potassium usually decreased.
- *Thyroid Function.* Abnormal (especially in stimulant users).
- *Glucose.* May be increased or decreased; further evaluation by HgbAlC or GTT may be indicated.
- *Stool.* Occult blood present.

Sedatives-Hypnotics. Sedative-hypnotic abuse may be detected by symptoms similar to a state intoxication followed by drowsiness. Withdrawal from sedatives (benzodiazepines)-hypnotics can be fatal. Detoxification from sedatives-hypnotics should always be in an inpatient setting. Many times there are no obvious physical findings, except in an overdose. Clients who overdose are seen in the emergency room.

Cannabis. Cannabis abuse may be detected by means of physical examination, with close attention to the eyes, and an electrocardiogram.

Physical Examination

- *General Appearance.* Dreamlike state.
- *Skin.* Burns on fingers or around mouth if cannabis is smoked.
- *Eyes.* Conjunctival injection often the only objective sign.
- *Vascular System.* Tachycardia and hypertension (especially if multiple drugs are used). A diagnostic electrocardiogram may show non-specific ST-T wave changes related to rate.

Opiates. Opiates can be taken orally (oxycodone, hydromorphone), injected intravenously (IV) (heroin, morphine, or merperidine), or smoked (heroin). Unlike alcohol, opiates do not produce serious organ pathology. Clients may have constipation, respiratory depression, and anorexia from the substances used to cut the heroin. The use of IV injection via shared needles places the client at risk for hepatitis B, human immunodeficiency virus (HIV) infection, endocarditis, local injection site infections, and other problems associated with contaminated IV injection.

Cocaine. Cocaine can be smoked, snorted, or injected IV. Cocaine abuse may be detected by examining the nose, chest, and cardiovascular system and by carrying out various diagnostic tests.

Physical Examination

- *Nose.* Nasal bleeding, erythematous nostrils, nasal septal atrophy with perforation.
- *Chest.* Increased respiratory rate, abnormal breath sounds.
- *Vascular System.* Increased heartrate, palpitations, cardiac arrhythmias, hypertension (possibly), elevated body temperature.
- *Extremities.* Track marks.
- *Neurological.* Jitteriness, symptoms of depression.

Tobacco. Tobacco is consumed in a variety of products. It can be snuffed, chewed, and smoked. Tobacco can be easily detected by smell. Tobacco and cigarette stains can be seen on the teeth and fingers. Use can cause sore throat, cough, dyspnea, and frequent respiratory infections. Cough may be the only indication of cancer. Bloody sputum is a serious complaint.

Physical Examination

- *HEENT.* Irritation of the nasal passages, postnasal exudate on the posterior pharynx, tenderness of the sinuses, bad breath, stained teeth.
- *Chest.* Increased respiratory rate, dyspnea, orthopnea, inspiratory and expiratory wheezes, rhonchi and increased A-P diameter of the chest, angina.
- *Vascular System.* Evidence of peripheral vascular disease may be observed; claudication may occur. Clubbing of the finger may have occurred.

Diagnostic Tests

- Hepatitis panel
- Rapid plasma reagin (RPR)
- HIV infection
- Urine toxicology (for cocaine, cannabis, sedatives)
- See Chapter 21 for respiratory disease tests.

Nursing Implications

The primary health care provider's role is to help the client recognize and accept the negative relationship between her substance abuse and the consequences of abuse (Stenchever et al., 2001). If substance use causes problems (physical, mental, legal, or financial), then use is abuse. The client needs to be told that a problem exists and given evidence to support this conclusion. Subsequently, the client should be directed to the proper resources. Primary care providers should also be familiar with symptoms of withdrawal for each of the substances abused. Treatment should be individualized, multifaceted, and continue indefinitely for maximum success. If, on the other hand, substance use is detected, the woman should be educated about the potential problem of abuse to prevent it.

Differential Medical Diagnoses

Excessive stress, depression, anxiety, hyperthyroidism, viral or bacterial gastroenteritis, upper respiratory infection, chronic sinusitis, lower respiratory tract illness, emphysema not caused by smoking.

Plan

Psychosocial Interventions. Involve others close to the client in the treatment plan and inform them about the disease process. Use a positive approach and emphasize that the disease is treatable. Physician/psychiatric consultation is recommended for evaluation for dual-diagnosis disorders.

Dealing with denial is critical. Review all physical, emotional, financial, spiritual, and psychological effects of the substance abused to date. The first priority is to stop substance use, not to determine the cause of abuse. Total abstinence is the ideal; however, ability to abstain does not mean elimination of the problem. The inability of a woman to use a substance in moderation indicates that a problem may exist.

Contracts with self may be useful if the client is motivated to change her behavior. A contract should have realistic goals within a definite time. One way to help a woman realize that she has a problem is to have her contract to use a limited amount of substance (within reason) for a set time (3 months) in her usual pattern. If she finds she is using more than she contracted to use, then a potential problem exists. Four *A* activities are advised by the National Cancer Institute to help people stop smoking:

*A*sk all women if they smoke; ask routinely.

*A*dvise smokers to stop and give reasons.

*A*ssist the woman in stopping. Give self-help suggestions, a quit date, a plan, suggest nicotine gum/patch.

*A*rrange follow-up to review progress.

Smoking cessation success may be enhanced by using behavioral therapy alone or in conjunction with nicotine replacement products or even a nonnicotine anti-depressant. First, assess the woman's readiness to quit, then help her plan a specific quit program. The provider must prepare her for withdrawal symptoms that may sabotage her earnest attempts. Assure her it takes most people several attempts. A partial list of withdrawal symptoms includes irritability, restlessness, hunger, drowsiness, difficulty concentrating, sleep disturbances, and strong cravings for nicotine (Schaffer, 2002). Direct nicotine absorption into the circulation in concentrations sufficient to alleviate symptoms can occur through buccal (gum), nasal mucosa (spray), or skin (patch). Available nicotine replacement systems include nicotine inhalation system (Nicotrol inhaler), nicotine nasal spray (Nicotrol NS), nicotine polacriliex (Nicorette gum), and nicotine transdermal system (Nicoderm, Nicotrol, Prostep, Habi-trol, etc). In the heaviest smokers, the nicotine nasal spray seems to be most effective (Fiore, Bailey, Cohen, et al., 2000)

The FDA has not approved nicotine replacement therapy for pregnant women; however, continued heavy smoking during pregnancy may have higher associated risks than the short-term use of nicotine replacement, providing replacement is followed by complete nicotine abstinence. Lower nicotine levels in replacement therapy may mean less uterine vasoconstriction (Schrefer, 2001).

A nonnicotine alternative antidepressant to aid in smoking cessation has recently become available. Bupro-pion hydrochloride (Zyban) has been shown to be effective for smoking cessation while having minimal side effects along with reduced weight gain. Bupropion is not recommended for pregnant or lactating women (FDA Category B in pregnancy). Risks and benefits of use with the individual smoker must be weighed, (Schaffer, 2002).

Readers are urged to read Schaffer (2002) carefully for more detailed information and resources on helping smokers with this difficult addiction. This is an area in which providers can have a real impact.

Medication. Disulfiram is recommended for alcohol abuse; the use of sedatives is not desirable. Disulfiram 500 mg, administered orally daily (after abstention for 12 hours) and reduced to 250 mg after one week, may be a deterrent. Disulfiram blocks metabolism of alcohol with acetaldehyde buildup, resulting in headaches, flushing, and nausea. Extreme side effects include hypertension, shock, and coma. The client must be taught about the medication and its potential danger. Side effects, without concomitant alcohol use, include impotence, liver damage, drowsiness, and fetal anomalies if taken by pregnant

women. Contraindications are pregnancy, cardiac disease, and psychoses (Gorroll, May, & Mulley, 2000).

To avoid withdrawal symptoms, nicotine is available in a gum or transdermal patch for those trying to stop smoking. Many of these products are now available without a prescription. Other agents that are used include Clondine, a centrally acting adrenergic blocking agent; Lobeline, nicotine imposter; and antidepressants, especially if smokers also exhibit symptoms of depression (Schaffer, 2002).

Since detoxification from alcohol and other substances may require hospitalization (Martin, 2000b), specific drugs and therapies are not discussed in this chapter. The health care provider who is required to manage in-client detoxification or outpatient treatment should consult psychiatric and pharmacotherapeutics references.

Follow-Up

Refer the client for psychiatric consultation or other mental health services. Along with mental health resources, a client often needs help accessing financial aid, job training, and insurance benefits. Women in all socioeconomic groups may face legal problems with child custody, drug theft, and driving infractions; therefore, they may need information about the legal system. Encourage the client to become involved in Alcoholics Anonymous or a similar group, especially those clients who have little family or friend support to help with behavior changes. Significant others should become involved in a support group that deals with enabling behaviors. Biofeedback and relaxation training may also be helpful.

At first, the client should be followed closely. A minimum of one weekly visit is recommended, with additional phone contact if necessary.

Tobacco Addiction. Continuous monitoring of the client who is trying to quit is essential (Office of the Surgeon General, 2002). Clients should be told the symptoms of nicotine withdrawal, prescribed a nicotine withdrawal agent if no contraindications, and scheduled for a visit at two weeks. Women may find it more difficult to quit than men because of a lack of social support and more reliance on cigarettes to cope with stress, anxiety, and fear of weight gain. Relapses in women occur in situations involving negative mood states such as excessive stress, conflicts, especially with others, and loss. Repeat visits, as necessary, should be made up to one year to reinforce and support the client's efforts. Structured programs for smokers have been shown to be the most effective.

Weight gain averages about 5 pounds. Support clients with ways to avoid high calorie foods and encourage them to increase exercise as needed.

MENTAL HEALTH PROBLEMS

DEPRESSION

The DSM-IV-TR (*Diagnostic and Statistical Manual of Mental Disorders*, APA, 2000) classification of depression is descriptive, considering clinical features of the depressive disorder. Depression, classified as a mood disorder, includes major depression and dysthymic disorder.

Major depression occurs as a single episode or recurrent condition independent of life events. The client either has a depressed mood or loses interest or pleasure in all or almost all her usual activities and experiences four of the following conditions: significant weight loss or gain or changes in appetite, sleep disturbances, psychomotor agitation or retardation, fatigue or loss of energy, feelings of worthlessness or inappropriate guilt, diminished ability to concentrate, recurrent thoughts of death. Symptoms must have been present during the same two-week period and represent a change from previous functioning (APA, 2000).

Dysthymia is a chronic, less acute mood disorder. The client must experience depressed mood for more than two years without being symptom free for more than two months and have two of the following conditions: poor appetite or overeating, sleep disturbance, low self-esteem, fatigue, poor concentration or difficulty making decisions, feelings of hopelessness. (APA, 2000). Dysthymia is frequently a consequence of a preexisting, chronic nonmood disorder, such as anorexia nervosa, psychoactive substance dependence, or anxiety disorder.

Everyone may experience some depressive symptoms following some traumatic or notable life event. Mild depressive episodes are usually related to some type of loss and are often accompanied by anger and guilt. The symptoms are usually self-limited and no treatment is necessary.

Epidemiology

Etiology. Biological, social, and psychological hypotheses have been developed to explain why depression occurs more frequently in women (Martin, 2000a).

Psychological models include psychosocial stresses and developmental problems (personality defects, childhood events). Sense of loss, failure to live up to one's ego ideal, and a sense of hopelessness and helplessness are all important concepts in the etiology of depression. Often, loss or perceived loss precedes the onset of depression. Loss may involve a person, expectation, or job. Common ideals are to be loved, to be good and kind, to be recognized for achievements, and to attain goals. With disappointments and failures comes the feeling of not living up to one's ego ideals. Guilt felt because of failure can lead to anger and self-hatred with feelings of hopelessness and helplessness. These feelings are related to one's negative self-concept, negative interpretation of one's experiences, and negative view of the future.

Other factors thought to affect the incidences of depression in women are environmental factors, other biologic and genetic components, and interpersonal processes (Martin, 2000a). Sexual discrimination, victimization, and sexual abuse occur more frequently in women than in men. Women are still the primary caretakers for their families and often must juggle the demands of home and work simultaneously. Difficulties in interpersonal relationships (West, Rose, Spreng et al., 1999), decreased self-esteem (Beeber, 1999; Roberts & Kendler, 1999), neuroticism (Roberts & Kendler, 1999), positive family history of depression (Bierut, Health, Bucholz, et al., 1999), and declines in physical health (Heidrich, 1998) are thought to increase the risk for depression. Ethnic differences in the rates of depression in women have also been noted. African American women and Hispanic women report higher levels of depressive symptoms than white women (Martin, 2000a; Rickert, Wiemann & Berenson, 2000).

A strong genetic basis has been implicated in the development of a depressive illness; a family history of depression increases a person's risk for depression. In addition, neurochemical dysregulation and changes in brain function are all thought to play a role (McCance & Huether, 2002). Decreases in the level of monoamines, norepinephrine, and serotonin are thought to cause symptoms with support evidenced by the decrease in symptoms with use of pharmacotherapy. Antidepressants, monoamine oxidase inhibitors (MAOIs), tricyclic antidepressants, and selective seritonin reuptake inhibitors (SSRIs) increase the level of monamines (norepinephrine and serotonin), albeit through different mechanisms. However, just increasing the level of MAOIs, is unlikely to be the only mechanism in reducing depressive symptoms (McCance & Huether, 2002; Stuart & Laraia, 2001). Clinically, there is a delay from when the drug is administered and the detection of improved mood by the clients. Over time, these various medications are about equal in effectiveness, suggesting that other mechanisms play a role.

In addition to a dysfunction in the MAOI system, the hypothalamic-pituitary-adrenal (HPA) axis also may be involved in depression. The HPA axis manages the body's response to stress by increasing hypothalamic production of corticotropin-releasing factor (CRF), which induces pituitary secretion of adrenocorticotropic hormone (ACTH), which in turn, stimulates adrenal release of cortisol. These changes provoke the "fight-or-flight response" (McCance & Huether, 2002). Chronic stimulation of this system is associated with depression.

Complex interactions between the monamines and acetylcholine systems suggest the need for further research on the diversity of neurotransmitters, their functions and response to antidepressant medications, and their interactions with other neurotransmitter systems (McCance & Huether, 2002). In addition, changes in the prefrontal and limbic regions of the brain are posited to be associated with the development of depression. There is significant correlation between cerebrovascular disease, specific brain injury (50 percent of clients develop poststroke depression) and depressive disorders (McCance & Huether, 2002). Further research may lead to other therapies to reduce depressive symptoms by treating these neuroanatomic and functional abnormalities.

Risk Factors. Risk factors include childhood adversity (Harkness & Monroe, 2002) a family history of depression, poor self-concept or self-esteem, female gender, chronic nonmood disorders, substance abuse, loss or death, and stressful life event. Suicidal risk factors include previous attempted suicide, depression, dysfunctional family, battering, alcoholism, and chronic illness.

Incidence. Women continue to have higher rates of depression than do men despite improvement in their economic status and opportunities for self-development. (Narrow, 1998). Nearly twice as many women (6.5 percent) as men (3.3 percent) suffer from major depression each year (Narrow, 1998). Reproductive events, such as menarche, menopause, childbirth, and infertility, are often associated with women's depression (Freeman, 2002). These data suggest that ovarian steroids may play an important role in the greater vulnerability to depression in women. The World Health Organization developed a single measure called the Disability Adjusted Life years (DALYs), which ranked major depression second only to

ischemic heart disease in the magnitude of disease burden in established market economies (Murray & Lopez, 1996).

Subjective Data

Women frequently report somatic symptoms rather than depression, and several conditions are typically revealed in history taking, including chronic illness and substance abuse.

Symptoms that the depressed woman frequently reports include headaches, constipation, sleep disturbance, loss of energy, change in appetite with weight loss or gain, decreased libido, and chronic pain. These symptoms are somatic complaints, and a woman will more often present with them than complaints of depression. Unidentifiable somatic complaints frequently indicate depression and fatigue, but often women with these symptoms are labeled hypochondriacal or neurotic (Stuart & Laraia, 2001). When asked about her feelings, a woman may admit to sadness; crying spells; feelings of guilt, worthlessness, or hopelessness; loss of interest in daily events; or withdrawal from work and recreation. She may complain of difficulty concentrating and thinking or an inability to make decisions.

History incorporates five areas: medical, family medical, gynecologic obstetric, social, and psychological.

Medical history is taken with the realization that any illness may cause depression, but chronic illness is the most likely cause. Questions regarding hospitalizations and injuries may provide important clues, especially if injuries are related to events such as violence or numerous accidents. Substance use should be included in the history, as it is often related to depression. In addition, include prescription and over-the-counter medications that are being taken, because some are associated with symptoms of depression. Stimulants can cause depression during withdrawal; certain antihypertensive agents, oral contraceptives, and corticosteroids may also cause depression.

Family medical history includes questions about the family's history of depression, mental illness, suicide, and substance abuse.

Gynecologic obstetric history includes the date of the previous menstrual period and cycle length to determine the possibility of premenstrual syndrome (PMS); PMS is associated with depression.

Social history includes marital status, family satisfaction, past or present violence or abusive home or work problems, job changes, economic status, and support systems. Recent losses and major stressors should be assessed (Stuart & Laraia, 2001).

Psychological history includes information about previous psychiatric illness, suicide attempts, and cognitive abilities (memory and thought process). Always ask about suicidal ideation, what means would be used, if a plan has been established, and when the plan is to be carried out (Stuart & Laraia, 2001).

Objective Data

A physical examination is done, as are several diagnostic tests, including those ruling out substance abuse.

Physical Examination. Begins with evaluation of the client's general appearance. She may be over-or under-weight, be unkempt, have poor affect, or move sluggishly.

- *Skin, Nails, and Hair.* Hair may be dirty and uncombed, and nails brittle and dry. Scars may be visible on the wrist or other parts of body.
- *Eyes.* The eyes may appear dull with fixed gaze, poor eye contact, circles under eyes from lack of sleep, and pale conjunctiva and mucosa.
- *Mouth.* Oral hygiene may be poor.
- *Neck.* Thyroid may be palpable or with nodules.
- *Nervous System.* See Substance Abuse and Violence sections. Mental status may require qualitative scales to determine degree of depression.

Diagnostic Tests. Vary according to presentation. Hematocrit and hemoglobin tests rule out anemia. The thyroid panel rules out thyroid disease. See Substance Abuse section for specific tests.

Nursing Implications

The health care provider must give full attention to the client in the privacy of an office. If the client does not feel comfortable, she will probably not be honest about her problem. A nurse practitioner may provide care for a mildly depressed woman usually in collaboration with a physician, but referral should be made to a qualified mental health professional for a seriously depressed woman. It is critical to know when to refer. *Always refer a client if suicidal ideation is expressed.*

Differential Medical Diagnoses

Chronic illness, hypothyroidism, depressive side effects from medication, premenstrual syndrome, substance abuse.

Plan

Psychosocial Intervention. The type of intervention depends on the type of depression. Individuals with major depression may benefit from antidepressant medication, education, supportive counseling, psychotherapy, and family therapy (Stuart & Laraia, 2001). Individuals with dysthymia are often given antidepressant medication for symptom relief, but they are not as helpful in alleviating symptoms as they are for a client with major depression. The client with dysthymia should also receive psychotherapy or supportive counseling. The client with reactive depression usually requires no antidepressant medication but responds well to education, supportive counseling, and family therapy. When precipitated by an illness, depression often resolves as the illness improves.

Client education should include information about depression and the relationship of its symptoms to medical illness, stressors, and situational crisis. It should be stressed that depression is a medical illness, not a character defect or weakness. Treatments are effective, and there are many treatment options. An effective treatment can be found for nearly every client. Recovery is the rule, not the exception. The goal is complete symptom remission. Recurrence is a risk; therefore, the client should be encouraged to return with any recurrent signs and symptoms. Teaching stress reduction, coping styles, and assertiveness may be beneficial (Martin, 2000a). Help the client identify and express her feelings of anger, hostility, sadness, and anxiety.

Supportive counseling focuses on encouraging the client to develop a social network and increase her activity. Participation in support groups may be beneficial for the client and her family. When appropriate, always involve persons who are important in the client's life.

Family counseling may be beneficial because episodes of depression have been associated with family dysfunction. Psychotherapy's goal is to correct specific aspects of depression, including thoughts, behavior, and affect. Its purpose is not to change the client's personality.

Treatment of Depression. Psychopharmacotherapeutics are frequently required in the treatment of mental health problems. Depression is no exception. Providers should be aware of certain principles of psychopharmacotherapy and adhere as closely as possible to these recommendations (see Table 23–1). Acute treatment (6 to 12 weeks) aims at remission of symptoms. When medication is used, it should be individualized to the client to optimize treat-

TABLE 23–1. Adverse Effects of Antidepressants

Drugs	Sedation	Anticholinergic	Orthostatic hypotension	Cardiac effects
Heterocyclics				
Amitriptyline	High	High	Moderate	High
Clomipramine	High	High	Low	Moderate
Desipramine	Low	Low	Low	Moderate
Doxepin	High	Moderate	Moderate	Moderate
Imipramine	Moderate	Moderate	High	High
Maprotiline	Moderate	Moderate	Low	Moderate
Nortriptyline	Moderate	Moderate	Low	Moderate
Protriptyline	Low	Moderate	Low	Moderate
Trimipramine	High	High	Moderate	High
Selective Serotonin Reuptake Inhibitors				
Fluoxetine	Low	None	None	None
Paroxetine	Low	Low	None	None
Sertraline	Low	None	None	None
Fluvoxamine	Low	None	None	None
Citalopram	Low	None	None	None
Selective Norepinephrine Reuptake Inhibitors				
Reboxetine	Low	Low	Low	Low
Dibenzoxazepines				
Amoxapine	Low	Moderate	Low	None
Phenylpiperazines				
Trazodone	High	Low	Moderate	Low
Nefazodone	Low	Low	Low	Low
Aminoketones				
Bupropion	High	Very low	Very low—none	Low
Serotonin and Norepinephrine Reuptake Inhibitors				
Venlafaxine	Low	Very low	Very low	Low
Serotonin and Norepinephrine Receptor Activity				
Mirtazapine	Moderate	Low	Low	Low
Monoamine Oxidase Inhibitors				
Isocarboxazid	Low	None	High	None
Phenelzine	Low	Low	High	None
Tranylcypromine	High	Very low	Very low	None

Source: Janiak, 2001.

ment benefits and lower risk. Considerations in choosing a medication include short- and long-term side effects, past experience with medications, possible drug interactions, presence of other conditions, and age. Acute treatment should be monitored every one to two weeks. Evaluation at six weeks determines if the client is responding. If the desired response occurs, continue treatment for six weeks. If the client experiences some improvement, but not the desired response, consider adjusting the dosage. If there is no response, the treatment may need to be changed. Continue to monitor every one to two weeks. Consult if the desired response does not occur.

Continuation treatment (4 to 9 months) aims at preventing relapse. Medication should be continued at full dosage.

Maintenance treatment aims at preventing recurrences in clients with prior episodes. Clients who have has three or more major depressive episodes should continue medication for at least one to two years. Current recommendations for clients who have had three or more episodes in five years is lifelong drug therapy (Goroll et al., 2000).

The objective throughout each treatment phase is attainment of a sustained asymptomatic state. The essential features of the plan should include education; regular monitoring of side effects, if mediation is prescribed, and depressive symptoms; and adjustment or changes in the plan if response is not timely or complete. While advances in psychopharmacology have reduced depressive symptoms in certain clients, health care providers should remember the need still remains to examine aspects of a woman's interpersonal relationships and resultant patterns of coping that may contribute to the development of and reoccurrence of major depression.

Medication. Medication includes antidepressant drugs, which work to elevate mood. Three major types are tricyclic antidepressants (TCAs), monoamine oxidase inhibitors (MAOIs), heterocyclic antidepressants and selective serotonin reuptake inhibitors (SSRIs). SSRIs are the most commonly prescribed antidepressant medication due to their low occurrence of side effects. Most antidepressants may take several weeks before clinical improvement. Consequently, tell the client not to expect sudden improvement. Stress compliance. Instruct the client to avoid alcohol and other mood altering substances. Table 23–1 provides an overview of the adverse effect profiles of antidepressants, and Table 23–2 gives common treatments by generic name, brand name, usual initial dose, titrated dose regimen, and the relative cost.

Caution clients to notify the provider if they have thoughts of suicide. Consultation with a physician is indicated.

Follow-Up

Initially, follow-up should be weekly, with telephone backup. The health care provider may counsel the reactive depressed client without referral for therapy. The client with major depression or dysthymia, however, should be referred for family counseling and psychotherapy. If a client exhibits a personality disorder or suicidal tendencies or the cause of depression is unidentifiable, a referral to a mental health professional should also be made. After medication is determined, collaboration with a physician and follow-up may be indicated.

The suicidal client should always be referred. If a client contacts the provider and states she is suicidal, find out her location, keep her on the line, and telephone

TABLE 23–2. Antidepressants

Generic Name	Brand Name	Customary Initial Dose	Titrate Dose Up To	Relative Cost
Selective Serotonin Reuptake Inhibitors				
Citalopram	Celexa	20 mg/d	20–40 mg/d	1.0
Fluoxetine	Prozac	20 mg/d	20–40 mg/d	1.25
Fluvoxamine	Luvox	50 mg/d	100–250 mg/d	1.25
Paroxetine	Paxil	20 mg/d	20–60 mg/d	1.25
Sertraline	Zoloft	50 mg/d	100–250 mg/d	1.1
Atypical Antidepressants				
Bupropion (sustained release)	Bupropion-SR	150 mg SR qam	150–200 mg bid	1.9
Mirtazapine	Remeron	15 mg qhs	30–45 mg qhs	1.1
Nefazodone	Serzone	50 mg bid	150–300 mg bid	0.8
Trazodone	Desyrel	50–100 mg qhs	200–600 mg/d	3.6
	Generic			0.2
Venlafaxine (extended release)	Effexor-XR	37.5 mg XR bid	75–150 mg bid	1.1
Tricyclic Antidepressants				
Amitriptyline	Elavil	25 mg qhs	150–300 mg qhs	1.1
	Generic			0.03
Clomipramine	Anafranil	25 mg qhs	150–200 mg qhs	1.3
Desipramine	Norpramin	25 mg qam	150–300 mg qam	1.9
	Generic			0.3
Doxepin	Adapin	25 mg qhs	150–300 gm qhs	
Imipramine	Tofranil	25 mg qhs	150–300 mg qhs	1.5
	Generic			0.03
Nortriptyline	Pamelor	10 mg qhs	50–150 mg qhs	1.8
	Generic			0.2
Protriptyline	Vivactil	10 mg qam	30–60 mg qam	0.35
Trimipramine	Surmontil	25 mg qhs	150–250 mg qhs	0.36
Monoamine Oxidase Inhibitors				
Phenelzine	Nardil	15 mg bid	45–90 mg/d	0.44
Tranylcypromine	Parnate	10 mg bid	40–80 mg/d	0.53
L-Deprenyl	Eldepryl	10 mg bid	30–40 mg/d	2.2

Source: Goroll, May, Mulley, 2000.

emergency medical services if another line is available. If she has not yet attempted suicide, try to persuade her to postpone suicide for a set period; if she has attempted suicide, try to find out what method was used.

ANXIETY

Anxiety may be defined as a normal emotional experience (part of normal stress reduction), a pathological cognitive/physiological symptom, or an abstract theoretical construct. (Stuart & Laraia, 2001). DSM-IV-TR classifies anxiety disorders as panic disorder, agoraphobia, social phobia, simple phobia, obsessive-compulsive disorder, post-traumatic stress disorder, and generalized anxiety disorder. The disorders may overlap. With striking regularity, concomitant medical illness occurs in psychiatric clients (APA, 2000). Indeed, medical illness may cause psychiatric symptoms or exacerbate underlying psychiatric symptomatology. In patients who suffered major depression and chronic disease, Katon (2001) noted four primary adverse impacts: (1) increased medical utilization and costs, (2) higher symptom burdens, (3) increased functional impairment and other morbidities, and (4) increased rates of mortality.

Types of Anxiety Disorders

Four types of anxiety are described below.

Panic disorders are short-lived, recurrent, unpredictable episodes of intense anxiety accompanied by physiological symptomatology. Episodes of apprehension, fear, and a sense of doom may be precipitated by a stimulus or may arise spontaneously (APA, 2000).

Generalized anxiety is defined as unrealistic or excessive anxiety and worry about two or more life circumstances occurring for six months or longer (APA, 2000). This disorder does not develop into panic attacks or phobias and is not due to physiological effects of a substance or a general medical condition (APA, 2000).

Phobic disorders use the mechanism of displacement. Clients transfer their feelings of anxiety from the true object to one that can be avoided (APA, 2000). Agoraphobia or a specific phobia can develop.

Obsessive-compulsive disorder involves an irrational idea or impulse that persistently intrudes into awareness (APA, 2000). The client recognizes its absurdity, but anxiety is relieved only with ritualistic performance, impulse, or entertainment of an idea.

Post-traumatic stress disorder is discussed later in this section.

Epidemiology

Risk Factors. Physical and mental illness, life situations or crises, and family history of anxiety disorders are risk factors for anxiety.

Incidence. Incidence varies among the four types of anxiety. Approximately 19.1 million Americans ages 18 to 54, or about 13.3 percent of people in this age group in a given year, have an anxiety disorder (Narrow, Rae, & Regier, 1998).

Panic Disorder. Ratio is 2:1 for prevalence among women; onset between late adolescence and mid-30s (late adulthood); affects between 1 to 2 percent with some studies reporting as high as 3.5 percent of the population (APA, 2000; NIMH, 2002).

Generalized Anxiety Disorder (GAD). Approximately 4.0 million U.S. adults ages 18 to 54, or about 2.8 percent of this age group in a given year, have GAD (Narrow et al., 1998). GAD can begin across the life cycle, though the risk is highest between childhood and middle age (NIMH, 2002).

Phobic Disorder. Depends on type of phobia (animal phobias and agoraphobia are more common among women). (APA, 2000). *Agoraphobia* involves intense fear and avoidance of any place or situation where escape might be difficult or help unavailable in the event of developing sudden panic-like symptoms. Approximately 3.2 million U.S. adults ages 18 to 54, or about 2.2 percent of people in this age group in a given year, have agoraphobia (Narrow et al., 1998). *Specific phobia* involves marked and persistent fear and avoidance of a specific object or situation. Approximately 6.3 million U.S. adults ages 18 to 54, or about 4.4 percent of people in this age group in a given year, have some type of specific phobia (Narrow et al., 1998).

Obsessive-Compulsive Disorder. Occurs equally in women and men. Community studies have estimated a lifetime prevalence of 2.5 percent; however, methodology problems reported with the assessment tool may have overestimated this rate, and the rate may, in fact, be lower than reported (APA, 2000).

Subjective Data

The client may report dyspnea, shortness of breath or smothering sensation, palpitations, tachycardia, chest pain, flushing, sweating or cold clammy hands, abdominal discomfort, diarrhea, nausea, dry mouth, difficult swallowing, urinary frequency, headache, muscle tension, aches, soreness, trembling, twitching, or shakiness (APA, 2000).

Psychological complaints may include restlessness, fatigue, sleep disturbances, irritability or edginess, exaggerated startle response, difficulty concentrating, fear of being in places or situations from which escape might be difficult.

Anxiety produces symptoms that involve multiple organ systems and causes confusion and frequent medical consultation and testing. Moreover, certain medical conditions and medication produce symptoms of anxiety disorders (APA, 2000). In taking a history, explore the client's chief complaint, including precipitating factors, duration of symptoms, and use and effectiveness of self-treatment.

Past medical history includes chronic disease, illness, hospitalizations, and surgeries.

Medication use includes present and past prescription medications and over-the-counter medicines. Medications such as bronchodilators, caffeine, thyroid preparations, and sedatives-hypnotics can cause anxiety states.

Habits include caffeine intake and use of tobacco, alcohol, and illicit substances.

Family medical history includes chronic diseases, substance abuse, and mental illness.

Gynecologic/obstetric history includes date of last (previous) menstrual period, cycle, and premenstrual symptoms.

Social history includes support systems, lifestyle, abusive home life, and job.

Psychiatric history includes previous depressive episode, peptic ulcer disease, migraine headaches, ulcerative colitis, or irritable bowel syndrome.

Objective Data

An extensive physical examination is done and a variety of diagnostic tests are performed.

Physical Examination

- *General Appearance.* The client may appear restless, trembling, or emotional.
- *Eyes.* Circles under the eyes indicate a lack of sleep. Nystagmus may be elicited with different maneuvers.
- *Ears.* Rule out otitis externa or media.
- *Mouth.* Rule out large tonsils, lesions, and polyps in throat causing difficult swallowing.
- *Neck.* Enlarged, tender, or nodular thyroid indicates thyroid disorder.
- *Skin.* Skin may be cold, clammy, sweaty, flushed, or pale.

- *Chest.* Respiratory rate may be increased. The client may hyperventilate. Wheezing may indicate asthma.
- *Vascular System.* Blood pressure and heartrate may be increased. A murmur, gallop, or click may indicate mitral valve prolapse or arrhythmias. Rule out heart disease with chest pain.
- *Abdomen.* The client may experience pain with palpation. Bowel sounds may be absent or hyperactive.
- *Musculoskeletal System.* Gait may be unsteady. Joints may be red and edematous and a source of pain. Muscle strength may be abnormal. Signs of trauma may be evident.
- *Nervous System.* Examination may reveal hyper-reflexia, positional vertigo, and abnormal cranial nerve findings.

Diagnostic Tests

- Electrocardiogram
- Electroencephalogram
- Urinalysis to rule out urinary tract infection and diabetes
- Thyroid panel as indicated
- Complete blood count to rule out anemia and infection
- Electrolytes as indicated
- Glucose tolerance test to rule out diabetes and hypoglycemia
- Upper and lower GI series if indicated

Nursing Implications

Showing genuine concern and empathy increases the chance that the client will perceive the health care provider as sympathetic to her problem. Use open-ended questions when interviewing to allow the client to disclose information she may not otherwise have revealed. Permit the client to ventilate her concerns and, at the same time, to prioritize them. Reassuring her may also be helpful.

Differential Medical Diagnoses

Hyperthyroidism, hypoglycemia, cancer, organic brain syndrome, depression, substance abuse, hypertension, side effects of prescription or over-the-counter medication, physical or sexual abuse.

Plan

Barlow (2002) has written a comprehensive treatment manual for anxiety disorders. Providers who are not familiar with these disorders and their treatment may benefit from reviewing this text.

Psychosocial Intervention. During an acute anxiety episode, stay with the client, decrease environmental stimuli, and, above all, remain calm. Counseling that focuses on the present, using reflection and clarification, is most effective. Deal with issues of fears, self-concept, self-esteem, problem solving, and coping mechanisms. Acknowledge and express acceptance of anxiety. Relaxation techniques and imagery may help decrease anxiety. Assist the client to identify sources of anxiety, to develop plans to deal with them, and to modify her lifestyle. Generally, it is important to emphasis healthy lifestyle behaviors; avoiding stress when possible, decreased caffeine, no alcohol or illicit drugs, proper exercise and sleep. Social support is known to be helpful in reducing anxiety symptoms. Knowing that she has a condition that is treatable provides immense relief, as many people think they are going crazy.

Medication. Medication categories include SSRIs, benzodiazepines, tricyclic antidepressants, monoamine oxidase inhibitors (MAOIs); and beta-adrenergic blocking agents. If the client's symptoms are not related to a specific syndrome other than anxiety, the client is usually treated with psychotropic medications. Benzodiazepines (BZDs) are the most widely used of the anxiolytics. Table 23–3 provides pharmacokinetic properties of commonly used BZDs. For single-dose use, the desirable pharmacokinetic properties are rapid onset and offset. For maintenance use, a drug's serum half-life is the important parameter. Short-acting BSDs increase the likelihood of anxiousness between doses (Goroll et al., 2000). If a primary care provider selects one of the BZDs, it should be considered only for clients with disabling or severe symptoms and for clients who are unlikely to abuse it. Duration of therapy should be short and dosage tailored to the individual. Progress must be monitored. Addiction and withdrawal are possible. Betaadrenergic blockers (propranolol) can be used to reduce peripheral somatic symptoms, but they are considered less effective than other anti-anxiety agents. SSRIs are often used as first-line agents in the treatment of anxiety. The major symptoms of panic disorder, social phobia, generalized anxiety disorder, PTSD, and OCD can often be alleviated by these drugs (Goroll et al., 2000). TCAs and MAOIs are generally used for refractory patients.

Common side effects of BZDs are dizziness, drowsiness, fatigue, confusion, disorientation, and, above all, psychological addiction. Contraindications are pregnancy, known hypersensitivity to BZDs, and use with alcohol and other central nervous system depressants. Weekly follow-up visits are encouraged. Discontinue medication as soon as possible. Provide information about side effects and contraindications and when to contact provider. Emphasize the need to use an effective contraceptive and avoid alcohol and other central nervous system depressants. Caution clients not to drive or use potentially dangerous equipment because of the sedative effects of anxiolytic agents.

Common side effects of beta blockers are masking of hypoglycemic symptoms in diabetics, bradycardia, and hypotension. They are contraindicated in clients who have congestive heart failure, greater than first-degree A-V block, and asthma. Tricyclic antidepressants can cause sedation, orthostatic hypotension, and anticholinergic effects. A small number of clients may experience a worsening of their anxiety symptoms while taking TCAs.

Another medication used as an anxiolytic, but unrelated to benzodiazepines or barbiturates, is busperone (Buspar). Buspar requires several weeks to achieve its full effect. The dosage is increased daily (by 5mg/day) to a maximum of 20 mg po every 8 hours. Dizziness, headaches, GI upset, nervousness are selected side effects. It is contraindicated if the women is receiving MAOIs. Advantages of Buspar are that it causes less sedation, and no withdrawal symptoms or tolerance are reported. Currently, it is the treatment of choice for generalized anxiety disorder (GAD).

Other Treatment. Psychotherapy is often helpful in the treatment of anxiety disorders. Interpersonal dynamic and cognitive-behavior therapies are used in conjunction with medication. Clients with dual diagnoses or personality disorders should be referred to a mental health specialist for consultation.

Follow-Up

Follow-up is weekly; however, during an acute episode, daily clinic visits may be necessary. Referral depends on the health care provider's expertise, the severity of the client's symptoms and functional impairment, her response to intervention, and her receptiveness and motivation. Consultation with a physician, referral, or both are indicated when medication is used or if signs of underlying physical or emotional problems are present. Immediately refer a client with any suicidal ideation.

POST-TRAUMATIC STRESS DISORDER

Epidemiologic survey studies have shown that post-traumatic stress disorder (PTSD) is twice as common in women as men (Brady, 2001). Gender differences may be related to the type of trauma exposure, presentation of ill-

TABLE 23–3. Half-Lives, Doses, and Preparations of Benzodiazepine Receptor Agonists and Antagonists

Drug	Dose Equivalents	Half-Life (h)	Rate of Absorption	Usual Adult Dosage	Dose Preparations
Agonists					
Clonazepam	0.5	Long (metabolite, > 20)	Rapid	1–6 mg/d b.i.d.	0.5 mg, 1.0 mg, and 2.0 mg tablets
Diazepam	5	Long (> 20) (Nordiazepam—long, > 20)	Rapid	4–40 mg/d b.i.d. to q.i.d.	2 mg, 5 mg, and 10 mg tablets (slow-release 15 mg capsules)
Alprazolam	0.25	Intermediate (6–20)	Medium	0.5–10 mg/d b.i.d. to q.i.d.	0.25 mg, 0.5 mg, 1.0 mg, and 2.0 mg tablets
Lorazepam	1	Intermediate (6–20)	Medium	1–6 mg/d t.i.d.	0.5 mg, 1.0 mg, and 2.0 mg tablets, 2 mg/mL, 4 mg/mL parenteral
Oxazepam	15	Intermediate (6–20)	Slow	30–120 mg/d t.i.d. or q.i.d.	10 mg, 15 mg, and 30 mg capsules (15 mg tablets)
Temazepam	5	Intermediate (6–20)	Medium	7.5–30 mg/d h.s.	7.5 mg, 15 mg, and 30 mg capsules
Chlordiazepoxide	10	Intermediate (6–20) (Demethylchlordiazepoxide—intermediate, 6–20) (Demoxapam—long, >20) (Nordiazepam—long, >20)	Medium	10–150 mg t.i.d. or q.i.d.	5 mg, 10 mg, and 25 mg tablets or capsules
Flurazepam	5	Short (<6) (N-hydroxyethylflurazepam—short, <6) (N-desalkylflurazepam—long, >20)	Rapid	15–30 mg h.s.	15 mg and 30 mg capsules
Triazolam	0.1–0.03	Short (<6)	Rapid	0.125 mg or 0.250 mg h.s.	0.125 mg or 0.250 mg tablets
Clorazepate	7.5	Short (<6) Nordiazepam—long, >20)	Rapid	15–60 mg b.i.d. or q.i.d.	3.75 mg, 7.5 mg, and 15 mg tablets (slow release 11.25 mg and 22.5 mg tablets)
Halazepam	20	Short (<6) (Nordiazepam—long, >20)	Medium	60–160 mg/d t.i.d. or q.i.d.	20 mg and 40 mg tablets
Prazepam	10	Short (<6) (Nordiazepam—long, >20)	Slow	30 mg/d (20–60 mg/d) q.i.d. or t.i.d.	5 mg, 10 mg, or 20 mg capsules
Estazolam	0.33	Intermediate (6–20) (4-hydroxyestazolam—intermediate 6–20)	Rapid	1.0 or 2.0 h.s.	1 mg and 2 mg tablets
Quazepam	5	Long (>20) (2-oxoquazepam-N-desalkylflurazepam—long, >20)	Rapid	7.5 or 15 mg h.s.	7.5 mg and 15 mg tablets
Midazolam	1.25–1.7	Short (<6)	Rapid	5 to 50 mg parenteral	5 mg/mL parenteral, 1 mL, 2 mL, 5 mL, and 10 mL vials
Zolpidem	2.5	Short (<6)	Rapid	5 mg or 10 mg h.s.	5 mg and 10 mg tablets
Zaleplon	?	Short (1)	Rapid	10 mg h.s.	5 mg and 10 mg capsules
Antagonist					
Flumazenil	0.05	Short (<6)	Rapid	0.2 to 0.5 mg/min injection over 3–10 min (total, 1–5 mg)	0.1 mg/mL (5 mL and 10 mL vials)

Source: Kaplan & Sadock, 2000.

ness, and presence of other psychiatric disorders (Brady, 2001). Alteration in biologic systems in PTSD may be related to the influences of sex hormones (Yehuda, 2001).

Symptoms of post-traumatic stress disorder (PTSD) develop following a psychologically distressing event that is outside the range of usual human experience (APA, 2000). The affected client reexperiences the traumatic event, avoids stimuli associated with the event, and exhibits a numbed general responsiveness and increased arousal (APA, 2000). The trauma that is experienced may be a serious threat to life or physical integrity, a serious threat or harm to someone close to the client, sudden destruction of one's home or community, or recently seeing someone injured or killed (APA, 2000).

Subjective Data

According to DSM-IV-TR (APA, 2000), a client must meet the following diagnostic criteria for PTSD: A person must have experienced a traumatic event in which both of the following were true: (1) the person experienced, observed, or was involved with an event(s) where harm or death were threatened and (2) intense fear, helplessness or horror were the primary affects. Symptoms may include any of the following: (1) persistent distressing memories of the event, (2) recurrent upsetting dreams, (3) reliving the experience as if it were happening now, (4) psychological distress following cues that remind the client of the event, (5) persistent avoidance of specific things that remind the client of the event, and (6) symptoms of increased arousal, e.g., insomnia, exaggerated startle response.

Objective Data and Differential Medical Diagnoses

See Anxiety, Depression, and Substance Abuse sections.

Plan

Figure 23–1 describes the treatment strategies recommend for anxiety related disorder.

Psychosocial Intervention. Focus on counseling that emphasizes the here and now and strengthens existing defenses. Helping clients to clarify the problem allows them to begin viewing it within its proper context and facilitates decision making. Instructing clients about stress reduction techniques and encouraging them to develop relaxation and exercise programs may help them to reduce stress by providing other outlets for their feelings.

Medication. Selective serotonin reuptake inhibitors (SSRIs) are efficacious in the treatment of PTSD (Brady, Pearlstein, Asnis, et al., 2000; Davidson, Pearlstein, Londborg, et al., 2001; Davidson, Rothbaum, Van der Kolk, Sikes, & Farfel; 2001).

Follow-Up

Group and individual psychotherapy are usually needed for PTSD. Refer the client to a psychiatrist or mental health counselor for psychotherapy and medication. As with anxiety, referral for other manifestations of stress depends on the health care provider's expertise, the severity of symptoms and functional impairment, the client's response to intervention, and her receptiveness and motivation (Goroll et al., 2000).

EATING DISORDERS

Eating disorders are complex psychological problems that have genetic, neurochemical, developmental, sociocultural, behavioral, and familial component. Table 23–4 describes the American Psychiatric Association's diagnostic criteria for the three major eating disorders. For additional information about the developmental aspects of an eating disorder, see Chapter 3. Disorders discussed in this chapter are anorexia nervosa, bulimia, and binge-eating disorder; these are the most common eating disturbances of adolescents and adults (Goroll et al., 2000).

The largest percentage of clients with eating disorders are female (APA, 2000). The contemporary American body is seen as lean, strong, feminine, and graceful. The focus on this ideal has led many women to strive for unrealistic goals for their body shape.

A client's symptoms of an eating disorder can vary throughout the disease course. For example, a client may exhibit behaviors seen in different types of eating disorders, or her behavior may change over time from behavior more typical of anorexia to that which is typical of bulimia.

Several characteristics, however, are frequently reported by women with an eating disorder. For example, one or both parents or a sibling is preoccupied with weight and food. Or a crisis, such as loss, may precipitate an eating disorder; loss may be real (death) or psychological (breakup of a relationship or a move from familiar surroundings).

Another characteristic is family chaos, such as alcoholism drug addiction, violence, sexual abuse (Wonderlich, Crosby, Mitchell, et al., 2001) compulsive gambling, affective disorder, or depression. The client's behavior is a symptom of the family's ineffective coping style, not the cause of it. She has learned that unpleasant emotions, such as anger, disappointment, sorrow, and loss, are to be avoided. Consequently, she becomes accomplished at denial and may be unable to recognize the normal range and expression of human emotions.

In addition, a client's independence or autonomy from her family may have been stifled, allowing little control over her life. Control of her body is control of something. Finally, the common denominators of any eating disorder are low self-esteem and a distorted body image.

Eating disorders include a wide spectrum of gross disturbances in eating behaviors. Generally, however,

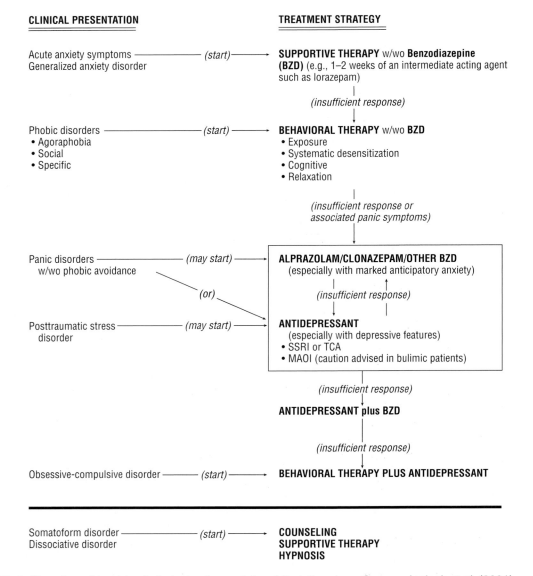

FIGURE 23–1. Overview of treatment strategies for anxiety-related disorders. *Source: Janicak et al. (2001).*

anorexics control weight by restricting food intake and by excessive exercise; bulimics alternate strict dieting with episodes of binging and purging; binge eaters also alternate strict dieting with binges but do not purge. It is important to differentiate binge-eating disorder from obesity: Although the two have similar long-term health risks, *obesity* is a term based on weight that does not address psychological issues.

Unfortunately, predictors of outcome and prognosis for clients with anorexia and bulimia vary considerably

because of diverse methodology, inconsistent utilization of diagnostic criteria, and lack of specifically defined criteria for recovery, relapse, and recurrence. It is important to note that eating disorders can be fatal, and even if they are not, they can cause significant physical and psychological complications.

DSM-IV-TR also includes the category Eating Disorders Not Otherwise Specified. Binge-eating disorder is one example of such a disorder. It is characterized by normal or excess weight in a person who has binge eating

TABLE 23–4. Eating Disorders: Characteristics That Aid in Diagnosis

Bulimia Nervosa

Concern about personal weight or shape of body is excessive; weight usually in normal range though may fluctuate widely

Binge eating is recurrent and uncontrolled followed by purging, fasting, laxative abuse, diuretic use, or excessive exercising

Socially, very outgoing, but frequently evidences symptoms of depression

Anorexia Nervosa

Obsessed with maintaining low weight; is less than 85 percent of expected body weight or BMI is less than 17.5 kg/m^2; appearance is emaciated

Personal perception of body weight, size, or shape is distorted; socially withdrawn

Obsessed with food and very fearful of gaining weight even when extremely thin

Evidences a rigorous need to control weight; fasting, dieting, purging, excessive exercising, repeated laxative use are examples of methods

Lack of menses (amenorrhea) is common and may be the symptom/sign that brings the woman to see the provider

Binge-Eating Disorder

Stress, dysphoric mood, hunger trigger bingeing

Bingeing is recurrent more than once a week for six months or more

Evidences extreme distress plus at least three of the following: eating alone; very rapid eating; eating until so full as to be uncomfortable; eating when no hunger is felt

Does not purge, exercise excessively, or fast

Sources: Adapted from APA (2000); Goroll et al. (2000); Landis & Bryant (1999).

episodes but does not engage in purging behaviors (APA, 2000). One consistent finding of studies is that the prevalence of eating disorders is increasing (APA, 2000).

Palmer (2002) has written a clinical guide describing the assessment and treatment of eating disorders. Providers not as familiar with these disorders may find it helpful.

Anorexia Nervosa

Essential features of anorexia nervosa according to *DSM-IV-TR* criteria are refusal to maintain body weight above minimal normal weight for age and height; intense fear of gaining weight or becoming fat, even though underweight; distorted body image ("feeling fat" when obviously underweight or even emaciated); and amenorrhea (absence of at least three consecutive menstrual cycles when otherwise expected to occur or menstruation that occurs only following hormone administration) (APA, 2000).

The DSM-IV-TR specifies two types of anorexia nervosa: the restricting type in which clients do not regularly engage in binge eating or purging behavior and the binge-eating/purging type in which clients do engage in binge-eating or purging behavior.

The client is preoccupied with food, weight, and diet (e.g., she counts the calories in one Life-saver candy when keeping a food diary) and weighs herself more than once a day. She exhibits compulsive behaviors and low self-esteem. The client hoards food, has bizarre eating behaviors, and limits selections to a few low calorie foods. She may overexercise to the point of exhaustion or injury.

Epidemiology

Risk Factors. Among the risk factors are female gender (20:1 female:male ratio); rarely occurs over age 40; age range of 15 to 50 (APA, 2000); career choice that stresses thinness, competition, perfection, or self-discipline (modeling, theater, ballet, competitive athletics); parent or sibling with eating disorder, affective disorder, or substance abuse problem; psychiatric illness or depression; or being achievement oriented, compliant, "model" child, or perfectionist. A tremendous toll is taken on the families and clients affected by this illness. Mortality from anorexia nervosa is estimated to be between 6 and 10 percent; in a hospitalized population, it is estimated to be over 10 percent. Death usually results from starvation, suicide, or electrolyte imbalance (APA, 2000).

Incidence. Approximately 0.5 percent of the female population will develop anorexia nervosa usually between the ages of 13 to 18 (APA, 2000). Onset is usually early to late adolescence. Anorexia nervosa usually occurs among white females of middle-upper socioeconomic status.

Subjective Data. The client may report feeling bloated, fatigue, constipation, diarrhea, decreased libido, cold intolerance, insomnia, sore tongue, frequent upper respiratory infections, muscle weakness and cramps, dizziness, social isolation, nausea, fainting spells. She may deny hunger or exhaustion. Amenorrhea or infertility is associated with anorexia and bulimia (APA, 2000). Women often hide their symptoms so the provider should maintain a high index of suspicion especially if menstral irregularities exist (Goroll et al., 2000). An evaluation should begin when clients report missing three to six menstrual cycles.

Subtle clues may be detected by a health care provider who is attuned to the client. For example, the client may be oversensitive when weighed or have excessive concerns about being overweight, even if she appears normal or under normal weight. She may request advice about fad diets and weight loss programs, may claim she "does not have enough time to eat," may dress in oversized clothes or layers of clothing to hide weight or health (yet she denies a problem), and may be compulsive about exercise. A wide discrepancy may exist in caloric intake and expenditure, leading to caloric deficit and subsequent weight loss.

Thorough medical and psychosocial histories are of utmost importance. Various screening tools are available and most often used in psychotherapy: *Eating Attitudes Test* (EAT), *Diagnostic Survey for Eating Disorders* (DSED), *Eating Disorder Inventory* (EDI), and *Bulimia Test* (BULIT). A pertinent history that is applicable to any eating disorder addresses five topics.

Attitude. Weight attitudes and problems may be detected by asking several questions. Do you like yourself at current weight? What would you like to weigh? What was your weight in the past month? The past six months? What are your highest and lowest weights? Have you always been over/underweight? Are other family members over/underweight?

Diet History. Ask the client to complete a 24-hour dietary intake record of the previous day including breakfast, lunch, dinner, snacks; caffeine (sodas, tea, coffee); alcohol, recreational drugs, and tobacco; and medications (prescription and over the counter). Ask the client the following: What constitutes a binge? A reasonable meal? Note her reluctance or resistance to respond during the diet history. Assign the client the task of keeping a food/mood diary for several days: time of day eating occurred, food or beverage consumed, amount eaten, calories, food group supplied, how quickly meal was eaten, degree of hunger, feelings and circumstances that prompted eating, where eating took place, names of persons who ate with client, activities while eating (e.g., sitting, standing, walking, lying down).

Exercise. Describe frequency (per day or week) and type of exercise. Differentiate compulsive exercise and athletic exercise. The athlete participates in purposeful training with an athletic goal and has high exercise tolerance, good muscle development, body fat within normal limits, and, most importantly, an accurate body image. The pressure to excel, especially among elite athletes, has brought attention to the "female athlete triad": disordered eating, amenorrhea, and osteoporosis. This is especially common among athletes competing in appearance or endurance sports. Parents, coaches, athletic trainers, team physicians, and athletic association administrators must also recognize their roles in the development of this pattern and consider the lifelong consequences for the athlete. If the client is a competitive athlete, she must learn at what point exercise loses its beneficial quality and becomes harmful. Reasons for excessive exercise should be evalu-

ated: Is it the demand of a coach or sport or is it compulsive behavior to manage anxiety or purge the effects of eating? Also, can the athlete with an eating disorder stop dieting, bingeing, or purging when the season is over? Does the athlete realize that the behavior may compromise, rather than enhance, performance?

Menstrual History. At what age did menarche occur and at what age did regular menses begin? Is the client currently menstruating? Has the client experienced a recent change in menstrual pattern (in many anorexics, this may be the first sign before low body weight)? What contraceptive method does she use? How many pregnancies? Abortions?

Social History. Does the client live alone? Does she cook or eat alone? Have friends and family complained of a change in her behavior? Ask the client to describe the number and character of her relationships. How many hours per week does she devote to school, work, or both?

Psychological History. Has she undergone a recent crisis? Has she ever had psychological counseling? Is she now undergoing counseling? Does she have symptoms of depression or anxiety? History of substance abuse? Does she exhibit symptoms of a personality disorder?

Bingeing/Purging History. Does she vomit frequently or use laxatives, diuretics, or appetite suppressants? Does she use syrup of ipecac? Ipecac is an inexpensive, over-the-counter drug that can be lethal. Repeated use results in chronic absorption causing myopathy, which is reversible on discontinuation of the drug. Potentially fatal cardiomyopathy, however, may also be a consequence of chronic use.

Objective Data. Data are determined by means of specific calculations to measure body fat and mass, physical examination, and several diagnostic tests to identify anemia and rule out imbalances in body chemistry and other metabolic reasons for weight loss.

Measurements. Measure frame size and compare height and weight with standardized height/weight tables (see Chapter 5 for discussion of ideal body weight). Measure percentage of body fat using skin fold calipers. Plot body mass index [weight (kg)/height cm^2]; indexes greater than 25.2 and 29.9 indicate obesity in men and women, respectively (Goroll et al., 2000). A BMI below 22 should raise a suspicion; a BMI of 15 means starvation.

Physical Examination

- *General Appearance.* The client appears pale and emaciated and manifests delayed sexual maturation.
- *Skin.* The client may have lanugo (fine, downy hair that covers extremities and face), brittle nails, dry skin, hair loss or thinning, and carotenemia evidenced by yellowing palms and soles.
- *Throat.* Buccal mucosa may be erythematous.
- *Breasts.* Breasts may be atrophied or poorly developed.
- *Vascular System.* Arrhythmias (secondary to electrolyte abnormalities) and peripheral edema may be detected.
- *Abdomen.* The abdomen may appear scaphoid. Bowel sounds may be hypoactive.
- *Genitalia and Reproductive Tract.* The client may have primary or secondary amenorrhea, irregular menses (may not be identified if she takes oral contraceptives), and decreased fertility. Preterm birth and stillbirth are associated with anorexia and pregnancy.
- *Rectal Area.* Hemorrhoids (secondary to constipation) may be present.
- *Musculoskeletal System.* The client may exhibit overuse injuries (stress fractures, joint or tendon problems). A client with severe anorexia is at risk for osteoporosis.
- *Nervous System.* Determine if the client is suicidal.
- *Endocrine System.* Thyroid abnormalities may be detected.

Diagnostic Tests

- *Urinalysis.* A urinalysis is done to evaluate carbohydrate metabolism and specific gravity. Elevated ketones and protein indicate low carbohydrate metabolism (due to poor intake). Specific gravity is increased if the client is dehydrated and decreased if she is drinking excessive water (common before being weighed). A urine pregnancy test is done if amenorrhea is a symptom and the client is sexually active.
- *Blood Chemistry.* A complete blood count is done to determine anemia and neutropenia. A full set of electrolytes are evaluated. Individuals who vomit and use laxatives and/or diuretics usually will have significant and sometimes life-threatening electrolyte imbalances. Decreased potassium may cause arrhythmia, then death. In addition, decreased calcium, magnesium, chloride, sodium, albumin, and globulin and increased BUN are typical with anorexia nervosa.

- *Liver Function Tests.* To help rule out other causes of weight loss, some values may be affected by malnutrition.
- *Endocrine Tests.* Levels of follicle-stimulating hormone and luteinizing hormone may be decreased. Prolactin, thyroid-stimulating hormone, and thyroxine levels may be normal. Thyroid function tests may be borderline low.
- *Electrocardiogram.* An electrocardiogram is indicated to determine the presence of arrhythmias, especially if the health care provider suspects poor follow-up or severe disease.
- If amenorrhea is persistent and weight loss marked, obtain a bone mineral density measure to rule out osteoporosis.

Differential Medical Diagnoses Weight loss: rule out hyperthyroidism, malabsorption syndrome, mesenteric artery syndrome, Addison's disease, Alzheimer's disease, Crohn's disease, depression, ischemic heart disease, carcinoma, other chronic diseases.

Amenorrhea, primary: rule out pituitary adenoma, ovarian failure, genital tract obstruction. (See Chapter 8.) Amenorrhea, secondary: rule out pregnancy, pituitary failure, weight loss or decreased body fat due to body building or sports. (See Chapter 8.)

Plan

Psychosocial Interventions. It is vital that a trusting relationship be established between the primary health care provider and the client; this process takes time. Support the client, and remain nonjudgmental if she reveals bizarre food habits. Help the client to find appropriate alternative coping behaviors and reestablish a healthy attitude regarding food and weight. In addition, act as role model by accepting your body size and weight and by maintaining healthy eating and exercise habits. Villapiano and Goodman (2001) have written a comprehensive workbook that providers may find helpful in work with clients suffering from eating disorders.

Since the woman with anorexia nervosa is at risk for serious health consequences, consultation with a mental health professional and a primary care physician is advised. Coordination of care between providers is critical. Other resources are essential, for example, individual and/or group therapy (group therapy reduces secrecy and allows sharing of concerns), assertiveness training, self-esteem and body image groups, family therapy.

Medication. Psychotropics are not usually used in treating anorexia nervosa but a SSRI, such as fluoxetine (up to 60 mg per day) can help prevent relapse if weight is within 15 percent of normal (Goroll et al., 2000).

Diet. Diet modification includes psychological measures, as well as careful nutritional planning, preferably by a nutritionist. Goals are to help the client understand basic nutritional education, her own nutritional requirements, and the relationship between dieting and disordered eating patterns. A computer nutritional analysis is helpful in comparing the client's intake with healthy percentages of fat, carbohydrates, and protein. Estimate her basal metabolic rate. This method provides reality-based information to help dispel the client's nutritional myths.

Contract negotiation between client and health care provider focuses on an acceptable weight range and plan for exercise, food intake, and follow-up. Self-contract enhances the client's control in that she is responsible both for changing her behavior and identifying the reward to reinforce health-promoting behavior. The ultimate responsibility for recovery lies with the client. If, however, the provider feels the client is endangering herself (low weight, excessive purging, refusing to eat, suicidal gestures), the provider must recommend inpatient therapy, which requires breaking confidentiality.

The food pyramid is used in nutritional planning (Villapiano & Goodman, 2001). The client chooses foods in all food groups. Urge her to use servings, *not* calories, as a basis for planning: no fewer than 2 or 3 servings of meat or other protein, 6 to 11 of grains, 2 to 4 of fruits, 3 to 5 of vegetables, and 2 to 3 of milk. Smaller, more frequent meals may be more acceptable to a client who "feels full" quickly. Incorporate previously "forbidden" foods, that is, carbohydrates, into plan. Increase calories enough to elicit a 1- to 2- pound per week increase in weight.

Exercise. Exercise should be modified. Encourage the client to decrease the amount and intensity; for example, change from high-impact aerobics to strengthening/stretching, low-impact aerobics, or walking several times a week. If the client refuses to decrease exercise, she must substantially increase her food intake.

Follow-Up. Monitor the client's well-being. Assess weight weekly; the client should wear similar clothes each time. If the client weighs herself several times daily, encourage her to limit weighing to once a day or less.

Hospitalization criteria are made clear to client at her initial visit. This places the responsibility for control on the client.

Medical Indications for Hospitalization.

- Loss of more than 40 percent of premorbid or ideal weight (or 30 percent if within three months)

- Rapid progression of weight loss
- Presence of cardiac arrhythmias
- Persistent hypokalemia unresponsive to outpatient treatment
- Symptoms of inadequate cerebral perfusion or mentation (syncope, severe dizziness, listlessness) (Goroll et al., 2000)

Psychiatric Indications for Hospitalization.

- Moderate to severe depression (suicide risk)
- Inability to function at home, work, or school
- Inability of family or current living arrangement to provide adequate psychological environment for improvement to occur
- Lack of improvement in outpatient treatment

The prognosis for recovery from anorexia nervosa is poor, thus requiring long-term treatment and follow-up. Some clients may fully recover after one incidence, others may recover and relapse many times, still others continue to have symptoms over a number of years with gradual physical deterioration. The long-term mortality is estimated to be 5 percent (Goroll et al., 2000).

Bulimia

Specific criteria characterize bulimia (APA, 2000). Most characteristic, perhaps, are the recurrent episodes of binge eating. A binge is described as the rapid consumption of a large amount of food in a discrete period. To be diagnosed with bulimia, a client must have had, on average, a minimum of two binge-eating episodes per week for at least three months. During binges, clients often consume high-calorie, sweet, salty, or starchy food (junk food) that is easily and rapidly eaten. The binge is terminated by abdominal discomfort, sleep, social interruption, or induced vomiting. The client feels a lack of control over eating behavior during binges. Moreover, the client is often self-critical and depressed following a binge.

In addition, self-induced vomiting, use of laxatives or diuretics, strict dieting or fasting, or vigorous exercise is used to prevent weight gain. The client is persistently overconcerned with body shape and weight. Frequent weight fluctuations (10 pounds per month) due to alternating binges and fasts are common; most bulimics are within the normal weight range. Bulimics also exhibit poor impulse control (promiscuity, shoplifting, self-mutilation) and may be multiple substance abusers (most frequently sedatives, amphetamines, cocaine, or alcohol).

Epidemiology. Bulimia occurs most often among females aged 13 to 50 and can affect up to 15 percent of college women (Goroll et al., 2000).

Risk Factors. Obesity during adolescence (may have started restrictive diet, now out of control), substance abuse, depression, and family history of alcoholism or affective disorder are risk factors.

Incidence. The condition is estimated to occur among 1 to 3 percent of adolescent and young women; the rate in males is estimated to be approximately one-tenth of that in females (APA, 2000).

Onset occurs in adolescence and early adulthood or during developmental transitions (college, marriage, breakup of relationship). Mortality is rare. It is usually related to unintended aspiration of vomitus or electrolyte abnormalities that cause cardiac arrhythmias or sudden death.

Subjective Data. The client usually acknowledges and is disturbed by her abnormal eating behavior. Negative thoughts, routine stress, and diet hunger can lead to binges. She usually feels shame and self-loathing afterwards. She may report abdominal distention, cramping, and constipation secondary to chronic laxative abuse. She may seek advice or prescriptions for laxatives, diuretics, or diets. The client may also describe muscle weakness and fatigue, depression, chronic pharyngitis, difficulty swallowing, esophageal irritations, frequent dental problems, shortness of breath, palpitations, and chest pain. She may spontaneously regurgitate food, may skip heartbeats, and may be able to consume large amounts of food that are inconsistent with her weight.

She may be secretive and plan binges. Family or roommates report that the client is frequently in the bathroom after meals with the shower or water running. She may steal money to buy food or steal food or laxatives. Binges may cost significant amounts of money; consequently, the woman is always without funds.

Weight fluctuations occur as a result of binges, which vary from 1000 to 5000 calories. Bingeing and purging may be carried out from a few times per month to twenty times per day. Injuries result from excessive exercise (3 to 5 hours per day); the client may be an aerobics instructor at more than one fitness center. She may be a high achiever, but passive and nonassertive.

Objective Data. A complete physical examination is done as are several diagnostic tests.

Physical Examination

- *General Appearance.* The client appears to be of normal weight for her height, although she may be slightly overweight.

- *Skin.* There may be scars on the dorsum of the hand from induced vomiting.
- *Head.* Examination may reveal bilateral parotid gland enlargement and "chipmunk" appearance.
- *Eyes.* Conjunctival hemorrhages may result from forceful vomiting.
- *Throat.* The dental enamel on inner aspects of the teeth may be eroded.
- *Chest.* Aspiration pneumonia from vomitus is most likely to occur with concomitant alcohol or drug ingestion.
- *Breasts.* Striae may be the result of weight fluctuations.
- *Vascular System.* Examination may reveal arrhythmias and peripheral edema secondary to laxative withdrawal (related to electrolyte disturbances). Sudden death may result from the cumulative ingestion of syrup of ipecac.
- *Abdomen.* There may be esophageal tears or rupture. Abdominal striae and poor musculature are due to rapid weight changes.
- *Genitalia and Reproductive Tract.* Pregnancy is a risk if the client vomits after taking oral contraceptives. In pregnancy, severe electrolyte imbalance can be lethal to the fetus. Other associated reproductive complications are low birthweight, low APGAR scores, stillbirth, cleft palate, and abnormal presentation during labor.
- *Rectum.* Tearing and fissures may be caused by frequent enemas or hemorrhoids.
- *Musculoskeletal System.* Overuse injuries may be evident.
- *Nervous System.* Convulsions may be due to electrolyte imbalances.
- *Endocrine System.* Menstrual irregularities may be experienced. Conceiving may be difficult. The client who is an insulin-dependent diabetic is at risk for hyper- or hypoglycemia and ketoacidosis.

Diagnostic Tests

- Urinalysis
- Complete blood count (anemia neutropenia).
- Electrolytes (calcium, potassium, magnesium, sodium, phosphorus, chloride, total protein decreased due to laxative abuse).
- Liver function tests (especially with alcohol or substance abuse).
- Electrocardiogram (indicated especially with ipecac use, prolonged use can cause a reversible proximal myopathy and a potentially fatal cardiomyopathy

- ◆ Amylase test (differing reports use it as an indication of bulimia).
- ◆ Chest x-ray (may be indicated to rule out aspiration pneumonia).

Differential Medical Diagnoses. Digitalis or pilocarpine toxicity, gastrointestinal carcinoma, malignant hypertension, pyloric obstruction, mesenteric artery syndrome, metabolic alkalosis, migraine, pinealoma, postconcussive syndrome, posterior fossa tumor.

Plan

Psychosocial Intervention. Psychotherapy is required for treatment. Mental health professionals often use cognitive-behavior therapy to modify eating and weight control behaviors and promote changes in attitudes that contribute to the disordered eating. For interventions appropriate for the primary care provider, see the Anorexia section.

Medication. Fluoxetine is the only drug approved by the FDA for use in the treatment of bulimia. Tricyclics (desipramine and imipramine, dosages of up to 300 mg per day) have been shown to be helpful (Goroll et al., 2000).

Diet. Dietary intervention includes identifying "triggers." In addition, the client should be instructed in several steps toward recovery: to keep binge foods out of sight (or not purchase them), to be with other people at times known to be vulnerable (weekends, evenings) or to change her environment; to learn to nurture self in ways other than eating (taking bubble baths, reading, pursuing hobbies, telephoning a friend). The client should plan three to four regularly scheduled meals per day and eat them regardless of binges and purges. Nonemaciated bulimics should be encouraged to maintain weight or to gain gradually by consuming no fewer than 1800 to 2400 calories per day.

Lifestyle Changes. See Anorexia.

Follow-Up. Follow-up is weekly or every two weeks to assess the client's weight. More crucial than weight evaluation, however, is monitoring the frequency of binge/purge behavior, exercise, and abuse of laxatives, appetite suppressants, and diuretics.

Hospitalization criteria are described under Anorexia. Hospitalization is not usual for bulimia unless bingeing and purging are almost totally interfering with the woman's life. Suicidal ideation requires hospitalization. Severity of the eating disorder, financial resources, and ability to manage the client in an outpatient setting will influence the decision to hospitalize a client with bulimia. Morbidity and mortality rates associated with this disorder are not known.

Binge-Eating Disorder

Binge-eating disorder is presently listed in the section on criteria sets and axes provided for further study in the DSM-IV-TR (APA, 2000). It is characterized by clients who eat large quantities of food and calories, but do not attempt to prevent weight gain by purging, fasting, or excessive exercise (APA, 2000). Previous description of this problem included compulsive overeating and pathological overeaters. The binge eating occurs, on average, at a minimum of two days a week for six months. Food is used to cope with stress, emotional conflicts, daily problems, boredom, depression, anxiety, loneliness, and anger (APA, 2000).

Not all clients diagnosed with binge-eating disorder are overweight. Many are of normal weight, from any race, and are all ages. They frequently can be diagnosed with other psychiatric problems, such as anxiety or mood disorders.

Epidemiology. Binge-eating disorder is thought to begin during early childhood when eating patterns are developed. The condition continues through life. A parent may comfort an infant by feeding; a family may use eating as an escape from feelings or as an activity when bored. The client as a consequence responds to external cues (sight or smell of food) rather than internal cues (hunger or satiation following eating). Weight gain may be unremarkable until metabolic needs decrease as a young adult.

Studies drawn from weight-control programs have shown the overall prevalence to be 15 percent to 50 percent (with a mean of 30 percent), with females 1.5 times more likely to meet diagnostic criteria for this disorder than males (APA, 2000).

Subjective Data. From the client's history, it becomes evident that she reports a lack of control over her eating; she eats little in public, yet high weight is maintained due to private binges. Obese women who failed to lose weight often underreported their actual calorie intake and overestimated their physical activity. The client binges on any available food, most likely at night or on weekends. She has a long history of unsuccessful diets and restricts social activities because she is embarrassed about her weight (inability to fit in normal size seats). The client may attribute social and career failures to weight (false belief that she would be a better person if thin) and may fear medical complications such as diabetes, hypertension, and heart disease.

Objective Data. A physical examination and several diagnostic tests are done.

Physical Examination

- *General Appearance.* The client appears healthy, but has excessive body fat on the extremities as well as the trunk.
- *Vital Signs.* Tachycardia and hypertension (use appropriately sized blood pressure cuff) are possible.
- *Skin.* Skin breakdown is observed at intertriginous areas (beneath abdomen, vulva, groin, breasts, axillae); wound healing is poor. If obesity is accompanied by androgen excess, acne and hirsutism of the face, lower abdomen, thighs, and chest may be observed.
- *Chest.* Respirations are increased. There is dyspnea on exertion.
- *Breasts.* Hair surrounds the areolae in women with androgen excess.
- *Vascular System.* Varicosities and thrombophlebitis may be present.
- *Abdomen.* Abdomen is protuberant.
- *Genitalia and Reproductive Tract.* There may be a history of pregnancy or delivery complications, newborn complications, or male hair pattern in females (if androgen excess).
- *Musculoskeletal System.* Examination may reveal osteoarthritis (especially of the hips and knees), sciatica, and lower extremity injuries.
- *Nervous System.* Depression may be revealed.
- *Endocrine System.* Hyperglycemia and amenorrhea are possible findings.

Diagnostic Tests

- Complete blood count
- Glucose and lipid profiles (cholesterol, high density and low density lipoproteins, fasting triglycerides)
- Electrolyte analysis (especially if using fad diets)
- Urinalysis
- Electrocardiogram
- Endocrine studies when indicated (follicle-stimulating hormone, thyroid-stimulating hormone, prolactin, luteinizing hormone, free testosterone, dehydroepiandrosterone sulfate)

Differential Medical Diagnoses. Obesity with amenorrhea—rule out polycystic ovary syndrome/anovulation; obesity due to compulsive eating disorder; complications of obesity, such as hypertension, gallbladder disease, hyperlipidemia, and non-insulin-dependent diabetes.

Plan

Psychosocial Interventions. See Anorexia section. Suggest to the client that she join a support group, such as Overeaters Anonymous.

Medication. Since many clients will also have an Axis I diagnosis, antidepressants may be indicated (see Depression). Desipramine has shown the most promise (Goroll et al., 2000). Medical therapy should not be used, however, without appropriate education and lifestyle and nutritional changes. Regain of weight is a consistent problem after drug therapy is stopped and long-term therapy should be considered for women who have a history of repeated losses and gains.

Diet. Dietary interventions are numerous (also see Anorexia). No fewer than 1,200 calories should be consumed per day; otherwise, essential nutrients are restricted and metabolism decreased, possibly prompting a binge.

Suggest to the client that she replace problem behaviors with alternative behaviors. Provide accurate information regarding weight loss programs, including the risks involved with fad diets or powdered-formula diets. The following questions are helpful in evaluation of weight loss programs.

- Is this a diet the client could live with indefinitely?
- What is the recommended rate of weight loss?
- Does the program take individual differences into account to determine caloric needs?
- To what extent does the plan educate the client about nutrition, behavior modification, and the importance of exercise?
- Does the program put the client in contact with professionals such as physicians, registered dietitians, and psychotherapists?
- What percentage of clients reach goal weight and maintain their losses?
- Does the program offer a maintenance plan once weight is lost?
- What is the nature of the advertisements and endorsements?
- How much does the program cost?

Exercise. Exercise needs to be incorporated into lifestyle. Inform the client about the health benefits of regular exercise. Exercise increases basal metabolic rate, which increases calorie use and promotes weight loss. Exercising at least four times per week for 20 to 30 minutes is recommended.

Devise a mutually acceptable plan for aerobic exercise; calculate the target heartrate (Goroll et al., 2000). Weight loss cannot occur and be maintained if the client is unwilling to continue exercise and reasonable caloric restriction.

Explain to the client that weight may not change drastically; rather, she should use as a guide how she feels physically and how her clothes fit. Encourage the client to wear flattering clothing to boost self-esteem.

Follow-up. Follow-up visits are scheduled for every two weeks or monthly to evaluate weight and blood pressure and review exercise, dietary goals, and compliance problems. Self-monitoring, setting goals, social support, and the length of treatment are associated with successful loss of weight, whereas physical activity, continuing in a program, and self-monitoring are important to successfully keeping the weight off (Goroll et al., 2000).

HOMELESSNESS

Approximately 250,000 to 3 million men, women, and children are homeless at some time each year (Graves, 1999). The number of women and children living without a permanent place of dwelling is the fastest growing population among the homeless. Exactly how many women are homeless is not known. Women often remain out of sight to protect themselves against the possibility of violence.

Reasons for homelessness are complex; poverty, violence, substance abuse and mental illness are often cited as major causes (Anderson & Imle, 2001). The Stewart B. McKinley Homeless Act (Public Law 100-77) defined the homeless person as one who does not have a fixed, regular, and adequate nighttime dwelling. This dwelling may be (1) a supervised or publicly operated shelter designed for temporary living quarters, (2) an institution serving as temporary residence for those requiring institutionalization, or (3) any public or private place not intended for regular sleeping quarters. (Institute of Medicine, 1988).

Rarely does the literature on homeless persons distinguish health problems of women from those of men. According to Tessler, Rosenheck, and Gamache (2001), women cite eviction, interpersonal conflict, and loss of social support as the most common reasons for their homelessness. In contrast, men cite loss of a job, discharge from an institution, mental health problems, and substance abuse as the most common reasons. Women who are homeless are at risk for the same health problems as women who are not homeless. Due to their poverty, sense of powerlessness, and inability to access health care, however, women are particularly at risk for conditions and diseases that might be preventable if detected earlier. Pregnant women are particularly vulnerable to complications during pregnancy, labor and the postpartum periods (Stein, Lu, & Gelberg 2000). It is important for primary care providers to note that the use of screening tests is correlated more with access to preventive health care than to income or minority status (Lane, Polednak & Burg, 1992). Homeless women are likely to experience malnutrition and related problems such as anemia. Other common health problems are infections, communicable diseases, skin complaints, poorly managed diabetes, and hypertension. Exposure to the elements, especially hypothermia, is also common (Drapkin, 1990).

Along with physical problems, women who are homeless experience stress, anxiety, and depression. They are also at risk for abuse and trauma, both physical and psychological (Wenzel, Leake, & Gelberg, 2001). Use of drugs and alcohol are common (Kilbourne, Herndon, Andersen, Westzel, & Gelburg, 2002). These psychological problems are complicated by a lack of resources. Homeless women often do not have health insurance and are unable to pay for many of the traditional treatments for mental health problems.

Primary care providers must work with community agencies to devise practice models that improve accessibility to care and follow-up. Systems of care that improve access to care are located in many urban areas throughout our country. Funding, especially for health care services, continues to be a problem. Any system of care should focus on early identification of the at-risk population, provision of services that are required to reduce morbidity and mortality from acute and chronic diseases, and follow-up. Practices located near homeless shelters and streets where homeless women and their families are likely to be found will increase access to preventive health care services. Primary providers must also examine their attitudes and beliefs regarding homeless women and look for ways to create therapeutic client-provider relationships and implement health care services.

REFERENCES

American College of Obstetrics and Gynecology (ACOG) Practice Bulletin. (2001). Clinical Management Guidelines for Obstetricians-Gynecologists. *Emergency oral contraception,* No. 25. Washington, DC: ACOG.

American Medical Women's Association. (2002). *Domestic violence.* Retrieved on 3-24-02 from http://www.dvcme.org/

American Nurses Association (ANA). (2002). *Position statement: Sexual harassment.* Retrieved 3-21-02 from http://www.nursingworld.org/readroom/position/workplac/wkharass.htm.

American Psychiatric Association. (2000). *Diagnostic and statistical manual of mental disorders* (DSM-IV-TR) (4th ed.). Washington, DC: Author.

Anderson, D.G., & Imle, M.A. (2001). Families of origin of homeless and near-homeless women. *Western Journal of Nursing Research, 23*(4), 394–413.

Bailey, C. (1998). Assessing health during pregnancy. In Youngkin, E. & Davis, M. Women's health: A primary care clinical guide (2nd ed). Stamford, CT: Appleton & Lange.

Barlow, D. (2002). Anxiety and its disorders: The nature and treatment of anxiety and panic (2nd ed). New York: Guilford Press.

Barnes, M.D., Pase, M., Van Leeuwen, D. (1999). The relationship of economic factors and stress among employed, married women with children. *American Journal of Health Promotion, 13*(4), 203–206.

Becker, K.L. & Walton-Moss, B. (2001). Detecting and addressing alcohol abuse in women. *Nurse Practitioner, 26*(10), 13–16, 19–25.

Beeber, L.S. (1999). Testing an explanatory model of the development of depressive symptoms in young women during a life transition. *Journal of American College Health, 47*(5), 227–234.

Bierut, L.J., Health, A.C., Bucholz, K., et al. (1999). Major depressive disorder in a community-based twin sample: Are there different genetic and environmental contributions for men and women? *Archives General Psychiatry, 56*(6), 557–563.

Brady, K.T. (2001). Pharmacotherapeutic treatment for women with PTSD. Program and abstracts of the 154th annual Meeting of the American Psychiatric Association, May 5–10, 2001. New Orleans: Lousiana Symposium 12 E.

Brady, K.T., & Randall, C.L. (1999). Gender differences in substance use disorders. *Psychiatric Clinics of North America, 22*(2), 241–252.

Brady, K., Pearlstein, T., Asnis, G.M., et al. (2000). Efficacy and safety of sertraline treatment of posttraumatic stress disorder: A randomized controlled trial. *Journal of the American Medical association, 283,* 1837–1844.

Burgess, A. W. (January 31, 2002). Overview and summary: Domestic violence: How many steps forward? How many steps back? *Online Journal of Issues in Nursing, 7*(1). Retrieved from *http://www.nursingworld.org/ojin/topic17/tpc17ntr.htm.*

Busfield, J. (1996). *Men, women and madness: Understanding gender and mental disorder.* London: Macmillan Press Ltd.

Campbell, J.C. (1998). Making the health care system an empowerment zone for battered women: Health consequences, policy recommendations, introduction, and overview. In J.C. Campbell (Ed.), *Empowering survivors of abuse: Health care for battered women and their children* (pp. 241–258). Thousand Oaks, CA: Sage.

Campbell, J.C., Pliska, M.J., Taylor, W., & Sheridan, D. (1994). Battered women's experiences in the emergency department. *J Emerg Nursing, 204,* 280–288.

Centers for Disease Control and Prevention (CDC). *Journal of Emergency Nursing* (2001). National Vital Statistics Report. Vol. 48, No. 1, February 7, 2001, 33.

Crowe, M. (2000). Constructing normality: A discourse analysis of the DSM-IV, *Journal of Psychiatric and Mental Health Nursing, 7,* 69–77.

Davidson, J., Pearlstein, T., Londborg, P., et al. (2001). Efficacy of sertaline in preventing relapse of post traumatic stress disorder: Results of a 28-week double-blind, placebo-controlled study. *American Journal of Psychiatry, 158,* 1974–1981.

Davidson, J.R., Rothbaum, B.O., Van der Kolk, B.A., Sikes, C.R., & Farfel, G.M. (2001). Multicenter, double-blind comparison of sertraline and placebo in the treatment of posttraumatic stress disorder. *Archives of General Psychiatry, 58,* 485–492.

Drapkin, A., (1990). Medical problems of the homeless. In C.L. Canton (Ed.), *Homeless in America.* New York: Oxford University Press.

Draucker, C.B. (January 31, 2002). Domestic violence: The challenge for nursing. *Online Journal of Issues in Nursing, 7*(1), Manuscript 1. Retrieved from *http://www.nursingworld.org/ojin/topic 17/tpc17 1.htm.*

Feldhaus, K.M., Houry, D., & Kamisky, R. (2000). Life-time sexual assault prevalence rates and reporting practices in an emergency department population. *Annals of Emergency Medicine, 36,* 2327.

Fiore M.C., Bailey W.C., Cohen S.J., et al. (2000). *Treating Tobacco Use and Dependence. Clinical Practice Guideline.* Rockville, MD: U.S. Department of Health and Human Services, Public Health Service.

Freeman, S. (2002). *Women and primary care conference coverage.* Retrieved 3-20-02 from *http:www.medscape.com/viewarticle/420192.*

Golding, J. (1996). Sexual assault history and limitations in physical functioning in two general population samples. *Research in Nursing and Health, 19,* 33–44.

Goroll, A., May, L., & Mulley, A. (2000). *Primary care medicine* (4th ed.). Philadelphia: Lippincott.

Graves, S. (1999). Migrant and homeless populations. In E. Youngkin, K. Sawin, J. Kissinger, & D. Israel (Eds.). *Pharmacotherapeutics: A primary care clinical guide.* Stamford, CT: Appleton & Lange.

Griffin, M., & Koss, M. (2002, January 31). Clinical screening and intervention in cases of partner violence. *Online Journal of Issues in Nursing, 7*(1), Manuscript 2. Retrieved from *http://www.nursingworld.org/ojin/topic17/tpc17 2.htm.*

Harkness, K., & Monroe, S. (2002). Childhood adversity and the endogenous versus non-endogenous distinction in women with major depression. *American Journal of Psychiatry, 159*(3), 387–393.

Heidrich, S.M. (1998). Older women's lives through time. *Advances in Nursing Science, 20*(3), 65–75.

Holmes, M.M., Resnick, H.S., Kilpatrick, D.G., & Best, C.L. (1996). Rape-related prequency: Estimates and descriptive characteristics from a national sample of women American Journal of Obstetics & Gynecology, 175(2), 320–324.

Houry, D., Sachs, C.J., Feldhaus, K.M., & Linden, J. (2002). Violence-inflicted injuries: Reporting laws in the fifty states. *Annals of Emergency Medicine, 39*(1), 56–60.

Institute of Medicine. (1988). *Homelessness, health, and human needs.* Washington, DC: National Academy Press.

Institute of Medicine. (2001). *Health and behavior: The interplay of biological, behavioral and societal influences.* Washington, DC: National Academy Press.

Janicak, P., Davis, J., Preskorn, S., & Ayd, F. (2001). *Principles and practice of psychopharmacotherapy* (3rd ed.). Philadelphia: Lippincott, Williams & Wilkins.

Jorgenson, L.M., & Wahl, K.M. (2000). Workplace sexual harassment: Incidence, legal analysis, and the role of the psychiatrist. *Harvard Review of Psychiatry, 8*(2), 94–98.

Kaplan, H.I. & Sadock, U.A. (2000). Kaplan and Sadock's pocket handbook of psychiatric drug treatment. Philadelphia: Lippincott, Williams & Wilkins.

Katon, W.J. (2001, May 5–10). *The depressed patient with co-morbid illness. Program and abstracts of the 154th Annual Meeting of the American Psychiatric Association.* New Orleans, LA: Industry Symposium, Part 2, 43B.

Kenney, J.W., & Bhattacharjee, A. (2000). Interactive model of women's stressors, personality traits and health problems. *Journal of Advanced Nursing, 32*(1), 249–258.

Kilbourne, A.M., Herndon, B., Andersen, R.M., Wenzel, S.L., & Gelberg, L. (2002). Psychiatric symptoms, health services and HIV risk factors among homeless women. *Journal of Health Care Poor Underserved, 13*(1), 49–65.

Kilpatrick, A.O., & White, A.W. (2000). Unwanted advances: Sexual harassment in the workplace. *Emergency Medicine Services, 29*(6), 64–68.

Kopp, W.J. (1999). Chronic and acute psychological risk factors for clinical manifestations of coronary artery disease. *Psychosomatic Medicine, 61,* 476–487.

Lane, D., Polednak, A., & Burg, M.A. (1992). Does breast cancer screening differ between users of county-funded health canters and women in the entire community? *American Journal of Public Health, 82.* 199–203.

Lester, S.J., Baggott, M., Welan, S., Schiller, N.B., Jones, R.T., Foster, F., & Mendelson, J. (2000). Cardiovascular effects of 3,4-methylenedioxymethamphetamine: A double-blind, placebo-controlled trial. *Annals of Internal Medicine, 133*(12), 969–973.

Mahoney, P., Williams, L.M., & West, C.M. (2001). Violence against women by intimate relationship partners. In C.M. Renzetti, J.L. Edleson, & R.K Bergen (Eds.), *Sourcebook on violence against women* (pp. 143–178). Thousand Oaks, CA: Sage.

Malamut, A.B., & Offermann, L.R. (2001). Coping with sexual harassment: Personal, environmental, and cognitive determinants. *Journal of Applied Psychology, 86*(6), 1152–1166.

Martin, A. (2000a). Major depressive illness in women: Assessment and treatment in the primary care setting. *Nurse Practitioner Forum, II*(3), 179–186.

Martin, A. (2000b). Protocol for alcohol outpatient detoxification. *Lippincott's Primary Care Practice, 4*(2), 221–227.

Martin, A. (2002). It's never too late to start: Seven steps toward good health. *Topics in Advanced Practice Nursing eJournal, 2*(1). Retrieved 3-20-02 from *http://www.medscape.com/ viewarticle/421471 print.*

McAllister, M. (2000). Domestic violence: A life-span approach to assessment and intervention. *Primary Care Practice, 4*(2), 174–189.

McCance, K.L., & Huether, S.E. (2002). *Pathophysiology: The biologic basis for disease in adults and children* (4th ed.). St. Louis: Mosby.

McConkey, T.E., Sole, M.L., & Holcomb, L. (2001). Assessing the female sexual assault survivor. *Nurse Practitioner, 26*(7 Pt 1), 28–30, 33–34, 37–39; quiz 40–41.

McNutt, A., Carlson, B., Gagen, D., & Winterbauer, N. (1999). Reproductive violence screening in primary care: Perspectives and experiences of patients and battered women. *Journal of American Medical Women's Association, 54*(2), 85–90.

Medscape. (2002). *Date violence, rape experienced by 9% of girls, 6% of boys.* Retrieved on 3-20-02 from *http://www.medscape.com/viewarticle/411331.*

Murray, C.J.L. & Lopez, A.D. (Eds.). (1996). *The global burden of disease and injury series, Volume 1: A comprehensive assessment of mortality and disability from diseases, injuries, and risk factors in 1990 and projected to 2020.* Cambridge, MA: Published by the Harvard School of Public Health on behalf of the World Health Organization and the World Bank, Harvard University Press. Retrieved on 3-17-02 from *http://www.who.int/msa/mnh/ems/dalys/intro.htm.*

Narrow, W.E. (1998). *One-year prevalence of depressive disorders among adults 18 and over in the U.S.: NIMH ECA prospective data.* Population estimates based on U.S. Census estimated residential population age 18 and over on July 1, 1998. Unpublished.

Narrow, W.E., Rae, D.S., & Regier, D.A. (1998). *NIMH epidemiology note: Prevalence of anxiety disorders.* One-year prevalence best estimates calculated from ECA and NCS data. Population estimates based on U.S. Census estimated residential population age 18 to 54 on July 1, 1998. Unpublished.

National Institutes of Mental Health (NIMH). (2002). *The numbers count: Mental health disorders in America.* Retrieved 3-17-02 from http://www.nimh.nih.gov/publication/numbers.cfm.

Office of the Surgeon General. (2002). *Treating tobacco use and dependence: Quick reference guide for clinicians.* Retrieved from http:www.surgeongeneral.gov/tobacco/.

Palmer, B. (2002). *Helping people with eating disorders: A clinical guide to assessment and treatment.* New York: John Wiley & Sons, Ltd.

Patel, M., & Minshall, I. (2001). Management of sexual assault. *Emergency Medical Clinics of North America, 19*(3), 817–831.

Raj, A., Silverman, J.G., Wingood, G.M., & DiClemente, R.J. (1999). Prevalence and correlates of relationship abuse among a community-based sample of low-income African American women. *Violence Against Women, 5*(3), 272–291.

Rickert, V.I., & Wiemann, C.M. (1998). Date rape among adolescents and young adults. *Journal of Pediatric Adolescent Gynecology; 11,* 167–175.

Rickert, V.I., Wiemann, C.M., & Berenson, A.B. (2000). Ethnic differences in depressive symptomatology among young women. *Obstetrics Gynecology, 95*(1), 55–60.

Riggs, W., Houry, D., Long, G., Markovchick, V., & Feldhaus, K.M. (2000). Analysis of 1076 cases of sexual assault. *Annals of Emergency Medicine, 35*(4), 358–362.

Roberts, S.B., & Kendler, K.S (1999). Neuroticism and self-esteem as indices of the vulnerability to major depression in women. *Psychological Medicine, 29*(5), 1101–1109.

Ryan, M., & Houry, D. (2000). Clinical forensic medicine. *Annals of Emergency Medicine, 36*(3), 271–273.

Schaffer, S. (2002). Cleaning the air: Brief strategies for smoking cessation. *Topics in Advanced, Practice in Nursing & Journal, 2*(1). Retrieved 3-20-02 from http://www.medscape.com/viewarfede/421476_print

Schrefer J., ed. (2001). *Mosby's GenRx: A Comprehensive Reference for Generic and Prescription Brand Drugs,* 11th ed. St. Louis, MO: Mosby.

Snow, D. (2000). Managing patients with alcohol use disorders. *Lippincott's Primary Care Practice, 4*(2), 133–148.

Stein, J.A., Lu, M.C., & Gelberg, L. (2000). Severity of homelessness and adverse birth outcomes. *Health Psychology, 19*(6), 524–534.

Stenchever, M., Mishell, D., Herbst, A., & Droegemueller, M. (2001). *Comprehensive gynecology* (4th ed.). St. Louis: Mosby.

Stuart, G.W., & Laraia, M.T. (2001). *Principles and practice of psychiatric nursing.* St. Louis: Mosby.

Substance Abuse and Mental Health Services Administration (SAMHSA). (2001). *Summary of findings from the 2000 National Household Survey on Drug Abuse.* Office of Applied Studies, NHSDA Series H-13, DHHS Publication No. (SMA) 01-3549. Rockville, MD: Author.

Tessler, R., Rosenheck, R., & Gamache, G. (2001). Gender differences in self-reported reasons for homelessness. *Journal of Social Distress & the Homeless, 10*(3), 243–254.

Thomas, S.P. (1997). Distressing aspects of women's roles, vicarious stress and health consequences. *Issues in Mental Health Nursing, 18*(6), 539–557.

Tjaden, P., & Thomas, N. (1998, November). *Prevalence, incidence, and consequences of violence against women: Findings from the National Violence Against Women Survey.* Pub. No.NCJ 172837. Washington, DC: National Institute of Justice, Centers for Disease Control and Prevention.

Urbano-Marquez, A., Estruch, R., Fernandez-Sola, J., Nicholas, J., Pare, J.C., & Rubin, E. (1995). The greater the risk of alcoholic cardiomyopathy and myopathy in women compared with men. *Journal of American Medical Association, 274,* 149–154.

U.S. Department of Health and Human Services (USDHHS) (2000). *Healthy people 2010: Understanding and improving health.* Washington, DC: Author.

U.S. Equal Opportunities Commission. (2002). *Facts about sexual harassment.* Retrieved 3-24-02 from http://www.lloc.gov/facts/fs-sex.html

Villapiano, M., & Goodman, L. (2001). *Eating disorders: Time for a change.* New York: Brunner-Routledge: Taylor & Francis Group.

Waalen J, Goodwin MM, Spitz AM, Petersen R, Saltzman LE. (2000) Screening for intimate partner violence by health care providers: a review of barriers and interventions. American Journal of Preventive Medicine; 19(4):230–237.

Walker, L.E. (1984). *The battered woman syndrome.* New York: Springer.

Warshaw, C., & Ganley A.I. (1998). *Improving the health care response to domestic violence: A resource manual for health care providers.* San Francisco, CA: Family Violence Prevention Fund.

Wenzel, S.L., Leake, B.D., & Gelberg, L. (2001). Risk factors for major violence among homeless women. *Journal of Interpersonal Violence, 16*(8), 739–752.

West, M., Rose, S.M., Spreng, S., et al. (1999). Anxious attachment and severity of depressive symtomatology in women. *Women & Health, 29*(1), 47–56.

Wonderlich, S.A., Crosby, R.D., Mitchell, J.E., Thompson, K.M., Redlin, J., Demuth, G., Smyth, J., & Haseltine, B. (2001). Eating disturbances and sexual trauma in childhood and adulthood. *International Journal of Eating Disorders, 30*(4), 401–412.

Wright, N., & Owen, S. (2000). Feminist conceptualizations of women's madness: A review of the literature. *Journal of Advanced Nursing, 36*(1), 143–150.

Yeager, K., & Seid, A., (2002). Primary care and victims of domestic violence. *Primary Care, 29*(1), 125–150, vii–viii.

Yehuda, R. (2001). *Immune neuroanatomic neuroendocrine gender differences in PTSD.* Program and abtracts of the 15th Annual Meeting of the American Psychiatric Association, May 5–10, 2001. New Orleans, LA: Symposium 12A.

Zoellner, L.A., Feeny, N.H., Albarez, J., Watlington, C., O'Neil, M.L., Zager, R., & Foa, E.B. (2000). Factors associated with completion of the restraining order process in female victims of partner violence. *Journal of Interpersonal Violence, 15*(10), 1081–1099.

CHAPTER 24

HEALTH CARE CONCERNS FOR WOMEN WITH PHYSICAL DISABILITY AND CHRONIC ILLNESS

Kathleen J. Sawin ◆ *Janet C. Horton*

*B*eing disabled does not contradict responsible, effective parenting, yet judgmental attitudes continue.

Highlights

- Discrimination
- Culture and Disability
- Negative Attitudes Among Health Care Providers
- Women Who Are Lesbians
- Health Promotion
- Access Issues/Barriers
- Sexuality
    Communication
    Body Image
    Service Animals
    Spasticity
    Spinal Cord Injury
    Joint Inflexibility and Pain
    Multiple Sclerosis
    Diabetes Mellitus
    Epilepsy
    Urinary and Bowel Appliances
    Pelvic Radiotherapy
    Cystic Fibrosis
    Cognitive Impairment
    Visual/Hearing Impairment
    Menarche
    Personal Attendant
    Sexual Activity
    Abuse
- Issues of Aging/Menopause
- History/Medical Examination
- Management of Contraception
- Pregnancy and Parenting
- Future Research
- Resources

❖   INTRODUCTION

The unmet needs of women with physical disabilities include accessibility to gynecologic care, sexuality and birth control counseling, and accessibility to pro-

fessionals with a knowledge of how disability impacts primary care.

DISCRIMINATION

The discrimination that women with disabilities and chronic illness face is twofold: First, they are women, and second, they are individuals with disabilities. Narrow negative social attitudes set unnecessary barriers to the optimal growth and development of these women and the health care they obtain (Groce, 1999). An example is the stereotypic image of American women as having two major functions—caretaker and object of beauty. The ideal woman is physically "perfect" (Blackwell-Stratton, Breslin, Mayerson, & Bailey, 1988; Nosek, Howland, Young, et al., 1994), but women with disabilities are seen as dependent and nonproductive and are judged incompetent to perform women's work or seen as invisible (Bauer, 2001; Gill, 1996).

The Americans with Disabilities Act (ADA) became law in 1990. Discrimination in employment against qualified persons with disabilities is against the law, enforced by the U.S. Equal Employment Opportunity Commission and related agencies. As of July 26, 1994, this law applied to all employers with fifteen or more employees.

IMPACT OF DISABILITY

Specific disabilities (spinal cord injury, cerebral palsy, multiple sclerosis, or disabling arthritis) prevent women, it is thought, from meeting society's major functions. Attractive women who use wheelchairs are seen as less than whole. For example, a comment overheard in a family planning clinic concerned a very attractive 19-year-old woman who had recently sustained a spinal cord injury and now used a wheelchair for mobility: "She used to be so pretty." In fact, the accident left no scar but changed only her mode of mobility. However, opportunities to establish romantic relationships are limited for women with disabilities (Nosek, Howland, Rintala, Young, & Chanpong, 1997).

ECONOMICS

Women experience greater effects from disability than do men in that they earn less, work less, and are studied less. When rehabilitation services are provided, women are more likely to be rehabilitated for homemaking and much less likely to be rehabilitated for competitive employment (U. S. General Accounting Office, 1993). High divorce rates are associated with disability; the highest rates are when the woman is the disabled spouse (Drew, 1990). Nearly half live alone (Iezzoni, McCarthy, Davis, & Siebens, 2000; McNewil, 1993). Economic status may even have an impact on a women's adaptation to disability. In addition, women with disability face extraordinary barriers in accessing health insurance (Nosek, Young, Rintala, et al., 1995). Women around the world are more limited by prevailing social, cultural and economic factors than by physical, psychosocial, sensory, or cognitive impairments (Groce, 1999).

CULTURE AND DISABILITY/ILLNESS

Culture shapes women's experience with disabilities. The prevalence of disability is higher among minority women (Anderson & Brownson, 2000), yet little is written about the experience of disability for women in diverse cultures. The more the disability experience is divergent from the societal norm of the referent culture group, however, the more issues women will face. For women who are immigrants, the experience is more difficult as the woman must deal with her marginality, social isolation, and alienation in a foreign culture (Anderson, 1991). The devaluation of self is not only rooted in the chronic illness experience but also from the definition of self that is constructed in dealing with the migration experience.

For African American women with disabilities, there may be issues of identity, role conflict, employment, and sexuality (Alston, Bell, & Feist-Price, 1996; Alston & McCowan, 1994). African American women may experience greater difficulty with multiple role conflict. They tend to have more roles, more children, greater environmental stress and may be more likely to be single parents. The kinship network of the African American woman, however, is a positive protective factor. If the disability causes collapse of that network, health care providers need to aggressively assist the woman to repair or renew her support network. Employment is a challenge for African American women. Women of color with disabilities have lower employment income levels than all other men and women. They earn $.22 for every dollar earned by a white nondisabled man (Alston & McCowan, 1994). The evidence indicates that many African American women are traditional in their sexual practices. If the woman is hesitant to participate in oral sex behaviors, masturbation, or experiment with alternative methods of sexual intimacy, she may be at risk for sexual dissatisfaction. Health professionals need to assess the woman for the discrepancy between her ideal and real experiences. Assistance that helps decrease the discrepancy will optimize the woman's adjustment. Further, emphasis needs to be placed on conditions that unequally affect African American women, such as sickle cell. Lupus strikes most during the childbearing age, and African American women are overrepresented (Brown, 1996).

Activists and scholars writing about the civil rights movement of individuals with disabilities reject the traditional view of disability as physically defective and needing to be fixed. Instead, these activists are asserting that individuals with disabilities are a legitimate cultural minority. This philosophy is based on the belief that most of the problems faced by individuals with disabilities are not caused by the body "but by a society that refuses to accommodate our differences." This culture proposes that medical needs are only a small part of the disability experience, with the larger, more pressing problems being social and political (Gill, 1996; Hahn & Beaulaurier, 2001; Yoshida, Li, & Odette, 1999).

NEGATIVE ATTITUDES AMONG HEALTH CARE PROVIDERS

Women with disabilities face multiple barriers to quality reproductive health care services (Becker, Stuifbergen, & Tinkle, 1997) and receive fewer services (MMWR, 1998). Health care providers have negative attitudes toward women with disabilities (Nosek et al., 1995; Welner, 1993), expect less of them (Muir & Ogden, 2001), and overestimate the negative impact of disability on family life (Gill, 1996; Saxton, 1996). Often, health care providers speak without sensitivity. They are frequently unaware of how many adults with disabilities live independently in the community, use adaptive equipment, modify homes, and use attendant care (Kirshbaum,

1988). Health care providers' perception of issues such as appearance, ease of communication, and autonomy can influence their response to women (Muir & Ogden, 2001). Moreover, professionals are more aware of predominately male disabilities and underestimate the frequency of disabilities among women (Nosek, 1992; Nosek et al., 1994, 1995).

Health care providers have strong influence on knowledge, beliefs, and expectations of women with physical disabilities and chronic illness as they strive to maintain reproductive health (Nosek et al., 1995). Forging partnership is vital (Stewart & Reutter, 2001). Inservice training sessions for primary care providers and women's centers are needed to address access and attitudinal barriers (Sawin & Conti, 1994).

INVISIBLE ASEXUAL MISPERCEPTION

Women with disabilities, especially those growing up with a disability, are seen by health care providers as asexual (Howland & Rintala, 2001; Nelson, 1995; Nosek, Rintala, Young, et al., 1996). To the contrary, these women have numerous needs. Thirty-two women with disabilities reported, unanimously, their need for health care providers to see them as sexual beings (Sawin, 1982). Denying the sexuality of a woman limits the services that are provided for her (Nosek et al., 1994, 1995, 1996).

LOWERED EXPECTATIONS

Health care providers are among those who often send the message that a woman's body is unacceptable (Boston Women's Health Book Collective, 1992; Nelson, 1995). Expectations are that women with disabilities are less likely to marry or have children; they may be seen as more dependent, weak, and less able to care for themselves or a child (Blackwell-Stratton et al., 1988; Nelson, 1995). In fact, a significant factor in whether young women with disabilities have active social lives was their parent's expectations (Howland & Rintala, 2001; Nelson, 1995). Unfortunately, although these parents had educational goals for their daughters, only a small, percentage expected their daughters to be socially active (Nelson, 1995).

- Adolescents with cognitive impairments often face barriers accessing the traditional rites, roles, and rituals of adulthood not encountered by their peers without disabilities (Jordan & Dunlap, 2001).

◆ School nurses given the same vignette about young adolescents with and without disabilities starting their menstrual period for the first time at school held different expectations for knowledge, self-care, and independence based only on the adolescents' use of a wheelchair for mobility (Tsy & Opie, 1986).

◆ Women with disabilities are often not considered for driver's education in high school although youth with disabilities believe driving would increase freedom, independence, and improve employment and recreational choices (McGill & Vogtle, 2001).

SURMISED RETARDATION

Often women are treated as if physical disability means mental retardation, especially if their speech is impaired. Characteristically, clinic and hospital personnel talk to the person who is accompanying the individual with a disability, not to the individual herself. In addition, they frequently "talk down" or use language patterns appropriate for a child (Nosek, 1992). Frequently, inebriation is assumed in addition to low IQ. Talking more loudly or more simply is a frequent reaction to speech disability.

PERCEIVED PARENTHOOD CONFLICT

Conflict is perceived between carrying out the responsibilities of parenthood and complying with a medical regimen. Mothers report that health care providers seem unable to recognize the profound interrelationship between their mothering responsibilities and chronic illness or disability. Many women hold the opinion that it is a contradiction to be both an effective mother and a "good patient" (Thorne, 1990).

WOMEN WHO ARE LESBIANS

If women with disabilities/chronic illnesses experience double discrimination, women in the lesbian community are even more disadvantaged. Although literature exploring issues for lesbians with disabilities is very limited, a few recent authors help us understand these women's experiences. (Marshall, 1995; O'Toole, 1996; O'Toole & Bregante, 1993; Stevens, 1994). Themes identified include (1) a sense of voicelessness in social and political arena, (2) difficulties in dealing with health care professionals, (3) discrimination in the workplace, (4) anger at public ignorance and injustice, and (5) physical abuse.

One women with a stroke who had two prior experiences with physical attacks and "gay bashing" indicated "I feel even more vulnerable in a wheelchair" (Marshall, 1995). Further, the family, a source of support for many individuals, may not be a positive factor for some women as they report the overwhelming feelings of powerlessness being both disabled and lesbian within the traditional family. Women report discriminatory practices in the workplace, which frequently seem insurmountable. Thus, economic dependence complicates the situation. This economic issue may be a factor in some of the anger voiced by women who had worked hard to escape poverty only to have a chronic illness/disability "pulling me back" (Marshall, 1995). Women report both negative and positive experiences when relating to health care providers, although the overwhelming reaction is one of "not being listened to" and "not feeling safe or respected." Both of these lead to "health care hopping" and lack of continuity of care. Women report how powerful the acceptance is when they can introduce their girlfriend to their health care provider and "it's ok" (Marshall, 1995; Stevens, 1994). Many lesbians with disabilities experience negative repercussions, however, when they "come out" with health care providers (Lehmann, Lehmann, & Kelly, 1998; Stevens, 1994).

Lesbians with disabilities indicate that their "safe haven" is the lesbian community. They report total acceptance and caring here that they do not find in the disability or conventional communities (O'Toole, 1996). They indicate a pervasive able-bodyism in the feminist movement that excludes women with disabilities. According to these authors, feminists are reluctant to encompass women with disabilities because they perceive them as dependent, passive, and needy. They are seeking to portray a more powerful, competent, appealing female image.

Some lesbians with disabilities report a spiritual experience from the community support and others report religion itself used as a coping mechanism. The women interviewed by Marshall indicated that their partners figured most prominently in how they dealt with their disabilities (Marshall, 1995). Lesbians with disabilities are diverse, and their needs will need to be individually heard. The health care provider can "give all women a voice," listen and convey acceptance to women's diversity, and affirm women's moving on to action from anger. The provider can do none of this, however, if lesbians with disabilities remain "invisible." Unapproachable health care providers add to the unaddressed health care needs of this population. For example, more than 50 percent of lesbians have not had a Pap smear in the last twelve months

(Stevens, 1994). Contrary to popular beliefs, these women are at risk for acquiring sexually transmitted diseases, including HIV infection, and for transmitting them to their female partners (Leu, Welker, & Haines, 1999).

The interventions addressed for all lesbians (see Chapter 7) are core to establishing a message of effective communication, approachability, and effectiveness when working with women with disability. To do this, providers need to increase their sensitivity. As one women indicated,

> The pious compassion shown to disabled people cannot be demonstrated to lesbians and gays. Conversely, the violent hostility shown gays and lesbians is hidden due to our disability. In a word, we are different. However, we are proud of our nonstereotypical multi-identities, and this power will force our communities to expand their own horizons of the "acceptable." All disabled people are viewed as asexual, but we challenge that oppression twice. Our social challenge is that our sameness and our difference are included. We are in the struggle and we are OUT about it (Hevey, 1993, cited in O'Toole & Bregante, 1993).

Health care providers need to create an environment where women feel safe to voice their concerns and have their unique health care needs met (Eliason, 1996). REGARD, a self-advocacy organization for disabled lesbians and gays, works to establish knowledgeable providers. In addition, disabled lesbians have been totally excluded from the small numbers of studies that have explored lives of women with disabilities especially motherhood (O'Toole & D'aoust, 2000). In order to achieve optimal health, lesbians need to be included—in our expectations and our research (Hevey, 1993 cited in O'Toole & Bregante, 1993; Spinks, Andrews, & Boyle, 2000).

INEFFECTIVE TERMINOLOGY

Language is a powerful communicator of negative attitudes. Communication needs to be inclusive; Limiting, stereotypic terms must be avoided. See Table 24–1.

HEALTH PROMOTION

A Healthy People 2000 priority goal is to reduce health disparities among Americans. "The health promotion and disease prevention needs of people with disabilities are not nullified because they were born with an impairing condi-

tion or have experienced a disability or injury that has long-term consequences. In fact, the need for health promotion is accentuated (USDHHS, 1992). Identifying interventions to support health promoting behaviors in persons with disabilities is the top priority of researchers in rehabilitation nursing (Gordon, Sawin, & Basta, 1996). There is a growing emphasis both from clinicians/researchers (Gordon, Sawin, & Basta, 1996; Krotoski, Nosek, & Turk, 1996; Murphy, Molnar, & Lankasky, 1995; Stuifbergen, 1996) and National Institutes of Health to generate knowledge about an area ignored until recently—health promotion or wellness needs of women with disabilities/chronic illnesses (Iezzoni et al., 2001). The Center for the Study of Women with Disabilities has been created at Baylor University, NIH has held a consensus conference on the Health of Women with Disabilities, and organizations such as the Spina Bifida Association and the American Epilepsy Society have created an organizational committee or task force to address the unique needs of this population.

Nosek et al. (1994) interviewed 31 women about wellness issues. The concepts of coherence, self-regulation, competence, resilience, empowerment, and health awareness have been cited in existing models of wellness. These women's experience indicated that resilience was the relevant concept in their lives. Their lines of defense emerged as an important part of this resilience as their boundaries were continually threatened by insensitive behaviors of medical professionals and overwhelming overprotectiveness by family. Women who were identified as high in wellness tended to be assertive, resourceful, and proactive in their search for knowledge and answers to the barriers they experienced.

Health promotion in women with disabilities embraces all activities traditionally encompassed in health promotion programs (Nosek et al., 1996) but also may include complementary therapies and programs aimed at specific disabilities such as Stay Well! The Polio Network's Manual for a Health Promotion Program (Roller, 1996). Exercise may be a crucial component (Yoshida, Li, & Yodette, 1999). A majority of women with conditions such as lupus, multiple sclerosis, rheumatoid arthritis, and osteoporosis did not view themselves as disabled in spite of immense physical limitations (Gordon, Feldman, & Crose, 1999). Wellness is the lens of their self-perception.

NUTRITION

Optimal health promotion, including adequate nutrition, is essential for women with chronic conditions. Relatively little is known about the nutritional status and need of women

TABLE 24–1. Language Guidelines for Use When Interacting with Women Who Have a Disability

1. Where possible, emphasize an individual, not a disability. Say "people or persons with disabilities" or "person who is blind" rather than "disabled persons" or "blind person." (Many individuals prefer to use the words *physically challenged* to describe this population.)
2. When speaking of people with disabilities always choose words that accurately describe the disability. Avoid using emotional descriptors such as unfortunate, pitiful, and so on. Do not refer to or focus on a disability unless crucial for the purpose of communication.
3. Talk directly to the person with a disability. If using an interpreter, speak facing the person with hearing impairment.
4. Avoid labeling persons into groups, as in "the disabled," "the deaf," "retardate," and "the arthritic"; instead, say "people who are deaf," "person with arthritis," and "persons with disabilities."
5. Do not sensationalize a disability by saying "afflicted with," "victim of," and so on. Instead, say "person who has multiple sclerosis" or "person who has polio."
6. Avoid portraying persons with disabilities who succeed as superhuman. This implies that persons who are disabled have no talents or unusual gifts.
7. Avoid use of "confined to wheelchair." Instead, consider "wheelchair user." Indeed, many individuals are liberated by a wheelchair rather than limited by the chair.
8. Emphasize abilities, such as "walks with a cane (braces)," rather than "is crippled"; "is partially sighted" rather than "partially blind." Never use the term "normal" in contrast.
9. After an initial greeting, sit down so that a person using a wheelchair won't have to crane his or her neck to make eye contact.
10. Shake whatever a person offers in greeting—a hand, prosthesis, or elbow.
11. When speaking with a person with a hearing loss, try to keep your face out of the shadows and your hands away from your mouth as you speak.
12. If someone's ability to read, write, or handle documents is limited, be prepared to provide assistance in completing paperwork.
13. When someone with a disability enters your clinic, don't assume she needs your help. Greet the person and tell her you're available for assistance.
14. Always speak directly to a person with a disability. Don't assume a companion is a conversational go-between.
15. When you offer to assist someone who is visually impaired, allow the person to take your arm so you can guide, rather than propel her.
16. Act naturally. Do not be afraid to use expressions such as "Would you like to see that?" or "Let me run over there." On the other hand, don't ask personal questions you wouldn't ask someone without a disability.
17. When speaking with a person with speech difficulty, talk normally. Don't pretend to understand when you don't. If necessary, ask the person to repeat. She has experienced this before and knows problems can arise.

Specific Language Guidelines

Disability (disabled, physically disabled). General term used for a (semi)permanent condition that interferes with a person's ability to do something independently—walk, see, hear, learn, lift. It may refer to a physical, mental, or sensory condition. Preferred usage is as a descriptive noun or adjective, as in persons who are disabled, people with disabilities, or disabled persons. Terms such as the disabled, crippled, deformed, and invalid are inappropriate.

Handicap. Often used as a synonym for disability. Usage, however, has become less acceptable (one origin is from "cap in hand," as in begging). Except when citing laws or regulations, *handicap* should not be used to describe a disability. This word can be used to describe the society or environment that limits accessibility.

Mute or Person Who Cannot Speak. Preferred terms to describe persons who cannot speak. Terms such as *deaf-mute* and *deaf* and *dumb* are inappropriate. They imply that persons without speech are always *deaf*.

Nondisabled. In a media portrayal of persons with and without disabilities, *nondisabled* is the appropriate term for persons without disabilities. Able-bodied should not be used, as it implies that persons with disabilities are less able. *Normal* is appropriate only in reference to statistical norms.

Seizure. Describes an involuntary muscular contraction symptomatic of the brain disorder epilepsy. Rather than saying "epileptic," say a "person with epilepsy" or "person with a seizure condition." The term *convulsion* should be reserved for seizures involving contractions of the entire body. The term *fit* is used by the medical profession in England, but it has strong negative connotations.

Spastic. Describes a muscle with sudden, abnormal involuntary spasms. It is not appropriate for describing a person with cerebral palsy. *Muscles* are spastic; people are not.

Speech Impaired. Describes persons with limited or difficult speech patterns.

Cesarean Birth. Should be used to describe a surgical birth. Avoid "section," it depersonalizes. Grapefruits get sectioned; women give birth.

Source: Adapted from Guidelines for reporting and writing about people with disabilities. (1987). Media Project, Research and Training Center on Independent Living (348 Haworth Hall, University of Kansas, Lawrence, KS 66045); Sawin, K. J. (1986). Physical disability in contemporary women's health. Menlo Park. CA: Addison-Wesley; and Disability etiquette. Virginia Commonwealth University: Office of EEO/Affirmative Action Services. Dajani, K. F. (2001). What's in a name? Terms used to refer to people with disabilities. Disability Studies Quarterly, 21(3), 196–209.

with disabilities—this needs to be a focus for future research (Nosek et al., 1997). We need to better understand the health promotion practices of women with disability that may assist them in dealing with their chronic conditions. Women with MS were found to consume inadequate (10% lower than recommended) carbohydrates, fiber, calcium, and zinc and higher than recommended Vitamin C, A, fat, protein, and iron (Timmerman & Stuifbergen, 1999). Vitamin D and calcium supplementation is important because women with epilepsy are at increased risk for osteoporosis with long-term AED treatment (Brodie & French, 2000). Evidence (MMWR, 1991) supports that 0.4 mg (400 micrograms) per day of folic acid will significantly reduce the number of cases of neural tube defects (NTDs). Because NTDs occur in the early days of pregnancy before women are even aware of even being pregnant, the USPHS recommends that ALL women of childbearing age in the United States who are capable of becoming pregnant should take a multivitamin containing 0.4 of folic acid a day to reduce the risk of having a pregnancy affected with spina bifida or NDT. Women who have had a prior pregnancy affected by NTDs are considered high risk, should be placed on higher daily doses of folic acid (4 mg), and need to plan with their health care provider for any anticipated pregnancies. Providers need to be aware that high doses of folic acid may mask vitamin B_{12} deficiency (MMWR, 1991). Obesity may put women at two to four times higher risk for NTD despite folic acid supplementation (Shaw, Velie, & Schaffer, 1996). Thus, preconceptual counseling for weight reduction has even more impact if the client seeks conception (Murphy, 1996).

Efforts need to be made to broadly disseminate this information to the general public and to those using contraception services (Stengel, 1996). In a recent survey identifying that over 50 percent of at-risk women are not taking a multivitamin, women acknowledged that they would be more likely to take the multivitamin if it was recommended by their health care provider (Modlin, 2000). One such model is the "train the trainer" model used in select public health departments. One professional in each agency participates in training and is then responsible to document educating others in the home agency. This work, underwritten by the March of Dimes at the local level, may be an effective model using agencies, organizations, and schools.

PHYSICAL ACTIVITY/SPORTS

Individuals with disabilities have demonstrated physiological responses to exercise similar to women without disabilities. In addition, exercise has been shown to yield positive overall fitness and psychological outcomes (Ashton-Shaeffer, Gibson, Autry, & Hanson, 2001). Although most of the studies have been done on men, the data suggest normal wheelchair propulsion is not sufficient to maintain physical condition, and training programs yield positive changes in physical conditioning (DePauw, 1996). African American women with disabilities engaged in very low levels of exercise and participation in unstructured physical activities was almost absent (Rimmer, Rubin, & Braddock 2000). Research is needed that explores the responses of women with disability to a variety of recreational and sports programs and the interaction of women's health status with these programs (Blinde & Mcallister, 1999). The opportunities for physical activity or women with disabilities need to be expanded (Henderson & Bedini, 1995). This is particularly important for girls in physical education classes who are experiencing segregation inclusion and social isolation (Place & Hodge, 2001).

ACCESS ISSUES/BARRIERS

The characteristics of medical systems sometimes constitute barriers to women with physical disabilities. Several women report dissatisfaction with services they receive from their provider, such as a different provider each time, procedures in some offices that prohibit staff from offering assistance to women in mounting an exam table, staff unwilling to offer assistance with dressing, and appointments denied because the women use wheelchairs (Nosek et al., 1995). A recent study (Persaud, 2000) of women with spinal cord injuries indicated three barriers to preventive health: (1) inadequate knowledge regarding health risk, (2) reliance on caregivers to facilitate preventive health practices, and (3) perceived problems with access to competent health care providers.

Health care clinics that have architectural barriers limit the independence of women with mobility limitations. Access to buildings via appropriately constructed ramps and to elevators is critical to quality care, as is easy access to bathrooms, examination rooms, and scales. Most medical facilities have numerous architectural barriers such as nonelevating exam tables and lack of platform scales to weigh persons who use a wheelchair (Welner, 1996). Even if the facility is architecturally accessible, furniture placement can make the examination room functionally unaccessible. Women experience difficulty obtaining reliable information regarding contraception and often get conflicting recommendations. A truly accessible environment regards women with disabilities as experts on the functioning of their own bodies and is sensitive to histories of traumatic interactions with medical environments. These settings actively develop policies that will increase access to reproductive health services for women with disabilities (Nosek et al., 1995).

In addition, very little attention has been given to determining if access issues for women are different than for men. For mothers, daycare access, school, public playgrounds, and affordable housing are all fundamental access issues that are usually not on the list for "assessing accessibility" for most organizations (DePauw, 1996).

SPECIAL PROBLEMS
General Considerations

Specific educational resources are listed prior to the References at the end of this chapter.

Providers may feel that once a woman experiences a disability, she should return to the homemaker role, even when the disability is not severe. Women who report that their sense of self-esteem is tied to work are least likely to report a specific disability (Mudrick, 1993).

Sight and Hearing Impairment

Deaf or blind clients are limited in their ability to communicate with providers if interpreters are not available. If a woman provides an interpreter, she loses the option of having private interaction with the provider. If sign language is used in relating issues of sexuality and sexual intercourse, it should be remembered that sign communication is easily interpreted "across the room"; therefore, attention must be given to interview area (Henderson & Bedini, 1995).

Severe Disability

Women institutionalized with severe multiple disabilities, including cognitive impairment, may have such clinical problems as vaginal discharge, menstrual cycle dysfunction, and oligomenorrhea. Sensitive onsite management is essential (Furman, 1989). The severity of physical impairment, however, is not a good predictor of the impact of a disability on a woman (DePauw, 1996; Mudrick, 1993; Stengel, 1996).

Providers need to assess the assumptions they hold. They may be surprised to learn that the severity of physical impairment is not a good predictor of impact of the disability on women (Harrison, Glass, & Soni, 1995). In fact, fatigue and pain have been found to be better predictors of health outcomes even after the impact of functional ability has been taken into consideration.

SEXUALITY

COMMUNICATION AND EDUCATION

Communicating and obtaining information about sexuality are among a woman's greatest concerns. The subject of sexuality and disabled women has been studied little, perhaps because of the erroneous assumption that among clients with a disability, sexuality adjustment is less an issue for women than for men (Drew, 1990). Women report that professionals rarely initiate discussion of sexuality issues (Meeropol, 1991; Nosek et al., 1996).

The health care provider needs to take responsibility for initiating discussions of sexuality, but also important is offering "assistance rather than avoiding or overemphasizing the issue" (Drew, 1990; Guest, 2000). Assumptions should not be made at either extreme: None of these

women has sexuality issues, or all of them do. Instead, assess each individual. Do not neglect to screen for STDs.

Some authors propose that the primary barriers to full expression of sexuality are the negative attitudes of others, especially family members and medical and rehabilitation professionals. The attitude that the disability has somehow "neutered" the woman interferes with her belief in her right to sexual feelings and expression (Blackwell-Stratton et al., 1988; DePauw, 1996; Nelson, 1995; Nosek et al., 1994, 1996).

From their in-depth qualitative interviews, researchers (Nosek et al., 1994) identified tasks important to developing a wellness perspective of sexuality among women with physical disabilities (see Table 24–2). These characteristics of being a "well woman," however, are not all of the story. The study found that examination of wellness cannot focus only on the individual and cannot be framed in a deficiency model if solutions are to be found. It is important to study the context. These researchers concluded that the roots of problems are to be found in the macro system that insists on a normative group against which all others are to be compared and found deficient. The way a social problem is defined determines policy, strategies for change, and criteria for evaluation.

In the quantitative portion of this study, 475 women with disabilities were compared with a population of 425 women without disabilities. There was no difference between groups in sexual desire. Further, there was no impact of the severity of disability on sexual activity. Women with disabilities did report lower amounts of sexual activity, sexual response, and sexual satisfaction. Women with disabilities since childhood had more sexual thoughts and higher desire. No differences were found in sexual frequency, arousal, or satisfaction. The psychological factors predicted the greatest amount of sexual variance, 35 percent of variance in sexual satisfaction and 40 percent of the variance in sexual activity (Nosek et al., 1994). Other researchers agree, reporting decreased function without changes in interest or importance of sexual activity (Harrison et al., 1995).

In a study of adolescents with disabilities, Meeropol found that few of the adolescents or their parents ever talked to a nurse or physician for sexuality information, and one-quarter of the adolescents and 40 percent of their parents wished that a health care professional had offered this information. (Meeropol, 1991).

As long as women with disabilities are viewed as deviant from the social norm based only on disability, they will continue to be invisible (Nosek et al., 1994). The Sydney Manifesto, a statement of the World Assembly of

TABLE 24–2. Wellness Perspective of Sexuality among Women with Physical Disabilities

Having a Positive Sexual Self-Concept
She appreciates her own value.
She asserts her right to make a choice.
She feels ownership of her body.
She is able to restrict the limitations resulting from her disability to physical functioning only and does not impose those limitations to her sexual self.
She is accepting, not ashamed, of her body.

Having Sexual Information
She has general information about sexuality and is able to apply to herself.
She actively seeks information about how her disability affects her sexuality.

Having Positive, Productive Relationships
She feels generally satisfied with her relationships.
She is able to communicate effectively with others.
She feels stability in her relationships.
She is able to control the amount and nature of contact with others.

Managing Barriers
She is able to recognize psychological, physical, and sexual abuse and its exploitation and take action to reduce or eliminate it or neutralize its impact.
She has learned to reduce her vulnerability.
She understands her disability-related environmental needs and seeks information on how to meet these needs.
She recognizes her right to live in a barrier-free environment and takes action to achieve it.
She confronts societal barriers by using good communication skills to educate her partner, friends, and family.

Maintaining Optimal Health and Physical Sexual Functioning
She participates in health maintenance activities and engages in health-promoting behaviors.
She feels congruity between her values/desires and her sexual behaviors.
She manages her environment to optimize privacy for intimate activities.
She is satisfied with the frequency and quality of sexual activity.
She is able to communicate freely with her partner about limitations and devices and about what pleases her sexually.

Source: Adapted from Nosek, M. A., Howland, C. A., Young, M. E., Georgiou, D., Rintala, D. H., Foley, C. C., Bennett, J. L., & Smith, Q. (1994). Wellness models and sexuality among women with disabilities. Journal of Applied Rehabilitation Counseling (25), 50–57.

Disabled Peoples International held in Sydney in 1994, summarizes the rights of women with disabilities. This Manifesto asserts that each time issues for women are considered, the woman with disabilities needs to be included.

Conditions that Impact Sexuality

The specific effects of a disability on sexual activity need to be communicated to a woman. For example, in some conditions spasticity might be experienced with orgasm (Berhard, 1989).

The PLISSIT Model. This model, used to order levels of intervention for clients with sexual issues, is helpful for health care providers (see Chapter 6). PLISSIT is derived from "Permission giving, provision of Limited Information and Specific Suggestions, Intensive Therapy." All providers need to be skilled in permission giving, reinforcing the ability for a woman with a disability to be a sexual person and to be involved in sexual activities. The professional needs to understand and convey to women with disabilities that any manifestation of sexuality that is acceptable and satisfying to the individual or individuals involved is normal.

Body Image

Concerns about body image exist for some women with disabilities. The reactions of others may suggest to a woman that her body is unacceptable (Nelson, 1995).

Perceived Lack of Control. Issues such as physical dependency, bladder incontinence, spasticity, or other involuntary movements, which are not seen as adult conditions, may make the woman with a disability seem like an infant. The lack of control can lead to a mind-body split. "It was like my body belonged to the doctors, it wasn't mine any more." "Once I put my feet up in the stirrups, I had no control—my body belonged to them [examiners]" (Sawin, 1982).

Appliances. The need to use appliances or equipment may interfere with a woman's sense of self as sexually desirable.

Source of Trouble. The body may have a history of "causing" trouble. If a child grew up with a disability, her body may have caused parents trouble and could have become the "enemy."

Service Animals

The use of service animals is growing in popularity. These animals, most often dogs or monkeys, assist their owners in a wide variety of tasks from alerting a woman with hearing impairment that someone is at the door to retrieving objects for a woman with mobility impairment. Women report they feel less vulnerable if their service animal is a large dog that barks loudly at strangers. In addition, the relationship with the service animal has been found to impact outcome (Modlin, 2000).

Spasticity

Spasticity can be elicited by a variety of tactile stimulations. Each woman needs to determine the ability of a variety of sexual activities to produce this response. Slow-building stimulation may produce less spasticity than more intense stimulation. Women with spasticity might experience spasticity with orgasm (Mudrick, 1993). The knee-chest position during sexual activities may facilitate decrease in spasticity.

SPINAL CORD INJURY

Because a women's fertility is not affected in a spinal cord injury, many providers and researchers have assumed no sexuality problems exist. Spinal cord injury precipitates specific physiological changes that reflect the level of cord injury and the completeness of the lesion. Some authors categorize lesions as above thoracic 10, between thoracic 10 and 12, and distal to thoracic 12 (Berhard, 1989). Women with SCI have identified three areas of highest need: personal care, activities of daily living, and general health and sexuality (Schopp, Kirkpatrick, Hagglund, Meyer, & Meyer, 2001). Their major secondary conditions included fatigue, mobility, physical deconditioning, spasticity, and joint pain (Coyle, Santiago, Shank, Ma, & Boyd, 2001). Women with complete lesions experience neither traditional orgasm nor clitoral or vaginal sensation (Kettl, Zarefoss, Jacoby, et al., 1991; Mudrick, 1993; Yarkony & Chen, 1995); however, women with spinal cord injury do report satisfying pleasurable orgasm-like sensations from stimulation of the breasts, ears, or other sensitive areas (Whipple, Gerdes, & Kopmisarut, 1996). Even women with complete lesions report psychological and even physical sensations of orgasm or "intense pleasure" during sex (Donohue & Gebhard, 1995; Kettl et al., 1991; Sipski, Alexander, & Rosen, 1995; Yang, 2000) Preliminary data support the ability of women with SCI as high at T-6 to experience physiological organisms with self-stimulation (Whipple, Gerdes, & Komisarut, 1996). These orgasm experiences are not related to type or level of SCI (Donohue & Gebhard, 1995). In addition, menstrual discomfort may remain, even if altered. Vaginal lubrication may occur via reflex for women with lesions at T9–T11 or above (Boone, 1995; Sipski et al., 1995; Yarkony & Chen, 1995) and has also been reported in relation to masturbation unrelated to level of lesion (Donohue & Gebhard, 1995). In addition, some women report cervical and vaginal pressure (Whipple, Richard, et al., 1996). Arousal was present in women regardless of level of lesion and not correlated with type of stimulation (vaginal, cervical, or hypersensitive area). Clearly, the mechanism of sexual response in women with spinal cord injuries does not totally follow the traditional physiological model. Further research is needed to understand the

physical and cognitive processes women experience (Charlifue, Gerhart, Menter, Whiteneck, & Manley, 1992; Sipski et al., 1995). In addition, although women with mobility problems were unlikely to get immunization (pneumonia and influenza), they were less likely to receive Pap tests and mammograms (Iezzoni et al., 2000).

Change in Patterns

Adjustment in the first years after injury are most difficult. Some women report issues revolving around physical problems (bladder control, dry vagina), but issues regarding social interaction (attitudes of others) are numerous (Drew, 1990). Changes in the reproductive system are listed:

- Temporary cessation of menses is normal for 60 to 90 percent of women for several months following injury. Cessation of menses may persist for up to two years, with the average duration being six months. For 89 percent of women, menses returns by one year (Boone, 1995; Whipple et al., 1996: Yarkony & Chen, 1995).
- Patterns of sexual activity for women with a disability may be decreased. Many women report the lack of a partner. It is important, however, to remember that the problem is universal. Participants in a Sexual Attitude Reassessment (SAR) workshop reported they were not as active as they wished (women without disability 56 percent, women disabled 57 percent) (Harrison et al., 1995).
- Alternative areas of sexual stimulation and strategies for sexual expression need to be identified, including alternative positions, such as side-lying, knee-chest positions, and chair sitting, for paraplegics and quadriplegics and the stuffing technique (of flaccid penis) for women whose partner is paraplegic. If graphic depiction of positions for sexual intercourse would be helpful, the health care provider needs to communicate the appropriate resources (Page, Cheng, Pate, et al., 1987).
- The normal sexual responses that may occur are opening of the labia, contraction of the outer third of the vagina, expansion of the inner two-thirds of the vagina, and uterine contraction.
- Resumption of ovulation is unpredictable. It may occur before menstruation (Whipple et al., 1996)
- Women at or approaching climacteric may become menopausal (Yarkony & Chen, 1995)

◆ Many women (69 percent in a large SCI follow-up study) are satisfied with postinjury sexual experience, although many were not satisfied with information provided in rehabilitation SCI (Charlifue et al., 1992)

Autonomic Dysreflexia

A potentially fatal complication for women with spinal cord injury, autonomic dysreflexia, occurs if the lesion is complete and above T-6 and can lead to a stroke (Zasler, 1991).

Autonomic dysreflexia is a physiological reflex response to stimulation. Stimulation may be caused by conditions such as skin breakdown, bladder hyperdistention often due to kinked tubing, bowel distention, severe constipation, pelvic examination, labor, or intercourse positions.

Patterns of response vary among individuals; however, among all who have a complete lesion, the pathway within the cord that transmits sensations to higher levels is blocked. So, too, is the mechanism that relays messages downward from the brain. Consequently, blood pressure is not suppressed, and blood pressure rises with sustained reflex. As long as the sensation continues, the blood pressure continues to rise. Normal blood pressure for women with spinal injury is often lower than normal, for example, 90/60. Blood pressure in early dysreflexia might be 140/83. At this level, a woman could have significant symptoms of dysreflexia.

Dysreflexia is often overlooked by health care providers who do not know about the altered blood pressure norm. Headache, sweating, goose flesh above the level of lesion, flushed face, and nasal stuffiness are other signs of this potentially lethal complication.

Sources of stimulation can be additive. For example, if a client is slightly constipated or sitting or lying on an object, or her urine drainage system is slightly kinked, an additional stimulation such as a pelvic exam, sexual intercourse, or labor contraction could trigger dysreflexia. If dysreflexia occurs, the total situation must be assessed for hidden problems.

◆ If dysreflexia occurs during a procedure, *have the client sit up immediately.* Blood pressure increases when a person is lying down. A semi-sitting position is helpful to prevent dysreflexia during pelvic exams. Labor in that position might be helpful if it is comfortable.

◆ Monitor blood pressure during labor contractions.

◆ Assist the client in establishing effective bowel and bladder routines, which can prevent or reduce acci-

dents and decrease the chance of additive dysreflexia episodes.

◆ Take extreme care to protect skin when transferring the client to an examining table.

◆ May need medication for acute episodes or on a long-term basis. Unresponsive dysreflexia is a medical emergency.

A woman with a spinal cord injury who is educated about the symptoms of autonomic dysreflexia needs to be listened to. She may have a card with treatment outlined or a hotline for contacting a rehabilitation consultant. Discuss the pattern of autonomic dysreflexia with all women with spinal cord injury before high risk situations (pelvic examination, labor, catheter change, etc.) occur (Nosek et al., 1995). Ask the client about the frequency of the symptoms, triggering factors, and usual treatment. Were there any episodes in which she did not respond? Does she take medications routinely?

Latex Allergy

Since 1991, the Centers for Disease Control and Prevention (CDC) have been receiving an increasing number of reports of latex related allergy. Individuals (especially children) with spina bifida or myelomeningocele (a congenital spinal cord injury) have the highest incidence of latex allergy, varying from 12 percent to 40 percent of the population (Banta, Bonanni, & Prebluda, 1993; Gleeson, 1995; Pearson, Cole, & Jarvis, 1994). This condition also occurs in some women with multiple congenital malformations, especially multiple urinary anomalies, and in some health care providers with increased latex exposure. Reaction varies from mild wheal and flare episodes to anaphylatic reactions (Barton, 1993; Hatcher et al., 1998; Sussman & Beezhold, 1995; Tosi, Slater, Shaer, & Mostello, 1993). The latter are most frequently related to surgery. In addition, 3 to 17 percent of health care workers develop latex allergy (Taylor & Praditsuwan, 1996).

Most children/adolescents who have developed this allergy have reacted to balloons and gloves; however, condoms, dental dams, and urinary catheters have also created allergic response. Women with spina bifida are considered high risk and should be tested for latex allergy (RAST—radioallergosorbent testing) (Fisher & Sawin, 1998; Shaer & Meeropol, 1995). Health care providers need to be alert to the possibility of latex sensitivities in their clients. Avoidance of latex materials (condoms, diaphragms, latex gloves) may be recommended for all individuals with spina bifida. Many settings that provide services to at-risk patients have converted to a nonlatex environment (Gleeson, 1995). Staff in hospitals, clinics, dentists' offices, and especially ORs need to be well versed in precautions. The Spina Bifida Association of America has a comprehensive list of nonlatex options, which is updated every six months (Shaer & Meeropol, 1995) and a short-well done video useful to both families and professionals (see Resource list). Individuals with a confirmed allergy should wear a medic alert bracelet and carry an epinephrine autoinjector kit (Crotty, McFarlane, Brooks, et al., 1994). The issue of latex allergy in the workplace can be an important barrier to full employment (NIOSH, 2002).

JOINT INFLEXIBILITY AND PAIN

Arthrogryposis congenita, sickle cell anemia with joint involvement, arthritis, severe scoliosis, amputation, and dwarfism may result in joint inflexibility and pain. With respect to sexual activity, careful assessment of physical parameters, such as range of motion, is helpful. Discussion about alternative positioning may follow. The importance of extended foreplay, possible gentle warming up and stretching, warm showers, and use of vibration, massage, or masturbation to achieve orgasm may also be considered. Prolonged rest should be avoided in order to decrease likelihood of joint stiffness. Sexual activity may augment an overall sense of comfort, as orgasm releases endorphins. The client may profit from some helpful suggestions.

- Choose the time of day for sexual activity relative to pain history.
- Consider a warm shower or compress in foreplay if effective in pain relief.
- Consider medicine for pain relief before intercourse if pain is limiting.
- Consider referral to a physical therapist for comprehensive muscle assessment in complex cases.

Assess social support. Data indicate that after controlling for physical limitations and social integration, social support was found to influence the outcome in women with arthritis (Brown & Williams, 1995; Crotty et al., 1994; Dale, 1996).

Encourage a positive, proactive attitude. Self-assessed health status is a powerful predictor of function (joint inflex) (Becker et al., 1998).

MULTIPLE SCLEROSIS

MS is the most common neurologic disease among young adults. Women are affected twice as often as men. Female sex hormones, estrogen and progesterone, may be involved. Clinical symptoms often appear during changes in hormonal balance during the menstrual cycle, after pregnancy, and during the climacteric.

The symptoms of multiple sclerosis may vary greatly and may include spasticity, dry vagina, fatigue, muscle weakness, pain, bladder and bowel incontinence, and difficulty achieving orgasm (Hatzichristou, 1996; Lundberg & Hulter, 1996; Mattson, Petrie, Srivastave, & McDermott, 1995). No change, however, occurs in fertility or menstruation. Balance and fatigue may necessitate energy sparing sexual activities and positions for intercourse. A water-soluble lubricant may be used if the vagina is dry. Vibrators have been found to be helpful to those who tried them, as a way to increase stimulation and achieve orgasm (Mattson et al., 1995).

Data indicate that about half of women who have multiple sclerosis report changes in their sexual life (McCabe, McDonald, Deeks, Vowels, & Cobain, 1996; Yang, 2000). The duration of MS, degree of disability, number of exacerbations in the last year, disability score, and presence of bowel problems or fatigue have little impact on the presence of sexual dysfunction, although the amount of sexual activity may decrease. Corticosteroids are most often used to reduce sexual malfunction but improved function in one study in only 24 of 60 subjects (Mattson et al., 1995).

Mattson reports that most women were interested in lovemaking, although interest did vary with disease activity. Eighty-eight percent of women in his study were satisfied and 95 percent of their partners were satisfied with sexual activity. Few women indicated dysfunction caused marital problems (Mattson et al., 1995). Some clients have irregular ovulation. This may lead to an abnormal secretion of hormones within the pituitary-gonadal axis, which in turn results in irregular menses and possible infertility. Corticosteroids started for other symptoms have resulted in improved sexuality for many women (Hatzichristou, 1996; Lundberg & Hulter, 1996; Mattson et al., 1995).

Life stressors, in addition to the disease, have a significant impact on women's sense of mastery. Thus, it might be helpful to have a shift from the emphasis of managing the physical condition to managing the uncertainty and assisting people with MS to achieve a better sense of mastery (Crigger, 1996). Professional help is rarely sought for dysfunction. Sensitive professionals need to address this subject openly with women and their partners. A recent study indicates that a home-based resistance exercise intervention may be possible without increasing fatigue, which may increase women's health and sense of well-being (Slawta et al., 2002).

DIABETES MELLITUS

The effect of diabetes on the sexuality of women is unclear, although sexual changes have been identified among men who have diabetes. Therefore genitosexual innervation appears to be analogous in males and females (Kolodny, 1980). In a recent study, more women with diabetes had sexual dysfunction than controls, with women with diabetes reporting a significant difference only for decreased lubrication. While age, BMI, length of diabetes, medication, or menopausal status were not related to sexual dysfunction, lower marital quality and depression were. Those with more complications reported more dysfunction and altered treatment satisfaction (Enzlin, Mathieu, Van Den Bruel, et al., 2002).

Spontaneous remission of sexual dysfunction reported on 6-year follow-up was related to improvement in the overall marital and social situations. Acceptance of illness (as judged by interviewer) and psychological distress were strong predictors of sexual function (Jensen, 1986). Clearly, sexuality issues need to be aggressively assessed and addressed to optimize quality of life for women with diabetes function.

EPILEPSY

Women with epilepsy (WWE) have normal fertility. Several concerns exist for these women, however, including the effect of their hormones and menstrual cycle on seizures, contraception, fertility, and sexuality issues (Callanan & Stalland, 1996). Some experts now estimate up to 50 percent of WWE, experience variations in seizure frequency with hormonal changes (Liporace, 1997). There is minimal data on adolescents and epilepsy. Epilepsy does not substantially alter puberty in adolescents. Approximately 70 percent will have no change in seizure frequency, 15 percent experience increase, and 15 percent experience a decrease in seizure frequency, with more seizures at ovulation and imediately before and after the menstrual flow (Liporace, 1997). Many of the antiepilepsy drugs (AEDs) taken to control seizures have teratogenic potential, especially if the young woman is on more than one medication (Dodson 1996). Infant malformations occur more in women using polytherapy rather than monotherapy. Safer sex becomes critical as the best outcomes of pregnancy are when the pregnancy is planned. The greatest risk for seizure recurrence when women attempt to withdraw from AEDs occurs in the first six months. Thus, if women have been seizure-free for two to five years and wish to consider withdrawal in collaboration with their neurologist, it is desirable that a slow taper be used and withdrawal be completed at least six months before any planned conception (AAN, 1998). After the pregnancy, it is too late to change medications or try to reduce the number as the risk of prolonged convulsions is also a risk for the fetus (Callanan & Stalland, 1996).

Callanan and Stalland recommend that women chart their seizures in relation to their menstrual cycle and/or ovulation to see if a pattern emerges. Some women would benefit from supplemental hormonal therapy. Puberty, a time of severe hormonal changes, should be monitored closely. The adolescent developmental tasks and emotional status further complicate the health care providers ability to identify patterns or cycles. All WWE, including adolescents, capable of becoming pregnant should be taking 0.4 mg of folic acid. Select AEDs have been shown to lower folic acid levels, which increases the risk for neural tube conditions. Genetic counseling may be helpful to determine patterns of birth defects in the family (Yang, 2000).

A healthy development of sexuality has been affected for some. These women report problems with self-image and self-confidence with occasional social isolation. Women report these issues relate to the frequency of their seizures (Callanan & Stalland, 1996). Some sexuality issues may be related to AEDs. A major initiative focusing on women has been underway in the organizations serving individuals with epilepsy. Focus groups of WWE identify the same issues of concerns as other women with disabilities: to be taken seriously and considered equal partners in health care, to have options in treatment and lifestyle, and to have a more informed public and health care provider (Shafer, Austin, Callanan, & Clerico, 1996).

URINARY AND BOWEL APPLIANCES

Apparatus may discourage sexual activity. Steps, however, can be taken to ease discomforts.

◆ Foley catheters can be taped out of the way or removed, but may need to be reinserted soon after sexual activity; individuals using intermittent catheterizations should catheterize before sexual activity to prevent urine leakage.

◆ Stomal appliances can be ignored, changed, covered, or removed before sexual activity, based on what has been ordered and individual preference.

◆ Clients should be told that masturbation and coitus may stimulate bladder or bowel incontinence.

◆ Discussing how to tell potential partners about bladder and bowel issues may be critical. Role-playing may be helpful.

PELVIC RADIOTHERAPY

Radiation may cause vaginal constriction, resulting in dyspareunia.

CYSTIC FIBROSIS

Young women with cystic fibrosis are living into their third decade and beyond. Their pattern is parallel to other women with disabilities, however. Many adolescents with cystic fibrosis have delayed menarche. Weight has been shown to be the major predictor. It is interesting to note that up to 20 percent of girls may menstruate even though they had not reached the critical 17 percent criterion of body fat. Edenborough (2001) suggest that if this body mass is not reached in time, other factors, unclear at this time, may come into play. Single women with cystic fibrosis start dating at a later age, have dated less often, felt less attractive, had less sexual desire, and had more sexual issues than a comparison group of women without cystic fibrosis (Coffman, Levine, Althof, & Stern, 1994). These authors conclude the tendency to overprotect these women may interfere with their sense of autonomy and self-worth. In addition, women who had a defiant attitude toward their chronic illness did better. This attitude is an example of "healthy denial" defined by this author not as denial of the illness but denial of the illness to impact normal function despite challenges. Women who were married differed from their single peers; they had later onset of illness, better physical health, and better sexual health. There is little evidence that fertility is impaired in healthy women with CF. Although pregnancy was well tolerated in women with mild disease, those with poor lung function, severe disease and diabetes had increased risk of prematurity and decline after delivery (Edenborough, 2001). Eighty-one percent of pregnancies progress after 20 weeks, although one-fourth of these delivered prematurely.

COGNITIVE IMPAIRMENT

It is difficult for women with cognitive impairment or developmental delays to achieve sexual options available to other women with disabilities (Gill & Brown, 2000; Walsh, Heller, Schupf, van Schrojenstein Lantman-de Valk, 2001). Women with severe cognitive impairments are often seen as nonadults and as unequal to their peers without disabilities (Jordan & Dunlap, 2001). Issues of sexual education, effective birth control, sexual expression, and pregnancy are complex (Sulpizi, 1996). Even when parents verbalize the opinion that young adults with cognitive impairment should have sexual options, it is difficult for the same parents to prepare their own children to make sexual decisions (Shepperdson, 1995), consider teaching their teen the appropriate use of masturbation (Blackburn, 1995), or teach abuse prevention skills. Better understanding of the needs of young women who grow up with cognitive delay or developmental disabilities is crucial to provision of effective care (Evenhuis, Henderson, Beange, Lennox, & Chicoine, 2001; Walsh et al., 2001).

VISUAL/HEARING IMPAIRMENT

Many women who are deaf/blind enter adulthood sexually unaware but with normal sexual drives and desires. They often lack basic sexual information such as physical differences between the sexes, information related to reproduction and contraceptive options, and knowledge of sexually transmitted diseases (STDs). This deficit in sexual and reproductive education created by parents' and health care providers' lack of alternate methods of communication is compounded by the deaf/blind youth's inability to learn about sexuality by watching others model appropriate and inappropriate sexual behaviors. Sexuality education for women who are deaf-blind should be taught throughout their life span. The better informed the women are, the less likely they will be sexually maladjusted or abused (Ingraham, Vernon, Clemente, & Olney, 2000).

CHANGES IN MENARCHE

It appears that some variations in menarche occur among women with select disabilities. For example, individuals with Down syndrome and spinal bifida experience menarche eleven months earlier than a comparison group of nondisabled subjects; however, others with genetic disabilities may have delayed menarche (Furman, 1989). Individuals with blindness experience menarche earlier than normal. Head injury is also associated with precocious puberty (Sockalosky & Kriel, 1987). Most women with spinal cord injury report the same or more discomfort with their menses after injury (Kettl et al., 1991). For some women with mobility impairments, lack of manual dexterity and difficulty transferring can impair independence and may lead a woman to seek a means to reduce or eliminate the menstrual cycle. Nosek (1992) indicates the practice is widespread in well-meaning parents of women with cognitive impairment. Her point is that no research exists on the long-term effects of these drugs for women with decreased mobility. Depo-Provera, for example, may have serious cardiovascular side effects such as thrombophlebitis and pulmonary embolisms. Women and their families must carefully weigh the risks and benefits of interventions to manage menstrual hygiene with potential long-term effects. However, some conditions, such as epilepsy, asthma, rheumatoid arthritis, irritable bowel syndrome, and diabetes, have menstrual-related changes. Medical suppression of ovulation using gonadotropin-releasing hormone agonists may be useful for either diagnosis or treatment of severe, recurrent menstrual cycle-related disease exacerbations (Case & Reid, 1998).

PERSONAL CARE ATTENDANT

Many women with mobility or sensory limitations employ a personal care attendant. She may address some unique sexuality issues; for example, she may place the cervical cap or diaphragm and carry out the bowel or bladder program before sexual activity. Spouses and significant others often function as personal care attendants, but it can be difficult to be both care provider and lover. Each couple needs to address this issue. If both the woman and her partner are disabled, the attendant may assist in positioning the couple. The political issues surrounding reimbursement, regulation, and licensing of personal care attendants may dramatically affect the quality of life for women with disabilities (Nosek, 1993).

PLANNING SEXUAL ACTIVITY

Women report a need to avoid spontaneity and instead plan for sexual activity. This need, however, can be seen as a benefit: Because many disabled persons must communicate with their partners about sexual possibilities and restrictions, this opens up avenues for communica-

tion in other areas of the relationship. Unfortunately, many people who are totally physically independent may never experience such communication (Bogle & Shaul, 1981).

ABUSE

Women with physical and cognitive disabilities may be at higher risk for abuse (Curry, Hassouneh-Phillips, & Johnston-Silverberg, 2001; Gill, 1996; Hassouneh-Phillips & Curry, 2002; Nosek, 1995; Powers, Curry, Oschwald, et al., 2002; Young, Nosek, Howland, et al., 1997). Abuse is a serious problem for women with disabilities because they have even fewer options for escaping or resolving the abuse than women in general (Nosek et al., 1997).

There is combined cultural devaluation of women, devaluation based on age, and devaluation of disability. The woman with disability often has experienced overprotection and has internalized social expectations. Combine this with a lack of knowledge, overcompliance, an unrealistic view that everyone is a friend, limited social opportunity, constant negative feedback (women with disability are ugly, worthless, etc.), low self-esteem, and limited or no assertiveness or refusal skills, and it is understandable this population has a high incidence of abuse (Elvik, Berkowitz, Nichols, & Inkelis, 1990; Nelson, 1995). Women may not report abuse because of fear of not being believed due to their devalued status (Cole, 1993). If a disabled teenager or adult feels undesirable, she may become vulnerable to exploitation, particularly in sexual relations (Welner, 1993). In a national survey of over 800 women, Nosek (1994) found women with disabilities one and one-half times more likely to have been abused than their nondisabled peers; 50 percent of women with disability and 34 percent of women without disability reported abuse. These researchers proposed that women who get little information regarding sexuality are vulnerable to exploitation. Children who undergo frequent physical examinations or therapy can come to feel that their body causes pain or is connected with unpleasant experiences. This feeling may yield a child or teen who feels disconnected from her body, at risk for abuse (Nelson, 1995). In a qualitative study of 31 women with disabilities, the disability itself did not seem to be related to the abuse experience (Nosek, 1995). These researchers concluded that it is the asexual, dependent, passive stereotype of women with physical disability that may be the root of the vulnerability to sexual abuse rather than the disability itself.

It is important that the health care provider acknowledge the sexuality of women with disabilities, teach healthy sexuality in the context of family, reinforce a positive sense of self, learn to recognize signs of abuse, listen to the patient, and act on reports of abuse. Assessment of abuse and treatment interventions for women with disabilities will be the same as their peers without disabilities. In order to increase services, considerably more needs to be known about interventions that are most effective for this population (Nosek, Howland, & Hughes, 2001). Prevention, however, is the major key (Elvik et al., 1990).

Educational programs need to be developed to address skill building in coping with potential or real abuse and orientation to sexuality rights and responsibilities (Elvik et al., 1990).

In addition, health care providers need to include sexual assertiveness skills in sex education or family life education curricula. The optimal time for this education is in childhood or adolescence. The vast majority of shelters for women who have been abused are unaccessible (Nosek, 1995). Professionals need to seek out opportunities to act as a consultant to schools and community groups that serve this population (YWCA, local school districts, and schools). These women may need a myriad of specialized services for treatment (Gilson, Cramer, & DePoy, 2001). Agencies such as independent living centers may be useful partners in these endeavors (Swedlund & Nosek, 2001).

ISSUES OF AGING/MENOPAUSE

People with disabilities are now living into "old age." Postpolio syndrome is a reality for many women in their 50s. We do know that the major causes of death to persons with spinal cord injuries are respiratory infections, urinary tract infections and external causes such as suicide. There is little data, however, explaining why most other people with lifelong disabilities die. Individuals with disabilities and chronic illness are asking questions such as the following: What are the implications of aging to 60 if you have had osteoarthritis since 20? What is menopause like for women with disabilities (Nosek, 1992), or what are the implications on joint health of walking for many years with altered gait or of the early transition to wheelchair as primary source of mobility? Even though a majority of persons with disabilities are female, there is very little research that examines the im-

pact of aging on women with disabilities (Pentland, Trembly, Spring, & Rosenthal, 1999).

Women with disabilities may experience unique changes in addition to or independently from the customary aging processes (Brown & Murphy, 2002). We know that the use of long-term steroids in women with lupus may compound osteopenia and that calcium supplementation with vitamin D needs to be included unless creatinine clearance or calcium excretion is impaired (Julkunen, Kaaja, & Friman, 1993). Further, women with physical disabilities are less likely to ambulate, participate in physical exercise, and are more likely to have a history of phlebitis. They enter menopause with fewer years of weight bearing and little or no participation in aerobic activity (Welner, 1996). Thus, they are at risk for obesity, cardiovascular deconditioning, and cardiovascular illnesses. Women with disabilities have a sevenfold increased risk of osteoporosis with some already diagnosed in their 30s, and as of yet we have no data or treatment to delay the onset in this population (Nosek et al., 1997).

Menopause can also bring decreased skin turgor and strength, loss of elasticity and decreased blood supply. This can put a woman with disability at increased risk for skin breakdown (Julkunen et al., 1993). It is also clear that menopause may occur earlier in women with Down syndrome and women with epilepsy (Brown & Murphy, 2002; Carr & Hollins, 1995). Women with Down syndrome may also experience sensory, adaptive, or cognitive losses earlier than other women (Brown & Murphy, 2002).

Women who may benefit from estrogen replacement have often been eliminated from consideration due to concerns over thrombotic events. The transdermal estrogen therapy, however, may be a safer option for many, especially if the thrombosis history is old (Stampfer, Colditz, Willett, et al., 1991). Nevertheless, with recent research findings related to hormone replacement therapy and stroke, MI, and deep vein thrombosis, management in collaboration with gynecologist, geriatrician, and physiatrist consultants is advised to optimize care for older women with disabilities. (see Chapter 15 for more information.)

Children or young women who survived polio may experience postpolio syndrome characterized by increased joint weakness and joint stiffness when they reach midlife (40 to 60 years of age). We need further research to know how the aging trajectory differs for people with disabilities since childhood or young adult. In addition, we know little about the impact of lifelong disability or chronic illness on menopause or about sexuality issues in those aging with disability (Pitzele, 1996). What we do know is the emotional vitality decreases a wide range of negative outcomes and substantial number of women with even the most severe disabilities can be described as vital (Penninx, Guralink, Bandem-Roche, et al., 2000).

PHARMACOLOGICAL AGENTS

A number of drugs may have a negative impact on sexual function. A full assessment of both prescription and over-the-counter drugs is critical when addressing issues of sexuality with women who have a disability (Zasler, 1991).

HISTORY

INSPECTION OF SELF

Examiners should look at their own attitudes and expectations to determine potential problems before eliciting a history from women with disabilities. Do not vary the history protocol to omit potential issues. If you usually ask about first sexual experiences, birth control, episodes of unwanted intercourse, or satisfaction with intimate relationships, also ask women with disabilities. In doing so, it is important to watch your "handicapism" terms and use inclusive and sensitive language (see Table 24–1).

SEXUAL EDUCATION HISTORY

The woman's knowledge of sexuality is pertinent. What was her family life while in school? Does she understand what implications her disability has for sexuality, contraception, birth control, and routine health needs? Ask if sexual information given either in adolescence or during rehabilitation was sufficient. From discussions with the client, determine knowledge deficits. In addition, identify unmet sexual and health needs. Include review of condition specific issues such as dysreflexia for women with spinal cord injury, latex allergy for women with spina bifida, or spasticity issues for women with cerebral palsy. Ask all women about any allergy-type reactions to latex products (balloons, rubber products, and condoms, for example).

PROBLEMS PRESENTED

Ask the client what problems the disability has presented and how she has overcome these barriers.

PHYSICAL EXAMINATION

PHYSICAL ACCESSIBILITY OF CLINIC

Physical Layout

In assessing the physical layout of a clinic, determine wheelchair accessibility, for example, ramp dimensions, bathrooms, and doorways. Using a wheelchair may be helpful in assessing the environment. Lack of accessibility promotes the dependence of clients (Nosek, 1992; Nosek et al., 1995; Welner et al., 1999)

The Americans With Disabilities Act, enacted in 1990, mandates that all new buildings meet minimal accessibility standards. Section 504 of the Persons With Disabilities Act of 1978 applies to all facilities receiving any federal funds. The regulations do not require that a facility have special programs or services. The regulations do, however, require that the same services offered to women without disabilities must be offered to women with disabilities (Federal Register, 1990). For example, if women without disabilities are weighed, accurate mechanisms are needed to weigh women with disabilities. Wheelchair-accessible scales can be used to weigh ambulating women as well. If the clinic offers Pap smears and pelvic examinations, it needs to offer women with disabilities the same services and to make necessary accommodations.

Accessible Supportive Examination Table

A table at wheelchair height facilitates transfer of women with motor disabilities. One such table (Welner, 1999) adjusts to wheelchair height to facilitate transfer to the table; it provides armrests to support women with cerebral palsy and spasticity who may fear falling off the table when severe or unexpected spasms occur. The absence of leg support, however, may be a major drawback for women with leg weakness or paralysis. Examination tables that have leg support but are not at wheelchair height may be preferred in some settings. Each setting needs to assess its target population for services and provide the most accessible examination table (Welner, Foley, Nosek, & Holmes, 1999).

Client's Equipment

The health care provider must realize that the wheelchair, crutches, and/or other equipment are part of the client's personal space. *Ask permission from the client before sitting or leaning on the equipment or moving it, particularly when the client is in it or on the examination table, where she may want her equipment close by.* The use of service animals needs the same sensitivity. *Do not approach, speak to, or pet these animals without their owners' permission.* Such activities only detract the animals from their jobs—caring for the person with a disability.

Special Equipment.

Equipment such as nonlatex gloves, plastic catheters, and nonlatex pads needs to be available.

PSYCHOLOGICAL ACCESSIBILITY

It has been suggested that the client may find it more difficult to gain psychological accessibility to the health care provider than physical accessibility to the clinic. Providers must limit stereotypes, actively pursue optimal communication procedures, value mutual problem solving and goal setting, and use every opportunity to reaffirm normalcy. In a clinical setting, guidelines are needed to enhance accessibility, beginning with the first telephone contact. Proposed guidelines have been delineated by the Task Force on Concerns of Physically Disabled Women (1978). When the first appointment is made, clients should be asked the following:

- ◆ Do you have a physical disability? If so, ask the client to specify if it is difficult getting around, hearing, or seeing, and so on.
- ◆ What accommodations will be necessary for your visit to the clinic? Arrangements may need to be made that will allow for a longer visit.

Altered Pelvic Examination

Mutual Problem Solving. A health care provider must be aware that a client with disabilities may need an altered pelvic examination (Sawin, 1986). Discussion with the client should attempt to solve problems she might have had during previous pelvic exams. Ask what positions caused problems and what worked best for her. Additional personnel may be needed to assist in supporting the client (e.g., holding legs) during the exam. The client should collaborate in deciding the need. She may prefer to bring a family member or friend with her to the exam.

- ◆ *Altered Range of Motion.* A side-lying position or speculum exam with "handle up" may be necessary because of alterations in range of motion.
- ◆ *Spasticity.* Women with cerebral palsy report spasms, especially adductor spasms, which may be controlled if the woman takes the knee-chest position, with an assistant "hugging" her or the side-lying position, with the bottom leg flexed and upper leg on the examiner's shoulder (similar to left lateral delivery position) (Carty, Tali, & Hall, 1990). Keeping the woman's extremities close to the body decreases movement that may stimulate additional spasms.
- ◆ *Amputation and Decreased Range of Motion.* The client may be examined in a semisitting position. She may choose to hold the stump herself and place the other leg on the examiner's shoulder or she may choose to have assistance with holding her stump so she can hold a mirror and participate in the examination.
- ◆ *Specific Examination.* Examination of the genitalia must include inspection of the vaginal walls for atrophic changes, determination of intravaginal tone, and assessment of hair distribution in the genital region to help rule out possible endocrinopathies (Zasler, 1991). Some examiners find a handle-up technique helpful for women with limited range of motion. This handle-up technique may also make viewing a midposition or anteverted cervix easier.

In patients who have a history of autonomic dysreflexia, spasticity, or pain on insertion of the speculum, xylocaine gel applied generously to the perineal area can make the exam more effective and comfortable if the gel will not interfere with any specimens needed. All movements in the examination should be gradual to allow patient accommodation.

Some authors suggest select use of the Q-Tip Pap smear for the rare woman with disabilities who is unable to tolerate a speculum examination. This technique is much less accurate, however, and every effort should be made to assist the client and her family to understand the implications of its use (Ware, Muram, & Gale, 1992).

Reaffirming Normalcy. During the pelvic examination, reaffirm the client's identified normalcy and healthy status. This makes a strong positive impact on her perception of self.

BREAST SELF-EXAMINATION

In some rehabilitation and primary care settings, breast self-examination is not discussed with women with disabilities, even when they present for gynecologic examinations. Clinical breast exam is especially important for older women with arthritis or neuropathies (Rodin, 2000). Women with intact manual dexterity and sensation, however, can be taught breast self-examination. Moreover, some women with impaired sensation can perform a modified examination, or an attendant or partner can perform it. If neither of these plans is acceptable, more frequent examination by a health care provider should be considered (Sawin, 1986).

CONTRACEPTION

LACK OF INFORMATION

Information on contraception is often not offered to women with disabilities (Meeropol, 1991; Nosek et al., 1996; Pope & Tarlov, 1991). It is important, however, for health care providers to examine the options with clients. The choice may be a balance of risk factors, (Pope & Tarlov, 1991), for example, the risk of pregnancy versus the risk of the contraceptive method. If oral contraception or an intrauterine device (IUD) is considered and the method carries risk, consultation with or referral to a gynecologic specialist needs to be initiated.

Discussion of alternatives needs to take place with the woman who is allergic or whose partner is allergic to latex. Contraceptive options may be significantly restricted for women with mobility impairment or with a latex allergy. Joint management with a physician colleague is indicated.

ADOLESCENTS

To prove that they are normal, adolescents with chronic illness or disability often increase their sexual behavior. Consequently, they are at increased risk of pregnancy, sexually transmitted diseases, and abuse. Primary care of all adolescent women with chronic illness and disability must include assessment of the potential for sexual activity or actual sexual activity and the need for contraception.

Blum, Kelly, and Ireland (2001) identify myths related to sexuality and disability in adolescents:

1. Young people with disabilities are not sexually active.
2. The social and sexual aspirations of adolescents with disabilities and chronic conditions are different from those of peers.
3. Parents of teenagers with disabilities provide sufficient sex education.
4. Young people with chronic conditions are not sexually vulnerable.
5. Problems of sexual expression are a function of the chronic condition or disability.

Sawin, Buran, Brei, and Fastenau (2002) concur, finding that adolescents with spina bifida had low family/peer access to spina bifida and specific sexuality information. They also reported low romantic appeal and only moderate knowledge of sexuality, including fertility.

TIMING OF DISABILITY

It is not clear what impact the timing of disability onset has on a woman's satisfaction with contraception and sexuality information. Women whose onset of disability is after menarche are identified by some as having special needs for contraception and sexuality (Harrison et al., 1995). Other data suggest that women who grow up with their disability do not have adequate sexuality and contraception counseling (Sawin, 1986). The need for sexuality and contraception counseling must be assessed regardless of the time of onset.

BARRIER METHODS

Barrier methods are often an optimal choice. If a client has manual limitations and, consequently, difficulty manipulating a barrier device, it is important to determine the availability of a partner or personal care attendant and their roles. A client may need to explore ways to ask her partner to assist with a barrier method. Many women have not considered asking a personal care attendant to assist with placement of a contraceptive device before sexual activity.

♦ *Condoms.* Condoms, which also provide protection against AIDS and other sexually transmitted diseases, are an option. Water-soluble lubricants can ease vaginal dryness. Caution should be taken to identify women who have, or whose partners have, latex allergies. A nonlatex condom (Avante) is now available. Testing is still underway to determine effectiveness against STDs and HIV, and FDA approval is pending for these purposes. Another nonlatex condom (Tactylon) is currently under development and being tested with release expected in the near future.

◆ *Cervical Cap.* For some women, a cervical cap is attractive, as it can be inserted in the morning by a personal care attendant and removed 24 hours later, eliminating the need for assistance during lovemaking (Sawin, 1986).

◆ *Diaphragm.* An increase in urinary infections is associated with the arch diaphragm. It may present particular problems and not be appropriate for women with urinary stasis. Caution should be taken to identify women who have, or whose partners have, latex allergies.

IMPLANTED AND INJECTED HORMONAL CONTRACEPTIVES

Norplant may be an option for some women if memory or manual dexterity is an issue. The presence of erratic bleeding, however, may be problematic for these women (Welner, 1993). Depo-Provera widely used in other countries. This contraceptive has been prescribed for women, including adolescents, with cognitive impairment; 5,105 woman-months of experience were reported without pregnancy or side effects (Neinstein & Katz, 1986).

Parents of youth with cognitive impairment reported high satisfaction with this method. The World Health Organization (WHO) has found no evidence that Depo-Provera is harmful (Hatcher et al., 1998). For teens with moderate or severe retardation, the benefits probably outweigh the risks.

An additional benefit of injected hormones is derived by women with severe mobility restrictions. If these women are dependent on others for menstrual hygiene care, the possible lack or decreased frequency of menstrual periods may increase their functional status (Welner, 1993). Depo-Provera can be associated with decreased circulating estradiol and thus may cause vaginal dryness. More serious is the hypothetical concern about the effect of decreased estradiol on bone mass (Pitzele, 1996).

Women with disability who are active in the political arena warn that we do not have enough data on either of these methods to be clear about their long-term impact for women with disabilities and recommend cautious use until more data are available (Nosek, 1992).

SEXUALLY TRANSMITTED DISEASES

Little is written about how women with disabilities/chronic illness experience STDs. If sensation is impaired, however, women may have special issues with STDs. For example, if women with disabilities have HSV, they may have limited ability to promptly respond to a prodome if it is tingling or itching in the affected area. Inability to identify developing "painful" lesions may have severe consequences to these women. These women will need to learn to identify and monitor more subtle cues. Many of these women may be in the habit of frequent visual skin inspection but may need to include genital area in this visual check (Welner, 1993).

SPECIFIC CONDITIONS AND CONTRACEPTIVE NEEDS

Although research is limited, the data that are available for the most frequent disabilities and chronic illnesses are reported here and may be presented in discussions with clients. Because women with disabilities are considered high risk medically, joint management with a physician colleague or referral for a form of contraception other than a barrier method is recommended.

Spinal Cord Injury

The fertility of women with spinal cord injury is unaffected. Their decreased mobility and the increased incidence of deep vein thrombosis place them at high risk with respect to hormonal contraceptives, especially those containing estrogen. Birth control pills and Norplant are absolutely contraindicated if the woman is receiving antihypertensive medication or if she is known to have circulatory problems (Boston Women's Health Book Collective, 1992).

Many women have healthy pregnancies and vaginal births. Some complications (urinary tract infections, immobility, skin breakdown) do occur, but in studies that have been conducted, the incidence is low (Dangoor & Florian, 1994; U. S. General Accounting Office, 1993).

Intrauterine devices pose a risk because of the woman's decreased sensation and ability to determine warning signs of infection. Some women, however, indicate that dysreflexia is triggered by the "pain" that the patient is unable to perceive. The women may thus be able to "identify" infection with the occurrence of dysreflexia. In addition, they propose that checking the IUD string placement could be carried out by their partners. In a large follow-up study of women with spinal cord injury, the IUD was actually the preferred method (Charlifue et al., 1992).

Most women with paraplegia can usually manage barrier methods with no or minimal assistance in positioning legs for effective insertion. Women with higher spinal cord lesions require assistance from a partner or an attendant.

Multiple Sclerosis

The menstrual and fertility patterns of women with multiple sclerosis rarely change (Boston Women's Health Book Collective, 1992). Oral contraceptive use has no effect on the risk of developing multiple sclerosis. Smoking, however, may be a risk factor (Cook, Troiano, Bansil, & Dowling, 1994; Swain, 1996).

The risk of pregnancy is not totally clear. Data are conflicting. Some studies show no effect on multiple sclerosis; others indicate exacerbation of the condition during pregnancy and postpartum (Hatcher et al., 1998). A series of recent studies indicate pregnancy does not influence long-term prognosis (Cook et al., 1994; Stenager, Stenager, & Jensen, 1994; Villard-Makintosh & Vessey, 1993). In fact, Verdu, in a study of 200 women with multiple sclerosis, found women who had one pregnancy after onset of multiple sclerosis were dependent on a wheelchair after 18.6 years versus 12.5 for other women without pregnancy (Verdru, Pol, D'Hooghe, & Carton, 1994). Cook et al. found the pregnancy year may be a higher risk, but it did not have a negative impact on the long-term rate of problems. There was an exacerbation of multiple sclerosis symptoms, however, in 20 to 40 percent of patients in the first three months postpartum (Cook et al., 1994).

At present, there is significant evidence that hormonal therapy alters the course of multiple sclerosis (Neinstein & Katz, 1986). Such therapy is contraindicated only for women with paralysis or restricted mobility. Of concern is one study that reported 54 percent of subjects used no contraception because of fear of side effects (Task Force on Concerns of Physically Disabled Women, 1978).

Cystic Fibrosis

Women with cystic fibrosis now live until their 30s, and with increasing technology, the age of survival may increase even further in the next few years. Pregnancy can be a significant risk for both mother and infant.

Data on hormonal contraception are conflicting. The method may cause bronchial mucus to become scant, and it may support the development of endocervical polyps (Neinstein & Katz, 1986). Pulmonary function and respiratory symptoms were not affected in a small study of 10 young women 15 to 24 years old. Nevertheless, hormonal contraception should be used only with extreme caution and very close monitoring of pulmonary status. There is no contraindication to the use of barrier methods among women with cystic fibrosis (Neinstein & Katz, 1986a & b).

Rheumatoid Arthritis

Rheumatoid arthritis is known to improve during pregnancy. Recently lactation and prolactin have been studied as predictors of onset, flare, or relapse of arthritis (Hampl & Papa, 2001). Some evidence is reported that the onset of arthritis may be delayed by hormonal contraceptives (Hatcher et al., 1994). Hormonal therapy, however, has not been shown to affect active disease.

Barrier methods may be difficult for some women to use if they experience weakness and decreased manual dexterity (Neinstein & Katz, 1986). An intrauterine device may worsen existing anemia. Among some women who may be genetically susceptible, breastfeeding is associated with an increased risk of rheumatoid arthritis, particularly after the first pregnancy (Hampl & Papa, 2001). The use of oral contraceptive pills (OCPs) seems to have a protective effect on disease progression, while having several children appears to predict a more severe disease progression in women with rheumatoid arthritis (Hatcher et al., 1998; Jorgensen, Picot, Bologna, & Sany, 1996).

Cerebral Palsy

The effect of cerebral palsy on contraception varies greatly. If the client is paralyzed or has decreased mobility, hormonal contraception is risky. Independent use of barrier methods, especially the diaphragm or cervical cap, may be troublesome for women with spasticity; however, these methods are viable with partner participation.

Epilepsy

Estrogen levels are related to seizure threshold in WWE. Seizures vary during the menstrual cycle: Incidence is highest during the estradiol spike before ovulation and the rapid drop in progesterone immediately before and during menstruation.

The relationship between oral hormonal therapy and seizures is less evident; however, no strong evidence has been found against the use of hormonal contraception (Hatcher et al., 1998; Neinstein & Katz, 1986a & b). Most reports of interaction between hormonal agents and seizure medication indicate accelerated breakdown of estrogens and recommend the use of 50 mg estrogen (Altman, 1996; Hatzichristou, 1996; Hatcher et al., 1998), and the risk of contraceptive failure should be discussed and documented (AAN, 1998). Breakthrough bleeding is a common sign that the anti-epileptic drug is lowering the effect of the BCP and a signal that a higher dose pill needs to be considered. No studies were found that supported the use of either levonorgestral implants or medroxyprogesterone in WWE (AAN, 1998). Levonorgestral is a progestin-only formulation, its efficacy is reduced, and it is contraindicated (AAN, 1998, Brodie & French, 2000). IM medroxyprogesterone has higher doses of progestin but has not been evaluated for effectiveness in WWE (AAN, 1998). Counseling for the potential of tetraogenic effects secondary to AEDs, seizure changes during pregnancies, and close follow-up during pregnancies are critical for WWE (AAN, 1998).

The WHO does not recommend restricting the use of copper-bearing intrauterine devices because of epilepsy (Hatcher et al., 1998); however, infection potentially caused by an IUD may decrease medication control.

Inflammatory Bowel Disease

Data are limited on the relationship between inflammatory bowel disease and use of contraception. It is known, however, that the majority of women with inflammatory bowel disease worsen with pregnancy (Neinstein & Katz, 1986). It is, therefore, important that the disease be stable for a year before pregnancy is even considered.

Barrier methods are recommended for contraception. A review of the literature indicates that the use of oral hormonal contraceptives is advised only with reservations; that is, low-dose estrogen or progestin-only oral contraceptives may be taken with close monitoring of the disease by the consulting physician. With active disease or in the presence of malabsorption, hormonal therapy may be ineffective or dangerous (Neinstein & Katz, 1986).

Down Syndrome

Fertility is unaffected. For many women with Down syndrome, the choice of contraception is affected by mobility, chronic illness, and cognitive factors. In the use of contraception, informed consent is a critical aspect.

- Oral hormonal contraception requires that a woman's memory skills be adequate for the regimen.
- Implants may be attractive to some.
- Women who have multiple disabilities (motor and cognitive) may not be able to manage a diaphragm.
- Adolescents and young women need comprehensive ongoing sex education and accessible adults to assist with problem solving and skill development.

Women with Sickle Cell Disease

Contraception for women with sickle cell disease is important for two reasons: (1) Women with this condition can get pregnant and (2) their pregnancies are high risk and need careful planning. All barrier methods, most low dose pills, Norplant and Depo-Provera are options to consider for women with this condition. An IUD is contraindicated because of its association with infections and the complications of infections in women with sickle cell condition (Earles, Lessing, & Vichinsky, 1994).

Women with this condition need to consider genetic counseling before pregnancy is attempted. The transmission risk may be as high as 100 percent or as low as 0 percent. All children of women with sickle cell disease will have the sickle cell trait (Earles et al., 1994).

Women with Lupus

Oral contraceptives increase risk of hypertension, thrombosis, and disease exacerbation. Barrier method in combination with spermicide is safest. Permanent sterilization may be an option chosen by some women.

PREGNANCY

CONFRONTING NEGATIVE ATTITUDES AND BARRIERS

Disability is not a contraindication to responsible, effective parenting, yet judgmental attitudes continue (Carty et al., 1990; Earles et al., 1994; Wasser, Killoran, & Bansen, 1993). Moreover, few agencies exist to assist the increasing number of pregnant women and mothers with disabilities. The majority (81 percent) of registered nurses, nurse practitioners, and occupational and physical therapists indicate that their experience, education, and training have not prepared them adequately for this high risk population (Carty et al., 1990). Resources for perinatal educators need to provide specific information on pregnancy in disability (Rogers, 1993).

Education of Health Care Providers

Programs must be developed to address health care providers' lack of information about the needs of mothers with disabilities. (Sawin & Metzger, 2002). Parents report insufficient and inadequate information in prenatal education (Blackford, Richardson, & Grieve, 2000). Furthermore, many adolescents get their sexuality education from professionals and even then report deficits in specific information (Sawin et al., 2002). Information that is modified to answer questions about the unique situation of women with disabilities is needed. What are the emotional and physical changes of pregnancy? What are the special demands of labor and delivery? What are the adaptive parenting skills and equipment necessary for responsible parenting?

Consumer Guidance

Little information is provided to parents by professionals. One study found that women with rheumatoid arthritis depended on lay resources rather than on health professionals for guidance in nutrition; use of alcohol, tobacco, and nonprescription drugs; sexuality; consequences of a pregnancy on their disability or disease; and infant care techniques, equipment, and devices (Carty et al., 1990). Health care providers who are involved in coordinating care and have no disability-related experience must consult with others. For example, consideration should be given to speaking with a colleague in rehabilitation or an experienced, active consumer with disabilities. A qualitative study (Lipson & Rogers, 2000) concluded that women's experiences were influenced by their own perspectives and the characteristics of the health care system when they were receiving care.

Case Management

During pregnancy, case management may be indicated for a woman with disabilities. The case manager is responsible for assuring that the client's unique health care needs are being met, especially if numerous agencies are involved.

Partner Preparation

It is important for the health care provider to assess whether a woman's partner needs preparation. The partner may require information from the provider about the woman's special needs in order to give realistic support and avoid unnecessary restrictions. A typical concern of any couple experiencing pregnancy—hesitancy to have sexual relations for fear of hurting the baby—may be expanded for couples in which the woman has a disability; they may be afraid of hurting the woman (Carty et al., 1990).

Although it is especially important for health care providers to interact with partners, data indicate that women with disabilities feel their partners are unwanted by health care providers during labor and delivery (Craig, 1990; Wasser et al., 1993). A prenatal care provider or case manager may need to initiate educational sessions to discuss attitudinal barriers. These activities should be organized well before delivery. If the partner also has a disability, special considerations may be needed to facilitate his involvement.

ACCESSIBILITY TO LABOR AND DELIVERY FACILITIES

Several questions should be asked about the structure of health care facilities and their accessibility to women with mobility and sensory impairment. Are labor and delivery rooms and bathrooms large enough to transfer women from a wheelchair? Are large showers available without a raised lip, which would prevent a woman from rolling her wheelchair into the shower? Are select rooms large enough to accommodate wheelchairs, consumer-owned specially padded commode chairs, leg braces, crutches, and other equipment? Can a woman in a wheelchair be weighed in prenatal, labor, and delivery settings (Nosek et al., 1997)?

Specific Adaptive Needs of Client

Determine what the client needs with respect to her condition. Is a pressure relief mattress or raised toilet seat needed? Does she want to bring equipment from home? Plan a tour of the hospital during the fifth or sixth month of pregnancy so that the need for special equipment can be identified and the equipment ordered.

Accessibility to Equipment

Having necessary equipment within reach is critical to the well-being and comfort of the client (Carty et al., 1990).

Education for All Staff

Housekeeping personnel may need to know that a wheelchair positioned in a particular way next to a bed allows a woman to be independent. To move the chair makes the woman essentially a prisoner, as it removes her independence. Nursing staff may need to review prevention of skin shearing, management of dysreflexia, and implications of contraction monitoring.

PRENATAL AND PERINATAL PERIODS

The effects of a disability on the course of pregnancy are summarized in Table 24–3. Generally, in perinatal management, a health care provider needs to determine if a woman with a disability has access to a role model who has the same disability as she or if the client needs case management services.

Self-Assessment

The client should be able to identify the stressors and fears, both general and specific, that are related to her disability.

Staff Assessment

A woman's muscle strength, activities of daily living, and child care skills must be assessed. Determinations may be made by direct observation, reports of activities, and a child care activity assessment tool (Connie, 1988; Kirshbaum, 1988). Or, referral may be made to a physical or occupational therapist, depending on resources and the severity of the woman's limitations. Assessment needs to be made early in pregnancy in order to design adaptive equipment. For example, one woman with minimal distal muscle strength who wished to breastfeed was able to place the child at the breast and initiate nursing but did not have the strength to hold the child throughout nursing. Believing that she could not breastfeed, she switched to formula. If she had been assessed early in pregnancy, her strength deficiency might have been identified and referral made to a rehabilitation engineer to design or modify a fabric infant carrier that would support the child during nursing. Most women with a disability are able to nurse their newborns. Indeed, the convenience of breastfeeding can be an advantage for women with mobility limitations (Asreal, 1987).

Dependency Increase

If a woman's dependency increases during pregnancy, there is a need to assess her specific level of function. Similarly, assess the body image issues generated by pregnancy.

Normal Emotional Changes

Reassure the client of the normalcy of emotional fluctuations during pregnancy.

Cesarean Birth

If cesarean birth is a possibility, discuss the options available, including father participation (Kirshbaum, 1988).

Breastfeeding

This normal and healthy method in infant feeding is preferred by an increasing number of women with disability and chronic illness despite being discouraged by many health care providers. Breastfeeding is generally not contraindicated for women with spinal cord injury, multiple sclerosis, arthritis or epilepsy (Callanan & Stalland, 1996; Charlifue et al., 1992; Cook et al., 1994; Santilli, 1996) but is contraindicated for women with sickle cell disease (Earles et al., 1994). Women with lupus taking immunosuppressive medications should not breastfeed (Buchanan et al., 1992). Women with lupus not on these medications need to have close monitoring of their child's growth while breastfeeding (Sala, 1993). Some women may need adaptive equipment or counseling about specific strategies to make breastfeeding successful (Thomson, 1995).

PARENTING

Health care providers unfamiliar with the adaptive skills of women with disabilities often question the ability of these women to care for their babies (Kirshbaum, 1996; Reinelt & Fried, 1993). In fact, there are over 8 million families with children in which one or both parents has a disability (Farber, 2000; O'Toole & D'aoust, 2000). Many social institutions, however, such as family court, social services, and health care providers continue to have discriminary attitudes. Availability of a role model with a disability similar to the woman's can be very helpful to both the health care provider and the client. The roles of the parents and other caregivers must be assessed. Moreover, for the provider without expertise in infant care issues, consultation with a pediatric nurse practitioner, pediatrician, occupational therapist, rehabilitation consultant, or rehabilitation engineer may be helpful. In addition, an independent living center or a program that focuses on promoting positive parenting for women with disabilities, such as Through the Looking Glass, may be consulted (Kirshbaum, 1988).

ADAPTATION OF THE FAMILY

Videotaped Evidence

A videotape study of parents with disabilities was conducted and several findings were reported (Kirshbaum, 1988).

TABLE 24–3. Effect of Disability on Course of Pregnancy and Labor/Delivery/Postpartum

Disability/Condition	Pregnancy	Labor/Delivery/Postpartum
Spinal Cord Injury	May increase risk for skin problems. Women with SCI have the same problems as nondisabled women (UTIs, constipation, incontinence). (Crosby, St-Jean, Reid, & Elliot, 1992; Cross, Meythaler, Tuel, & Cross, 1992; Sauer & Harvey, 1993). Data is scarce. Recent evidence indicates frequency of these problems is increased in women with SCI (Crosby et al., 1992; Sauer & Harvey, 1993). Some women do report having to change their regular urinary management during pregnancy (Jackson, 1996; Nosek et al., 1997). Anemia, cardiac irregularity and toxemia may occur (Charlifue et al., 1992). Management of anemia with iron may increase constipation. Consider this possibility proactively and take action to prevent it (Yarkony & Chen, 1995). Assess women's ability to catherize and perform self-care as pregnancy progresses. May need temporary assistance (Sauer & Harvey, 1993). It is not clear if patients with asymptomatic bacteriuria are at high enough risk of pyelonephritis to warrant antibiotic suppression or whether suppressive therapy would be more effective than frequent cultures. To decrease the risk of bacteriuria, SCI women should minimize residual volume and avoid continuous bladder catheterization (Cross et al., 1992). Nausea/vomiting can be especially uncomfortable with limited mobility (Charlifue et al., 1992). Women who are wheelchair users may already experience orthostatic edema that may be accentuated increasing not only edema but also risk of skin problems. Frequency of weight shifts/position changes may need to increase. Need close monitoring of skin daily (Sauer & Harvey, 1993). Autonomic dysreflexia increased (Sauer & Harvey, 1993; Sipski et al., 1995b; Yarkony & Chen, 1995). Eighty-five percent of clients with SCI at T=6 or above will experience autonomic dysreflexia at some time (Sauer & Harvey, 1993). Medication may be needed to control. Weekly exam after 28 weeks and antepartum anesthesia consultation for epidural block to prevent dysreflexia (Crosby et al., 1992; Sauer & Harvey, 1993). Psychosocial issues common in pregnancy similar to psychosocial issues generally experienced in pregnancy. Report feelings of powerlessness (Carty et al., 1990).	No premature deliveries, infant outcomes were near normal weight, no major complications (Charlifue et al., 1992; Cross et al., 1991, 1992) although relatively high rates of autonomic dysreflexia (32%) and preeclampsia (35%) have been reported (Nosek et al., 1997). Vaginal delivery the norm. Cesarean birth reserved for obstetrical indications. Lochial flow and sanitary pads put skin at risk. Frequent perinatal care necessary (Corbin, 1987). Silk sutures should be considered for women having episiotomies. Reabsorbable sutures should not be used for episiotomy since denervated regions do not absorb catgut suture (Cross et al., 1991). Bladder/bowel, skin circulatory problems improve in postpartum (Sauer & Harvey, 1993). If environment not accessible, may need extra assistance in transferring (Sauer & Harvey, 1993). Labor/birth in semi-sitting position (Charlifue et al., 1992; Craig, 1990). Women with high lesions may need help in positioning. Autonomic dysreflexia increased in second stage labor (Yarkony & Chen, 1995). Early identification and treatment essential for maternal/fetal health. Can lead to subarachnoid hemorrhage (Cross et al., 1992). Aggressive labor management is critical. Epidural anesthesia often effective (Crosby et al., 1992; Yarkony & Chen, 1995). If does not respond to regional, potent short-acting hypotensive appropriate (Cross et al., 1992). Blood pressure monitoring frequently is not continuously. Take BP during contraction. Critical to avoid known causes. Often misinterpreted as preeclampsia. Unlike toxemia, the BP increases with contractions and falls between contractions (Cross et al., 1991, 1992; Yarkony & Chen, 1995). Treatment is different. Mothers with dysreflexia have no response to magnesium sulfate (Yarkony & Chen, 1995). Can be triggered by catheterization, enema, insertion of uterine catheter if fetal monitor used, contractions or insertion of IV lines (Cross et al., 1992). May also occur if woman sits on episiotomy or during breastfeeding. Need to assess carefully for rebound hypotension in postpartum period (Sauer & Harvey, 1993). Assess labor/delivery bed/table for skin risks. Pad delivery tables. Stirrups not recommended if woman has spasticity (Cross et al., 1991). Respiratory rate less than 12 or greater than 16 indicates abnormal bleeding patterns and needs further evaluation. Pulse oximetry in labor and administration of supplemental oxygen may be necessary. Women with high lesions or above may be at risk for respiratory insufficiency (Sauer & Harvey, 1993). At risk for unattended labor (Sauer & Harvey, 1993), although 66 percent are aware of onset of labor (Charlifue et al., 1992). Report being victims of inadequate environmental design that hindered mobility (Wasser et al., 1993). Increased powerlessness if partner blocked from participation in labor and delivery (Carty et al., 1990). Breastfeeding is possible. Women with high lesions and above may need special assistance with positioning and feeding. Women with SCI above T=6 may experience decreased milk production six weeks after delivery (Charlifue et al., 1992; Cross et al., 1991; Westgren, Hultling, Levi, & Westgren, 1993). Early mobilization is recommended to prevent DVT (Yarkony & Chen, 1995).

TABLE 24–3. (*cont.*)

Disability/Condition	Pregnancy	Labor/Delivery/Postpartum
Rheumatoid Arthritis	Seventy-five percent will experience remission of disease. ADL easier to perform due to decreased joint stiffness, swelling, increase in grip strength (Neinstein & Katz, 1986). May have overwhelming fatigue. Need to continue supervised exercise routine. For those with hand/shoulder involvement, dressing may become difficult (Crotty et al., 1994; Dale, 1996).	Joint contracture may limit positioning. Pain needs to be carefully assessed. Ninety-five percent will experience flare up to symptoms (Dale, 1996; Crotty et al., 1994). No increased risk for complications, low birthweight or birth defects (Mueller, Zhang & Critchlow, 2002).
Multiple Sclerosis	Pregnancy and postpregnancy stress may increase symptoms but do not influence long-term prognosis (Cook et al., 1994; Villard-Makintosh & Vessey, 1993).	Risk for exacerbation of symptoms may be greater in the postpartum. Twenty to 40 percent of patients may have exacerbations in first three months postpartum (Cook et al., 1994). Women who have been on long-term corticosteroids at the time of delivery may have relative adrenal insufficiency and should be given supplemental corticosteroid for 24 hours (Cook et al., 1994; Confavreaux et al., 1998). Some experts believe women who have been on interferon beta should resume it soon after birth (Whitaker, 1998). No contradiction to breastfeeding unless drugs are toxic to the baby. Limb weakness or gait disturbances may necessitate assistance with child care (Cook et al., 1994).
Impaired Vision	Changing body may dramatically affect ability to function (center of gravity changes may alter her relation to object). Use tactile models. Assist to palpate abdomen. Lack of material in braille or on audiotape necessitates increased individual teaching. Birth rehearsal in labor room helps orient self to room, bed, bathroom.	Needs lots of labeling of people/equipment. Introduce self and identify function. Get women's input on amount of light needed in labor/delivery areas. Important to describe baby and his/her specific reactions/behaviors/facial expressions. Will assist mom to attach. May use tactile calibrated bottle (Carty et al., 1990).
Impaired Hearing	Talk to woman even if interpreter used eye to eye contact; get attention before proceeding.	Visual interaction critical. Assess light needed. Assess if needs to be in room where nurses station can be seen (Federal Register, 1990).
Systemic Lupus	Lupus the great imitator so diagnosis difficult. Placenta impairment can be a direct result of disease inflammatory process or the thrombotic effects of lupus. Exacerbations of SLE first trimester or first 6 weeks postpartum. Drug therapy is individualistic and somewhat controversial. May experience fewer relapses during pregnanacy (Cortinovis-Tourniaire, & Moreau, 1998). Most women can achieve successful pregnancy. Fetal (fetal loss, preterm birth) and maternal (lupus flares, worsening renal function) morbidity remain major problems. Needs frequent monitoring, frequent assessment and control of maternal lupus activity. May need to adjust medication to avoid fetal tetratogenicity. Assess for interuterine problems (MacMullen & Dulski, 1996). Corticosteroid treatment is continued for many women without negative effect on the fetus. Needs close collaboration among specialists (internist, rheumatologist, obstetrican and neonatologist (Tincani, Faden, Tarantini, et al., 1992). Careful management and close monitoring have substantially improved fetal outcomes. A series of studies suggest adding doppler flow assessment of placental perfusion after the fourteenth week of pregnancy and treatment with heparin for women with antiphosphlipid syndrome and previous history of thrombotic event. Pregnancy loss was significantly reduced (Derkesen, 1991).	There is increased risk of spontaneous abortion and premature birth in women with SLE. Premature births occur most often with the lupus flares (Sala, 1993). Intrapartum major goal to prevent infections—meticulous hand washing, limiting the number of vaginal exams and paying strict attention to sterile technique for any invasive procedure. Potential renal involvement requires frequent BP monitoring (screen at least hourly—more if any abnormal findings), hourly urinary protein, abnormal DTRs and clonus, and women's affect to assess for superimposed preeclampsia (Derkesen, 1991). At risk for postpartum exacerbation. Intensive nursing care for 24 to 48 hours. Infant care complicated by fatigue (Derkesen, 1991). Newborns need to be assessed for neonatal lupus and congenital cardiac problems (Zurier et al., 1987). Cesarean birth is needed only for obstetrical issues. Mothers who are being treated by immunosuppressive drugs should not breastfeed (Buchanan et al., 1992). If breastfeed follow infant growth closely (Sala, 1993).
Sickle Cell	While a women with this condition can have a healthy baby, there are risks, thus preconceptual and prenatal care are critical (Smith, Espeland, Bellevue, et al., 1996). Women may have to discontinue some medications and consider treatment options. Emotional support as well as aggressive treatment of acute events optimizes outcomes (Helman, 1990; Koshy, 1995).	Women with this condition have a higher rate of preterm deliveries, preeclampsia, pain crisis and pulmonary complications and SGA babies (Seoud, Cantwell, Nobles, & Levy, 1994). Neonates have more jaundice, anemia, and respiratory distress (Brown, Sleeper, Pegelow, et al., 1994; Koshy, 1995; Larrabee & Cowan, 1995). Newborn screening should be standard in all settings (Sickle Cell Disease Guideline Panel, 1993). Emotional support as well as aggressive treatment of acute events optimize outcomes (Koshy, 1995).

Epilepsy

Although many women with epilepsy have been pressured to terminate a pregnancy because of the provider's or family's assumption that they could not have a healthy baby, over 90 percent of women with epilepsy will have normal healthy infants. (Foy, Penney, & Greer, 2000). However, women with suboptimal health care have been reported to have more birth defects, including craniofacial abnormalities and neural tube deficits (Fairgrieve, Jackson, Jonas, et al., 2000). Prenatal folic acid, monotherapy, and close monitoring are essential (Rochester & Kirchner, 1997).

In over half of women studied, seizure frequency does not change during pregnancy. When the frequency did change, roughly half of the women had increases in frequency and half had decreases. If seizures increased, they occurred most often in the end of the first trimester and the beginning of the second. Women taking valproate (depakote, depakene) or carbamazepine (Tegretol) during the first trimester have a 0.5 to 2 percent risk of having a child with neural tube disease. The drugs most likely to cause severe congenital problems, Trimethadione (Tridione) and paramethadione (paradione), are rarely prescribed today (Callanan & Stalland, 1996).

It is recommended that women with epilepsy see their neurologist monthly during pregnancy (Yarby & Lannon, 1992).

The following recommendations were proposed as practice options by the AAN Guidelines:

- Non-protein-bound AED levels should be monitored during pregnancy. For the stable patient, levels should be ascertained before contraception, at the beginning of each trimester, and in the last month of pregnancy. Additional levels should be drawn with increased seizures, side effects or suspected nonadherence.
- AED levels should be monitored through the eighth postpartum week. Decrease in AEDs may often be necessary if the drug had to be increased during pregnancy and may be critical to avoid toxicity.
- Vitamin K, 10 mg per day, should be prescribed in the last month of pregnancy if WWE is taking enzyme-inducing AEDs.
- Pregnant WWE should be encouraged to participate in the pregnancy registries (See EFA in resources) with enzyme-inducing AEDs such as carbamazepine (Tegretol).

Women with seizures have a 2 to 3 percent higher rate of birth defects with cleft lip, cleft palate, heart defects, and spina bifida. All AEDs appear to increase the risk. There is an increased risk of seizures in the immediate postlabor and delivery phase. There is a slight chance of increased infant bleeding in the neonatal period.

If parental vitamin K was not given prenatally, it should be administered as soon as possible after the onset of labor. This should not change the ACOG/AAP recommendations for 1 mg vitamin K for the neonate (AAN, 1998).

Mothers taking AEDs can breastfeed. It may be helpful to have the father give a nighttime bottle as fatigue is related to increased seizure activity. Growth and sedation of the infant needs to be closely monitored and a 2-week checkup is critical (AAN, 1998; Callanan & Stalland, 1996).

Diabetes (see Chapter 21 on medical problems)

Preconception control is critical in women with diabetes. High maternal glucose levels are related to spontaneous abortions and major malformations of newborns. Unfortunately, two-thirds of pregnancies in this population are unplanned. All women of childbearing age should be carefully counseled, take folic acid at all times, and pursue effective contraception (American Diabetes Association, 2002).

♦ Infants adapt extremely early to their mothers who have physical disabilities.

♦ Mothers develop the ability to read their infants' states and teach them to assist with necessary movement.

♦ Children differentiate between care providers. For example, an active toddler lies still during a long diapering by the blind father but resists and struggles from the outset with the sighted mother.

Equipment as Part of the Environment

It is common for children to consider a parent's equipment, such as wheelchairs and reachers, as ordinary parts of their environment without negative connotations. A toddler was overheard talking with her mom during a basketball tournament in which there was a wheelchair division. While observing a game played by nondisabled college students, she said, "Mom, what are they doing?" "Playing basketball, Honey." "But Mom, where are their wheelchairs?" Frequently, support services in both the health and social service arena are uninformed about resources that would make parenting and caretaking more effective for women with disabilities. Consultation with agencies that are knowledgeable in this area is critical to success.

Animals

If a woman with a disability uses a guide dog or other animal to assist with impaired mobility, close assessment must be made of its impact on child care (Modlin, 2000).

Equipment Adaptation for Child Care

A woman with impaired mobility can alter equipment or procedures to assist with child care (Carty et al., 1990).

♦ Women with mobility impairment may face special adaptation needs as parents (Carty et al., 1990). Women who previously used a manual wheelchair may choose to use an electric wheelchair to free hands for child care.

♦ Furniture may need to be altered so that the woman can wheel up to the crib, changing table, or reclined stroller and be able to change the baby without moving her or him. Furniture may also be altered to create firm raised edges for infant safety and to assist the woman with decreased hand or arm strength.

♦ Velcro can be sewn on the clothes of both mother and baby for necessary alterations. For example, breastfeeding may be made easier if the mother's bra and blouse have Velcro fasteners. Also, Velcro fasteners on the infant's clothes assist the mother in dressing her baby (Earles et al., 1994).

♦ Bottle holders and bottle devices, such as a tactile calibrated bottle, may be helpful, as may adapting a breastfeeding position in the wheelchair (Carty et al., 1990).

Impaired Vision and Hearing

A woman with impaired vision or hearing can also adapt procedures for child care (Carty et al., 1990). The provider may need to facilitate the mother's interaction with her infant. The Brazelton tool is used to teach a mother about the states of the infant (Brazelton, 1973). For a woman with impaired vision, the focus is on her hearing and touching and how they increase interaction with the infant. On the other hand, for women with hearing impairment, a visual role model, tactile stimulation, and musical toys are used. If both parents have sensory impairment, referral to an infant stimulation program should be considered.

Monitoring devices in a room or on a child can be helpful. Audiovisual resources may be useful.

Epilepsy

Infant care is often more of a concern of the family and friends than of the woman with epilepsy. The health professional needs to evaluate the real risks with the woman based on the type of seizure she experiences. Women with seizures at night may not need to adjust their daytime activities dramatically. Developing a reality-based concrete safety plan is recommended (Shafer et al., 1996). Women can change the baby on a mat on the floor, use plastic bottles and containers, have two adults when giving an infant or child a bath, always feed the child in an infant seat, highchair, or appropriate chair, use a playpen for a safe play area, keep extra clothes on each level of the house to avoid stair climbing, use disposable diapers, move the child by stroller instead of being hand carried, and use microwave rather than conventional stove (Stalland & Shafer, 1996).

FUTURE RESEARCH NEEDED

Several major official and voluntary organizations now have initiatives to explore the experiences of women with disabilities. This work, however, is early in its development. The research agenda developed by the National Center for Medical Rehabilitation Research, which called for "urgent and immediate need for development of an appropriate model of rehabilitation that addresses woman's unique role physically and also addresses the needs within the structure of her own environment," is still a timely call to action (Gordon, 1996). The current work raises as many questions as it answers. Researchers call for major initiatives in the significant area affecting the lives of people with disabilities. They identify the major focus areas as childhood, sexuality, contraception, sexually transmitted diseases, fertility, marriage, pregnancy, labor and delivery, parenting, decision to become a parent, parenting abilities, and influences of parent with disability on children (Graves, 1993; Gray & Schimmel, 1993). The near future, it is hoped, will bring answers to many of the questions currently being raised.

SUMMARY

Women with disabilities are women first. Their similarities with other women are more common than their differences. One woman writes the following:

> We want to know that you value us as people and not just as examples of cultural diversity. We want you to know that life with a disability can be just fine. Sure, there are attitudinal and environmental barriers that make life difficult for us sometimes, but those obstacles are out there, not inside of us. Just imagine for a moment a woman in a wheelchair carrying a tiny baby. This woman is not being discharged from a maternity hospital where every woman must ride in a wheelchair. She is at the grocery store with her baby in an infant carrier and a cart full of groceries. Imagine her getting herself, her baby, her wheelchair, and her groceries into the car alone and driving away. Imagine her independent, sexual, competent, mature, busy, happy, and, like all new parents, exhausted! To you she may be an amazement, but to me, I just feel like myself (Craig, 1990).

If approached with

- a willingness to listen and hear the issues and concerns of these women
- a willingness to see the woman as a true participant/partner in planning and one who may have more medical information about her disability than the provider does

- an awareness of one's own comfort level with uncertainty and individuals with disability
- a nonjudgmental approach

the sensitive clinician can create a quality experience for the individual and build a new reality for women with disabilities and chronic illnesses.

RESOURCES FOR WOMEN, THEIR FAMILIES, AND PROFESSIONALS

INTERNET RESOURCES/ ORGANIZATIONS

Multiple Internet resources have been developed, and one study found that using web sites aimed at women with disabilities was effective in increasing knowledge (Pendergrass, Nosek, & Holcomb, 2001).

Antiepileptic Drug and Pregnancy Register (888-233-2334): www.efa.org/services/wei/registry.html

Coalition on Sexuality and Disability (212-242-3900)

CROWD, The Center for Research on Women with Disabilities (Fact Sheet, Research Summary and Bibliography): www.bem.tmc.edu/crowd

Easter Seals: www.easter-seals.org

Epilepsy Foundation: Information packet for women with disabilities (800-332-1000), Antiepileptic Drug Pregnancy Registry (888-233-2334). www.efa.org

Guidelines for management of pregnancy in women with epilepsy: www.show.scot.nhs.uk/sign/sogap.1.htm

Multiple Sclerosis Foundation: www.msfacts.org

National Clearinghouse on Women and Girls with Disabilities: www.edequity.org/welcome.html

National Information Center for Children with Youth and Disabilities (800-999-5599): www.nichy.org

National Organization on Disability (NOD) (800-248-2253): www.nod.org

National Women's Health Information Center, Women with Disablities. (NICHY) information and referral services (800-695-0285): www.4women.gov/wwd

Parents with Disabilities Online! www.disabledparents.net

Siecus: Multiple annotated bibliographies on sexuality issues including disability. www.seicus.org

Spina Bifida Association of America (800-621-3141): www.sbaa.org

Through the Looking Glass: Information for parents with disabilities. www.lookingglass.org.

UCP (United Cerebral Palsy): www.ucpa.org

There are national groups for most chronic illness or disability conditions. Contact your local library for current addresses or toll free numbers.

GENERAL

Krotoski, D., Nosek, M. A., & Turk, M. A. (Eds.). (1996). *Women with physical disabilities.* Baltimore: Paul H. Brookes Publishing Co.

PHYSICAL ACCESSIBILITY OF HEALTH CARE SETTING

Mace, R. L. (1998). *Removing barriers to health care: A guide for health care providers.* Booklet from the North Carolina Office on Disability and Health. University of North Carolina at Chapel Hill, Campus Box 89185, Chapel Hill, NC 27599. (919) 966-0868. $3.00/copy.

PARENTING AND INFANT CARE

Campion, M.J. (1990). *The baby challenge: A handbook on pregnancy for women with a physical disability.* New York: Tavistock/Routledge.

Cheatham, D., King, E., Bartz, A. (1995) *Childbirth education for women with disabilities and their partners: A training manual for professionals.* Columbus, OH: Nisonger Center Publications.

Conine, T.A., Carty, E., & Safarik, P. (1988). *Aids and adaptations for disabled parents: An illustrated manual for service providers and parents with physical or sensory disabilities* (2nd ed.). Vancouver: School of Rehabilitation Medicine, University of British Columbia.

Disability, Pregnancy and Parenthood International (1996, April) *Learning to adapt.* London: Arrowhead Publications [On-line]. Available: http://www.healthworks.co.uk/dacess/D-Acess_digf/dpp.html

Family challenges: Parenting with a disability. 25-minute video that explores family relationships when a parent has a disability, for children, teens, and adults. Aquarious Health Care Videos. 888-440-2963. email:aqvideo@tiac.net

Rogers, J., Matsumura, M. (1991) *Mothers to be: A guide to pregnancy and birth for women with disabilities.* New York: Demos Publication.

ABUSE

Blackburn, M. (1995). Sexuality, disability, and abuse: Advise for life . . . not just for kids. *Child Care, Health and Development, 2*(1), 1–7.

SEXUALITY AND WOMEN'S HEALTH EDUCATION

American Academy of Pediatrics (AAP). (1996). Sexuality education of children and adolescents with developmental disabilities. Policy Statement (RE9303). *Pediatrics, 97*(3), 275–278.

Breast Health Access for Women with Disabilities—San Francisco area, but serves as good model. http://www.cancerlynx.com/breast_health.html

Kroll, K., & Klein, E.L. (1992). *Enabling romance: A guide to love, sex, and relationships for the disabled (and the people who care about them).* New York: Harmony Books.

Managing menustration for children with spina bifida and family planning for teenagers with spina bifida. Appendix to Furman, L. & Mortimer, J. C. (1994). Menarche and menstrual function in patients with myelomeningocele. *Developmental Medicine and Child Neurology, 36,* 910–917.

Smith, K., Wheeler, B., Pilecki, P., & Parker, T. (1995). The role of the pediatric nurse practitioner in educating teens with mental retardation about sex. *Journal of Pediatric Health Care, 9*(2), 59–66.

Whitaker, V., & LaVerne, A. (1993). A breast self-examination program for adolescent special education students. *Family & Community Health, 16*(2), 30–40.

Whole issues for 1993 of the journal *Sexuality and Disability* dedicated to sexual counseling for people with disabilities (includes a SIECUS annotated bibliography).

FOR TEENS AND THEIR FAMILIES

Kaufman, M. (1995). *Easy for you to say. Questions and answers for teens living with chronic illness or disability.* Toronto: Key Porter Books, Ltd. A frank and explicit question and answer book addressing issues teens with disabilities or chronic illness and their families face. Includes sections on overprotectiveness, sexuality, coping with medical personnel, work, school, and peers.

Kriegsman, K.H., Zaslow, E.L., & D'Zmura-Rechsteiner, M.A. (1992). *Taking charge: Teenagers talk about life and physical disability.* Bethesda, MD: Woodbine House. Available from the American Spina Bifida Association. Much acclaimed primer for older school-age and teenage patients.

Ochs, V. (1995). *Protecting your child in an unpredictable world.* New York: Penguin Books.

Lollar, D.J. (Ed.). (1994). *Preventing secondary conditions associated with spina bifida or cerebral palsy.* Washington, DC: Spina Bifida Association of America (800-621-3141)

NEWSLETTERS (AVAILABLE WITHOUT CHARGE AND OF INTEREST TO PROVIDERS AND FAMILIES)

Resourceful Woman, a free newsletter distributed via print, e-mail, or audiotape provides current information and in-depth analysis of issues relevant to women with disabilities. From the Rehabilitation Institute of Chicago. Contact the Development Office at (312) 238-6013.

COLLEGE INFORMATION

Albrecht, A. (1996, September). School daze: What I wish I had known before I started college. *Exceptional Parent,* 64–67.

Back to School. (1996, May/June) *Sports 'N Spokes,* 11–17. An article listing financial assistance available to students with disabilities at colleges or universities across the country. Also describes characteristics of a school that may be of interest to young women with disabilities (disabled student services, wheelchair sports, attendant care).

How to choose a college: Guide for the student with a disability. One free copy is available from HEATH Resource Center, One Dupont Circle, Suite 800, Washington DC 20036. 1-800-544-3284. (HEATH is a newsletter addressing postsecondary education for persons with disabilities).

POPULAR PRESS ARTICLES

Mairs, N. (1996, March). Young and disabled: What it's like to seek friendship and love, work and happiness if you are young and disabled. *Glamour, 94,* 196–199.

Perry-Sheridan, N. (1995, October). I was told not to have children. *Parents, 70,* 121–122+.

EQUIPMENT/LATEX-FREE PRODUCTS

Patented wheelchair accessible Powermate™ exam table, models #4450, 4453, Hausmann Industries, Inc. 103 Union Street, Northvale, N.L. 07647. Tel: 201-767-0255. Fax: 201-767-1369. Toll Free 1-888-Hausman. Information on accessible GYN exam table: www.hausmann.com

Avanti brand polyurethane condom (Schmid Laboratories). Has had limited testing that supports the prevention of pregnancies and STDs. A 1995 *Consumer Reports* article questioned how much protection is offered. To date the FDA has not allowed the manufacturer to make any effectiveness claims.

Reality Female Condom (The Female Health Company). Made of polyurethane. Laboratory testing showed that Reality was an effective barrier to HIV and also to a virus particle that is smaller than the hepatitis B virus, the smallest virus known to cause an STD. May be covered by Medicaid. Call to check in your state (1-800-643-0844): www/femalehealth.com

Latex Allergy List—a very useful list: updated yearly. SBAA: www.sbaa.com

Latex Allergy: A video. Available from the Spina Bifida Association of America, 4590 MacArthur Blvd NW, Suite 250. Washington, DC 20007-4226. (12-minute video suitable for professional and lay audiences) For an extensive list of products updated every six months contact: Spina Bifida Association of America: www.infohiway.com/spinabifida/

Sawin, K., & Fisher, D. (1998) Latex allergy: Pearls for practice in the primary care setting. *Journal of the American Academy of Nurse Practitioners, 10*(5), 203–208.

REFERENCES

Alston, R. J., Bell, T. L., & Feist-Price, S. (1996). Racial identity and African Americans with disabilities: Theoretical and practical considerations. *The Journal of Rehabilitation, 62*(2), 11–16.

Alston, R. J., & McCowan, C. J. (1994). African American women with disabilities: Rehabilitation issues and concerns. *Journal of Rehabilitation, 60,* 36–40.

Altman, B. M. (1996). Causes, risks and consequences of disability among women. In D. M. Krotoski, M. A. Nosek, & M. A. Turk (Eds.), *Women with physical disabilities.* Baltimore, Paul H. Brookes Publishing Co.

American Academy of Neurology (AAN). (1998). Practice parameter: Management issues for women with epilepsy. *Neurology, 51,* 944–948.

American Diabetes Association. (2002). Preconception care of women with diabetes. (Position Statement). *Diabetes Care, 25*(1), S82–85.

Anderson, E. M., & Brownson, R. C. (2000). Disability and health status: Ethnic differences among women in the United States. *Journal of Epidemiology and Community Health, 54*(3), 200–206.

Anderson, J. M. (1991). Immigrant women speak of chronic illness: The social construction of the devalued self. *Journal of Advanced Nursing, 16*(6), 710–717.

Asreal, W. (1987). The rehabilitation team's role during the childbearing years for disabled women. *Sexuality and Disability, 8,* 47–62.

Ashton-Shaeffer, C., Gibson, H. J., Autry, C. E., & Hanson, C. S. (2001). Meaning of sport to adults with physical disabilities: A disability sport camp experience. *Sociology of Sport Journal, 18*(1), 95–114.

Banta, J. V., Bonanni, C., & Prebluda, J. (1993). Latex anaphylaxis during spinal surgery in children with myelomeningocele. *Developmental Medicine and Child Neurology, 35*(6), 543–548.

Barton, E. C. (1993). Latex allergy: Recognition and management of a modern problem. *Nurse Practitioner, 18*(11), 54–85.

Bauer, A. M. (2001). "Tell them we're girls": The invisibility of girls with disabilities. In P. O'Reilly & E. M. Penn, (Eds.). *Educating young adolescent girls* (pp. 29–45). Mahwah, NJ: Lawrence Erlbaum Associates.

Becker, H., Stuifbergergen, A., & Tinkle, M. (1997). Reproductive health care experiences of women with physical disabilities: A qualitative study. *Archives of Physical Medicine and Rehabilitation, 78*(5), 26–33.

Berhard, E. J. (1989). The sexuality of spinal cord injured women: Physiology and pathophysiology. A review. *Paraplegia, 27* (2), 99–112.

Blackburn, M. (1995). Sexuality, disability and abuse: Advice for life . . . not just for kids. *Child Care, Health and Development, 21*(5), 351–361.

Blackford, K. A., Richardson H., & Grieve S. (2000). Prenatal education for mothers with disabilities. *Journal of Advanced Nursing, 32*(4), 898–904.

Blackwell-Stratton, M., Breslin, M. L., Mayerson, A. B., & Bailey, S. (1988). Smashing icons: Disabled women and the disability women's movements. In M. Eine & A. Asch (Eds.), *Women with disabilities: Essays in psychology, culture, and politics* (pp. 306–332). Philadelphia: Temple University Press.

Blinde, E. M., & McCallister, S. G. (1999). Women, disability, and sport and physical fitness activity: The intersection of gender and disability dynamics. *Research Quarterly for Exercise and Sport, 70*(3), 303.

Blum, R. W., Kelly, A., & Ireland, M. (2001). Health-risk behaviors and protective factors among adolescents with mobility impairments and learning and emotional disabilities. *Journal of Adolescent Health, 28*(6), 481–490.

Bogle, J. E., & Shaul, S. L. (1981). Body image and the woman with a disability. In D. G. Bullard & S. E. Knight (Eds.), *Sexuality and physical disability.* St. Louis: C. V. Mosby.

Boone, T. (1995). The physiology of sexual function in normal individuals. *Physical Medicine and Rehabilitation: State of the Art Reviews, 9*(2), 313–323.

Boston Women's Health Book Collective. (1992). *The new our bodies, ourselves.* New York: Simon & Schuster.

Brazelton, T. B. (1973). *Neonatal behavioral assessment scale.* Philadelphia: J. B. Lippincott.

Brodie, M. J., & French, J. A. (2000). Management of epilepsy in adolescents and adults. *Lancet, 356,* 323–329

Brown, A. A., & Murphy, L. (2002). *Aging and developmental disabilities: Women's health issues.* Available [online] http://thearc.org/faqs/whealth.html.

Brown, A. K., Sleeper, L. A., Pegelow, C. H., Miller, S. T., Gill, F. M., & Waclawiw, M. A. (1994). The influence of infant and maternal sickle cell disease on birth outcome and neonatal course. *Archives of Pediatric and Adolescent Medicine, 148*(11), 1156–1162.

Brown, C. N. (1996). Pregnancy and women with lupus: Answering questions and dispelling myths. Unpublished paper. Virginia Commonwealth University.

Brown, S., & Williams, A. (1995). Women's experience of rheumatoid arthritis. *Journal of Advanced Nursing, 21,* 695–701.

Buchanan, N. M., Khamashta, M. A., Morton, K. E., Kerslake, S., Baguley, E. A., & Hughes, G. R. (1992). A study of 100 high risk lupus pregnancies. *American Journal of Reproductive Immunology, 28,* 192–194.

Callanan, M., & Stalland, N. (1996). Issues for women with epilepsy. In N. Santilli (Ed.), *Managing seizure disorders.* Landover, MD: Lippincott-Ravin Publishers.

Carr, J., & Hollins, S. (1995). Menopause in women with learning disabilities. *Journal of Intellectual Disabilities Research, 39,* 137–139.

Carty, E. M., Tali, C. A., & Hall, L. H. (1990). Comprehensive health promotion for the pregnant woman who has disabilities. *Journal of Nurse-Midwifery, 35*(3), 133–190.

Case, A. M., & Reid, R. L. (1998). Effects of the menstrual cycle on medical disorders. *Archives of Internal Medicine, 158*(13), 1405–1413.

Charlifue, S. W., Gerhart, K. A., Menter, R. R., Whiteneck, G. G., & Manley, M. (1992). Sexual issues of women with spinal cord injury. *Paraplegia, 30,* 192–199.

Coffman, C. B., Levine, S. B., Althof, S. E., & Stern, R. (1994). Sexual adaptation among single young adults with cystic fibrosis. *Chest, 86*(3), 412–418.

Cole, S. S. (1993). Facing the challenges of sexual abuse in persons with disabilities. In M. Nagler (Ed.), *Perspectives in disability* (2nd ed., pp. 273–282). Palo Alto, CA: Health Markets Research.

Confavreux, C., Hutchinson, M., Hours, M. M., Cortinovis-Tourniaire, P., & Moreau, T. (1998). Rate of pregnancy-related relapse in multiple sclerosis. *The New England Journal of Medicine, 339*(5), 285–292.

Connie, T. A. (1988). *Aids and adaptations for disabled parents: An illustrated manual for service providers and parents with physical or sensory disabilities* (2nd ed.). Vancouver: School of Rehabilitation Medicine, University of British Columbia.

Cook, S. D., Troiano, R., Bansil, S., & Dowling, P. C. (1994). Multiple sclerosis and pregnancy. *Advanced Neurology, 64,* 83–95.

Corbin, J. M. (1987). Women's perceptions and management of pregnancy complicated by chronic illness. *Health Care Women International, 8*(5–6), 317–337.

Coyle, C. P., Santiago, M. C., Shank, J. W., Ma, G. X., & Boyd, R. (2000). Secondary conditions and women with physical disabilities: A descriptive study. *Archives of Physical Medicine and Rehabilitation, 81*(10), 1380–1387.

Craig, D. I. (1990). The adaptation to pregnancy of spinal cord injured women. *Rehabilitation Nursing, 15*(1), 6–9.

Crigger, N. J. (1996). Testing an uncertainty model for women with multiple sclerosis. *Advanced Nursing Science, 18*(34), 37–47.

Crosby, E., St-Jean, B., Reid, D., & Elliot, R. (1992). Obstetrical anesthesia and analgesia in chronic spinal cord-injured women. *Canadian Journal of Anaesthia, 39,* 487–494.

Cross, L. L., Meythaler, J. D., Tuel, S. M., & Cross, A. L. (1991). Pregnancy following SCI. *Western Journal of Medicine, 154*(5), 607–611.

Cross, L. L., Meythaler, J. D., Tuel, S. M., & Cross, A. L. (1992). Pregnancy, labor and delivery post spinal cord injury. *Paraplegia, 30,* 890–902.

Crotty, M., McFarlane, A., Brooks, P. M., Hopper, J. L., Bieri, D., & Taylor, S. L. (1994). The psychosocial and clinical status of younger women with early rheumatoid arthritis: A longitudinal study with frequent measures. *British Journal of Rheumatology, 33,* 754–760.

Curry, M. A., Hassouneh-Phillips, D., & Johnston-Silverberg, A. (2001). Abuse of women with disabilities: An ecological model and review. *Violence Against Women, 7*(1), 60–79.

Dajani, K. F. (2001). What's in a name? Terms used to refer to people with disabilities. *Disability Studies Quarterly, 21*(3), 196–209.

Dale, G. D. (1996). Intimacy and rheumatic disease. *Rehabilitation Nursing, 231,* 38–40.

Dangoor, N., & Florian, V. (1994). Women with chronic physical disabilities: Correlates of their long-term psychosocial adaptation. *International Journal of Rehabilitation Research, 17,* 159–168.

DePauw, K. P. (1996). Adapted physical activity and sport. In D. M. Krotoski, M. A. Nosek, & M. A. Turk (Eds.), *Women with physical disabilities.* Baltimore, Paul H. Brookes.

Derkesen, R. H. (1991). Systemic lupus erythematosus and pregnancy. *Rheumatology International, 11*(3), 121–125.

Dodson, W. E. (1996). Issues in the comprehensive management of epilepsy in children and young adults. In N. Santilli (Ed.), *Managing seizures disorders.* Landover, MD: Lippincott-Raven Publishers.

Donohue, J., & Gebhard, P. (1995). The Kinsey Institute/Indiana University report on sexuality in spinal cord injury. *Sexuality and Disability, 13*(1), 7–85.

Drench, M. E. (1992). Impact of altered sexuality and sexual function in spinal cord injury: A review. *Sexuality and Disability, 10,* 3–14.

Drew, J. (1990). *Implications for nursing practice: A five-year review of recent spinal injury research.* Paper presented at 16th Annual Conference, Association of Rehabilitation Nursing, Phoenix, AZ.

Earles, A., Lessing, S., & Vichinsky, E. (Eds.). (1994). *A parents' handbook for sickle cell disease, Part II.* Sacramento: State of California Department of Health Services, Genetic Disease Branch.

Edenborough, F. P. (2001). Women with cystic fibrosis and their potential for reproduction. *Thorax, 56*(8), 649.

Eliason, M. J. (1996). Lesbian and gay family issues. *Journal of Family Nursing, 2*(1), 10–29.

Elvik, S. L., Berkowitz, C. D., Nichols, E. L., & Inkelis, S. H. (1990). Sexual abuse in the developmentally disabled: Dilemmas of diagnosis. *Child Abuse Neglect, 14*(4), 497–502.

Enforcement of nondiscrimination on the basis of the handicap in federally assisted programs. (1990). *Federal Register, 55*(244), 52136.

Enzlin, P., Mathieu, C., Van Den Bruel, A., Bosteels, J., Vanderschueren, D., & Demyttenaere, K. (2002). Sexual dysfunction in women with type I diabetes. *Diabetes Care, 25,* 672–677.

Evenhuis, H., Henderson, C. M., Beange, H., Lennox, N., & Chicoine, B. (2001). Healthy aging—Adults with intellectual disabilities: Physical health issues. *Journal of Applied Research in Intellectual Disabilities, 14*(3), 175–194.

Fairgrieve, S. D., Jackson, M., Jonas, P., Walshaw, D., White, K., Montgomery, T. L., Burn, J., & Lynch, S. A. (2000). Population based, prospective study of the care of women with epilepsy in pregnancy. *British Medical Journal, 321*(7262), 674.

Farber, R. S. (2000). Mothers with disabilities: In their own voice. *American Journal of Occupational Therapy, 54*(3), 260–268.

Fisher, D., & Sawin, K. (1998). Latex allergy: Pearls for practice in the primary care setting. *Journal of the American Academy of Nurse Practitioners, 10*(5), 203–208.

Foy, R., Penney, G., & Greer, I. (2000) Scottish group is developing guideline for managing pregnant women with epilepsy (statistical data included) (Letter to the Editor). *British Medical Journal, 320*(7242), 1146.

Furman, L. M. (1989). Institutionalized disabled adolescents: Gynecologic care. *Clinical Pediatrics, 28,* 163–170.

Gill, C. J. (1996). Becoming visible: Personal health experiences of women with disabilities. In D. M. Krotoski, M. A. Nosek, & M. A. Turk (Eds.), *Women with physical disabilities.* Baltimore, Paul H. Brookes.

Gill, C. J., & Brown, A. A. (2000). Overview of health issues of older women with intellectual disabilities. *Physical and Occupational Therapy in Geriatrics, 18*(1), 23–36.

Gilson, S. F., Cramer, E. P., & DePoy, E. (2001). Redefining abuse of women with disabilities: A paradox of limitation and expansion. *Affilia-Journal of Women and Social Work, 16*(2), 220–235.

Gleeson, R. M. (1995). Use of non-latex gloves for children with latex allergies. *Journal of Pediatric Nursing, 10*(1), 65–66.

Gordon, D. (1996). Foreword to D. M. Krotoski, M. A. Nosek, & M. A. Turk (Eds.), *Women with physical disabilities.* Baltimore: Paul H. Brooks.

Gordon, D. L., Sawin, K. J., & Basta, S. M. (1996). Developing research priorities for rehabilitation nursing. *Rehabilitation Nursing Research, 5*(2), 60–66.

Gordon, P. A., Feldman, D., & Crose, R. (1998). The meaning of disability: How women with chronic illness view their experiences. *The Journal of Rehabilitation, 64*(3), 5–7.

Graves, W. H. (1993). Future directions in research and training in reproduction issues or persons with physical disabilities. In F. P. Haseltine, S. S. Cole, & D. B. Gray (Eds.), *Reproductive issues for persons with physical disability.* Baltimore: Paul H. Brooks.

Gray, D., & Schimmel, A. B. (1993). Future directions for research on reproductive issues for people with physical disabilities. In F. P. Haseltine, S. S. Cole, & D. B. Gray (Eds.), *Reproductive issues for persons with physical disability.* Baltimore: Paul H. Brooks, Publishing Co.

Groce, N. E. (1999). Disability in cross-cultural perspective: Rethinking disability. *Lancet, 354*(9180), 756–757.

Guest, G. V. (2000). Sex education: A source for promoting character development in young people with physical disabilities. *Sexuality and Disability, 18*(2), 137–142.

Hahn, H., & Beaulaurier, R. L. (2001). Attitudes toward disabilities: A research note on activists with disabilities. *Journal of Disability Policy Studies, 12*(1), 40–46.

Hampl, J. S., & Papa, D. J. (2001). Breastfeeding-related onset, flare, and relapse of rheumatoid arthritis. *Nutrition Reviews, 59*(8), 264.

Harrison, C. A., Glass, R. G., & Soni, B. (1995). Factors associated with sexual functioning in women following spinal cord injury. *Internal Medical Society of Paraplegia, 33,* 687–692.

Hassouneh-Phillips, D., & Curry, M. A. (2002). Abuse of women with disabilities: State of the science. *Rehabilitation Counseling Bulletin, 45*(2), 96–104.

Hatcher, R. A., Trussel, J., Stewart, F. Stewart, G. K., Kowal, D., Guest, F., & Cates, W. (1994). *Contraceptive technology* (16th rev. ed.). New York: Irvington.

Hatcher, R. A., Trussel, J., Stewart, F. Stewart, G. K., Kowal, D., Guest, F., & Cates, W. (1998). *Contraceptive technology* (17th rev. ed.). New York: Irvington.

Hatzichristou, D. G. (1996). Preface to the special issue: Management of voiding, bowel and sexual dysfunction in multiple sclerosis: Towards a holistic approach. *Sexuality and Disability, 14*(1), 3–7.

Helman, N. S. (1990). Sickle cell disease and pregnancy. *NAACOGS' Clinical Issue Perinatal Women's Health Nursing, 1*(2), 194–201.

Henderson, K. A., & Bedini, L. A. (1995). I have a soul that dances like Tina Turner, but my body can't: Physical activity and women with mobility impairments. *Research Quarterly on Exercise and Sport, 66,* 151–161.

Howland, C., & Rintala, D. H. (2001). Dating behaviors of women with physical disabilities. *Sexuality & Disability, 19*(1), 41–70.

Iezzoni, L. I., McCarthy, E. P., Davis, R. B., & Siebens, H. (2002). Mobility impairments and use of screening and preventive services. *American Journal of Public Health, 90*(6), 955–961.

Ingraham, C. L., Vernon, V., Clemente, B., & Olney, L. (2000). Sex Education for Deaf-Blind Youths and Adults. *The Journal of Visual Impairment and Blindness. 94* (12), 756–764.

Jackson, A. B. (1996). Pregnancy and delivery. *Sexuality and Disability, 14*(3), 211–219.

Jordan, B., & Dunlap, G. (2001) Construction of adulthood and disability. *Mental Retardation, 39*(4), 286–296.

Jorgensen, C., Picot, M. C., Bologna, C., & Sany, J. (1996). Oral contraception, parity, breast feeding, and severity of rheumatoid arthritis. *Annals of the Rheumatic Diseases, 55*(2), 94–99.

Julkunen, H. A., Kaaja, R., & Friman, C. (1993). Contraceptive practice in women with systemic lupus erythematosus. *British Journal of Rheumatology, 32,* 227–230.

Kettl, P., Zarefoss, S., Jacoby, K., German, C., Hulse, C., Rowley, F., Corey, R. Sredy, M., Bixler, E., & Tyson, K. (1991). Female sexuality after spinal cord injury. *Sexuality and Disability, 9,* 287–295.

Kirshbaum, M. (1988). Parents with physical disabilities and their babies. *Zero to Three, 8*(5), 7–11.

Kirshbaum, M. (1996). Mothers with physical disabilities. In D. M. Krotoski, M. A. Nosek, & M. A. Turk (Eds.), *Women with physical disabilities.* Baltimore: Paul H. Brooke.

Kolodny, R. C. (1980). Sexual problems in diabetes and selected endocrine disorders. Paper presented at 1st Annual conference on sexuality and physical disabilities: Medical Aspects and Clinical Care, Ann Arbor, MI.

Koshy, M. (1995). Sickle cell disease and pregnancy. *Blood Rev, 9*(3), 157–164.

Krotoski, D., Nosek, M. A., & Turk, M. A. (1996). *Women with physical disabilities.* Baltimore: Paul H. Brookes.

Larrabee, K., & Cowan, M. (1995). Clinical nursing management of sickle cell disease and trait during pregnancy. *Journal of Perinatal Neonatal Nursing, 9*(2), 29–41.

Lehmann, J. B., Lehmann, C. U., & Kelly, P. J. (1998). Development and health care needs of lesbians. *Journal of Women's Health, 7*(3), 379–387.

Leu, M., Welker, M. J., & Haines, D. J. (1999). A perspective on lesbian health care for the primary care physician. *Family Practice Recertification, 21*(13), 89–92, 95–96, 99–100.

Liporace, J. D. (1997). Women's issues in epilepsy: Menses, childbearing, and more (includes related information). (Symposium: Second of Four Articles on Seizure Management.) *Postgraduate Medicine, 102*(1), 123–132.

Lipson, J. G., & Rogers, J. G. (2000). Pregnancy, birth, and disability: Women's health care experiences. *Health Care for Women International, 21*(1), 11–26.

Lundberg, P. O., & Hulter, B. (1996). Female sexual dysfunction in multiple sclerosis: A review. *Sexuality and Disability, 14*(1), 65–72.

MacMullen, N. J., & Dulski, L. A. (1996). Systemic lupus erythematosus what are the perinatal implications? *Mother Baby Journal, 1*(5), 7–10, 20–22.

Marshall, A. (1995). *Disability within the lesbian community.* Unpublished manuscript. Virginia Commonwealth University.

Mattson, D., Petrie, M., Srivastave, D., & McDermott, M. (1995). Multiple sclerosis, sexual dysfunction and its response to medications. *Archives of Neurology, 52,* 862–868.

McCabe, M. P., McDonald, E., Deeks, A. A., Vowels, L. M., & Cobain, M. J. (1996) The impact of multiple sclerosis on sexuality and relationships. *The Journal of Sex Research, 33*(3), 241–249.

McGill, T., & Vogtle, L. K. (2001). Driver's education for students with physical disabilities. *Exceptional Children, 67*(4), 455–466.

McNewil, J. M. (1993). *Current population reports, Americans with disabilities 1991–1992.* Washington, DC: U.S. Bureau of the Census.

Meeropol, E. (1991). One of the gang: Sexual development of adolescents with physical disabilities. *Journal of Pediatric Nursing, 6*(4), 243–249.

MMWR. (1991). Use of folic acid for prevention of spina bifida and other neural tube deficits, 1983–1991. *Morbidity and Mortality Weekly Report, 40*(30), 513–516.

MMWR. (1998). Use of cervical and breast cancer screening among women with and without functional limitations—United States, 1994–1995. *Morbidity and Mortality Weekly Report, 47*(40), 53–56.

Modlin, S. (2001). From puppy to service dog: Raising service dogs for the rehabilitation team. *Rehabilitation Nursing, 26*(1), 12–17.

Modlin, S. J. (2000). Service dogs as interventions: State of the science. *Rehabilitation Nursing, 25*(6), 212–219.

Mudrick, N. R. (1993). Predictors of disability among midlife men and women: Differences by severity of impairment. *Community Health, 13*(2), 70–84.

Mueller, B. A., Zhang, J., & Critchlow, C. W. (2002). Birth outcomes and need for hospitalization after delivery among women with multiple sclerosis. *American Journal of Obstetrics and Gynecology, 186*(3), 446–453.

Muir, E. H., & Ogden, J. (2001). Consultations involving people with congenital disabilities: Factors that help or hinder giving care. *Family Practice, 18*(4), 419–424.

Murphy, F. A. (1996). Commentary. *APNSCAN: Literature Review for the Advanced Practice Nurse, 12,* 3.

Murphy, K. P., Molnar, G., & Lankasky, K. (1995). Medical and functional status of adults with cerebral palsy. *Dev Med Child Neurol, 37*(12), 1075–1084.

National Institute of Occupational Safety and Health (NIOSH). (2002). *Preventing reactions to natural rubber latex in the workplace.* (NHHS Publication No. 97–135). Washington, DC: US Government Printing Office.

Neinstein, L. S., & Katz, B. (1986a). Contraceptive use in the chronically ill adolescent female: Part I. *Journal of Adolescent Health Care, 7,* 123–133.

Neinstein, L. S., & Katz, B. (1986b). Contraceptive use in the chronically ill adolescent female: Part II. *Journal of Adolescent Health Care, 7,* 350–360.

Nelson, M. R. (1995). Sexuality in childhood disability. *Physical Medicine and Rehabilitation: State of the Art Reviews, 9*(2), 451–462.

Nosek, M. (1992). Primary care issues for women with severe physical disabilities. *Journal of Women's Health, 1*(4), 245–248.

Nosek, M. A. (1993). Personal assistance: It's on the long-term health of a rehabilitation hospital population. *Archives of Physical Medicine and Rehabilitation, 74*(3), 127–133.

Nosek, M. A. (1995). Sexual abuse of women with physical disabilities. *Physical Medicine and Rehabilitation: State of the Art Reviews, 9*(2), 487–501.

Nosek, M. A., Howland, C. A., & Hughes, R. B. (2001). The investigation of abuse and women with disabilities: Going beyond assumptions. *Violence Against Women, 7*(4), 477–499.

Nosek, M. A., Howland, C., Rintala, D. H., Young, M. E., & Chanpong, G. F. (1997). *National study of women with physical disabilities: Final report.* Houston, TX: Center for Research on Women with Disabilities.

Nosek, M. A., Howland, C. A., Young, M. E., Georgiou, D., Rintala, D. H., Foley, C. C., Bennett, J. L., & Smith, Q. (1994). Wellness models and sexuality among women with physical disabilities. *Journal of Applied Rehabilitation Counseling, 25*(1), 50–58.

Nosek, M. A., Rintala, D., Young, M. E., Howland, C. A., Foley, C. C., Rossi, D., & Chanpong, G. (1996). Sexual functioning among women with physical disabilities. *Archives of Physical Medicine and Rehabilitation, 77,* 107–115.

Nosek, M. A., Young, M. E., Rintala, D. H., Howland, C. A., Foley, C. C., & Bennett, J. (1995). Barriers to reproductive health maintenance among women with physical disabilities. *Journal of Women's Health, 4,* 505–518.

O'Toole, C. J. (1996). Disabled lesbians: Challenging monocultural constructs. *Sexuality and Disability, 14*(3), 221–235.

O'Toole, C. J., & Bregante, J. L. (1993). Disabled lesbians: Multicultural realities. In M. Nagler (Ed.), *Perspectives on disability.* Palo Alto, CA: Health Markets Research.

O'Toole, C. J., & D'aoust, V. (2000). Fit for motherhood: Towards a recognition of multiplicity in disabled lesbian mothers. *Disability Studies Quarterly, 4*(2), 145–154.

Page, R. C., Cheng, H., Pate, T. C., Mathus, B., Pryor, D., & Ko, J. (1987). The perception of spinal cord injured persons toward sex. *Sexuality and Disability Journal, 8*(2), 112–132.

Pearson, M. L., Cole, J. S., & Jarvis, W. R. (1994). How common is latex allergy? A survey of children with myelodysplasia. *Developmental Medicine and Child Neurology, 36,* 64–69.

Pendergrass, S., Nosek, M. A., & Holcomb, J. D. (2001). Design and evaluation of an internet site to education women with disabilities on reproductive health. *Sexuality and Disability. 19*(1) 71–83.

Penninx, B. W. J., Guralnik, J. M., Bandeen-Roche, K., Kasper, J. D., Simonsick, E. M., Ferrucci, L., & Fried L. P. (2000). The protective effect of emotional vitality on adverse health outcomes in disabled older women. *Journal of the American Geriatrics Society, 48*(11), 1359–1366.

Pentland, W., Tremblay, M., Spring, K., & Rosenthal, C. (1999). Women with physical disabilities: Occupational impacts of aging. *Journal of Occupational Science (Australia), 6*(3), 111–123.

Persaud, D. (2000). Barriers to preventive health practices in women with spinal cord impairments. *SCI Nursing, 17*(4), 168–175.

Pitzele, S. K. (1996). Chronic illness, disability and sexuality in people older than fifty. *Sexuality and Disability, 139*(4), 309–311.

Place, K., & Hodge, S. R. (2001). Social inclusion of students with physical disabilities in general physical education: A behavioral analysis. *Adapted Physical Activity Quarterly, 18*(4), 389–404.

Pope, A. M., & Tarlov, A. R. (1991). *Disability in America: Summary and recommendations: Toward a national agenda for prevention.* Washington, DC: National Academy Press.

Powers, P. E., Curry, M. A., Oschwald, M., Maley, S., Saxton, M., & Eckels, K. (2002). Barriers and strategies in addressing abuse: A survey of disabled women's experiences (PAS Abuse Survey). *The Journal of Rehabilitation, 68*(1), 4–10.

Reinelt, C., & Fried, M. (1993). "I am this child's mother": A feminist perspective on mothering with a disability. In Nagler, M. (Ed.), *Perspectives on disability.* Palo Alto, CA: Health Markets Research.

Rimmer, J. H., Rubin, S. S., & Braddock, D. (2000). Barriers to exercise in African American women with physical disabilities. *Archives of Physical Medicine and Rehabilitation, 81*(2), 182–188.

Rochester, J. A., & Kirchner, J. T. (1997). Epilepsy in pregnancy (includes patient information). *American Family Physician, 56*(6), 1631–1638.

Rodin, M. B. (2000). Annual clinical breast exam especially important for older women with arthritis or neuropathies. Position Statement. *Journal of the American Geriatrics Society, 55*(9), 30.

Rogers, J. G. (1993). Perinatal education for women with physical disabilities. AWHONNS Clinical Issues. *Perinatal Womens Health Nursing, 4*(1), 141–147.

Roller, S. (1996). Health promotion for people with chronic neuromuscular disabilities. In D. M. Krotoski, M. A. Nosek, & M. A. Turk (Eds.), *Women with physical disabilities.* Baltimore: Paul H. Brookes.

Sala, D. J. (1993). Effects of systemic lupus erythematosus on pregnancy and the neonate. *Journal of Perinatal Nursing, 7*(3), 39–48.

Santilli, N. (1996). Selection and discontinuation of antiepileptic drugs. In N. Santilli (Ed.), *Managing seizure disorders.* Landover, MD: Lippincott-Raven Publishers.

Sauer, P. M., & Harvey, C. J. (1993). Spinal cord injury and pregnancy. *Journal of Perinatal and Neonatal Nursing, 7*(1), 22–24.

Sawin, K. J. (1982). *Disabled women's perception on a health care visit for a physical examination.* Paper presented at 8th annual conference, Association of Rehabilitation Nursing, Denver, CO.

Sawin, K. J. (1986). Physical disability. In J. Griffith-Kinney (Ed.), *Contemporary women's health.* Reading, MA: Addison-Wesley.

Sawin, K. J, Buran, C. F., Brei, T. J., & Fastenau, P. S. (2002). Sexuality issues in adolescents with chronic neurological condition. *The Journal of Perinatal Education, 11*(1), 22–34.

Sawin, K. J., & Metzger, S. G (2002). *Development of an "Access" curriculum for PCPs with emphasis on well women's care for women with disabilities.* Unpublished manuscript. Virginia Commonwealth University.

Saxton, M. (1996). Teaching providers to become our allies. In D. M. Krotoski, M. A. Nosek, & M. A. Turk (Eds.), *Women with physical disabilities.* Baltimore: Paul H. Brookes.

Schopp, L. H., Kirkpatrick, H. A., Hagglund, K. J., Meyer, T. M., & Meyer, L. (2001). Serving rural women with spinal cord injury: Training needs assessment of health professionals in rural settings. *SCI Psychosocial Process, 14*(3), 132–141.

Seoud, M. A., Cantwell, C., Nobles, G., & Levy, D. L. (1994). Outcome of pregnancies complicated by sickle cell and sickle-C hemoglobinopathies. *American Journal of Perinatology, 11*(3), 187–191.

Shaer, C., & Meeropol, E. (1995). *Latex (natural rubber) allergy in spina bifida patients.* Spina Bifida Insights. Included in the latex packet along with a list of latex containing products. Packet available from the Spina Bifida Association of America 1-800-621-3141.

Shafer, P. O. (1996). Women's issues: Momentum growing in search for answers. *Epilepsy USA, 6.*

Shafer, P. O., Austin, D. R., Callanan, M., & Clerico, C. M. (1996). Safety and activities of daily living for people with epilepsy. In N. Santilli (Ed.), *Managing seizures disorders.* Landover, MD: Lippincott-Raven Publishers.

Shaw, G. M., Velie, E. M., & Schaffer, D. (1996). Risk of neural tube defect-affected pregnancies among obese women. *Journal of the American Medical Association, 275*(14), 1093–1096.

Shepperdson, B. (1995). The control of sexuality in young people with Down's syndrome. *Child Care, Health and Development, 21*(5), 333–349.

Sickle Cell Disease Guideline Panel. (1993). *Sickle cell disease: Screening, diagnosis, management and counseling in newborns and infants. Clinical Practice Guideline No. 6* (AHCPR Pub No. 93–0562). Rockville, MD: Agency for Health Care Policy and Research, Public Health Service, U.S. Department of Health and Human Services.

Sipski, M. L., Alexander, C. J., & Rosen, R. C. (1995a). Orgasm in women with spinal cord injuries: A laboratory-based assessment. *Archives of Physical Medicine and Rehabilitation, 76,* 1097–1102.

Sipski, M. L., Alexander, C. J., & Rosen, R. C. (1995b). Physiological parameters associated with psychogenic sexual arousal in women with complete spinal cord injuries. *Archives of Physical Medicine and Rehabilitation, 76,* 811–818.

Slawta, J. N., McCubbin, J. A. Wilcox, A. R., Fox, S. D., Nalle, D. J., Anderson, G. (2002). Coronary heart disease risk between active and inactive women with multiple sclerosis. *Medicine and Science in Sports and Exercise, 34*(6), 905–912.

Smith, J. A., Espeland, M., Bellevue, R., Bonds, D., Brown, A. K., Koshy, M. (1996). Pregnancy in sickle cell disease: Experience of the cooperative study of sickle cell disease. *Obstetrics and Gynecology, 87*(2), 199–204.

Sockalosky, J. J., & Kriel, R. L. (1987). Precocious puberty after traumatic brain injury. *Journal of Pediatrics, 100,* 373.

Spina Bifida Association of America. (2001). Parents with Disabilities. *Insights into Spina Bifida, 8*(3), 1, 6–7.

Spinks, V. S., Andrews, J., & Boyle, J. S. (2000). Providing health care for lesbian clients. *Journal of Transcultural Nursing, 11*(2), 137–143.

Stalland, N., & Shafer, P. O. (1996). When the parent has epilepsy. In N. Santilli (Ed.), *Managing seizures disorders.* Landover, MD: Lippincott-Raven Publishers.

Stampfer, M. J., Colditz, G. A., Willett, W. C., et al. (1991). Postmenopausal estrogen therapy and cardiovascular disease. *New England Journal of Medicine, 325,* 756–762.

Stenager, E., Stenager, E. N., & Jensen, K. (1994). Effect of pregnancy on the prognosis for multiple sclerosis. A 5-year follow up investigation. *Acta Neurology Scandinavia, 90*(5), 305–308.

Stengel, P. J. (1996). *A train the trainer project on preconceptional counseling the role of folate in the prevention of neural tube defects.* Thesis. Virginia Commonwealth University.

Stevens, P. (1994). Lesbians' health-related experiences of care and noncare. *Western Journal of Nursing Research, 16*(6), 639–659.

Stewart, M. J., & Reutter, L. (2001). Fostering partnerships between peers and professionals. *Canadian Journal of Nursing Research, 33*(1), 97–116.

Stuifbergen, A. K. (1996). Health promotion services and research: Opportunities for rehabilitation nursing. *Rehabilitation Nursing Research, 5*(2), 34, 42.

Sulpizi, L. K. (1996). Issues in sexuality and gynecologic care of women with developmental disabilities. *Journal of Obstetrics and Gynecology Neonatal Nursing, 7,* 609–614.

Sussman, G. L., & Beezhold, D. H. (1995). Allergy to latex rubber. *Annals of Internal Medicine, 122*(1), 43–46.

Swain, S. E., (1996). Multiple sclerosis, primary health care implications. *Nurse Practitioner, 21,* 40–54.

Swedlund, N. P., & Nosek, M. A. (2000) An exploratory study on the work of independent living centers to address abuse of women with disabilities. *The Journal of Rehabilitation, 66*(4), 57.

Task Force on Concerns of Physically Disabled Women. (1978). *Within reach: Providing family planning services to physically disabled women.* New York: Human Sciences Press.

Taylor, J. S., & Praditsuwan, P. (1996). Latex allergy. Review of 44 cases including outcome and frequent association with allergic hand eczema. *Archives of Dermatology, 132,* 265–271.

Thomson, V. M. (1995). Breastfeeding and mothering one-handed. *Journal of Human Lactation, 11*(3), 211–215.

Thorne, S. E. (1990). Mothers with chronic illness: A predicament of social construction. *Health Care Women International, 11*(2), 209–221.

Timmerman, G. M., & Stuifbergen, A. K. (1999). Eating patterns in women with multiple sclerosis. *Journal of Neuroscience Nursing, 31*(3), 152.

Tincani, A., Faden, D., Tarantini, M., Lojacono, A., Tanzi, P., Gastaldi, A., DiMario, C. Spatola, L., Cattaneo, R., & Balestrieri, G. (1992). Systemic lupus erythematosus and pregnancy: A prospective study. *Clinical Exp Rheumatology, 10*(5), 429–431.

Tosi, L., Slater, J. E., Shaer, C., & Mostello, L. A. (1993). Latex allergy in spina bifida patients: Prevalence and surgical implications. *Journal of Pediatric Orthopedics, 13*(6), 709–712.

Tsy, A. M., & Opie, N. D. (1986). Menarche in the severely disabled adolescent: School nurses' attitudes, perceptions and perceived teaching responsibilities. *Journal of School Health, 56*(10), 443–447.

U. S. General Accounting Office. (1993). *Vocational rehabilitation: Evidence for federal program's effectiveness is mixed.* (GAO Pub. No: PEMD-93-19).

USDHHS, PHS. (1992). *Healthy people 2000: National health promotion and disease prevention objectives.* Boston: Jones and Bartlett.

Verdru, P., Pol, T., D'Hooghe, M., & Carton, H. (1994). Pregnancy and multiple sclerosis: The influence on long term disability. *Clinical Neurology and Neurosurgery, 96,* 38–41.

Villard-Makintosh, L., & Vessey, M. P. (1993). Oral contraceptives of reproductive factors in multiple sclerosis incidence. *Contraception, 47*(2), 161–168.

Walsh, P. N., Heller, T., Schupf, N., van Schrojenstein Lantman-de Valk, H. (2001). Healthy aging—Adults with intellectual disabilities: Women's health and related issues. *Journal of Applied Research in Intellectual Disabilities, 14*(3), 195–217.

Ware, L., Muram, D., & Gale, C. L. (1992). Q-Tip Pap smear: Should it be done routinely in patients who have developmental disabilities? *Sexuality and Disability, 10,* 189–192.

Wasser, A. M., Killoran, M. M., & Bansen, S. S. (1993). Pregnancy and disability. *AWOHNNS' Clinical Issues in Perinatal and Women's Health, 4*(2), 328–337.

Welner, S. (1996). Contraception, sexually transmitted diseases and menopause. In D. M. Krotoski, M. A. Nosek, & M. A. Turk (Eds.), *Women with disabilities.* Baltimore: Paul H. Brooks.

Welner, S. L. (1993). Gynecologic care of the disabled woman. *Contemporary OB/GYN, 38*(1), 55–67.

Welner, S. L., Foley, C. C., Nosek, M. A., & Holmes, A. (1999). Practical considerations in the performance of physical examinations on women with disabilities. *Obstet Gynecol Surv, 54*(7), 457–462.

Westgren, N., Hultling, C., Levi, R., & Westgren, M. (1993). Pregnancy and delivery in women with a traumatic spinal cord injury in Sweden, 1890–1991. *Obstetrics & Gynecology, 81,* 926–930.

Whipple, B., Gerdes, C. A., & Komisarut, R. (1996). Sexual response to self-stimulation in women with complete SCI. *The Journal of Sex Research, 33*(3), 231–241.

Whipple, B., Richard, E., Tepper, M., & Komisaruk, R. (1996). Sexual response in women with complete spinal cord injury. In D. M. Krotoski, M. A. Nosek, & M. A. Turk (Eds.), *Women with physical disabilities.* Baltimore: Paul H. Brookes.

Yang, C. C. (2000). Female sexual function in neurologic disease. *The Journal of Sex Research, 37*(3), 205.

Yarby, M. S., & Lannon, S. L. (1992). *Epilepsy, pregnancy and parenting.* Morris Plains, NJ: Park Davis.

Yarkony, G. M., & Chen, D. (1995). Sexuality in patients with spinal cord injury. *Physical Medicine and Rehabilitation: State of the Art Reviews, 9*(2), 325–344.

Yoshida, K. K., Li, A., & Odette, F. (1999). Cross-cultural views of disability and sexuality: Experiences of a group of ethnoracial women with physical disabilities. *Sexuality and Disability, 17*(4), 321–337.

Young, M. E., Nosek, M. A., Howland, C. A., Changong, G., & Rintala, D. H. (1997). Prevalence of abuse of women with physical disabilities. *Archives of Physical Medicine and Rehabilitation, 78*(Supp), S34–S38.

Zasler, N. D. (1991). Sexuality in neurologic disability: An overview. *Sexuality and Disability, 9,* 11–27.

Zurier, R., et al. (1987). *Systematic lupus erythematosus.* New York: Wiley.

U. S. Dept. of Health and Human Services (HHS) (2000). *Disability and Secondary Conditions in Health People 2010: Understanding and Improving Health, Vol. 1* (2nd Ed.) Washington DC: Office of Disease Prevention and Health Promotion (ODPHP), pp 6.1–6.28.

EMERGENCY CHILDBIRTH

Brenda T. Brickhouse

INTRODUCTION

When a woman presents complaining of labor, the health care provider must quickly perform an assessment appropriate to the specific needs of the client; that is, the provider must determine whether delivery of the infant is imminent or if there is time for further assistance to be obtained. The nature of the assessment and interventions depends on the resources available. Arrangements should be made for car or ambulance transportation to the nearest facility equipped for maternal and newborn care (Bidwell, 1990; Cunningham et al., 2001; Norwitz, 2002; Varney, 1997).

ASSESSMENT OF LABOR STATUS

MOTHER'S HISTORY AND SUBJECTIVE ASSESSMENT OF CURRENT STATUS

Ask the client her due date, gravida, and para. If she has had previous pregnancies, were they vaginal or cesarean births? Has she been receiving regular prenatal care, and has she had any complications during this pregnancy? Ask if she has medical problems or if special tests were done for her or the fetus during pregnancy. Some complications that can impact delivery are not viewed as such by women, especially if they do not feel ill (i.e., hypertension, urinary tract infection, twins, fetal abnormalities). Ask the client the time of the onset of contractions and the status of the fetal membranes. If her membranes have ruptured, did she note the color? Was the amniotic fluid clear or meconium stained? Brownish-green amniotic fluid indicates the fetus has been stressed and passed meconium; the infant may need airway clearance and resuscitation immediately after birth. How long have her membranes been ruptured? Membranes ruptured longer than 24 hours place mother and infant at risk for infection and sepsis. Ascertain the presence or absence of vaginal bleeding, fetal activity, history of allergies, and use of any medications or drugs. Has she had an ultrasound during her pregnancy; if so, was she told she had a placenta previa? If she has a placental previa, vaginal examination is contraindicated and immediate transport by ambulance is indicated. Ask the client if she feels the urge to bear down or have a bowel movement during contractions; this would indicate that the fetal presenting part is in the vaginal vault (putting pressure on the wall of the rectum) and birth is imminent.

ANXIETY LEVEL

Determine the client's ability to cooperate during examination and delivery by her response to questions and directions, degree of physical relaxation (resting between contractions) versus tension and fear (thrashing, uncontrolled bearing down), and tone of verbalizations (calm versus frantic).

The authors wish to acknowledge the contribution of Mary Beth Bryant McGurin, who prepared this Appendix for the 1st edition.

PHYSICAL ASSESSMENT

Examination of the client should include her vital signs, notation of fetal position and presentation, fetal heart rate and the duration, and quality of uterine contractions. If there are no contraindications to pelvic examination, the degree of cervical dilatation, effacement, status of the membranes, and type and station of the presenting part should be determined.

1. *Is the infant's head visible?* Inspect the vulva: bulging of the perineum, anal sphincter, or both, with separation of labia, revealing protruding membranes or crowning of the fetal head, indicates that birth is imminent.

2. *Is amniotic fluid or blood present?* Leaking amniotic fluid, bloody show (blood-tinged mucus), or both indicate only that labor is in progress, not necessarily that birth is imminent. As discussed earlier, note the color of the amniotic fluid if the sac appears to have ruptured. Frank vaginal bleeding (blood flowing like a menstrual period) or dried blood on the legs indicates a possible abnormality of the placenta. *Do not* insert the fingers, a speculum, or any other object into the vagina (see Abnormal Bleeding later in this appendix).

3. *Are uterine contractions effectively dilating the cervix?* Palpate the abdomen. Uterine contractions that begin every 2 minutes, last 60 to 90 seconds, and are hard (indentation is not elicited by fingertips pressing on abdomen during peak of contraction) indicate that active labor is in progress. If the client is bearing down and pushing with contractions, the fetal head is probably already out of the uterus (i.e., the cervix is fully dilated) and into the vaginal vault. Delivery is probably imminent. If sterile gloves are available and there is no frank vaginal bleeding, perform a vaginal exam, after receiving the client's permission, gently insert the index and middle fingers of one hand into the vagina until the fetal presenting part or cervix is palpable. Instruct the client to breathe slowly during the exam and to relax her buttocks; tell her what you are checking for. A gravid cervix is very soft, often indiscernible from the vaginal wall, but easily distinguishable from the fetal presenting part, which is firmer. If the cervix can be felt between your fingers and surrounding the fetal presenting part, then you may have time to attempt transportation by ambulance to the closest facility offering maternity services. If only the fetal head is palpable deep in the vagina close to the perineum, the cervix is completely dilated, and delivery is imminent.

4. *Is the fetus tolerating the intrauterine environment?* Fetal well-being is assessed to ascertain measures that need to be taken before birth, to decrease stress to the fetus, and after delivery, to facilitate the transition to extrauterine life. If not already known, ask when the infant is due to be born and if there are any known or suspected problems with the infant. The gestational age of the fetus and any physical challenges will determine how much stress the infant can tolerate. (*Note:* Estimation of the gestational age of the fetus by measurement of fundal height is not accurate during the late stages of labor.) Between contractions, perform Leopold's maneuvers to determine which side of the abdomen to listen to for fetal heart sounds; that is, the side where you can feel a smooth, firm fetal back. Listen with the bell side of the stethoscope in the lower abdomen on that side. Count heartbeats for 15 to 30 seconds and multiply to obtain the beats per minute. If the fetal heartrate is less than 100 bpm or if amniotic fluid is meconium stained (green or brown), the fetus is or has been stressed; be prepared to resuscitate the infant immediately after birth. If birth does not seem imminent, turn the client onto her side (preferably left) to allow better blood flow to her uterus and the fetus. Auscultate the fetal heartbeat every 5 to 10 minutes. Also ask the client if the fetus has been moving in the last few hours, another measure of fetal well-being. A stressed, compromised fetus will not be as active as usual.

PROVISION OF EMOTIONAL SUPPORT AND RELAXATION COACHING

Enhance the client's ability to cooperate during the examination and delivery by teaching her how to gain some measure of control with her breathing. Encourage her to open her mouth and pant or blow slowly during contractions and to breathe normally between contractions. She is probably frightened and uncomfortable. Acknowledge that everything possible will be done to help her. Ask her to keep her eyes open and to watch for directions. Maintain eye contact, speak calmly, and give simple directions. Have any available support person stay by her upper body to hold her hands and assist with instructions. Give frequent feedback and reassurance that they are both doing a good job. Ideally, transport of the laboring woman should be done by emergency service providers. However, if you are transporting the woman and delivery of the fetus begins, stop the vehicle; this facilitates balance and concentration for you and mother.

PREPARATION FOR DELIVERY

ASSEMBLY OF AVAILABLE SUPPLIES

Where delivery is taking place will determine the type and amount of assistance and equipment available. If a readymade delivery kit is available, open it and place it to one side within easy reach. If no kit is readily available, have someone get the following items for you if possible: eight or more towels, sheets, or blankets (warm two of them); bulb syringe; sterile scissors; three cord clamps, kelly clamps, or shoestrings; two pair of sterile gloves; bowl or sealable plastic bag; sanitary pads; 3 cc syringe with needle; alcohol wipes; 1000 mL 5% dextrose in half-normal saline or in lactated Ringer's; intravenous catheters; intravenous tubing; other intravenous start supplies; two vials oxytocin (Pitocin, 10 units each) or 0.2 mg (1 cc) of methylergonovine maleate (Methergine); hot water bottle (filled) or heat pack. *Note:* If no supplies are available, use whatever cloth is available to protect your hands from contact with body fluids.

POSITIONING OF MOTHER AND DRAPING

Wash hands. Position the client lying on her back on a firm surface, with her knees bent and spread apart and her upper body elevated if possible. (This position provides maximum control in an emergency situation.) Observe the perineum while maintaining intermittent eye contact with the client and her support person.

INTRAVENOUS INFUSION

Start an intravenous infusion at a keep-vein-open rate; draw up both vials of oxytocin to be added to the intravenous fluid immediately following delivery of placenta.

DELIVERY OF THE INFANT

DELIVERY OF PRESENTING PART AND CLEARANCE OF AIRWAY

To ensure gradual and slow delivery of the head, have the client pant or blow during contractions and give gentle, short pushes only between contractions. Place the hand most comfortable for you on the presenting part, usually the crown of the head, as it protrudes from the vagina during each contraction. Most practitioners use their nondominant hand, leaving their dominant hand to handle equipment or supplies. With your fingers, keep the fetal head flexed by maintaining gentle, even pressure on the head as it advances. Allowing the head to slide out of the vagina slowly minimizes perineal tearing. (It may take several contractions to complete delivery of the head.) If the amniotic sac is intact over the infant's face, remove it with your fingers. As soon as the head is born, place the fingertips of one of your hands on the back of the baby's head and then slide them down the neck, sweeping them in both directions feeling for the umbilical cord. If found, pull the cord gently over the head. If the loop is too tight, have the mother pant or blow while you clamp the cord in two places; cut between the two clamps. Wipe the baby's face and head and wipe off fluid from the nose and mouth with a soft absorbent cloth. Gently suction the baby's mouth and nose with a soft rubber bulb syringe. With the next contraction, the head will align with the infant's body and externally rotate.

DELIVERY OF BODY

Shift slightly toward the back of the infant's head. Place your hands on each side of the head so that your fingers point toward the face, with the little fingers closest to the perineum. With a contraction, or gentle pushes from the mother, exert downward and outward pressure on the side of the head with your top hand until the infant's anterior shoulder has slipped out from under the mother's symphysis pubis bone and can be seen. Then apply upward and outward pressure on the sides of the head with your bottom hand, and with both hands lift the infant's head toward the ceiling. As the infant is being born, slide your bottom hand down close to the perineum so that the shoulder, arm, elbow, and hand are held close to the infant's body, controlled, and born into the palm of your hand. The thumb on your bottom hand will be on the infant's back, your fingers will be across the infant's chest, and the infant's head will be resting on your wrist. Slide your top hand down the infant's back, slip your index finger between the infant's legs as the buttocks clear the perineum, and grasp the infant by the ankles. Of primary importance is simple support of each part of the infant as it delivers. *Note the time of delivery.*

IMMEDIATE INFANT CARE

Move the infant in a smooth arc into a football hold by allowing the head and shoulders to pivot in your hand while swinging the legs and torso around; the infant's back is supported by your lower arm, and the lower half of the infant's body is tucked between your upper arm and side. Keep the infant's head in a downward position and turned to the side. Stay close enough to the mother so that there is no tension on the umbilical cord. The infant may rest between the mother's legs for observation.

Observe the infant for normal respiration and aspiration. Dry the infant. Drying promotes normal respiration and provides tactile stimulation. Keep the infant warm and, if indicated, bulb suction the infant's mouth and nose gently or wipe out with a cloth. It is usually not necessary to clamp and cut the cord. However, if the cord is cut, first clamp the umbilical cord in two places about 6 inches from the infant's body and cut between the clamps. If clamps are not available, tie with shoestrings. (Not with thread!) If the infant does not breathe spontaneously and start to cry, dry the skin vigorously, rub the back, and flick the foot with your finger. Initiate infant CPR (rescue breathing and chest compressions) if necessary. When the infant does cry, place her or him on the mother's chest or abdomen, skin to skin, and cover with warm blankets so that the infant's scalp is covered but the face can be seen. If necessary, use a hot water bottle or heat pack covered with a towel to keep the infant warm. Observe the infant for cyanosis or lethargy; stimulate as above if needed. Assign APGAR scores at 1 and 5 minutes. (Refer fo Appendix B.)

DELIVERY OF PLACENTA

Observe the vaginal opening for lengthening of the cord or increased bleeding, which indicate placental separation. Do *not* pull on the cord; instead, wait for uterine contractions to push out the placenta with attached membranes, and place it in a bowl or plastic bag. Transport to the hospital with the infant. Note any tears in the perineum.

IMMEDIATE POSTDELIVERY CARE OF MOTHER

CONTROL OF BLEEDING

Locate the grapefruit-sized uterine fundus under the umbilicus and assess for firmness. If not firm, massage it with one hand while supporting the uterus with the other hand just above the symphysis pubis. If oxytocin is available and an IV is running, introduce 20 units of oxytocin into the bag, and allow the IV to run open for about 5 minutes or until the uterus remains firm. If no IV is running, give 10 units (1 cc) oxytocin or 0.2 mg (1 cc) methylergonovine maleate IM into the buttocks or thigh. Even if medications are not available, vaginal bleeding should be minimal if the infant is put to breast, and the uterus is kept well contracted with massage every 10 to 15 minutes. The uterus should be assessed for firmness every 15 minutes. Place a sanitary pad or folded cloth firmly against the perineum. Record blood pressure, pulse, and respirations every 15 minutes; the urinary bladder should be checked for distention and emptied if needed. If the uterus is soft or is above the umbilicus, it has lost its muscle tone and is full of clots. The fundus needs to be massaged (with support from the opposite hand just above the pubic bone to prevent eversion of the uterus into the vagina) until clots are expelled and the fundus is firm. If the uterus is displaced to one side of the midline, the urinary bladder is distended and needs to be emptied.

PHYSICAL AND EMOTIONAL RECOVERY

If the mother experiences severe shaking chills, reassure her that this reaction is normal after the hard work and anxiety of delivery. Slow, deep breathing may help alleviate the "shakes" and increase relaxation. Cover her with available blankets. Reinforce what a wonderful job she did during her labor and delivery. Encourage her to interact with her infant and support person. Assist the mother to breastfeed. Notify the receiving health care facility of the impending arrival and condition of the mother and infant.

ABNORMAL CONDITIONS

BREECH PRESENTATION

When initially assessing the client's vaginal opening, note that instead of the top of the infant's head, the buttocks may present first (breech presentation), often accompanied by meconium. This delivery should only occur in a hospital. Only attempt a breech delivery if there are no other alternatives. Immediately activate Emergency Medical Services (EMS). Prepare the client and supplies as usual; allow the infant's legs, buttocks, and trunk to deliver spontaneously. When the baby is born up to the umbilicus, the remainder of the baby needs to be delivered in 3 to 5 minutes to prevent anoxia. In this event, gently pull down a loop of cord to prevent tension on the cord. If the arms do not deliver spontaneously, reach up for the hands, one at a time, and sweep them down over the face. The body will turn to one side and the shoulders will deliver, the top shoulder followed by the bottom shoulder. The head is ready to deliver when the back is up (toward the ceiling). Put two fingers in the vagina below the head and press downward to make enough room for the baby to breathe. Have the mother push until the face starts to deliver. Then she should pant and the back of the head can be delivered slowly. Support the body in the palm of your gloved hand and on your lower arm, if unable to deliver the head transport to the nearest hospital's obstetric unit with the mother's buttocks elevated; be prepared to resuscitate the infant if the head does deliver en route. Alert the receiving facility of impending arrival.

OTHER ABNORMAL PRESENTATION SITUATIONS

If the infant's arm protrudes from the vagina, transport the mother immediately to the nearest hospital's obstetric unit. This woman will not deliver spontaneously.

If a loop of umbilical cord protrudes from the vagina, cover it with moistened cloth (preferably with normal saline). Have the client assume the knee-chest position on the stretcher or car seat. (This is difficult to do, and the client and her support person will need much reassurance!) Insert your gloved hand into the vagina, and attempt to hold the presenting part off the prolapsed cord until you reach the delivery room, where staff are prepared to perform a cesarean delivery.

If the mother is carrying more than one fetus, deliver subsequent infants just as the first. Remember that twin babies are likely to be smaller and in need of warmth and possible resuscitation.

ABNORMAL BLEEDING

If, before or during delivery, you observe blood flow rather than blood-tinged mucus, suspect a placental abnormality. Transport the client to the nearest hospital's obstetric unit while maintaining her in shock position (head down, hips elevated, covered with blankets). Record blood pressure, pulse, respirations, and fetal heart rate every 10 minutes. Monitor contractions and deliver the infant as indicated, being prepared to resuscitate the infant as needed and to treat the mother for shock if pulse rises and blood pressure drops. If the mother bleeds after delivery despite breastfeeding or nipple stimulation and your best efforts to keep her fundus firm, look for perineal lacerations, and apply a peripad or folded cloth snugly to the vulva. Bring all blood-soaked pads or material to the hospital. Always call the receiving facility to alert them of the arrival time and condition of the client and infant.

REFERENCES

Bidwell, D. (1990). Congratulations—It's a baby! *Emergency Medical Services, 19*(10), 21–24.

Cunningham, F.G., Gant, N.F., Gilstrap, L.C., Hauth, J.C., Leveno, K.J., & Wenstrom, K. D. (Eds.), (2001) *Williams obstetrics* (21st ed., pp. 309–329). New York, NY: McGraw-Hill.

Norwitz, E.R. (2002). Labor and delivery. In S. G. Gabbe, J. R. Neibyl, & J. L. Simpson, (Eds.), *Obstetrics: Normal and problem pregnancies* (4th ed., pp. 353–394). Philadelphia, PA: Churchill Livingstone.

Varney, H. (1997). *Varney's midwifery* (3rd ed.). Sudbury, MA: Jones and Bartlett Publishers.

IMMEDIATE ASSESSMENT OF THE NEWBORN

Marcia Szmania Davis

INTRODUCTION

Newborn assessment is an ongoing process incorporating the basic principles of health care and promotion.

- *Purposes*
  a. To provide baseline information.
  b. To identify problems with transition from intra- to extrauterine life.
  c. To document individual variation and reactivity.
- *Principles*
  a. Follow a systematic approach, progressing from noninvasive to invasive, clean to dirty, and head to toe.
  b. Anticipate, on the basis of history.
  c. Do no harm.
  d. Attend to instinctive feelings that something may be wrong.
- *General Guidelines*
  a. Maintain universal precautions and neutral thermal environment.
  b. Focus on ABCs of cardiopulmonary resuscitation.
  c. Assess symmetry.
  d. If an external abnormality is visible, closely assess internal organs.
  e. Measure lesions, graph vital statistics, and document and interpret findings.

REVIEW OF HISTORY FOR RISK FACTORS (SEE CHAPTER 12)

- *Maternal*. Age; past medical history; social, developmental, and occupational history.
- *Obstetric*. Parity; last menstrual period (LMP); previous menstrual period (PMP); history of prematurity; medical complications and outcome of previous or current pregnancy.
- *Perinatal*. Intrapartum events; gestational age; condition at birth.

APGAR SCORES

EVALUATION OF INITIAL NEONATAL TRANSITION PERIOD

The acronym *APGAR* facilitates assessment of five components of neonates' responses: appearance, pulse, grimace, activity, and respiration.

INTERPRETATION

- The APGAR is scored at 1 and 5 minutes of life.
- Five signs are evaluated and scored 0, 1, or 2.
- *10–10, Best Possible Condition*. As most healthy newborns are acrocyanotic, expect a score of 8 or 9.

APGAR SIGNS

Signs	0	1	2
Appearance (color)	Blue/pale	Body pink Extremities blue	Completely pink
Pulse (heart rate)	Absent	< 100	> 100
Grimace (reflex irritability)	No response	Grimace	Cough, sneeze, cry
Activity (muscle tone)	Limp	Some flexion	Flexed, active motion
Respiration (breathing efforts)	Absent	Weak, irregular gasping	Strong cry

♦ When the 5-minute score is 6 or less, some states require a 10-minute score. It is useful to obtain additional scores every 5 minutes until 20 minutes has passed or until two successive scores of 7 or higher are obtained.

♦ *0–2, Severe Asphyxia.* Infant is at high risk; requires resuscitation and further evaluation.

♦ *3–4, Moderate Asphyxia.* Infant is at moderate risk; probable resuscitation and further evaluation.

♦ *5–7, Mild Asphyxia.* Infant is at risk; possible intermittent resuscitation, and with or without further evaluation.

♦ *8–10, No Asphyxia.* Infant is at minimal risk; routine elective procedures.

PHYSICAL EXAMINATION

Abnormal findings are noted in parentheses.

GENERAL SURVEY

♦ *State.* Deep or light sleep; drowsy; quiet or active alert; crying.

♦ *Reactivity.* State changes, interactive capacity, self-consolability.

♦ *Color.* Pink, acrocyanosis; mottling (plethora, pallor, jaundice, cyanosis).

♦ *Posture.* Flexed (asymmetry, restricted movement).

♦ *Skin.* Smooth, elastic, warm, moist; vernix; lanugo; desquamation; Mongolian spots; milia; nevi; edema or petechiae over presenting part (pustules, lacerations, ecchymosis, rashes, café-au-lait spots, hemangiomas, meconium staining, pitting edema, poor turgor, scaling, sweating).

♦ *Respirations at Rest.* Rate = 30–60; symmetric; diaphragmatic or abdominal (flaring; grunting; intercostal, supraclavicular, or substernal retractions).

HEENT, MOUTH, AND NECK

♦ *Head.* Occipitofrontal circumference: 32.5–37 cm. Round; symmetric; molding; overriding or slightly open sutures; caput succedaneum = scalp edema, may cross suture line; cephal hematoma = subperiosteal hemorrhage, does not cross suture line (irregularities; craniotabes; depressions; asymmetry; fracture; fixed widely spaced/closed sutures). Fontanelles soft, flat, may bulge with crying; anterior = diamond; posterior = triangle (sunken; bulging at rest; enlarged; absent anterior; third fontanelle).

♦ *Face.* Symmetric; intact (asymmetry with movement, micrognathia; clefts).

♦ *Eyes.* Symmetric; lids easily open; positive blink; pupils round, equal, and reactive to light; positive red reflex; blue-gray or brown iris; no discharge; cornea and lens clear and intact; sclera bluish white; minor hemorrhages; pale pink conjunctiva; subconjunctival hemorrhage; chemical conjunctivitis; nystagmus; strabismus (asymmetry; short palpebral fissures; hypertelorism; fused edematous, drooping, or inflamed lids; setting sun sign; unequal, constricted, or poorly reactive pupils; pinkish or clefted iris; blue or jaundiced sclera; corneal opacities or ulcerations; purulent discharge; persistent uncoordinated movements).

♦ *Ears.* Well formed; symmetric; upper pinna at or above outer canthus of eye; curved pinna, firm cartilage; patent canals; positive response to noise (asymmetric; low-set; rotated; very large or small; malformed; preauricular, auricular skin tags, sinuses).

♦ *Nose.* Midline; intact; no discharge; bilateral nasal patency; obligatory nose breather (flattened nasal bridge; flaring; clefts; chloanal atresia).

♦ *Mouth and Throat.* Pink, moist mucosa; sucking blisters; positive suck, root, and gag reflexes; transient circumoral cyanosis; midline mobile tongue; well-formed palate and gums; Epstein's pearls; inclusion cysts; teeth; scant saliva (clefts; thrush; tongue protrusion; long frenulum; macroglossia; high arched palate; excessive mucus).

- *Neck.* Short, straight, full range of motion; intact clavicles (webbing; masses; edema, venous distention; limited range of motion; torticollis; crepitation; fractures; opisthotonus).

CHEST

- *Thorax.* Symmetric; cylindrical; circumference at nipple line = 30–33 cm (bulging, depressed sternum; retractions; tachypnea; apnea).
- *Nipples.* Present; symmetric placement; supernumerary; enlarged; milky secretion (asymmetry; purulent drainage).
- *Breath Sounds.* Auscultate for vesicular or clear bilaterally (expiratory grunting; rales/crackles; rhonchi/wheezes; decreased, unequal).
- *Heart Sounds.* Rate = 120–160; auscultate for two clear, distinct sounds: S_2 slightly sharper, higher pitched than S_1; regular rhythm; point of maximal impulse (PMI) = lower left sternal border (displaced, distant, muffled, extra sounds; bradycardia/tachycardia; irregular rhythm; hyperactive precordium).

ABDOMEN

- *Contour.* Protuberant; symmetric; cylindrical shape; diastasis recti; prominent superficial veins (asymmetry; distention; flat; scaphoid; masses; visible peristalsis).
- *Bowel Sounds Present in All Four Quadrants.* Intermittent tinkling (hyperactive or absent).
- *Liver.* Palpate 1–2 cm below right costal margin; sharp edge (enlarged; round edge).
- *Kidneys.* Palpate oval structure in posterior flanks 1–2 cm above umbilicus; often difficult to palpate (enlarged; absent).
- *Umbilical Cord and Umbilicus.* Two arteries; one vein; gelatinous, bluish-white; skin clear and dry; umbilical hernia (two vessels; thin cord; foul odor; discharge; meconium stained).
- *Femoral Pulses and Lymph Nodes.* Palpate strong, regular pulses bilaterally (absent, irregular, weak, bounding, absent pulses; enlarged nodes).
- *Rectum and Anus.* Patent; positive anal wink (imperforate anus; fistulas; decreased tone); document passage and character of stools; meconium = dark green, tarry, thick viscous; mucus plug (foul odor; diarrhea; mucus; blood).

GENITOURINARY TRACT

- *Urination.* Confirm; clear; yellow; full stream (bladder distention; abnormal stream; blood-tinged).
- *External Genitalia.* Confirm appropriate for given gender (ambiguous; fecal urethral discharge).
  - *Male:* Observe urinary stream; meatus at tip of penis, glans covered by prepuce (epispadias = dorsal; hypospadias = ventral surface; phimosis); scrotum—pink to brown; symmetric; pendulous; rugation; testes descended or descending bilaterally; edema or bruising if breech (hydrocele = positive transillumination; hernia = negative transillumination; undescended or absent testes).
  - *Female:* Observe presence and position of urethra; introitus posterior to clitoris; labia majora meet midline; labia minora prominent; edema; hymenal tags; pseudomenstruation; mucoid, milky discharge (absent vagina or meatus).

BACK

- *Back and Spine.* Midline; straight; intact; easily flexed; symmetric; lanugo; pilonidal dimple (asymmetry; abnormal curvature; masses; pilonidal cyst, sinus, dimple, hair tufts; spina bifida).
- *Buttocks.* Symmetry; Mongolian spots (asymmetric gluteal folds).

EXTREMITIES

- *General.* Appearance, symmetry, size, length, and range of motion.
- *Fingers and Toes.* All present.
- *Hands and Feet.* Palmar and plantar creases; fisted hands (simian crease; dysplastic nails; tightly fisted hands, obligatory palmar thumb; metatarsus varus; club feet; rocker-bottom feet; absent digits, abnormal spacing).
- *Arms.* Occasional tremors; easily adduct from trunk; full range of motion at elbow (fracture; palsy; paralysis).
- *Legs.* Mild medial rotation; transient in utero positioning = breech, "frogs' legs"; symmetry of medial thigh skinfolds (asymetric size/appearance; limited range of motion).
- *Hips.* Tests to evaluate:
  - *Ortolani's Maneuver—Abduct, Up and Out.* Flex knees and hips, placing fingers bilaterally on greater trochanters, thumbs gripping medial aspect

of femurs; adduct and abduct (positive jerking motion as femur passes over acetabulum).

- *Barlow's Test—Up and Back, "Piston."* Flex hip and knee 90 degrees; gently attempt to slip femur head onto posterior tip of acetabulum by lateral pressure of thumb and by rocking knee medially with knuckle of index finger (palpable or audible hip click; movement is not normally felt).

- *Peripheral Pulses.* Present; symmetric; strong (absent; varied strength).

NERVOUS SYSTEM

- *Character of Cry.* Strong, lusty (weak, high-pitched, constant or none).
- *Reflexes.* Assess symmetry and strength of responses.
  - *Asymmetric Tonic Neck ("Fencing").* With the infant supine, turn head to one side. The infant may extend arm and leg on side head is turned toward with flexion of opposite arm and leg.
  - *Moro or Startle.* Abrupt position change or noise elicits extension and abduction of arms and extension of fingers with subsequent flexion or drawing in; infant may habituate or diminish response with repeated attempts.
  - *Rooting.* Stroke side of cheek, lips, or mouth with finger or nipple and head turns toward the stimulus, mouth opens, and sucking begins.
  - *Sucking.* Finger or nipple in mouth elicits sucking movements.
  - *Swallow.* Assess coordination of suck or swallow with first oral feeding.
  - *Extrusion.* Solid object placed on tongue causes tongue to push outward to remove it.
  - *Palmar and Plantar Grasp.* Finger placed in palm and base of toes elicits grasp of finger and brief downward curling of toes.
  - *Babinski.* Stroke up lateral aspect of feet and toes fan up and out.
  - *Pull to Sit or Traction.* With the infant supine, grasp the arms and pull to sitting position; the head lags, then is brought up and held briefly; note position and tone.

- *Glabellar or Blink.* Tap forehead at bridge of nose with finger to elicit bilateral blink.
- *Galant or Trunk Incurvation.* With infant in ventral suspension over examiner's hand, gently stroke, with finger of other hand, paravertebral portion of spine to elicit curvature toward stimulus.
- *Placing or Stepping.* Holding infant upright on flat surface elicits "stepping" movements with alternating flexion and extension of feet (may also elicit this response by stroking dorsum of foot while holding infant upright).

ESTIMATION OF GESTATIONAL AGE

Use Dubowitz or Ballard clinical assessments of physical characteristics and neuromuscular maturity to classify neonates by gestational age and to determine potential mortality and morbidity risks.

REFERENCES

Aldoretta, P. W., & Spedale, S. B. (1997). Care of the newborn. In G. R. Merenstein, D. W. Kaplan, & A. A. Rosenberg (Eds.), *Handbook of pediatrics,* (18th ed.). Stamford, CT: Appleton & Lange.

Apgar, V. (1996). The newborn (APGAR) scoring system: Reflections and advice. *Pediatric Clinics of North America, 13,* 645.

Ballard, J. L., Khoury, J. C., Wedig, K., Wang, L., Eilers-Walsman, B. L., Lipp, R. (1991). New Ballard score, expanded to include extremely premature infants. *Journal of Pediatrics, 3,* 417.

Brazelton, T. B. (1973). *Neonatal behavioral assessment scale.* Philadelphia: J. B. Lippincott/Spastics International Medical Publishers.

Dubowitz, L. M. S., Dubowitz, V., & Goldberg, C. (1970). Clinical assessment of gestational age in the newborn infant. *Journal of Pediatrics, 77,* 1.

NAACOG. (1991). *OGN Nursing Practice Resource: Physical assessment of the neonate.* Washington, DC: Author.

Parks, D. K., Montgomery, D., & Yetman, R. J. (2000). Perinatal conditions. In C. E. Burns, M. A. Brady, A. M. Dunn, & N. B. Starr, (Eds.), *Pediatric primary care: A handbook for nurse practitioners* (2nd ed). Philadelphia: W. B. Saunders Co.

BIBLIOGRAPHY

Coody, D., et al. (1996). Perinatal Conditions. In *Pediatric Primary Care: A Handbook for Nurse Practitioners*. Philadelphia: W. B. Saunders.

Reimann, D. & Coughlin, M. (1996). Newborn Adaptation to Extrauterine Life. In *Perinatal Nursing*. AWHONN Philadelphia: Lippincott.

Witt, P. (1993). Physical Assessment of the Newborn. In *Core Curriculum for Neonatal Intensive Care Nursing*. AWHONN Philadelphia: W. B. Saunders.

SELECTED LABORATORY VALUES[a]

Ellis Quinn Youngkin

Comprehensive metabolic panel (1,2)

Sodium	135–145 mEq/L (mmol/L)
Potassium	3.5–5.0 mEq/L (mmol/L)
Chloride	101–111 mEq/L (mmol/L)
Carbon dioxide	22–30 mEq/L (mmol/L)
Glucose (fasting)	70–105 mg/dL
Blood urea nitrogen	6–19 mg/dL
Creatinine	0.5–1.4 mg/dL
Calcium	8.4–10.2 mg/dL
Albumin	3.5–5.0 g/dL
Bilirubin (total)	0.1–1.0 mg/dL
Alkaline phosphatase	31–97 IU/L
AST (SGOT)[b]	10–37 IU/L
ALT (SGPT)[b]	10–40 IU/L
Protein (total)	6–8.3g/dL

Lipid Profile (1,3,4)

Cholesterol	140–199 mg/dL
Triglycerides	35–160 mg/dL
LDL-CHO[b]	< 130 mg/dL
HDL-CHO[b]	40–80 mg/dL
Cholesterol/HDL ratio (1)	≤ 4.4
Apolipoprotein[a]	10–20 mol/dL (119–240 mg/dL)

Thyroid Profile (1,5,6,7)

TSH[b]	0.5–5.6 µIU/mL
T_3 uptake[b]	25–35%
T_4 (total)[b]	4–12.2 µg/dL
FTI (calc)[b](6)	4.6–11.2
Free T_4 (6)	0.8–2.7 ng/dL
T_3 (total)	60–190 ng/dL

Other Values

Prolactin (1,6)	3.34–26.72 ng/mL (premenopausal)
FSH (1,6)	2.74–19.64 ng/mL (postmenopausal)
Follicular	3.85–8.78 mIU/mL
Luteal	1.79–5.12 mIU/mL
Midcycle	4.54–22.51 mIU/mL
Postmenopausal	16.74–113.59 mIU/mL
LH (1,6)	(mIU/mL)
Follicular	2.12–10.89 mIU/mL
Luteal	1.20–12.86 mIU/mL
Midcycle peak	19.18–103.03 mIU/mL
Postmenopausal	10.87–58.64 mIU/mL
Estradiol (serum)(1)	
Follicular	1.8–2.4 ng/dL
Midcycle	16.6–23.2 ng/dL
Luteal	6.3–7.3 ng/dL
Progesterone (serum)(1)	
Follicular	37–57 ng/dL
Midcycle	Rising
Luteal	330–1198 ng/dL
Testosterone (4)	20–75 ng/dL (adult females)
Free testosterone (4)	100–200 pg/dL
DHEA-SO_4[b]	80–350 µg/dL (decreases with age)
Androstenedione (4)	< 250 ng/dL
17-Hydroxyprogesterone (4)	15–70 ng/dL (follicular phase)
	35–290 ng/dL (luteal phase)
Cortisol (4)	
8:00 AM	5–25 µg/dL
4:00 PM	3–12 µg/dL
10:00 PM	< 50% of AM value

After ACTH stimulation test: plasma cortisol should increase 2–3 times over baseline at 30 and 60 minutes (4)

Dexamethasone suppression test	5+ µg/dL cortisone = test failure
Albumin (1,4)	3.5–5.0 g/dL

Anemia Workup (1,4,6)

Complete blood count	
Red blood cells	4.2–5.4 million/mm^3
Hemoglobin	12–16 g/dL
Hematocrit	36–47%
MCV	78–102 µm^3
MCH	25–35 µg
MCHC	31–37 g/dL
White blood cells	4,800–10,800 cells/mm^3 (4.8–10.8 K/mL)
Differential	
Neutrophils	45–79%
Lymphocytes	13–46%
Monocytes	3–11%
Eosinophils	0–8%

Basophils	0–3%
Bands or stabs (young neutrophils)	0–5%
Reticulocyte count	0.5–2.5%
Iron	30–160 µg/dL
Total iron binding capacity	250–420 µg/dL
Transferrin	200–400 µg/dL
Transferrin saturation	20–50%
Ferritin	20–400 ng/mL
Hemoglobin electrophoresis	
Hgb A$_1$	95–98%
Hgb A$_2$	2–3%
Hgb F	0.8–2%
Hgb S	0%
Hgb C	0%
Platelet count	130,000–400,000/µL
Folic acid	3.1–17.5 ng/dL
Vitamin B$_{12}$	> 250 pg/dL

[a]Values vary from laboratory to laboratory and among clinicians and upon method used for calculation.

[b]AST(SGOT), aspartate aminotransferase (serum glutamic-oxaloacetic transaminase); ALT(SGPT), alanine aminotransferase (serum glutamic–pyruvic transaminase); LDL-CHO, low-density lipoprotein cholesterol; HDL-CHO, high-density lipoprotein cholesterol; TSH, thyroid-stimulating hormone; T$_3$, triiodothyronine; T$_4$, thyroxine; FTI (calc), free thyroxine index (calculated); FSH, follicle-stimulating hormone; LH, luteinizing hormone; DHEA-SO$_4$, dehydroepiandrosterone sulfate; MCV, mean corpuscular volume; MCH, mean corpuscular hemoglobin; MCHC, mean corpuscular hemoglobin concentration; Hgb, hemoglobin.

1. Sacher, R. A., McPherson, R. A., & Campos, J. M. (2000). *Widmann's clinical interpretation of laboratory tests* (11th ed.). Philadelphea, PA: F.A. Davis Co.

2. The basic metabolic panel is comprised of the first seven tests.

3. McCauley, K. M. (June 25, 2002). Women and heart disease: Risk factor modification. AWHONN Convention 2002, p. 23–24 Session Resources.

4. Pagana, K. D., & Pagana, T. J. (1997). *Mosby's diagnostic and laboratory test reference* (3rd ed.). St. Louis: Mosby.

5. Arem, R. (1999). *The thyroid solution.* New York: Ballentine Books.

6. Corbett, J. V. (2000). *Laboratory tests and diagnostic procedures with necessary diagnoses* (5th ed.). Upper Saddle River, New Jersey: Prentice Hall Health.

7. Shames, R. L., & Shames, K. H. (2001). *Thyroid power: 10 steps to total health.* New York: Harper Collins.

INDEX